STROKE AND CEREBROVASCULAR DISEASE IN CHILDHOOD

Edited by

Vijeya Ganesan and Fenella J. Kirkham

INTERNATIONAL REVIEW OF CHILD NEUROLOGY SERIES

INTERNATIONAL REVIEW OF CHILD NEUROLOGY SERIES

STROKE AND CEREBROVASCULAR DISEASE IN CHILDHOOD

Edited by

VIJEYA GANESAN

Senior Lecturer in Paediatric Neurology, University College London, Institute of Child Health; Neurology Department, Great Ormond Street Hospital for Children NHS Trust, Great Ormond Street, London

and

FENELLA J. KIRKHAM

Professor of Paediatric Neurology, University College London, Institute of Child Health, London; Consultant Paediatric Neurologist, Department of Child Health, Southampton General Hospital, Southampton; Honorary Professor of Paediatric Neurology, University of Southampton

2011
MAC KEITH PRESS
for the
INTERNATIONAL CHILD NEUROLOGY ASSOCIATION

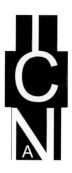

© 2011 Mac Keith Press
6 Market Road, London N7 9PW

Editor: Hilary Hart
Managing Director: Caroline Black
Production Manager: Udoka Ohuonu
Project Manager: Mirjana Misina

First published in this edition 2011

British Library Cataloguing-in-Publication data
A catalogue record for this book is available from the British Library

ISBN: 978-1-898683-34-6

Typeset by Graphicraft Limited, Hong Kong
Printed by TJ International, Padstow, Cornwall, UK

Cover image courtesy of Dr John Millar, Consultant Neuroradiologist, Wessex Neurological Centre, Southampton General Hospital,
Southampton, UK (see Fig. 16.4, p. 237)

Mac Keith Press is supported by Scope

CONTENTS

AUTHORS' APPOINTMENTS   ix

1. CHILDHOOD STROKE – THE UNKINDEST CUT OF ALL: A HISTORY OF
   CEREBROVASCULAR DISEASE IN CHILDHOOD   1
   Andrew N. Williams and Fenella J. Kirkham

2. DEVELOPMENT OF THE BRAIN CIRCULATION   17
   Chao Bao Luo, Marina Sachet Ferreira, Hortensia Alvarez, Georges Rodesch and
   Pierre L. Lasjaunias

3. THE EPIDEMIOLOGY OF CHILDHOOD STROKE   22
   Gabrielle deVeber

4. CLINICAL AND IMAGING FEATURES OF CHILDHOOD STROKE   27
   4.1 CLINICAL SYNDROMES   27
       4.1.1 ANTERIOR CIRCULATION STROKE   27
             Fenella J. Kirkham
       4.1.2 POSTERIOR CIRCULATION STROKES IN CHILDREN   38
             Bhuwan P. Garg
       4.1.3 SPINAL CORD STROKE   43
             Bettina Harms, Jason MacDonald and Fenella J. Kirkham
   4.2 NEUROIMAGING   48
       4.2.1 IMAGING OF PAEDIATRIC STROKE   48
             Dawn E. Saunders and W.K. Kling Chong
       4.2.2 RECENT ADVANCES IN MAGNETIC RESONANCE IMAGING   57
             Fernando Calamante, Jacques-Donald Tournier and Alan Connelly

5. RISK FACTORS AND TRIGGERS FOR CRYPTOGENIC (AND SYMPTOMATIC) STROKE   84
   5.1 CEREBROVASCULAR DISEASES FROM INFECTIOUS/INFLAMMATORY ORIGIN   84
       Guillaume Sébire and Benedict Michel (with a section on human immunodeficiency
       virus by Nomazulu Dlamini and Fenella J. Kirkham)
   5.2 THROMBOPHILIA AND CHILDHOOD STROKE   91
       Ulrike Nowak-Göttl and Ronald Sträter
   5.3 HYPERTENSION AND CHILDHOOD STROKE   94
       Juan C. Kupferman, Fenella J. Kirkham and Steven Pavlakis
   5.4 TRAUMA   96
       Fenella J. Kirkham
   5.5 IRON DEFICIENCY   96
       Fenella J. Kirkham

5.6 PATENT FORAMEN OVALE AND PARADOXICAL EMBOLISM 96
Vijeya Ganesan and Fenella J. Kirkham

6. ARTERIAL ISCHAEMIC STROKE AND VASCULAR DISEASE IN CHILDHOOD 107

6.1 CERVICOCEPHALIC ARTERIAL DISSECTIONS IN CHILDHOOD AND ADOLESCENCE 107
Göran Darius Hildebrand and Stéphane Chabrier

6.2 TRANSIENT CEREBRAL ARTERIOPATHY 115
Guillaume Sébire

6.3 MOYAMOYA SYNDROME IN CHILDHOOD 120
Vijeya Ganesan and Brian G.R. Neville

6.4 CEREBRAL VASCULITIS 127
Russell C. Dale

6.5 VASOSPASM 131
Fenella J. Kirkham

6.6 TORTUOSITY AND DOLICHOECTASIA 132
Katharine M.L. Forrest

6.7 DEVELOPMENTAL VENOUS ANOMALIES 133
Mara Prengler and Fenella J. Kirkham

7. CEREBAL SINOVENOUS (VENOUS SINUS) THROMBOSIS 145
Gabrielle deVeber

8. HAEMORRHAGIC STROKE 160

8.1 NON-TRAUMATIC INTRACRANIAL HAEMORRHAGE IN CHILDREN 160
Vijeya Ganesan and Dawn E. Saunders

8.2 SURGICAL TREATMENT OF HAEMORRHAGIC STROKE IN CHILDREN 169
Joan P. Grieve and Neil D. Kitchen

8.3 INTERVENTIONAL NEURORADIOLOGY IN THE MANAGEMENT OF ANEURYSMS 172
AND ARTERIOVENOUS SHUNTS IN CHILDREN

*Chao Bao Luo, Marina Sachet Ferreira, Hortensia Alvarez, Georges Rodesch,
Pierre L. Lasjuanias and Stefan K. Brew*

8.4 STEREOTACTIC RADIOSURGERY IN THE MANAGEMENT OF ARTERIOVENOUS
MALFORMATIONS IN CHILDREN 177

M.W.R. Radatz and A.A. Kemeny

9. NEONATAL STROKE 183

9.1 PERINATAL ARTERIAL STROKE 183

Frances Cowan and Eugenio Mercuri

9.2 INTRACRANIAL HAEMORRHAGE IN THE NEWBORN 194

Fenella J. Kirkham and Frances Cowan

10. VEIN OF GALEN ANEURYSMAL MALFORMATION 204

*Chao Bao Luo, Marina Sachet Ferreira, Hortensia Alvarez, Georges Rodesch, Pierre L.
Lasjaunias and Stefan K. Brew*

11. STURGE-WEBER SYDROME   212
     Sarah Aylett

12. HEMPILEGIC MIGRAINE   217
     Sarah Benton, Michel D. Ferrari, Fenella J. Kirkham and Peter J. Goadsby

13. ALTERNATING HEMIPLEGIA OF CHILDHOOD   225
     Jean Aicardi and Fenella J. Kirkham

14. INBORN METABOLIC DISEASE AND ACUTE FOCAL NEUROLOGY   233
     Robert Surtees and Fenella J. Kirkham

15. SYMPTOMATIC STROKE   245

     15.1 CARDIAC DISORDERS   245
           Vijeya Ganesen

     15.2 GENETICALLY DETERMINED VASCULOPATHIES AND STROKE SYNDROMES
           WITHOUT NEUROCUTANEOUS STIGMATA   251
           Fenella J. Kirkham and Nomazulu Dlamini

     15.3 GENETICALLY DETERMINED VASCULOPATHIES AND STROKE SYNDROMES
           WITH NEUROCUTANEOUS SYNDROMES   256
           Fenella J. Kirkham

     15.4 CONGENITAL AND ACQUIRED ANAEMIAS   261
           Dimitrios Zafeiriou, Mara Prengler, Steven Pavlakis and Fenella J. Kirkham

     15.5 IMMUNODEFICIENCY AND BONE MARROW TRANSPLANTATION   287
           Fenella J. Kirkham

     15.6 PREMATURE AGEING SYDROMES (PROGERIAS)   287
           Fenella J. Kirkham

     15.7 STROKE IN CHILDREN WITH CANCER   288
           Fenella J. Kirkham

     15.8 INFLAMMATORY VASCULOPATHIES   293
           Fenella J. Kirkham

16. ACUTE MANAGEMENT   319
     Rebecca Ichord, Anne Yardumian, Fenella J. Kirkham and Gabrielle DeVeber

17. RECURRENCE, OUTCOME AND REHABILITATION   337

     17.1 RECURRENCE AND SECONDARY PREVENTION   337
           Vijeya Ganesan and Fenella J. Kirkham

     17.2 OUTCOME AFTER STROKE IN CHILDHOOD   340
           *Anne Gordon, Lucinda Carr, Vijeya Ganesan, Fenella J. Kirkham and
           Gabrielle deVeber*

     17.3 ONTOGENETIC SPECIALIZATION OF HEMISPHERIC FUNCTION   354
           Faraneh Vargha-Khadem, Elizabeth Isaacs, Kate Watkins and Mortimer Mishkin

     17.4 NEURODEVELOPMENTAL OUTCOME IN CHILDREN WITH CONGENITAL HEART DEFECTS 362
           Amy Savage, Catherine Hill, Fenella J. Kirkham and Alexandra Hogan

17.5 SICKLE CELL DISEASE: COGNITIVE AND BEHAVIOURAL OUTCOME   370
   Alexandra Hogan

17.6 REHABILITATION AFTER STROKE IN CHILDREN   380
   Anne Gordon and Lucinda Carr

18. FUTURE DIRECTIONS   398
   Vijeya Ganesan and Fenella J. Kirkham

INDEX   403

Colour plates fall between pages 212 and 213.

AUTHORS' APPOINTMENTS

Jean Aicardi	Neurosciences Unit, UCL Institute of Child Health, The Wolfson Centre, London, UK
Hortensia Alvarez	Service de Neuroradiologie Diagnostique et Thérapeutique, Hôpital Bicêtre, Le Kremlin Bicêtre, France
Sarah Aylett	Neurosciences Unit, UCL Institute of Child Health, Great Ormond Street Hospital for Children NHS Trust, London, UK
Sarah Benton	Previously at Neurology Department, Great Ormond Street Hospital for Children NHS Trust, London, UK (deceased)
Stefan K. Brew	National Hospital for Neurological Diseases, Queen Square and Great Ormond Street Hospital for Children NHS Trust, London, UK
Fernando Calamante	Brain Research Institute, Neurosciences Building, Heidelberg West, Victoria, Australia
Lucinda Carr	Department of Neurology, Great Ormond Street Hospital for Children NHS Trust, London, UK
Stéphane Chabrier	Service de pédiatrie et génétique, Hôpital Nord, Saint-Etienne Cedex, France
W.K. Kling Chong	Radiology Department, Great Ormond Street Hospital for Children NHS Trust, London, UK
Alan Connelly	Radiology and Physics Unit, Institute of Child Health, University College London, London, UK; Brain Research Institute, Neurosciences Building, Heidelberg West, Victoria, Australia
Frances Cowan	Department of Paediatrics, Imperial College (Hammersmith Hospital), London, UK
Russell C. Dale	Neuroimmunology Group, Institute of Neuroscience and Muscle Research, The Children's Hospital at Westmead, University of Sydney, Australia
Gabrielle deVeber	Division of Neurology, Hospital for Sick Children, Toronto, Canada
Nomazulu Dlamini	Neurosciences Unit, Institute of Child Health, University College London, and the Evelina Children's Hospital, Guy's and St Thomas' NHS Trust, London, UK
Michel D. Ferrari	Department of Neurology, Chair, Leiden Centre for Translational Neuroscience, Leiden University Medical Centre, The Netherlands
Marina Sachet Ferreira	Service de Neuroradiologie Diagnostique et Thérapeutique, Hôpital Bicêtre, Le Kremlin Bicêtre, France
Katharine M.L. Forrest	Department of Paediatric Neurology, Southampton General Hospital, Southampton, UK
Vijeya Ganesan	Neurosciences Unit, University College London, Institute of Child Health; Neurology Department, Great Ormond Street Hospital for Children NHS Trust, London, UK
Bhuwan P. Garg	Division of Pediatric Neurology, Department of Neurology, Indiana University School of Medicine, Indianapolis, Indiana, USA
Peter J. Goadsby	Headache Group, Department of Neurology, University of California, San Francisco, California, USA and Hospital for Sick Children, Great Ormond Street Hospital for Children NHS Trust, London, UK

Anne Gordon	Department of Paediatric Neuroscience, Evelina Children's Hospital, London, UK; Murdoch Children's Research Institute, Royal Children's Hospital, Melbourne, Australia
Joan P. Grieve	Victor Horsley Department of Neurosurgery, National Hospital Queen Square, UCLH NHS Foundation Trust, London, UK
Bettina Harms	Department of Child Health, Southampton University Hospitals NHS Trust, Southampton, UK
Göran Darius Hildebrand	King Edward VII Hospital, Windsor; Royal Berkshire Hospital NHS Trust, Reading; University of Oxford, Oxford, UK
Catherine Hill	Department of Child Health, Southampton University Hospital NHS Trust, Southampton, UK
Alexandra Hogan	Developmental Cognitive Neuroscience Unit, UCL Institute of Child Health, University College London, UK
Rebecca Ichord	Department of Neurology, Children's Hospital of Philadelphia, Philadelphia, USA
Elizabeth Isaacs	Developmental Cognitive Neuroscience Unit, UCL Institute of Child Health, University College London and Great Ormond Street Hospital for Children NHS Trust, London, UK
A.A. Kemeny	National Centre for Stereotactic Radiosurgery, Royal Hallamshire Hospital, Sheffield, UK
Fenella J. Kirkham	Neurosciences Unit, University College London, Institute of Child Health, The Wolfson Centre, London; Department of Child Health, Southampton General Hospital, Southampton, UK
Neil D. Kitchen	Victor Horsley Department of Neurosurgery, National Hospital Queen Square, UCLH NHS Foundation Trust, London, UK
Juan C. Kupferman	Maimonides Infants and Children's Hospital, State University of New York, Downstate, New York, USA
Pierre L. Lasjaunias	Previously at Service de Neuroradiologie Diagnostique et Thérapeutique, Hôpital Bicêtre, Le Kremlin Bicêtre, France (deceased)
Chao Bao Luo	Service de Neuroradiologie Diagnostique et Thérapeutique, Hôpital Bicêtre, Le Kremlin Bicêtre, France
Jason MacDonald	Neuroradiology Department, Wessex Neurological Centre, Southampton University Hospital NHS Trust, Southampton, UK
Eugenio Mercuri	Department of Paediatrics, Imperial College (Hammersmith Hospital), London, UK and Rome, Italy
Benedicte Michel	Département de Pédiatrie, Cliniques Universitaires St-Luc, Bruxelles, Belgium
Mortimer Mishkin	Laboratory of Neuropsychology, National Institute of Mental Health, Bethesda, Maryland, USA
Brian G.R. Neville	Emeritus Professor of Paediatric Neurology, UCL-Institute of Child Health, London, UK
Ulrike Nowak-Göttl	Department of Paediatric Haematology/Oncology, University of Münster, Berlin, Germany
Steven Pavlakis	Maimonides Infants and Children's Hospital, Mount Sinai School of Medicine, New York, USA
Mara Prengler	Neurosciences Unit, UCL Institute of Child Health, University College London, London, UK
M.W.R. Radatz	National Centre for Stereotactic Radiosurgery, Royal Hallamshire Hospital, Sheffield, UK
Georges Rodesch	Service de Neuroradiologie Diagnostique et Thérapeutique, Hôpital FOCH, Suresnes, France
Dawn E. Saunders	Radiology Department, Great Ormond Street Hospital for Children NHS Trust, London, UK
Amy Savage	Department of Child Health, Southampton University Hospitals NHS Trust, Southampton, UK

Guillaume Sébire   Service de neuropédiatrie, CHU Fleurimont, Université de Sherbrooke, Canada

Ronald Sträter   Department of Paediatric Haematology/Oncology, University of Münster, Germany

Robert Surtees   Previously at Neurosciences Unit, UCL Institute of Child Health, University College London, London, UK (deceased)

Jacques-Donald Tournier   Radiology and Physics Unit, UCL Institute of Child Health, University College London, London, UK; Brain Research Institute, Neurosciences Building, Heidelberg West, Victoria, Australia

Faraneh Vargha-Khadem   Developmental Cognitive Neuroscience Unit, UCL Institute of Child Health, University College London and Great Ormond Street Hospital for Children NHS Trust, London, UK

Kate Watkins   Developmental Cognitive Neuroscience Unit, Institute of Child Health, University College London, Great Ormond Street Hospital for Children NHS Trust, London; University of Oxford, Oxford, UK

Andrew N. Williams   Virtual Academic Unit, Child Development Centre, Northampton General Hospital, Northampton, UK

Anne Yardumian   Department of Haematology, North Middlesex Hospital NHS Trust, London, UK

Dimitrios Zafeiriou   1st Department of Pediatrics, Aristotle University of Thessaloniki, Greece

1

CHILDHOOD STROKE – THE UNKINDEST CUT OF ALL: A HISTORY OF CEREBROVASCULAR DISEASE IN CHILDHOOD

Andrew N. Williams and Fenella J. Kirkham

For rightly is truth called the daughter of time, not of authority

Francis Bacon, 1620[1]

The course and the result of cerebral paralysis depend upon the extent of injury to the brain, its nature and the age at which it is inflicted – all these being conditions which are beyond the power of the physician to modify or control. The treatment of cerebral palsy is therefore extremely unsatisfactory

L. Emmett Holt, 1899[2]

Perhaps the main social responsibility of physicians is hard thinking in our daily work . . . Sometimes the doctor finds no cause and goes on to say "there's nothing wrong". He was answering his own question . . . forgetting to ask why the patient got it, we shall never arrive at prevention.

Ronnie Mac Keith, 1971[3]

Introduction

Depictions and descriptions of children who have had a stroke (or apoplexy or acute hemiplegia) have been around for millennia.[4–8] The concept of children at any age suffering and even dying from a stroke appears anachronistic, given our own experiences that it is typically a disease of the elderly. It is perhaps this very incongruity that has made the occurrence of stroke in childhood the more striking to medical observers often better known for other contributions.[9] Understanding of aetiology had to await the development of the concepts of the systemic and cerebrovascular circulation in adults from the seventeenth century onwards,[10–17] the distinction between upper and lower motor lesions and therefore between spinal (usually poliomyelitis) and cerebral paralysis,[4] the emergence of the concept of childhood[18] and the later twentieth century focus on differences between diseases of children and those of adults and therefore their needs in terms of investigation and rehabilitation.[19,20] The increase in research into childhood health and disease in general has at long last started to redress the deficiency.

History of childhood stroke

THE FIRST DESCRIPTION?
The very earliest medical literature (Table 1.1) provides an account suggestive of childhood stroke in the context of convulsions.

OTHER EARLY CLINICAL DESCRIPTIONS
In some ancient cultures, for example the Egyptian, the early historical record may only be pictorial,[4] probably at least in part because of a lack of practical experience with the body's anatomy, while others, including ancient Greece or Renaissance Italy, tolerated anatomical dissection and physiological empiricism and made scientific advances which are the basis of our current understanding. We should not be dismissive of these frameworks for thought, for to their practitioners they were, and indeed are, rational, causal and predictive. Traditional Chinese medicine is a contemporary example, which is constructed upon a completely different understanding from Western medicine. Ischaemic stroke is categorized under apoplexy and is mainly related to wind, fire, phlegm, stasis and deficiency.[21] There would not appear to be any specific case reports of childhood stroke within its vast historical canon – in present practice, cases would be managed as cerebral palsy (Professor Virginia Wong, personal communication, 2003).

Hippocrates (c.430BC) delineated sudden collapse, typically with aphasia and often hemiparesis, as apoplexy and recognized that it was more common in males and older people (although he did describe a boy),[22] as well as the relatively poor

---

TABLE 1.1
The earliest known reference to a movement disorder and aphasia after childhood convulsions, found in a Mesopotamian library of the 1st millennium BC. It may well be a copy of an earlier Sumerian work[8] (translated by M. Coleman and J. Scurlock)

DIšLÚ.TUR MU1.KÁM MU2.KÁM MU.3, KÁM MU.4.KÁM šu-ub-bu-us-ma te-be-a ù ú zu-uz-za la i-le- ´ -e NINDA a-ka-la la i-le- ´ -e KA-šú su ub-bu-ut-ma da-ba-ba la i-le- ´ -e re-hu-ut (DIǴER) Šùl-pa-è-a NU SI.SÁ	If an infant of one year, two years, three years, four years writhes in contortion so he is not able to get up and stand, his mouth is 'seized' so that he is not able to talk. [It is] 'spawn of Sulpaea'; he will not straighten up.

TABLE 1.2
'The Sacred Disease': Hippocrates (translated by Chadwick and Lloyd[7])

Infants who suffer from this disease usually die if the phlegm is copious and if the weather is southerly. Their little blood vessels are too narrow to absorb a large quantity of inspissated phlegm and so the blood is at once chilled and frozen, thus causing death. If the amount of phlegm is small and enters both main vessels, or if it enters but one of them, the patient survives but bears the stigmata. Thus the mouth may be distorted, or an eye, a hand or the neck: according to the part of the body in which some blood vessel become filled and obstructed with phlegm and thus rendered inadequate. As a result of this damage to the blood vessel, the corresponding part of the body must necessarily be weakened.

Taking a long view such a happening is generally a good thing because a child is not liable to another attack after an attack which has produced some permanent damage. The reason for this is that the strain of the attack causes injury to and some narrowing of the remaining blood vessels. As a result of this they will no longer admit the entry of phlegm to the same extent, although they will admit air. It is, however only to be expected that such deterioration in the condition of the blood vessels will lead to some weakening of the limbs.

Those who have a very small discharge at a time when the weather is northerly recover without any permanent injury, but there is a danger in such cases that the disease will remain with the child as he grows older.

prognosis for mild as well as severe cases. The term apoplexy was understood by the general public and appeared in the literature until the twentieth century. In adults the distinction between cardiovascular, cerebrovascular and other causes of collapse and coma became clearer during the nineteenth and twentieth centuries, but confusion has remained over how best to separate the aetiologies of the acute neurological presentations of childhood.[23] In 'The Sacred Disease', Hippocrates describes the motor outcome for epilepsy in children which we would recognize as hemiparesis (Table 1.2). Confusion about the overlap between the sequelae of acute convulsions (or hemiseizure-hemiplegia-epilepsy)[24] and childhood stroke secondary to cerebrovascular disease remains to this day, at least in part because so many children with a vascular aetiology present with seizures, although access to emergency imaging has improved the distinction between aetiologies in the majority of cases.

Galen distinguished paralysis, a deficit restricted to part of the body, from epilepsy, stupor, drowsiness and stiffness, and from apoplexy, which implied generalized loss of movement and sensation, but covered a number of non-neurological, as well as catastrophic neurological diagnoses.[25] He considered that apoplexy was caused by at least two mechanisms: an excess of abnormal phlegm in the ventricles and an excess of blood in the vessels.[25] He recognized the potential importance of the cerebral arteries and vessels of the rete mirabile, whose description he attributed to Herophilus, in the animals he was dissecting. However, he considered that the veins transported blood and nutrients while the vital pneuma was drawn up through the arteries to the rete mirabile where it spent enough time to be transformed into psychic or animal pneuma, in an analogy with the formation of breast milk, or of semen in the similar but less complex plexus of the testis.[26] He ascribed higher

cerebral functions to the rete mirabile but does not appear to have realized that this vascular structure did not exist in Man. In addition, although he linked haemoptysis to vascular rupture, there is no evidence that he linked apoplexy to the rupture of cerebral sex.[25] Galen commented on the association of apoplexy with lack of exercise,[25] and the different pulse seen in paralysis, suggesting that he may have recognized the link with cardiac dysrhythmia.[27] He mentions the protective effect of female sex,[25] the aetiology of which is still an active issue, attributing it to the loss of blood at menstruation, which remains a potentially important hypothesis, but did not refer directly to childhood stroke.

Within traditional Indian Medicine,[28] ailments that would today be described as the effects of stroke are usually classified as various types of paralysis, convulsion and spasm.[29] The existence of the heart and various ducts was acknowledged, but because it was taboo for high caste individuals to touch the dead, anatomical knowledge could only be gained by observing the decomposition of a body in flowing water, which meant that the anatomy of the bones was better understood than that of the soft tissues. The four humours, including blood, were recognized, and were considered to be carried by a multitude of vessels arising from the navel, while consciousness was considered to reside in the heart, the brain was considered insignificant and the causes of neurological illness were speculative. Diseases specific to children were well recognized[30] and there is a reference in the work of the Ayurvedic canon of Susrata (fifth century AD) to children being a vulnerable group, susceptible (in Sanskrit *Ardita*) to facial palsy,[29] attributed by some interpreters as indicating apoplexy and others as Bell's palsy (Table 1.3). We might recognize this condition now as poliomyelitis or perhaps as posterior reversible encephalopathy syndrome (PRES). The

TABLE 1.3
Description of acute focal neurology in the Sanskrit Ayurvedic canon of Susrata (SUŚRUTA; 5th century AD; in Wujastyk)[29]

The wind reaches the junctions of the head, nose lips, chin, forehead, and eyes, and hurts the face. Then it brings about lateral palsy of the face. This can happen to pregnant women, recently delivered women, children, old or emaciated people, or to those who have lost blood. One half of the mouth becomes crooked and the neck is twisted away. The head shakes and the speech is slurred, and the eyes and so on are disfigured. And the neck, chin and teeth hurt on that side.

distinction between upper and lower motor neurone facial palsy is not always easy to make in children even now and facial weakness is well recognized in hypertension, which is probably the most common cause of PRES. The emphasis was on treatment with several medi-cines to cover all possibilities, with psychological support in addition.

Ibn Sina, known in the West as Avicenna, distilled the previous Egyptian, Greek, Indian and Arab work in the Al-Qanum fi al-Tibb.[31,32] He published his observations on Laqve or facial paralysis, clearly distinguishing between upper and lower motor neurone facial palsy.[33,34] His work was translated into Latin as the Canon of Medicine; this and other Arabian and arabicized ancient texts were used in European universities until the seventeenth century, and were crucial for the transmission of ancient knowledge through the Dark Ages in Europe,[35] when there was little empirical work but many theories linking apoplexy to the brain or the vessels but not specifically to the cerebral vessels.[36,37]

There is little clinical material specific to neonatal and childhood stroke in the historical record until the nineteenth century, although parallel developments in anatomy[38] and the scientific method[39] laid the groundwork from the Renaissance onwards which led eventually to the concepts of the systemic and cerebrovascular circulation which we recognize today.[10–17] In 1605 Francis Bacon (1561–1626) in his Advancement of Learning defined the problem:

> In the enquiry which is made by anatomy I find much deficience: for they enquire of the parts, and the substance, figures and collocations: but they enquire not of the diversities of the parts, the secrecies of the passages, and the seats or nestling of the humours.
>
> *Bacon*[39]

ANATOMY

The return to human dissection with illustration in the universities of Renaissance Italy, particularly Padua, led by the Flemish Andreas Vesalius,[38] was of fundamental importance in challenging Greek and medieval misconceptions, and soon afterwards, the anastomotic circle at the base of the brain was described by Gabriele Fallopius in the *Observationes Anatomica* (1561),[40] published with humility as corrections to Vesalius' work but without illustrations, probably because it was at his own expense. Understanding of the cerebral circulation followed on from the key observation by William Harvey that the blood circulated through the body in response to the pumping of the heart.[10] Although medicine in Europe remained part of the Aristotelian and Galenic tradition, passed down through Ibn Sina's canon, as well as having a basis in alchemy, the Cartesian split between body and mind, the intellectual challenge to describe the limits of knowledge characteristic of the development of the Enlightenment in Europe and the preference for experiment opened up the possibility of describing new mechanisms for neurological diseases such as apoplexy.[41–43] Harvey's work spread by

way of the printing press to Padua, where Johann Wepfer (1620–1690) was studying[44] as well as to Thomas Willis (1621–1675); both accepted Harvey's findings, and independently injected dye into the cerebral circulation,[14,16] documenting the functional anastomoses of the circle which eventually led to further understanding of the vascular territories involved in stroke and the discrepancies between diseased vessels and cerebral pathology.

CONNECTING APOPLEXY TO THE BRAIN AND CEREBRAL VESSELS IN ADULTS AND CHILDREN

Despite the improved understanding of anatomy, progress on the pathology of disease was relatively slow as there were relatively few autopsies correlated to the clinical symptoms of the patient in life. The earliest unambiguous case descriptions of vascular causes of apoplexy (i.e. strokes) in adults and children, with confirmation that there was vascular pathology in the brain, were published in the seventeenth century. Jakob Wepfer described cases of cerebral haemorrhage in adults with apoplexy.[11,12,44] Thomas Willis invented the term neurology and also cared for children.[14,45,46] He described intracranial haemorrhage in an infant at post mortem but there is a good case for considering that this was subdural haemorrhage secondary to child abuse rather than a stroke.[47] The earliest childhood case of venous sinus thrombosis was described by Willis in *De anima brutorum* in 1672 (Table 1.4).

Recent comments on this case felt the history and post-mortem findings were in keeping with a venous infarction of the brain following a septic thrombosis of the vein of Galen or the straight sinus.[48,49] However, Willis's own reasoning was that 'without doubt in this case the headaches and subsequent delirium were caused by the incursion of the effervescent blood into the meninges and its accumulation there which caused a phlegmon', another in a long list of hypothesese for this condition.

Many of these cases were collected together with appropriate attribution in the Swiss Théophile Bonet's *Sepulchretum sive Anatomia Practica* (1679),[50,51] which was widely used by physicians during the seventeenth and eighteenth centuries. Morgagni, working in Padua in the Anatomical tradition of his predecessors, published his magnum opus *De Sedibus et causis morborum per anomem indagatis* as letters to a younger disciple at the end of his life in 1761, which was widely read in Latin and translated into English 8 years later.[52] Morgagni recognized subarachnoid haemorrhage as a cause of death in a 14-year-old boy but although he considered that cerebral aneurysms might be relevant, he did not report any in his cases and as a 'solidist' rather than a 'humourist' considered that the sudden onset of apoplexy was related to brain compression.[53] Whereas Bonet had included a number of patients who had sustained head injury prior to their apoplexy, Morgagni's series is mainly of spontaneous cases; whether or not to include post-traumatic cases of stroke, for example secondary to arterial dissection, remains a problem in the twenty-first century.

TABLE 1.4
**The first unambiguous description of childhood stroke by Thomas Willis in 1672 (translated by the late Professor
Alfred Moritz). Contemporary sources (Aubrey*) relate to boys attending Oxford and Cambridge from their early teens**

Olim juvenis Academicus cum per duas septimas de gravissimo capitis dolore ipsum incessanter affligente conquestus, erat tandem febre aucta, mox vigiliae, motus convulsivi, ac confabulatio delira succedebant: quo tempore medicus accersitus, phlebotomia, enematis, emplastris, revulsivis, vesicatoriis, item remediis internis, quae fluxionem sanguinis, ac humorunia capite devocent, sedulo adhibitis, nihil proficere potuit, quin mors brevi successerit. Calvaria aperta, vasa meningas obducentia erant sanguine replenta et plurimum distenta, quasi cruoris massa illuc tota confluxerat, ita ut sinibus dissectis et apertis, cruor affatim erumpens, ad plures uncias, supra lib. Fs. Pondus effexerit: porro ipsae membrane, tumore phlegmonide per totum affectae, discolores apparebant. Willis, 1672	Once a young scholar complained for two weeks of being incessantly afflicted by the most severe headache. This was eventually aggravated by a fever, and succeeded by insomnia, convulsive movements and delirious talk. At that time a doctor was called in and industriously applied phlebotomy, enemas, plasters, emetics and blistering and also internal remedies to divert the flow of blood and humours from the head. But he could make no progress to prevent the quick onset of death. When the skull was opened the vessels leading towards the meninges were full of blood and greatly distended as if all the arterial blood had flowed together there. When the sinuses were dissected and opened the blood burst out in abundance to the weight of several ounces above half a pint. In addition the membranes themselves, affected throughout by an inflamed swelling, appeared discoloured. When these coverings were removed all the bends of the brain and its ventricles were full of water and its substance, inasmuch as it was excessively watered was soaked and insufficiently firm.

* Aubrey, *Brief Lives*, edited Barber R.W. Boydell and Brewer, 1982.

Occasionally, survivors of acute paralysis in childhood were also reported; for example, Wepfer described a stroke in a child with hemiplegic migraine published posthumously in 1727.[12] The next 200 years continued in this vein with parallel descriptions of surviving cases with putative clinical triggers including infection and more convincing pathology in case series of those who died.

SPECULATION ON AETIOLOGY: CASE SERIES OF CHILDHOOD HEMIPLEGIA

The first case series of ischaemic stroke presenting in infancy was published by Cazauvieilh in 1827,[6] which was acknowledged as being an important landmark.[7]

> L'espèce de paralysie décrite dans ce mémoire, survenue chez le foetus ou dans la première enfance, dépend de deux états différens de l'encéphale. Le premier est un défaut de développement sans altération de tissu: le second est une altération de tissu, accompagnée d'un défaut de développement de la partie affectée et des parties environnantes.
>
> *Cazauvieilh, 1827*[6]

> Cerebral palsy as presented in this thesis and originating in fetal life or infancy is associated with two distinct forms of brain defect: firstly a primary developmental defect – i.e. without any focal damage – and secondly an acquired focal brain insult with secondary developmental effects.
>
> *Cazauvieilh, 1827*[6]

In Cazauvieilh's footsteps, many of the giants of nineteenth century medicine followed.[7,9,54] Jules Cotard induced cerebral atrophy by the experimental embolization of cerebral arteries in animals and suggested that this might be a mechanism in children as well as in adults, although he also noted some differences, for example in the likelihood of aphasia following apoplexy.[55] The work of Virchow shed considerable light on the pathology of thrombosis and embolus in vessels and was recognized to be of importance in adult stroke,[56] although its relevance to infantile hemiplegia continued to be an area of controversy.

In the latter half of the nineteenth century, debates raged about the apparently better outcome for apoplexy sustained in childhood and about the aetiology of congenital and acquired hemiplegia in the quest to find a single universal cause. Charles West (1816–1898), who founded Great Ormond Street Hospital in London in the middle of the nineteenth century, noted in 1852 that:

> Disturbance of the nervous system shows itself in children as well by loss of the motor power as by the occurrence of involuntary movements; and such an accident as the palsy of a limb naturally occasions parents the greatest anxiety. In the adult, a paralytic seizure is generally the result of a very serious disease either in the brain or spinal cord, and the sign of the commencement of a series of morbid processes which issue sooner or later in the destruction of the patient's life. Non-professional persons are aware of this fact, and suppose that the same rule holds good in the case of a child as in that of the adult; but you may in most instances quiet their fears with the assurance that paralysis in infancy and childhood seldom betokens any peril to life, though the affection is often very slow in disappearing, and sometime is quite incurable.
>
> *West, 1852*[57]

Interest in the subject during the late nineteenth century was stimulated by similar observations on outcome and the interest in cerebral localization in adults[58–60] alongside the further addition to the pathological literature of cases with porencephaly by Richard Heschl and Hans Kundrat, the suggestion by Joseph Parrott, a pioneering paediatrician in Paris, that venous congestion was important and Ernst Von Strümpell's (Fig. 1.1) unifying theory invoking a post polioencephalitic cause.[54,61] Several physicians in Europe and North America, including Thomas Barlow, Aletta Jacobs, Ernest Gaudard, Otto Huebner, Pierre Marie, L. Emmett Holt (Fig. 1.1), Sarah McNutt, William Osler, Bernard Sachs and Frederick Peterson (Fig. 1.2), published their experience with congenital, infantile and childhood hemiplegias between 1875 and 1900.[7,62–74]

Osler, who had trained with Virchow and had conducted large numbers of autopsies as part of his research at McGill University, wrote his monograph after moving to Philadelphia, where his interest turned to clinical follow-up of various

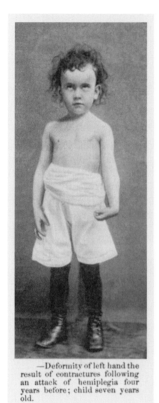

"It is of use from time to time to take stock ... of a particular disease, to see exactly where we stand in regard to it, to enquire to what conclusions the accumulated facts seem to point and to ascertain in what direction we may look for fruitful investigations in the future."
OSLER

—Deformity of left hand the result of contractures following an attack of hemiplegia four years before; child seven years old.

Fig 1.1. A case of childhood stroke reported by L.E. Holt in 1897.

conditions including the cerebral palsies, a term that he coined.[73] Both before and after he was President of the Clinical Section of the Royal Society of Medicine in London, cases were presented in various sections[75–78] in the era when the majority of children were cared for by general physicians and neurologists before paediatrics became a separate speciality.[79]

Sigmund Freud, who had described hemianopia in association with childhood hemiplegia, in *Infantile Cerebral Paralysis*,[7] undertook an extensive literature review and produced what can be regarded as a definitive nineteenth century opinion on childhood stroke. Reading this mighty work today, although we may have a greater understanding of the pathophysiology leading to a stroke in terms of practical effective management for the majority of cases, there has been little real progress beyond supportive care.

> Lack of therapy does not mean there is no chance for improvement or therapy. We know it is typical for many forms of infantile cerebral paralyses to tend to improvement, that there are light cases of the disease, and that even a complete recovery has occurred in a number of cases. An active interference on the part of the physician that can affect the process appears to be possible ... ... yet even under such conditions one must consider successful treatment as questionable.
>
> *Freud, 1897*[7]

It was clear to most authors that there were multiple risk factors for infantile hemiplegia, rather than a single cause. Sarah McNutt, whose work was recognized by Osler and Gowers

as being important and was the first female member of the American Association for Neurology, described hemiplegia after traumatic delivery with meningeal haemorrhage.[65–68] Osler mentions trauma as a trigger in older children in addition.[72] There was general agreement that infection was an important association but skepticism about the relationship with the flaccid paralysis of poliomyelitis. In 1860, Jacob von Heine had described hemiplegia after scarlet fever and after vaccination.[7] Gibotteau, who reported milder cases with improvement as well as those left with a residual hemiparesis, considered that all cases had an infectious aetiology.[71] Osler mentions measles, scarlet fever, diphtheria and whooping cough while Freud discusses congenital syphilis and smallpox (but not chickenpox)[7] and these infectious aetiologies were noted as triggers throughout the twentieth century. Interestingly, poliovirus was documented in the motor cortex of patients dying of the paralytic form of the disease[54,80] but the protagonists lost interest in the controversy once the disease was eradicated by the same author and his rival in the development of a safe vaccine.[81] Most of these diseases have either been eradicated or considerably reduced in prevalence at least in Western medicine through public health measures, immunization and antibiotics but children have continued to develop acute hemiplegia after infections. Ford and Schaffer in 1927 cited previously reported cases of focal encephalitis and monoplegia post-chickenpox and reported a case of their own.[82] The development of ventilation for patients with paralytic poliomyelitis has had benefits for the management of children presenting acutely with other neurological disorders including convulsions, coma and hemiplegia which, although it is difficult to prove, has probably improved outcome alongside emergency protocols for status epilepticus of any cause.

Acquired was clearly separated from congenital hemiplegia in the early nineteenth century French literature[6] and in the writings of Osler, Sachs and Freud.[7,72,74] In the field of neonatal stroke, clinical descriptions were typically included as 'congenital hemiplegia' as part of works on the outcome for birth asphyxia or the aetiology of cerebral palsies.[4,7,54,65–69,72–74,83] Many conditions presenting as acquired hemiplegia now known to have separate aetiologies, such as unilateral status epilepticus,[82] were published in the same series until the 1970s,[84–91] as were patients who presented in coma.[23,92,93] Nevertheless, some of those presenting with convulsions or coma almost certainly had a vascular aetiology, reminding us of the importance of broad nosological terms unless we really understand the pathology.[83,94–98]

Otitis media as a cause of cerebral venous thrombosis with 'the infection being carried by the blood vessels'[99] was previously well recognized as a cause of childhood and adolescent stroke. Interestingly, the debate as to the relative importance of arterial disease and venous thrombosis as a cause of childhood stroke is equally longstanding. In 1887 Abercrombie[70] was disputing Gowers' opinion[69] that 'thrombosis in arteries is a very rare lesion in childhood, far more rare than combined thrombosis in sinuses and veins', feeling instead that arterial

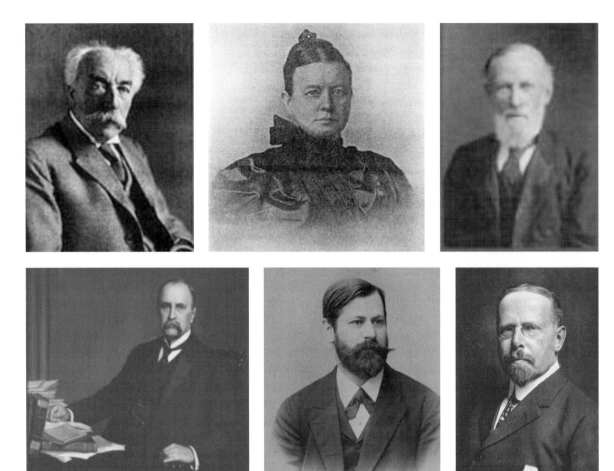

Fig. 1.2. The debate on aetiology of infantile hemiplegia in the late nineteenth century. Top row: Ernst Von Strümpell, Sarah McNutt, William Gowers. Bottom row: William Osler, Sigmund Freud and Bernard Sachs.

obstruction 'will hold good in the great majority in the other cases'. Although cerebral venous sinus thrombosis continues to be underdiagnosed in the twenty-first century, unless transient thrombosis in the venous circulation turns out to be common when sensitive imaging becomes available for all neurological emergencies in childhood, the passage of time has probably vindicated Abercrombie's judgement for the present day but it is impossible to obtain a clear answer for his own time or for the twentieth century.[100] Otitis media is frequently cited as the most common cause of cerebral venous thrombosis in the pre-antibiotic era, but as late as the 1960s venous occlusive disease made up 60% of cases in some autopsy series.[101] As antibiotics are prescribed less in the twenty-first than in the twentieth century, we need to maintain vigilance for this important and treatable cause of childhood death and disability.

These series of cases presenting to adult or paediatric neurologists rarely included children with underlying conditions that we consider common aetiologies now, such as sickle cell disease or cardiac disease. The importance of sickle cell disease[102] as an aetiological factor for childhood stroke went largely unrecognized for decades.[103–107] MacKenzie in the first volume of *Brain*[108] reported a case of cerebral embolus in a girl who appears to have endocarditis, probably secondary to rheumatic heart disease. He mentions the work of Kossuchin,

a Russian pathologist who published on the pathology of cerebral embolus in *Virchow's Archives* in 1874.[109] In addition to the recognition of the association of cerebral aneurysm with coarctation,[110] reports of stroke in congenital heart disease appeared,[76,82,111–113] although whether the mechanism was embolic remained controversial even when pathological studies were available. Interestingly Wood's case of a child with pulmonary stenosis and an atrial septal defect with severe cyanosis mentions venous congestion and the occipital softening may well have been secondary to venous thrombosis,[112] anticipating the current interest in the wide range of stroke syndromes in children with pre-existing problems.

EPIDEMIOLOGY

Over the last century, the epidemiology of childhood stroke appears to have changed with a decline in childhood stroke mortality being seen during the latter half of the twentieth century. Children less than 1-year old consistently have the highest mortality rate, the majority of deaths being due to haemorrhagic stroke.[114,115] This understanding has come about because there has been increased recognition of cerebral haemorrhage, at least in part because population-based studies have been undertaken and have included children who died.[116–121] Sachs[74] emphasized the relative rarity of intracerebral haemorrhage as a cause of stroke, whilst Broderick[121] demonstrated that it made up to 50% of cases seen. The fall in childhood stroke mortality seen during the late twentieth century has been mainly due to a fall in haemorrhagic stroke as opposed to other stroke subtypes. It could well be a reflection of changing aetiological factors that have been sustained now through several generations. On the other hand, the aggressive management of seizures has led to a marked reduction in cases of postictal hemiplegia and the severe and irreversible brain damage seen as a result.[24] However, iatrogenic causes have become more important as a consequence of medical advances allowing management to extend beyond supportive care.

Scientific Contributions from Anatomy and Pathology

Scientific advance was largely dominated by post-mortem studies until the middle of the twentieth century (Fig. 1.3), with increasingly accurate descriptions of the arterial and venous anatomy by meticulous neuropathologists and embryologists including Helena Riggs, Charles Rupp and Dorcas Padget.[122–127] Dorcas Padget's career is of particular interest as she originally trained as an illustrator and worked for many years with Walter Dandy, a pioneer of paediatric neurosurgery.[125,126] There were also steady advances in the understanding of cryptogenic and symptomatic arterial and venous stroke, periventricular leukomalacia, central pontine myelinolysis, hypertensive encephalopathy, Sturge–Weber syndrome and vein of Galen anomaly from the use of histopathological techniques and their detailed illustration or photography by Wilfred Le Gros Clark and Dorothy Russell, Morgan Berthrong, Betty Banker, Jeanne-Claudie Larroche, Dorcas Padget, Lucy Balian Rorke, Gilles Lyon and Ronald Norman amongst others.[23,101,128–152] Betty Banker pointed out the importance of cerebrovascular pathology as a cause of death in childhood as this was present in nearly 9% of 555 consecutive autopsies at the Children's Hospital of Philadelphia.[101] She re-emphasized the importance of cerebral venous pathology, particularly in those with congenital heart disease,[101] and separated out those with periventricular leukomalacia,[101,133] who only occasionally had demonstrable venous pathology, although she pointed out that the distribution of lesions suggested that these vessels were involved in aetiology, a subject of interest in the twenty-first century. When pathology could only be confirmed at autopsy, either in the acute phase or many years after the event, the timing of focal injury in infancy could only be guessed at, and many conditions, including cerebral venous sinus thrombosis[142,153] and arterial dissection,[141] were considered to have a poor prognosis because they may leave little trace after recovery so autopsy descriptions were considered representative. Even now we may not have the tools to exclude these conditions in settings in which its diagnosis and appropriate management might reduce childhood disability.

Outcome: Relation to Age at Injury

There have been relatively few long-term prospective follow-up studies of motor or cognitive outcome after childhood stroke before the twenty-first century (see chapter 17) and some potentially important material is not currently available in English.[154] As part of a series looking at aetiology and outcome of 334 children with spastic hemiplegia,[155,156] Philip Hood undertook statistical analyses for his doctorate under the supervision of Harold Westlake of the School of Speech at Northwestern University in Chicago and published the findings with Meyer Perlstein, who had a longstanding interest in cerebral palsy.[9] They looked at motor and language development[156] and at intelligence,[155] finding no difference in mean intelligence quotient between left and right hemiparesis or between congenital and postnatally acquired hemiparesis, although the developmental milestones were achieved a little earlier in the latter group. When computed tomography (CT) became available, several series were published linking presence, size and site of lesion to motor and cognitive outcome for congenital and acquired hemiplegia.[50,157–161]

Interest in the effect of age on outcome for focal damage to the hemisphere dates back to the nineteenth century when,

Fig. 1.3. Post mortem sequelae of acute hemiplegia. (From Le Gross Clark WE, Russell DS. Atrophy of the thalamus in a case of acquired hemiplegia associated with diffuse porencephaly and sclerosis of the left cerebral hemisphere. J Neurol Psychiatry 1940; 3:123–140; with permission from the BMJ Publishing Group.[128])

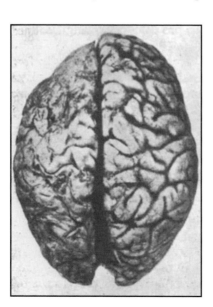
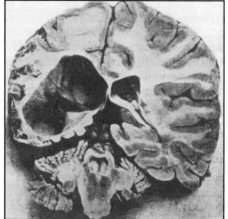

soon after the description of cerebral lateralization in adults, Felix Vulpian described experiments in young animals that appeared to move on both sides despite focal decortication.[162,163] Otto Soltmann hypothesized that motor function in the neonatal period was not reliant on the cerebral cortex and undertook experiments in dogs which showed that electrical stimulation in the cortex in the neonate did not lead to movement in the limbs and that unilateral lesions lead to late walking but not spasticity.[164,165] It became established that aphasia in adults typically resulted from lesions in the left hemisphere,[59,60] but the publication of an apparently transient case of aphasia from Great Ormond Street in a child with a right and then a left hemiplegia[62,63] led to the development of theories about equipotentiality and the development of specialization (see Chapter 17) which continue to be influential today.

Margaret Kennard worked at Yale during the 1930s and was undertaking experiments to look at the effects of cortical ablation in primates when she developed a collaboration with her obstetric colleagues which allowed her to study neonatal animals in addition. She and her colleagues were very surprised to realize that neonatal animals with focal cortical lesions did not develop spasticity and that this age effect persisted when lesions were performed in one- and two-year-old animals, although those operated on at later ages did worse than the neonates but less badly than the animals operated on as adults. Kennard's work was very influential[163,166–168] and was interpreted rather overenthusiatically to mean that outcome after focal lesions was generally better in the young. However, permanent aphasia may follow focal lesions sustained at a young age[169] and many children grow into their cognitive deficits even if language and motor function are relatively spared. The effect of age on motor and neuropsychological function after focal injury continues to be an area of controversy to the present day.

The advent of imaging

The twentieth century marked a decisive change in the visualization of cerebrovascular disease and its consequences in terms of haemorrhage or infarction. When previously only clinical acumen and craniotomy or trephination for extradural or subdural haematoma could reveal the cause of apoplexy in the living child,[170] imaging the living brain marked a decisive step,[149] even if this was initially only gross pathology.[171] Some of these techniques, such as pneumoencephalography,[172] although groundbreaking in their day, have become redundant and are now forgotten outside an historical review.[98] A limited understanding of ventricular size could be obtained from a skiagram[173] or pneumoencephalogram[24] (Fig. 1.4) and occasional series of unselected cases of acute hemiplegia in childhood were published, although the results were not necessarily illuminating except in showing atrophy independent of any vascular territory after status epilepticus[24] and unilateral brain swelling in the acute phase of hemiplegia.[90,95,174–176]

Understanding of the relative importance of various cerebrovascular pathologies improved with the advent of contrast

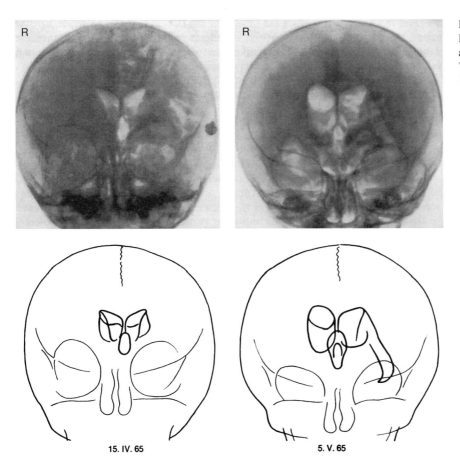

Fig. 1.4. Air encephalogram. (From Isler W. Post ictal hemiplegia. In: Acute Hemiplegias and Hemisyndromes in Childhood. London: William Heinemann Medical Books, 1971; 139; with permission.[217])

cerebral arteriography during the 1920s and 1930s.[177] Moniz included an 11-year-old girl with a tumour in an early series[178] but for stroke, the technique was used mainly in adults and only occasionally in children[179–185] unless surgery, for example for intractable epilepsy[186–188] or to prevent recurrence,[189–194] was considered, because of the perceived risk of the procedures after the experience with pneumoencephalography[195–200] and the perception that childhood stroke had a good prognosis and rarely recurred. However, the series of Charles Poser and Juan Taveras in New York, Kenneth Till and Dick Hoare in London and Edwin Bickerstaff in Birmingham, UK, John Shillito in Boston, Mark Dyken in Indianapolis and Derek Harwood Nash in Toronto, amongst others, made it clear that the test was commonly abnormal when haemorrhagic or ischaemic stroke was suspected clinically and that the benefit of making an ante-mortem diagnosis probably outweighed the relatively small risk for arteriography in their experienced hands.[98,195,201–205] Werner Isler in his series, published as a book,[98] acknowledged his debt to his predecessors and particularly to the participants at the Spastics Society meetings on Congenital Hemiplegia in Bristol[83] (Fig. 1.5) and on Acquired Hemiplegia in Clevedon in 1961,[97] which brought together clinicians and pathologists as well as the renowned anatomist Alf Brodal. Arteriography was felt to be safer and more useful in establishing a diagnosis than pneumoencephalography, so that even before cross-sectional imaging was available, case series

including the systematic use of vascular imaging in ischaemic stroke in childhood with clinical and laboratory information began to appear with the series of Hugh Greer and Arthur Waltz from the Mayo Clinic,[206] Jean Aicardi, Françoise Goutières and Jean-Jacques Chevrie in Paris,[90,207] Gail Solomon[85] and Sadek Hilal[86,208] from Arnold Gold's department at Colombia Prebyterian in New York, Tibbles and Brown from Canada,[209] Janaki[210] and Malik[211] from India, and Gösta Blennow[212] and Orvar Eeg-Olofsson from Scandinavia.[213] Systematic use of conventional angiography also allowed the distinction of cases with acute hemiplegia without cerebrovascular disease,[94,96] facilitating the diagnosis in life of venous sinus thrombosis,[207] which had been deduced previously,[100] the distinction of alternative diagnoses such as alternating hemiplegia[214] and the exclusion of hemiconvulsion-hemiplegia-epilepsy,[215,216] which had been previously included in many case series of acute hemiplegia in childhood.[90,94,98,217] These remain important issues as there is an important proportion of childhood stroke cases without vascular occlusion who must be excluded from any treatment trials to be conducted, for example of clot-busting drugs.

The advent of less invasive ultrasound, CT and magnetic resonance imaging (MRI)[106,160,218–234] has led to a renaissance of interest in the subject. Our perspective on childhood stroke has been revolutionized, allowing new perspectives including accurate identification of high risk groups with sickle cell disease[235–237], the diagnosis of silent or covert infarction[227] and

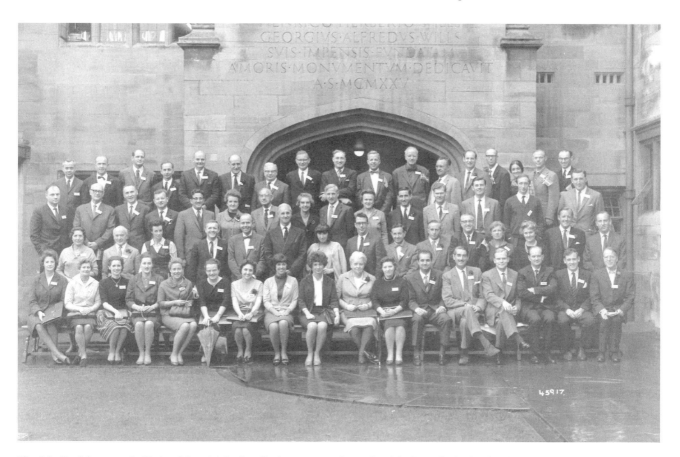

Fig. 1.5. Participants at the National Spastics Society Study group meeting on hemiplegic cerebral palsy in children and adults, held at the Wills Hall, University of Bristol, 1961. Ronnie Mac Keith is in the front row on the extreme right.[83]

comparisons with adults as well as giving us a greater understanding of the whole realm of cerebrovascular disease.

THE DAWN OF PHYSIOLOGY AND PATHOPHYSIOLOGY

Once investigation of the cerebrovascular circulation in life became possible, some workers began to explore the physiology as well as the anatomy associated with cerebrovascular disease in childhood. Cerebral blood flow was found to be much higher in normal children than in adults[238] using the nitrous oxide clearance method of Kety and Schmidt[239] and these data have proved useful in understanding the pathophysiology of sickle cell anaemia.[240,241] Using the Kety-Schmidt technique, Dyken found evidence that the least damaged hemisphere received blood from the contralateral carotid system in people who were long-term inpatients because they had sustained infantile hemiplegia[242] but these data are unlikely to be representative as most patients who have had a childhood stroke live independently as adults. Chronic focal perfusion deficits have been shown using other techniques,[243–245] but the relevance of these studies to outcome awaits less invasive methodologies which can be used in all children in the acute and chronic phases of stroke.

Although electroencephalography (EEG) was a breakthrough for the management of epilepsy, it was not a particularly sensitive technique for demonstrating the effect of focal infarction.[246] Attempts to use it for the diagnosis of paediatric neurological problems,[247] including congenital[248–250] and acute hemiplegia[94,251] did not bear fruit as it did not distinguish aetiology or predict prognosis. However, monitoring EEG during cardiopulmonary bypass using single channel devices such as the cerebral function monitor did lead to understanding of the role of intra-operative microembolization in the aetiology of poor neurological outcome in children as well as adults and thus to the introduction of filters which reduced the incidence.[252]

Interest in the physiology of sleep in the young dates back at least to the work of the Russian Maria Mikhaiovna Manasseina-Korkunov, also known as Marie von Manassein and Marie de Manacéïne, one of the first women doctors in Europe. In a paper presented at a meeting in Italy, she reported that depriving puppies of sleep led to reduced red cell counts and to death, with the youngest animals dying earliest, typically with localized intracerebral haemorrhage and abnormal blood vessels.[253–255] Her findings were followed up and largely replicated by Italian scientists,[254] but although links between sleep physiology and stroke have been reported in adults[256] and children, particularly those with sickle cell anaemia,[257,258] relatively little attention has been paid to the effects of duration since then, although this might be important in the preterm neonates vulnerable to intraventricular haemorrhage, in addition to the effect of nocturnal hypoxia on endothelial function. Interaction with haematologists and other laboratory scientists has been increasingly important in understanding the pathophysiology of childhood stroke, particularly as Maureen Andrew showed very clearly that haemostasis is affected by a number of factors, including age and hypoxia.[259,260] Like many

of the pioneers, she also trained up a number of distinguished clinical academics who continue to try to understand these complex problems.

Conclusion

The change in attitude is reflected in the increased medical literature devoted to this topic. Additionally there have been important changes in nomenclature. Osler's book gives a useful list of terms previously used in the nineteenth century,[72] while works from the mid-twentieth century tended to use his term 'cerebral palsy'[4,54] or, following Freud, 'hemiplegia', as did the early volumes of the Clinics in Developmental Medicine series supported by the Medical Advisory Committee of the National Spastics Society.[83,97,98] The different titles to the volumes published by key players based in Toronto, San Francisco, Chicago, Dallas and Paris in the 1980s and 1990s[261–264] reflect a more recent and wider understanding of the vascular nature of the majority of these conditions, as well as changing public attitudes. The definition of what we are including in clinical research has both hardened and widened in this period from that first suggested 40 years ago, when hemiplegia lasting less than one week was not included at Ronnie Mac Keith's insistence.[97] In contrast, most contemporary authors include not only patients with clinical stroke on the World Health Organization (WHO) criteria of a focal event lasting >24 hours with no cause other than vascular, but also those with transient ischaemic attacks lasting <24 hours (WHO) if there is a new lesion on cross-sectional imaging, and carefully clinically defined episodes lasting any length with reversible neuroimaging changes.

Arnold Gold and his colleagues attempted to examine the implications for treatment 50 years ago but it is only now that the challenges of running interventional studies are at last being met. The first large case controlled studies are now being published, examining the role of aetiological factors, often genetically controlled, which may not be obvious clinically at initial presentation, for example prothrombotic states. In preparation for, and subsequent to, the first international symposium on childhood stroke in 1998,[265,266] attempts have been made to develop a consensus, create a critical mass for research and to set a future research agenda. The conference on childhood cerebrovascular disease at the National Institutes of Health (NIH) in 2000 reviewed the available evidence on aetiology, risk factors for recurrence and outcome,[267] and in 2005 this was followed by an NIH-funded international meeting 'Towards the Establishment of Pediatric Stroke Trials'.[268] The development of guidelines and an international registry are stepping stones towards the trials needed for an evidence base for management. Re-inventing the wheel[269] is not an option.

A historical review merely provides pointers, restates unsolved questions and cautions against simplistic thinking.[270] Historians are sometimes asked from their understanding of the past to predict future developments. This we would hesitate to do, but would add that an examination of the changing management of other previously incurable conditions, for example childhood leukaemia, illustrates future possibilities as well as the difficulties, both in the short and long term, which have to be overcome. Already for stroke, authors have started to consider future therapeutic possibilities including neuronal regeneration and its limitations.

Childhood cerebrovascular disease has been described, if not recognized, since the dawn of medical literature and we can recognize its stigmata in art and literature. We are clearly seeing a sea change in attitudes to the investigation and management of childhood stroke and cerebrovascular disease on a background to changing attitudes to disability in childhood. For childhood cerebrovascular disease we appear at long last to be finally crossing from an era of 'one long hypothesis' through to an era of action based on sound theory.

We should not be complacent. At the beginning of the twenty-first century, we are still at an early stage in the medical evolution of the management of this condition. Single case reports and relatively small case series still inappropriately dominate the present day literature. Studies with matched controls have now been published which lay the groundwork for the future. The Stroke Prevention in Sickle Cell Anaemia (STOP) trial demonstrates the effectiveness of targeted intervention.[237] At the time of writing large international interventional studies are actively being considered. One hundred years after Freud's comprehensive review of this field the majority of cases still have little beyond general supportive care, but L. Emmett Holt's then contemporary gloomy thesis can no longer be supported. Our greater understanding and the new will of international cooperation raise the possibility that within our working lifetime, evidence-based acute and rehabilitative treatments for the acute stages of childhood cerebrovascular disease will become a realistic prospect for the majority.

Dedication
We would like to dedicate this chapter to the memory of Dr Stuart H. Green, MA (Cantab) MRCS, FRCP, FRCPCH consultant paediatric neurologist, children's physician, inspirational teacher and friend.

Acknowledgements
A.N.W. would like to thank the late Professor Alfred Moritz for his translation of Willis, Dr D. Wujastyk, Dr M. Miles, Professor Robert Arnott, Professor W. Wong, Mr H.J.R. Wing, Rabbi L. Tann and Professor Kitchen for their comments and the History of Medicine Unit, Medical School Birmingham, UK for their unstinting support. F.J.K. would like to thank her history teachers, particularly Pauline Churcher, Michael Hoskin and Karl Figlio. Thanks are also due to Miss Naomi Wills and Mrs Janine Smith for their assistance in obtaining the references.

REFERENCES

1. Bacon F. The New Organon or True Directions Concerning the Interpretation of Nature: 1620; Aphorism lxxxiv.

2. Holt L.E., Section VII, Chapter 1. Diseases of Infancy and Childhood Diseases of the Nervaus System. Thomas Lewin, London, 1899:750.
3. Mac Keith R. Social Responsibility. Dev Med Child Neurol 1971;13(1):1–2.
4. Christensen E, Melchior J. Cerebral Palsy – a clinical and neuro-pathological study. London: William Heinemann Medical Books, 1967.
5. Hippocrates. The Sacred Disease. In: Hippocratic Writings, 1st edn (ed GE Lloyd). London: Penguin Classics, 1983; 244–245.
6. Cazauvieilh J. Memoires et Observations. Recherches sur l'agenesie cerebrale et la paralysie congeniale. Arch Gen de Med 1827; 5.
7. Freud S. Infantile Cerebral Paralysis. Coral Gables: University of Miami Press, 1968.
8. Bax M. Fifty Years on – Editorial. Dev Med Child Neurol 1996; 38:755–756.
9. Ashwal S. The Founders of Child Neurology. San Francisco: Norman Publishing, 1990.
10. Harvey W. The Circulation of the Blood and Other Writings. Dent Dutton, 1628.
11. Wepfer JJ. Observations Anatomicae, ex cadaveribus eorum, qus sustulit apoplexia, cum exerciatione de ejus loco affecto. Schaffhausen: Joh Caspari Suteri, 1658.
12. Pearce JM. Johann Jakob Wepfer (1620–95) and cerebral haemorrhage. J Neurol Neurosurg Psychiatry 1997; 62(4):387.
13. Willis T. De anima brutorum quae hominis vitalis ac sensitiva est. Oxford: Richard Davis; 1672.
14. Williams AN. Thomas Willis' understanding of cerebrovascular disorders. J Stroke Cerebrovasc Dis 2003; 12(6):280–284.
15. Thomas Willis: the first Oxford neuropathologist. In: Neuroscience Across the Centuries (ed F Rose). London: Smith-Gordon, 2009; 93–94.
16. Fields WS, Lemak NA. A history of Stroke, its Recognition and Treatment. New York: Oxford University Press, 1989.
17. Gurdjian ES, Gurdjian ES. History of occlusive cerebrovascular disease. II. After Moniz, with special reference to surgical treatment. Arch Neurol 1979; 36(7):427–432.
18. Aries P. Centuries of Childhood, 1st edn. New York: Knopf, 1962.
19. Holt KS. Developmental pediatrics: definitions, scope and nature. In: Developmental Pediatrics (ed J Apley). London: Butterworths, 1977; 1–2.
20. Eisenberg L. Cross-cultural and historical perspectives on child abuse and neglect. Child Abuse Negl 1981; 5:299–308.
21. Keji C, Jun S. Progress of research on ischemic stroke treated with Chinese medicine. J Tradit Chin Med 1992; 12(3):204–210.
22. Clarke E. Apoplexy in the hippocratic writings. Bull Hist Med 1963; 37:301–314.
23. Lyon G, Dodge PR, Dams RD. The acute encephalopathies of obscure origin in infants and children. Brain 1961; 84:680–708.
24. Aicardi J, Baraton J. A pneumoencephalographic demonstration of brain atrophy following status epilepticus. Dev Med Child Neurol 1971; 13(5):660–667.
25. Karenberg A. Reconstructing a doctrine: Galen on apoplexy. J Hist Neurosci 1994; 3(2):85–101.
26. Hankinson RJ. The Cambridge Companion to Galen. Cambridge: Cambridge University Press, 2008.
27. Singer PN. Galen – Selected Works. Oxford: Oxford University Press, 1992.
28. Kutumbiah P. The Hindu medical theories. Indian J Hist Med 1956; 1(2):6–16.
29. Susrata. The Roots of Ayurveda: selections from the Ayurvedic Classics. London: Penguin Classics, 1998.
30. Kutumbiah P. Pediatrics (kaumara bhrtya) in ancient India. Indian J Pediatr 1959; 26:328–337.
31. Ibn Sina. Al-Qanum fi al-Tibb The Canon of Medicine. Tehran: Soroush Press, 1997.
32. Sarrafzadeh AS, Sarafian N, von GA, Unterberg AW, Lanksch WR. Ibn Sina (Avicenna). Historical note. Neurosurg Focus 2001; 11(2):E5.
33. Resende LA, Weber S. Peripheral facial palsy in the past: contributions from Avicenna, Nicolaus Friedreich and Charles Bell. Arq Neuropsiquiatr 2008; 66(3B):765–769.

34. Aciduman A, Arda B, Gunaydin A, Belen D. Laqve (wry mouth) considered in Avicenna's renowned treatise the Canon of Medicine. Neurocirugia (Astur) 2008; 19(3):267–271.

35. Karenberg A, Hort I. Medieval descriptions and doctrines of stroke: preliminary analysis of select sources. Part III: multiplying speculation – the high and late Middle Ages (1000–1450). J Hist Neurosci 1998; 7(3):186–200.

36. Karenberg A, Hort I. Medieval descriptions and doctrines of stroke: preliminary analysis of select sources. Part I: The struggle for terms and theories – late antiquity and early Middle Ages. J Hist Neurosci 1998; 7(113 Pt 2):162–173.

37. Karenberg A, Hort I. Medieval descriptions and doctrines of stroke: preliminary analysis of select sources. Part II: between Galenism and Aristotelism – Islamic theories of apoplexy (800–1200). J Hist Neurosci 1998; 7(3):174–185.

38. Vesalius A. De humani corporus fabrica. Basel: Johannes Oporinus, 1543.

39. Bacon F. The Two Books on the Profocience and the advancement of Learning Divine and Human. Printed by J. McCreery, for T. Payne, Pall Mall, 1808; 223.

40. Fallopius G. Observationes anatomicae. Venice: Marcum Antonium Ulmum, 1561.

41. Figlio KM. Theories of perception and the physiology of mind in the late eighteenth century. Hist Sci 1975; 13(3):177–212.

42. Martensen RL. The Brain Takes Shape: an early history. Oxford University Press, 2004.

43. Whitaker H, Smith CUM, Finger S. Brain, Mind and Medicine: essays in eighteenth century neuroscience. Springer; 2007.

44. Karenberg A. Johann Jakob Wepfer (1620–1695). J Neurol 2004; 251(4):501–502.

45. Williams AN, Sunderland R. Thomas Willis: the first paediatric neurologist? Arch Dis Child 2001; 85(6):506–509.

46. Williams AN. Thomas Willis's practice of paediatric neurology and neurodisability. J Hist Neurosci 2003; 12(4):350–367.

47. Williams AN. Too good to be true? Thomas Willis – neonatal convulsions, childhood stroke and infanticide in seventeenth century England. Seizure 2001; 10(7):471–483.

48. Hughes JT. Thomas Willis- the first Oxford Neuropathologist. In: Neuroscience Across the Centuries, 1st edn (ed F Clifford-Rose). London: Smith-Gordon, 1989; 93.

49. Williams AN. Cerebral venous thrombosis: the first reported case of adolescent stroke? J R Soc Med 2000; 93(10):552–553.

50. Bonet T. Sepulchretum sive Anatomia practica ex Cadaveribus Morbo Denatus. Geneva, 1679.

51. Schutta HS, Howe HM. Seventeenth century concepts of 'apoplexy' as reflected in Bonet's'Sepulchretum'. J Hist Neurosci 2006; 15(3):250–268.

52. Morgagni GB. On the Seats and Causes of Diseases Investigated by Anatomy. London: Miller & Cadell, 1769.

53. Schutta HS. Morgagni on apoplexy in De Sedibus: a historical perspective. J Hist Neurosci 2009; 18(1):1–24.

54. Ingram TTS. Pediatric Aspects of Cerebral Palsy. Edinburgh: Churchill Livingstone, 1964.

55. Cotard S. Etude sur l'Atrophie Cerebrale. Paris, 1868.

56. Safavi-Abbasi S, Reis C, Talley MC, Theodore N, Nakaji P, Spetzler RF et al. Rudolf Ludwig Karl Virchow: pathologist, physician, anthropologist, and politician. Implications of his work for the understanding of cerebrovascular pathology and stroke. Neurosurg Focus 2006; 20(6):E1.

57. West C. Lectures on the Diseases of Infancy and Childhood, 2nd edn. London: Longman, Brown, Green and Longmans, 1852; 145.

58. Gross CG. The discovery of motor cortex and its background. J Hist Neurosci 2007; 16(3):320–331.

59. Finger S, Roe D. Gustave Dax and the early history of cerebral dominance. Arch Neurol 1996; 53(8):806–813.

60. Buckingham HW. The Marc Dax (1770–1837)/Paul Broca (1824–1880) controversy over priority in science: left hemisphere specificity for seat of articulate language and for lesions that cause aphemia. Clin Linguist Phon 2006; 20(7–8):613–619.

61. von Strümpell AG. Uber die akute Encephalitis der Kinder (Polioencephalitis acuta, cerebrale Kinderlähmung). Jahrbuch Kinderheilkunde 1885; 22:173–178.

62. Barlow T. On a case of double hemiplegia, with cerebral symmetrical lesions. Br Med J 1877; 2:103–104.

63. Hellal P, Lorch MP. The validity of Barlow's 1877 case of acquired childhood aphasia: case notes versus published reports. J Hist Neurosci 2007; 16(4):378–394.

64. Eling P. Cerebral localization in the Netherlands in the nineteenth century: emphasizing the work of Aletta Jacobs. J Hist Neurosci 2008; 17(2):175–194.

65. McNutt SJ. Double infantile spastic hemiplegia, with the report of a case. Am J Med Sci 1885; 89:58–79.

66. McNutt SJ. Apoplexia neonatorium. Am J Obstet 1886; 18:73–81.

67. Horn SS, Goetz CG. The election of Sarah McNutt as the first woman member of the American Neurological Association. Neurology 2002; 59(1):113–117.

68. Accardo P. William John Little and cerebral palsy in the nineteenth century. J Hist Med Allied Sci 1989; 44(1):56–71.

69. Gowers WR. Clinical lecture on birth palsies. Lancet 1888; 1:709–711, 759–760.

70. Abercrombie J. Clinical lecture on hemiplegia in children. Br Med J 1887; 1:1323–1325.

71. Gibotteau A-M. Les paralysies d'origine cerebrale chez les enfants. Paris, 1889.

72. Osler W. The Cerebral Palsies of Children: a clinical study from the infirmary for nervous diseases. Philadelphia: Blakiston, 1889.

73. Longo LD, Ashwal S. William Osler, Sigmund Freud and the evolution of ideas concerning cerebral palsy. J Hist Neurosci 1993; 2(4):255–282.

74. Sachs B. A Treatise on the Nervous Diseases of Children. Infantile Cerebral Paralysis. Coral Gables: University of Miami Press, 1895; 159.

75. Guthrie LG, Mayou S. Right hemiplegia and atrophy of left optic nerve. Proc R Soc Med 1908; 1(Clin Sect):180–184.

76. Wright JA. Congenital heart disease (pulmonary stenosis); cerebral hemiplegia. Proc R Soc Med 1911; 4(Sect Study Dis Child):190.

77. Humphrey L. Case of post-diptheretic paralysis and hemiplegia. Proc R Soc Med 1927; 196–197.

78. Rolleston JD. Hemiplegia following scarlet fever. Proc R Soc Med 1927; 213–214.

79. Forfar JO, Jackson ADM, Laurence BM. The British Paediatric Association 1928–1988. London: The British Paediatric Association, 1989.

80. Sabin AB, Ward R. The natural history of human poliomyelitis: I. Distribution of virus in nervous and non-nervous tissues. J Exp Med 1941; 73(6):771–793.

81. Pearce JM. Salk and Sabin: poliomyelitis immunization. J Neurol Neurosurg Psychiatry 2004; 75(11):1552.

82. Ford FR, Schaffer AJ. The etiology of infantile acquired hemiplegia. Arch Neurol Psychiatry 1927; 18(3):323–347.

83. The National Spastics Society Study Group. Hemiplegic Cerebral Palsy in Children and Adults. London: Medical Advisory Committee of the National Spastics Society, 1961.

84. Carter S, Gold AP. Acute infantile hemiplegia. Pediatr Clin North Am 1967; 14(4):851–864.

85. Solomon GE, Hilal SK, Gold AP, Carter S. Natural history of acute hemiplegia of childhood. Brain 1970; 93(1):107–120.

86. Hilal SK, Solomon GE, Gold AP, Carter S. Primary cerebral arterial occlusive disease in children. I. Acute acquired hemiplegia. Radiology 1971; 99(1):71–86.

87. Gold AP, Challenor YB, Gilles FH, Kilal SP, Leviton A, Rollins EI. Report of Joint Committee for Stroke Facilities: IX. Strokes in Children (Part 1). Stroke 1973; 4:835–894.

88. Gold AP, Carter S. Acute hemiplegia of infancy and childhood. Pediatr Clin North Am 1976; 23(3):413–433.

89. Golden GS. Strokes in children and adolescents. Stroke 1978; 9(2):169–171.

90. Aicardi J, Amsili J, Chevrie JJ. Acute hemiplegia in infancy and childhood. Dev Med Child Neurol 1969; 11(2):162–173.

91. Aicardi J, Chevrie JJ. Consequences of status epilepticus in infants and children. Adv Neurol 1983; 34:115–125.

92. Seshia SS, Seshia MM, Sachdeva RK. Coma in childhood. Dev Med Child Neurol 1977; 19(5):614–628.

93. Seshia SS, Johnston B, Kasian G. Non-traumatic coma in childhood: clinical variables in prediction of outcome. Dev Med Child Neurol 1983; 25(4):493–501.

94. Majewska Z. The aetiology of acute hemiplegia in childhood. In: Acute Hemiplegia in Childhood (eds M Bax, RG Mitchell). London: William Heinemann Medical Books, 1962.

95. Evans P. Some clinical features of acute hemiplegia in childhood. In: Acute Hemiplegia in Childhood (eds M Bax, RG Mitchell). London: William Heinemann Medical Books, 1962.

96. Sandifer P. Non-vascular causes of acute idiopthic hemiplegia. In: Acute Hemiplegia in Childhood (eds M Bax, RG Mitchell). London: William Heinemann Medical Books, 1961.

97. Bax M, Mitchell RG (eds). Acute Hemiplegia in Childhood. London: William Heinemann Medical Books, 1962.

98. Isler W. Acute Hemiplegias and Hemisyndromes in Childhood Clinics. London: William Heinemann Medical Books Ltd, 1971.

99. Holt LE. Section VII. Diseases of the Nervous System. London: Thomas Lewin, 1899; 749.

100. Mitchell RG. Venous thrombosis in acute infantile hemiplegia. Arch Dis Child 1952; 27(131):95–104.

101. Banker BQ. Cerebrovascular disease in infancy and childhood. 1. Occlusive vascular disease. J Neuropathol Exp Neurol 1961; 21:127–134.

102. Herrick JB. Peculiar elongated and sickle-shaped red blood corpuscles in a case of severe anemia. 1910. Yale J Biol Med 2001; 74(3):179–184.

103. Bridgers WH. Cerebrovascular disease accompanying sickle cell anemia. Am J Pathol 1939; 15:353–361.

104. Adeloye A, Odeku E. Nervous system in sickle cell disease. Afr J Med Sci 1970; 1:33.

105. Portnoy BA, Herion JC. Neurological manifestations in sickle-cell disease, with a review of the literature and emphasis on the prevalence of hemiplegia. Ann Intern Med 1972; 76(4):643–652.

106. Powars D, Wilson B, Imbus C, Pegelow C, Allen J. The natural history of stroke in sickle cell disease. Am J Med 1978; 65(3):461–471.

107. Osuntokun BO. Neurological syndromes management and prognosis in sickle-cell anaemia. Trop Doct 1981; 11(1):2–7.

108. MacKenzie S. Embolic hemiplegia with optic neuritis. Brain 1877; 1: 400–409.

109. Kossuchin. Zur Lehre von dem embolischen infarcte. Virchows Arch 1874; 449.

110. Reifenstein GH, Levine SA, Gross RE. Coarctation of the aorta; a review of 104 autopsied cases of the adult type, 2 years of age or older. Am Heart J 1947; 33(2):146–168.

111. Palmer FS. Congenital heart disease and hemiplegia. Proc R Soc Med 1914; 7(Clin Sect):48–49.

112. Wood P. Congenital pulmonary stenosis with left ventricular enlargement associated with atrial septal defect. Br Heart J 1942; 4(1–2):11–16.

113. Corner B, Perry B. Hemiplegia in cyanotic congenital heart disease. Br Heart J 1942; 4(4):121–123.

114. Mallick AA, Genesan V and O'Callaghan FJK. Mortality from childhood stroke in England and Wales, 1921–2000. Arch Dis Child 2010; 95:12–19.

115. Fullerton HJ, Chetkovich DM, Wu YW, et al. Deaths from stroke in US children, 1979 to 1998, Neurology 2002;59:34–9.

116. Alter M, Christoferson L, Resch J, Myers G, Ford J. Cerebrovascular disease: frequency and population selectivity in an upper midwestern community. Stroke 1970; 1(6):454–465.

117. Abraham J, Rao PS, Inbaraj SG, Shetty G, Jose CJ. An epidemiological study of hemiplegia due to stroke in South India. Stroke 1970; 1(6):477–481.

118. Gudmundsson G. Primary subarachnoid hemorrhage in Iceland. Stroke 1973; 4(5):764–767.

119. Gudmundsson G, Benedikz JE. Epidemiological investigation of cerebrovascular disease in Iceland, 1958–1968 (ages 0–35 years): a total population survey. Stroke 1977; 8(3):329–331.

120. Schoenberg BS, Mellinger JF, Schoenberg DG. Cerebrovascular disease in infants and children: a study of incidence, clinical features, and survival. Neurology 1978; 28(8):763–768.

121. Broderick J, Talbot GT, Prenger E, Leach A, Brott T. Stroke in children within a major metropolitan area: the surprising importance of intracerebral hemorrhage. J Child Neurol 1993; 8(3):250–255.

122. Padget DH. The circle of Willis-its embryology and anatomy. In: Intracranial Arterial Aneurysms (ed WE Dandy). Ithaca, NY: Comstock Publishing, Cornell University, 1944; 67–90.

123. Padget DH. The development of the cranial arteries in the human embryo. Contrib Embryol 1948; 31:207–261.

124. Padget DH. The cranial venous system in man in reference to development, adult configuration, and relation to the arteries. Am J Anat 1956; 98(3):307–355.

125. Sugar O. Dorcas Hager Padget: artist and embryologist. Surg Neurol 1992; 38(6):464–468.

126. Kretzer RM, Crosby RW, Rini DA, Tamargo RJ. Dorcas Hager Padget: neuroembryologist and neurosurgical illustrator trained at Johns Hopkins. J Neurosurg 2004; 100(4):719–730.

127. Riggs HE, Rupp C. Variation in form of circle of Willis. The relation of the variations to collateral circulation: anatomic analysis. Arch Neurol 1963; 8:8–14.

128. Le Gros Clark WE, Russell DS. Atrophy of the thalamus in a case of acquired hemiplegia associated with diffuse porencephaly and sclerosis of the left cerebral hemisphere. J Neurol Psychiatry 1940; 3:123–140.

129. Geddes JF. A portrait of 'The Lady': a life of Dorothy Russell. J R Soc Med 1997; 90(8):455–461.

130. Berthrong M, Sabiston DC. Cerebral lesions in congenital heart disease. J Neuropathol Exp Neurol 1951; 10(1):98–99.

131. Berthrong M, Sabiston DC, Jr. Cerebral lesions in congenital heart disease, a review of autopsies on 162 cases. Bull Johns Hopkins Hosp 1951; 89(5):384–406.

132. Banker BQ. Occlusive vascular disease affecting the central nervous system in infancy and childhood. Trans Am Neurol Assoc 1959; 84:38–46.

133. Banker BQ, Larroche JC. Periventricular leukomalacia of infancy. A form of neonatal anoxic encephalopathy. Arch Neurol 1962; 7:386–410.

134. Banker BQ. The neuropathological effects of anoxia and hypoglycemia in the newborn. Dev Med Child Neurol 1967; 9(5):544–550.

135. Chester EM, Agamanolis DP, Banker BQ, Victor M. Hypertensive encephalopathy: a clinicopathologic study of 20 cases. Neurology 1978; 28(9 Pt 1):928–939.

136. Lyon G. The neuropathology of childhood cerebral hemiplegia. Rev Electroencephalogr Neurophysiol Clin 1972; 2(1):87–94.

137. Harvey FH, Alvord EC, Jr. Juvenile cerebral arteriosclerosis and other cerebral arteriopathies of childhood – six autopsied cases. Acta Neurol Scand 1972; 48(4):479–509.

138. Norman RM. Infantile cerebral palsies: pathology and aetiology. Proc R Soc Med 1953; 46(8):627–631.

139. Smith HV, Norman RM, Urich H. The late sequelae of pneumococcal meningitis. J Neurol Neurosurg Psychiatry 1957; 20(4):250–259.

140. Norman RM, Urich H, McMenemey WH. Vascular mechanisms of birth injury. Brain 1957; 80(1):49–58.

141. Norman RM, Ulrich H. Dissecting aneurysm of the middle cerebral artery as a cause of acute infantile hemiplegia. J Path Bact 1957; 73:580.

142. Dekaban AS, Norman RM. Hemiplegia in early life associated with thrombosis of the sagittal sinus and its tributary veins in one hemisphere. J Neuropathol Exp Neurol 1958; 17(3):461–470.

143. Norman RM, Urich H, Woods GE. The relationship between prenatal porencephaly and the encephalomalacias of early life. J Ment Sci 1958; 104(436):758–771.

144. Alexander GL, Norman RM. The Sturge–Weber Syndrome. Bristol: John Wright, 1960.

145. Norman RM. The neuropathology of status epilepticus. Med Sci Law 1964; 4:46–51.

146. Cadman TE, Rorke LB. Central pontine myelinolysis in childhood and adolescence. Arch Dis Child 1969; 44(235):342–350.

147. Crosley CJ, Rorke LB, Evans A, Nigro M. Central nervous system lesions in childhood leukemia. Neurology 1978; 28(7):678–685.

148. Sladky JT, Rorke LB. Perinatal hypoxic/ischemic spinal cord injury. Pediatr Pathol 1986; 6(1):87–101.

149. Ashwal S, Rorke LB, Epstein MA, Sladky JL, Zimmermann RA. Rapid deterioration in a three-year-old with left hemiparesis. Pediatr Neurosci 1988; 14(3):124–133.

150. Rorke LB. Pathology of cerebral vascular disease in children and adolescents. In: Cerebral Vascular Disease in Children and Adolescents (eds MSB Edwards, HJ Hoffman). Baltimore: Williams and Wilkins, 1989; 95–138.

151. Epstein MA, Packer RJ, Rorke LB, Zimmerman RA, Goldwein JW, Sutton LN et al. Vascular malformation with radiation vasculopathy after treatment of chiasmatic/hypothalamic glioma. Cancer 1992; 70(4):887–893.

152. Rorke-Adams LB. Lucy Balian Rorke-Adams, MD: an autobiography. J Child Neurol 2008; 23(6):674–682.

153. Byers RK, Hass GM. Thrombosis of dural sinus in infancy and childhood. Am J Dis Child 1933; 45(6):1161–1183.

154. Majewska Z, Radecka G. [Long-term follow-up in acquired hemiplegia in children.] Pol Tyg Lek 1980; 35(50):1953–1955.

155. Perlstein MA, Hood PN. Infantile spastic hemiplegia. III. Intelligence. Pediatrics 1955; 15(6):676–682.

156. Hood DPN, Perlstein MA. Infantile spastic hemiplegia. V. Oral language and motor development. Pediatrics 1956; 17(1):58–63.

157. Kotlarek F, Rodewig R, Brull D, Zeumer H. Computed tomographic findings in congenital hemiparesis in childhood and their relation to etiology and prognosis. Neuropediatrics 1981; 12(2): 101–109.

158. Claeys V, Deonna T, Chrzanowski R. Congenital hemiparesis: the spectrum of lesions. A clinical and computerized tomographic study of 37 cases. Helv Paediatr Acta 1983; 38(5–6):439–455.

159. Levine SC, Huttenlocher P, Banich MT, Duda E. Factors affecting cognitive functioning of hemiplegic children. Dev Med Child Neurol 1987; 29(1):27–35.

160. Uvebrant P. Hemiplegic cerebral palsy. Aetiology and outcome. Acta Paediatr Scand Suppl 1988; 345:1–100.

161. Banich MT, Levine SC, Kim H, Huttenlocher P. The effects of developmental factors on IQ in hemiplegic children. Neuropsychologia 1990; 28(1):35–47.

162. Vulpian A. Leçons sur la Physiologie Générale and et Comparée du Système Nerveux. Paris, 1866.

163. Finger S, Wolf C. The 'Kennard effect' before Kennard. The early history of age and brain lesions. Arch Neurol 1988; 45(10): 1136–1142.

164. Soltmann O. Experimentalle studien über der functionen des grosshirns der neugeborenen. Jahrbuch Kinderheilkunde 1876; 9: 106–148.

165. Finger S, Beyer T, Koehler PJ. Dr. Otto Soltmann (1876) on development of the motor cortex and recovery after its removal in infancy. Brain Res Bull 2000; 53(2):133–140.

166. Kennard MA. Age and other factors in motor recovery from precentral lesions in monkeys. Am J Physiol 1936; 115:138–146.

167. Kennard MA. Factors affecting the electroencephalogram in children and adolescents. J Nerv Ment Dis 1948; 108(5):442–448.

168. Finger S. Margaret Kennard on sparing and recovery of function: a tribute on the 100th anniversary of her birth. J Hist Neurosci 1999; 8(3):269–285.

169. Guttmann E. Aphasia in children. Brain 1942; 65:205–219.

170. Wisoff HS, Rothballer AB. Cerebral arterial thrombosis in children. Review of literature and addition of two cases in apparently healthy children. Arch Neurol 1961; 4:258–267.

171. Shepherd GM. Creating Modern Neuroscience: the revolutionary 1950s. Oxford University Press; 2009.

172. Dandy WE. Rontgenography of the brain after the injection of air into the spinal canal. Ann Surg 1919; 70(4):397–403.

173. Weber FP. Right-sided hemi-hypotrophy resulting from right-sided congenital spastic hemiplegia, with a morbid condition of the left side of the brain, revealed by radiograms. J Neurol Psychopathol 1922; [s1–3]:134–139.

174. Garofalo E. [Pneumoencephalography in infantile hemiplegia.] Fracastoro 1966; 59(4):329–373.

175. Dyken ML, Nelson G. Cerebral circulatory and metabolic studies related to pneumoencephalography. Acta Neurol Scand 1968; 44(2):148–155.

176. Abraham J, Sheety G, Jose CJ. Strokes in the young. Stroke 1971; 2(3):258–267.

177. Moniz E. L'angiographie cerebrale. Paris: Masson, 1931.

178. Moniz E. Diagnostic des Tumeurs Cérébrales et Épreuve de l'encephalographie artérielle. Paris: Masson, 1931.

179. Litchfield HR. Carotid artery thrombosis complicating retropharyngeal abscess. Arch Pediatr 1938; 55:36–41.

180. Knight GC. Infantile hemiplegia. Cerebral angioma. Subarachnoid haemorrhage. Proc R Soc Med 1939; 32(3):224.

181. Ingraham FD, Cobb CA, Jr. Cerebral angiography; a technique using dilute diodrast. J Neurosurg 1947; 4(5):422–434.

182. Picaza JA. Cerebral angiography in children; an anatomoclinical evaluation. J Neurosurg 1952; 9(3):235–244.

183. Carrea R. Cerebral angiography in a child. Arch Pediatr Urug 1952; 23(2):130.

184. Faure C, Lefebvre J, Lepintre J, Perez J. Results of cerebral angiography in cerebral hemiplegia in children. Acta Radiol 1956; 46(1–2): 456–465.

185. Duffy PE, Portnoy B, Mauro J, Wehrle PF. Acute infantile hemiplegia secondary to spontaneous carotid thrombosis. Neurology 1957; 7(9):664–666.

186. Krynauw RA. Infantile hemiplegia and its treatment by hemispherectomy. Sem Hop 1951; 27(25):1091–1097.

187. Wilson PJ. Cerebral hemispherectomy for infantile hemiplegia. A report of 50 cases. Brain 1970; 93(1):147–180.

188. Torma T, Donner M. Hemispherectomy in early hemiplegia and intractable epilepsy. Acta Paediatr Scand 1971; 60(5):545–552.

189. Christensen E, Brandt S. Recurrent acute infantile hemiplegia caused by a deep hemispheric angioma. Nord Med 1959; 62: 1574–1576.

190. Laitinen L. Arterial aneurysm with subarachnoid hemorrhage in children. Nord Med 1964; 71:329–333.

191. Matson DD. Intracranial arterial aneurysms in childhood. J Neurosurg 1965; 23(6):578–583.

192. Kudo T. Spontaneous occlusion of the circle of Willis. A disease apparently confined to Japanese. Neurology 1968; 18(5):485–496.

193. Suzuki J, Takaku A. Cerebrovascular "moyamoya" disease. Disease showing abnormal net-like vessels in base of brain. Arch Neurol 1969; 20(3):288–299.

194. Gold AP. Cerebral arteriovenous malformations. Dev Med Child Neurol 1973; 15(1):84–87.

195. Poser CM, Taveras JM. Clinical aspects of cerebral angiography in children. Pediatrics 1955; 16(1):73–80.

196. Czochanska-Kruk J, Kmiolek W, Losiowski Z. [Reactions and complications following pneumoencephalography in children.] Pediatr Pol 1966; 41(11):1277–1282.

197. Daute KH. EEG changes following pneumoencephalography in childhood. Psychiatr Neurol Med Psychol Beih 1967; 6:64–70.

198. Bordiuk JM, Gelband H, Steeg CN, Tasker W. Electrocardiographic changes in children undergoing pneumoencephalography. Neurology 1969; 19(12):1217–1222.

199. Iivanainen M, Collan R, Donner M. Adverse effects of pneumoencephalography performed under general anaesthesia in children. Ann Clin Res 1970; 2(1):71–78.

200. Seshia SS. Subdural haematoma: a complication of lumbar pneumoencephalography (a case report). Neurol India 1971; 19(4): 207–211.

201. Taveras JM, Poser CM. Roentgenologic aspects of cerebral angiography in children. Am J Roentgenol Radium Ther Nucl Med 1959; 82:371–391.

202. Bickerstaff ER. Aetiology of acute hemiplegia in childhood. Br Med J 1964; 2(5401):82–87.

203. Dyken M. Angiographic study of the middle cerebral artery in chronic infantile hemiplegia. J Neurol Neurosurg Psychiatry 1964; 27:326–331.

204. Shillito J, Jr. Carotid arteritis: a cause of hemiplegia in childhood. J Neurosurg 1964; 21:540–551.

205. Harwood-Nash DC, McDonald P, Argent W. Cerebral arterial disease in children. An angiographic study of 40 cases. Am J Roentgenol Radium Ther Nucl Med 1971; 111(4):672–686.

206. Greer HD, III, Waltz AG. Acute neurologic disorders of infancy and childhood. Dev Med Child Neurol 1965; 7(5):507–517.

207. Aicardi J, Goutieres F. Intracranial venous thromboses. Complication of acute dehydration in infants. Arch Fr Pediatr 1973; 30(8):809–829.

208. Hilal SK, Solomon GE, Gold AP, Carter S. Primary cerebral arterial occlusive disease in children. II. Neurocutaneous syndromes. Radiology 1971; 99(1):87–94.

209. Tibbles JA, Brown BS. Acute hemiplegia of childhood. Can Med Assoc J 1975; 113(4):309–314.

210. Janaki S, Baruah JK, Jayaram SR, Saxena VK, Sharma SH, Gulati MS. Stoke in the young: a four-year study, 1968 to 1972. Stroke 1975; 6(3):318–320.

211. Malik GK, Sharma B, Misra PK, Chhabra DK, Tandon SC. A study of acute hemiplegia in children. Indian Pediatr 1979; 16(10): 867–872.

212. Blennow G, Cronqvist S, Hindfelt B, Nilsson O. On cerebral infarction in childhood and adolescence. Acta Paediatr Scand 1978; 67(4):469–475.

213. Eeg-Olofsson O, Ringheim Y. Stroke in children. Clinical characteristics and prognosis. Acta Paediatr Scand 1983; 72(3):391–395.

214. Verret S, Steele JC. Alternating hemiplegia in childhood: a report of eight patients with complicated migraine beginning in infancy. Pediatrics 1971; 47(4):675–680.

215. Gastaut H, Poirier F. The electroencephalogram in cerebrovascular diseases. Neurology 1961; 11(4)(Pt 2):110–111.

216. Gastaut H. ACTH, adrenocortical hormones and juvenile epilepsy. Introduction. Epilepsia 1961; 2:343–344.

217. Isler W. Post ictal hemiplegia. In: Acute hemiplegias and hemisyndromes in Childhood (ed EH Burrows). London: William Heinemann Medical Books, 1971; 139.

218. Ambrose J, Hounsfield G. Computerized transverse axial tomography. Br J Radiol 1973; 46(542):148–149.

219. Kramer DM, Schneider JS, Rudin AM, Lauterbur PC. True three-dimensional nuclear magnetic resonance zeugmatographic images of a human brain. Neuroradiology 1981; 21(5):239–244.

220. Kendall BE, Claveria LE. The use of computed axial tomography (CAT) for the diagnosis and management of intracranial angiomas. Neuroradiology 1976; 12(3):141–160.

221. Schrager GO, Cohen SJ, Vigman MP. Acute hemiplegia and cortical blindness due to moya moya disease: report of a case in a child with Down's syndrome. Pediatrics 1977; 60(1):33–37.

222. Kingsley DP, Kendall BE. Cranial computed tomography in leukaemia. Neuroradiology 1978; 16:543–546.

223. Kingsley DP, Kendall BE, Moseley IF. Superior sagittal sinus thrombosis: an evaluation of the changes demonstrated on computed tomography. J Neurol Neurosurg Psychiatry 1978; 41(12):1065–1068.

224. Ito M, Konishi Y, Okuno T, Nakano Y, Yamori Y, Hojo H. Computed tomography of cerebral palsy: evaluation of brain damage by volume index of CSF space. Brain Dev 1979; 1(4):293–298.

225. Pellock JM, Kleinman PK, McDonald BM, Wixson D. Childhood hypertensive stroke with neurofibromatosis. Neurology 1980; 30(6):656–659.

226. Wilimas J, Goff JR, Anderson HR, Jr, Langston JW, Thompson E. Efficacy of transfusion therapy for one to two years in patients with sickle cell disease and cerebrovascular accidents. J Pediatr 1980; 96(2):205–208.

227. Hindmarsh PC, Brozovic M, Brook CG, Davies SC. Incidence of overt and covert neurological damage in children with sickle cell disease. Postgrad Med J 1987; 63(743):751–753.

228. Baumann RJ, Carr WA, Shuman RM. Patterns of cerebral arterial injury in children with neurological disabilities. J Child Neurol 1987; 2(4):298–306.

229. Fischer AQ, Anderson JC, Shuman RM. The evolution of ischemic cerebral infarction in infancy: a sonographic evaluation. J Child Neurol 1988; 3(2):105–109.

230. Sran SK, Baumann RJ. Outcome of neonatal strokes. Am J Dis Child 1988; 142(10):1086–1088.

231. Smith CD, Baumann RJ. Clinical features and magnetic resonance imaging in congenital and childhood stroke. J Child Neurol 1991; 6(3):263–272.

232. el Gammal T, Adams RJ, Nichols FT, McKie V, Milner P, McKie K et al. MR and CT investigation of cerebrovascular disease in sickle cell patients. AJNR Am J Neuroradiol 1986; 7(6):1043–1049.

233. Wiklund LM, Uvebrant P, Flodmark O. Morphology of cerebral lesions in children with congenital hemiplegia. A study with computed tomography. Neuroradiology 1990; 32(3):179–186.

234. Wiklund LM, Uvebrant P. Hemiplegic cerebral palsy: correlation between CT morphology and clinical findings. Dev Med Child Neurol 1991; 33(6):512–523.

235. Adams R, McKie V, Nichols F, et al. The use of transcranial ultrasonography to predict stroke in sickle cell disease. N Engl J Med. 1992;326:605–610.

236. Adams RJ, McKie VC, Carl EM, et al. Long-term stroke risk in children with sickle cell disease screened with transcranial Doppler. Ann Neurol. 1997;42:699–704.

237. Adams R, McKie V, Hsu L, Files B, Vichinsky E, Pegelow C, et al. Prevention of a first stroke by transfusion in children with abnormal results of transcranial Doppler ultrasonography. N Engl J Med. 1998;339:5–11.

238. Kennedy C, Sokoloff L. An adaptation of the nitrous oxide method to the study of the cerebral circulation in children; normal values for cerebral blood flow and cerebral metabolic rate in childhood. J Clin Invest 1957; 36(7):1130–1137.

239. Kety S, Schmidt C. Nitrous oxide method for the quantitive determination of cerebral blood flow in man: theory, procedure and normal values. J Clin Invest 1948; 27:476–483.

240. Huttenlocher PR, Moohr JW, Johns L, Brown FD. Cerebral blood flow in sickle cell cerebrovascular disease. Pediatrics 1984; 73(5):615–621.

241. Herold S, Brozovic M, Gibbs J, Lammertsma AA, Leenders KL, Carr D et al. Measurement of regional cerebral blood flow, blood volume and oxygen metabolism in patients with sickle cell disease using positron emission tomography. Stroke 1986; 17(4):692–698.

242. Dyken M, Nelson G. Changes in local blood flow characteristics in chronic unilateral brain damage. Acta Neurol Scand 1964; 40: 361–368.

243. Sztriha L, Al Suhaili AR, Prais V, Nork M. Regional cerebral blood perfusion in children with hemiplegia: a SPECT study. Neuropediatrics 1996; 27(4):178–183.

244. Gordon I. Cerebral blood flow imaging in paediatrics: a review. Nucl Med Commun 1996; 17(12):1021–1029.

245. Powars DR, Conti PS, Wong WY, Groncy P, Hyman C, Smith E et al. Cerebral vasculopathy in sickle cell anemia: diagnostic contribution of positron emission tomography. Blood 1999; 93(1):71–79.

246. Epstein JA, Lennox MA, Noto O. Electroencephalographic study of experimental cerebro-vascular occlusion. Electroencephalogr Clin Neurophysiol 1949; 1(4):491–502.

247. Kennard MA, Rabinovitch R, Wexler D. The abnormal electroencephalogram as related to reading disability in children with disorders of behaviour. Can Med Assoc J 1952; 67(4):330–333.

248. Gibbs FA, Gibbs EL, Perlstein MA, Rich CL. Electroencephalographic and clinical aspects of cerebral palsy. Pediatrics 1963; 32:73–84.

249. Dyken ML, White PT, Nelson G. Electroencephalographic lateralization in chronic infantile hemiplegia. Electroencephalogr Clin Neurophysiol 1964; 17:693–695.

250. Roger J, Bureau M, Dravet C, Dalla BB, Tassinari CA, Revol M et al. Cerebral hemiplegias in children. EEG data and epileptic manifestations related to childhood cerebral hemiplegia in children. Rev Electroencephalogr Neurophysiol Clin 1972; 2(1):5–28.

251. Pampiglione G, Cooper M. Neurophysiological studies of the cerebral circulation. In: Acute Hemiplegia in Childhood (eds M Bax, RG Mitchell). London: William Heinemann Medical Books, 1962.

252. Branthwaite MA. Detection of neurological damage during open-heart surgery. Thorax 1973; 28(4):464–472.

253. de Manacéïene M. Quelques observations expérimentales sur l'influence de l'insomie absolue. Arch Ital de Biol 1894; 21:322–325.

254. Bentivoglio M, Grassi-Zucconi G. The pioneering experimental studies on sleep deprivation. Sleep 1997; 20(7):570–576.

255. Kovalzon VM. Some notes on the biography of Maria Manasseina. J Hist Neurosci 2009; 18(3):312–319.

256. Partinen M, Palomaki H. Snoring and cerebral infarction. Lancet 1985; 2(8468):1325–1326.

257. Robertson PL, Aldrich MS, Hanash SM, Goldstein GW. Stroke associated with obstructive sleep apnea in a child with sickle cell anemia. Ann Neurol 1988; 23(6):614–616.

258. Davies SC, Stebbens VA, Samuels MP, Southall DP. Upper airways obstruction and cerebrovascular accident in children with sickle cell anaemia. Lancet 1989; 2(8657):283–284.

259. Andrew M, O'Brodovich H, Sutton J. Operation Everest II: coagulation system during prolonged decompression to 282 Torr. J Appl Physiol 1987; 63(3):1262–1267.

260. Andrew M, Paes B, Milner R, Johnston M, Mitchell L, Tollefsen DM et al. Development of the human coagulation system in the full-term infant. Blood 1987; 70(1):165–172.

261. Cerebral Vascular Disease in Children and Adolescents. Baltimore: Williams and Wilkins, 1989.

262. Biller J and Love BB (eds) Stroke in Children and Young Adults. 1 ed. Newton: Butterworth-Heinemann; 1994.

263. Roach ES, Riela AR (eds). Pediatric Cerebrovascular Disorders. Armonk: Futura Publishing Company, 1995.

264. Lasjaunias P, in collaboration with Karel ter Brugge. Vascular Diseases in Neonates, Infants, and Children: interventional neuroradiology management. Berlin: Springer, 1997.

265. Cerebrovascular Disease and Stroke in Childhood. Pre-Satellite Symposium of the 8th International Child Neurology Association Meeting. Institute of Health and Great Ormond Street Hospital for Children, NHS Trust, London, 1998.

266. Kirkham FJ. Cerebrovascular disease and stroke in childhood: report from the London Satellite Symposium at the Institute of Health and Great Ormond Street Hospital for Children, NHS Trust, London, September 1998. In: New Developments in Child Neurology (ed MV Perat). Bologna: Monduzzi Editore, 1998; 279–289.

267. Lynch JK, Nelson KB, Curry CJ, Grether JK. Cerebrovascular disorders in children with the factor V Leiden mutation. J Child Neurol 2001; 16(10):735–744.

268. Pavlakis SG, Hirtz DG, deVeber G. Pediatric stroke: opportunities and challenges in planning clinical trials. Pediatr Neurol 2006; 34(6):433–435.

269. Williams AN. Childhood stroke – beyond re-inventing the wheel. Eur J Paediatr Neurol 2000; 4(3):103–107.

270. Miles M. Goitre, cretinism and iodine in South Asia: historical perspectives on a continuing scourge. Med Hist 1998; 42(1):47–67.

2
DEVELOPMENT OF THE BRAIN CIRCULATION

Chao Bao Luo, Marina Sachet Ferreira, Hortensia Alvarez, Georges Rodesch and Pierre L. Lasjaunias

General aspects of development of the arterial supply to the brain tissue

The development of the cerebral arteries involves continuous adaptation of the vasculature to changes in the shape, size and metabolism of the brain, with reciprocal interactions in which the blood supply is tailored to the metabolic requirements of cerebral activity. Secondary morphological changes of the neural tissue reshape the arterial tree.[1] At the earliest stage of development, initial nutritional support for the closed neural tube comes via diffusion through its external surface. Ventral to the rhombencephalon, two arterial channels can be recognized, one on each side of the midline, the ventral longitudinal neural arteries.[2] The caudal extremities communicate laterally with the carotid system through the first segmental artery, the proatlantal artery. At the level of the trigeminal nerve, another transient communication is established, the trigeminal artery. Additional transient anastomoses supply the ventral neural longitudinal arteries, in particular the hypoglossal artery at the level of the XIIth cranial nerve (Figs 2.1 and 2.2).

At the end of 5th to 6th week of gestation, the neural tube undergoes major modification from three primitive to five vesicles, associated with an accentuation of the previous flexures; these morphological change associated with the ongoing growth of the neural tube require adaptation of the vascular system to fulfill the metabolic needs of the parenchyma.[3] The most significant change in the arterial tree at this stage is the development at the ventral aspect of the prosencephalon of two branches from the carotid tree[2] (Fig. 2.3). The first is an anterior or rostral branch, creating an arterial ring around the neck of each telencephalic vesicle, this artery is called either the olfactory or the telencephalic artery. The second is the posterior or caudal branch, which reaches the cephalic end of the ipsilateral ventral longitudinal neural artery to constitute the posterior communicating artery (PCoA). This leads to

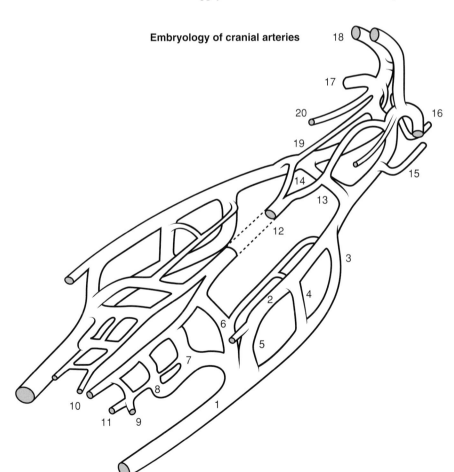

Embryology of cranial arteries

Fig. 2.1. Schematic view of the embryonic cranial arteries. 1, ventral aorta (VA); 2, dorsal aorta (DA); 3, first aortic arch (1AA); 4, second aortic arch (2AA); 5, third aortic arch (3AA); 6, hypoglossal artery (HA); 7, pro-atlantal artery, type I (PA 1); 8, pro-atlantal artery, type II (PA 2); 9, third cervical segmental artery; 10, longitudinal neural arteries (LNA); 11, para-ventral (lateral) neural artery; 12, basilar artery (fused ventral arteries) (BA); 13, trigeminal artery (Trig.A); 14, primitive maxillary artery (PMA); 15, dorsal ophthalmic artery (DOPHA); 16, ventral ophthalmic artery (VOPHA); 17, middle cerebral artery (MCA); 18, anterior cerebral artery (ACA); 19, internal carotid posterior (caudal) division (ICA Cd); 20, anterior choroidal artery (AChA}. (From Lasjaunias P. Segmental identity and vulnerability in cerebral arteries. Interv Neuroradiol 2000; 6:113–124, with permission.)

Internal carotid artery embryology early stage

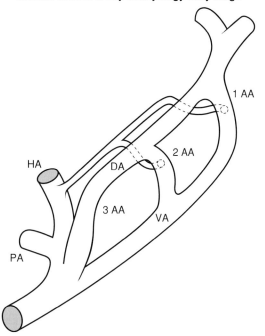

Fig. 2.2. Aortic arches. Internal carotid artery embryology: early stage. For definitions of abbreviations, see legend to Fig. 2.1. (From Lasjaunias P. Segmental identity and vulnerability in cerebral arteries. Interv Neuroradiol 2000; 6:113–124, with permission.)

regression of the preexisting transient anastomoses of trigeminal and hypoglossal arteries.[2] Simultaneously, the ventral longitudinal neural arteries tend to fuse at the midline to form the basilar artery, and therefore the posterior segment of the circle of Willis. The development of the tectum mesen-

cephalii and of the primitive cerebellar lips leads to the individualization of arterial channels which encircle the middle neural tube to constitute the mesencephalic and anterior superior cerebellar arteries. At this stage these arteries originate from the caudal division of the internal carotid system. During the 6th, 7th and 8th weeks, at the telencephalic level the preexisting arteries are incorporated and form a ring around the neck of the telencephalic vesicles. The anterior portion is the future anterior cerebral artery, the posterior portion is the future anterior choroidal artery, both belonging to the rostral division of the internal carotid artery (ICA), forming the telencephalic choroidal ring.

From the posterior branch of the ICA, another artery courses toward the choroid plexus of the 3rd ventricle and will become the posterior choroidal or diencephalic artery. At the level of the 4th ventricle, the arterial supply to the choroid plexus arises from the basilar artery, via the future anterior inferior cerebellar artery. The longitudinal anastomoses that are established at the same time at the cervical level, between the segmental arteries from the subclavian artery to the craniocervical junction, constitute the vertebral artery. Arising from the anterior branch of the telencephalic artery, vessels will grow on the medial and lateral surfaces of the telencephalic vesicles representing the future hemispheric territories of the anterior cerebral and middle arteries.

Analysis of embryology and evolution locates the ICA division at the level of the PCoA. The posterior or caudal division deserves that name more than that of posterior cerebral or posterior communicating artery. The anterior or rostral division of the ICA branches into two trunks: the anterior cerebral and middle cerebral arteries. The latter can be considered

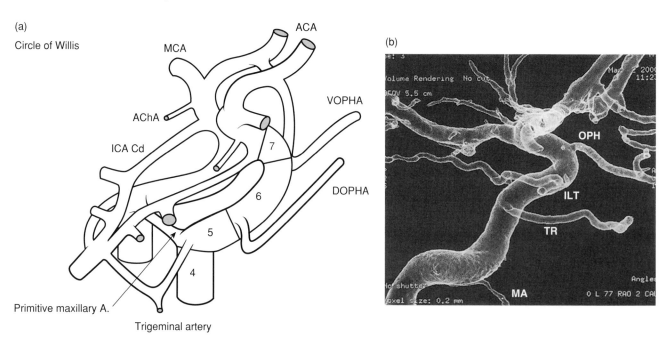

Fig. 2.3. (a) Intracranial segments (4 to 7) successively extending between the mandibular (not seen) and the trigeminal-primitive maxillary arteries, the dorsal ophthalmic artery, the ventral ophthalmic artery and the bifurcation. (b) Internal carotid angiography with the 5th cranial segments' arterial boundaries visible. ILT, infero-lateral trunk; MA, mandibular artery; OPH, ophthalmic artery; TR, trigeminal remnant. (From Lasjaunias P. Segmental identity and vulnerability in cerebral arteries. Interv Neuroradiol 2000; 6:113–124, with permission.)

as a branch of the former. The anterior choroidal artery has seen its territory change greatly throughout evolution. Its variable origin partially reflects this past role and remains unpredictable: one part belongs to the anterior division, whereas the other is fully linked to the posterior division.

When compared with the embryonic stage, the fetal period is characterized by intense cellular multiplication. As the neural tube thickens, diffusion from the meninx primitiva or from the ventricular fluid becomes inadequate. An intrinsic vascular system has to develop from the perineural vascular network. From the 24th to the 28th week, multiplication of lateral ramifications from the existing vessels and the development of penetrating superficial branches are seen. The density of the vasculature of the brain seems to depend on the number of synaptic connections that are established and the metabolic activity. The vascular density follows the increase in thickness of the cerebral tissue as well as its tangential growth.[4] Thus the density of the superficial vessels is explained both by the type of concentric increase in volume, and by the adaptation of the arterial supply to the sequential inside-out apposition of cellular layers on the brain surface.

As soon as the intracerebral vascularization develops the pial capillary network, which had provided the nutrition of the neural tube at the earlier stages of development, disappears. The arteries and veins of the surface are now connected to each other through the new system of arteriolo-capillary-venular loops which have developed within the parenchyma.

General and phylogenetic aspects of the cerebral vascularization

The principles governing the arterial supply to the brain are functional: consistency, economy of distribution and convenience of sources.[5] We have reviewed the vascular trees from fish to the amphibians, reptiles, birds and mammals. Options and solutions in the vascular arrangements summarize the evolution that the supply to the brain has undergone to reach the human pattern throughout this group of animals.

The ICA branches into two main trunks: the caudal and rostral divisions. The caudal division travels dorsally and branches into tectal and cerebellar arteries prior to anastomosis with its counterpart. It constitutes the basilar trunk and supplies the entire posterior fossa contents and part of the spinal cord.

PHYLOGENETIC STEPS

In fish, the rostral division gives off two branches which follow the olfactory system: (1) a medial branch supplies the olfactory nerve and rhinencephalic structures, this system can be considered as the primitive expression of the anterior choroidal artery (AChA) complex in man; and (2) a lateral branch follows the lateral root of the olfactory nerve and can be considered as representative of the future artery of Heubner and the AChA. In amphibians,[6] the lateral olfactory arterial system branches into: (1) a lateral striate artery, part of this lateral striate system belongs to the striate territory of

the future AChA; and (2) the posterior telencephalic artery that supplies the choroidal sac and the pineal region, the probable forerunner of the main trunk of the AChA.

In reptiles, regrouping of both the striate and cortical territories of the future AChA has occurred. However, the AChA system is called the inferior cerebral artery. The middle cerebral artery (MCA) is not a single vessel at this stage, but is represented by a series of small anastomotic channels within the lateral striate arteries.[5] The late appearance of the MCA constitutes the basis for multiple variation.[7,8]

In birds, the lateral striate artery is now individualized into an MCA whereas the medial olfactory artery has become the anterior cerebral artery (ACA); the inferior cerebral artery of the reptiles has become the posterior cerebral artery (PCA) which shows a midline fusion on the medial aspect of both hemispheres. In humans, the equilibrium between the medial and lateral striate arteries expresses the early origin of the striatal branches of the MCA. The MCA continued evolving through the mammals and primates to become the stem that we know in man. The MCA is therefore a recent acquisition, having developed from the lateral olfactory artery of the fish. Its representative in amphibians is the striate artery. The striatal territory of the anterior choroidal artery is reduced to the supply to the amygdaloid body and part of the medial pallidum.

THE DIVISION OF THE INTERNAL CAROTID ARTERY

At an initial stage of development the ventral aorta (VA) and dorsal aorta (DA) are anastomosed by a certain number of arterial structures, the aortic arches. The arches are numbered from 1 to 4 in the craniocaudal direction (Fig. 2.2). At a later stage of development, the ventral cephalic aorta has become the common carotid artery at this stage and is divided into two branches, the internal and external carotid arteries. Intracranially, the ICA branches into two: a cranial or rostral ramus (CrR), and a caudal or dorsal one (CaR). The CrR gives rise to a prominent ACA and AChA. Both supply the choroid plexus and anastomose at the interventricular foramen. In addition, they present telencephalic branches that anastomose on the surface of the vesicles. Caudally, the CaR gives rise to a diencephalic and a mesencephalic branch. The trunk fuses with its counterpart ventral to the mesencephalon and distal to the origin of the anterior superior cerebellar artery (ASCA) to constitute the basilar artery (BA). A posterior choroidal artery develops (PChA) from the diencephalo-mesencephalic trunk of the CaR and anastomoses at the atrium with the previous AChA from the rostral division.

Phylogeny has shown that the true division of the ICA is located at the PCoA origin. The basilar artery results from the cranio-caudal fusion of ventrally located paired arteries (longitudinal neural arteries). The remaining PCA (P2-P3-P4 segments) is similar to the pial network of the cord, linked to the previous system at the junction PcoA-P1. During the development of the intrinsic anastomoses, perforators arising from this system are in haemodynamic balance at the ventral portion of the mesencephalon and diencephalon.

At this stage, the division of the ICA clearly occurs at the CrR-CaR level. The flow is craniofugal in to the basilar system and the ASCA belongs to the unfused segment of the ICA caudal division. These stages, which correspond to the anterior choroidal nourishment of the developing vesicle, rapidly evolve by partial annexation of this territory by the posterior choroidal artery of the CaR. Additional changes occur simultaneously at the telencephalic level, by means of anastomosis and capture, regressions and changes in flow direction.

Internal carotid artery anterior division

The anterior or rostral division of the ICA can be considered as part of the ventral longitudinal arterial pial system, in which two main pial trunks (ACA-MCA) deserve specific attention. Embryologically, the ACA gives rise to a ventral ophthalmic artery that courses caudally and laterally to join the intracranial opening of the optic canal, medial to the supracavernous ICA. The proximal segment of the primitive ophthalmic artery rapidly regresses and the ophthalmic artery now arises from the ICA. Embryologically, a group of lateral striate arteries develop from the proximal ACA stems to supply the growing telencephalic vesicles. As seen in phylogeny, the recurrent artery of Heubner (RAH) develops from this system, as does the MCA and some other small vessels which penetrate the hemispheres at the anterior perforated substance. Therefore a natural balance will exist between these two vessels. In a simplified way, one can describe the MCA as a large RAH. In addition, the RAH shares a cortical territory, independent of the deep zone, and will be in balance with the MCA. Phylogenetic studies show how the ACA and AChA first provide the developing brain with the necessary sources of supply. Then a transfer of most cortical territories from the AChA to the PCA displaces the previous ACA-AChA balance to an ACA-PCA balance, in a more posterior location at the medial surface of the cerebral hemisphere. Finally, the developing MCA links together all these preexisting cortical arteries and establishes its own anastomotic channels at the convexity of the hemispheres with all the previous distributor systems.

The MCA is a recent phylogenetic acquisition and can be considered as a branch of the ACA.[9] Later in evolution, the MCA has surrendered some of its striated and paleo-olfactorial distribution. The central supply of the MCA is in equilibrium with the ACA striatal arteries.

Internal carotid artery posterior division

The AChA system consists of two parts: one belonging to the cranial division of the ICA and supplying the paleostriatum and piriform cortex, the other belonging to the caudal division and supplying the remainder of the anterior choroidal territories. The cranial component is mainly paleostrial in distribution and supplies, in addition to the piriform cortex, part of the head of the caudate nucleus and most of its tail, the posteromedial part of the amygdaloid nucleus and most of the globus pallidus. The caudal component supplies the optic tract and lateral geniculate body, the middle third of the crus cerebrii, the subthalamic region, the posterior two-thirds of the posterior limb of the internal capsule, the optic radiation, the antero-inferior part of the fascia dentata, the hippocampus and the choroid plexus.

The PCA belongs to the ICA system and constitutes its caudal terminal branch. The upper basilar artery distal to the trigeminal artery remnant is included in this system. Embryologically, the PCA is a diencephalomesencephalic artery, which gathers its telencephalic supply by distal annexation of the AChA territory. The caudal division of the ICA extends to the BA, the true PCA starts at P2. To be accurate as regards the human anatomy, the following terminology is the most appropriate: (1) PCoA + P1 becomes the caudal division of the ICA with its diencephalo-mesencephalic territory. It extends to the upper BA post-segmental portion and interferes with the ASCA pattern. (2) P2-P3-P4 are the true PCA system. (3) AChA remains as telencephalo-diencephalo-mesencephalic.

ARTERIAL SUPPLY TO THE POSTERIOR FOSSA

The arteries of the posterior fossa should be regarded as a transitional pattern between the simplified arrangement of the spinal cord and the complex cerebral pattern. The junction between both systems may be grossly located at the trigeminal remnant site on the basilar artery. Morphologically, three vesicles constitute the basis of the classical posterior derivatives: the mesencephalon, metencephalon and myelomeres. Phylogeny and ontogeny show that the BA derives from the caudal division of the ICA, which also includes the ASCA.

The BA results from the midline fusion of the paired ventral longitudinal arteries. The tectal derivatives of the mesencephalon have created a peculiar network which includes many branches on the colliculi, arising from the caudal division of ICA, the PCA system and the ASCA. ASCA represents the hypertrophy of one pial channel in relation to cerebellar development. AICA is the labyrinthine system and was only incidentally recruited to participate in cerebellar and choroidal supply. The posterior inferior cerebellar artery is the latest acquisition of this system in man. It represents a spinal cord artery which annexed cerebellar territory through the primitive meninx of the choroid plexus of the IV ventricles, when the cerebellum relocated over the myelencephalon.

Conclusion

The ACA is a terminal branch of the ICA. It presents various modalities of midline anastomoses:

1. The MCA is a branch of the ACA and belongs to the group of lateral striate arteries. It develops after the RAH. They both share territories and variations; and are in haemodynamic balance in their deep territory.
2. The AChA is an old artery which transiently vascularizes an extensive cortical territory, the majority of which will

be transferred to the tectal artery of the caudal division of the ICA, later to become the PCA.

3. The PCA prolongs the caudal division of the ICA. It only supplies the tectum and becomes the true PCA when it annexes most of the cortical territories from the AChA.

4. The BA results from a craniocaudal fusion, medial to the posterior division of the ICA. The initial fusion occurs caudal to the ASCA, at the level of the trigeminal remnant. The former belongs in most species to the supratentorial cerebral pathway.

5. The vertebrobasilar junction is a recent acquisition. The role played by each vertebral artery is unpredictable.

For the sake of accuracy in human anatomy and to be consistent with the above, we should adopt the following terminology:

1. The ICA distal to PCoA, with A1 and probably 5mm of A2 of ACA, is the cranial division of ICA with a diencephalo-telencephalic territory.

2. A2 (minus the first 5mm) + A3 and A4 of ACA are the true ACA system (telencephalic).

3. The MCA persists (purely telencephalic).

4. The AChA remains as such (telencephalo-diencephalo-mesencephalic).

5. PCoA + P1 is the caudal division of the ICA, a diencephalo-mesencephalic territory. It extends to the upper post-segmental portion of BA, and often interferes with the ASCA pattern.

6. P2 + P3 and P4 of PCA are the true PCA system.

REFERENCES

1. Raybaud C. Development of the vessels. In: Surgical Neuroangiography: clinical vascular anatomy and variations, vol 3 (eds P. Lasjaunias and A. Berenstein). Springer: Berlin, 1990.

2. Padget DH. The development of the cranial arteries in the human embryo. Contrib Embryol 1948; 31:207–261.

3. Streeter GL. The developmental alterations in the vascular system of the brain of the human embryo. Contrib Embryol 1918; 8:5–38.

4. Normal MG, O'Kusky JR. The growth and development of microvasculature in human cerebral cortex. J Neuropathol Exp Neurol 1986; 45(3):222–232.

5. Shellshear JL. The basal arteries of the forebrain and their functional significance. J Anat 1920; 55:27–35.

6. Gillilan LA. A comparitive study of the extrinsic and intrinsic arterial blood supply to brains of submammalian vertebrates. J Comp Neurol 1967; 130:175–196.

7. Hofmann M. Zur vergleichenden anatomie der Gehirn und Rückenmarksarterien der Vertebraten. Z Morph Anthrop 1900; 2:246–322.

8. Dandy WE. Concerning the cause of trigeminal neurolagia. Am J Surg 1934; 24:447–455.

9. De Vriese B. Sur la signification morphologique des arteres cerebrales. Arch Biol 1905; 21:357–365.

3
THE EPIDEMIOLOGY OF CHILDHOOD STROKE

Gabrielle deVeber

Introduction

Childhood stroke is seldom considered as a significant health care problem. However, among childhood diseases, stroke is not rare and the burden of illness related to the neurological damage and mortality from this disorder is significant. The incidence of first stroke probably exceeds 6 per 100 000 children[1] per year. Cerebrovascular disease is one of the top ten causes of death in childhood.[2] Adults with stroke have benefited from the development of evidence-based treatments as the result of clinical trials. By contrast, clinical trials of prevention or treatment have not been conducted in children with stroke, with the important exception of sickle cell disease.[3] There does appear to be a decline in the incidence of stroke in sickle cell disease[4–6] since the publication of the STOP primary prevention trial in 1998.[3] Although the death rate has decreased somewhat in the past 40 years,[7,8] mortality for ischaemic stroke has fallen at only half the rate of that for adults,[7] reflecting the lack of a coordinated approach to research.

Epidemiological data including incidence, stroke subtypes and outcomes from childhood stroke must be obtained in large populations of children with stroke. There are considerable age-related differences in the vascular, coagulation and nervous systems in neonates, older infants and children, compared with adults. There are also age-related differences in the pathophysiology and clinical features of stroke. The diagnosis of stroke in children is often delayed due to the relative infrequency of this disorder, and the lack of familiarity with this diagnosis. The risk factors for, and diseases underlying, stroke are very different from adults, in whom atherosclerosis is the cause in over two-thirds. The potential for recovery from stroke in infants and children may be different, perhaps because of increased plasticity in the immature brain. Finally, the burden of illness for children sustaining permanent disability through stroke will be increased related to their special educational needs, as well as the many decades of disability over a full life span. As a result of these age-related differences, the risks and benefits of specific therapies for stroke will differ. Even the design of childhood stroke trials will differ from adult trials. For example in studying adult stroke, data from tertiary care centres where only a minority of stroke patients are treated would result in significant referral bias. However over 90% of children with stroke are referred to tertiary care paediatric centres.[9]

Epidemiological data in children with stroke are critical to the design of effective trials for children with stroke. The required sample size, acceptability and safety of candidate therapies, relevant outcomes, and subgroups of children requiring the most aggressive therapies are all fundamental to the design of clinical trials. These data can only be developed from large population-based studies of children with stroke providing the incidence, stroke subtypes and outcomes of childhood stroke. This chapter reviews the epidemiology of stroke in infants and children, including the incidence and relative proportions of stroke subtypes. Ischaemic stroke includes *arterial ischaemic stroke* (cerebral arterial occlusion with focal cerebral infarction) and *cerebral sinovenus (venous sinus) thrombosis* (cerebral vein or venous sinus occlusion with or without accompanying cerebral infarction). Haemorrhagic stroke includes non-traumatic *intracerebral haemorrhage* with extravasation of blood into the brain parenchyma or *subarachnoid haemorrhage* with bleeding into the subarachnoid space; the underlying pathology may be arterial or venous. Although the population-based data on outcomes in childhood stroke will be briefly reviewed, more detail will be available in the related chapters in this book and other sources.[10]

Incidence and stroke subtypes

The original studies of childhood stroke found an incidence of around 2.5 per 100 000 in the USA[11,12] and Sweden[13] and around 3/100 000 in the UK[14] and Iceland.[15] Although some recent studies,[7,16–20] have found a similar incidence, others have reported higher rates[1,21–23] (Table 3.1). Data from Saudi Arabia suggest that the incidence is much higher there but the denominator appears to be hospital attendances rather than the whole childhood population.[24,25] A recent longitudinal population-based study from Cincinnati[8] found that the change in point estimate for later years, although higher, was not significantly different. Nevertheless, the diagnosis of stroke in children may have increased over the past 25 years. Several factors may have contributed to this observation. First, the methods of research studies into the incidence of childhood stroke have changed, and enabled the identification of increased numbers of children with stroke. Second, an increased number of children with stroke have come to diagnosis as the techniques for computed tomography (CT) and magnetic resonance imaging (MRI) have undergone refinement in sensitivity, and become increasingly available. Finally, the number of strokes may have increased as children with congenital heart disease, malignancy and other disorders which predispose to stroke have experienced prolonged survival. The increased

TABLE 3.1
Incidence of major subtypes of stroke in childhood

Author, year	Study 'N'	Ischaemic stroke incidence[a]	Haemorrhagic stroke incidence[a]	Ratio ischaemic to haemorrhagic	Combined incidence[a]
Gudmundsson, 1977 (Iceland)[15]					3.1
Schoenberg, 1978 (USA)[11]	4	0.6	1.9	0.33	2.5
Osuntokun, 1979 (Nigeria)[41]	4				2
Eeg-Olofsson, 1983 (Sweden)[13]					2.1
Bamford, 1988 (Oxford, UK)[14]	2				3.0
Satoh, 1991 (Tohoku, Japan)[43]	54	0.2			
Broderick, 1993 (Cincinnati 1988–9)[12]	16	1.2	1.5	0.78	2.7
Kleindorfer 2006 (Cincinnati 1999)[8]					6.4
Giroud, 1995 (Dijon, France)[21]	28	7.9	5.1	0.4	13.2
Merino Arribas, 1997 (Burgos, Spain)[45]	21	1.1	2.3	0.5	3.4
Earley, 1998 (Baltimore, USA)[16]	35	0.58	0.71	0.81	1.29
	Age>1 year		(excluded SAH)		
deVeber, 2000 (Canada)[46]	820	3.3	–	–	3.3
		AIS 2.6; SVT 0.7			
Lynch, 2002 (USA 1980–1998)[1]	1300	7.8	2.9	~ 2	13.5
Williams, 2002 (Birmingham, UK 1993–1998)[17]	120	1.17	0.89	1.31	2.06
Fullerton, 2003 (USA)[31]	2278	1.2	1.2 (0.8 intracranial, 0.4 subarachnoid)	1	2.3
Chung, 2004 (Hong Kong)[47]	94			2.57	2.1
Barnes, 2004 (Melbourne, Australia)[32]	98	1.8			
Williams, 2004 (UK 2001)[18]	239	1.05	0.5	2.19	1.94
Steinlin, 2005 (Switzerland)[20]	80	2.1			
Zahuranec, 2005 (USA)[23]	8				4.3
Simma 2007 (Voralberg, Austria)[48]	22	1.96	0.74	2.67	2.7
Fullerton, 2007 (California, USA)[49]	153		1.7		
Al Sulaiman 1999[b] (Eastern Saudi Arabia)[24]	31				(29.7)
Salih 2006[b] (Riyadh, Saudi Arabia)[25]	117				(27.1)

[a] Incidence = per 100 000 children per year.
[b] Figures compare stroke with total paediatric admissions, not paediatric population.

AIS, arterial ischaemic stroke; SAH, subarachnoid haemorrhage; SVT, sinovenous thrombosis.

survival from these primary diseases reflects the development of more effective treatments, which can themselves be risk factors for stroke.

Estimates of the incidence and relative proportions of stroke types in different studies are widely disparate, as shown in Table 3.1. Among the studies listed in Table 3.1, the inclusion criteria, methods of patient identification and geographical population evaluated have differed, with each study contributing differently to our understanding of incidence and subtypes of stroke. Stroke is undoubtedly more common in neonates with an incidence of at least 25–30 per 100 000 or 1 in 2300–4000 live births[1,26–28] and a recent study from Estonia had findings of 63/100 000.[29] Estimates depend on inclusion criteria: all ischaemic strokes or only arterial; patients with motor impairment as an outcome (17 per 100 000[30]) or all patients with focal ischaemia in an arterial distribution (20 per 100 000[26]). Whether neonates are excluded or not, the peak age for ischaemic stroke and intracerebral haemorrhage is the first year of life, with around one-third of cases presenting in this age group,[31,32] while subarachnoid haemorrhage is more common in teenagers.[31] Boys are at higher risk than girls in all studies, even when cases involving a history of trauma are

excluded.[31] There appears to be an excess of strokes in those of black ethnicity[31] which is not fully explained by the prevalence of sickle cell disease in this population.[16] Asians have a similar incidence, while the incidence in Hispanics appears to be lower.[31]

The first incidence data for childhood stroke appear similar whether studies were confined to children and based in single large cities,[11,12] or drew from a wider population base as part of a study which included adults.[14,15] However, numbers of cases reported were small (Table 3.1). For example, four cases were identified in the Rochester, Minnesota population, resulting in an overall incidence for childhood stroke of 2.5/100 000 children/year with haemorrhagic stroke three times more frequent than ischaemic stroke.[11] In the Rochester study, neonates, children older than 14 years, and children with head trauma were excluded. Sixteen strokes (nine haemorrhagic and seven ischaemic) were identified in metropolitan Cincinnati, Ohio, yielding an incidence of 2.7/100 000/year, with haemorrhagic stroke 1.25 times more frequent than ischaemic stroke.[12] This study reported that blacks were at increased risk for childhood stroke with an overall incidence rate of 3.1 per 100 000 children per year, compared with whites who had an incidence rate of 2.6.[12] Earley[16] reported 35 children with stroke identified from the central region of the state of Maryland and from Washington, DC. The diagnosis of stroke was confirmed by chart review in all cases. Excluding neonates and children older than 15 years, the incidence rate for all stroke was 1.29 per 100 000 children per year. Even excluding subarachnoid haemorrhage, haemorrhagic stroke was more frequent than ischaemic stroke. In the UK, regional and national studies have reported an incidence of about 2/100 000[17,18] (Fig. 3.1).

There may have been significant lack of recognition of ischaemic stroke in early studies, as the World Health Organization definition (focal neurological deficit lasting more than 24 hours) was used and neuroimaging was often not undertaken, so that infarction in children with seizures or focal deficits of short duration would have been missed. In Europe, Giroud reported 28 children with stroke in Dijon, France, resulting in an overall incidence rate of 13.02/100 000.[21] For the first time, the Dijon study reported that ischaemic stroke was more frequent than haemorrhagic stroke in children.[21] The explanation for the greatly increased stroke incidence rates reported in the latter study is not known, but may relate to the geography, with all patients in the region referred to one hospital where the stroke team was led by a dual-accredited paediatrician and neurologist, so that all study participants had their diagnosis confirmed by CT or MRI. In a single institutional study in Montreal, Canada, ischaemic strokes were more than twice as frequent as intracerebral haemorrhage, although subarachnoid haemorrhage was again excluded.[33] Paediatric ischaemic stroke is therefore likely to be an important health problem; in a study[34] based in Salt Lake City, Utah, children less than age 18 comprised 22% of ischaemic strokes in the 'young' (aged less than 40 years) despite the exclusion of neonates.

In recent years, data from large national studies looking specifically at stroke in children have become available. In the

Canadian Pediatric Ischemic Stroke Registry over 1000 children with ischaemic stroke (from term birth to 18 years) have been identified at all children's health care centres in the country during the initial 10 years, resulting in an estimated incidence rate of ischaemic stroke of at least 3.3 per 100 000 children per year (95% confidence intervals 3.02–3.63).[35] Diagnostic code searches with ICD-9 codes and standardized chart reviews were conducted in all cases to confirm the diagnosis. The Canadian Registry provides the first data on the incidence of cerebral venous sinus thrombosis.[36] In the Registry, neonates comprised 43% of cerebral venous sinus thrombosis and 25% of arterial ischaemic strokes. The sex distribution was similar to previous studies, with 54% of cerebral venous sinus thrombosis and 58% of arterial ischaemic stroke occurring in males.

In the largest study of childhood stroke to date, paediatric stroke cases were identified by hospital discharge diagnosis searches with ICD-9 codes in the US National Hospital Discharge Survey (NHDS).[1] The NHDS is a continuous nationwide sample survey of short-stay hospitals in the USA. The incidence of stroke for infants from birth (predominantly at term) to 30 days of age was 26.4/100 000. The rates for ischaemic stroke and haemorrhagic stroke were 17.8/100 000 and 6.7/100 000 live births per year respectively. The rates for children 0–18 years were 13.5/100 000 children per year for all stroke codes; 7.8/100 000 for ischaemic stroke codes (ICD-9 433–437, excluding 435 'transient cerebral ischaemia') and 2.9/100 000 for haemorrhagic stroke codes (ICD-9 430–431).[1] The latter study provides overall incidence rates which are similar to those from Dijon. It is possible that the rates of stroke were overestimated by the hospital ICD-9 coding, since confirmatory chart review to verify stroke diagnosis was not part of the study. In addition, the inclusion of codes for related cerebrovascular disease, including ICD-9 codes 436 (which includes 'cerebral seizure') and 437 (which includes moyamoya, hypertensive encephalopathy and unruptured aneurysms) may have resulted in an overestimate. However, the rates for neonates with ischaemic stroke are less than those from the Canadian Registry and the Estonian study. Lynch's study[1] has provided the most detailed information to date on the incidence rates for all subtypes of childhood cerebrovascular diseases and the stroke-related mortality rates, and over time will provide important race-specific stroke rates in children. A Northern California a study ascertained 205 validated pediatric ischemic strokes yeilding an incidence of 2.4/100000 children/year.[21]

Overall, the mean combined incidence rates for ischaemic and haemorrhagic stroke in children is 6.8 per 100 000 children per year. The relative proportion of ischaemic to haemorrhagic stroke is not entirely clear, and reported ratios of ischaemic to haemorrhagic strokes range from 0.33 to 2.0 with a mean rate of 0.86, which translates into haemorrhagic stroke being 1.2 times more common than ischaemic stroke. A recent study based on a large number of childhood strokes actually found a 1:1 ratio.[31]

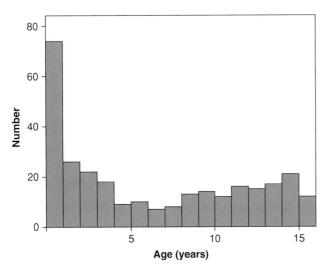

Fig. 3.1. Age distribution of 296 children with stroke (38 neonates) presenting in the UK and Eire in 2001 (median age 4.76 years).

Health care utilization

Incidence data only partially describe the impact of a given disease. For stroke, health care utilization costs and loss of productive years when significant neurological or psychological deficits result are significant contributors to the burden of the illness. In adults, the lifetime cost of a first stroke is estimated to be $90 981.[37] The types and magnitude of health care costs generated by childhood stroke have only recently been assessed.[38] In the US the cost per pediatric stroke acute admission ranges from $20 000 to $81 000 with 5-year costs of $51 000 for neonates and $135 000 for children[39,40]. The median cost for the first year after diagnosis is $43 212. In one study length of inpatient stay and degree of physical and social impairment correlated with higher cost so that stroke cost may act as an indicator of stroke severity. The cost of treating haemorrhagic stroke was higher than for ischaemic stroke care, but infarct volume did not correlate with cost. However children's inpatient stay is longer than that of adults. Part of the cost for health care utilization includes aetiological investigations and procedures which include multiple radiographic tests, laboratory tests and cardiac echocardiography. In children with stroke, in whom risk factors are heterogeneous and multiple, the extent and costs of investigations are likely to be increased compared with adults. In contrast, the costs of certain stroke treatments including t-PA and endarterectomy not currently utilized in children with stroke will be decreased. The costs of acute and chronic rehabilitation and the treatment of disease-related comorbid conditions add significant health care costs to the acute hospitalization costs. Finally, the cost of recurrent strokes over the lifetime of children with stroke may be considerably increased compared with adults.

Conclusion

Stroke in adults is preventable, and stroke in children may be preventable as well. However, in contrast to adults, evidence-based treatments for childhood stroke are not available because no clinical trials have been conducted. Health care priorities and the funding of stroke care programmes have not included childhood stroke to date. Until the true burden of illness and impact on the health care system of each initial and recurrent childhood stroke is appreciated, this situation will change only slowly.

The available epidemiological data indicate that the incidence of stroke in children is increasing and currently exceeds 6 per 100 000 children per year. Children with stroke face rates of adverse outcomes which include death in 10–40%, and in survivors, significant neurological disability, learning problems or seizures in least 50%. Since children with stroke are expected to live a full lifespan, the burden of illness per individual will last for 50–70 years.

However, the true impact of childhood stroke is unknown because large population-based studies on the incidence, health care utilization and outcomes for all subtypes of childhood stroke are sparse. In addition, there are very few population-based data from resource-poor countries,[41,42] where, in addition to the high prevalence of predisposing conditions such as sickle cell anaemia and the additional risk posed by Westernization, infections commonly causing stroke (see Chapter 5, Section 5.1) may not have been controlled. Osuntokun's[41] study from Nigeria quoted an incidence of 2 per 100 000, but there were no cases under the age of 10 years, probably because they likely presented with seizures and were not recognized.[43] Smadja's[42] study from Martinique found an incidence of 8 per 100 000 for those aged 0–34 years; their youngest patient was 3. It is important to develop global epidemiological data[50] in order to provide evidence of the importance of childhood stroke across populations, including the subtypes and outcomes of stroke. Multi national population-based studies are forming, and over time will provide these data, which will serve as the foundation for the first clinical trials in childhood stroke. Through clinical trials, evidence will be obtained which will direct treatment in individual patients, and reduce the current, unacceptably high cost of stroke in children.

REFERENCES

1. Lynch JK, Hirtz DG, deVeber G, Nelson KB. Report of the National Institute of Neurological Disorders and Stroke workshop on perinatal and childhood stroke. Pediatrics 2002; 109(1):116–123.
2. Mallick AA, Ganesan V, O'Callaghan FJ. Mortality from childhood stroke in England and Wales, 1921–2000. Arch Dis Child 2010; 95(1):12–19.
3. Adams RJ, McKie VC, Hsu L, Files B, Vichinsky E, Pegelow C et al. Prevention of a first stroke by transfusions in children with sickle cell anemia and abnormal results on transcranial Doppler ultrasonography. N Engl J Med 1998; 339(1):5–11.
4. Fullerton HJ, Adams RJ, Zhao S, Johnston SC. Declining stroke rates in Californian children with sickle cell disease. Blood 2004; 104(2):336–339.
5. Telfer P, Coen P, Chakravorty S, Wilkey O, Evans J, Newell H et al. Clinical outcomes in children with sickle cell disease living in England: a neonatal cohort in East London. Haematologica 2007; 92(7):905–912.
6. McCarville MB, Goodin GS, Fortner G, Li CS, Smeltzer MP, Adams R et al. Evaluation of a comprehensive transcranial doppler screening program for children with sickle cell anemia. Pediatr Blood Cancer 2008; 50(4):818–821.
7. Fullerton HJ, Chetkovich DM, Wu YW, Smith WS, Johnston SC. Deaths from stroke in US children, 1979 to 1998. Neurology 2002; 59(1):34–39.
8. Kleindorfer D, Khoury J, Kissela B, Alwell K, Woo D, Miller R et al. Temporal trends in the incidence and case fatality of stroke in children and adolescents. J Child Neurol 2006; 21(5):415–418.
9. deVeber G, Andrew M, Adams C, Bjornson B, Booth F, Buckley DJ et al. Cerebral sinovenous thrombosis in children. N Engl J Med 2001; 345(6):417–423.
10. Roach ES, Riela AR. Vasculopathies of the nervous system. In: Pediatric Cerebrovascular Disorders, 2nd edn (eds ES Roach, AR Riela AR). Aronk, New York: Futura Publishing Company, 1995; 163–180.
11. Schoenberg BS, Mellinger JF, Schoenberg DG. Cerebrovascular disease in infants and children: a study of incidence, clinical features, and survival. Neurology 1978; 28(8):763–768.
12. Broderick J, Talbot GT, Prenger E, Leach A, Brott T. Stroke in children within a major metropolitan area: the surprising importance of intracerebral hemorrhage. J Child Neurol 1993; 8(3):250–255.
13. Eeg-Olofsson O, Ringheim Y. Stroke in children. Clinical characteristics and prognosis. Acta Paediatr Scand 1983; 72(3):391–395.
14. Bamford J, Sandercock P, Dennis M, Warlow C, Jones L, McPherson K et al. A prospective study of acute cerebrovascular disease in the community: the Oxfordshire Community Stroke Project

1981–86. 1. Methodology, demography and incident cases of first-ever stroke. J Neurol Neurosurg Psychiatry 1988; 51(11):1373–1380.

15. Gudmundsson G, Benedikz JE. Epidemiological investigation of cerebrovascular disease in Iceland, 1958–1968 (ages 0–35 years): a total population survey. Stroke 1977; 8(3):329–331.

16. Earley CJ, Kittner SJ, Feeser BR, Gardner J, Epstein A, Wozniak MA et al. Stroke in children and sickle-cell disease: Baltimore-Washington Cooperative Young Stroke Study. Neurology 1998; 51(1):169–176.

17. Williams AN, Eunson PD, McShane MA, Lynn R, Green S, Kirkham F. Childhood cerebrovascular disease and stroke like illness in the United Kingdom and Eire, a descriptive epidemiological study. Arch Dis Child 2002; 86 supplement 1:A40(G113).

18. Williams AN, Kirkham FJ. Childhood stroke, stroke-like illness and cerebrovascular disease. Stroke 2004; 35 supplement 1:311.

19. Steinlin M, Pfister I, Pavlovic J, Everts R, Boltshauser E, Capone MA et al. The first three years of the Swiss Neuropaediatric Stroke Registry (SNPSR): a population-based study of incidence, symptoms and risk factors. Neuropediatrics 2005; 36(2):90–97.

20. Agrawal N, Johnston SC, Wu YW, Sidney S, Fullerton H. Imaging data reveal a higher pediatric stroke incidence than prior US estimates. Stroke 2009; 40(11):3415–3421.

21. Giroud M, Lemesle M, Gouyon JB, Nivelon JL, Milan C, Dumas R. Cerebrovascular disease in children under 16 years of age in the city of Dijon, France: a study of incidence and clinical features from 1985 to 1993. J Clin Epidemiol 1995; 48(11):1343–1348.

22. deVeber GA, MacGregor D, Curtis R, Mayank S. Neurologic outcome in survivors of childhood arterial ischemic stroke and sinovenous thrombosis. J Child Neurol 2000; 15(5):316–324.

23. Zahuranec DB, Brown DL, Lisabeth LD, Morgenstern LB. Is it time for a large, collaborative study of pediatric stroke? Stroke 2005; 36(9):1825–1829.

24. Al-Sulaiman A, Bademosi O, Ismail H, Magboll G. Stroke in Saudi children. J Child Neurol 1999; 14(5):295–298.

25. Salih MA, bdel-Gader AG, Al-Jarallah AA, Kentab AY, Alorainy IA, Hassan HH et al. Stroke in Saudi children. Epidemiology, clinical features and risk factors. Saudi Med J 2006; 27 Suppl 1:S12–S20.

26. Lee J, Croen LA, Lindan C, Nash KB, Yoshida CK, Ferriero DM et al. Predictors of outcome in perinatal arterial stroke: a population-based study. Ann Neurol 2005; 58(2):303–308.

27. Lee J, Croen LA, Backstrand KH, Yoshida CK, Henning LH, Lindan C et al. Maternal and infant characteristics associated with perinatal arterial stroke in the infant. JAMA 2005; 293(6):723–729.

28. Schulzke S, Weber P, Luetschg J, Fahnenstich H. Incidence and diagnosis of unilateral arterial cerebral infarction in newborn infants. J Perinat Med 2005; 33(2):170–175.

29. Laugesaar R, Kolk A, Tomberg T, Metsvaht T, Lintrop M, Varendi H et al. Acutely and retrospectively diagnosed perinatal stroke: a population-based study. Stroke 2007; 38(8):2234–2240.

30. Wu YW, March WM, Croen LA, Grether JK, Escobar GJ, Newman TB. Perinatal stroke in children with motor impairment: a population-based study. Pediatrics 2004; 114(3):612–619.

31. Fullerton HJ, Wu YW, Zhao S, Johnston SC. Risk of stroke in children: ethnic and gender disparities. Neurology 2003; 61(2):189–194.

32. Barnes C, Newall F, Furmedge J, Mackay M, Monagle P. Arterial ischaemic stroke in children. J Paediatr Child Health 2004; 40(7):384–387.

33. Lanthier S, Carmant L, David M, Larbrisseau A, de Veber G. Stroke in children: the coexistence of multiple risk factors predicts poor outcome. Neurology 2000; 54(2):371–378.

34. Kerr LM, Anderson DM, Thompson JA, Lyver SM, Call GK. Ischemic stroke in the young: evaluation and age comparison of patients six months to thirty-nine years. J Child Neurol 1993; 8(3):266–270.

35. deVeber GA, MacGregor D, Curtis R, Mayank S. Neurologic outcome in survivors of childhood arterial ischemic stroke and sinovenous thrombosis. J Child Neurol 2000; 15(5):316–324.

36. deVeber G, Andrew M, The Canadian Paediatric Ischemic Stroke Study group. The epidemiology and outcome of sinovenous thrombosis in pediatric patients. New Engl J Med 2001; 345(6):417–423.

37. Taylor TN, Davis PH, Torner JC, Holmes J, Meyer JW, Jacobson MF. Lifetime cost of stroke in the United States. Stroke 1996; 27(9):1459–1466.

38. Lo W, Zamel K, Ponnappa K, Allen A, Chisolm D, Tang M et al. The cost of pediatric stroke care and rehabilitation. Stroke 2008; 39(1):161–165.

39. Gardner MA, Hills NK, Sidney S, Johnston SC, Fullerton HJ. The 5-year direct medical costs of neonatal and childhood stroke in a population-based cohort. Neurology 2010; 74(5):372–378.

40. Perkins E, Stephens J, Xiang H, Lo W. The cost of pediatric stroke acute care in the United States. Stroke 2009; 40(8):2820–2827.

41. Osuntokun BO, Bademosi O, Akinkugbe OO, Oyediran AB, Carlisle R. Incidence of stroke in an African City: results from the Stroke Registry at Ibadan, Nigeria, 1973–1975. Stroke 1979; 10(2):205–207.

42. Smadja D, Cabre P, May F, Fanon JL, Rene-Corail P, Riocreux C et al. ERMANCIA: Epidemiology of Stroke in Martinique, French West Indies: Part I: methodology, incidence, and 30-day case fatality rate. Stroke 2001; 32(12):2741–2747.

43. Chadehumbe MA, Khatri P, Khoury JC, Alwell K, Szaflarski JP, Broderick JP et al. Seizures are common in the acute setting of childhood stroke: a population-based study. J Child Neurol 2009; 24(1):9–12.

44. Satoh S, Shirane R, Yoshimoto T. Clinical survey of ischemic cerebrovascular disease in children in a district of Japan. Stroke 1991; 22(5):586–589.

45. Merino Arribas JM, de Pablo CR, Grande GT, Sanchez MJ, Gonzalez de la Rosa JB. Nontraumatic hemorrhagic stroke in children after the neonatal period. An Esp Pediatr 1997; 47(4):392–396.

46. deVeber G, Chan A. Aspirin versus low-molecular-weight heparin for ischemic stroke in children: an unanswered question. Stroke 2002; 33(8):1947–1948.

47. Chung B, Wong V. Pediatric stroke among Hong Kong Chinese subjects. Pediatrics 2004; 114:e206–e212.

48. Simma B, Martin G, Muller T, Huemer M. Risk factors for pediatric stroke: consequences for therapy and quality of life. Pediatr Neurol 2007; 37(2):121–126.

49. Fullerton HJ, Wu YW, Sidney S, Johnston SC. Recurrent hemorrhagic stroke in children: a population-based cohort study. Stroke 2007; 38(10):2658–2662.

50. Mallick AA, O'Callaghan FJK. The epidemiology of childhood stroke. Eur J Paediatr Neurol 2010; 14(3):197–205.

4
CLINICAL AND IMAGING FEATURES OF CHILDHOOD STROKE

4.1 Clinical syndromes

4.1.1 Anterior circulation stroke

Fenella J. Kirkham

Introduction

Stroke and cerebrovascular disease can cause considerable anxiety to the paediatrician. There is a large number of individual conditions each of which is relatively rare,[1] the differential diagnosis includes a wide range of alternative pathologies[2–4] (Fig. 4.1) and protocols for investigation and treatment are not well worked out. For symptomatic stroke, the pre-existing diagnosis, and for cryptogenic stroke, the trigger(s) are often important clinical clues to diagnosis. In adults, as a result of controlled trials of thrombolysis and of stroke units, there is an increased awareness of the need for rapid assessment and appropriate management of acute stroke and the concept of 'brain attack' has received widespread publicity. Thrombolysis must begin within 4.5 hours, however, and even fewer children than adults are triaged this quickly.[2,5] Although in one study the median time at diagnosis was 22.7 hours,[6] in many children the correct diagnosis may not be made for days or even weeks.[2] Nevertheless, there is little doubt that stroke units save adult lives and improve outcome in survivors,[7] in part because a team's experience may lead to rapid diagnosis and appropriate management of common and rare stroke syndromes. Currently, services for children are not organized in this way in the UK, and it has not yet proved possible to conduct large randomized trials of treatment in groups of children with similar pathologies. Physicians have found an advisory service helpful,[8] although this type of service may be difficult to maintain because of issues of indemnity.

There is no universally recognized system for classifying stroke in childhood.[9–11] One of the main problems is that there is a wide differential diagnosis for acute focal neurological deficit in childhood.[2,3,12] There are a number of 'stroke mimics' which may be benign and require no treatment[3] while cerebrovascular disease may present without stroke. Emergency magnetic resonance imaging (MRI) studies may provide information to guide management.

Predisposing conditions

Cerebrovascular disease is at least as common as brain tumour in childhood, with an incidence of up to 13.0 per 100 000 per year.[13,14] At least 300 children present with stroke in the UK each year[15] Half of the events are haemorrhagic (Figs 4.2[column a] and 4.3), secondary to arteriovenous malformations, aneurysms, clotting disorders[16] or venous sinus thrombosis.[17] Sickle cell disease is probably the most common cause of childhood stroke world-wide[18,19] with a very wide variety of stroke syndromes[20] (see Chapter 15). Other predisposing conditions for arterial (Figs 4.2[columns b,c,d,f1] and 4.4) and venous (Figs 4.2[column e] and 4.5) ischaemic cerebrovascular accidents in children include congenital heart malformations (see Chapter 15), chromosomal disorders such as Down (see Chapter 15), neurocutaneous syndromes (see Chapter 15) and infections such as meningitis (see Chapter 5), but around half of such accidents occur in children who were previously well (cryptogenic stroke).[12]

Clinical presentation

Acute hemiparesis in childhood can be symptomatic of a variety of pathologies. The World Health Organization (WHO) definition of stroke is 'rapidly developing clinical signs of focal (or global) disturbance of cerebral function, with symptoms lasting 24 hours or longer, or leading to death, with no apparent cause other than of vascular origin'. Patients whose signs resolve within 24 hours have transient ischaemic attacks (TIA) by definition, but many have recent cerebral infarction or haemorrhage on imaging.[12] The rapidity of onset may help to decide which investigations should be undertaken first as an abrupt onset (<30 minutes to complete deficit) was documented in more than two-thirds of those subsequently found to have a non-arteriopathic arterial ischaemic stroke, for example embolism, compared with only 32% of children with arteriopathic stroke.[4] Coma is a well recognized presentation in children with large middle cerebral artery (MCA) territory infarction, vertebrobasilar circulation stroke, venous sinus thrombosis, bilateral borderzone ischaemia and reversible posterior reversible encephalopathy syndrome (PRES) as well as subarachnoid or intracerebral haemorrhage. Seizures[21,22] or headache are common presentations of stroke and cerebrovascular disease, particularly venous sinus thrombosis,[17] in

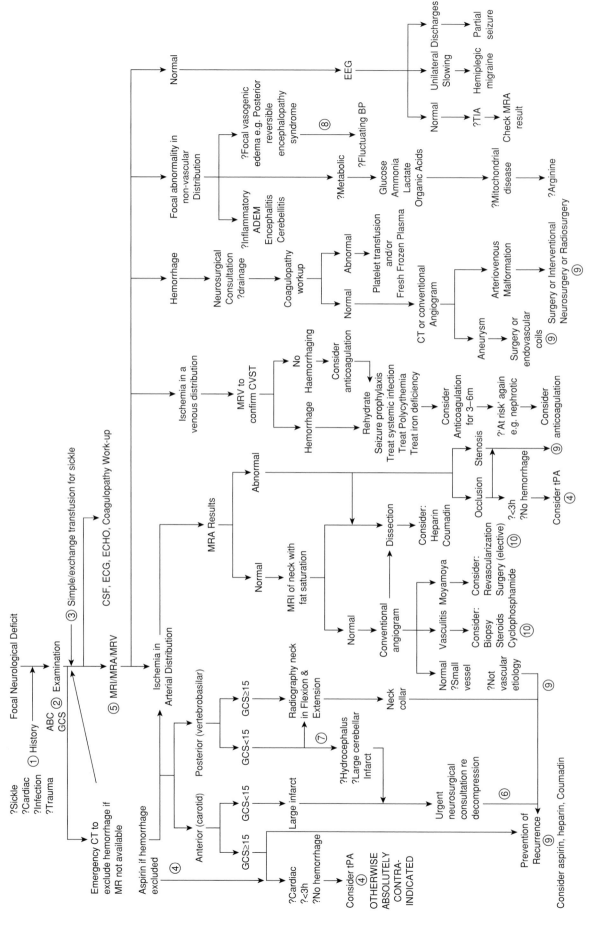

children. Covert or 'silent' infarction may be demonstrated on MRI in 'at risk' populations, particularly those with sickle cell disease (SCD), and may progress silently.[23,24] On the other hand, there may be potentially serious cerebrovascular disease, either venous or arterial, without infarction at presentation; timely intervention may prevent stroke. Comprehensive radiological investigation is therefore essential and there is increasing evidence that MRI studies provide provides information which may, in certain circumstances, guide management in the individual patient (Fig. 4.1).[25]

Children with stroke syndromes can present acutely sick in a variety of ways.[26] Unlike adult stroke, the vast majority of paediatric stroke victims will either present to or be rapidly referred to a tertiary centre. Paediatric intensive care involvement may thus commence at the stage of resuscitation and retrieval and will continue to facilitate elective or emergency intervention. Table 4.1 lists the common clinical presentations. The importance of the recognition of these as a medical/surgical emergency cannot be overstated.

Children may present with an immediate airway problem in coma, needing anaesthesia and intubation for airway protection, with status epilepticus resistant to first line therapy and requiring airway protection for second line therapy, for example barbiturate coma, or with a reduced level of consciousness either requiring regular observation or mandating airway protection for further investigation. They may also present with signs of intracranial hypertension or imminent central or uncal herniation.

Differential diagnosis (Table 4.1; Figs 4.1 and 4.2)
Haemorrhagic stroke, which may require urgent neurosurgical intervention, must be excluded by emergency CT or MRI (Fig. 4.2(column a)). If available, MRI is very useful in acute ischaemic stroke, either in excluding alternative pathologies or confirming arterial disease (Figs 4.1 and 4.2(rows 2,3,4)).

Venous sinus thrombosis may be accompanied by haemorrhagic or bland infarction, typically parietal;[27] MR venography or CT with and without contrast usually demonstrates the occluded sinus. Stroke mimics include acute disseminated encephalomyelitis (ADEM), post-streptococcal inflammation, reversible posterior leukoencephalopathy, border-zone ischaemia, hemiplegic migraine, hemispheric or focal oedema in a non-vascular distribution and degenerative conditions, such as Aicardi–Goutières syndrome (Figs 4.2(column f), 4.6 and 4.7).[3] Metabolic stroke, for example secondary to mitochondrial encephalopathy with lactic acidosis and stroke-like episodes or ornithine transcarbamylase deficiency, is relatively rare (see Chapter 14). There are often clinical clues, for example persistent vomiting, and on neuroimaging the infarcts are usually not in a typical vascular distribution. The electroencephalogram (EEG) in hemiplegic migraine usually shows unilateral slow background activity (see Chapter 12). Acute disseminated encephalomyelitis is usually obvious on MRI,[28] although post-streptococcal inflammation may not be (Fig. 4.7) and epilepsy (including benign Rolandic) with post-ictal hemiparesis may be diagnosed on EEG. In addition, it is important that the vascular pathology in arterial ischaemic stroke is defined so that conditions requiring urgent management, such as arterial dissection, are not missed.

Common ischaemic stroke syndromes in children

ARTERIAL STROKE (Fig. 4.2[columns b,c,d])
Up to 80% of children with arterial ischaemic stroke have cerebrovascular disease,[12,29] and accurate diagnosis may guide management to prevent recurrent stroke or TIA, which is more common in patients with vascular disease,[29] particularly those with moyamoya.[24,30] Magnetic resonance imaging (with fat saturation images in the neck to look for dissection; see below) and angiography in the acute phase is diagnostic in

Fig. 4.1. (*opposite*) Investigation and management for a child with acute focal neurological signs. (Adapted from Maria BL. Current Management in Child Neurology, 4th edn. People's Medical Publishing House, BC Decker, 2009.)
(1) A history of an underlying cause such as sickle cell disease, cardiac disease or meningitis may require urgent specific treatment.
(2) Examination should include an assessment of vital signs (airway, breathing and circulation (ABC)) and Glasgow Coma Scale (GCS). Complete neurological examination includes visual fields and acuity and retinal examination. General examination includes careful auscultation of the heart and neck, palpation of pulses and documentation of cutaneous abnormalities and dilated scalp veins.
(3) In sickle cell stroke, simple/exchange transfusion should be performed urgently. CSF, cerebrospinal fluid; ECG, electrocardiogram.
(4) In the exceptional circumstance that a patient >10 years has known cardiac disease (but no recent procedure) and no haemorrhage on CT, thrombolysis (e.g. tissue plasminogen activator [tPA]) may be considered within 3 hours of the onset of the focal deficit ('time last seen well'); otherwise it is absolutely contraindicated.
(5) MRI, magnetic resonance angiography (MRA) and magnetic resonance venography (MRV) should be obtained as soon as possible in all patients with suspected new onset cerebrovascular disease. Fluid attenuated inversion recovery, diffusion and perfusion-weighted MRI improve diagnostic accuracy.
(6) In a large anterior infarct, surgical decompression may prevent cerebral herniation and death. Non-communicating hydrocephalus may require CSF drainage via a ventricular drain.
(7) Vertebral body instability may be associated with vertebral dissection. If this is likely, the patient should wear a neck collar in the acute phase.
(8) Focal vasogenic oedema has been reported in hypertensive encephalopathy and with drugs, e.g. cyclosporin. Blood pressure must be reduced very slowly and may need raising first with volume expanders if it has fallen below previous baseline.
(9) Secondary prevention strategies should include advice on diet (including adequate vitamin intake, e.g. folate) and exercise, and the exclusion of obstructive sleep apnoea. Aspirin may be prescribed for non-neonates (or anticoagulation if studies indicate vascular dissection, venous sinus thrombosis or a prothrombotic state) but there are no controlled data evaluating safety or efficacy in preventing stroke recurrence in children.
(10) The decision about choice of treatment for aneurysms or arteriovenous malformations should be made by an experienced team with access to all options (surgical, gamma knife, endovascular). Referral should also be considered for patients with rare conditions with specific treatments, e.g. moyamoya or vasculitis. CVST, cerebral venous sinus thrombosis; ADEM, acute disseminated encephalomyelitis.

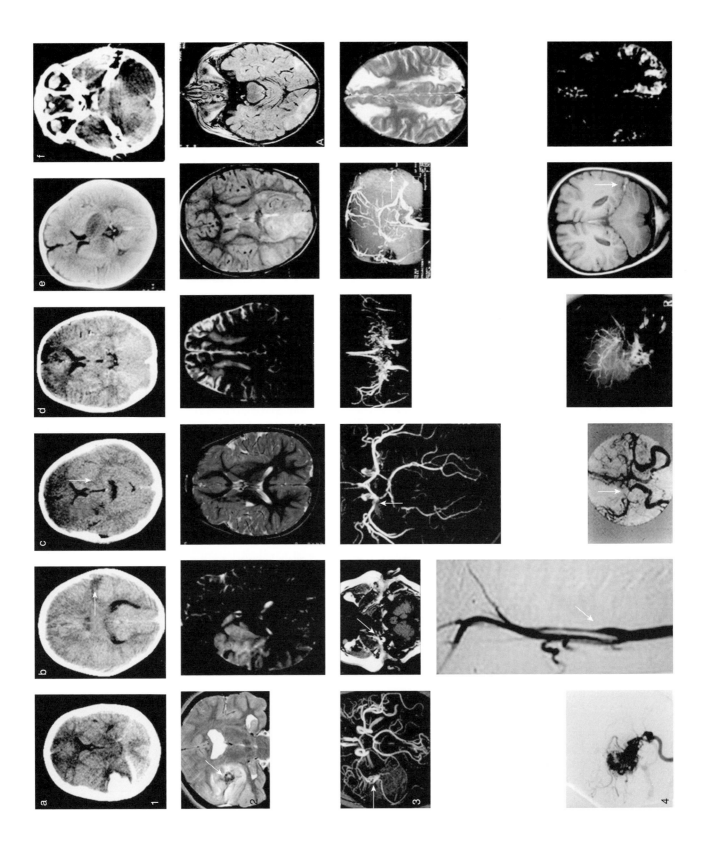

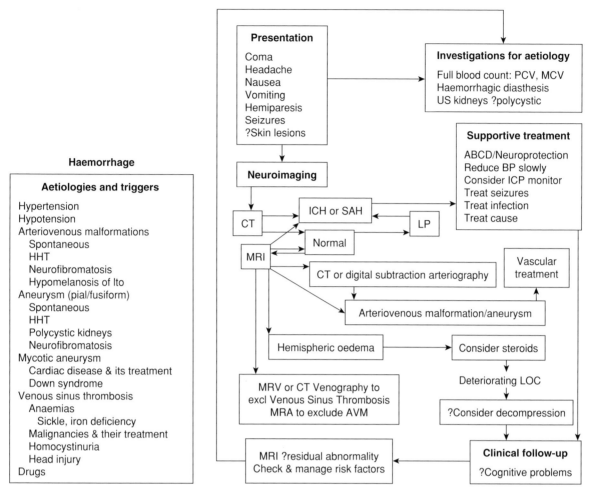

Fig. 4.3. Flow diagram for diagnosis and management of haemorrhagic stroke. ABCD, Airway Breathing Circulation Disability; AVM, arteriovenous malformation; BP, blood pressure; HHT, hereditary haemorrhagic telangiectasia; ICP, intracranial pressure; ICH, intracranial haemorrhage; LOC, level of consciousness; MCV, mean cell volume; MRA, magnetic resonance angiography; MRV, magnetic resonance venography; PCV, packed cell volume; SAH, subarachnoid haemorrhage; US, ultrasound.

Fig. 4.2. (*opposite*) Neuroimaging in children with stroke. (From Pappachan and Kirkham Arch Dis Child 2008.)
Row 1: CT scans. Row 2: T2-weighted MRI. Row 3: vascular imaging – a–d, MRA; e, MRV; f, watershed infarction. Row 4: additional imaging which may be useful in difficult cases – a–d, conventional angiography; e, venous thrombosis on coronal MRI; f, potentially reversible signal abnormality on diffusion weighted imaging.
(a) Haemorrhage: a1, Spontaneous intracerebral haemorrhage with midline shift; a2, MRI showing haemorrhage from mycotic aneurysm in a patient with subacute bacterial endocarditis; a3, mycotic aneurysm on magnetic resonance angiography; a4, digital subtraction arteriography showing arteriovenous malformation.
(b) Extracranial dissection: b1, infarct in a child who had suffered a minor head injury 24 hours before; b2, large cerebral infarct after head injury; b3, fat saturated T1 MRI of the neck showing haemorrhage in the vessel wall; b4, digital subtraction arteriography showing tapering 'rat's tail' appearance characteristic of extracranial dissection.
(c) Transient cerebral arteriopathy: c1, infarct in a child with stuttering stroke onset; c2, infarct in a child with recent varicella; c3, MRA from child in c2, short segment of middle cerebral artery stenosis; c4, digital subtraction arteriography from child in c1 showing longer segment of middle cerebral artery stenosis. The infarct had extended in size on the post-arteriography CT scan.
(d) Moyamoya: d1, bilateral frontal infarction in a child with livedo reticularis; d2, bilateral frontal infarction in a child with sickle cell anaemia; d3, bilateral middle cerebral artery stenosis with collateral formation obvious on MRA; d4, digital subtraction arteriography showing attenuation of major intracranial vessels and collaterals.
(e) Venous sinus thrombosis: e1, bilateral thalamic signal change in severe iron deficiency anaemia; e2, occipital signal change in nephrotic syndrome; e3, sagittal sinus thrombosis in systemic lupus erythematosus presenting with psychiatric symptoms; e4, transverse sinus thrombosis on plain MRI in child in e1.
(f) Posterior circulation stroke and stroke mimics: f1, cerebellar infarction in a boy with vertebral dissection; f2, bilateral occipital signal change suggestive of posterior leukoencephalopathy; f3, bilateral watershed infarction after facial infection in sickle cell anaemia, MRA and magnetic resonance venography were normal; f4, diffusion-weighted imaging shows potentially reversible pathology in a patient with hemiplegic migraine and normal T2-weighted MRI.

31

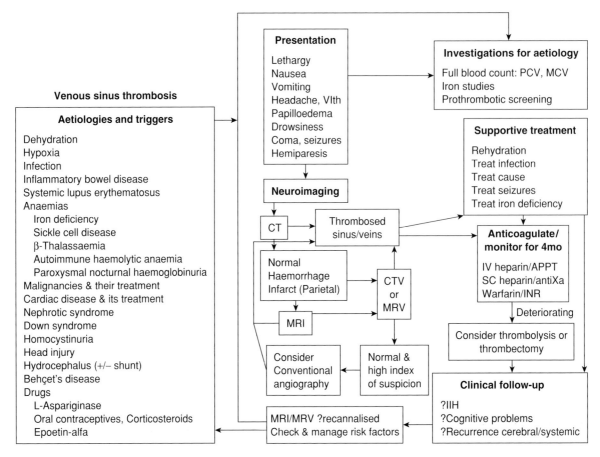

Fig. 4.4. Flow diagram for diagnosis and management of ischaemic stroke. CSVT, cerebral sinovenous thrombosis; PHACES, posterior fossa malformations, haemangiomas, arterial anomalies, cardiac defects, eye abnormalities, and sternal or ventral defects; SCD, sickle cell disease.

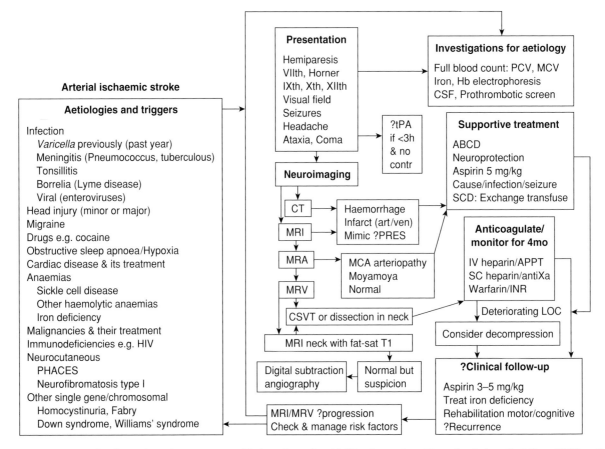

Fig. 4.5. Flow diagram for diagnosis and management of ischaemic stroke. ABCD, airway, breathing, circulation, disability; APPT, activated partial thromboplastin time; CSVT, cerebral venous sinus thrombosis; IIH, idiopathic intracranial hypertension; INR, international normalised ratio; LOC, level of consciousness; MCV, mean cell volume; MO, months; PCV, packed cell volume; PHACES, posterior fossa malformations, haemangiomas, arterial anomalies, cardiac defects, eye abnormalities, and sternal or ventral defects; SCD, sickle cell disease.

TABLE 4.1
Differential diagnosis in children presenting with acute focal neurological deficit

Acute ischaemic arterial stroke +/− haemorrhage +/− **mass effect**

Acute venous stroke +/− haemorrhage +/− venous infarction +/− **mass effect**

Primary haemorrhagic stroke +/− **mass effect**

Non-accidental injury
• Subdural haematoma
• Strangulation with compression of internal carotid artery

Posterior reversible encephalopathy syndrome (PRES) (hyper/hypotension or immunosupression)

Unilateral hemispheric cerebral oedema, e.g. secondary to diabetes, hyperammonaemia (ornithine carbamoyl transferase deficiency)

Hemiplegic migraine (but diagnosis of exclusion-migrainous symptoms seen in cerebrovascular disease)

Post-ictal (Todd paresis)
• Short duration so neuroimaging essential if persistent
• Children with prolonged seizures may develop permanent hemiparesis with seizures (hemiseizure-hemiplegia-epilepsy)

Acute disseminated encephalomyelitis

Brain tumour

Encephalitis, e.g. secondary to herpes simplex (usually have seizures)

Rasmussen encephalitis

Mitochondrial encephalopathy with stroke-like episodes

Alternating hemiplegia

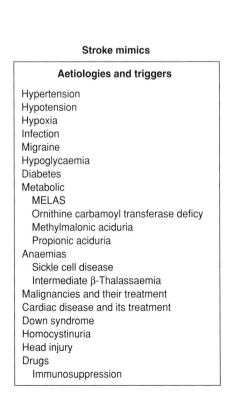

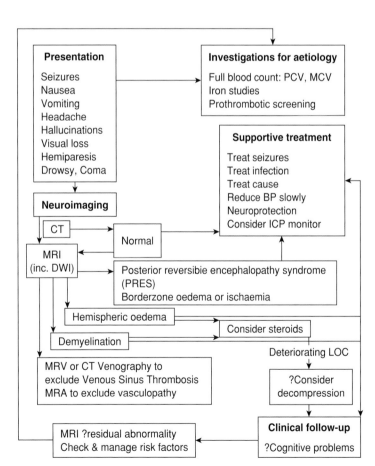

Fig. 4.6. Flow diagram for management of stroke mimics. DWI, diffusion-weighted imaging; ICH, intracranial haemorrhage; ICP, intracranial pressure; LOC, level of consciousness; MCV, mean cell volume; MRA, magnetic resonance angiography. MRV, magnetic resonance venography; PCV, packed cell volume.

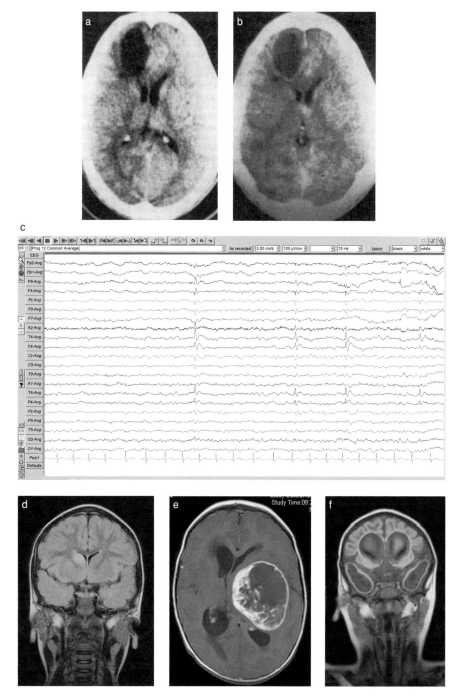

Fig. 4.7. Differential diagnosis of childhood stroke. (a,b) Axial CT before and after intravenous contrast 9 months after presentation in a 16-year-old boy who originally developed left hand numbness and weakness, severe left facial weakness, unsteadiness of gait,impaired hearing in his left ear, occipital headache and visual disturbance. The cerebrospinal fluid showed oligoclonal immunoglobulin G bands and high dose intravenous methylprednisolone was given with a working diagnosis of multiple sclerosis. Nine months later, he developed headache and vomiting with progressive disturbance of vision and balance and drowsiness. CT scan showed a large ring enhancing lesion with mass effect and some surrounding oedema in the right frontal lobe. Cerebral abscess was suspected, but on aspiration via a burr hole, the lesion was found to contain clear xanthochromic fluid and cytological study was negative for neoplastic cells. The cyst wall was removed, together with the surrounding abnormal tissue on the assumption that this was a glioma. Histological appearances were those of a subacute demyelinating lesion compatible with a plaque of multiple sclerosis. (c) An EEG showing discharges typical of benign Rolandic epilepsy from a child presenting with a persistent hemiparesis. (d) Coronal fluid attenuation inversion recovery (FLAIR) MRI in a child presenting with a mild hemiparesis and dystonic movements 1 week after an upper respiratory tract infection showing signal change in the basal ganglia not typical of infarction. She improved after a course of steroids. (e) Thalamic tumour in a boy presenting with very slowly progressive hemidystonia over a 6-month period. (f) Coronal FLAIR MRI showing bilateral destructive changes in a boy in whom the diagnosis of Aicardi–Goutières syndrome was confirmed at post mortem.

the majority of cases but conventional angiography may be required occasionally, for example to exclude dissection, particularly in the posterior circulation, or small vessel vasculitis. Previous varicella zoster infection, preceding trauma, hypertension, recent infection and anaemia are common in children with arterial ischaemic stroke, while previously undetected structural cardiac abnormalities are rare.[12] Inherited prothrombotic states, such as protein C deficiency or factor V Leiden, and disorders of lipid metabolism, for example raised lipoprotein(a) levels, are of variable frequency, depending at least in part on the population studied,[31] but importantly may be risk factors for recurrence.[24,32]

Carotid and vertebrobasilar dissection (Fig. 4.2(column B))
Dissection of the carotid or vertebrobasilar circulation (see Chapter 6) may be responsible for up to 20% of paediatric arterial ischaemic strokes[33] if emergency cerebrovascular imaging is performed. Many occur in the context of trauma or physical exertion but there may be an underlying vasculopathy. Recurrent stroke usually occurs on an embolic basis, and the risk may be reduced by early anticoagulation.

Intracranial arteriopathy

'Transient' cerebral arteriopathy in cryptogenic stroke
(Fig. 4.2[column c])
Chabrier et al[33,34] described transient cerebral arteriography (see Chapter 6) in previously healthy children presenting with acute hemiplegia. In up to a third, recurrence occurs within 3 months of the initial stroke. Cerebral imaging shows small subcortical infarcts located in the basal ganglia and internal capsule, and on digital subtraction arteriography there are multifocal lesions of the arterial wall, with narrowing in the distal internal carotid and the proximal anterior, middle or posterior cerebral arteries. Longitudinal arteriographic follow-up shows initial worsening of the arterial lesions for up to 7 months, followed by complete regression, improvement or stabilization of the lesions. One-third of the patients had mild or severe sequelae. The stabilization of arterial lesions and lack of late recurrence in the majority are in favour of a transient pathophysiological process involving the large intracranial arteries.

Intracranial arteriopathy in sickle cell disease
(see Chapter 15)
Involvement of the distal internal carotid and proximal middle and cerebral arteries is also characteristic of sickle cell disease, although in these patients, the initial narrowing often gradually progresses to occlusion.[35] Pathological examination of these arteries shows endothelial proliferation, fibroblastic reaction, hyalinization and fragmentation of the internal elastic lamina.[36] The majority of clinical and silent infarcts occur in the borderzones between the middle, anterior and posterior cerebral territories[36,37] or in the territory of the middle cerebral artery.[37]

Moyamoya (Fig. 4.2[column d])
In Japanese children with stroke, Suzuki described the arteriographic appearance of progressive occlusion of the distal internal carotid arteries with collateral formation, the appearance of which reminded him of 'a puff of smoke drifting hazily through the air' ('moyamoya' in Japanese;[38] see Chapter 6). Although the prevalence of moyamoya is higher in Japan, the arteriographic appearances have been described in children and adults of various races with ischaemic and haemorrhagic stroke. There may be differences in aetiology and natural history between primary, genetically determined, moyamoya disease in Japanese populations, and moyamoya syndrome secondary to conditions such as sickle cell disease. Idiopathic and syndromic moyamoya is seen sporadically in Europe and the USA,[39] and may also be associated with sickle cell disease.

VENOUS SINUS THROMBOSIS (Fig. 4.2[column e])
Venous sinus thrombosis may be the underlying pathology in infarctive or haemorrhagic stroke, coma or idiopathic intracranial hypertension (see Chapter 7). CT may not be adequate to exclude the diagnosis and there should be a low threshold for emergency MRI and venography in acute neurological presentations. This is important as although there are no randomized controlled trials in children, two trials in adults provided evidence that anticoagulation was of benefit and many paediatricians currently anticoagulate older children without haemorrhage, initially with heparin and then with warfarin.

POSTERIOR REVERSIBLE ENCEPHALOPATHY SYNDROME
(Fig. 4.2[column f2]) and borderzone ischaemia
(Fig. 4.2[column f3])
Posterior reversible encephalopathy syndrome (PRES) is a clinico-neuroradiological syndrome characterised by seizures, disorders of consciousness, altered mental status, visual abnormalities and headaches, associated with predominantly posterior white matter abnormalities on CT and MRI examinations[40] but without arterial or venous disease. PRES is a relatively common stroke mimic[3] and has been recognized in an increasing number of medical settings, including hypertensive encephalopathy, eclampsia, after acute chest crisis in sickle cell disease[41,42] and immunosuppression (e.g. with ciclosporin).[41] It may be difficult to distinguish from stroke in the acute phase; diffusion-weighted MRI may be helpful. As treatments are different, it is essential to distinguish PRES from posterior circulation embolic stroke secondary to vertebrobasilar dissection (Figs 4.8 and 4.9);[43] the latter typically presents 'out-of-the-blue', is much more common in boys and there is typically infarction in the cerebellum and/or brainstem as well as the occipito-parietal cortex, but MR and digital subtraction arteriography may be required to make a positive diagnosis.[43] It is also important to exclude sinovenous thrombosis, particularly of the sagittal and straight sinuses, which may be associated with venous infarction in the parietal and occipital lobes as well as the thalami.

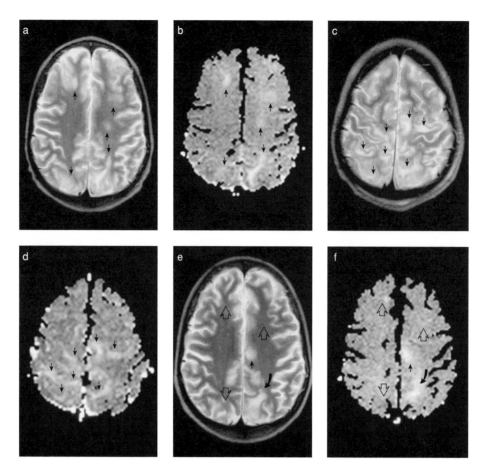

Fig. 4.8. Axial MR images of a 9-year-old patient with sickle cell disease and a viral-induced nephritic syndrome, who developed a generalized seizure 4 days after commencing ciclosporin therapy and experienced prolonged impairment of higher neurological function. Regions of increased diffusion matched all the areas of T2 signal change. Many of the areas resolved without any residual T2 or diffusion abnormality. These findings suggest that the neurotoxic effects of ciclosporin were associated with a partially reversible extravasation of fluid into the brain. (a) A T2-weighted image (day 2 after seizure) shows cortical and juxtacortical signal alteration within both frontal and parietal lobes (arrows). (b) The apparent diffusion coefficients (ADC) map (day 2) reveals increased diffusion in all areas of T2 abnormality (arrows). (Normal brain = 1.02, abnormal areas = 1.33.) (c) A T2-weighted image (day 6) shows new, more superior abnormalities (arrows). (d) The ADC map (day 6) again reveals that all of the T2-weighted abnorm-alities correspond to areas of increased diffusion. (Normal brain = 0.93, abnormal areas = 1.48.) (e) A T2-weighted image (day 49), obtained at the same level as the images presented in a and b, shows complete resolution of most of the lesions that were present on day 2 (open arrows). A new lesion is present in the left posterior frontal lobe (solid arrow). A preexisting abnormality in the left pari-etal lobe (curved arrow) is essentially unchanged. (f) The ADC map (day 49) reveals increased diffusion in the new area of T2 prolongation (solid arrow). No diffusion abnormality, however, is present where the lesions have resolved (open arrows). (Normal brain = 0.93, open arrows = 0.92, solid arrow = 1.34, curved arrow = 1.36.) (From Coley SC, Porter DA, Calamante F, Chong WK, Connelly A. Quantitative MR diffusion mapping and cyclosporine-induced neurotoxicity. AJNR Am J Neuroradiol. 1999 Sep;20(8):1507–10.

The rapid resolution of clinical and neuroradiological abnormalities in the majority of cases of PRES suggests vasogenic cerebral oedema, which is thought to result from impaired cerebrovascular autoregulation and endothelial injury. The majority of patients make a full clinical and radiological recovery after conservative measures, including slow reduc-tion of blood pressure and maintenance of normal oxygenation. Some patients with otherwise typical PRES have additional imaging abnormality anteriorly and/or in the grey matter, often in a distribution suggestive of borderzone ischaemia, and the changes are not necessarily reversible in all cases.[42] Patients with parieto-occipital infarction may have visual problems and epilepsy in the long term.[40]

ACUTE DISSEMINATED ENCEPHALOMYELITIS AND OTHER INFLAMMATORY DISORDERS (Fig. 4.7)
MRI may reveal demyelination in children presenting with acute focal neurological signs.[3,12] The incidence of acute disseminated encephalomyelitis is lower than that of stroke in childhood (0.2–0.4 per 100 000)[44] but presentation with focal as well as generalized weakness is not uncommon,[45,46] and it is a very important differential as management is different. As CSF oligo-clonal bands are rarely abnormal, the distinction is usually made on neuroimaging characteristics, with those with ADEM typic-ally having multifocal subcortical lesions. Other inflammatory conditions, including post-streptococcal chorea and paedia-tric autoimmune neuropsychiatric disorders associated with

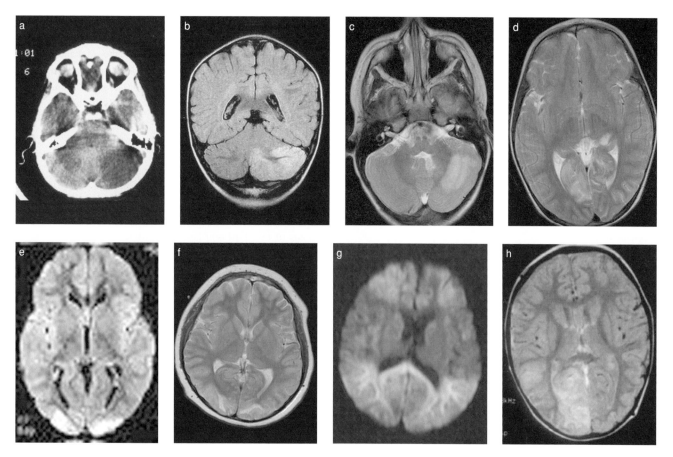

Fig. 4.9. CT (a), coronal fluid attanuated inversion recovery MRI (b), axial T2-weighted MRI (c,d,f,h) and diffusion-weighted MRI (e,g) showing infarcts in the posterior circulation associated with cerebrovascular pathology (a–d) as well as stroke mimics. e and f, posterior reversible encephalopathy syndrome; g, widespread bilateral borderzone ischaemia in the frontal as well as the parieto-occipital regions; h, occipital oedema secondary to straight sinus thrombosis.

streptococcal infections (PANDAS) (Fig. 4.1), may present with unilateral weakness. There is evidence that intravenous methyl prednisolone reduces the duration of the illness and perhaps improves long-term outcome. Immunoglobulin and plasmapheresis may also benefit some patients.[47]

METABOLIC STROKE (see Chapter 14)
Hypoglycaemia and inborn errors of metabolism can cause acute focal neurological symptoms and signs (metabolic stroke) either due to vascular injury or direct tissue injury, which may be permanent or transitory.[48]

Vascular injury

• Homocysteine is a highly chemically reactive thiol amino acid that can cause direct endothelial injury and measurement is justified in childhood stroke as high levels are not an uncommon association with childhood stroke[49] and may predict recurrence,[50] while dietary manipulation and vitamin supplementation may reduce levels. Inborn errors affecting three enzymes (or the synthesis of their vitamin co-factors) are known to cause homocystinuria: 5,10-methylenetetrahydrofolate reductase (MTHFR); methionine

synthase (MS); and cystathionine β-synthase (CBS) and may present with arterial or venous stroke in infancy or childhood.[51,52]

• Fabry disease is an X-linked lysosomal storage disorder caused by deficiency of the lysosomal hydrolase α-galactosidase A and is an important cause of cryptogenic stroke in young adults, particularly those with vertebrobasilar territory infarction. Proteinurea may be a useful screen but if there is a strong index of suspicion, exclusion should be by enzyme diagnosis, as replacement is available.

Non-vascular injury

• Hypoglycaemia is not an uncommon cause of hemiparesis, for example in diabetics.[53]
• Organic acidaemias, urea cycle disorders and other inborn errors of metabolism can cause metabolic stroke.
• Female carriers with ornithine carbamoyl transferase deficiency may present with focal signs; plasma ammonia is usually high.
• Mitochondrial disorders can cause stroke-like episodes (such as mitochondrial encephalopathy with lactic acidosis and stroke-like episodes, MELAS). The exact mechanisms

by which these occur are unknown. In the organic acidaemias and urea cycle disorders, it is likely that accumulation of a toxic metabolite causes infarction of a selectively vulnerable area of the brain. By contrast, mitochondrial disorders are liable to cause infarction because of deficient energy supply and by the generation of oxygen free radicals. As arginine supplementation may be beneficial,[54] it is important to exclude mitochondrial disorders.

4.1.2 Posterior Circulation Strokes in Children

Bhuwan P. Garg

Introduction

Posterior circulation strokes can often, but not always, be distinguished from strokes in the anterior circulation by clinical examination. The classic feature of a lesion in the brainstem is cranial nerve involvement, which is often secondary to stroke in the vertebrobasilar territory, although lower cranial nerve involvement is a feature of carotid dissection in children (see Chapter 6). There is usually an accompanying crossed hemiparesis. There may be a cerebellar deficit and sometimes a tremor is present which may be cerebellar or 'rubral'. Headache, vomiting, altered mental state, ataxia and visual field deficits are other common presenting symptoms.

Strokes in this vascular distribution are less common than those in the anterior or carotid circulation.[13,55] Eight per cent of strokes involved the posterior circulation in the London cohort,[12,43] and 18 and 37% of Taiwanese and Australian series had posterior circulation stroke[56,57] while of 124 children with ischaemic strokes presenting to our centre in Indianapolis, we found that 23% of the strokes were in the posterior circulation.[58] Nearly one-third (14/46) cryptogenic strokes were in the posterior circulation in a recent French series.[59]

There is considerable overlap in presentation with brain tumour[60] as well as cerebral venous sinus thrombosis[27] and stroke mimics, including complicated migraine,[3] PRES[3,61] (Figs 4.1, 4.2[column f], 4.8 and 4.9). PRES, which occurs in children with hypertension, ciclosporin toxicity and sickle cell disease,[40–42] may be difficult to distinguish from stroke in the acute phase.

Vascular anatomy

The posterior circulation is the vertebral-basilar arterial system. The vertebral arteries are often of unequal size and combine to form the basilar artery at the lower border of the pons. The posterior inferior cerebellar artery (PICA) is the distal most major branch of the vertebral artery. The basilar artery ends in the posterior cerebral arteries after giving off paired anterior inferior cerebellar arteries (AICA), superior cerebellar arteries and the internal auditory arteries. There are also penetrating paramedian and circumferential branches of the basilar artery. The PICA supplies the lateral part of the medulla oblongata, the inferior vermis, parts of the cerebellum and the choroid plexus of the 4th ventricle while the AICA supplies the caudal pontine tegmentum and parts of the cerebellum. There is an inverse relationship between the arterial supply of the AICA and the PICA with each supplementing the territory of the other so that together they cover the blood supply of the lateral and inferior cerebellum. The superior cerebellar arteries supply the superior vermis, the superior surface of the cerebellar hemispheres and the deep cerebellar nuclei. The paramedian and circumferential branches supply the pons and parts of the midbrain. The internal auditory artery supplies the cochlea and the labyrinth. The posterior cerebral arteries supply parts of the midbrain, thalamus, quadrigeminal plate, pineal gland, choroid plexus of the third and lateral ventricles, inferior surfaces of the temporal lobes, superior parietal lobes and the occipital lobes. There is considerable variation in the blood supply.

Vascular syndromes of the brainstem

The classic clinical picture of a brainstem vascular lesion is that of a cranial nerve deficit with alternating hemiplegia, a term introduced to the neurological literature by Adolphe Gubler.[62] Several classic syndromes affecting the brainstem have been described (Table 4.2). Many of these syndromes that are often due to vascular lesions were initially described in patients with space occupying lesions in the brainstem. For example, the case described by Gubler was that of a 44-year-old woman who probably had a pontine tuberculoma. Paediatric neurologists may be more interested in the case of a 4-year-old boy with tuberculosis that Moritz Benedikt discussed as a visiting professor in Paris in the spring of 1889.[62] These and some of the other syndromes are listed in Table 4.2. Typical symptoms include vertigo, dysarthria and ataxia. Pain in the head or neck is said to be a strong clinical indicator of dissection,[63] but this is not a consistent feature in childhood, possibly because young children may not be able to clearly localize pain.[43] Thalamic syndromes, extensively described in the adult literature, have been reported in children secondary to arterial disease;[64] venous sinus thrombois is an important differential.[27]

Risk factors

AGE AND SEX

The incidence of stroke increases with advancing age and children and young adults account for less than 5% of all stroke cases but posterior circulation stroke has been described in infancy.[43] While the reason for stroke in the elderly is usually atherosclerotic, the causes of stroke in the young are more diverse.[65] For posterior circulation stroke, there is a male predominance in many published case reports,[66,67] with 77% of boys in a series reporting a high prevalence of associated vertebrobasilar disease,[43,68] although this was not the case in our larger series.[58] Possible explanations for this include increased potential for trauma and also the increased incidence of structural abnormalities of the cervical spine in boys.[69] There

TABLE 4.2
Selected brainstem syndromes

Syndrome	Signs	Vessel involved
Mesencephalic syndromes		
Weber syndrome	Oculomotor palsy, Contralateral hemiplegia	Peduncular penetrating branches
Perinaud syndrome	Palsy of upgaze and accommodation	Quadrigeminal, Unreactive pupils branch
Claude syndrome	Oculomotor palsy, contralateral ataxia and tremor	Circumferential branch
Benedikt syndrome	Oculomotor palsy, contralateral hemiparesis, ataxia and tremor	Penetrating paramedian branches
Nothnagel syndrome	Oculomotor and gaze palsy, and contralateral ataxia	Thalamoperforating branches
Top of basilar syndrome	Upgaze palsy, oculomotor palsy, hemianopsia or cortical blindness	Basilar bifurcation
Dejerine–Roussy syndrome	Painful hemianaesthesia with chorea or other movement disorder	Thalamoperforant branches
Pontine syndromes		
Millard–Gubler syndrome	Ipsilateral VIth and VIIth nerve palsy with crossed hemiparesis	Short circumferential branch
Foville syndrome	Ipsilateral VIIth nerve and conjugate gaze palsy with crossed hemiparesis	Paramedian penetrating branches
Superior pontine syndrome	Ipsilateral Horner, ataxia and loss of facial sensation	Superior cerebellar artery
Medial longitudinal fasciculus (MLF) syndrome	Paralysis of ipsilateral ocular adduction during horizontal gaze and nystagmus of the abducting eye	Paramedian penetrating branches
Medullary syndromes		
Wallenberg syndrome	Ipsilateral Vth, IXth, Xth, XIth palsy (lateral medullary ataxia, Horner syndrome, with cerebellar artery syndrome), loss of contralateral pain and temperature	Posterior inferior
Dejerine syndrome	Ipsilateral XIIth palsy (medial medullary hemiparesis sparing face, deep perforaters syndrome) sensation loss	Contralateral paramedian

is some evidence that individuals who experience arterial dissection have abnormalities of collagen at the ultrastructural level.[70] The possibility of an X-linked condition, such as a collagen disorder or Fabry disease,[71] has not yet been excluded in series of childhood posterior circulation stroke, although there is no evidence for clinical features of this condition and controversy continues in the literature on cryptogenic stroke in young adults.[72]

CARDIAC DISORDERS
Cardiac disease is a leading risk factor for stroke in children. Heart disease may be congenital or acquired. Rheumatic heart disease is the most common acquired heart disease in the world. Infective endocarditis, prosthetic valves, cardiomyopathies whether metabolic or acquired, cardiac tumours, cardiac arrhythmias and myocardial infarction are other causes. Stroke following cardiac surgery remains an important cause in children.[73]

Patients with coarctation or aortic stenosis may have primary cerebrovascular disease involving the posterior as well as the anterior circulation.[74–77] Posterior circulation cardioembolic stroke usually occurs in the setting of a right to left shunt in children, for example after a Fontan procedure,[73,78,79] or with a patent foramen ovale;[80] right heart pressures are assumed to exceed those on the left side at the time of embolus. The stroke is usually abrupt, without prior warning in an awake child with the neurological deficit maximum at the onset. Embolic material may consist of fibrin, platelets, thrombi, micro-organizms, tumor cells or other calcific material. Multiple infarcts are typical[80] and evidence of systemic embolization reinforces the

diagnosis. In the posterior circulation, the posterior cerebral arteries or their branches and the basilar artery apex (top of basilar syndrome) are more often involved, athough pontine stroke from occlusion of the penetrating vessels is also seen.

Although 15% were cardioembolic in one series[56] there is little evidence for a cardiac aetiology in the majority of vertebrobasilar territory strokes in childhood. In one series of 22 paediatric posterior circulation strokes,[43] all patients had praecordial echocardiography (including bubble contrast in two cases) and six patients also underwent transoesophageal echocardiography. Eighteen had completely normal studies. Three patients (all girls) had evidence of poor ventricular function (secondary to septicemia, congenital heart disease and non-accidental poisoning with tricyclic antidepressants in one case each) and one boy with right vertebral artery stenosis with further irregularity in the basilar artery had a small secundum atrial septal defect without any evidence of a right to left shunt at atrial level.

VASCULOPATHIES
Vasculopathy is common in posterior circulation stroke[56] (Fig. 4.10), diagnosed in 20/22 patients in one series,[43] and may be atherosclerotic or non-atherosclerotic.

Atherosclerotic vasculopathies
Atherosclerotic vasculopathies are rare in children and may be seen in teenagers with severe hyperlipidaemic and dyslipidaemic syndromes, although cholesterol was high in only 1 patient of the 13 in whom it was measured in one series.[43]

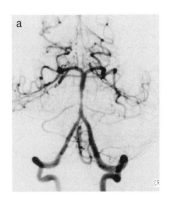
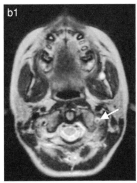
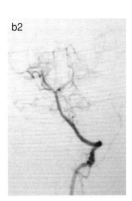

Fig. 4.10. (a) Magnetic resonance angiography (MRA) showing basilar stenosis in a 15-year-old boy with a previous pontine stroke. (b1) Vertebral dissection on axial T1 MRI of the neck and (b2) conventional cerebral angiogram (L vertebral artery injection) in another boy with a posterior circulation stroke.

Hyperhomocysteinaemia may also play a role in the pathophysiology of atherosclerosis and was seen in three of the eight patients in whom it was measured,[43] while three were homozygous for the thermolabile variant of the methylene tetrahydrofolate reductase gene, one of whom had a normal plasma homocysteine. Hypertension is probably also a risk factor for the progression of atherosclerosis and was common (9/22) in this series.[43]

Non-atherosclerotic vasculopathies

Cervicocephalic and intracranial arterial dissection
(see Chapter 6)
Cervicocephalic arterial dissection affecting the vertebral and basilar artery is an important cause of posterior, as well as anterior circulation stroke in children,[81] and was the final diagnosis in 10 out of 22 in one series.[43] Of the 12 with vasculopathies not finally diagnosed as definite dissection, the diagnosis was considered to be possible in three and not excluded in nine, mainly because vascular imaging had not been performed in the acute phase. It is well recognized that confidently excluding vertebrobasilar dissection using MR alone is difficult and that digital subtraction arteriography may be required (Fig. 4.10).[82,83]

Trauma
Trauma to the head and neck is frequently the reason for vertebrobasilar[68] and posterior cerebral dissection, although it may be mild in many cases and apparently spontaneous dissection occurs.[84] The intracranial or extracranial portion of the vessel or both may be affected. In traumatic dissection of the vertebral artery the C1–C2 segment is most commonly involved.[68] Traumatic dissection was the aetiology in 4 of 16 patients in whom the stroke was confined to the posterior circulation in our study[58] and in 5 of the 10 patients with definite dissection in the study reported by Ganesan et al.[43]

Mechanical factors in vertebrobasilar and posterior cerebral artery compression
Congenital or traumatic structural abnormalities of the cervical vertebrae, particularly of the atlas or the axis, may be associated with posterior circulation stroke in childhood.[85]

Congenital abnormalities include the spectrum of odontoid dysplasia and laxity of the ligamentum transversarium of the atlas, both of which result in instability of the atlanto-axial joint.[86] Odontoid aplasia,[69] os odontoideum[87] or subluxation at the antlanto-axial joint[43,88] may play a role in the forces required to cause vertebral compression and/or dissection in posterior circulation stroke in childhood.

Cushing et al[89] have described calcification of the arcuate ligament in a series of children with posterior circulation stroke. This means that the vertebral arteries traverse the upper cervical spine in a canal rather than a groove, with potential for the artery to become distorted or fixed within it. Compression of the vertebral artery due to head rotation is well recognized in adults with cervical spondylosis and osteophytes and has been reported in a child with thalamic stroke.[90] Physiological degrees of neck rotation may lead to occlusion of the vertebral arteries at the level of the atlantoaxial joint.[90] In this situation the territory supplied by the posterior circulation is dependent on an adequate circle of Willis or other collateral pathways for cerebral perfusion.

Particular movements which predispose to arterial injury or occlusion are traction, hyperextension and rotation.[68,85] Mechanisms which have been implicated include arterial stretching, intimal trauma with direct thrombosis (with or without embolization) and arterial dissection.[68,91,92]

Plain radiographs of the cervical spine in flexion and extension may reveal evidence of instability[68] or calcification of the arcuate ligament.[89] CT may, however, be required in order to demonstrate vertebral fractures in cases where there has been antecedent trauma.[93,94] The vertebral arteries are particularly vulnerable at the C1/C2 level (V3 segment of the artery),[68] but also more proximally (V1 segment), where they are traversed by fascial bands and skeletal muscle.[91] In one series, both patients who had cervical spine radiography acutely had a range of movement at the extreme limits of normal, and in one patient there were recurrent clinical symptoms until the neck was immobilized.[43]

For dissections of the posterior cerebral artery, which have been reported after mild trauma and typically occur at the P1–P2 junction, the free edge of the tentorium cerebelli may be the point at which the artery is caught.[95] This is a possible aetiology for stroke in the posterior cerebral artery territory after severe trauma,[96] although stretching and endothelial injury triggering thrombosis[97] and embolization from proximal injury is also likely.[98]

Infection
Beta haemolysing streptococcus group A throat infection may play a role in vertebrobasilar dissection.[99] Posterior cerebral artery occlusion of uncertain origin has also been reported after mycoplasma infection.[100]

Moyamoya (see Chapter 6)
Moyamoya disease is a chronic progressive non-inflammatory occlusive vasculopathy of unknown aetiology, most often presenting in childhood with carotid artery territory TIAs or ischaemic strokes. Presentation with vertebrobasilar ischaemic symptoms is unusual, although involvement of the extracranial vertebrobasilar circulation[101,102] and posterior cerebral arteries is often present as the disease progresses and may be associated with progressive reduction of cerebral blood flow on single photon emission computed tomography (SPECT).[103]

Vasculitis
Cerebral vasculitis may be infectious or non-infectious in nature.[104] Infectious vasculitis as seen in meningitis or fungal infection in the immunocompromised is probably more common and may cause large or small vessel stroke.[105,106] Thalamic stroke has been reported in meningitis,[64,90] although posterior cerebral artery territory stroke is more typical.[106] Non-infectious vasculitis may be idiopathic or due to a variety of systemic diseases and although it is an uncommon cause of stroke in children, both anterior and posterior circulations may be affected.[107,108] Schoenberg et al found no case of vasculitis in children younger than 14 years of age in their epidemiological study.[55] In our study of 92 children with ischaemic stroke, vasculitis was the aetiology in four.[9]

Anaemia
In one series reporting a total of 22 patients, three girls with posterior circulation stroke and poor ventricular function on echocardiography were also anaemic;[12] two had normal cerebral vasculature and one had occlusion of the right posterior cerebral artery in the context of recent varicella infection and a coagulopathy.

Sickle cell disease (see Chapter 15) is another predisposing factor. Most children have anterior circulation stroke, which may be predicted using transcranial Doppler and has a high risk or recurrence, so should prevented or treated with lifelong regular blood transfusions.[109–111] Posterior circulation or borderzone territory stroke may be an outcome for PRES in the context of hyperventilation, chest crisis and other complications such as nephrotic syndrome.[41,42,61,112]

Hypercoagulable states (see Chapter 5)
Under normal circumstances thrombophilic and thrombolytic factors are kept in fine balance in the circulating blood. A prothrombotic state is one in which the haemostatic equilibrium has shifted towards thrombosis, brought about because of deficiency of any of the many antithrombotic proteins or abnormality in the fibrinolytic system. Protein C, protein S, antithrombin III, heparin cofactor II deficiency and antiphospholipid syndrome may be inherited but are commonly acquired, for example with *Varicella*, liver disease, nephrotic syndrome, and administration of drugs such as L-asparaginase and oral contraceptives. Congenital and acquired protein S deficiency may contribute to posterior circulation stroke[43,113] and oral contraceptive use also may be associated.[114] Activated protein C resistance is most often due to factor V Leiden mutation, especially in children of Northern European ancestry, and may play a role in recurrent events after posterior circulation stroke, potentially preventable with anticoagulation.[115]

Migraine (see Chapter 12)
Migraine in children may be of the common, classic or complicated variety. Common migraine is characterised by paroxysmal headache associated with nausea, vomiting, abdominal discomfort, and photophobia or phonophobia. Classic migraine is common migraine preceded by transient neurological deficits such as scotomas representing migraine aura. Complicated migraine is a migraine in which the neurological symptoms outlast the headache by a sizable time. There is no temporally associated abnormality on neuroimaging and the neurological deficit resolves. Common migraine or migraine without aura is the most common variety of migraine seen in children.

Even though migraine is common in children, migrainous infarction is not.[61] Patients with acute confusional or hemiplegic migraine may have imaging evidence for ischaemia,[61,116] (Fig. 4.2[column f4]) even if infarction is not demonstrated after recovery. Criteria for the diagnosis of migrainous infarction include the presence of a fixed neurological deficit that is typical of a previous migraine attack and which arises during a migraine attack and is not explainable by another aetiology. In other words, migrainous infarction is a classic or complicated migraine in which the neurological deficit does not resolve.[117,118] Patients with migraine in whom the infarction is remote from the attack of migraine may be called to have migraine associated infarction. The latter may be more common than that in which the migraine is 'causal' and may be seen in children.[64] In all children with migrainous infarction or migraine-associated stroke, consideration should be given to thorough investigation for other risk factors to distinguish migraine from other conditions such as cerebral autosomal dominant arteriopathy with subcortical infarcts and leukoencephalopathy (CADASIL; see Chapter 15).[119–121]

Metabolic diseases
A variety of metabolic diseases are associated with strokes in children (see Chapter 14). Most of these strokes are in the carotid circulation, especially involving the deep nuclei. However mitochondrial diseases such as mitochondrial encephalomyopathy, lactic acidosis and stroke like episodes (MELAS)

may be associated with a stroke like picture typically affecting the occipital lobes.[122,123] The distribution of these 'strokes' does not correlate with an arterial distribution and this is often a useful distinguishing feature.

Management (Fig. 4.11)

INVESTIGATION

Children with posterior cerebral infarction require an organized, logical approach to arrive at an aetiology (Figs 4.1 and 4.11). History and physical examination often point to a likely cause such as cardiac disease or trauma. The majority of children with posterior circulation stroke are boys who have vertebrobasilar arterial abnormalities which are commonly multifocal; many have the radiological characteristics of arterial dissection. Some are recognized on early MRI with specific sequences, for example fat-saturated T1 of the neck, or on MRA (Fig. 4.10).[124] Although the sensitivity is less good for

vertebrobasilar than for carotid dissection,[125] the diagnostic rate will almost certainly improve with higher field strengths, but digital subtraction angiography is indicated if a definitive diagnosis is not made on MRI. Increased diffusion on diffusion-weighted MRI with swelling rather than infarction on T2-weighted sequences may be helpful in suggesting PRES (Fig. 4.8)[41,42] or MELAS.[126,127] In the remainder, dissection and embolism from an unidentified extra- or intracranial source are possible diagnoses.

Additional investigations should include echocardiography and cervical spine X-ray in flexion and extension. In some patients, a family history of prothrombotic states may direct appropriate investigations. It is important to recognize that more than one risk factor may be present in any given patient. Thus a child with a patent foramen ovale or cervicocephalic dissection may also have a prothrombotic state. We have been able to find a probable cause in more than 80% of children with a posterior circulation stroke.[58]

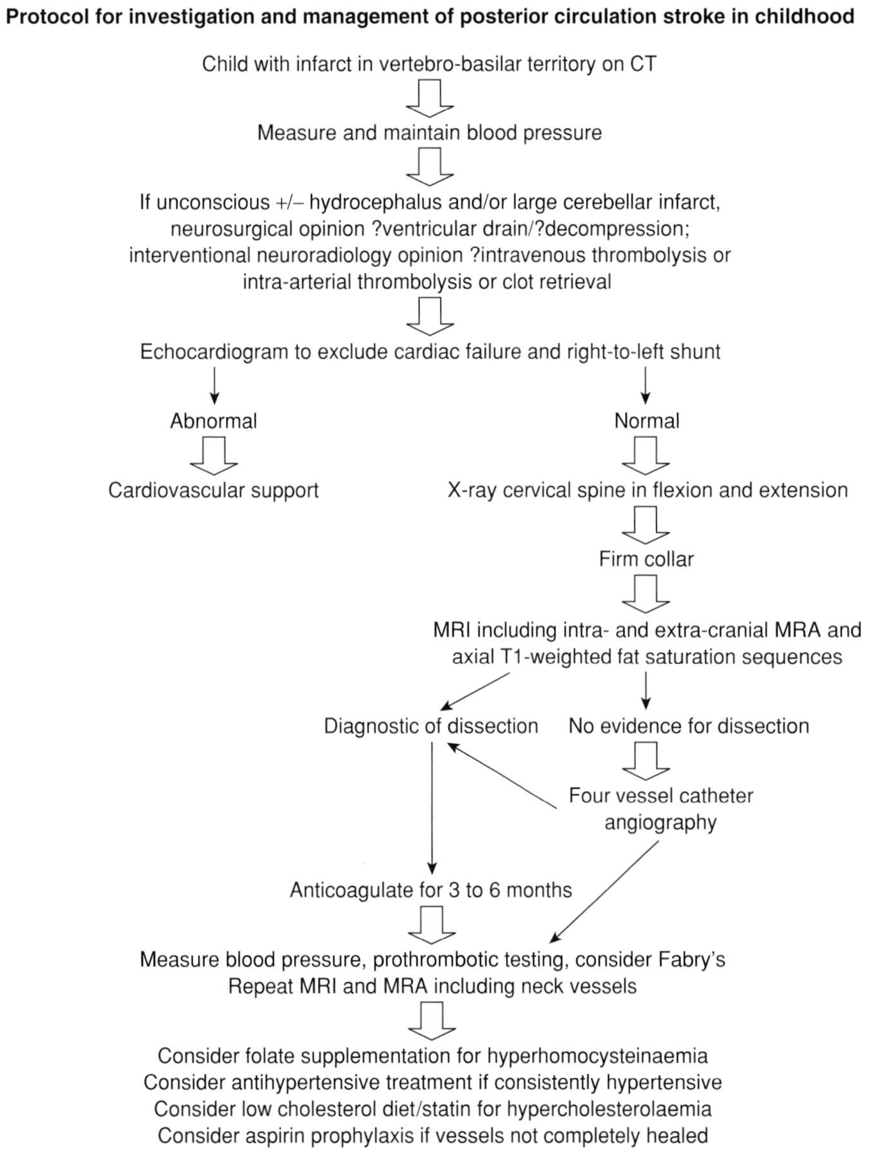

Protocol for investigation and management of posterior circulation stroke in childhood

Fig. 4.11. Flow chart for investigation and management of posterior circulation stroke. MRA, magnetic resonance angiography.

THERAPY

Therapy depends upon the presentation and any identified risk factors (Fig. 4.11). Basilar occlusion is life-threatening and thrombolysis, probably with mechanical clot lysis as well as urokinase or tissue plasminogen activator, may be reasonable as part of an audited study (see Chapter 16). Patients presenting in coma with cerebellar infarction may need external drainage of any associated hydrocephalus or surgical decompression.[128]

There is a substantial risk of recurrent stroke in patients with posterior stroke and vertebrobasilar pathology,[43,56,59] even in those treated with aspirin or anticoagulation.[59] If the neck is unstable in the acute phase, a collar is unlikely to be harmful and may reduce the strain on the damaged artery and therefore the chance of further thromboembolism. Anticoagulation may prevent recurrence in dissection. Aspirin, heparin, including low molecular weight heparins, and warfarin have been used to reduce the recurrence risk most frequently, athough there have not been any prospective double blind studies that have evaluated their efficacy in children. Folic acid and other vitamin supplementation and treatment of hyperlipidaemic states with diet and drugs may be indicated in some patients. Surgical revascularization may occasionally be required in patients with recurrent transient ischaemic attacks.[43]

Surgical correction of an identified cardiac defect may be important in preventing future events. Regular transfusion therapy in patients with sickle cell anaemia and stroke is currently mandated, although the risk of recurrence after posterior circulation strokes is not known.

Despite the high rate of recurrence, eventual outcome is good in the majority of cases,[43] although this does depend upon the site and extent of the infarct and to some extent on aetiology. Long-term cognitive problems have been reported after cerebellar stroke, often in those with a good motor recovery,[129,130] in addition to the mutism sometimes seen in the acute phase.[131]

4.1.3 Spinal Cord Stroke

Bettina Harms, Jason MacDonald and Fenella J. Kirkham

Introduction

Until emergency MRI of the spinal cord became the norm, ischaemic (Fig. 4.12) and haemorrhagic (Fig. 4.13) spinal cord stroke was rarely diagnosed in life. Before recommendations for terminology were published in 2002,[132] the term 'transverse myelitis' was used rather loosely even when a vascular, rather than an inflammatory, pathology was suspected,[133,134] and in rapidly progressive cases, Guillain–Barré syndrome has often been the initial diagnosis.[135,136] Although imaging of the spinal cord to make a definitive diagnosis is not easy, newer techniques may allow rapid diagnosis of spinal cord stroke so that evidence-based management strategies can be investigated.

Anatomy of the arterial supply to the spinal cord

The anterior spinal artery descends in the midline along the anterior cord and supplies 75% of the blood required by the cord. There are also two smaller posterior spinal arteries which ascend on either side of the spinal cord posteriorly and supply the other 25%. Thirty-one pairs of small segmental arteries arising from the aorta, vertebral and iliac arteries enter

Fig. 4.12. Ischaemic spinal cord stroke. Sagittal subjective texture image retrieval (STIR), T2- and T1-weighted MRI with axial T1-weighted MRI showing intrinsic high signal and swelling of the cervical cord secondary to an anterior spinal artery infarct.

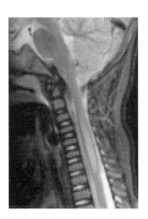
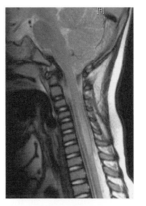
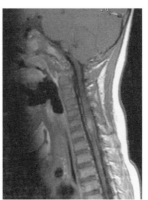
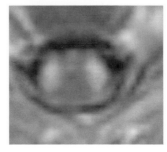

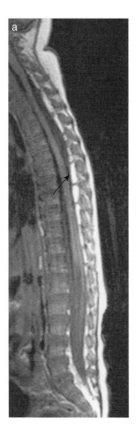
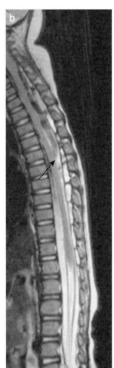
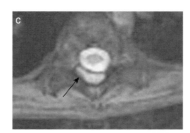
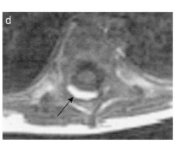
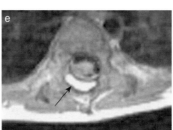

Fig. 4.13. (a) Spinal epidural haemorrhage in a child with haemophilia. (b–e) Same child 4 days after first 'episode' with second acute symptoms, previously treated conservatively. Sagittal T1- and T2-weighted MRI with axial T1-, T2-weighted and proton density MRI showing an extensive and loculated posterior subacute epidural haematoma without cord compression.

every intervertebral foramen supplying their corresponding nerve roots and then divide into radicular or medullary arteries which also supply the spinal cord with a rather variable anatomy. During development, five to eight of the anterior radicular arteries become dominant and provide most of the flow to the anterior two-thirds of spinal cord through the anterior spinal artery. These feeding vessels are known as radiculomedullary arteries. In most individuals, one of these anterior vessels, typically arising from the left intercostal arteries between T5 and L3, becomes notably larger and provides a major portion of the blood flow to anterior portions of the lower thoracic cord and the lumbar enlargement. If single, this artery is commonly known as the great anterior radiculomedullary artery or great artery of Adamkiewicz, although as many as a quarter of people undergoing angiography have more than one enlarged feeding artery. Arterioles from the anterior and posterior spinal arteries encircle the cord forming a fine pial plexus. The cervical portion of the cord receives blood from the vertebral, posterior inferior cerebellar and segmental radicular arteries at each intervertebral foramen. The thoracic region from C8 to T9 receives blood from the one or two dominant radiculomedullary arteries or directly from an intercostal vessel. The lower two-thirds of the spinal cord receives its blood supply from the anterior spinal artery via the great artery of Adamkiewicz, which usually supplies from T11 to L3. As there is extensive anastomosis, and the supply is from numerous feeding vessels, the posterior cord is less vulnerable to ischaemic infarction. However, the vascular anatomy of the supply to the anterior cord is variable and there are usually borderzones between the territories of the branches of the anterior spinal artery around the high thoracic and midlumbar regions, where the anastomoses are inadequate[137] and which may be vulnerable to hypoxic-ischaemic damage if the perfusion pressure or tissue oxygenation drop. In addition, the radiculomedullary feeding vessels, including the great artery of Adamkiewicz, are vulnerable to occlusion from bland or fibrocartilaginous embolus or at surgery to the spine or the aorta.

Ischaemic stroke

EPIDEMIOLOGY

Spinal cord infarction is a well-described aetiology of acute flaccid paralysis, and may not be as rare in children as previously thought, as it has been difficult to exclude definitively because of the difficulty in imaging the spinal cord and a reluctance to undertake conventional angiography. Although there are some clinical and laboratory clues (Table 4.3), the distinction from transverse myelitis[138–140] has not necessarily been easy to make with confidence,[141–144] so the figures for incidence are probably an underestimate. Differentiating between transverse myelitis and ischaemic stroke is particularly difficult when the underlying aetiology or trigger has been described with both, for example *Varicella*,[145] *Mycoplasma*,[146,147] *Borrelia*,[148,149] schistosomiasis,[150,151] systemic cancer and leukaemia,[152,153] Down syndrome[151] and systemic lupus erythematosus (Table 4.4).[148,154–156]

TABLE 4.3
Clinical, laboratory and imaging differences between transverse myelitis and spinal cord ischaemia

	Transverse myelitis	Spinal cord ischaemia
Time course	Neurological progression 4 hours to 21 days (mean time to maximum deficit 2 days)	Rapid evolution of full syndrome: minutes to hours
CSF cells	Pleocytosis or immunoglobulin G index	Normal
CSF protein	Raised in around half	Raised in around half
MRI	Non-vascular distribution	Vascular distribution
Diffusion imaging	May be abnormal in patchy distribution not confined to territory of one vessel	May be abnormal soon after presentation in distribution suggestive of infarction
Gadolinium	Enhancement inflammation	Normal

In Hong Kong, the acute flaccid paralysis notification rate consistently exceeds 1.0 per 100 000 population below 15 years of age.[157] The Australian Paediatric Surveillance study found an incidence of acute flaccid paraplegia of approximately 0.8 per 100 000 children <15 years of age per annum,[158] but another study in Victoria, Australia, used a two-source capture–recapture method to suggest an average annual incidence of 1.4 per 100 000 children aged under 15 years (95% CI=1.1–1.7).[159] Of 143 children presenting with non-polio acute flaccid paralysis in the Australian Paediatric Surveillance study,[158] four children had ischaemic damage of the spinal cord (attributable to complications of cardiac surgery in three) and the diagnosis was haemangioma adjacent to the spinal cord in one child. However, ischaemic mechanisms may not have been excluded in those with trauma (N=8), tumours (N=4), including neuroblastomas in two and transverse myelitis (N=27; 19%).[158] In the Hong Kong series of 120 patients with acute flaccid paralysis, 6.8% had a cardiovascular cause, 3.3% had miscellaneous causes including Kawaski disease, 7.5% remained undiagnosed and 67.5% (81) had neurological causes, 12 of which were diagnosed as transverse myelitis and 12 with encephalomyelitis, while three had meningitis; ischaemic stroke was not excluded in any of these cases. In a series from Wessex, UK, the incidence was approximately 1 per 100 000. Of 28 children (21 boys) presenting at a median age of 153 (range 19–197) months, final diagnoses were traumatic spinal cord injury in nine, transverse myelitis in five (although none had CSF evidence of inflammation), ischaemic stroke in four, epidural haematoma in two, tumour in four and other spinal pathology in four (one subluxation with atlantoaxial instability, one anterior cervical arachnoid cyst, one bony narrowing of spinal canal with underlying syndrome and one demyelination).[144]

ANTERIOR SPINAL ARTERY SYNDROME
The most common syndrome, anterior spinal artery syndrome (ASAS), is caused by interruption of blood flow to the anterior spinal artery, producing ischaemia in the anterior two-thirds of the cord, with sudden onset of flaccid weakness of the legs (and of the arms if the cervical cord is involved) and dissociated sensory loss, often accompanied by back pain.[137] The levels typically involved are C4–5 and L2–3, which are considered to be the borderzone areas of the spinal cord, although as discussed above, there is considerable variation in anatomy and embolus to a feeding artery cannot be excluded.

Patients usually present with sudden (minutes to hours) onset of flaccid paraparesis or quadriparesis, loss of pain and temperature sensation one or two levels below the level of injury with preservation of vibration, position and touch modalities, and bladder and bowel involvement.[137] There is often also burning pain.[137,143] Clinically, the rapid onset suggests spontaneous spinal cord infarction[143] rather than transverse myelitis.[138–140] Laboratory features compatible with spinal cord infarction include normal CSF, including absence of oligoclonal bands and low IgG index. Although there is clearly overlap,[160] in spinal cord stroke MR abnormality is typically in an anterior distribution involving mainly grey matter,[161] visible early on diffusion imaging[162] (Table 4.3), without the gadolinium enhancement suggestive of patchy inflammation in transverse myelitis.[163] Sagittal T2-weighted images appear most sensitive for detecting acute ischaemic change, with a hyperintense appearance typically in the shape of a pencil, which may be visible as early as 2 hours after onset of symptoms.[164] In around two-thirds of adult patients, MRI demonstrates a T2-weighted abnormality, but a normal study does not exclude a spinal cord infarction, which then becomes a diagnosis of exclusion.

RISK FACTORS FOR SPINAL CORD INFARCTION (Table 4.4)
Aortic disease is a cause of ASAS, typically coarctation in children,[165,166] although ASAS due to aortic dissection has been described in an 18 year old.[167] Spinal cord ischaemia is a dreaded complication of interventional radiological procedures as well as surgery, for example for scoliosis, particularly if there is an underlying condition predisposing to vascular disorders, such as Ehlers–Danlos syndrome[168,169] or neuroblastoma.[170] Other iatrogenic causes (Table 4.4) include umbilical artery catheterization,[171] bronchial artery embolization in cystic fibrosis[133] and sclerotherapy for oesophageal varices.[172]

TABLE 4.4
Risk factors for ischaemic spinal cord injury in childhood

Trauma
• Fibrocartilaginous emboli from the nucleus pulposus of the intervertebral disc

Infections
Meningitis[182,191,192]
• *Escherichia coli*
• *Haemophilus influenzae*
• Pneumococcus
• Meningococcus
• *Mycobacterium tuberculosis*

Atlanto-axial instability
• Down syndrome[151]
• Achondroplasia[174]
• I-cell disease[175]
• Choreo-athetoid cerebral palsy[173]
• Marfan syndrome[176]
• Klippel–Trenaunay syndrome

Past medical history
• Haemoglobinopathy[189,190]
• Haemolytic uraemic
• Post-streptococcal glomerulonephritis

Post-intervention
• Scoliosis (spontaneous and Harrington rods)
• Ehlers–Danlos[168]
• Coarctation of the aorta[165,166,184–188]
• Thoracic neuroblastoma[170]
• Umbilical artery catheterization[171]
• Oesophageal varices (sclerotherapy)[172]
• Bronchial artery embolization in cystic fibrosis[133]
• Interventional neuroradiology

Prothrombotic disorders[179–183]
Anaemia[188–190]

Patients with atlanto-axial instability, such as those with choreo-athetoid cerebral palsy,[173] achondroplasia[174] and I-cell disease,[175] are at risk of spontaneous spinal cord infarction (Table 4.4). Of 513 patients with Marfan syndrome, two had spinal cord infarction.[176] Other risk factors include sepsis, hypotension[177,178] and thromboembolic disorders. Protein S deficiency,[179] the thermolabile methylene tetrahydrofolate reductase,[143] prothrombin G20210A[180,181] and factor V Leiden[182] mutations and primary antiphospholipid syndrome[183] may be prothrombotic risk factors for spinal cord infarction.

Aortic coarctation and its repair
Spinal cord ischaemia is a complication of untreated and otherwise previously asymptomatic coarctation of the aorta.[184] In addition it is a well recognized sequel of surgical repair,[165,166,185] with an incidence of up to 1.5% in series from the 1970s, although in later series from the 1980s and 1990s it is very rare indeed in patients with simple coarctation or coarctation with ventricular septal defect.[186] The typical neurological deficit, with a sensory level, a flaccid paraplegia and bladder and bowel involvement, usually indicates focal ischaemia or stroke in the distribution of the anterior spinal artery.[166] Risk factors for this type of injury include the

following: (1) hypotension; (2) long duration of aortic cross clamping;[187] (3) anaemia;[188] and (4) infection and/or inflammation which, together with high temperature itself, tends to exacerbate ischaemic damage.

Sickle cell disease
Symptoms and signs attributable to spinal cord involvement in sickle cell disease may be secondary to osteomyelitis and epidural abscess, extramedullary haematopoiesis and vertebral collapse. Spinal cord infarction has been described in sickle cell anaemia[189] and sickle cell trait.[190]

Meningitis
Symptoms and signs of spinal cord injury are occasionally seen in purulent meningitis in neonates, usually with *Escherichia coli*, and in older children with *Haemophilus influenzae*, pneumococcal[191] and meningococcal infections.[192] Tuberculous meningitis is also a cause. Although ischaemic stroke is rarely demonstrated on MRI and there are few reports of vascular imaging, arterial disease is the likely pathology in many of these cases from the clinical presentation and the available autopsy data.[192] Many have signs compatible with anterior spinal artery involvement. Reduced perfusion probably plays a significant role.[192] The cervical cord may be at particular risk if there is cerebellar tonsillar descent in the context of a Chiari malformation or after lumbar puncture.[192] Epidural haemorrhage or abscess are also possible mechanisms which should be excluded on MRI.[192]

Traumatic spinal cord infarction of the artery of Adamkiewicz
Spinal cord injury without radiological abnormality (SCIWORA) has only been described in children, typically affects the cervical, and less often the thoracic, spinal cord,[193,194] and usually presents acutely at the time of the trauma. Deforming strains are involved in the pathogenesis of SCIWORA. This entity was initially described in the era previous to the availability of MRI but the majority of those with signs consistent with partial transection of the cord have no abnormality on acute MRI, while those with haemorrhage or oedema on MRI usually have complete transection and a very poor prognosis.[195,196]

Delayed presentation, hours to days after trauma,[193,197,198] is also very likely to have a vascular pathophysiology, particularly if the thoracic or lumbar cord is involved,[199] perhaps involving hypotension[200] or thrombosis or dissection of one of the large radiculomedullary branches. These patients are usually hypotensive and neurologically intact at admission after blunt thoracic or abdominal trauma, and then after a latent period, they develop a profound neurological deficit, usually paraplegia, which rarely shows signs of recovery. MRI may show spinal cord infarction located in the territory of the great artery of Adamkiewicz.[199]

Cervical cord infarction has been described after very minor trauma in young children in the era before MRI.[201] The pathophysiology is uncertain but may involve spasm. Spinal cord infarction may also be caused by stabbing involving the great artery of Adamkiewicz.[202,203]

Fibrocartilaginous emboli from the nucleus pulposus of the intervertebral disc

This is recognized in veterinary medicine, as well as from post-mortem studies in humans, with positive staining for fibrocartilaginous emboli within the vascular supply of the necrotic cord. It is not possible to diagnose this entity definitively in surviving patients but the presence of degenerative disease of the spine, with or without Schmorl's nodes, in a patient with a very sudden onset of paralysis and MRI abnormality in a distribution compatible with anterior spinal artery ischaemia is suggestive.[141–143,204] Schmorl's nodes are probably the end result of ischaemic necrosis beneath the cartilaginous endplate. This mechanism may explain the typical association of rapid paralysis and sphincter involvement in patients with a recent history of mild trauma. There is general agreement that emboli originate from the intervertebral disc, but the mechanism whereby disc fragments enter the vessels is poorly understood.

Spinal cord haemorrhage

Intramedullary haemorrhage may occur secondary to cavernomas,[205] arteriovenous malformations, aneurysms[206] and haemorrhaging disorders (see Chapter 8) in neonates,[207] infants and children. In addition, epidural, subdural[208–210] and subarachnoid haematomas[211] are well recognized.[212] Subdural and subarachnoid haemorrhages usually occur in the context of trauma, often severe, and epidural haemorrhage may also be traumatic. Although rare, spontaneous spinal epidural haematoma is probably a more common cause for acute cord compression in children.[213–216]

Spinal Epidural Haematoma

Initial presentation of spontaneous spinal epidural haematoma (SSEH) can be non-specific. Presenting symptoms of epidural haemorrhage are usually pain, either local or radicular, followed by progressive bilateral motor weakness. Sensory loss develops hours or even days later.[215,217] Less frequently patients may present with slowly progressing chronic or relapsing symptoms or with neurological signs that mimic an acute intervertebral disc prolapse. SSEH has also been described as mimicking Guillain–Barré syndrome[136] or tumour in a child.[218] Predisposing factors, most commonly coagulopathy (haemophilia, leukaemia), arteriovenous malformation, anticoagulation, and procedures such as lumbar puncture and epidural anaesthesia,[136] are only found in 50–60% of cases. Spinal epidural haematomas may have a traumatic origin.[219–222] Recurrence is unusual.[223,224]

Epidural haematomas may be secondary to, or even the presentation of, haemorrhaging disorders such as factor VIII,[225–228] factor IX deficiency,[229,230] factor XIII deficiency[231] or thrombocytopaenia. Spinal haemorrhage has been reported after lumbar puncture in neonates[232] and children,[233] including

those with leukaemia.[234,235] Spinal epidural haematomas have been reported in the context of surgery, for example for scoliosis,[236] mediastinal lymphangioma[237] and epidermal naevus syndrome.[238] MRI is the neuroimaging modality of choice. On T2-weighted MRI, they are hyperintense and are usually located posterolaterally.[239–241]

The pathogenesis is unclear, but the haemorrhaging is mostly believed to be venous in origin. The reason for this assumption is that there are few, if any, arteries in the normal epidural space.[242] The lack of valves in the epidural venous plexus makes it especially vulnerable to any intrinsic change in pressure. Activities causing sudden fluctuation in the intra-abdominal and intra-thoracic pressure or prolonged Valsalva manoeuvres have been described to precede neurological symptoms, including whooping cough, voiding, weight lifting, trumpet playing,[217] sneezing, bending, coughing and coitus.[215] Vascular cases make up less than 10% of all spinal epidural haematomas.[243,244] In the absence of other causes for the haemorrhage, spinal arteriovenous malformations have to be considered, even where there is no MRI evidence. In such cases the blood clot found at operation should be examined histologically.[245]

Treatment of epidural spinal haematomas is either conservative (with close observation) or surgical evacuation, usually as an emergency. Conservative management may only be considered in mild cases with early resolution of the haematoma and neurological deficits and provided that the patient is followed neurologically and with repeated MRI imaging.[246] Recognition of the symptoms and rapid diagnostic evaluation are essential to minimize delay in surgery. Factors predicting recovery are the location of the haematoma, preoperative neurological deficit and operative interval.[247] The outcome is good if evacuation is performed before the onset of complete sensorimotor paralysis. Recovery is significantly better when surgical decompression is performed within 36 hours in patients with complete sensorimotor and within 48 hours in patients with incomplete sensorimotor deficit.[221,247] Complete neurological recovery has been described in approximately 50% of patients and partial recovery in 44%.[217]

Spinal cord arteriovenous malformations

Spinal arteriovenous fistulae and malformations occur in children[248] and may present with neurological or systemic ischaemic symptoms referable to their localization.[249–256] Children may present with symptoms refereable to vascular steal,[251] including chest pain.[253] Brown–Séquard syndrome has been described,[250] as has intracranial hypertension[255] and scoliosis when the spine was involved.[256] Patients with unexplained myelopathy and an MRI showing increased T2 signal or flow voids may have an arteriovenous malformation[257] and should be referred to a centre which can undertake diagnostic, and if appropriate, interventional conventional angiography. Hereditary haemorrhagic telangiectasia should be considered in children presenting with spinal arteriovenous malformation.[258] Patients with skin lesions, such as those seen in the Klippel–

Trenauny–Weber[259–261] or Cobb syndromes,[262,263] may be at risk of spinal cord ischaemia secondary to the associated spinal arteriovenous malformation.

Management of spinal cord stroke

PREVENTION AND MANAGEMENT OF ISCHAEMIC SPINAL CORD STROKE

In addition to monitoring of somatosensory evoked potentials, assessment of the anatomy of the artery of Adamkiewicz with MR[264] or CT angiography[265] may inform the surgical or interventional approach to scoliosis repair or other procedures which put the spinal cord at risk. Immobilization in a rigid collar and restriction of sporting activities prevents the majority of late presentations after SCIWORA involving the cervical cord.[266]

Although there is no class A evidence of benefit and the trials in traumatic cord injury were flawed,[267] reports of good outcome for transverse myelitis in children after intravenous methylprednisolone[268,269] means that this treatment is usually initiated as soon as possible after presentation. If a stroke is considered clinically likely, aspirin 3–5mg/kg/day is a reasonable option. Spinal epidural haematoma is a risk when using tissue plasminogen activator,[270] which cannot be recommended at the present time, although as the prognosis is poor, randomized controlled trials of early treatment[271] might be considered.

MANAGEMENT OF HAEMORRHAGIC SPINAL CORD STROKE

Epidural haemorrhage is a neurosurgical emergency as the spinal cord injury secondary to compression may be reversible if the haematoma is removed rapidly. Neurological outcome is correlated with preoperative neurological deficits and delay before surgery.[247,272,273] Some patients may do well with conservative management and this has been preferred in some patients on anticoagulants[274] or with haemorrhaging disorders,[275,276] but prediction of those who do not require surgery is not perfect.[246]

It is important to consider prophylaxis for deep vein thrombosis, for example with compression stockings and/or subcutaneous heparin, for all immobile patients. Rehabilitation may require specialist spinal services, although the setup may not be appropriate for young children. Particular attention must be paid to the management of the neuropathic bladder.[277,278]

MANAGEMENT OF SPINAL ARTERIOVENOUS MALFORMATIONS (see Chapter 8)

As for intracerebral arteriovenous malformations and aneurysms, these patients should be referred to an experienced team. Endovascular management may be an option for spinal cord aneurysms[279] and arteriovenous malformations.[252,280–284] An underlying diagnosis such as hereditary haemorrhagic telangiectasia does not necessarily preclude interventional treatment.[285] A combined surgical and endovascular approach may be appropriate in some cases.[286]

4.2 Neuroimaging

4.2.1 Imaging of Paediatric Stroke

Dawn E. Saunders and W.K. Kling Chong

Introduction

The radiological evaluation of paediatric patients following cerebral infarction has dramatically improved over the last decade. By challenging traditional views regarding stroke, imaging has led to a greater understanding of the pathophysiology of the underlying diseases. The role of imaging in paediatric stroke is to confirm the diagnosis and exclude other causes, demonstrate an underlying vascular cause and thereby guide treatment and monitor progress of the condition.

CT scanning has been the primary modality of brain imaging in acute stroke but has been surpassed by increased availability and recent developments in MRI techniques. CT remains the imaging method of choice for the detection of acute haemorrhage and is the mainstay of imaging in acute trauma, neurosurgical complications and subarachnoid haemorrhage. Although MRI is more sensitive than CT in the imaging of acute stroke, CT is still performed as it is more widely available in general hospitals and can be useful in excluding other causes of stroke.

This chapter reviews the imaging modalities including ultrasound, CT, MRI, conventional angiography and nuclear medicine used for the evaluation of paediatric stroke. Imaging modalities available to the neuroradiologist have not changed for over a decade but developments in both software and hardware have resulted in significant advances in data acquisition and post-processing. The most significant advances have occurred in the field of MRI and the development of new techniques, such as diffusion and perfusion imaging, has transformed its role in the evaluation of children with cerebral infarction. The MRI features relevant to ischaemic and haemorrhagic stroke are discussed and other causes of stroke are briefly considered at the end of the chapter.

Imaging modalities in paediatric stroke

ULTRASOUND

Ultrasound is an established non-invasive bedside imaging modality used in the neonatal period to diagnose germinal matrix and intraventricular haemorrhage, and periventricular leukomalacia. A variable 5–8MHz probe is used to image the neonatal brain via the anterior fontanelle and an 8–12MHz linear array probe is used for the examination of superficial abnormalities, such as subdural haemorrhage and hygromas. Cerebellar haemorrhage can be detected via the posterolateral fontanelle of the posterior fossa in neonates.

The transcranial Doppler (TCD) examination allows the measurement of blood flow velocities within the major intracranial arteries of the circle of Willis. The examination is carried out using a low frequency (2MHz) pulsed Doppler transducer and produces either a spectral waveform or a colour Doppler display of the blood flow (duplex ultrasound). Power Doppler imaging has recently been developed and measures the strength of the Doppler-shifted echoes without providing direction of flow.[287] Access to the intracranial arteries is obtained via the transtemporal, transorbital, suboccipital and submandibular approach. The intracranial arteries of the circle of Willis are detected via standard transtemporal and suboccipital approaches and the ophthalmic artery and siphon of the internal carotid artery can be visualized by a transorbital approach.[288] The identification of the arteries is based on the depth of sample volume, the angle of the transducer, the direction of flow and spatial relationship of one Doppler signal to another.

The mean velocity calculated by the TCD method is based on the time average of the velocity. The pulsatility index is calculated (peak systolic velocity minus end diastolic velocity divided by mean velocity) and reflects either obstruction or resistance proximal and distal to these points of the artery. Intracranial arterial velocities are determined by the volume of flow over time and the cross-sectional area of the artery. Cerebral blood flow (CBF) is influenced by the age of the patient, haematocrit, partial pressure of $p\text{CO}_2$, $p\text{O}_2$, temperature, blood pressure, cardiac output, raised intracranial pressure, proximal arterial obstruction, distal arterial stenosis and arteriovenous malformation.

Clinical applications of TCD in the assessment of paediatric stroke patients include screening for vasculopathy in sickle cell disease[289,290] (see Chapter 15 and colour plate 6). Although less well-established, assessment of intracranial vasculature in children with stroke;[291–293] and diagnosis of cerebrovascular disease such as moyamoya is feasible.[294–297] Duplex ultrasound is feasible can be used to evaluate the extracranial internal carotid artery in the detection of an arterial dissection and work has been carried out in neonates and infants[298] and adults[299] in its use in venous sinus thrombosis.

COMPUTERIZED TOMOGRAPHY
CT images are obtained by the projection of a high kilovoltage collimated beam of X-rays through the brain. A standard examination of the head consists of a series of contiguous sections, usually 5cm thickness through the posterior fossa and then 10cm thickness to the vertex. The orbitomeatal line is used as the plane of section to avoid radiation dose to the eyes. Although widely available for the exclusion of intracerebral haemorrhage, one of the main disadvantages of CT is that ischaemic stroke is often not obvious on CT within the first 24 hours.

CT angiography
In the past decade, advances in slip ring technology have made helical CT possible which has resulted in faster scans and the development of CT angiography (CTA) which requires imaging at the time of the arterial phase of the contrast injection and provides a 3D reconstruction of the intracranial or

extracranial anatomy. More recently, advances in the number of detectors and type of solid state detectors lining the gantry have led to faster spiral imaging with simultaneous data from multiple (up to 4), thinner (down to 0.5mm) slices. This allows for greater temporal and spatial resolution without additional radiation dose.[300] CTA may avoid digital subtraction arteriography for the anatomical definition of cerebral vascular lesions requiring neurosurgery in childhood.[301]

3D CTA has been proposed as the method of choice for diagnosis and follow-up of dissection as differences in the attenuation of blood and contrast can be used to distinguish the true and false lumens[302] while allowing assessment of the overall external diameter of the vessel. After blunt trauma, multidetector-row computed tomography is probably the method of choice for excluding vascular pathologies including extracranial dissection[303] and, given the high risk of ischaemic stroke and death,[304] should probably be used more widely in children in the emergency setting if MR or digital subtraction arteriography are not immediately available. There are few data in children,[304] however, presumably reflecting reluctance to utilize this modality in this age group in view of the relatively high radiation dose.

CT cerebral blood flow measurements
Stable xenon CT allows the measurement of local CBF by scanning a selected slice between 6 and 10 times whilst the subject breathes a xenon/oxygen mixture via an inhalation system. Xenon has a high atomic number which makes it a good contrast medium and an increase in the tissue xenon causes an increase in the density measured. The arterial xenon content is determined from the end-tidal air and the patient's haematocrit. Quantitative CBF measurements in mL/min/100g can be calculated using a two-parameter fit method which links the CT arterial xenon content and the arterial xenon input.[305] Although the technique has been successfully applied in the adult population, it is not used in our institution and its use in children is very limited as the procedure is unpleasant and poorly tolerated and a general anaesthetic is required.

Relative CBF and relative cerebral blood volume (CBV) have been calculated using the first pass bolus technique of CT perfusion with conventional water soluble contrast agents.[306] The passage of contrast laden blood is tracked by serial 1- to 2-second scans and time density curves are plotted. The area under the curve is used to estimate the amount of blood delivered to a particular area of the brain. Time of first arrival of contrast, time to peak and arteriovenous transit time measurements can also be made. There are advantages for this technique in terms of comparison with normals[307] and availability in the emergency situation.[307]

MAGNETIC RESONANCE IMAGING
During the past decade, tremendous progress has been made in MRI due to the development of new imaging methods such as diffusion and perfusion imaging as well as the development

of faster imaging techniques such as echo-planar imaging. The new techniques demand higher hardware specification; higher field strength, typically 1.5T, echo planar capability and rapid gradients.

Our protocol for the evaluation of the paediatric stroke patient includes standard T2-weighted axial images which show tissue contrast well, and sagittal and coronal T1-weighted images which maximize contrast between the cerebral tissue and CSF and which provide morphological information and detect early haemorrhage. In addition, we obtain fluid-attenuated inversion recovery (FLAIR) sequences in which suppression of the signal from the CSF increases the visibility of periventricular lesions. To assess the intracranial vasculature we obtain a magnetic resonance angiography (MRA) centred on the circle of Willis, and perfusion images to assess the more distal CBF. In addition, we acquire an extracranial MRA and axial fat-saturated T1-weighted images through the neck for the detection of carotid and vertebral artery dissection.

There is some controversy as to whether conventional MRI can detect hyperacute haemorrhage (<24 hours)[308] or whether more sensitive sequences are required. Gradient echo imaging uses a T2* image to detect the paramagnetic qualities of haemoglobin found in different stages of haemorrhage and is useful in the detection of haemorrhagic change within an infarct, as well as the detection of germinal matrix or parenchymal haemorrhage. Gradient echo T2* images are more sensitive than the more commonly used diffusion weighted images in the detection of petechial haemorrhage within cerebral infarcts and it has been proposed that gradient echo images should be acquired in all cases of acute stroke.[309]

Magnetic resonance angiography and venography
MRA and magnetic resonance venography (MRV) sequences use the inherent contrast of flowing blood and do not require the injection of contrast. The two main sequence types used are 2D or 3D time of flight and phase contrast imaging and can be adjusted to look at either the arterial or venous system. Time of flight imaging uses the difference in magnetization between the excited flowing blood and the suppressed background signal from the brain and is the preferred method for both intra- and extracranial MRA, whilst phase contrast imaging is the preferred method for MRV.

MRA is sensitive to turbulent flow caused by either vessel narrowing or anaemia which results in signal drop and an overinterpretation of the degree of stenosis. This can be overcome by acquiring the MRA sequence following the injection of gadolinium contrast agents and more recently an 'angiographic' sequence has been developed which acquires a series of consecutive MRAs from the arterial through the venous phase in less than 20 seconds.[309] These techniques can be applied to both the intra- and extracranial vasculature.

Diffusion imaging
Diffusion imaging is able to detect ischaemic regions of the brain before any changes are detectable on conventional

MRI.[310] It uses the Brownian motion, or diffusion, of water molecules to detect changes in tissue contrast. In the normal brain, the random motion of water molecules results in small displacement distances comparable to cellular dimensions and is therefore a method of probing cellular integrity. An increase in the cellular dimension (cytotoxic oedema) occurs early in cerebral infarction and results in a reduction in the distance the water molecules can move (restricted diffusion). It is thought to result from both a reduction in mobile extracellular water and an alteration in the intracellular proteins and is followed by vasogenic oedema, when the cell membrane is broken down and diffusion is free.[310] There are some uncertainties related to the precise biophysical mechanisms underlying the diffusion changes in acute stroke but the view that these changes are associated with cytotoxic oedema have been substantiated by several groups.[311] Although, as in adults, in the majority of patients scanned a few hours after presentation, diffusion imaging abnormality is associated with T2-weighted abnormality in a similar distribution, diffusion imaging abnormality in the absence of infarction has been documented in hemiplegic migraine in a child.[116]

Perfusion imaging
Perfusion imaging allows the demonstration of blood flow within the arterioles and capillaries of the brain. There are two general MRI approaches to the assessment of cerebral perfusion.[312] The most commonly used technique is the bolus tracking method which involves the injection of a paramagnetic contrast agent intravenously and the tracking of transient changes of signal intensity observed by a series of rapid images obtained at intervals of 1 to 2 seconds. Compromise of the arterial supply to the brain is detected as either a delay in arrival of the contrast agent or attenuation of the signal change due to the arrival of less contrast agent. Computer modelling techniques convert the transient signal changes into maps that reflect CBV, CBF and mean transit time.

The second approach involves the magnetic labelling of inflowing water protons within the blood and is known as arterial spin labelling.[313,314] The advantage of this technique is that it is a completely non-invasive and can provide quantitative measurements of perfusion. There are various technical problems in the implementation of the technique and there has been very limited use of this method in clinical practice.

A more detailed approach to diffusion and perfusion imaging can be found in Chapter 4, 2.2.

Magnetic resonance spectroscopy
Magnetic resonance spectroscopy (MRS) is a non-invasive method that allows the in vivo investigation of biochemical changes in both animals and humans. The application of MRS to the study of stroke has made possible dynamic studies of intracellular metabolism in cerebral ischaemia but to date remains a research tool. The concentration of cerebral metabolites in the brain is many magnitudes lower (2–20mM) than that of water (41.7M of water or 83.4M of protons). The

nuclear magnetic resonance signal from the metabolite is therefore very much smaller than the signal from water used to generate an anatomical display in MRI. Hence, the minimum voxel size required for MRS is larger and data acquisition times are longer than in MRI. Multi-section proton MRS is a technique which enables the sampling of a large area of the brain to be divided into relatively small regions of interest and then displayed as a low resolution metabolite map.[315] Despite the relatively low signal-to-noise ratio of spectroscopy, improvements in magnet and gradient design, and the wider availability of magnets at higher field strength (1.5T), now enable good quality brain proton MRS spectra to be recorded on most modern clinical instruments. Within an infarct, MRS demonstrates a reduction of *N*-acetylaspartate, a neuronal marker, and the appearance of lactate, not normally detected in the brain and a marker of anaerobic metabolism.[316] As well as having prognostic value in paediatric traumatic and non-traumatic coma,[317,318] and after cardiopulmonary bypass,[319] similar changes have been demonstrated in sickle cell disease[320] and acute stroke in a few children.[321,322] However, because of limited access to emergency MRS, this technique has been restricted to the diagnosis and management of metabolic stroke including ornithine carbamoyl transferase deficiency,[323–325] mitochondrial disease[326,327] and disorders of glycosylation.[327,328]

Cerebral Angiography

Although cerebral angiography is the criterion standard for the imaging of vascular anatomy and pathology, its role has changed in the last decade. Improvements in Doppler ultrasound techniques, MRA and CTA have allowed these techniques to compete with more invasive cerebral angiography.[82,329,330] In our institution, angiography is performed in patients with cerebral infarction and no obvious aetiology provided by medical history and cardiac echocardiography and normal vascular imaging determined by MRA. It may also be performed in children with suspected dissection not demonstrated on MRI and extracranial MRA.

Cerebral angiography is performed under general anaesthetic and parental consent is required. Although the procedure is invasive, the risk of stroke is low and quoted as 0.5–1%[331] but appears to be lower in children.[332] There is also a risk of local complications, such as groin haematoma complicating arterial access acquired through the common femoral artery.[332]

A 4F sheath and catheter are used to catheterize the common carotid and vertebral arteries, and in some patients the internal carotid arteries are catheterized to improve the concentration of contrast and allow better visualization of the basal and small arteries. Patients with a suspected dissection have arch angiography performed to visualize the origins of the cerebral vessels prior to catheterization. Biplane imaging is desirable for the examination of children because of restrictions in terms of volume of iodinated contrast and radiation dose. The volume of non-ionic iodinated contrast agents depends on body weight, surface area and renal function. Images are acquired in both the arterial (2 frames/s for 4 seconds) and the venous phase (1 frame/s for 20 seconds).

Nuclear Medicine

Radionucleotide imaging through SPECT offers the potential for semi-quantitation of cerebral perfusion in paediatric stroke. SPECT has replaced the use of the more invasive positron emission tomography in the measurement of cerebral blood flow in children. The ideal brain SPECT pharmaceutical has not been developed and the modality competes with dynamic CT and MRI. The commonly used radionucleotides are technetium (Tc-99m)- and iodo-amines including hexemethylpropyleneamine oxide (HMPAO) bicasate.[333] Tc-99m labelled HMPAO is the most readily available agent and is of value in imaging regions of reduced cerebral blood flow in patients with chronic hypoperfusion, for example in children with moyamoya disease,[334] hemiplegia[335] and occasionally acute stroke.[336]

Sedation of children for neuroimaging

Children undergoing all imaging modalities other than ultrasound require either sedation or general anaesthesia (GA). All children require GA for cerebral angiography as it is an invasive procedure and there is an inherent necessity for the child to keep very still. In our institution, infants less than 3 months of age and 5kg weight are fed prior to CT and MRI, and then scanned whilst asleep. Eligible children over 3 months of age (Fig. 4.14) are sedated in the department of radiology following a period of sleep deprivation. Chloral hydrate is used for children under 10kg and temazepam and droperidol are given to those over 10kg. The child is scanned asleep whilst oxygen saturation is monitored and a parent is expected to be present throughout the procedure. We have a nurse-led sedation unit and 95% of children are successfully scanned following sedation. Children who fail are given a GA on a separate hospital visit.

In the acute stroke period, MRI is performed under GA in the young child, and is considered in older children if it is felt they will not tolerate the scan awake. CT is more often performed in the emergency situation without an anaesthetic.

Neuroimaging of paediatric stroke

CT of Cerebral Infarction

Contrast determined by CT is due to the absorption of the X-ray beam through the tissues through which it passes. Pathological changes in cerebral tissue result in an increase in the water content of the tissue and a resultant alteration in the absorption properties. Neurons are the cells most sensitive to ischaemia and they are located in the grey matter, which is usually denser than white matter. The first sign of cerebral ischaemia is the loss of density of grey matter, with an overall result of loss of grey–white matter differentiation. The decline in grey–white matter differentiation results in four signs of early

- Sedation advised for children over 3 months – 5 years of age
- Sedation considered for children >5 years with developmental delay, cerebral palsy and epilepsy.
- General aneasthetic for children with an acute stroke, those that fail sedation and for children undergoing conventional angiography
- Common relative contraindications to sedation
  - Airways problems e.g. snoring or stridor, small mandible, large tongue
  - Apnoeic episodes
  - Respiratory disease: <94% O_2 saturation in air, respiratory failure
  - Raised intracranial pressure
  - Epilepsy in children with
    - Generalised convulsions within 24 hours
    - Generalised convulsions more then once/day
    - Convulsions <4 hours prior to sedation
  - Associated with major neuromuscular disease or neurological disease such as encephalitis
  - Failure to regain full conscious level after a recent convulsion
  - Risk of pulmonary aspiration e.g. abdominal distention, severe vomiting
  - Severe metabolic, liver or renal disease
  - Sickle cell disease

Fig. 4.14. Sedation guidelines. (From Great Ormond Street Hospital, London, UK.)

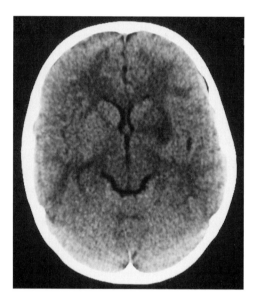

Fig. 4.15. Axial CT scan at the level of the internal capsule acquired, of a 7-year-old boy with a history of chickenpox. Low density change of the lentiform nucleus on the left and loss of clarity of the adjacent internal capsule is evident on the day of symptom onset.

cerebral infarction: (1) loss of clarity of the internal capsule; (2) loss of visibility of the insular ribbon; (3) loss of differentiation between white and cortical grey matter;[337] and (4) gyral swelling seen as sulcal effacement (Fig. 4.15).[338] Further increase in tissue water results in the typical appearance of an area of low density on CT but these changes occur later and may not be visible on the early CT scan.[338] Although blood–brain barrier breakdown occurs early in cerebral infarction, the use of intravenous contrast agents in CT does not increase the detectability of infarcts within the first 24 hours and is not necessary in the evaluation of children with cerebral infarction although venous sinus thrombosis may be detected.[339]

An infrequently seen sign on CT scans of children with cerebral infarction is the 'hyperdense MCA' sign which indicates thrombus present in the vessel. A similar appearance can also be seen in the basilar artery following occlusion.

MRI OF CEREBRAL INFARCTION

MRI is sensitive to changes in the relaxation properties and diffusion of water protons affected by their microscopic environment. Cerebral ischaemia is characterised by changes in electrolyte and water balance that result in alterations in this environment and these differences are exploited to increase contrast and therefore the sensitivity of MRI. Acute infarcts are more visible on MRI than CT, with over 80% of MRI's positive within the first 24 hours compared with only 60% visible on CT.[338] MRI is particularly superior in the detection of infarcts within the posterior fossa where CT is limited by beam hardening artefact from the skull base. In addition, lacunar infarcts and small cortical infarcts are seen with greater conspicuity by MRI.[338,340]

In acute stroke, before any change on the T2-weighted images has occurred, there is an initial reduction in an apparent diffusion coefficient (ADC) associated with cytotoxic oedema.[341] This is seen as an area of reduced signal on an ADC map but as increased signal on a diffusion-weighted image. At 6–12 hours, with the onset of vasogenic oedema, increased T2-weighted signal intensity may be seen. As the cell membrane breaks down and necrosis starts, there is a gradual reversal of the ADC change because the diffusion of water becomes less restricted. At around 3–10 days when the T2 value is high, the ADC achieves its original normal value, a process known as 'pseudonormalization'. As diffusion becomes more free, the ADC value will increase further and be seen as an area of increased signal on an ADC map. Because a diffusion-weighted image is a modified T2-weighted image, the effect of the underlying T2-weighted signal change will be seen (known as T2 shine through) in the later stages of infarction. The advantage of an ADC map over the diffusion-weighted image is that the T2 shine through is eliminated and the time from onset of the cerebral infarct can be roughly determined, allowing the distinction of infarcts occurring at different times.

To illustrate these points, Fig. 4.16 shows T2-weighted, diffusion-weighted and the ADC map of the 7-year-old child scanned within 3 days of stroke onset. (CT performed on the

Fig. 4.16. MRI of the child whose CT is shown in Fig. 4.15. Axial T2-weighted images (a,d), diffusion-weighted images (b,e) and the ADC map (c,f) at two levels through the basal ganglia acquired 3 days from symptom onset. On T2-weighted and diffusion-weighted images, focal abnormalities are seen in the basal ganglia and in the posterior territory of the middle cerebral artery. The apparent diffusion coefficient (ADC) map indicates that the medial basal ganglia infarction (arrowheads) and the posterior abnormalities are new (low ADC) (short arrows) but the lateral basal ganglia change (long arrow) is similar to background brain, i.e. is pseudonormalizing, and is likely to have occurred at least 3 days previously implying an embolic cause. See text for further explanation.

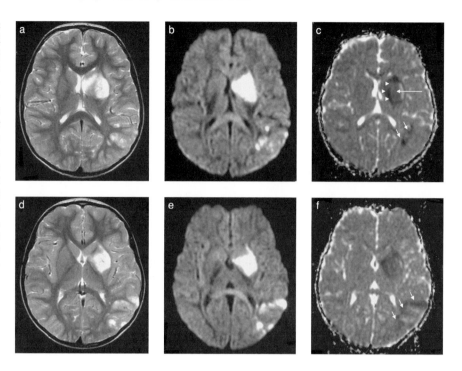

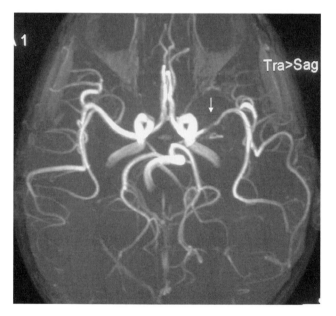

Fig. 4.17. Time-of-flight magnetic resonance angiography of the child whose MRA is shown in Fig. 4.16, demonstrating narrowing of the proximal left middle cerebral artery (MCA), presumed source of emboli (arrow), and preserved flow in the distal MCA branches.

day of admission is shown in Fig. 4.15 and the MRA demonstrates a narrowing of the proximal MCA in Fig. 4.17.) On T2- and diffusion-weighted images, focal abnormalities are seen in the basal ganglia and in the posterior territory of the MCA. The ADC map indicates that the medial basal ganglia infarction and the posterior abnormalities are new (low ADC) but the lateral basal ganglia change is similar to background brain, i.e. is psuedonormalizing, and is likely to have occurred at least 3 days previously. This implies an embolic rather than

haemodynamic aetiology of the infarction, likely to have arisen from the abnormal MCA. Similar appearances may be seen in patients with arterial dissection.[341]

Measurements of the ADC on a pixel by pixel basis may be used in the future to predict the potential recovery of the ischaemic tissue. Recent studies in animals and man have shown that the extent of the fall in ADC is greater in regions where the tissue progressed to infarction compared with those regions in which the tissue recovered (ischaemic penumbra).[342]

The conspicuity of both cortical and lacunar cerebral infarcts can be improved by using an inversion recovery sequence that suppresses signal from CSF whilst maintaining the T2-weighting, known as the FLAIR sequence.[343] Vascular enhancement of infarcts can be seen 75% of the time within the first week following cerebral infarction, thought to be related to slow flow and known as luxury perfusion.[344] The enhancement does not improve the visibility of the infarct and normally contrast is reserved for patients who have perfusion imaging.

MRA AND CEREBRAL ANGIOGRAPHY IN CEREBRAL INFARCTION

The most common angiographic findings in children with cerebral infarction is a focal and regular stenosis of the proximal middle or anterior cerebral arteries[34] which have been shown to be related to recent varicella zoster infection.[345] Follow-up angiographic studies have demonstrated improvement and complete resolution of the lesions in the majority of children and worsening of the lesion in around a quarter of children studied (Fig. 4.18).[346] Other findings include complete occlusion of large vessels, the 'string of beads' appearance typical of fibromuscular dysplasia, and small vessel abnormalities compatible with primary angiitis of the central nervous system.

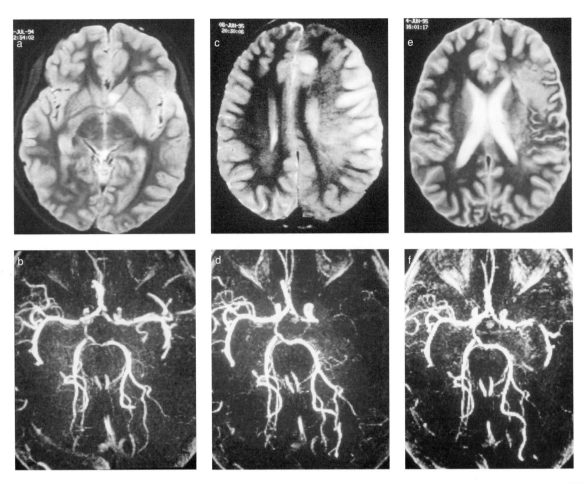

Fig. 4.18. Axial T2-weighted images and magnetic resonance angiography (MRA) at presentation, 2 days later and 2 weeks later in a child found to have both factor V Leiden and methylenetetrahydrofolate reductase deficiency. (a,b) The left middle cerebral artery (MCA) territory infarct at presentation is associated with irregularity of the proximal left MCA. (c,d) Two days later, the infarct extended to involve the periventricular white and cortical grey matter and the MRA demonstrated an occluded MCA. (e,f) Two weeks later, there is less swelling and increased signal in the left MCA territory and the MCA is narrowed but with evidence of flow in the distal MCA branches.

Which of these commonly reported angiographic features predict progressive vasculopathy and recurrent stroke has not yet been clarified as to date, the data are either cross-sectional[347] or where longitudinal data are available, a simple classification has been used.[346] Patients with chronic stenosis of the distal internal carotid arteries and its branches as a result of moyamoya or sickle cell disease may demonstrate the classical 'puff of smoke' appearance due to the presence of multiple leptomeningeal collateral vessels (Fig. 4.19).[38] Children with dissection of the carotid or vertebral arteries may have have the typical findings on MRA but when this is inconclusive a conventional angiogram is required (see section 'Carotid and vertebral artery dissection' below).

In a study comparing conventional angiography and MRA, the latter was diagnostic in children with large vessel occlusion, stenosis or moyamoya disease, but 50% of children with a normal MRA had diagnoses of dissection or vasculitis made on conventional cerebral angiography.[82] As a result of the study, the authors propose a role for cerebral angiography in the identification of potentially treatable cerebrovascular abnormalities in ischaemic stroke which included moyamoya syndrome, arterial dissection and vasculitis, and devised a clinical algorithm for neuroimaging of ischaemic stroke in children (Fig. 4.20).[82]

Other angiographic abnormalities observed in cerebral infarction are slow antegrade flow with prolonged circulation time and delayed 'wash out' of arterial contrast agent. Areas of non-perfused brain distal to an arterial occlusion are seen in some cases. Angiography performed within a few days of stroke onset may demonstrate 'luxury perfusion', which is a vascular blush of contrast in the ischaemic brain. The pathophysiology of this phenomenon is not completely understood and proposed mechanisms include arteriolar-venular shunting, capillary dilatation and increased flow though preserved vascular channels.[348]

PERFUSION IMAGING IN CEREBRAL ISCHAEMIA/INFARCTION
Perfusion imaging (PI) is currently not routinely performed outside the research setting (see below). Perfusion abnormalities reflect abnormalities of large vessels, and of particular

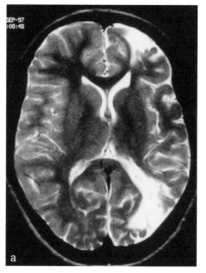
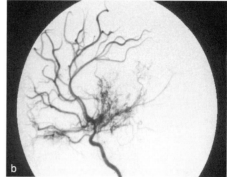

Fig. 4.19. (a) Axial T2-weighted image of a patient with sickle cell disease and long-standing atrophy in the anterior and posterior watershed region. (b) Conventional internal carotid artery angiogram showing a leash of leptomeningeal collateral vessels and absent middle cerebral artery branches characteristic of moyamoya syndrome.

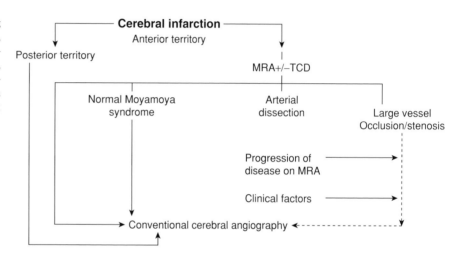

Fig. 4.20. An algorithm for the imaging investigation of paediatric stroke. MRA, magnetic resonance angiography; TCD, transcranial Doppler. (Adapted from Ganesan V, Savvy L, Chong WK, Kirkham FJ. Conventional cerebral angiography in children with ischemic stroke. Pediatr Neurol 1999; 20(1):38–42.)

interest in patients with acute stroke are regions of reduced perfusion which are greater in extent than diffusion abnormalities and are believed to represent potentially salvageable tissue.[349,350] In children, there is little published data on what is referred to as diffusion-perfusion mismatch in acute stroke.[351] In a study of children with sickle cell disease, perfusion/diffusion mismatch was demonstrated in more than half of the symptomatic patients with perfusion deficits and was statistically more likely to occur in the presence of large vessel abnormality on MRA or TCD.[352] PI can also detect abnormalities not visible using other MRI techniques and has detected reduced perfusion in the watershed territory of a child with sickle cell disease, headaches and increased flow velocity in the internal carotid and middle cerebral arteries determined by TCD.[341,352] Diffusion-perfusion mismatch has also been demonstrated in children with chromic cerebral ischaemia resulting from moyamoya disease and is consistent with a haemodynamic mechanism for ischaemia.[353]

MRI OF CEREBRAL HAEMORRHAGE
Intracerebral haemorrhage is the cause of stroke in about 20% of children. CT has demonstrated nearly a 100% sensitivity to the detection of intraparenchymal haemorrhage, except in very anaemic patients. Although MRI is a sensitive method of detecting intracranial haemorrhage,[354] so that MRI can be used for imaging of acute stroke, the main value is in the detection of the underlying lesion (see Chapter 8).

Diagnostic difficulties in stroke

CAROTID AND VERTEBRAL ARTERY DISSECTION
Dissection of the cervical and intracranial portions of the carotid arteries and vertebral arteries may occur spontaneously or as a result of trauma and should be considered in all children presenting with cerebral infarction of unknown cause, particularly if it is in the posterior territory. Dissection is most common in young adults but is well documented in children as young as 3 months of age[84,355,356] and should be considered in all children with arterial occlusion with no predisposing cause and a history of preceding trauma[33,357,358] (Chapter 6). The ratio of extracranial carotid to extracranial vertebral artery dissection is similar in adults and children, but intracranial carotid dissection may be more common in children,[355,357] although this diagnosis is difficult to make in life[359] and there is controversy

over the overlap with transient cerebral arteriopathy.[360] The most common site for vertebral artery dissection in children is at the level of the C1–C2 vertebral body[357] and a recent study has suggested that there may be a causal association between the presence of an arcuate foramen and tethering of the vertebral artery at this site.[89]

The neuroradiological diagnosis of an arterial dissection can be made using ultrasound, CTA, MRI, MRA or conventional angiography. Conventional angiography was originally the diagnostic criterion standard[361] but has been supplanted by MRI and MRA, which have the advantage of being non-invasive.[362] Recent studies suggest that although MRI and MRA are said to be 84% sensitive and 99% specific in the detection of carotid arterial dissection,[363] conventional angiography is still of value in the detection of vertebral artery dissection.[43,364,365]

Findings on MRI include absence of the normal flow void or altered luminal signal intensity, and narrowing of the arterial lumen with haematoma within the arterial wall. Fat saturated T1-weighted imaging of the neck and base of skull aid in the visualization of haematoma within the lumen (Fig. 4.21). MRA may show a tapered narrowing or occlusion of the dissected vessel (Fig. 4.22), an extraluminal pouch or pseudoaneurysm, a coiled spring appearance of fibromuscular dysplasia of the vessel or branch occlusions.[366] Findings on conventional angiography include those seen on MRA but also demonstrate the classical 'rat's tail' deformity and may even demonstrate the intimal flap. Colour flow Doppler ultrasound directly visualizes the intimal flap in less than 15% of cases.[366] CT and CTA may be helpful in patients not able to tolerate MR and in extracranial dissections where there are no significant artefacts from the skull base. Findings are similar to MRI and include low attenuation thrombus in the arterial wall, intimal flap, vascular stenoses and pseudoaneursyms.[367]

The authors recommend MRI, intra- and extracranial MRA and fat-saturated T1-weighted axial images of the neck in children with suspected dissection in the first instance, followed by cerebral angiography if there is any diagnostic uncertainty.

VENOUS SINUS THROMBOSIS
Cerebral venous sinus thrombosis (CVST) in children is a rare disorder but is increasingly diagnosed because of greater clinical

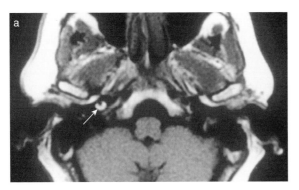
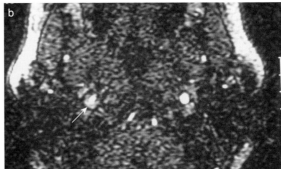

Fig. 4.21. The radiological appearance of cresentic high signal (arrows) within the wall of the right internal carotid artery (ICA) in the neck on both the (a) fat saturated T1-weighted axial images at the skull base and (b) source images of extracranial magnetic resonance angiography of a right ICA dissection.

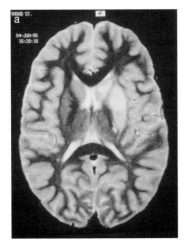
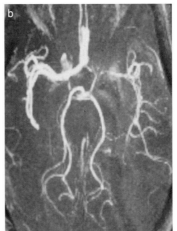
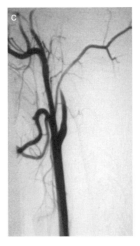

Fig. 4.22. (a) Axial T2-weighted, (b) intracranial time-of-flight magnetic resonance angiography (MRA) and (c) conventional left common carotid angiogram from a child with left basal ganglia and internal capsular infarct and narrowing of the proximal left middle cerebral artery demonstrated on the MRA indistinguishable from the vasculopathy of sickle cell disease. Imaging of the neck vessels reveals the typical 'rat tail' narrowing of the internal carotid artery indicative of a carotid dissection.

awareness and sensitive neuroimaging techniques.[368–370] In the acute phase of the illness, high density thrombus may be clearly demonstrated on unenhanced CT. As the thrombus becomes less dense, contrast may demonstrate lack of enhancement of the sagittal sinus known as the 'empty delta' sign.

MRI and MRV are important in both the demonstration of the characteristic cortical haemorrhagic infarct and the clot within the venous sinuses. Expansion of the sinus due to clot is an important radiological feature of venous sinus thrombosis. On MRI, the thrombus is readily recognizable in the subacute phase when it is high signal on a T1-weighted scan. In the acute phase the thrombus is isodense on T1-weighted imaging and of low signal on T2-weighted imaging and can be mistaken for flowing blood but MRV will demonstrate an absence of flow in the thrombosed sinus. MRI and MRV are techniques prone to flow artefacts and in equivocal cases an endoluminal technique such as CT venography or conventional angiography may be required as a final arbiter.

The Canadian Paediatric Stroke Registry study recently reviewed the imaging of 104 children who had both CT and MRI/MRV, and CT demonstrated a thrombosed venous sinus in only 84% of children in which the radiological diagnosis was made on MRI and MRV.[17] The location of the thrombosis was superficial in 86% and deep in 38% of children, with no significant difference between neonates and non-neonates. In neonates, power Doppler ultrasound is a valuable non-invasive bedside test for the diagnosis and monitoring of venous sinus thrombosis[371] and does not suffer from false positive results seen with CT in this age group due to increased haematocrit and slow venous flow.[372]

STROKE MIMICS

Subarachnoid haemorrhage (SAH) is uncommon in children but can result from arterial or venous pathology and can lead to cerebral ischaemia or infarction secondary to vasospasm. Although MRI is able to detect fresh subarachnoid blood,[373] acute SAH is best seen on CT.[308] Intracerebral tumours may be detected in children presenting with a stroke-like syndrome on both MRI and CT. Focal cortical dysplasia may be the underlying cause in epilepsy patients who present with a Todd's paresis and may be visualized only on high resolution MRI. Symmetrical involvement of the deep grey structures and brainstem seen on MRI are compatible with a metabolic disease, such as a mitochondrial disorder, whilst a step like progression of the neurological deficit and multiple infarcts of the parietal and occipital lobes and basal ganglia should raise the suspicion of MELAS. Children with the reversible posterior leukoencephalopathy syndrome or posterior reversible encephalopathy, often due to hypertension or ciclosporin toxicity (Fig. 4.8),[40,374] present with sudden onset of blindness and seizures, but the characteristic diffusion imaging appearances of vasogenic oedema in the posterior fossa exclude cerebral infarction as the cause.[41,42,375] This condition has multiple names[40] and reversible posterior leukoencephalopathy is a misnomer, as the condition may affect grey matter in posterior and anterior regions and may lead to infarction but its importance is as a differential for acute neurological presentations in various groups of patients (see Chapter 15), including those with sickle cell disease.[41,42,112]

4.2.2 Recent Advances in Magnetic Resonance Imaging

Fernando Calamante, Jacques-Donald Tournier and Alan Connelly

Introduction

As described in the previous section, MRI (where available) has become the imaging modality of choice in many centres for the investigation of children with ischaemic stroke and cerebrovascular disease. This is due not only to the high information content of MR images, but also to the absence of ionizing radiation, which is particularly important in paediatric studies. Major advances in hardware and data acquisition software have enabled the implementation on clinical scanners of techniques previously confined to the study of experimental models. In particular, the availability of echo-planar imaging (an extremely rapid image acquisition technique[376]) has in turn allowed the development of practical MR methods of diffusion and perfusion imaging. These techniques arguably constitute the most significant recent advances in imaging of patients with cerebral ischaemia, and are becoming increasingly significant in the investigation of such patients. This section therefore describes the technical background to these methods, and summarizes the applications to date in patients with stroke and cerebrovascular disease.

Principles of MR diffusion imaging

DIFFUSION

The term 'diffusion' describes the random thermal motion of molecules on a microscopic scale (also referred to as Brownian motion). This effect is distinct from flow in that there is no bulk motion of the molecules: their average displacement remains zero. In a large population of freely diffusing molecules, such as in a liquid, the molecules would be expected to diffuse equally in all directions. This can be represented by a spherical 'diffusion volume' (Fig. 4.23a), the radius of which increases in proportion to the square root of the diffusion time (the time that diffusion is allowed to evolve). Diffusion behaviour in an *in vivo* environment, however, is more complex, and is dependent on the nature and arrangement of any obstacles to the movement of the diffusing molecules.

Diffusion-weighted imaging

The signal intensity on an MR image can be made dependent on the rate of water diffusion in the brain by the addition of appropriate magnetic field gradients (e.g. two identical gradients, one either side of the refocusing pulse in a spin echo sequence[377]). Diffusion of water in the presence of these

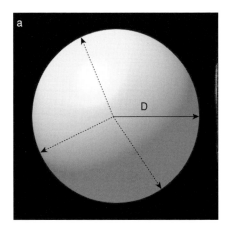

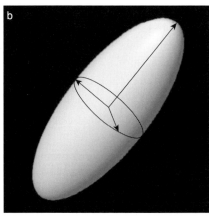

Fig. 4.23. (a) Isotropic diffusion. In this case, the diffusion *D* is the same in all directions, the 'diffusion volume' is described by a sphere, and diffusion weighted images weighted in a single direction are enough to characterize the diffusion properties; i.e. to obtain the diffusivity, *D*. (b) Anisotropic diffusion. When diffusion is not the same in all directions (e.g. diffusion of water in white matter), the measured value of *D* will depend on the direction with respect to the local structure. For example, diffusion inside axons would be larger in the direction parallel to the axon than in the direction perpendicular to the cylinder. Therefore, the 'diffusion volume' is not described by a sphere, but by an ellipsoid.

gradients introduces signal loss in the image. The resulting MR image intensity will be weighted according to the rate of water diffusion (hence the name diffusion-weighted imaging (DWI)), with high diffusivity regions giving relatively low signal intensity, while regions of restricted or hindered diffusion would give relatively high signal intensity.

The diffusion-weighted signal is extremely sensitive to the effects of brain motion, and even microscopic movements will introduce large random phase errors. These errors preclude the use of conventional multi-shot imaging methods for DWI: images produced by such methods suffer severe degradation when diffusion-weighting gradients are added. Although there are several potential solutions to this problem, single-shot diffusion weighted echo-planar imaging (EPI) is by far the most common method in use at present,[378] with the concomitant limitations of image distortions in regions of high magnetic susceptibility gradients (e.g. in the region of temporal lobes or the frontal sinuses) and low spatial resolution (typically of the order of 2mm).

The degree of diffusion weighting in an MR image is dependent on a combination of the strength of the diffusion gradient, the length of time the diffusion gradient is on and the time between the pair of diffusion gradients.[377] These contributions to diffusion weighting are collectively described by a '*b*-value'; the higher the value of *b*, the greater the degree of diffusion weighting.

Quantitative diffusion mapping

In DWI, the image intensity is weighted not only by water diffusivity, but also by the proton density and the relaxation times, T1 and T2. The contribution of diffusion can be isolated by means of quantitation, i.e. by calculation of what is usually referred to as the ADC. This term is used since the measured diffusion is dependent not only on water diffusivity, but also on factors such as barrier permeability and diffusion time.

What is required to properly quantify diffusion is dependent on the nature of the local environment. Diffusion that is the same in all directions (*isotropic diffusion*) can be described by a scalar quantity, *D* (the diffusion coefficient; *in vivo*, this would

be the ADC). *D* can be determined by acquiring DW images at two different *b* values, with the diffusion weighting applied in any arbitrary direction (since diffusion is isotropic) (Fig. 4.23a). This is not the case for *anisotropic diffusion*, where the water diffusivity varies according to the direction of the applied diffusion weighting gradient; this can confound data reproducibility but may also provide further information, as discussed below. Diffusion in an *anisotropic system* cannot be described by a simple number (as above), but is characterised by a diffusion tensor matrix, **D** (denoted using a bold font to identify it as a matrix). Again, *in vivo* this would be an apparent diffusion tensor. In effect, rather than diffusivity being characterised by a sphere (as in the isotropic case), anisotropic diffusion is characterised by the *size, shape* and *orientation* of a *diffusion ellipsoid* (see Fig. 4.23b), with three potentially non-equal axes representing different diffusivities in three orthogonal (i.e. mutually perpendicular) directions. Characterisation of this ellipsoid requires at least seven DW images (diffusion weighting in six independent directions, plus one measurement with low diffusion weighting, typically *b*=0).[379] This form of DWI is usually referred to as diffusion tensor imaging (DTI).

In tissues with randomly oriented microstructure, water diffusivity appears to be the same in all directions (i.e. there appears to be isotropic diffusion). However, in tissues with highly organized microstructure, such as brain white matter, the measured diffusivity of tissue water varies with the tissue's orientation relative to the diffusion weighting gradient (anisotropic diffusion). Therefore, to obtain a reproducible measure of diffusion in the brain, it is not meaningful to calculate the ADC in a single direction. The axes of the cells (or their diffusion ellipsoids) will be arbitrarily oriented with respect to the fixed *x*, *y* and *z* axes of the magnet, resulting in a misleadingly inhomogeneous DW signal intensity that is furthermore dependent on the direction of the applied diffusion weighting gradient. It has therefore become common practice in the investigation of acute stroke to average the ADC in three orthogonal directions (ADC$_{AV}$) to remove the confounding effects of diffusion anisotropy (Fig. 4.24). Note, however, that

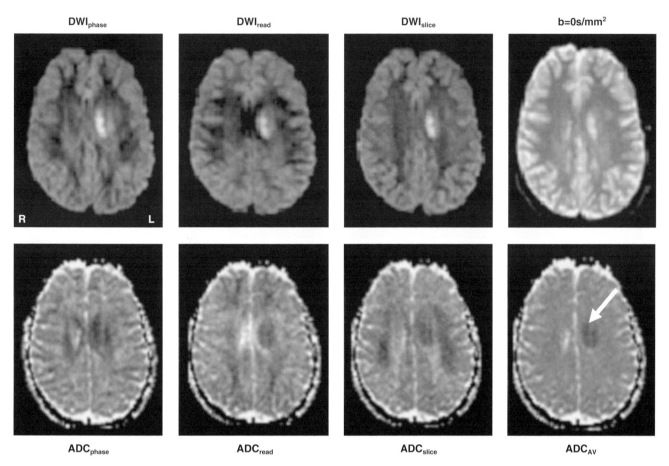

Fig. 4.24. Effect of diffusion anisotropy on lesion delineation in stroke. Diffusion weighted images (DWI's; diffusion along phase (vertical), read (horizontal) and slice (perpendicular to the page) directions), un-weighted image (b=0s/mm^2) and corresponding apparent diffusion coefficient (ADC) maps acquired approximately 24 hours after the onset of stroke in a 10-year-old girl. There is a region of hyperintensity in the left hemisphere (right side of the images) clearly seen in the DWIs and the unweighted image (top row). The single directional ADC maps show this affected region as an area of reduced diffusion. However, there are also areas with apparently similar diffusion reduction due to the anisotropy properties of the tissue. Therefore, it is not possible to distinguish these areas from the ischaemic region. The confounding effects of diffusion anisotropy on lesion delineation are eliminated in the average ADC map (bottom right). In this map, the small ischaemic area is clearly seen as a hypointense region (white arrow).

this approach (using three orthogonal directions) cannot be used to obtain diffusion anisotropy information that is orientation independent; as mentioned above, DTI is required to properly characterise an appropriate diffusion ellipsoid for each voxel of an imaging volume.[380]

From the diffusion tensor, **D**, it is possible to calculate new quantitative scalar and vector-valued parameters that characterise specific features of the diffusion process. These scalar quantities are designed to be rotationally invariant, i.e. independent of the coordinate system in which the MR measurement is made, and the orientation of subjects in the magnet. The most commonly used rotationally invariant scalar measure that characterises the bulk diffusion properties of the tissue, independent of the orientation of the fibres, is the *Trace* of the diffusion tensor (*Trace*(**D**))[380] (The trace of a matrix is the sum of the diagonal elements; i.e. $Trace(\mathbf{D}) = D_{xx} + D_{yy} + D_{zz}$). This quantity is proportional to the orientationally averaged diffusion coefficient (an average of diffusion coefficients measured in all spatial directions). Note that the ADC$_{AV}$ described above is generally a good approximation

to *Trace*(**D**), and since the former is simpler to acquire, it is commonly used in the clinical imaging of ischaemia. However, the most fundamental rotationally invariant quantities are the three principal diffusivities (or *eigenvalues*) of D, which are the principal diffusion coefficients along the three coordinate directions that constitute the local axes of the ellipsoid in each voxel (Fig. 4.23b). Other widely used rotationally invariant scalar measures that can be suitably applied in anisotropic systems include indices of the Relative- and Fractional-Anisotropy.[381] These provide measures of the degree to which the diffusion ellipsoid's shape deviates from being spherical, with high values typically found in white matter regions with parallel arrangement of fibres (e.g. the corpus callosum, the pyramidal tract, etc.) (Fig. 4.25. See also colour plate 1).

Each of the three eigenvalues is also associated with a direction (*eigenvector*) that is intrinsic to the tissue. These eigenvectors are mutually perpendicular and define a local fibre frame of reference. They are typically sorted according to the magnitude of their corresponding eigenvalue (λ_1 = highest diffusivity, λ_2 = intermediate diffusivity, and λ_3 = lowest

FA   Trace(D)   DEC

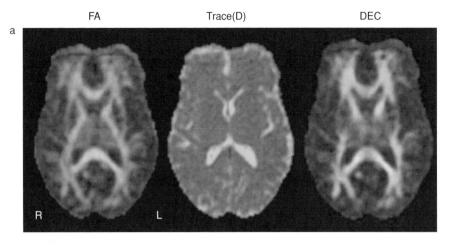

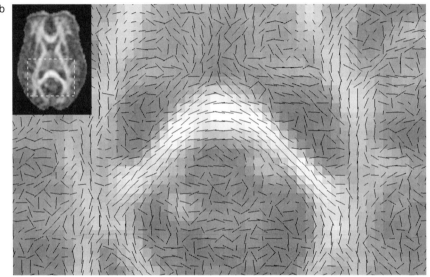

Fig. 4.25. (a) Fractional anisotropy (FA) map (top left), trace of the diffusion tensor (Trace(D), top middle) and directionally encoded colour (DEC) map (top right) calculated from diffusion tensor imaging in a normal volunteer. The contrast of the FA and Trace(D) maps is very different. While the FA map has very high grey/white matter contrast, that is not the case for the Trace(D). Three different diffusion properties can be identified in the brain: (1) high anisotropy and moderate average diffusivity (white matter); (2) low anisotropy and moderate average diffusivity (grey matter); (3) low anisotropy and high average diffusivity cerebrospinal fluid). The DEC map is created by colouring each voxel in the FA map according to the direction of the eigenvector associated with the largest eigenvalue of the diffusion tensor ((λ_1) (red, left–right; green, anterior–posterior; blue, inferior–superior). (b) Expansion of a portion of the FA map (see dotted white insert in left inset image) showing in each voxel the projection of the eigenvector associated with the largest eigenvalue. As can be seen, the direction of the eigenvector is a good representation of the white matter fibre direction. (See colour plate 1.)

diffusivity). In anisotropic tissues consisting of ordered parallel bundles, the largest eigenvalue, λ_1, represents the diffusion coefficient along the direction parallel to the fibres, while λ_2 and λ_3 represent the diffusion coefficients in the transverse directions.[380] Therefore, the eigenvectors of the diffusion tensor provide unique directional information that can be used to infer interesting features of living tissue. In particular, measurements of the eigenvector associated with the largest eigenvalue (λ_1) in each voxel have been used to construct maps of white matter fibre direction within an imaging volume (Fig. 4.25. See also colour plate 1). This information can also be encoded in the anisotropy map by colouring each voxel according to the direction of this eigenvector; this map is often referred to as a directionally encoded colour (DEC) map (Fig. 4.25. See also colour plate 1). These maps provide contrast between different white matter structures that cannot be differentiated using any other imaging modality.

The white matter orientation information that can be obtained using DWI also provides the potential for non-invasive fibre tractography in the brain.[382] Tractography or fibre-tracking methods attempt to infer the path of white matter bundles of fibres through the brain, by following the local direction of the white matter step by step. These techniques have been used successfully to delineate known major white matter pathways such as the corticospinal tracts and the superior longitudinal fasciculus.[383] There are however a number of technical limitations with the methods most commonly used that can introduce significant bias into the results.[384] These stem principally from the inadequacy of the diffusion tensor model to describe multiple fibre orientations within any given voxel.[385–388] At the resolutions typically achievable using DWI (approximately 2mm), many voxels will contain contributions from more than a single fibre bundle; in other words there will be partial volume effects between adjacent or intermeshing white matter tracts (these are commonly referred to as 'crossing fibre' effects). In these voxels, the estimate of white matter orientation provided by the diffusion tensor model will be severely biased (Fig. 4.26. See also colour plate 2). This will often cause tractography algorithms that rely on this model to deviate from the true path of the tract, and thereby to infer connections with adjacent unrelated structures.[384] It has recently been estimated that as many as one-third of white matter voxels are affected by this problem.[389] It is therefore a serious problem, especially considering that the vast majority of white matter tracts will probably traverse at least one such voxel along their path.

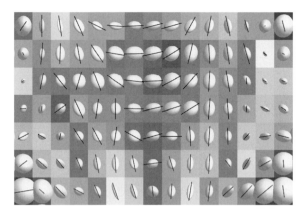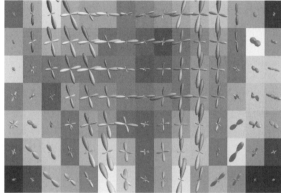

Fig. 4.26. Diffusion tensor (left) and constrained spherical deconvolution (right) results displayed as a coronal slice through the pons, in a region known to contain crossing fibres. The principal direction of diffusion (i.e. the eigenvector with the largest eigenvalue) is shown overlaid on the diffusion tensor ellipsoid to aid visualization of the estimated white matter orientations. It can readily be appreciated that the diffusion tensor model fails to adequately characterize the complex arrangement of the fibre tracts in this region. These erroneous orientations have obvious deleterious consequences for fibre tractography results. Constrained spherical deconvolution, on the other hand, is robust to crossing fibre effects, and provides a much more adequate estimate of the fibre orientations present in this region. In particular, the corticospinal tracts and transverse pontine fibres can easily be identified. (See colour plate 2.)

Although most commonly available tractography algorithms are based on the diffusion tensor model, a number of alternative approaches have recently been proposed to address this issue, such as Q-ball imaging,[387] persistent angular structure (PAS) MRI[385] and constrained spherical deconvolution[390] (Fig. 4.26. See also colour plate 2). These methods typically require a larger amount of DWI data to be collected, using a large number of uniformly distributed DW directions (a so-called high angular resolution DW imaging (HARDI) acquisition). Another important development has been the introduction of probabilistic tractography methods to take into account the effects of image noise.[391] Although these new methods are promising and do provide more reliable results than can be achieved using the tensor model, it should be emphasized that tractography methods in general have not been fully validated; any unexpected findings such as 'new' tracts should therefore be interpreted with appropriate caution.

Principles of MR perfusion imaging

In the context of MR, the terms *perfusion* and *cerebral blood flow* (CBF) are often used indistinguishably. They refer to the volume of blood delivered to the capillary bed of a block of tissue in a given period of time, and the units are therefore ml/100g/min. It is important to distinguish between perfusion at the capillary level and bulk flow through major vessels (such as is visualized on MRA). In the latter there is no exchange of oxygen and nutrients between blood and tissue. It is this exchange, at the capillary level, which will determine the adequate survival of the tissue, and thus the interest in measuring perfusion with good spatial resolution, such as that available with MRI.

There are two general MR approaches to the assessment of perfusion;[312] they differ with regard to their respective use of an exogenous and endogenous MR-visible tracer. However, it is worth noting that neither requires ionizing radiation, and therefore they have, in principle, advantages over other perfusion techniques such as PET and SPECT. The first MRI approach, *dynamic susceptibility contrast* (DSC) MRI or '*bolus tracking*', relies on bolus injection of a paramagnetic contrast agent. The second approach involves magnetic labelling of inflowing water protons in blood using MR techniques that are known collectively as *arterial spin labelling* (ASL).

Dynamic Susceptibility Contrast MRI (DSC-MRI)

If a bolus of paramagnetic contrast agent (e.g. gadolinium-DTPA) is injected intravenously, its passage through the brain produces a transient decrease in signal intensity on a series of gradient-echo or spin-echo images (Fig. 4.27).[392] Assuming a linear relationship between the change in relaxation rate (calculated from the signal intensity time curve) and the concentration of contrast agent ($C(t)$, usually referred to as the 'peak' due to its shape), $C(t)$ can be calculated on a pixel by pixel basis. The tissue contrast concentration is not only affected by CBF (the quantity of interest) but also by the time-dependent *delivery* of the contrast agent to the tissue (the so-called arterial input function, AIF). For example, an area with a small and wide 'peak' could represent tissue with low CBF and/or tissue to which the contrast agent was delivered very slowly. Similarly, a region with a large and narrow 'peak' could represent tissue with high CBF and/or tissue to which the bolus was delivered very fast. Therefore, to quantify CBF one must remove the contribution to the 'peak' shape from the *delivery* of the bolus, a mathematical process known as deconvolution.[312,393] Therefore, CBF quantification requires measurement of the AIF.

The analysis of DSC-MRI data can produce not only information about CBF, but also about two other important physiological parameters: CBV and the mean transit time (MTT) through the tissue. Therefore, within a very short acquisition time (approximately 1 min), DSC-MRI provides considerable (clinically relevant) information.

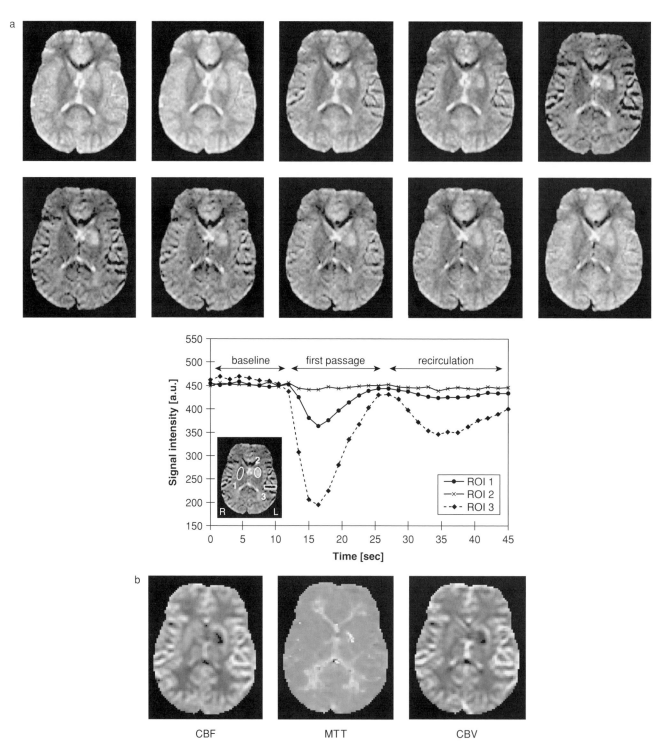

Fig. 4.27. (a) Magnetic resonance perfusion data in a 4-year-old child 12 hours after a stroke involving the left basal ganglia (right side of the images). Sequential SE echo-planar images during the first passage of a bolus of contrast agent (TR=1.5s), together with the signal intensity time course (in arbitrary units) for three regions of interest (ROI) (ROI 1: right basal ganglia; ROI 2: left basal ganglia; ROI 3: peripheral branch of the right middle cerebral artery). The top left and bottom right images correspond to t=12s and 25.5s, respectively. The images show the signal intensity decrease associated with the passage of the bolus. Three different periods can be identified in the time-course data: the baseline (before the arrival of the bolus), the first passage of the bolus and the recirculation period (in this case, a second smaller peak, more clearly seen in the arterial region (ROI 3)). Note that the affected region (ROI 2) shows almost no contrast agent passage because of the very low cerebral blood flow (CBF) to that area. (b) CBF, mean transit time (MTT) and cerebral blood volume (CBV) maps obtained from the dynamic data shown in (a). The focal ischaemic region is clearly seen on the perfusion maps. ((a) previously published in Thomas DL, Lythgoe MF, Pell GS, Calamante F, Ordidge RJ. The measurement of diffusion and perfusion in biological systems using magnetic resonance imaging. Phys Med Biol 2000; 45(8):R97–138, Copyright © 2000, IOP Publishing Ltd.)

There are two main concerns regarding the accuracy of the deconvolution approach in stroke patients. First, it is generally believed to produce only relative measurements of perfusion.[394,395] Although there have been some studies reporting absolute measurements in healthy volunteers which are consistent with expected CBF,[396–398] a full validation under various physiological conditions is still required.[399–401] Until then, absolute values of perfusion should be interpreted with caution. The second concern is related to the measurement of the AIF. This is generally estimated from the signal time curve from pixels within a major artery (e.g. middle cerebral artery). The measured AIF can be further delayed and dispersed in time on its transit from that artery to the tissue of interest. This is sometimes observed in cases of abnormal vascular distribution, such as in occlusion, stenosis, or in the presence of collateral flow.[402] This extra delay and dispersion is interpreted by the model as occurring *within* the tissue and leads to errors in CBF, which can be as large as 70% underestimation in some patients.[402,403] The errors due to bolus delay can be avoided by shifting the curves to a common time origin,[403–405] or by using a deconvolution method that is insensitive to the presence of delay;[406–408] any of these methods is therefore recommended when studying patients with vascular abnormalities (where bolus delay is highly likely). In contrast, the errors due to bolus dispersion are more difficult to correct,[409] and require the use of a so-called *local* AIF: an AIF measured in the vicinity of the tissue of interest (i.e. the local AIF varies throughout the brain and accounts for the time spread of the bolus in its transit to the different brain regions). Methods to define a local AIF have been recently proposed,[410–412] but they are not currently widely available. Therefore, special care must be taken when interpreting perfusion data in the presence of delays and dispersion.

It should be noted that since the transit time of the bolus through the tissue is only a few seconds, a fast imaging technique is required to properly characterise the peak. The most commonly used technique is EPI, which allows several slices to be acquired with a time resolution of 1–2 seconds.[376] However, EPI suffers from several drawbacks such as low resolution and image distortions.[413] Therefore, image quality is commonly sacrificed to achieve the necessary time resolution for the analysis of DSC data.

ARTERIAL SPIN LABELLING (ASL)

MRI can also measure perfusion without requiring the use of any exogenous contrast agent, by using blood itself as an endogenous agent. An MRI can be sensitized to the effect of inflowing blood spins if those spins are in a different magnetic state to that of the static tissue. ASL techniques use this idea by magnetically labelling blood flowing into the slices of interest[414,415] (Fig. 4.28). Labelled blood flowing into the imaging slice exchanges with tissue water, altering the tissue magnetization. A perfusion-weighted image can be generated by the subtraction of an image in which inflowing spins have been labelled (the so-called 'labelled image') from an image in which spin labelling has not been performed (the 'control image'). Absolute quantification of perfusion can be obtained if other parameters (such as tissue T1, the efficiency of spin labelling and the transit time from the labelling site to the tissue) also are measured.[312,416,417]

Under the general heading of ASL, two distinct subgroups exist, although both share a similar basis: continuous ASL (CASL) and pulsed ASL (PASL). In the first subgroup, CASL, the arterial spins are magnetically labelled as they flow through an inversion plane by continuous inversion using a long off-resonance radio-frequency (RF) pulse[415] (Fig. 4.28a).

Fig. 4.28. The images in the top row schematically show the continuous arterial spin labelling (CASL) and pulsed arterial spin labelling (PASL) methods. In CASL, the blood magnetization is inverted when it flows through an inversion plane (indicated by the dashed line). In PASL, the blood magnetization is inverted in a spatially defined region (a slab inferior to the slice of interest, in the particular example shown). The bottom row shows typical control and labelled images, and the difference image obtained by image subtraction. Note that, for visualization purposes, the windowing in the difference image is not the same as that used for the control and labelled images.

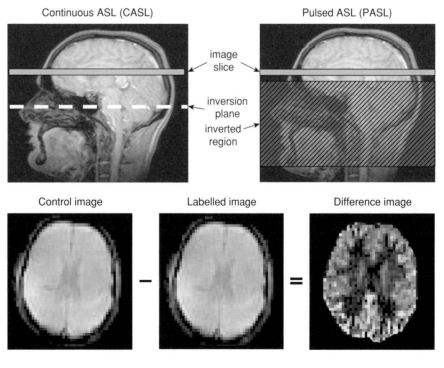

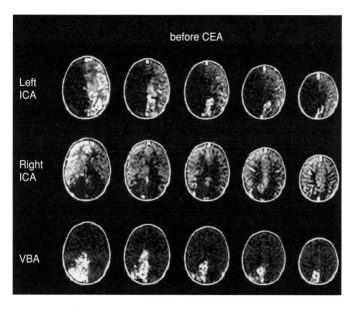
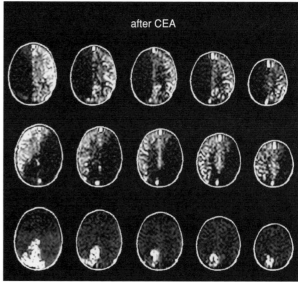

Fig. 4.29. Transverse perfusion territory images in a patient with symptomatic left-sided internal carotid artery (ICA) stenosis of 90% before and after carotid endarterectomy (CEA) of left ICA. When labeling the left ICA before CEA, signal is observed in left middle cerebral artery (MCA) territory and left posterior part of the imaging sections. After CEA, perfusion territory of left ICA has extended into ipsilateral anterior cerebral artery (ACA) territory. When labeling the right ICA before CEA, signal is detected in both the left and right MCA and ACA territories. After CEA, perfusion territory is restricted to the right ACA and MCA territories. When labelling vertebrobasilar artery (VBA) before CEA, signal is only present in the right posterior part of the imaging sections. The left posterior part of the imaging sections is supplied by left ICA via left-sided fetal-type posterior cerebral artery. After CEA, no change in perfusion territory of VBA is observed. (Image kindly provided by Dr Peter Jan van Laar, and previously published in van Laar PJ, van der Grond J, Hendrikse J. Brain perfusion territory imaging: methods and clinical applications of selective arterial spin-labeling MR imaging. Radiology 2008; 246(2):354–364. (Copyright © 2008, RSNA.))

A steady state develops where the regional magnetization in the brain is directly related to CBF.[312,415] In the other subgroup, PASL, the arterial labelling is achieved by using a short (typically ~10ms) RF pulse to label simultaneously a spatially defined region (Fig. 4.28b),[418–420] and CBF can be obtained from the time dependent signal change created by the exchange of the labelled blood and brain tissue water.[312,421]

There are several limitations of ASL techniques, as well as sources of artefact, that have contributed to its slow incorporation into the clinical setting.[312,417] One of the main limitations is low signal-to-noise ratio (SNR), since the relative signal difference in the perfusion-weighted image mentioned above is approximately 1% at the field strength of most clinical scanners. Therefore, many image averages are often required to generate high quality images (typically ~30 averages), making the typical ASL scan time 5–10 times longer than for DSC-MRI. Furthermore, during the same measurement time DSC-MRI can also provide information regarding CBV and MTT, while ASL only measures CBF. A second limitation of ASL techniques is due to possible long (and unknown) transit times from the labelling site to the tissue; this can be particularly problematical in stroke patients. In the presence of cerebrovascular abnormalities, the transit times from the labelling site to the tissue can be particularly long and the magnetic labelling of the blood is lost (due to T1 relaxation). Various methods have been proposed to minimize this effect,[422,423] but they require a careful selection of the ASL sequence parameters; these may become impractical if the

transit time is very long, such as in patients with cerebrovascular abnormalities.[424] The main drawback of these techniques is that the ASL sequence modifications required to reduce the sensitivity to transit time effects[422,423] reduce even further the perfusion signal. Moreover, a fundamental problem with ASL methods in patients with very prolonged transit times is the possibility of not being able to differentiate between no flow (CBF=0, no signal in the ASL image) and very long transit times (full relaxation of the labelled blood, no signal in the ASL image regardless of CBF). Although DSC-MRI cannot measure CBF accurately in such situations,[395] it can still differentiate these cases, which have different clinical implications.

There are a number of further limitations that are particularly relevant to paediatric studies. First, the high RF power deposition using CASL (due to the long (~2–3 seconds) RF required for arterial labelling) may limit its practical utility in children. Second, the extra parameters required for CBF quantification (e.g. T1, labelling efficiency, etc.) are usually not measured in each patient: to maintain acquisition time to a minimum, these parameters are often assumed from literature values, usually from adult values. The problem with this approach is that these parameters can vary with age, introducing errors in CBF quantification, particularly in neonates and young children.[425,426]

Since exogenous contrast agents are not used in ASL techniques, the perfusion measurement is completely non-invasive; it can be repeated therefore as often as required. This has made ASL particularly applicable to longitudinal studies, such as studies of brain activation (fMRI),[427] and in animal models of stroke.[312] On the other hand, given the relatively low SNR (and therefore correspondingly relatively long acquisition time) ASL has not been used routinely in clinical investigations to date. Recent improvements in MRI hardware (e.g. better receiver coils and higher magnetic field strength) and sequence modifications to improve the efficiency of ASL (e.g. background suppression[428] and pseudo-continuous labelling[429]) are now allowing good quality ASL data with large coverage to be acquired in a more clinically relevant acquisition time.[430] These advances, and other recent technical improvements (e.g. velocity selective labelling[431] and multi-inversion time Look-Locker acquisitions[432]), should contribute to promoting the use of ASL in clinical studies. Furthermore, the completely non-invasive nature of ASL also makes it ideally suited for paediatric studies,[426] where it is expected to play an increasingly relevant role in the coming years.

ASL also has the (arguably unique) ability to *selectively* label individual arteries (and therefore characterise individual arterial territories) in vivo and non-invasively.[433] This application of ASL is expected to play a significant role in the study of cerebrovascular disease. Figure 4.29 illustrates an example of selective ASL acquired before and after carotid endarterctomy (CEA).

Applications of diffusion and perfusion imaging
The main area of interest to date for the application of DWI is in the field of stroke.[311] DWI provides the opportunity not only to identify the very early tissue changes following a stroke, but also to investigate the underlying pathophysiology.[311,434,435] The interpretation of the diffusion and perfusion findings in clinical studies are based on the understanding gained from experimental animal models of cerebral ischaemia. The following sections, therefore, describe some of the significant findings to date, firstly in experimental animal models, then in patients with stroke.

EXPERIMENTAL MODELS
In this section we describe briefly some important features of DWI in the context of cerebral ischaemia, such as the mechanisms of signal change, CBF thresholds, and temporal evolution of diffusion change in experimental models of stroke and following reperfusion.

Diffusion-weighted imaging
For a clinician investigating a patient with stroke, an accurate early diagnosis is essential. However, ischaemic changes on CT or on standard MRI are not observed until approximately 6–12 hours following the initial event. The introduction of DWI[434] allowed the identification of ischaemic tissue in an animal model within minutes of an initial event, with the opportunity to monitor the development of lesions over time. The current interpretations of the change in water diffusion are discussed below.

Mechanisms of DWI changes following a stroke
The DWI changes in cerebral ischaemia have been shown to be associated with a shift of extracellular water to intracellular compartments, as a result of a disruption of ion homeostasis.[434] This is believed to occur due to the following chain of events: a decreased blood supply following an initial insult reduces the amount of oxygen and glucose delivered to the tissue, and this is accompanied by a decrease in the available adenosine triphosphate (ATP), the main source of cellular energy. ATP normally provides energy to pump Na^+ out of and K^+ into the cell to maintain ionic homeostasis. When the supply of ATP ceases, there is an accumulation of intracellular Na^+, causing an influx of water into the cell by osmosis, which leads to cell swelling (cytotoxic oedema) and, in time, cell death. Later work[436] supported Moseley's early hypothesis, and it is now generally accepted that a drop in the tissue water ADC in ischaemic tissue is associated with the development of cytotoxic oedema. (Note that a reduction in water ADC corresponds to *high signal* in the DW image, but *low signal* in an ADC map (e.g. see Fig. 4.24).)

Despite considerable work in this field, the underlying biophysical mechanisms of the observed water ADC reduction in ischaemia remain unclear, although several further hypotheses have been suggested. These include:[311,437,438] a reduction in extracellular diffusion due to an increase in the tortuosity of the extracellular space that occurs after cell swelling; a reduction in cell membrane permeability; a decrease in intracellular diffusivity (as evidenced by intracellular metabolites), either by a decrease in the intracellular circulation or an increase in viscosity. It is possible that more than one of these mechanisms makes some contribution to the observed reduction in ADC, since there is some evidence for each. However, there is general agreement that common to all is the presence of cell swelling, and that DWI is able to detect very early cellular disturbances at a time when such changes are thought to be potentially reversible.

DWI and cerebral blood flow
A number of studies have indicated that a reduction of blood flow to brain tissue does not necessarily result in a reduction in ADC, but that there is a critical CBF threshold, possibly associated with energy failure. For example, Busza et al found that DWI signal enhancement only occurred when the CBF fell below ~20ml/100g/min (i.e. ~70% reduction), using a gerbil model of forebrain ischaemia.[439] This is similar to the flow threshold for the maintenance of tissue high-energy metabolites necessary for normal cellular ion homeostasis.[440] Subsequent work corroborated that there is a threshold level of CBF below which an ADC decrease will occur, but also indicated that the actual threshold is dependent upon species, as well as the duration and degree of the reduction in CBF.[311,437,441] It is therefore not possible to give a single CBF value that would describe the threshold in every circumstance; nevertheless, it is important to note in principle that such a threshold exists, since it has crucial

implications for the characterisation of tissue status in patients with stroke.

Ischaemic lesion development

Following occlusion of a cerebral artery, the resultant ischaemic lesion in both rat and cat expands primarily during the first 2 hours.[311,437] However, the ADC value continues to decrease for up to 48 hours (to around 50% of control). In the chronic stages of cerebral ischaemia, the ADC of water exhibits a different pattern. In animal models, at approximately 24–48 hours after a vessel occlusion, the ADC rises and slowly returns to normal at around 3 days. Following this 'pseudonormalization' (so-called since the ADC returns to normal only in transition from abnormally low to abnormally high ADC), a subsequent increase in the diffusion of water above control values can be observed approximately after 1 week after occlusion. This elevated ADC of tissue water is associated with cell lysis, the loss of cellular barriers and vasogenic oedema.

(NB: Following a stroke in humans, a reduced ADC has been observed as early as 11 minutes after the initial onset[435] and as with the animal studies, a pseudo-normalization occurs, although with a different timescale (between 4 and 10 days),[311] followed by an elevation in ADC. The large timing variation in human results may be dependent on the both the site/size of the lesion, and depth of ischaemia).

Restoration of blood flow following cerebral ischaemia

It is of obvious interest whether ADC changes have any prognostic role in the investigation of stroke. This has been the case particularly following the demonstration in 1991 that the hyperintense regions of the ischaemic brain seen on DWI could be reversed if the occlusion was removed sufficiently soon after vessel occlusion (approximately 30 minutes after middle cerebral artery occlusion (MCAO) in the rat[442]). A later study showed that the size of the lesion based on DWI's declined if the blood flow was restored 1 hour following occlusion, but not after 2 hours.[443] The introduction of quantitative measures of the ADC of water allowed the exploration of potential thresholds for reversibility of lesions.[311,437,438] These and further data suggest that there is potential prognostic information in the measurement of ADC values, but that reversibility is likely to have a complex dependence on both the duration and the degree of ADC reduction.

As discussed above, animal models have indicated that, after reperfusion of a previously ischaemic region, the low ADC values can return to normal levels. However, more recent studies have reported a secondary decline in ADC following reperfusion, which is not well understood as yet. This secondary decline had been termed 'secondary' or 'delayed' energy failure. Initial reports using MR spectroscopy in infants suffering a hypoxic/ischaemic insult during birth (birth asphyxia) demonstrated a delayed fall in the concentration of phosphocreatine/inorganic phosphate at 24–48 hours.[444] This hypoxic-ischaemic condition has been modelled in piglets and a

secondary decline has also been observed in ADC values.[445] This effect is not limited to a hypoxic-ischaemic insult, since a delayed ADC decrease, following normalization, has been observed at 24 hours post-reperfusion in a rat MCAO model.[446] Hypoperfusion following reperfusion produces gradual changes in ADC, where the ADC normalizes for a short period then gradually declines over a prolonged period of several hours.[447]

In summary, animal studies suggest that there are three ADC patterns that might be expected on restoration of CBF following a period of ischaemia:

1. ADC remains decreased at the ischaemic level, followed by ADC increasing chronically (see "Ischaemic lesion development" above)
2. ADC normalizes and remains normal
3. ADC normalizes (temporarily reversible) followed by a secondary decline, then proceeds as in (1) above.

The time-course observed in practice will be dependent on a number of factors, including the degree of hypoperfusion, whether reperfusion occurs, and if so how soon after the onset of hypoperfusion.

ACUTE STROKE IN HUMANS

The role of diffusion MRI

The main finding of diffusion MRI in experimental animal models of stroke, namely its sensitivity to cerebral ischaemia, has contributed extensively to the investigation of stroke in adults (Fig. 4.30).[311,448] However, this important application has not been fully exploited in the paediatric population, since the concept of 'brain attack' is less recognized in this patient group because of the relatively lower stroke incidence. It is very uncommon for a child to present in a MR unit for stroke diagnosis within the hyperacute period (first ~6 hours after symptom onset), when conventional MRI (T2- and T1-weighted MRI) is normal, although some studies have been reported.[426,449,450] Furthermore, studies in adults[451] have confirmed findings from animal models regarding the potential reversibility of diffusion MR changes (when conventional MRI is still normal) with appropriate treatment. Therefore, it may be important to extend the concept of 'brain attack' to the paediatric population, who could potentially benefit disproportionately from minimization of the degree of disability following a stroke.

Despite the lack of data during the 'hyperacute' period of stroke, there are many other interesting applications of diffusion MRI for the investigation of stroke in children. The time evolution of the ADC (low in the acute stage, reflecting cytotoxic oedema, and high in the chronic stage, reflecting vasogenic oedema and final cell necrosis) can offer important information.[452] First, it can be used to differentiate between acute and chronic lesions, as well as to identify the presence of a new lesion in the case of recurrent stroke (Fig. 4.31). Furthermore, it can also help to identify the presence of multiple acute lesions suggestive of a source of multiple

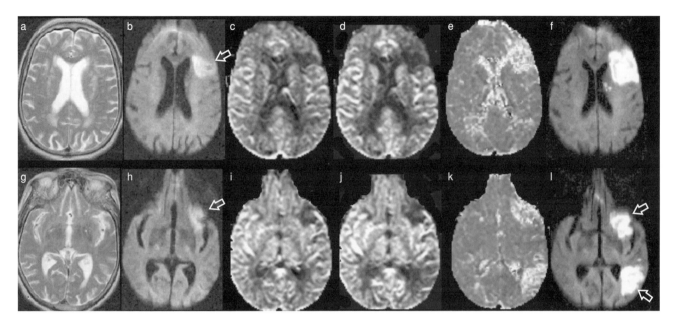

Fig. 4.30. MR diffusion-perfusion mismatch in acute ischaemia. Axial images at two anatomical levels from a 78-year-old female. a–e and g–k were obtained 3 hours after the onset of aphasia that occurred during cardiac catherization. Upper anatomical section: (a) T2-weighted image (no abnormality); (b) diffusion-weighted image (hyperintensity in the left frontal lobe, see arrow), haemodynamic images (slightly larger abnormality); (c) cerebral blood volume (CBV); (d) cerebral blood flow (CBF); (e) mean transit time (MTT); (f) follow-up diffusion-weighted image obtained at 5 days depicts infarction. Lower anatomical section: (g) T2-weighted image (no abnormality); (h) diffusion-weighted image (inferior frontal lobe hyperintensity, see arrow), haemodynamic images (two abnormal regions: a slightly larger abnormality in the front and a further area of normal T2 and diffusion, but abnormal CBF and MTT); (i) CBV; (j) CBF; (k) MTT. (l) Follow up diffusion-weighted image obtained at 5 days depicts infarction in both areas (see arrows). (Image kindly provided by Dr A. Greg Sorensen, and previously published in Sorensen AG, Copen WA, Ostergaard L, Buonanno FS, Gonzalez RG, Rordorf G et al. Hyperacute stroke: simultaneous measurement of relative cerebral blood volume, relative cerebral blood flow, and mean tissue transit time. Radiology 1999; 210(2):519–527. Copyright © 1999, Radiological Society of North America, Inc.)

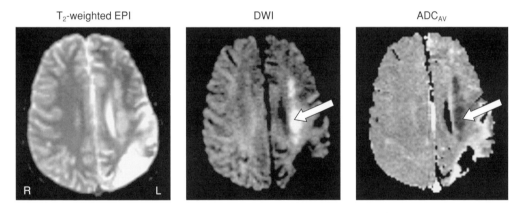

Fig. 4.31. Acute and chronic lesions in a 12-year-old child. MRI (EPI) was performed 2 days after the last event. Axial T2-weighted echoplanar image (left), diffusion-weighted image (DWI, middle) and average apparent diffusion coefficient (ADC) map (ADC_{AV}, right). There is a clear differentiation between the chronic (increased diffusion) and the acute (decreased diffusion, hyperintensity in the DWI (see arrows)) lesions. (Note low fluid signal (e.g. cerebrospinal fluid) on the ADC_{AV} map is due to a fluid attenuation inversion recovery preparation used in the DWI sequence to suppressed fluid signal.)

emboli (e.g. arterial dissection), which represents a high risk of further events if no action is taken (Fig. 4.32). Finally, the different diffusion properties of cytotoxic and vasogenic oedema can be exploited to rule out ischaemia as the source of symptoms in certain situations. For example, MR diffusion studies suggested that the oedema induced by ciclosporin-neurotoxicity (with increased ADC) is due to passive extravasation of fluid into the interstitium due to the disruption of the blood–brain barrier (vasogenic oedema), and not due to acute ischaemia (a widely accepted alternative hypothesis);[41] this finding was of particular value in the clinical management of one of the children in this study, where cerebral ischaemia secondary to sickle cell disease was considered as an alternative explanation for the observed T2-weighted signal hyperintensity.

The high sensitivity of diffusion MRI to cerebral ischaemia has also been used in the investigation of hypoxic-ischaemic

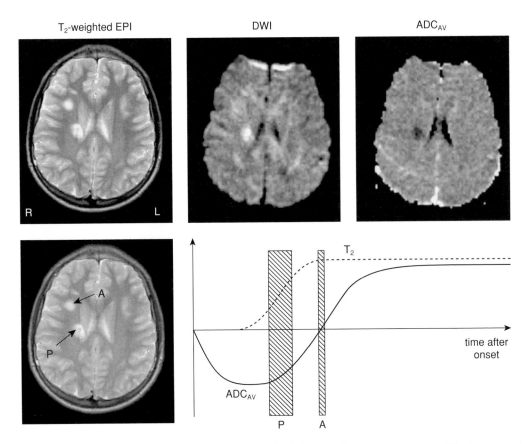

Fig. 4.32. Multiple acute events. MRI performed on a 15-year-old child 4 days after symptoms onset. The top row shows the axial T2-weighted Turbo-SE image (left), diffusion-weighted image (DWI, middle) and average apparent diffusion coefficient (ADC) (ADC_{AV}, right). Two regions of increased T2 can be seen in the right basal ganglia (left side of the images). While the more posterior (P) has decreased diffusion, the anterior (A) has already 'pseudonormalized', consistent with a further clinical event after the initial insult. The bottom graph shows a schematic diagram with the time-course of the T2 (dotted line) and ADC_{AV} (solid line) in the lesions, with the approximate time points of the two lesions. (Note low signal on the ADC_{AV} map is due to a fluid attenuation inversion recovery preparation used in the DWI sequence to suppressed fluid signal.) (Modified from a figure previously published in Connelly A, Calamante F, Porter DA, Gadian DG. Case study on diffusion and perfusion magnetic resonance imaging in childhood stroke. Electromedica 2000; 68:2–8. Copyright © 2000, Siemens AG).

injury in neonates and infants.[453–455] These studies have shown that brain lesions in neonates can be detected by diffusion MRI in the first days of life, when they can be less well seen with conventional MRI. However, due to the temporary normalization of the ADC (pseudonormalization), diffusion MRI should be interpreted always in combination with conventional MRI to avoid misinterpretation of the data. Although pseudonormalization typically occurs towards the end of the first week of life, this can be observed earlier, especially if some of the lesions originated during the prenatal period.

In the context of acute stroke, it should be noted not only that decreased diffusion does not necessarily lead to permanent damage (reversibility has been shown[116]), but also that normalization of the ADC in the context of normal structural MRI does not necessarily imply permanent tissue recovery. Several studies have shown that a secondary decline (usually referred to as 'secondary energy failure') can develop even days after the temporary recovery of the ADC,[451] consistent with findings from animal experiments (see "Restoration of blood flow following cerebral ischaemia" above).

The role of diffusion anisotropy and fibre tractography
Measurements of diffusion anisotropy have been generally applied to the investigation of white matter disease since grey matter is observed to be isotropic (except in the early neonatal period[456]). Diffusion anisotropy has been used to study many brain abnormalities including multiple sclerosis,[457] leukoaraiosis,[458] CADASIL,[459] and Wallerian degeneration.[384,460] However, it has not played a major role in the investigation of acute stroke so far. In adults, the areas of reduced ADC during acute stroke are generally seen to have decreased anisotropy in the sub-acute and chronic stages,[441,461–463] but increased anisotropy in the hyper-acute phase has also been reported.[441,462] As with the ADC, the mechanisms underlying the increased anisotropy in hyper-acute stroke are thought to be related to axonal swelling resulting from cytotoxic oedema,[441] although this remains to be demonstrated. On the other hand, the decreased anisotropy in sub-acute and chronic stroke are thought to be related to axonal degeneration.[441,462] Since the time-course of anisotropy changes differs somewhat from that of the ADC, these measures (in combination with ADC and T2) could potentially

be used to provide a more accurate estimate of the time of insult,[441] although the intrinsic heterogeneity of the anisotropy makes quantification difficult.

Diffusion anisotropy and fibre tractography have also been used in chronic stroke to assess the level of involvement of major tracts such as the motor-sensory tract (Fig. 4.35. See also colour plate 4),[464–466] or the arcuate fasciculus.[467] These have also been used to study Wallerian degeneration of the affected white matter tracts at locations remote from the lesion.[384,468] A common finding is of an association between a diffusion parameter measured for the relevant tract and clinical outcome. For example, such associations have been found between anisotropy in the posterior limb of the internal capsule (PLIC) and response to upper limb motor rehabilitation,[465] or between the overlap of the lesion with the motor pathways.[464,466]

There are very few reports of diffusion anisotropy measurements in acute stroke in children; some perinatal hypoxic ischaemia studies however have observed elevated anisotropy in the vicinity of the lesion within the first 10 days of life.[469,470] Diffusion anisotropy has been used more extensively to study brain development in healthy neonates,[471] preterm neonates[472,473] and preterm children with periventicular leukomalacia.[456,474–476] In normal development, there is a rapid decrease in ADC, accompanied by an increase in anisotropy that is tract dependent; for example, fibres underlying the visual cortex show a more rapid increase in anisotropy, thought to be associated with earlier myelination.[456] In periventricular leukomalacia, there is a common finding of decreased anisotropy in affected white matter pathways, even at locations remote from the lesions. This is thought to be due to Wallerian degeneration, or in more severe cases to actual white matter loss such as porencephalic cysts.[476] Fibre tractography has also been used to show abnormal patterns of white matter organization in some of these patients.[470,474,476]

Although the methods are very promising, there are still a number of issues that limit their interpretation. Most of the studies mentioned above have made use of the diffusion tensor model (with the exception of Newton et al[464]), and may therefore contain significant artefacts due to crossing fibre effects (see "Quantitative diffusion mapping" above). This makes it difficult to interpret any observed changes in anisotropy: although they may reflect real disruption of the white matter tissue, they may also reflect differences in the organization of the white matter pathways through this area; for example, an increase in anisotropy could be ascribed to a reduction in the contribution from one of the fibre bundles in a crossing fibre region, rather than disruption to the white matter at the microscopic level. Nonetheless, there are regions that may be assumed relatively free of crossing fibres (e.g. the PLIC) where changes in fractional anisotropy may truly reflect differences at the microscopic level. In the same way, any disruption to a particular tract of interest observed using fibre tractography may also be due to differences in crossing fibre effects; the selective loss of a dominant pathway may allow another pathway with a different orientation to become

dominant, leading the tractography algorithm to deviate from the true course of the tract,[384] or in some cases to terminate early because of a reduction in anisotropy.[470] The recent introduction of new fibre tracking methods robust to these artefacts will allow many of these issues to be resolved.

The role of perfusion MRI
Despite its high sensitivity, diffusion MRI has been shown to be negative in some patients (both children and adults) with acute ischaemic symptoms who later developed infarcts.[341,477,478] This is consistent with the concept of a flow 'threshold' for diffusion changes from animal models (see 'DWI and cerebral blood flow' above). The perfusion to certain areas of the brain can be low enough to affect brain function but with enough supply of oxygen and nutrients to maintain ionic homeostasis. Perfusion MRI is therefore believed to play an essential role in the investigation of stroke.[311,435,437,448,479] Many studies in adults have been concerned with predicting the eventual infarct volume in patients who have suffered an ischaemic insult, a major aim being to select the most appropriate patients for possible therapeutic intervention.[435,479] A large number of these studies have shown a regional mismatch between the diffusion abnormality and the perfusion deficit (e.g. see Fig. 4.30),[350,461,480–482] while others have shown the presence of perfusion abnormalities even in the absence of any abnormality on structural or diffusion MRI.[477,478] Although these areas of mismatch are generally believed to be 'at risk' of infarction,[311] their fate is evidently quite variable.[482–486] Recent studies in adults have focused on improving the characterisation of this mismatch area, with the aim of differentiating tissue that will eventually infarct from tissue that will remain viable.[486] This may be the area appropriate for therapeutic intervention.[435,479]

As previously mentioned, there have been very few MR studies of acute stroke in children.[341,351,426,449,450,487] Some of these studies have shown the presence of similar patterns of diffusion-perfusion mismatch (see Fig. 4.33 for an example of DSC-MRI and Fig. 4.34 for an example of ASL). Furthermore, these areas of mismatch have been observed not only during acute stroke, but also in patients with chronic hypoperfusion. These studies involved children with high stroke incidence such as those with sickle cell disease (see Chapter 15),[352,488,489] and moyamoya syndrome.[353,490–492] Extensive areas of decreased perfusion (in many cases with normal structural and diffusion imaging[352,353]) have been reported. These studies suggest that areas of decreased perfusion can persist for long periods of time, although it is not clear how long such compromised tissue could survive, since the flow 'thresholds' for energy failure are expected to increase with time (see 'DWI and cerebral blood flow' above). Similar areas of chronic hypoperfusion also have been reported in adults with internal carotid artery stenosis and occlusion.[397,493,494]

The use of these MR techniques has a potential role not only in the identification of tissue 'at risk' of infarction, but also in monitoring the efficacy of interventional strategies in rehabilitation and prevention, for example assessing the effect

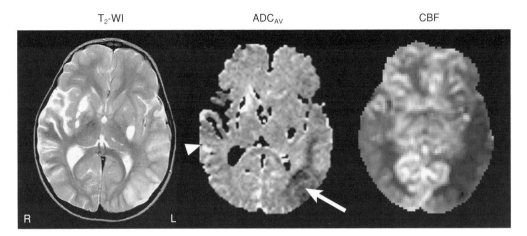

Fig. 4.33. Diffusion-perfusion mismatch and multiple acute events. Images obtained from a 3-year-old boy with a history of cardiac disease. From left to right: T2-WI, T2-weighted Turbo-SE image; ADC_{AV}, average apparent diffusion coefficient (ADC) map; CBF, cerebral blood flow perfusion map. This child suffered multiple cerebral insults as a result of multiple emboli associated with cardiac disease. The images shown illustrate a number of features of combined T2/diffusion-perfusion MRI. Firstly, the presence of chronic lesions in both the left and right basal ganglia regions, as evidence by hyperintensity on the T2-weighted images in conjunction with free diffusion (note low signal on the ADC_{AV} map is due to a fluid attenuated inversion recovery preparation used in the diffusion weighted image sequence to suppressed fluid signal). Second, two cortical regions of relatively recent infarction, but corresponding to different acute events (see Fig. 4.32): while both regions have signal hyperintensity in the T2-weighted image, the ADC_{AV} has 'pseudonormalized' on the right region (see arrowhead) but is still decreased on the left (see arrow). Third, the area of perfusion deficit on the left is larger than the diffusion abnormality (diffusion-perfusion mismatch). (Modified from a figure previously published in Connelly A, Calamante F, Porter DA, Gadian DG. Case study on diffusion and perfusion magnetic resonance imaging in childhood stroke. Electromedica 2000; 68:2–8. Copyright © 2000, Siemens AG).

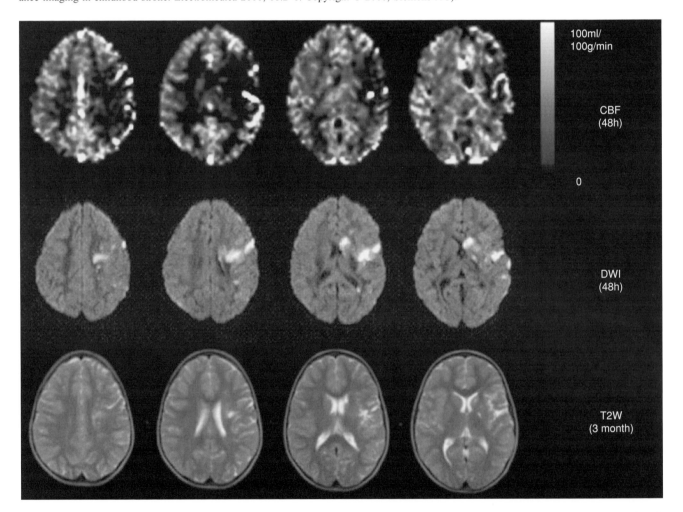

Fig. 4.34. Pulsed arterial spin labelling perfusion MRI and diffusion weighted images (DWI) acquired at 48 hours from symptom onset in a 6-year-old boy who presented with *varicella* vasculopathy and stroke. The follow-up T2-weighted images at 3 months are also shown. A mismatch between the deficits in the cerebral blood flow (CBF) and DWI is observed, akin to the ischaemia penumbra pattern in adult stroke. In this particular case, the final infarct did not expand beyond the initial DWI abnormality. The bright intraluminal artefact in the vicinity of the hypoperfused region results from markedly delayed arterial transit times to this region.[424] (Image kindly provided by Dr. Jiongjiong Wang, and modified from a figure previously published in Wang J, Licht DJ. Pediatric perfusion MR imaging using arterial spin labeling. Neuroimaging Clin N Am 2006; 16(1):149–167. Copyright © 2006, Elsevier Inc.)

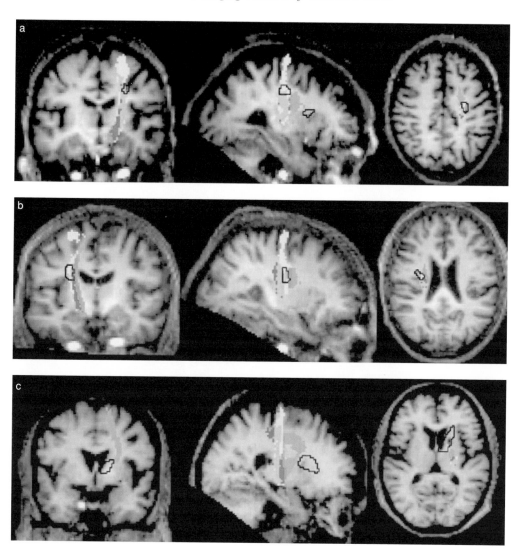

Fig. 4.35. An example of the application of fibre tractography to stroke recovery, showing the location of the lesion in three stroke patients (as identified by the area of low diffusion anisotropy) in relation to the path of different corticofugal pathways, identified in a group of healthy controls using fibre tractography. The inferred disconnections were found to explain enhanced hand-grip-related responses as assessed using functional MRI. (From a figure previously published in Newton JM, Ward NS, Parker GJ, Deichmann R, Alexander DC, Friston KJ et al. Non-invasive mapping of corticofugal fibres from multiple motor areas – relevance to stroke recovery. Brain 2006; 129(Pt 7):1844–1858. Copyright © 2006, Jennifer M Newton, published by Oxford University Press). (See colour plate 4.)

of blood transfusion therapy on brain perfusion in patients with sickle cell disease (see Chapter 15),[352] or the effectiveness of surgical revascularization in moyamoya syndrome.[353] Perfusion MRI can be also helpful in determining the presence and extent of recanalization (either spontaneous or due to thrombolysis).[451] For example, Fig. 4.36 shows a case of a newborn stroke showing hyperperfusion in the area of diffusion and structural abnormality.

Although applications of ASL to cerebrovascular disease are much more limited than DSC-MRI studies, several studies have been reported.[424,430,481,495–497] However, special care must be taken to account for the presence of long transit times in this patient group[497] to avoid misinterpreting the ASL images.

MRI can provide information not only about the 'resting' tissue perfusion status, but also about the cerebrovascular reserve capacity. It has been suggested that measurements

of regional cerebrovascular reactivity in response to carbon dioxide, breath holding or acetazolamide could potentially identify the subgroup of patients with carotid artery stenosis or occlusion who may be at increased risk of stroke.[498] Perfusion MRI provides a non-invasive means to obtain such information, with good spatial resolution, by comparing the measurement before to that after the vasodilatory stimulus.[313,314,397,493] It should be noted that studies of cerebrovascular reserve require repeated injections of contrast agent in DSC-MRI. Therefore, there is a particular advantage in using ASL approaches in these cases.[313,314]

Conclusion

As described above, MR diffusion and perfusion imaging are capable already of contributing significantly to the investigation of patients with ischaemic stroke and cerebrovascular

DWI ADC

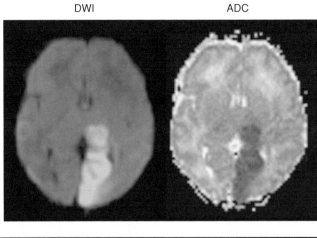

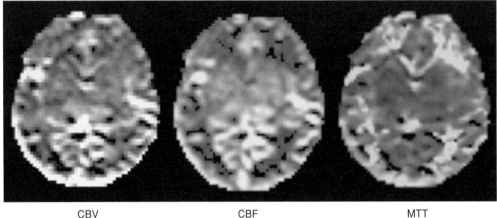

CBV CBF MTT

Fig. 4.36. Neonatal stroke presenting with seizures at 2 days of life and imaged at 3 days of life. There is a region of hyper-intensity on the diffusion-weighted image (DWI) and decreased diffusion on the apparent diffusion coefficient (ADC) map. This region of abnormality corresponds to a region of increased cerebral blood volume (CBV) and cerebral blood flow (CBF) compared with a similar region in the contralateral normal hemisphere, suggesting early reperfusion of the affected area. (Image kindly provided by Dr. P. Ellen Grant.)

disease. Moreover, this is currently a particularly active area of research, and substantial further advances are likely in the near future, including increased precision, improved image quality, ease of data acquisition and post-processing in a clinical environment, and the development of new applications. Therefore, there is a high expectation that diffusion and perfusion imaging, in combination with conventional MRI and MR angiography, will play an important role in the diagnosis and management of ischaemic disease.

REFERENCES

1. Calder K, Kokorowski P, Tran T, Henderson S. Emergency department presentation of pediatric stroke. Pediatr Emerg Care 2003; 19(5):320–328.
2. Braun KP, Kappelle LJ, Kirkham FJ, deVeber G. Diagnostic pitfalls in paediatric ischaemic stroke. Dev Med Child Neurol 2006; 48(12):985–990.
3. Shellhaas RA, Smith SE, O'Tool E, Licht DJ, Ichord RN. Mimics of childhood stroke: characteristics of a prospective cohort. Pediatrics 2006; 118(2):704–709.
4. Braun KP, Rafay MF, Uiterwaal CS, Pontigon AM, deVeber G. Mode of onset predicts etiological diagnosis of arterial ischemic stroke in children. Stroke 2007; 38(2):298–302.
5. Gabis LV, Yangala R, Lenn NJ. Time lag to diagnosis of stroke in children. Pediatrics 2002; 110(5):924–928.
6. Rafay MF, Pontigon AM, Chiang J, Adams M, Jarvis DA, Silver F et al. Delay to diagnosis in acute pediatric arterial ischemic stroke. Stroke 2009; 40(1):58–64.
7. Stroke Unit Trialists' Collaboration. Collaborative systematic review of the randomized trials of organized inpatient (stroke unit care after stroke). BMJ 1997; 314(7088):1151–1159.
8. Kuhle S, Mitchell L, Andrew M, Chan AK, Massicotte P, Adams M et al. Urgent clinical challenges in children with ischemic stroke: analysis of 1065 patients from the 1–800-NOCLOTS pediatric stroke telephone consultation service. Stroke 2006; 37(1):116–122.
9. Williams LS. Health-related quality of life outcomes in stroke. Neuroepidemiology 1998; 17(3):116–120.
10. Wraige E, Hajat C, Jan W, Pohl KR, Wolfe CD, Ganesan V. Ischaemic stroke subtypes in children and adults. Dev Med Child Neurol 2003; 45(4):229–232.
11. Wraige E, Pohl KR, Ganesan V. A proposed classification for subtypes of arterial ischaemic stroke in children. Dev Med Child Neurol 2005; 47(4):252–256.
12. Ganesan V, Prengler M, McShane MA, Wade AM, Kirkham FJ. Investigation of risk factors in children with arterial ischemic stroke. Ann Neurol 2003; 53(2):167–173.
13. Giroud M, Lemesle M, Gouyon JB, Nivelon JL, Milan C, Dumas R. Cerebrovascular disease in children under 16 years of age in the city of Dijon, France: a study of incidence and clinical features from 1985 to 1993. J Clin Epidemiol 1995; 48(11):1343–1348.
14. Mallick AA, O'Callaghan FJ. The epidemiology of childhood stroke. Eur J Paediatr Neurol. 2009; 30 Oct 2010; 14(3):197–205.

15. Williams AN, Eunson PD, McShane MA, Lynn R, Green S, Kirkham F. Childhood cerebrovascular disease and stroke like illness in the united kingdon and eire, a descriptive epidemiological study. Arch Dis Child 2002; 86(1):A40(G113).

16. Al-Jarallah A, Al-Rifai MT, Riela AR, Roach ES. Nontraumatic brain hemorrhage in children: etiology and presentation. J Child Neurol 2000; 15(5):284–289.

17. deVeber G, Andrew M, Adams C, Bjornson B, Booth F, Buckley DJ et al. Cerebral sinovenous thrombosis in children. N Engl J Med 2001; 345(6):417–423.

18. Earley CJ, Kittner SJ, Feeser BR, Gardner J, Epstein A, Wozniak MA et al. Stroke in children and sickle-cell disease: Baltimore–Washington Cooperative Young Stroke Study. Neurology 1998; 51(1):169–176.

19. Ohene-Frempong K, Weiner SJ, Sleeper LA, Miller ST, Embury S, Moohr JW et al. Cerebrovascular accidents in sickle cell disease: rates and risk factors. Blood 1998; 91(1):288–294.

20. Prengler M, Cox TC, Klein NJ, Evans JP, Bynevelt M, Chong WK et al. Progressive cerebrovascular disease in childhood stroke: associations and effect on recurrent risk. Dev Med Child Neurol 2000; 85:42–47.

21. Lee JC, Lin KL, Wang HS, Chou ML, Hung PC, Hsieh MY et al. Seizures in childhood ischemic stroke in Taiwan. Brain Dev 2009; 31(4):294–299.

22. Chadehumbe MA, Khatri P, Khoury JC, Alwell K, Szaflarski JP, Broderick JP et al. Seizures are common in the acute setting of childhood stroke: a population-based study. J Child Neurol 2009; 24(1):9–12.

23. Pegelow CH, Macklin EA, Moser FG, Wang WC, Bello JA, Miller ST et al. Longitudinal changes in brain magnetic resonance imaging findings in children with sickle cell disease. Blood 2002; 99(8):3014–3018.

24. Ganesan V, Prengler M, Wade A, Kirkham FJ. Clinical and radiological recurrence after childhood arterial ischemic stroke. Circulation 2006; 114(20):2170–2177.

25. Kirkham FJ. Therapy insight: stroke risk and its management in patients with sickle cell disease. Nat Clin Pract Neurol 2007; 3(5):264–278.

26. Jordan LC, van Beek JG, Gottesman RF, Kossoff EH, Johnston MV. Ischemic stroke in children with critical illness: a poor prognostic sign. Pediatr Neurol 2007; 36(4):244–246.

27. Sébire G, Tabarki B, Saunders DE, Leroy I, Liesner R, Saint-Martin C et al. Cerebral venous sinus thrombosis in children: risk factors, presentation, diagnosis and outcome. Brain 2005; 128(Pt 3):477–489.

28. Stonehouse M, Gupte G, Wassmer E, Whitehouse WP. Acute disseminated encephalomyelitis: recognition in the hands of general paediatricians. Arch Dis Child 2003; 88(2):122–124.

29. Fullerton HJ, Wu YW, Sidney S, Johnston SC. Risk of recurrent childhood arterial ischemic stroke in a population-based cohort: the importance of cerebrovascular imaging. Pediatrics 2007; 119(3): 495–501.

30. Dobson SR, Holden KR, Nietert PJ, Cure JK, Laver JH, Disco D et al. Moyamoya syndrome in childhood sickle cell disease: a predictive factor for recurrent cerebrovascular events. Blood 2002; 99(9):3144–3150.

31. Ganesan V, McShane MA, Liesner R, Cookson J, Hann I, Kirkham FJ. Inherited prothrombotic states and ischaemic stroke in childhood. J Neurol Neurosurg Psychiatry 1998; 65(4):508–511.

32. Sträter R, Becker S, von EA, Heinecke A, Gutsche S, Junker R et al. Prospective assessment of risk factors for recurrent stroke during childhood – a 5-year follow-up study. Lancet 2002; 360(9345):1540–1545.

33. Chabrier S, Lasjaunias P, Husson B, Landrieu P, Tardieu M. Ischaemic stroke from dissection of the craniocervical arteries in childhood: report of 12 patients. Eur J Paediatr Neurol 2003; 7(1):39–42.

34. Chabrier S, Rodesch G, Lasjaunias P, Tardieu M, Landrieu P, Sebire G. Transient cerebral arteriopathy: a disorder recognized by serial angiograms in children with stroke. J Child Neurol 1998; 13(1):27–32.

35. Kandeel AY, Zimmerman RA, Ohene-Frempong K. Comparison of magnetic resonance angiography and conventional angiography in sickle cell disease: clinical significance and reliability. Neuroradiology 1996; 38(5):409–416.

36. Rothman SM, Fulling KH, Nelson JS. Sickle cell anemia and central nervous system infarction: a neuropathological study. Ann Neurol 1986; 20(6):684–690.

37. Adams RJ, Nichols FT, McKie V, McKie K, Milner P, Gammal TE. Cerebral infarction in sickle cell anemia: mechanism based on CT and MRI. Neurology 1988; 38(7):1012–1017.

38. Suzuki J, Kodama N. Moyamoya disease – a review. Stroke 1983; 14(1):104–109.

39. Yilmaz EY, Pritz MB, Bruno A, Lopez-Yunez A, Biller J. Moyamoya: Indiana University Medical Center experience. Arch Neurol 2001; 58(8):1274–1278.

40. Pavlakis SG, Frank Y, Chusid R. Hypertensive encephalopathy, reversible occipitoparietal encephalopathy, or reversible posterior leukoencephalopathy: three names for an old syndrome. J Child Neurol 1999; 14(5):277–281.

41. Coley SG, Porter DA, Calamante F, Chong WK, Connelly A. Quantitative MR diffusion mapping and cyclosporin-induced neurotoxicity. AJNR Am. J. Neuroradiol 1999; 20:1507–1510.

42. Henderson JN, Noetzel MJ, McKinstry RC, White DA, Armstrong M, DeBaun MR. Reversible posterior leukoencephalopathy syndrome and silent cerebral infarcts are associated with severe acute chest syndrome in children with sickle cell disease. Blood 2003; 101(2):415–419.

43. Ganesan V, Chong WK, Cox TC, Chawda SJ, Prengler M, Kirkham FJ. Posterior circulation stroke in childhood: risk factors and recurrence. Neurology 2002; 59(10):1552–1556.

44. Banwell B, Kennedy J, Sadovnick D, Arnold DL, Magalhaes S, Wambera K et al. Incidence of acquired demyelination of the CNS in Canadian children. Neurology 2009; 72(3):232–239.

45. Leake JA, Albani S, Kao AS, Senac MO, Billman GF, Nespeca MP et al. Acute disseminated encephalomyelitis in childhood: epidemiologic, clinical and laboratory features. Pediatr Infect Dis J 2004; 23(8):756–764.

46. Weng WC, Peng SS, Lee WT, Fan PC, Chien YH, Du JC et al. Acute disseminated encephalomyelitis in children: one medical center experience. Acta Paediatr Taiwan 2006; 47(2):67–71.

47. Khurana DS, Melvin JJ, Kothare SV, Valencia I, Hardison HH, Yum S et al. Acute disseminated encephalomyelitis in children: discordant neurologic and neuroimaging abnormalities and response to plasmapheresis. Pediatrics 2005; 116(2):431–436.

48. Pavlakis SG, Kingsley PB, Bialer MG. Stroke in children: genetic and metabolic issues. J Child Neurol 2000; 15(5):308–315.

49. van Beynum IM, Smeitink JA, den Heijer M, te Poele Pothoff MT, Blom HJ. Hyperhomocysteinemia: a risk factor for ischemic stroke in children. Circulation 1999; 99(16):2070–2072.

50. Prengler M, Ganesan V, Dick MC. Risk factors for recurrent transient ischaemic event and stroke in sickle cell disease. Dev Med Child Neurol 2001; 43:27.

51. Cardo E, Campistol J, Caritg J, Ruiz S, Vilaseca MA, Kirkham F et al. Fatal haemorrhagic infarct in an infant with homocystinuria. Dev Med Child Neurol 1999; 41(2):132–135.

52. Kelly PJ, Furie KL, Kistler JP, Barron M, Picard EH, Mandell R et al. Stroke in young patients with hyperhomocysteinemia due to cystathionine beta-synthase deficiency. Neurology 2003; 60(2):275–279.

53. Kossoff EH, Ichord RN, Bergin AM. Recurrent hypoglycemic hemiparesis and aphasia in an adolescent patient. Pediatr Neurol 2001; 24(5):385–386.

54. Koga Y, Akita Y, Junko N, Yatsuga S, Povalko N, Fukiyama R et al. Endothelial dysfunction in MELAS improved by l-arginine supplementation. Neurology 2006; 66(11):1766–1769.

55. Schoenberg BS, Mellinger JF, Schoenberg DG. Cerebrovascular disease in infants and children: a study of incidence, clinical features, and survival. Neurology 1978; 28(8):763–768.

56. Mackay MT, Prabhu SP, Coleman L. Childhood posterior circulation arterial ischemic stroke. Stroke. 2010 Oct;41(10):2201–9.

57. Lee YY, Lin KL, Wang HS, Chou ML, Hung PC, Hsieh MY et al. Risk factors and outcomes of childhood ischemic stroke in Taiwan. Brain Dev 2008; 30(1):14–19.

58. Sokol DK, Williams L, Miller JH, Biller J, Garg BP. Ischemic strokes in the vertebro-basilar artery distribution in children. Ann Neurol 1997; 42:519.

59. Toure A, Chabrier S, Plagne M-D, Presles E, des Portes V, Rousselle C. Neurological outcome and risk of recurrence depending on the anterior vs posterior arterial distribution in children with stroke. Neuropediatrics 2009; 40(3):126–128.

60. Halevy A, Konen O, Straussberg R, Michowitz SD, Shuper A. Vertebral artery dissection and posterior stroke in a child. J Child Neurol 2008; 23(5):568–571.

61. Nezu A, Kimura S, Ohtsuki N, Tanaka M, Tada H. Alternating hemiplegia of childhood: report of a case having a long history. Brain Dev 1997; 19(3):217–221.

62. Wolf JK. The Classical Brainstem Syndromes. Springfield, Illinois: Charles C Thomas, 1971.

63. Mokri B, Houser OW, Sandok BA, Piepgras DG. Spontaneous dissections of the vertebral arteries. Neurology 1988; 38(6):880–885.

64. Garg BP, DeMyer WE. Ischemic thalamic infarction in children: clinical presentation, etiology, and outcome. Pediatr Neurol 1995; 13(1):46–49.

65. Walsh LE, Garg BP. Ischemic strokes in children. Indian J Pediatr 1997; 64(5):613–623.

66. Papp J, Dorsey ST. A preschool-age child with first-time seizure and ataxia. J Emerg Med 2009; 36(1):30–33.

67. Lin JJ, Chou ML, Lin KL, Wong MC, Wang HS. Cerebral infarct secondary to traumatic carotid artery dissection. Pediatr Emerg Care 2007; 23(3):166–168.

68. Garg BP, Ottinger CJ, Smith RR, Fishman MA. Strokes in children due to vertebral artery trauma. Neurology 1993; 43(12):2555–2558.

69. Phillips PC, Lorentsen KJ, Shropshire LC, Ahn HS. Congenital odontoid aplasia and posterior circulation stroke in childhood. Ann Neurol 1988; 23(4):410–413.

70. Brandt T, Hausser I, Orberk E, Grau A, Hartschuh W, Anton-Lamprecht I et al. Ultrastructural connective tissue abnormalities in patients with spontaneous cervicocerebral artery dissections. Ann Neurol 1998; 44(2):281–285.

71. Rolfs A, Bottcher T, Zschiesche M, Morris P, Winchester B, Bauer P et al. Prevalence of Fabry disease in patients with cryptogenic stroke: a prospective study. Lancet 2005; 366(9499):1794–1796.

72. Brouns R, Sheorajpanday R, Braxel E, Eyskens F, Baker R, Hughes D et al. Middelheim Fabry Study (MiFaS): a retrospective Belgian study on the prevalence of Fabry disease in young patients with cryptogenic stroke. Clin Neurol Neurosurg 2007; 109(6):479–484.

73. Day RW, Boyer RS, Tait VF, Ruttenberg HD. Factors associated with stroke following the Fontan procedure. Pediatr Cardiol 1995; 16(6):270–275.

74. Tyler HR, Clark DB. Cerebrovascular accidents in patients with congenital heart disease. Trans Am Neurol Assoc 1956; (81st Meeting):26–30.

75. Benson LN, Freedom RM, Wilson GJ, Halliday WC. Cerebral complications following balloon angioplasty of coarctation of the aorta. Cardiovasc Intervent Radiol 1986; 9(4):184–186.

76. Schievink WI, Mokri B, Piepgras DG, Kuiper JD. Recurrent spontaneous arterial dissections: risk in familial versus non-familial disease. Stroke 1996; 27:622–624.

77. Schievink WI, Mokri B, Piepgras DG, Gittenberger-de Groot AC. Intracranial aneurysms and cervicophalic arterial dissections associated with congenital heart disease. Neurosurgery 1996; 39:685–690.

78. du Plessis AJ, Chang AC, Wessel DL, Lock JE, Wernovsky G, Newburger JW et al. Cerebrovascular accidents following the Fontan operation. Pediatr Neurol 1995; 12(3):230–236.

79. Hutto RL, Williams JP, Maertens P, Wilder WM, Williams RS. Cerebellar infarct: late complication of the Fontan procedure? Pediatr Neurol 1991; 7(4):293–295.

80. Jauss M, Wessels T, Trittmacher S, Allendorfer J, Kaps M. Embolic lesion pattern in stroke patients with patent foramen ovale compared with patients lacking an embolic source. Stroke 2006; 37(8):2159–2161.

81. Schievink WI, Mokri B, Piepgras DG. Spontaneous dissections of cervicophalic arteries in childhood and adolescence. Neurology 1994; 44:1607–1612.

82. Ganesan V, Savvy L, Chong WK, Kirkham FJ. Conventional cerebral angiography in children with ischemic stroke. Pediatr Neurol 1999; 20(1):38–42.

83. Ganesan V, Ng V, Chong WK, Kirkham FJ, Connelly A. Lesion volume, lesion location, and outcome after middle cerebral artery territory stroke. Arch Dis Child 1999; 81(4):295–300.

84. Patel H, Smith RR, Garg BP. Spontaneous extracranial carotid artery dissection in children. Pediatr Neurol 1995; 13(1):55–60.

85. Pitter JH, French JH, PeBenito R, Hotson GC. Vertebrobasilar occlusion complicating nonpenetrating craniocervical trauma in a child. J Child Neurol 1990; 5(3):219–223.

86. Greenberg AD. Atlanto-axial dislocations. Brain 1968; 91(4):655–684.

87. Maruyama K, Mishima K, Saito N, Fujimaki T, Sasaki T, Kirino T. Radiation-induced aneurysm and moyamoya vessels presenting with subarachnoid haemorrhage. Acta Neurochir (Wien) 2000; 142(2):139–143.

88. Bhatnagar M, Sponseller PD, Carroll C, Tolo VT. Pediatric atlantoaxial instability presenting as cerebral and cerebellar infarcts. J Pediatr Orthop 1991; 11(1):103–107.

89. Cushing KE, Ramesh V, Gardner-Medwin D, Todd NV, Gholkar A, Baxter P et al. Tethering of the vertebral artery in the congenital arcuate foramen of the atlas vertebra: a possible cause of vertebral artery dissection in children. Dev Med Child Neurol 2001; 43(7):491–496.

90. Garg BP, Edwards-Brown MK. Vertebral artery compression due to head rotation in thalamic stroke. Pediatr Neurol 1995; 12(2):162–164.

91. Teiken S, Akyut-Bingol C, Aktan S. Case of cerebral artery dissection in young age. Pediatr Neurol 1997; 16:67–70.

92. Zimmerman AW, Kumar AJ, Gadoth N, Hodges FJ, III. Traumatic vertebrobasilar occlusive disease in childhood. Neurology 1978; 28(2):185–188.

93. Tulyapronchote R, Selhorst JB, Malkoff MD, Gomez CR. Delayed sequelae of vertebral artery dissection and occult cervical fractures. Neurology 1994; 44(8):1397–1399.

94. Parent AD, Harkey HL, Touchstone DA, Smith EE, Smith RR. Lateral cervical spine dislocation and vertebral artery injury. Neurosurgery 1992; 31(3):501–509.

95. Sherman P, Oka M, Aldrich E, Jordan L, Gailloud P. Isolated posterior cerebral artery dissection: report of three cases. AJNR Am J Neuroradiol 2006; 27(3):648–652.

96. Lin PJ, Chang YT, Lai CL. Ischemic stroke following multiple traumas in a child: a case report. Kaohsiung J Med Sci 2006; 22(4):189–193.

97. Kieslich M, Fiedler A, Heller C, Kreuz W, Jacobi G. Minor head injury as cause and co-factor in the aetiology of stroke in childhood: a report of eight cases. J Neurol Neurosurg Psychiatry 2002; 73(1):13–16.

98. Kelkar AS, Karande S, Chaudhary V, Kulkarni MV. Traumatic posterior cerebral artery occlusion in a 14-month-old child. Pediatr Neurol 2002; 27(2):147–149.

99. Bacigaluppi S, Rusconi R, Rampini P, Annoni F, Zavanone ML, Carnelli V et al. Vertebral artery dissection in a child. Is "spontaneous" still an appropriate definition? Neurol Sci 2006; 27(5):364–368.

100. Antachopoulos C, Liakopoulou T, Palamidou F, Papathanassiou D, Youroukos S. Posterior cerebral artery occlusion associated with *Mycoplasma pneumoniae* infection. J Child Neurol 2002; 17(1):55–57.

101. Miyamoto S, Kikuchi H, Karasawa J, Nagata I, Ikota T, Takeuchi S. Study of the posterior circulation in moyamoya disease. Clinical and neuroradiological evaluation. J Neurosurg 1984; 61(6):1032–1037.

102. Hackel M, Neumann J, Benes V, Jr. Extracranial vertebral artery stenosis in a patient with moyamoya disease. Acta Neurochir (Wien) 1999; 141(3):323–324.

103. Yamada I, Murata Y, Umehara I, Suzuki S, Matsushima Y. SPECT and MRI evaluations of the posterior circulation in moyamoya disease. J Nucl Med 1996; 37(10):1613–1617.

104. Lopez-Yunez A, Garg BP. Non-infectious cerebral vasculities in children. Semin Cerebrovasc Dis Stroke 2001; 1:249–263.

105. Snyder RD, Stovring J, Cushing AH, Davis LE, Hardy TL. Cerebral infarction in childhood bacterial meningitis. J Neurol Neurosurg Psychiatry 1981; 44(7):581–585.

106. Rickert CH, Greiner C, Rellensmann G, Kehl HG, Scheld HH, Paulus W et al. Mycotic cerebral vasculitis in a paediatric cardiac

transplant patient excludes misadventure. Int J Legal Med 2002; 116(4):233–237.

107. Barron TF, Ostrov BE, Zimmerman RA, Packer RJ. Isolated angiitis of CNS: treatment with pulse cyclophosphamide. Pediatr Neurol 1993; 9(1):73–75.

108. Abe T, Maruyama T, Nagai Y, Kamida T, Wakabayashi Y, Ishii K et al. Severe postoperative vasculitis of the central nervous system in a child with arteriovenous malformation: case report. Surg Neurol 2007; 68(3):317–321.

109. Pegelow CH, Adams RJ, McKie V, Abboud M, Berman B, Miller ST et al. Risk of recurrent stroke in patients with sickle cell disease treated with erythrocyte transfusions. J Pediatr 1995; 126(6):896–899.

110. Adams RJ, McKie VC, Hsu L, Files B, Vichinsky E, Pegelow C et al. Prevention of a first stroke by transfusions in children with sickle cell anemia and abnormal results on transcranial Doppler ultrasonography. N Engl J Med 1998; 339(1):5–11.

111. Adams RJ, Brambilla D. Discontinuing prophylactic transfusions used to prevent stroke in sickle cell disease. N Engl J Med 2005; 353(26):2769–2778.

112. Kirkham FJ. Therapy insight: stroke risk and its management in patients with sickle cell disease. Nat Clin Pract Neurol. 2007; 3(5):264–78.

113. Barinagarrementeria F, Cantu BC, Izaguirre R, De La PA. Progressive intracranial occlusive disease associated with deficiency of protein S. Report of two cases. Stroke 1993; 24(11):1752–1756.

114. Malm J, Kristensen B, Carlberg B, Fagerlund M, Olsson T. Clinical features and prognosis in young adults with infratentorial infarcts. Cerebrovasc Dis 1999; 9(5):282–289.

115. Cardo E, Campistol J, Kirkham F. The role of resistance to C active protein (R-APC) in a pediatric stroke. Rev Neurol 1997; 25(146): 1589–1591.

116. Connelly A, Chong WK, Johnson CL, Ganesan V, Gadian DG, Kirkham FJ. Diffusion weighted magnetic resonance imaging of compromised tissue in stroke. Arch Dis Child 1997; 77(1):38–41.

117. Classification and diagnostic criteria for headache disorders, cranial neuralgias and facial pain. Headache Classification Committee of the International Headache Society. Cephalalgia 1988; 8(Suppl 7):1–96.

118. Wober-Bingol C. Migraine in childhood and adolescence. Cephalalgia 1998; 18(6):304–305.

119. Hutchinson M, O'Riordan J, Javed M, Quin E, Macerlaine D, Wilcox T et al. Familial hemiplegic migraine and autosomal dominant arteriopathy with leukoencephalopathy (CADASIL). Ann Neurol 1995; 38(5):817–824.

120. Golomb MR, Sokol DK, Walsh LE, Christensen CK, Garg BP. Recurrent hemiplegia, normal MRI, and NOTCH3 mutation in a 14-year-old: is this early CADASIL? Neurology 2004; 62(12): 2331–2332.

121. Granild-Jensen J, Jensen UB, Schwartz M, Hansen US. Cerebral autosomal dominant arteriopathy with subcortical infarcts and leukoencephalopathy resulting in stroke in an 11-year-old male. Dev Med Child Neurol. 2009; 51(9):754–757.

122. Koo B, Becker LE, Chuang S, Merante F, Robinson BH, MacGregor D et al. Mitochondrial encephalomyopathy, lactic acidosis, stroke-like episodes (MELAS): clinical, radiological, pathological, and genetic observations. Ann Neurol 1993; 34(1):25–32.

123. Ito H, Mori K, Harada M, Minato M, Naito E, Takeuchi M et al. Serial brain imaging analysis of stroke-like episodes in MELAS. Brain Dev 2008; 30(7):483–488.

124. James CA, Glasier CM, Angtuaco EE. Altered vertebrobasilar flow in children: angiographic, MR, and MR angiographic findings. AJNR Am J Neuroradiol 1995; 16(8):1689–1695.

125. Khurana DS, Bonnemann CG, Dooling EC, Ouellette EM, Buonanno F. Vertebral artery dissection: issues in diagnosis and management. Pediatr Neurol 1996; 14(3):255–258.

126. Oppenheim C, Galanaud D, Samson Y, Sahel M, Dormont D, Wechsler B et al. Can diffusion weighted magnetic resonance imaging help differentiate stroke from stroke-like events in MELAS? J Neurol Neurosurg Psychiatry 2000; 69(2):248–250.

127. Kolb SJ, Costello F, Lee AG, White M, Wong S, Schwartz ED et al. Distinguishing ischemic stroke from the stroke-like lesions of MELAS using apparent diffusion coefficient mapping. J Neurol Sci 2003; 216(1):11–15.

128. Raco A, Caroli E, Isidori A, Salvati M. Management of acute cerebellar infarction: one institution's experience. Neurosurgery 2003; 53(5):1061–1065.

129. Kalashnikova LA, Zueva YV, Pugacheva OV, Korsakova NK. Cognitive impairments in cerebellar infarcts. Neurosci Behav Physiol 2005; 35(8):773–779.

130. Steinlin M. The cerebellum in cognitive processes: supporting studies in children. Cerebellum 2007; 6(3):237–241.

131. Baillieux H, Weyns F, Paquier P, De Deyn PP, Marien P. Posterior fossa syndrome after a vermian stroke: a new case and review of the literature. Pediatr Neurosurg 2007; 43(5):386–395.

132. Proposed diagnostic criteria and nosology of acute transverse myelitis. Neurology 2002; 59(4):499–505.

133. Fraser KL, Grosman H, Hyland RH, Tullis DE. Transverse myelitis: a reversible complication of bronchial artery embolization in cystic fibrosis. Thorax 1997; 52(1):99–101.

134. Muranjan MN, Deshmukh CT. Acute transverse myelitis due to spinal epidural hematoma-first manifestation of severe hemophilia. Indian Pediatr 1999; 36(11):1151–1153.

135. Hui AC, Wong KS, Fu M, Kay R. Ischaemic myelopathy presenting as Guillain–Barré syndrome. Int J Clin Pract 2000; 54(5):340–341.

136. Cakir E, Karaarslan G, Usul H, Baykal S, Kuzeyli K, Mungan I et al. Clinical course of spontaneous spinal epidural haematoma mimicking Guillain–Barré syndrome in a child: a case report and literature review. Dev Med Child Neurol 2004; 46(12):838–842.

137. Blennow G, Starck L. Anterior spinal artery syndrome. Report of seven cases in childhood. Pediatr Neurosci 1987; 13(1):32–37.

138. Knebusch M, Strassburg HM, Reiners K. Acute transverse myelitis in childhood: nine cases and review of the literature. Dev Med Child Neurol 1998; 40(9):631–639.

139. Defresne P, Hollenberg H, Husson B, Tabarki B, Landrieu P, Huault G et al. Acute transverse myelitis in children: clinical course and prognostic factors. J Child Neurol 2003; 18(6):401–406.

140. Pidcock FS, Krishnan C, Crawford TO, Salorio CF, Trovato M, Kerr DA. Acute transverse myelitis in childhood: center-based analysis of 47 cases. Neurology 2007; 68(18):1474–1480.

141. Wilmshurst J, Walker MC, Pohl KR. Rapid onset transverse myelitis in adolescence: implications for pathogenesis and prognosis. Arch Dis Child 1999; 80:137–142.

142. Davis GA, Klug GL. Acute-onset nontraumatic paraplegia in childhood: fibrocartilaginous embolism or acute myelitis? Childs Nerv Syst 2000; 16(9):551–554.

143. Nance JR, Golomb MR. Ischemic spinal cord infarction in children without vertebral fracture. Pediatr Neurol 2007; 36(4):209–216.

144. Harms B, Goodwin F, Whitney A, Sykes K, Nicolin G, Kennedy CR et al. Acute spinal cord lesions in children. Dev Med Child Neurol 2009; 51(Suppl 1):1.

145. McCarthy JT, Amer J. Postvaricella acute transverse myelitis: a case presentation and review of the literature. Pediatrics 1978; 62(2): 202–204.

146. Mills RW, Schoolfield L. Acute transverse myelitis associated with *Mycoplasma pneumoniae* infection: a case report and review of the literature. Pediatr Infect Dis J 1992; 11(3):228–231.

147. Candler PM, Dale RC. Three cases of central nervous system complications associated with *Mycoplasma pneumoniae*. Pediatr Neurol 2004; 31(2):133–138.

148. Linssen WH, Gabreels FJ, Wevers RA. Infective acute transverse myelopathy. Report of two cases. Neuropediatrics 1991; 22(2): 107–109.

149. Huisman TA, Wohlrab G, Nadal D, Boltshauser E, Martin E. Unusual presentations of neuroborreliosis (Lyme disease. in childhood. J Comput Assist Tomogr 1999; 23(1):39–42.

150. Boyce TG. Acute transverse myelitis in a 6-year-old girl with schistosomiasis. Pediatr Infect Dis J 1990; 9(4):279–284.

151. Nazer H, Hugosson C, Posas H. Transverse myelitis in a child with Down's syndrome and schistosomal colitis. Ann Trop Paediatr 1993; 13(4):353–357.

152. Lewis DW, Packer RJ, Raney B, Rak IW, Belasco J, Lange B. Incidence, presentation, and outcome of spinal cord disease in children with systemic cancer. Pediatrics 1986; 78(3):438–443.

153. Yavuz H, Cakir M. Transverse myelopathy: an initial presentation of acute leukemia. Pediatr Neurol 2001; 24(5):382–384.

154. Olfat MO, Al-Mayouf SM, Muzaffer MA. Pattern of neuropsychiatric manifestations and outcome in juvenile systemic lupus erythematosus. Clin Rheumatol 2004; 23(5):395–399.

155. Al-Mayouf SM, Bahabri S. Spinal cord involvement in pediatric systemic lupus erythematosus: case report and literature review. Clin Exp Rheumatol 1999; 17(4):505–508.

156. Avcin T, Benseler SM, Tyrrell PN, Cucnik S, Silverman ED. A followup study of antiphospholipid antibodies and associated neuropsychiatric manifestations in 137 children with systemic lupus erythematosus. Arthritis Rheum 2008; 59(2):206–213.

157. Lam RM, Tsang TH, Chan KY, Lau YL, Lim WL, Lam TH et al. Surveillance of acute flaccid paralysis in Hong Kong: 1997 to 2002. Hong Kong Med J 2005; 11(3):164–173.

158. Morris AM, Elliott EJ, D'Souza RM, Antony J, Kennett M, Longbottom H. Acute flaccid paralysis in Australian children. J Paediatr Child Health 2003; 39(1):22–26.

159. Whitfield K, Kelly H. Using the two-source capture-recapture method to estimate the incidence of acute flaccid paralysis in Victoria, Australia. Bull World Health Organ 2002; 80(11):846–851.

160. Tartaglino LM, Croul SE, Flanders AE, Sweeney JD, Schwartzman RJ, Liem M et al. Idiopathic acute transverse myelitis: MR imaging findings. Radiology 1996; 201(3):661–669.

161. Shimizu M, Hamano S, Nara T, Eto Y, Maekawa K. MRI findings of anterior spinal artery syndrome in childhood. No To Hattatsu 1996; 28(5):438–442.

162. Beslow LA, Ichord RN, Zimmerman RA, Smith SE, Licht DJ. Role of diffusion MRI in diagnosis of spinal cord infarction in children. Neuropediatrics 2008; 39(3):188–191.

163. Andronikou S, Buquerque-Jonathan G, Wilmshurst J, Hewlett R. MRI findings in acute idiopathic transverse myelopathy in children. Pediatr Radiol 2003; 33(9):624–629.

164. Weidauer S, Nichtweiss M, Lanfermann H, Zanella FE. Spinal cord infarction: MR imaging and clinical features in 16 cases. Neuroradiology 2002; 44(10):851–857.

165. Puntis JW, Green SH. Ischaemic spinal cord injury after cardiac surgery. Arch Dis Child 1985; 60(6):517–520.

166. Servais LJ, Rivelli SK, Dachy BA, Christophe CD, Dan B. Anterior spinal artery syndrome after aortic surgery in a child. Pediatr Neurol 2001; 24(4):310–312.

167. Garland H, Greenberg J, Harriman DG. Infarction of the spinal cord. Brain 1966; 89(4):645–662.

168. Vogel LC, Lubicky JP. Neurologic and vascular complications of scoliosis surgery in patients with Ehlers–Danlos syndrome. A case report. Spine 1996; 21(21):2508–2514.

169. Akpinar S, Gogus A, Talu U, Hamzaoglu A, Dikici F. Surgical management of the spinal deformity in Ehlers–Danlos syndrome type VI. Eur Spine J 2003; 12(2):135–140.

170. Boglino C, Martins AG, Ciprandi G, Sousinha M, Inserra A. Spinal cord vascular injuries following surgery of advanced thoracic neuroblastoma: an unusual catastrophic complication. Med Pediatr Oncol 1999; 32(5):349–352.

171. Munoz ME, Roche C, Escriba R, Martinez-Bermejo A, Pascual-Castroviejo I. Flaccid paraplegia as complication of umbilical artery catheterization. Pediatr Neurol 1993; 9(5):401–403.

172. Seidman E, Weber AM, Morin CL, Ethier R, Lamarche JB, Guerguerian AJ et al. Spinal cord paralysis following sclerotherapy for esophageal varices. Hepatology 1984; 4(5):950–954.

173. Amess P, Chong WK, Kirkham FJ. Acquired spinal cord lesion associated with os odontoideum causing deterioration in dystonic cerebral palsy: case report and review of the literature. Dev Med Child Neurol 1998; 40(3):195–198.

174. Wieting JM, Krach LE. Spinal cord injury rehabilitation in a pediatric achondroplastic patient: case report. Arch Phys Med Rehabil 1994; 75(1):106–108.

175. Goodman ML, Pang D. Spinal cord injury in I-cell disease. Pediatr Neurosci 1988; 14(6):315–318.

176. Wityk RJ, Zanferrari C, Oppenheimer S. Neurovascular complications of Marfan syndrome: a retrospective, hospital-based study. Stroke 2002; 33(3):680–684.

177. Singh U, Silver JR, Welply NC. Hypotensive infarction of the spinal cord. Paraplegia 1994; 32(5):314–322.

178. Novy J, Carruzzo A, Maeder P, Bogousslavsky J. Spinal cord ischemia: clinical and imaging patterns, pathogenesis, and outcomes in 27 patients. Arch Neurol 2006; 63(8):1113–1120.

179. Ramelli GP, Wyttenbach R, von der WN, Ozdoba C. Anterior spinal artery syndrome in an adolescent with protein S deficiency. J Child Neurol 2001; 16(2):134–135.

180. Young G, Krohn KA, Packer RJ. Prothrombin G20210A mutation in a child with spinal cord infarction. J Pediatr 1999; 134(6):777–779.

181. Hakimi KN, Massagli TL. Anterior spinal artery syndrome in two children with genetic thrombotic disorders. J Spinal Cord Med 2005; 28(1):69–73.

182. Almasanu BP, Owensby JR, Pavlakis SG, Edwards JH. Spinal cord infarction in meningitis: polygenic risk factors. Pediatr Neurol 2005; 32(2):124–126.

183. Hasegawa M, Yamashita J, Yamashima T, Ikeda K, Fujishima Y, Yamazaki M. Spinal cord infarction associated with primary antiphospholipid syndrome in a young child. Case report. J Neurosurg 1993; 79(3):446–450.

184. Darwish H, Archer C, Modin J. The anterior spinal artery collateral in coarctation of the aorta. A clinical angiographic correlation. Arch Neurol 1979; 36(4):240–243.

185. Serfontein SJ, Kron IL. Complications of coarctation repair. Semin Thorac Cardiovasc Surg Pediatr Card Surg Annu 2002; 5:206–211.

186. Quaegebeur JM, Jonas RA, Weinberg AD, Blackstone EH, Kirklin JW. Outcomes in seriously ill neonates with coarctation of the aorta. A multiinstitutional study. J Thorac Cardiovasc Surg 1994; 108(5):841–851.

187. Krieger KH, Spencer FC. Is paraplegia after repair of coarctation of the aorta due principally to distal hypotension during aortic cross-clamping? Surgery 1985; 97(1):2–7.

188. Amitay M, Welch RW, Byrne PJ, Robertson MA, Penkoske PA. Neonatal spinal cord syndrome associated with hypoplastic aortic arch and anemia. Ann Thorac Surg 1993; 56(3):568–70.

189. Rothman SM, Nelson JS. Spinal cord infarction in a patient with sickle cell anemia. Neurology 1980; 30:684–690.

190. Wolman L, Hardy AG. Spinal cord infarction associated with the sickle cell trait. Paraplegia 1970; 7(4):282–291.

191. Haupt HM, Kurlinski JP, Barnett NK, Epstein M. Infarction of the spinal cord as a complication of pneumococcal meningitis. Case report. J Neurosurg 1981; 55(1):121–123.

192. Moffett KS, Berkowitz FE. Quadriplegia complicating *Escherichia coli* meningitis in a newborn infant: case report and review of 22 cases of spinal cord dysfunction in patients with acute bacterial meningitis. Clin Infect Dis 1997; 25(2):211–214.

193. Pang D, Pollack IF. Spinal cord injury without radiographic abnormality in children – the SCIWORA syndrome. J Trauma 1989; 29(5):654–664.

194. Grabb PA, Pang D. Magnetic resonance imaging in the evaluation of spinal cord injury without radiographic abnormality in children. Neurosurgery 1994; 35(3):406–414.

195. Dare AO, Dias MS, Li V. Magnetic resonance imaging correlation in pediatric spinal cord injury without radiographic abnormality. J Neurosurg 2002; 97(1 Suppl):33–39.

196. Liao CC, Lui TN, Chen LR, Chuang CC, Huang YC. Spinal cord injury without radiological abnormality in preschool-aged children: correlation of magnetic resonance imaging findings with neurological outcomes. J Neurosurg 2005; 103(1 Suppl):17–23.

197. Walsh JW, Stevens DB, Young AB. Traumatic paraplegia in children without contiguous spinal fracture or dislocation. Neurosurgery 1983; 12(4):439–445.

198. Choi JU, Hoffman HJ, Hendrick EB, Humphreys RP, Keith WS. Traumatic infarction of the spinal cord in children. J Neurosurg 1986; 65(5):608–610.

199. Robles LA. Traumatic spinal cord infarction in a child: case report and review of literature. Surg Neurol 2007; 67(5):529–534.

200. Mulligan JM, Miller T, McGuffie AC, Graham CA. Spinal cord injury without radiographic abnormality in a 4-year-old child: hypoperfusion injury or direct trauma? Eur J Emerg Med 2007; 14(4):216–218.

201. Ahmann PA, Smith SA, Schwartz JF, Clark DB. Spinal cord infarction due to minor trauma in children. Neurology 1975; 25(4):301–307.

202. Rogers FB, Osler TM, Shackford SR, Wald SL. Isolated stab wound to the artery of Adamkiewicz: case report and review of the literature. J Trauma 1997; 43(3):549–551.

203. Feld RS. Spinal cord infarction from an isolated stab wound to the artery of Adamkiewicz. J Trauma 1998; 44(2):418–419.

204. Beer S, Kesselring J. Fibrocartilaginous embolization of the spinal cord in a 7-year-old girl. J Neurol 2002; 249(7):936–937.

205. Mottolese C, Hermier M, Stan H, Jouvet A, Saint-Pierre G, Froment JC et al. Central nervous system cavernomas in the pediatric age group. Neurosurg Rev 2001; 24(2–3):55–71.

206. Gupta SK, Dhir JS, Khosla VK. Traumatic spinal subarachnoid hematoma: report of a case with MRI. Surg Neurol 1997; 48(2):189–192.

207. Mutoh K, Ito M, Okuno T, Mikawa H, Minami S, Asato R et al. Nontraumatic spinal intramedullary hemorrhage in an infant. Pediatr Neurol 1989; 5(1):53–56.

208. Kotwica Z, Stawowy A, Polis L. Spinal chronic subdural haematoma in a 7-year old girl. Eur J Pediatr 1989; 148(8):779–780.

209. Hung R, Chan AK, deVeber GA. Aspirin therapy for prevention of recurrent cerebral thrombo-embolic events in children: a prospective cohort study. Ann Neurol 2002; 52:S123.

210. Eftekhar B, Ghodsi M, Ketabchi E, Bakhtiari A, Mostajabi P. Spinal subdural hematoma revealing hemophilia A in a child: A case report. BMC Blood Disord 2003; 3(1):2.

211. Handa T, Suzuki Y, Saito K, Sugita K, Patel SJ. Isolated intramedullary spinal artery aneurysm presenting with quadriplegia. Case report. J Neurosurg 1992; 77(1):148–150.

212. Kreppel D, Antoniadis G, Seeling W. Spinal hematoma: a literature survey with meta-analysis of 613 patients. Neurosurg Rev 2003; 26(1):1–49.

213. Ghanem Q, Ivan LP. Spontaneous spinal epidural hematoma in an 8-year-old boy. Neurology 1978; 28(8):829–832.

214. Caldarelli M, Di RC, La MF. Spontaneous spinal epidural hematoma in toddlers: description of two cases and review of the literature. Surg Neurol 1994; 41(4):325–329.

215. Patel H, Boaz JC, Phillips JP, Garg BP. Spontaneous spinal epidural hematoma in children. Pediatr Neurol 1998; 19(4):302–307.

216. Chang CW, Lin LH, Liao HT, Hung KL, Hwan JS. Spontaneous spinal epidural hematoma in a 5-year-old girl. Acta Paediatr Taiwan 2002; 43(6):345–347.

217. Ravid S, Schneider S, Maytal J. Spontaneous spinal epidural hematoma: an uncommon presentation of a rare disease. Childs Nerv Syst 2002; 18(6–7):345–347.

218. Kirwan R, Saigal G, Faingold R, O'Gorman A. Nontraumatic acute and subacute enhancing spinal epidural hematoma mimicking a tumor in a child. Pediatr Radiol 2004; 34(6):499–502.

219. Alva NS. Traumatic spinal epidural hematoma of a 10-month-old male: a clinical note. Pediatr Neurol 2000; 23:88–89.

220. Epstein NE, Gilder M, Black K. Anterior thoracic extradural hematoma in a 5-year-old child. Pediatr Neurosci 1989; 15(1):48–52.

221. Fountas KN, Kapsalaki EZ, Robinson JS. Cervical epidural hematoma in children: a rare clinical entity. Case report and review of the literature. Neurosurg Focus 2006; 20(2):E6.

222. Guillaume D, Menezes AH. Retroclival hematoma in the pediatric population. Report of two cases and review of the literature. J Neurosurg 2006; 105(4 Suppl):321–325.

223. Cheng CJ, Fang W, Chen CM, Wan YL. Spontaneous spinal epidural hematomas with repeated remission and relapse. Neuroradiology 1997; 39:737–740.

224. Abram HS, DeLaHunt MJ, Merinbaum DJ, Hammond DN. Recurrent spontaneous spinal epidural hematoma in a child: first case report. Pediatr Neurol 2007; 36(3):177–180.

225. Abdelaal MA, McGuinness FE, Sagar G. Case report: spinal extra-dural haematoma in haemophilia-A – a diagnosis not to be missed. Clin Radiol 1994; 49(8):573–575.

226. Hutt PJ, Herold ED, Koenig BM, Gilchrist GS. Spinal extradural hematoma in an infant with hemophilia A: an unusual presentation of a rare complication. J Pediatr 1996; 128(5 Pt 1):704–706.

227. Chretiennot-Bara C, Guet A, Balzamo E, Noseda G, Torchet MF, Rothshild C et al. Epidural hematoma in a child with hemophilia: diagnostic difficulties. Arch Pediatr 2001; 8(8):828–833.

228. Heer JS, Enriquez EG, Carter AJ. Spinal epidural hematoma as first presentation of hemophilia A. J Emerg Med 2008; 34(2):159–162.

229. Balkan C, Kavakli K, Karapinar D. Spinal epidural haematoma in a patient with haemophilia B. Haemophilia 2006; 12(4):437–440.

230. Bisson EF, Dumont T, Tranmer B. Spontaneous spinal epidural hematoma in a child with hemophilia B. Can J Neurol Sci 2007; 34(4):488–490.

231. Ugur S, Uzel N, Dundar K, Kaya U, Ayan I, Gedikoglu G. Intraspinal hemorrhage in a child with factor XIII deficiency. Pediatr Emerg Care 1991; 7(4):231–233.

232. Tubbs RS, Smyth MD, Wellons JC, III, Oakes WJ. Intramedullary hemorrhage in a neonate after lumbar puncture resulting in paraplegia: a case report. Pediatrics 2004; 113(5):1403–1405.

233. Koch BL, Moosbrugger EA, Egelhoff JC. Symptomatic spinal epidural collections after lumbar puncture in children. AJNR Am J Neuroradiol 2007; 28(9):1811–1816.

234. Staebler M, Azzi N, Sekhara T, Delpierre I, Damry N, Christophe C. Complications of lumbar puncture in a child treated for leukaemia. Pediatr Radiol 2005; 35(11):1121–1124.

235. Lee AC, Lau Y, Li CH, Wong YC, Chiang AK. Intraspinal and intracranial hemorrhage after lumbar puncture. Pediatr Blood Cancer 2007; 48(2):233–237.

236. Chang JH, Hoernschemeyer DG, Sponseller PD. Delayed post-operative paralysis in adolescent idiopathic scoliosis: management with partial removal of hardware and staged correction. J Spinal Disord Tech 2006; 19(3):222–225.

237. McLoughlin GS, Nuchtern JG, Dauser RC, Sciubba DM, Gokaslan ZL, Wolinsky JP. Mediastinal lymphangioma presenting as an acute epidural hematoma. J Neurosurg Pediatr 2008; 1(6):474–476.

238. Kotulska K, Jurkiewcz E, Jozwiak S, Kuczynski D. Epidermal nevus syndrome and intraspinal hemorrhage. Brain Dev 2006; 28(8):541–543.

239. Nagel MA, Taff IP, Cantos EL, Patel MP, Maytal J, Berman D. Spontaneous spinal epidural hematoma in a 7-year-old girl. Diagnostic value of magnetic resonance imaging. Clin Neurol Neurosurg. 1989; 91(2):157–60.

240. Lonjon MM, Paquis P, Chanalet S, Grellier P. Nontraumatic spinal epidural hematoma: report of four cases and review of the literature. Neurosurgery 1997; 41(2):483–486.

241. Sklar EM, Post JM, Falcone S. MRI of acute spinal epidural hematomas. J Comput Assist Tomogr 1999; 23(2):238–243.

242. Beatty RM, Winston KR. Spontaneous cervical epidural hematoma. A consideration of etiology. J Neurosurg 1984; 61(1):143–148.

243. Foo D, Chang YC, Rossier AB. Spontaneous cervical epidural hemorrhage, anterior cord syndrome, and familial vascular malformation: case report. Neurology 1980; 30(3):308–311.

244. D'Angelo V, Bizzozero L, Talamonti G, Ferrara M, Colombo N. Value of magnetic resonance imaging in spontaneous extradural spinal hematoma due to vascular malformation: case report. Surg Neurol 1990; 34(5):343–344.

245. Bozzao A, Pierallini A, Ferone E, Di SD, Capanna G, Bozzao L. Association between spinal extradural and cerebral arteriovenous malformations appearing as acute paraplegia after epidural hemorrhage. Eur Radiol 1999; 9(5):1007–1008.

246. Groen RJ. Non-operative treatment of spontaneous spinal epidural hematomas: a review of the literature and a comparison with operative cases. Acta Neurochir (Wien) 2004; 146(2):103–110.

247. Groen RJ, van Alphen HA. Operative treatment of spontaneous spinal epidural hematomas: a study of the factors determining postoperative outcome. Neurosurgery 1996; 39(3):494–508.

248. Riche MC, Modenesi-Freitas J, Djindjian M, Merland JJ. Arteriovenous malformations (AVM) of the spinal cord in children. A review of 38 cases. Neuroradiology 1982; 22(4):171–180.

249. Eldridge PR, Holland IM, Punt JA. Spinal arteriovenous malformations in children. Br J Neurosurg 1989; 3(3):393–397.

250. O'Brien DP, Dias PS, Farrell MA, Toland JA, Singh J. Brown–Sequard syndrome and an intradural arteriovenous fistula in a child. Br J Neurosurg 1994; 8(5):611–615.

251. Bandyopadhyay S, Sheth RD. Acute spinal cord infarction: vascular steal in arteriovenous malformation. J Child Neurol 1999; 14(10):685–687.

252. Cullen S, Alvarez H, Rodesch G, Lasjaunias P. Spinal arteriovenous shunts presenting before 2 years of age: analysis of 13 cases. Childs Nerv Syst 2006; 22(9):1103–1110.

253. Chen CC, Wang CM, Chu NK, Wu KP, Tang SF, Wong AM. Spinal cord arteriovenous malformation presenting as chest pain in a child. Spinal Cord 2008; 46(6):456–458.

254. Niimi Y, Berenstein A, Fernandez PM, Brisman JL, Song JK. Pediatric nonvertebral paraspinal arteriovenous fistulas along the segmental nerve: clinical, imaging, and therapeutic considerations. J Neurosurg 2005; 103(2 Suppl):156–162.

255. Bassuk AG, Burrowes DM, Velimirovic B, Grant J, Keating GF. A child with spinal cord AVM presenting with raised intracranial pressure. Neurology 2003; 60(10):1724–1725.

256. Molina A, Martin C, Munoz I, Aguilar L, Serrano S, Ballester J. Spinal intraosseous arteriovenous malformation as a cause of juvenile scoliosis. A case report. Spine 1997; 22(2):221–224.

257. Strom RG, Derdeyn CP, Moran CJ, Cross DT, Esper GJ, Mazumdar A et al. Frequency of spinal arteriovenous malformations in patients with unexplained myelopathy. Neurology 2006; 66(6):928–931.

258. Mandzia JL, Terbrugge KG, Faughnan ME, Hyland RH. Spinal cord arteriovenous malformations in two patients with hereditary hemorrhagic telangiectasia. Childs Nerv Syst 1999; 15(2–3):80–83.

259. Djindjian M, Djindjian R, Hurth M, Rey A, Houdart R. Spinal cord arteriovenous malformations and the Klippel–Trenaunay–Weber syndrome. Surg Neurol 1977; 8(4):229–237.

260. Rodesch G, Malherbe V, Alvarez H, Zerah M, Devictor D, Lasjaunias P. Nongalenic cerebral arteriovenous malformations in neonates and infants. Review of 26 consecutive cases (1982–1992). Childs Nerv Syst 1995; 11(4):231–241.

261. Brunaud V, Delerue O, Muller JP, Destee A. Klippel–Trenaunay syndrome and ischemic neurologic complications. Rev Neurol (Paris) 1994; 150:50–54.

262. Pascual-Castroviejo I, Frutos R, Viano J, Pascual-Pascual SI, Gonzalez P. Cobb syndrome: case report. J Child Neurol 2002; 17(11):847–849.

263. Matullo KS, Samdani A, Betz R. Low-back pain and unrecognized Cobb syndrome in a child resulting in paraplegia. Orthopedics 2007; 30(3):237–238.

264. Yoshioka K, Niinuma H, Ehara S, Nakajima T, Nakamura M, Kawazoe K. MR angiography and CT angiography of the artery of Adamkiewicz: state of the art. Radiographics 2006; 26(Suppl 1):S63–S73.

265. Ou P, Schmit P, Layouss W, Sidi D, Bonnet D, Brunelle F. CT angiography of the artery of Adamkiewicz with 64-section technology: first experience in children. AJNR Am J Neuroradiol 2007; 28(2):216–219.

266. Pollack IF, Pang D, Sclabassi R. Recurrent spinal cord injury without radiographic abnormalities in children. J Neurosurg 1988; 69(2):177–182.

267. Tator CH. Review of treatment trials in human spinal cord injury: issues, difficulties, and recommendations. Neurosurgery 2006; 59(5):957–982.

268. Lahat E, Pillar G, Ravid S, Barzilai A, Etzioni A, Shahar E. Rapid recovery from transverse myelopathy in children treated with methylprednisolone. Pediatr Neurol 1998; 19(4):279–282.

269. Defresne P, Meyer L, Tardieu M, Scalais E, Nuttin C, De Bont B et al. Efficacy of high dose steroid therapy in children with severe acute transverse myelitis. J Neurol Neurosurg Psychiatry 2001; 71(2):272–274.

270. Connolly ES, Jr, Winfree CJ, McCormick PC. Management of spinal epidural hematoma after tissue plasminogen activator. A case report. Spine 1996; 21(14):1694–1698.

271. Restrepo L, Guttin JF. Acute spinal cord ischemia during aortography treated with intravenous thrombolytic therapy. Tex Heart Inst J 2006; 33(1):74–77.

272. Liao CC, Lee ST, Hsu WC, Chen LR, Lui TN, Lee SC. Experience in the surgical management of spontaneous spinal epidural hematoma. J Neurosurg 2004; 100(1 Suppl Spine):38–45.

273. Chang FC, Lirng JF, Luo CB, Yen YS, Guo WY, Teng MM et al. Evaluation of clinical and MR findings for the prognosis of spinal epidural haematomas. Clin Radiol 2005; 60(7):762–770.

274. Tailor J, Dunn IF, Smith E. Conservative treatment of spontaneous spinal epidural hematoma associated with oral anticoagulant therapy in a child. Childs Nerv Syst 2006; 22(12):1643–1645.

275. Narawong D, Gibbons VP, McLaughlin JR, Bouhasin JD, Kotagal S. Conservative management of spinal epidural hematoma in hemophilia. Pediatr Neurol 1988; 4(3):169–171.

276. Sheikh AA, Abildgaard CF. Medical management of extensive spinal epidural hematoma in a child with factor IX deficiency. Pediatr Emerg Care 1994; 10(1):26–29.

277. Batista JE, Bauer SB, Shefner JM, Kelly MD, Darbey MD, Siroky MB. Urodynamic findings in children with spinal cord ischemia. J Urol 1995; 154(3):1183–1187.

278. Ganesan V, Borzyskowski M. Characteristics and course of urinary tract dysfunction after acute transverse myelitis. Dev Med Child Neurol 2001; 43(7):473–475.

279. Lavoie P, Raymond J, Roy D, Guilbert F, Weill A. Selective treatment of an anterior spinal artery aneurysm with endosaccular coil therapy. Case report. J Neurosurg Spine 2007; 6(5):460–464.

280. Glasser R, Masson R, Mickle JP, Peters KR. Embolization of a dural arteriovenous fistula of the ventral cervical spinal canal in a nine-year-old boy. Neurosurgery 1993; 33(6):1089–1093.

281. Bjork A, Eeg-Olofsson O, Svendsen P, Mostrom U, Pellettieri L. Endovascular treatment of a spinal arteriovenous malformation in a 21-month-old boy. Acta Paediatr 1994; 83(12):1326–1331.

282. Ito M, Yamamoto T, Mishina H, Sonokawa T, Sato K. Arteriovenous malformation of the medulla oblongata supplied by the anterior spinal artery in a child: treatment by microsurgical obliteration of the feeding artery. Pediatr Neurosurg 2000; 33(6):293–297.

283. Rodesch G, Hurth M, Alvarez H, Tadie M, Lasjaunias P. Spinal cord intradural arteriovenous fistulae: anatomic, clinical, and therapeutic considerations in a series of 32 consecutive patients seen between 1981 and 2000 with emphasis on endovascular therapy. Neurosurgery 2005; 57(5):973–983.

284. Ioannidis I, Sfakianos G, Nasis N, Prodromou P, Andreou A. Successful embolization of a giant perimedullary arteriovenous fistula of the cervical spine in a 6-year-old child. Childs Nerv Syst 2007; 23(11):1327–1330.

285. Stephan MJ, Nesbit GM, Behrens ML, Whitaker MA, Barnwell SL, Selden NR. Endovascular treatment of spinal arteriovenous fistula in a young child with hereditary hemorrhagic telangiectasia. Case report. J Neurosurg 2005; 103(5 Suppl):462–465.

286. Sure U, Wakat JP, Gatscher S, Becker R, Bien S, Bertalanffy H. Spinal type IV arteriovenous malformations (perimedullary fistulas) in children. Childs Nerv Syst 2000; 16(8):508–515.

287. Postert T, Federlein J, Przuntek H, Buttner T. Comparison of transcranial power Doppler and contrast-enhanced color-coded sonography in the identification of intracranial arteries. J Ultrasound Med 1998; 17(2):91–96.

288. Hunter JV. New radiographic techniques to evaluate cerebrovascular disorders in children. Semin Pediatr Neurol 2000; 7(4):261–277.

289. Adams R, McKie V, Nichols F, Carl E, Zhang DL, McKie K et al. The use of transcranial ultrasonography to predict stroke in sickle cell disease. N Engl J Med 1992; 326(9):605–610.

290. Adams RJ, Nichols FT, Figueroa R, McKie V, Lott T. Transcranial Doppler correlation with cerebral angiography in sickle cell disease. Stroke 1992; 23(8):1073–1077.

291. Hoffman WH, Pluta RM, Fisher AQ, Wagner MB, Yanovski JA. Transcranial Doppler ultrasound assessment of intracranial hemodynamics in children with diabetic ketoacidosis. J Clin Ultrasound 1995; 23(9):517–523.

292. Nishimaki S, Seki K, Yokota S. Cerebral blood flow velocity in two patients with neonatal cerebral infarction. Pediatr Neurol 2001; 24(4):320–323.

293. Lowe LH, Morello FP, Jackson MA, Lasky A. Application of transcranial Doppler sonography in children with acute neurologic events due to primary cerebral and West Nile vasculitis. AJNR Am J Neuroradiol 2005; 26(7):1698–1701.

294. Muttaqin Z, Ohba S, Arita K, Nakahara T, Pant B, Uozumi T et al. Cerebral circulation in moyamoya disease: a clinical study using transcranial Doppler sonography. Surg Neurol 1993; 40(4):306–313.

295. Ipsiroglu OS, Eichler F, Stockler-Ipsiroglu S, Trattnig S. Cerebral blood flow velocities in an infant with moyamoya disease. Pediatr Neurol 1999; 21(4):739–741.

296. Lee YS, Jung KH, Roh JK. Diagnosis of moyamoya disease with transcranial Doppler sonography: correlation study with magnetic resonance angiography. J Neuroimaging 2004; 14(4):319–323.

297. Perren F, Meairs S, Schmiedek P, Hennerici M, Horn P. Power Doppler evaluation of revascularization in childhood moyamoya. Neurology 2005; 64(3):558–560.

298. Lam AH. Doppler imaging of superior sagittal sinus thrombosis. J Ultrasound Med 1995; 14(1):41–46.

299. Stolz E, Gerriets T, Bodeker RH, Hugens-Penzel M, Kaps M. Intracranial venous hemodynamics is a factor related to a favorable outcome in cerebral venous thrombosis. Stroke 2002; 33(6):1645–1650.

300. Atkinson DS, Jr. Computed tomography of pediatric stroke. Semin Ultrasound CT MR 2006; 27(3):207–218.

301. Gatscher S, Brew S, Banks T, Simcock C, Sullivan Y, Crockett J. Multislice spiral computed tomography for pediatric intracranial vascular pathophysiologies. J Neurosurg 2007; 107(3 Suppl):203–208.

302. Leclerc X, Lucas C, Godefroy O, Tessa H, Martinat P, Leys D et al. Helical CT for the follow-up of cervical internal carotid artery dissections. AJNR Am J Neuroradiol 1998; 19(5):831–837.

303. Borisch I, Boehme T, Butz B, Hamer OW, Feuerbach S, Zorger N. Screening for carotid injury in trauma patients: image quality of 16-detector-row computed tomography angiography. Acta Radiol 2007; 48(7):798–805.

304. Chamoun RB, Mawad ME, Whitehead WE, Luerssen TG, Jea A. Extracranial traumatic carotid artery dissections in children: a review of current diagnosis and treatment options. J Neurosurg Pediatr 2008; 2(2):101–108.

305. Kety S, Schmidt C. Nitrous oxide method for the quantitive determination of cerebral blood flow in man: theory, procedure and normal values. J Clin Invest 1948; 27:476–483.

306. Hunter GJ, Hamberg LM, Ponzo JA, Huang-Hellinger FR, Morris PP, Rabinov J et al. Assessment of cerebral perfusion and arterial anatomy in hyperacute stroke with three-dimensional functional CT: early clinical results. AJNR Am J Neuroradiol 1998; 19(1):29–37.

307. Wintermark M, Cotting J, Roulet E, Lepori D, Meuli R, Maeder P et al. Acute brain perfusion disorders in children assessed by quantitative perfusion computed tomography in the emergency setting. Pediatr Emerg Care 2005; 21(3):149–160.

308. Atlas SW. MR imaging is highly sensitive for acute subarachnoid hemorrhage . . . not! Radiology 1993; 186(2):319–322.

309. Lin DD, Filippi CG, Steever AB, Zimmerman RD. Detection of intracranial hemorrhage: comparison between gradient-echo images and b(0) images obtained from diffusion-weighted echo-planar sequences. AJNR Am J Neuroradiol 2001; 22(7):1275–1281.

310. Moseley ME, Kucharczyk J, Mintorovitch J, Cohen Y, Kurhanewicz J, Derugin N et al. Diffusion-weighted MR imaging of acute stroke: correlation with T2-weighted and magnetic susceptibility-enhanced MR imaging in cats. AJNR Am J Neuroradiol 1990; 11(3):423–429.

311. Baird AE, Warach S. Magnetic resonance imaging of acute stroke. J Cereb Blood Flow Metab 1998; 18(6):583–609.

312. Calamante F, Thomas DL, Pell GS, Wiersma J, Turner R. Measuring cerebral blood flow using magnetic resonance imaging techniques. J Cereb Blood Flow Metab 1999; 19(7):701–735.

313. Detre JA, Samuels OB, Alsop DC, Gonzalez-At JB, Kasner SE, Raps EC. Noninvasive magnetic resonance imaging evaluation of cerebral blood flow with acetazolamide challenge in patients with cerebrovascular stenosis. J Magn Reson Imaging 1999; 10(5):870–875.

314. Detre JA, Alsop DC. Perfusion magnetic resonance imaging with continuous arterial spin labeling: methods and clinical applications in the central nervous system. Eur J Radiol 1999; 30(2):115–124.

315. Barker PB, Gillard JH, Van Zijl PC, Soher BJ, Hanley DF, Agildere AM et al. Acute stroke: evaluation with serial proton MR spectroscopic imaging. Radiology 1994; 192(3):723–732.

316. Saunders DE, Howe FA, van den Boogaart A, McLean MA, Griffiths JR, Brown MM. Continuing ischemic damage after acute middle cerebral artery infarction in humans demonstrated by short-echo proton spectroscopy. Stroke 1995; 26(6):1007–1013.

317. Ashwal S, Holshouser BA, Tomasi LG, Shu S, Perkin RM, Nystrom GA et al. [1]H-magnetic resonance spectroscopy-determined cerebral lactate and poor neurological outcomes in children with central nervous system disease. Ann Neurol 1997; 41(4):470–481.

318. Hunter JV, Thornton RJ, Wang ZJ, Levin HS, Roberson G, Brooks WM et al. Late proton MR spectroscopy in children after traumatic brain injury: correlation with cognitive outcomes. AJNR Am J Neuroradiol 2005; 26(3):482–488.

319. Ashwal S, Holshouser BA, Hinshaw DB, Jr, Schell RM, Bailey L. Proton magnetic resonance spectroscopy in the evaluation of children with congenital heart disease and acute central nervous system injury. J Thorac Cardiovasc Surg 1996; 112(2):403–414.

320. Wang Z, Bogdan AR, Zimmerman RA, Gusnard DA, Leigh JS, Ohene-Frempong K. Investigation of stroke in sickle cell disease by ^{1}H nuclear magnetic resonance spectroscopy. Neuroradiology 1992; 35(1):57–65.

321. Kohli A, Gupta R, Kishore J. Anterior cerebral artery territory infarction in neurocysticercosis: evaluation by MR angiography and in vivo proton MR spectroscopy. Pediatr Neurosurg 1997; 26(2):93–96.

322. Imamura A, Matsuo N, Ariki M, Horikoshi H, Hattori T. MR imaging and [1]H-MR spectroscopy in a case of cerebral infarction with transient cerebral arteriopathy. Brain Dev 2004; 26(8):535–538.

323. Connelly A, Cross JH, Gadian DG, Hunter JV, Kirkham FJ, Leonard JV. Magnetic resonance spectroscopy shows increased brain glutamine in ornithine carbamoyl transferase deficiency. Pediatr Res 1993; 33(1):77–81.

324. Castillo M, Kwock L, Green C. MELAS syndrome: imaging and proton MR spectroscopic findings. AJNR Am J Neuroradiol 1995; 16(2):233–239.

325. Sperl W, Felber S, Skladal D, Wermuth B. Metabolic stroke in carbamyl phosphate synthetase deficiency. Neuropediatrics 1997; 28(4):229–234.

326. Wilichowski E, Pouwels PJ, Frahm J, Hanefeld F. Quantitative proton magnetic resonance spectroscopy of cerebral metabolic disturbances in patients with MELAS. Neuropediatrics 1999; 30(5):256–263.

327. Moller HE, Kurlemann G, Putzler M, Wiedermann D, Hilbich T, Fiedler B. Magnetic resonance spectroscopy in patients with MELAS. J Neurol Sci 2005; 229–230:131–139.

328. Pearl PL, Krasnewich D. Neurologic course of congenital disorders of glycosylation. J Child Neurol 2001; 16(6):409–413.

329. Rollins N, Dowling M, Booth T, Purdy P. Idiopathic ischemic cerebral infarction in childhood: depiction of arterial abnormalities by MR angiography and catheter angiography. AJNR Am J Neuroradiol 2000; 21(3):549–556.

330. Husson B, Rodesch G, Lasjaunias P, Tardieu M, Sebire G. Magnetic resonance angiography in childhood arterial brain infarcts: a comparative study with contrast angiography. Stroke 2002; 33(5):1280–1285.

331. Mani RL, Eisenberg RL. Complications of catheter cerebral arteriography: analysis of 5,000 procedures. III. Assessment of arteries injected, contrast medium used, duration of procedure, and age of patient. AJR Am J Roentgenol 1978; 131(5):871–874.

332. Fung E, Ganesan V, Cox TS, Chong WK, Saunders DE. Complication rates of diagnostic cerebral arteriography in children. Pediatr Radiol 2005; 35(12):1174–1177.

333. Ogasawara K, Ogawa A, Ezura M, Konno H, Doi M, Kuroda K et al. Dynamic and static ^{99m}Tc-ECD SPECT imaging of subacute cerebral infarction: comparison with ^{133}Xe SPECT. J Nucl Med 2001; 42(4):543–547.

334. Kuroda S, Houkin K, Kamiyama H, Abe H, Mitsumori K. Regional cerebral hemodynamics in childhood moyamoya disease. Childs Nerv Syst 1995; 11(10):584–590.

335. Sztriha L, Al Suhaili AR, Prais V, Nork M. Regional cerebral blood perfusion in children with hemiplegia: a SPECT study. Neuropediatrics 1996; 27(4):178–183.

336. Gordon I. Cerebral imaging in paediatrics. Q J Nucl Med 1998; 42(2):126–132.

337. Truwit CL, Barkovich AJ, Gean-Marton A, Hibri N, Norman D. Loss of the insular ribbon: another early CT sign of acute middle cerebral artery infarction. Radiology 1990; 176(3):801–806.

338. Bryan RN, Levy LM, Whitlow WD, Killian JM, Preziosi TJ, Rosario JA. Diagnosis of acute cerebral infarction: comparison

of CT and MR imaging. AJNR Am J Neuroradiol 1991; 12(4): 611–620.

339. Kuroiwa T, Seida M, Tomida S, Hiratsuka H, Okeda R, Inaba Y. Discrepancies among CT, histological, and blood–brain barrier findings in early cerebral ischemia. J Neurosurg 1986; 65(4): 517–524.

340. Wardlaw JM, Dennis MS, Warlow CP, Sandercock PA. Imaging appearance of the symptomatic perforating artery in patients with lacunar infarction: occlusion or other vascular pathology? Ann Neurol 2001; 50(2):208–215.

341. Gadian DG, Calamante F, Kirkham FJ, Bynevelt M, Johnson CL, Porter DA et al. Diffusion and perfusion magnetic resonance imaging in childhood stroke. J Child Neurol 2000; 15(5):279–283.

342. Desmond PM, Lovell AC, Rawlinson AA, Parsons MW, Barber PA, Yang Q et al. The value of apparent diffusion coefficient maps in early cerebral ischemia. AJNR Am J Neuroradiol 2001; 22(7): 1260–1267.

343. Alexander JA, Sheppard S, Davis PC, Salverda P. Adult cerebrovascular disease: role of modified rapid fluid-attenuated inversion-recovery sequences. AJNR Am J Neuroradiol 1996; 17(8):1507–1513.

344. Elster AD, Moody DM. Early cerebral infarction: gadopentetate dimeglumine enhancement. Radiology 1990; 177(3):627–632.

345. Lanthier S, Armstrong D, Domi T, deVeber G. Post-varicella arteriopathy of childhood: natural history of vascular stenosis. Neurology 2005; 64(4):660–663.

346. Danchaivijitr N, Cox TC, Saunders DE, Ganesan V. Evolution of cerebral arteriopathies in childhood arterial ischemic stroke. Ann Neurol 2006; 59(4):620–626.

347. Aviv RI, Benseler SM, Silverman ED, Tyrrell PN, deVeber G, Tsang LM et al. MR imaging and angiography of primary CNS vasculitis of childhood. AJNR Am J Neuroradiol 2006; 27(1):192–199.

348. Hurst RW. Angiography of non-atherosclerotic occlusive cerebrovascular disease. Neuroimaging Clin N Am 1996; 6(3):651–678.

349. Barber PA, Darby DG, Desmond PM, Yang Q, Gerraty RP, Jolley D et al. Prediction of stroke outcome with echoplanar perfusion- and diffusion-weighted MRI. Neurology 1998; 51(2):418–426.

350. Schlaug G, Benfield A, Baird AE, Siewert B, Lovblad KO, Parker RA et al. The ischemic penumbra: operationally defined by diffusion and perfusion MRI. Neurology 1999; 53(7):1528–1537.

351. Huisman TA, Sorensen AG. Perfusion-weighted magnetic resonance imaging of the brain: techniques and application in children. Eur Radiol 2004; 14(1):59–72.

352. Kirkham FJ, Calamante F, Bynevelt M, Gadian DG, Evans JP, Cox TC et al. Perfusion magnetic resonance abnormalities in patients with sickle cell disease. Ann Neurol 2001; 49(4):477–485.

353. Calamante F, Ganesan V, Kirkham FJ, Jan W, Chong WK, Gadian DG et al. MR perfusion imaging in Moyamoya syndrome: potential implications for clinical evaluation of occlusive cerebrovascular disease. Stroke 2001; 32(12):2810–2816.

354. Oppenheim C, Touze E, Hernalsteen D, Peeters A, Lamy C, Mas JL et al. Comparison of five MR sequences for the detection of acute intracranial hemorrhage. Cerebrovasc Dis 2005; 20(5):388–394.

355. Schievink WI, Mokri B, Piepgras DG. Spontaneous dissections of cervicocephalic arteries in childhood and adolescence. Neurology. 1994; 44(9):1607–1612.

356. Ganesan V, Kirkham FJ. Carotid dissection causing stroke in a child with migraine. BMJ 1997; 314(7076):291–292.

357. Fullerton HJ, Johnston SC, Smith WS. Arterial dissection and stroke in children. Neurology 2001; 57(7):1155–1160.

358. Hildebrand D, Prengler M, Chawda SJ, Chong WK, Cox TC, Wade A et al. Clinical predictors of dissection in a stroke cohort. Ann Neurol 2003; 54(S7):137.

359. Lin CH, Jeng JS, Yip PK. Middle cerebral artery dissections: differences between isolated and extended dissections of internal carotid artery. J Neurol Sci 2005; 235(1–2):37–44.

360. Kirkham F. Improvement or progression in childhood cerebral arteriopathies: current difficulties in prediction and suggestions for research. Ann Neurol 2006; 59(4):580–582.

361. Petro GR, Witwer GA, Cacayorin ED, Hodge CJ, Bredenberg CE, Jastremski MS et al. Spontaneous dissection of the cervical internal carotid artery: correlation of arteriography, CT, and pathology. AJR Am J Roentgenol 1987; 148(2):393–398.

362. Goldberg HI, Grossman RI, Gomori JM, Asbury AK, Bilaniuk LT, Zimmerman RA. Cervical internal carotid artery dissecting hemorrhage: diagnosis using MR. Radiology 1986; 158(1):157–161.

363. Levy C, Laissy JP, Raveau V, Amarenco P, Servois V, Bousser MG et al. Carotid and vertebral artery dissections: three-dimensional time-of-flight MR angiography and MR imaging versus conventional angiography. Radiology 1994; 190(1):97–103.

364. Brugieres P, Castrec-Carpo A, Heran F, Goujon C, Gaston A, Marsault C. Magnetic resonance imaging in the exploration of dissection of the internal carotid artery. J Neuroradiol 1989; 16(1):1–10.

365. Hasan I, Wapnick S, Tenner MS, Couldwell WT. Vertebral artery dissection in children: a comprehensive review. Pediatr Neurosurg 2002; 37(4):168–177.

366. Eljamel MS, Humphrey PR, Shaw MD. Dissection of the cervical internal carotid artery. The role of Doppler/Duplex studies and conservative management. J Neurol Neurosurg Psychiatry 1990; 53(5):379–383.

367. Vieco PT. CT angiography of the carotid artery. Neuroimaging Clin N Am 1998; 8(3):593–605.

368. Medlock MD, Olivero WC, Hanigan WC, Wright RM, Winek SJ. Children with cerebral venous thrombosis diagnosed with magnetic resonance imaging and magnetic resonance angiography. Neurosurgery 1992; 31(5):870–876.

369. Casey SO, Alberico RA, Patel M, Jimenez JM, Ozsvath RR, Maguire WM et al. Cerebral CT venography. Radiology 1996; 198: 163–170.

370. Connor SE, Jarosz JM. Magnetic resonance imaging of cerebral venous sinus thrombosis. Clin Radiol 2002; 57(6):449–461.

371. Bezinque SL, Slovis TL, Touchette AS, Schave DM, Jarski RW, Bedard MP et al. Characterisation of superior sagittal sinus blood flow velocity using color flow Doppler in neonates and infants. Pediatr Radiol 1995; 25(3):175–179.

372. Ludwig B, Brand M, Brockerhoff P. Postpartum CT examination of the heads of full term infants. Neuroradiology 1980; 20(3): 145–154.

373. Ogawa T, Inugami A, Shimosegawa E, Fujita H, Ito H, Toyoshima H et al. Subarachnoid hemorrhage: evaluation with MR imaging. Radiology 1993; 186(2):345–351.

374. Ozyurek H, Oguz G, Ozen S, Akyuz C, Karli OK, Anlar B et al. Reversible posterior leukoencephalopathy syndrome: report of three cases. J Child Neurol 2005; 20(12):990–993.

375. Covarrubias DJ, Luetmer PH, Campeau NG. Posterior reversible encephalopathy syndrome: prognostic utility of quantitative diffusion-weighted MR images. AJNR Am J Neuroradiol 2002; 23(6):1038–1048.

376. Stehling MK, Turner R, Mansfield P. Echo-planar imaging: magnetic resonance imaging in a fraction of a second. Science 1991; 254(5028):43–50.

377. Tanner JE, Stejskal EO. Restricted self-diffusion of protons in colloidal systems by the pulsed-gradient spin-echo method. J Chem Phys 1968; 49:1768–1778.

378. Turner R, Le Bihan D. Single shot diffusion imaging at 2 Tesla. J Magn Reson 1990; 86:445–452.

379. Basser PJ, Pierpaoli C. A simplified method to measure the diffusion tensor from seven MR images. Magn Reson Med 1998; 39(6): 928–934.

380. Basser PJ, Mattiello J, LeBihan D. MR diffusion tensor spectroscopy and imaging. Biophys J 1994; 66(1):259–267.

381. Pierpaoli C, Basser PJ. Toward a quantitative assessment of diffusion anisotropy. Magn Reson Med 1996; 36(6):893–906.

382. Mori S, Van Zijl PC. Fiber tracking: principles and strategies – a technical review. NMR Biomed 2002; 15(7–8):468–480.

383. Catani M, Howard RJ, Pajevic S, Jones DK. Virtual in vivo interactive dissection of white matter fasciculi in the human brain. Neuroimage 2002; 17(1):77–94.

384. Pierpaoli C, Barnett A, Pajevic S, Chen R, Penix LR, Virta A et al. Water diffusion changes in Wallerian degeneration and their dependence on white matter architecture. Neuroimage 2001; 13(6 pt 1): 1174–1185.

385. Jansons KM, Alexander DC. Persistent angular structure: new insights from diffusion MRI data. Dummy version. Inf Process Med Imaging 2003; 18:672–683.

386. Tournier JD, Calamante F, Gadian DG, Connelly A. Direct estimation of the fiber orientation density function from diffusion-weighted MRI data using spherical deconvolution. Neuroimage 2004; 23(3): 1176–1185.

387. Tuch DS. Q-ball imaging. Magn Reson Med 2004; 52(6):1358–1372.

388. Anderson AW. Measurement of fiber orientation distributions using high angular resolution diffusion imaging. Magn Reson Med 2005; 54(5):1194–1206.

389. Behrens TE, Berg HJ, Jbabdi S, Rushworth MF, Woolrich MW. Probabilistic diffusion tractography with multiple fibre orientations: what can we gain? Neuroimage 2007; 34(1):144–155.

390. Tournier JD, Calamante F, Connelly A. Robust determination of the fibre orientation distribution in diffusion MRI: non-negativity constrained super-resolved spherical deconvolution. Neuroimage 2007; 35(4):1459–1472.

391. Behrens TE, Johansen-Berg H, Woolrich MW, Smith SM, Wheeler-Kingshott CA, Boulby PA et al. Non-invasive mapping of connections between human thalamus and cortex using diffusion imaging. Nat Neurosci 2003; 6(7):750–757.

392. Villringer A, Rosen BR, Belliveau JW, Ackerman JL, Lauffer RB, Buxton RB et al. Dynamic imaging with lanthanide chelates in normal brain: contrast due to magnetic susceptibility effects. Magn Reson Med 1988; 6(2):164–174.

393. Ostergaard L, Weisskoff RM, Chesler DA, Gyldensted C, Rosen BR. High resolution measurement of cerebral blood flow using intravascular tracer bolus passages. Part I: Mathematical approach and statistical analysis. Magn Reson Med 1996; 36(5):715–725.

394. Sorensen AG. What is the meaning of quantitative CBF? AJNR Am J Neuroradiol 2001; 22(2):235–236.

395. Calamante F, Gadian DG, Connelly A. Quantification of perfusion using bolus tracking magnetic resonance imaging in stroke: assumptions, limitations, and potential implications for clinical use. Stroke 2002; 33(4):1146–1151.

396. Ostergaard L, Johannsen P, Poulsen PH, Vestergaard-Poulsen P, Asboe H, Gee AD et al. Cerebral blood flow measurements by magnetic resonance imaging bolus tracking: comparison with [O-15] H₂O positron emission tomography in humans. J Cereb Blood Flow Metab 1998; 18:935–940.

397. Schreiber WG, Guckel F, Stritzke P, Schmiedek P, Schwartz A, Brix G. Cerebral blood flow and cerebrovascular reserve capacity: estimation by dynamic magnetic resonance imaging. J Cereb Blood Flow Metab 1998; 18(10):1143–1156.

398. Shin W, Horowitz S, Ragin A, Chen Y, Walker M, Carroll TJ. Quantitative cerebral perfusion using dynamic susceptibility contrast MRI: evaluation of reproducibility and age- and gender-dependence with fully automatic image post-proessing algorithm. Magn Reson Med 2007; 58:1232–1241.

399. Mukherjee P, Kang HC, Videen TO, McKinstry RC, Powers WJ, Derdeyn CP. Measurement of cerebral blood flow in chronic carotid occlusive disease: comparison of dynamic susceptibility contrast perfusion MR imaging with positron emission tomography. AJNR Am J Neuroradiol 2003; 24(5):862–871.

400. Grandin CB, Bol A, Smith AM, Michel C, Cosnard G. Absolute CBF and CBV measurements by MRI bolus tracking before and after acetazolamide challenge: repeatabilily and comparison with PET in humans. Neuroimage 2005; 26(2):525–535.

401. Takasawa M, Jones PS, Guadagno JV, Christensen S, Fryer TD, Harding S et al. How reliable is perfusion MR in acute stroke? Validation and determination of the penumbra threshold against quantitative PET. Stroke 2008; 39(3):870–877.

402. Calamante F, Willats L, Gadian DG, Connelly A. Bolus delay and dispersion in perfusion MRI: implications for tissue predictor models in stroke. Magn Reson Med 2006; 55(5):1180–1185.

403. Calamante F, Gadian DG, Connelly A. Delay and dispersion effects in dynamic susceptibility contrast MRI: simulations using singular value decomposition. Magn Reson Med 2000; 44(3):466–473.

404. Ibaraki M, Shimosegawa E, Toyoshima H, Takahashi K, Miura S, Kanno I. Tracer delay correction of cerebral blood flow with dynamic susceptibility contrast-enhanced MRI. J Cereb Blood Flow Metab 2005; 25(3):378–390.

405. Rose SE, Janke AL, Griffin M, Finnigan S, Chalk JB. Improved prediction of final infarct volume using bolus delay-corrected perfusion-weighted MRI: implications for the ischemic penumbra. Stroke 2004; 35(11):2466–2471.

406. Smith AM, Grandin CB, Duprez T, Mataigne F, Cosnard G. Whole brain quantitative CBF and CBV measurements using MRI bolus tracking: comparison of methodologies. Magn Reson Med 2000; 43(4):559–564.

407. Wu O, Ostergaard L, Weisskoff RM, Benner T, Rosen BR, Sorensen AG. Tracer arrival timing-insensitive technique for estimating flow in MR perfusion-weighted imaging using singular value decomposition with a block-circulant deconvolution matrix. Magn Reson Med 2003; 50(1):164–174.

408. Smith MR, Lu H, Trochet S, Frayne R. Removing the effect of SVD algorithmic artifacts present in quantitative MR perfusion studies. Magn Reson Med 2004; 51(3):631–634.

409. Calamante F. Bolus dispersion issues related to the quantification of perfusion MRI data. J Magn Reson Imaging 2005; 22(6):718–722.

410. Calamante F, Morup M, Hansen LK. Defining a local arterial input function for perfusion MRI using independent component analysis. Magn Reson Med 2004; 52(4):789–797.

411. Lorenz C, Benner T, Lopez CJ, Ay H, Zhu MW, Aronen H et al. Effect of using local arterial input functions on cerebral blood flow estimation. J Magn Reson Imaging 2006; 24(1):57–65.

412. Gruner R, Bjornara BT, Moen G, Taxt T. Magnetic resonance brain perfusion imaging with voxel-specific arterial input functions. J Magn Reson Imaging 2006; 23(3):273–284.

413. Fischer H, Ladebeck R. Echo-planar imaging image artefacts. In: Echo-Planar Imaging. Theory, Technique and Application (eds F Schmitt, MK Stehling, R Turner). Berlin: Springer; 1998; 179–200.

414. Detre JA, Leigh JS, Williams DS, Koretsky AP. Perfusion imaging. Magn Reson Med 1992; 23(1):37–45.

415. Williams DS, Detre JA, Leigh JS, Koretsky AP. Magnetic resonance imaging of perfusion using spin inversion of arterial water. Proc Natl Acad Sci USA 1992; 89(1):212–216.

416. Barbier EL, Lamalle L, Decorps M. Methodology of brain perfusion imaging. J Magn Reson Imaging 2001; 13(4):496–520.

417. Petersen ET, Zimine I, Ho YC, Golay X. Non-invasive measurement of perfusion: a critical review of arterial spin labelling techniques. Br J Radiol 2006; 79(944):688–701.

418. Edelman RR, Siewert B, Darby DG, Thangaraj V, Nobre AC, Mesulam MM et al. Qualitative mapping of cerebral blood flow and functional localization with echo-planar MR imaging and signal targeting with alternating radio frequency. Radiology 1994; 192(2): 513–520.

419. Kim SG. Quantification of relative cerebral blood flow change by flow-sensitive alternating inversion recovery (FAIR) technique: application to functional mapping. Magn Reson Med 1995; 34(3): 293–301.

420. Kwong KK, Chesler DA, Weisskoff RM, Donahue KM, Davis TL, Ostergaard L et al. MR perfusion studies with T1-weighted echo planar imaging. Magn Reson Med 1995; 34(6):878–887.

421. Buxton RB, Frank LR, Wong EC, Siewert B, Warach S, Edelman RR. A general kinetic model for quantitative perfusion imaging with arterial spin labeling. Magn Reson Med 1998; 40(3):383–396.

422. Alsop DC, Detre JA. Reduced transit-time sensitivity in noninvasive magnetic resonance imaging of human cerebral blood flow. J Cereb Blood Flow Metab 1996; 16(6):1236–1249.

423. Wong EC, Buxton RB, Frank LR. A theoretical and experimental comparison of continuous and pulsed arterial spin labeling techniques for quantitative perfusion imaging. Magn Reson Med 1998; 40(3): 348–355.

424. Detre JA, Alsop DC, Vives LR, Maccotta L, Teener JW, Raps EC. Noninvasive MRI evaluation of cerebral blood flow in cerebrovascular disease. Neurology 1998; 50(3):633–641.

425. Miranda MJ, Olofsson K, Sidaros K. Noninvasive measurements of regional cerebral perfusion in preterm and term neonates by magnetic resonance arterial spin labeling. Pediatr Res 2006; 60(3): 359–363.

426. Wang J, Licht DJ. Pediatric perfusion MR imaging using arterial spin labeling. Neuroimaging Clin N Am 2006; 16(1):149–167.

427. Detre JA, Wang J. Technical aspects and utility of fMRI using BOLD and ASL. Clin Neurophysiol 2002; 113(5):621–634.

428. Ye FQ, Frank JA, Weinberger DR, McLaughlin AC. Noise reduction in 3D perfusion imaging by attenuating the static signal in arterial spin tagging (ASSIST). Magn Reson Med 2000; 44(1):92–100.

429. Wu WC, Fernandez-Seara M, Detre JA, Wehrli FW, Wang J. A theoretical and experimental investigation of the tagging efficiency of pseudocontinuous arterial spin labeling. Magn Reson Med 2007; 58(5):1020–1027.

430. Fernandez-Seara MA, Edlow BL, Hoang A, Wang J, Feinberg DA, Detre JA. Minimizing acquisition time of arterial spin labeling at 3T. Magn Reson Med 2008; 59(6):1467–1471.

431. Wong EC, Cronin M, Wu WC, Inglis B, Frank LR, Liu TT. Velocity-selective arterial spin labeling. Magn Reson Med 2006; 55(6):1334–1341.

432. Gunther M, Bock M, Schad LR. Arterial spin labeling in combination with a look-locker sampling strategy: inflow turbo-sampling EPI-FAIR (ITS-FAIR). Magn Reson Med 2001; 46(5):974–984.

433. van Laar PJ, van der GJ, Hendrikse J. Brain perfusion territory imaging: methods and clinical applications of selective arterial spin-labeling MR imaging. Radiology 2008; 246(2):354–364.

434. Moseley ME, Cohen Y, Mintorovitch J, Chileuitt L, Shimizu H, Kucharczyk J et al. Early detection of regional cerebral ischemia in cats: comparison of diffusion- and T2-weighted MRI and spectroscopy. Magn Reson Med 1990; 14(2):330–346.

435. Hjort N, Christensen S, Solling C, Ashkanian M, Wu O, Rohl L et al. Ischemic injury detected by diffusion imaging 11 minutes after stroke. Ann Neurol 2005; 58(3):462–465.

436. Benveniste H, Hedlund LW, Johnson GA. Mechanism of detection of acute cerebral ischemia in rats by diffusion-weighted magnetic resonance microscopy. Stroke 1992; 23(5):746–754.

437. Thomas DL, Lythgoe MF, Pell GS, Calamante F, Ordidge RJ. The measurement of diffusion and perfusion in biological systems using magnetic resonance imaging. Phys Med Biol 2000; 45(8):R97–138.

438. Sotak CH. The role of diffusion tensor imaging in the evaluation of ischemic brain injury – a review. NMR Biomed 2002; 15(7–8): 561–569.

439. Busza AL, Allen KL, King MD, van BN, Williams SR, Gadian DG. Diffusion-weighted imaging studies of cerebral ischemia in gerbils. Potential relevance to energy failure. Stroke 1992; 23(11):1602–1612.

440. Crockard HA, Gadian DG, Frackowiak RS, Proctor E, Allen K, Williams SR et al. Acute cerebral ischaemia: concurrent changes in cerebral blood flow, energy metabolites, pH, and lactate measured with hydrogen clearance and ^{31}P and ^{1}H nuclear magnetic resonance spectroscopy. II. Changes during ischaemia. J Cereb Blood Flow Metab 1987; 7(4):394–402.

441. Bhagat YA, Hussain MS, Stobbe RW, Butcher KS, Emery DJ, Shuaib A et al. Elevations of diffusion anisotropy are associated with hyper-acute stroke: a serial imaging study. Magn Reson Imaging 2008; 26(5):683–693.

442. Mintorovitch J, Moseley ME, Chileuitt L, Shimizu H, Cohen Y, Weinstein PR. Comparison of diffusion- and T2-weighted MRI for the early detection of cerebral ischemia and reperfusion in rats. Magn Reson Med 1991; 18(1):39–50.

443. Minematsu K, Li L, Sotak CH, Davis MA, Fisher M. Reversible focal ischemic injury demonstrated by diffusion-weighted magnetic resonance imaging in rats. Stroke 1992; 23(9):1304–1310.

444. Azzopardi D, Wyatt JS, Cady EB, Delpy DT, Baudin J, Stewart AL et al. Prognosis of newborn infants with hypoxic-ischemic brain injury assessed by phosphorus magnetic resonance spectroscopy. Pediatr Res 1989; 25(5):445–451.

445. Thornton JS, Ordidge RJ, Penrice J, Cady EB, Amess PN, Punwani S et al. Anisotropic water diffusion in white and grey matter of the neonatal piglet brain before and after transient hypoxia-ischaemia. Magn Reson Imaging 1997; 15(4):433–440.

446. van Lookeren CM, Thomas GR, Thibodeaux H, Palmer JT, Williams SP, Lowe DG et al. Secondary reduction in the apparent diffusion coefficient of water, increase in cerebral blood volume, and delayed neuronal death after middle cerebral artery occlusion and early reperfusion in the rat. J Cereb Blood Flow Metab 1999; 19(12):1354–1364.

447. Pell GS, Lythgoe MF, Thomas DL, Calamante F, King MD, Gadian DG et al. Reperfusion in a gerbil model of forebrain ischemia using serial magnetic resonance FAIR perfusion imaging. Stroke 1999; 30(6):1263–1270.

448. Beauchamp NJ, Jr, Barker PB, Wang PY, vanZijl PC. Imaging of acute cerebral ischemia. Radiology 1999; 212(2):307–324.

449. Zimmerman RA, Haselgrove JC, Wang Z, Hunter JV, Morriss MC, Hoydu A et al. Advances in pediatric neuroimaging. Brain Dev 1998; 20(5):275–289.

450. Liu AY, Zimmerman RA, Haselgrove JC, Bilaniuk LT, Hunter JV. Diffusion-weighted imaging in the evaluation of watershed hypoxicischemic brain injury in pediatric patients. Neuroradiology 2001; 43(11):918–926.

451. Kidwell CS, Saver JL, Mattiello J, Starkman S, Vinuela F, Duckwiler G et al. Thrombolytic reversal of acute human cerebral ischemic injury shown by diffusion-perfusion magnetic resonance imaging. Ann Neurol 2000; 47(4):462–469.

452. Welch KM, Windham J, Knight RA, Nagesh V, Hugg JW, Jacobs M et al. A model to predict the histopathology of human stroke using diffusion and T2-weighted magnetic resonance imaging. Stroke 1995; 26(11):1983–1989.

453. Cowan FM, Pennock JM, Hanrahan JD, Manji KP, Edwards AD. Early detection of cerebral infarction and hypoxic ischemic encephalopathy in neonates using diffusion-weighted magnetic resonance imaging. Neuropediatrics 1994; 25(4):172–175.

454. Johnson AJ, Lee BC, Lin W. Echoplanar diffusion-weighted imaging in neonates and infants with suspected hypoxic-ischemic injury: correlation with patient outcome. AJR Am J Roentgenol 1999; 172(1):219–226.

455. Robertson RL, Ben-Sira L, Barnes PD, Mulkern RV, Robson CD, Maier SE et al. MR line-scan diffusion-weighted imaging of term neonates with perinatal brain ischemia. AJNR Am J Neuroradiol 1999; 20(9):1658–1670.

456. Neil JJ, McKinstry RC, Schlaggar BL, Schefft GL, Shiran SI, Shimony JS et al. Evaluation of diffusion anisotropy during human cortical grey matter development. In: Proc ISMRM, 8th Annual Meeting (Denver, USA), 2000; 591.

457. Werring DJ, Clark CA, Barker GJ, Thompson AJ, Miller DH. Diffusion tensor imaging of lesions and normal-appearing white matter in multiple sclerosis. Neurology 1999; 52(8):1626–1632.

458. Jones DK, Lythgoe D, Horsfield MA, Simmons A, Williams SC, Markus HS. Characterisation of white matter damage in ischemic leukoaraiosis with diffusion tensor MRI. Stroke 1999; 30(2):393–397.

459. Chabriat H, Pappata S, Poupon C, Clark CA, Vahedi K, Poupon F et al. Clinical severity in CADASIL related to ultrastructural damage in white matter: in vivo study with diffusion tensor MRI. Stroke 1999; 30(12):2637–2643.

460. Horsfield MA, Jones DK. Applications of diffusion-weighted and diffusion tensor MRI to white matter diseases – a review. NMR Biomed 2002; 15(7–8):570–577.

461. Sorensen AG, Copen WA, Ostergaard L, Buonanno FS, Gonzalez RG, Rordorf G et al. Hyperacute stroke: simultaneous measurement of relative cerebral blood volume, relative cerebral blood flow, and mean tissue transit time. Radiology 1999; 210(2):519–527.

462. Yang Q, Tress BM, Barber PA, Desmond PM, Darby DG, Gerraty RP et al. Serial study of apparent diffusion coefficient and anisotropy in patients with acute stroke. Stroke 1999; 30(11):2382–2390.

463. Zelaya F, Flood N, Chalk JB, Wang D, Doddrell DM, Strugnell W et al. An evaluation of the time dependence of the anisotropy of the water diffusion tensor in acute human ischemia. Magn Reson Imaging 1999; 17(3):331–348.

464. Newton JM, Ward NS, Parker GJ, Deichmann R, Alexander DC, Friston KJ et al. Non-invasive mapping of corticofugal fibres from multiple motor areas – relevance to stroke recovery. Brain 2006; 129(Pt 7):1844–1858.

465. Stinear CM, Barber PA, Smale PR, Coxon JP, Fleming MK, Byblow WD. Functional potential in chronic stroke patients depends on corticospinal tract integrity. Brain 2007; 130(Pt 1):170–180.

466. Kunimatsu A, Itoh D, Nakata Y, Kunimatsu N, Aoki S, Masutani Y et al. Utilization of diffusion tensor tractography in combination with spatial normalization to assess involvement of the corticospinal tract in capsular/pericapsular stroke: feasibility and clinical implications. J Magn Reson Imaging 2007; 26(6):1399–1404.

467. Breier JI, Hasan KM, Zhang W, Men D, Papanicolaou AC. Language dysfunction after stroke and damage to white matter tracts evaluated using diffusion tensor imaging. AJNR Am J Neuroradiol 2008; 29(3):483–487.

468. Thomalla G, Glauche V, Koch MA, Beaulieu C, Weiller C, Rother J. Diffusion tensor imaging detects early Wallerian degeneration of the pyramidal tract after ischemic stroke. Neuroimage 2004; 22(4):1767–1774.

469. van Pul C, Buijs J, Janssen MJ, Roos GF, Vlaardingerbroek MT, Wijn PF. Selecting the best index for following the temporal evolution of apparent diffusion coefficient and diffusion anisotropy after hypoxic-ischemic white matter injury in neonates. AJNR Am J Neuroradiol 2005; 26(3):469–481.

470. van Pul C, Buijs J, Vilanova A, Roos FG, Wijn PF. Infants with perinatal hypoxic ischemia: feasibility of fiber tracking at birth and 3 months. Radiology 2006; 240(1):203–214.

471. Gilmore JH, Lin W, Corouge I, Vetsa YS, Smith JK, Kang C et al. Early postnatal development of corpus callosum and corticospinal white matter assessed with quantitative tractography. AJNR Am J Neuroradiol 2007; 28(9):1789–1795.

472. Berman JI, Mukherjee P, Partridge SC, Miller SP, Ferriero DM, Barkovich AJ et al. Quantitative diffusion tensor MRI fiber tractography of sensorimotor white matter development in premature infants. Neuroimage 2005; 27(4):862–871.

473. Partridge SC, Mukherjee P, Berman JI, Henry RG, Miller SP, Lu Y et al. Tractography-based quantitation of diffusion tensor imaging parameters in white matter tracts of preterm newborns. J Magn Reson Imaging 2005; 22(4):467–474.

474. Hoon AH, Jr, Lawrie WT, Jr, Melhem ER, Reinhardt EM, Van Zijl PC, Solaiyappan M et al. Diffusion tensor imaging of periventricular leukomalacia shows affected sensory cortex white matter pathways. Neurology 2002; 59(5):752–756.

475. Thomas B, Eyssen M, Peeters R, Molenaers G, Van HP, De CP et al. Quantitative diffusion tensor imaging in cerebral palsy due to periventricular white matter injury. Brain 2005; 128(Pt 11): 2562–2577.

476. Huppi PS, Dubois J. Diffusion tensor imaging of brain development. Semin Fetal Neonatal Med 2006; 11(6):489–497.

477. Wang PY, Barker PB, Wityk RJ, Ulug AM, Van Zijl PC, Beauchamp NJ, Jr. Diffusion-negative stroke: a report of two cases. AJNR Am J Neuroradiol 1999; 20(10):1876–1880.

478. Sunshine JL, Bambakidis N, Tarr RW, Lanzieri CF, Zaidat OO, Suarez JI et al. Benefits of perfusion MR imaging relative to diffusion MR imaging in the diagnosis and treatment of hyperacute stroke. AJNR Am J Neuroradiol 2001; 22(5):915–921.

479. Hjort N, Butcher K, Davis SM, Kidwell CS, Koroshetz WJ, Rother J et al. Magnetic resonance imaging criteria for thrombolysis in acute cerebral infarct. Stroke 2005; 36(2):388–397.

480. Beaulieu C, de CA, Tong DC, Moseley ME, Albers GW, Marks MP. Longitudinal magnetic resonance imaging study of perfusion and diffusion in stroke: evolution of lesion volume and correlation with clinical outcome. Ann Neurol 1999; 46(4):568–578.

481. Chalela JA, Alsop DC, Gonzalez-Atavales JB, Maldjian JA, Kasner SE, Detre JA. Magnetic resonance perfusion imaging in acute ischemic stroke using continuous arterial spin labeling. Stroke 2000; 31(3):680–687.

482. Kane I, Sandercock P, Wardlaw J. Magnetic resonance perfusion diffusion mismatch and thrombolysis in acute ischaemic stroke: a systematic review of the evidence to date. J Neurol Neurosurg Psychiatry 2007; 78(5):485–491.

483. Neumann-Haefelin T, Wittsack HJ, Wenserski F, Siebler M, Seitz RJ, Modder U et al. Diffusion- and perfusion-weighted MRI. The DWI/PWI mismatch region in acute stroke. Stroke 1999; 30(8): 1591–1597.

484. Neumann-Haefelin T, Wittsack HJ, Wenserski F, Li TQ, Moseley ME, Siebler M et al. Diffusion- and perfusion-weighted MRI in a patient with a prolonged reversible ischaemic neurological deficit. Neuroradiology 2000; 42(6):444–447.

485. Grandin CB, Duprez TP, Smith AM, Mataigne F, Peeters A, Oppenheim C et al. Usefulness of magnetic resonance-derived quantitative measurements of cerebral blood flow and volume in prediction of infarct growth in hyperacute stroke. Stroke 2001; 32(5):1147–1153.

486. Wu O, Koroshetz WJ, Ostergaard L, Buonanno FS, Copen WA, Gonzalez RG et al. Predicting tissue outcome in acute human cerebral ischemia using combined diffusion- and perfusion-weighted MR imaging. Stroke 2001; 32(4):933–942.

487. Connelly A, Calamante F, Porter DA, Gadian DG. Case study on diffusion and perfusion magnetic resonance imaging in childhood stroke. Electromedica 2000; 68:2–8.

488. Tzika AA, Massoth RJ, Ball WS, Jr, Majumdar S, Dunn RS, Kirks DR. Cerebral perfusion in children: detection with dynamic contrast-enhanced T2*-weighted MR images. Radiology 1993; 187(2): 449–458.

489. Oguz KK, Golay X, Pizzini FB, Freer CA, Winrow N, Ichord R et al. Sickle-cell disease: continuous arterial spin-labelling perfusion MR imaging in children. Radiology 2003; 227(2):567–574.

490. Tzika AA, Robertson RL, Barnes PD, Vajapeyam S, Burrows PE, Treves ST et al. Childhood moyamoya disease: hemodynamic MRI. Pediatr Radiol 1997; 27(9):727–735.

491. Tsuchiya K, Inaoka S, Mizutani Y, Hachiya J. Echo-planar perfusion MR of moyamoya disease. AJNR Am J Neuroradiol 1998; 19(2):211–216.

492. Adams WM, Laitt RD, Li KL, Jackson A, Sherrington CR, Talbot P. Demonstration of cerebral perfusion abnormalities in moyamoya disease using susceptibility perfusion- and diffusion-weighted MRI. Neuroradiology 1999; 41(2):86–92.

493. Guckel FJ, Brix G, Schmiedek P, Piepgras Z, Becker G, Kopke J et al. Cerebrovascular reserve capacity in patients with occlusive cerebrovascular disease: assessment with dynamic susceptibility contrast-enhanced MR imaging and the acetazolamide stimulation test. Radiology 1996; 201(2):405–412.

494. Kluytmans M, van der GJ, Viergever MA. Grey matter and white matter perfusion imaging in patients with severe carotid artery lesions. Radiology 1998; 209(3):675–682.

495. Siewert B, Wielopolski PA, Schlaug G, Edelman RR, Warach S. STAR MR angiography for rapid detection of vascular abnormalities in patients with acute cerebrovascular disease. Stroke 1997; 28(6): 1211–1215.

496. Ances BM, McGarvey ML, Abrahams JM, Maldjian JA, Alsop DC, Zager EL et al. Continuous arterial spin labeled perfusion magnetic resonance imaging in patients before and after carotid endarterectomy. J Neuroimaging 2004; 14(2):133–138.

497. Hendrikse J, van Osch MJ, Rutgers DR, Bakker CJ, Kappelle LJ, Golay X et al. Internal carotid artery occlusion assessed at pulsed arterial spin-labeling perfusion MR imaging at multiple delay times. Radiology 2004; 233(3):899–904.

498. Derdeyn CP, Grubb RL, Jr, Powers WJ. Cerebral hemodynamic impairment: methods of measurement and association with stroke risk. Neurology 1999; 53(2):251–259.

5

RISK FACTORS AND TRIGGERS FOR CRYPTOGENIC (AND SYMPTOMATIC) STROKE

5.1 Cerebrovascular Diseases from Infectious/Inflammatory Origin

Guillaume Sébire and Benedicte Michel (with a section on human immunodeficiency virus by Nomazulu Dlamini and Fenella J. Kirkham)

Introduction

A causal link between infection and ischaemic stroke in children has been discussed for decades,[1-8] as concurrent local or systemic infection is temporally associated with cerebral infarction in 20–60% of young patients. In contrast to the large number of case reports, few controlled studies have been undertaken but the available data show that infections of viral and/or bacterial origin (Table 5.1), often involving the respiratory system, occurred more frequently in children[9] and adults[10] with ischaemic strokes than in control individuals (e.g. 34% versus 11% in the paediatric series). Recent upper respiratory tract infection predicted the presence of vasculopathy in the International Paediatric Stroke Study.[11] However, defining the relationship between stroke and infectious diseases is not

an easy matter. The fact that one event bears a temporal relation to another event does not mean that one causes the other. In other studies, infectious events do not clearly appear among the main risk factors for stroke: for example, a non-specific concurrent or previous infection was found in only 10% of children with ischaemic strokes in the series from Montreal.[12] Inflammation located in the arterial wall and attributed to post-infectious mechanisms has been mentioned only rarely in anatomical studies.[1,13] Thus the link between infection and ischaemic stroke, i.e. fortuitous, causal or as a direct or indirect risk factor, remains to be determined.

Some epidemiological definitions must be kept in mind. For instance, to be considered as a cause of a disease, a phenomenon has to fulfil all the main following criteria: (1) temporal

TABLE 5.1
Infections reported as associated with stroke

	Adult	Previously well child	Sickle cell disease
Pneumococcal meningitis	+	+	+
Haemophilus influenzae meningitis	+	+	+
Fusobacterium necrophorum meningitis	+	+	?
Salmonella meningitis	?	+	?
Meningococcal meningitis	+	+	–
Tuberculous meningitis	+	+	+
Tonsillitis	–	+	?
Varicella zoster	+	+	–
Treponema pallidum (syphilis)	+	–	–
Plasmodium falciparum (cerebral malaria)	+	+	?
Amoeba	?	+	?
Cystercercosis	+	+	–
Paragnomiasis	?	+	?
Borrelia burgdorferi (Lyme disease)	+	+	–
Chlamydia pneumoniae	+	–	–
Mycoplasma pneumoniae	+	?	?
Helicobacter pylori	+/–	–	–
Cytomegalovirus	+/–	?	?
Parvovirus B19	–	?	?
Enterovirus	–	?	–
Influenza A	–	?	–
West Nile Virus	+	+	–
Human Immunodeficiency Virus	+	+	–

relationship; (2) biological coherence; (3) convincing differences in disease occurrence between exposed and unexposed patients, using case control or prospective controlled studies; and (4) in certain conditions, a dose–response relation and/or reversibility of the association. Theoretically, a cause is considered either as 'sufficient' if inevitably leading to the disease or as 'necessary' if the disease cannot occur in its absence. A sufficient cause can either be a unique phenomenon or result from the combination of several. For instance, bacterial meningeal infection is a necessary cause but not sufficient to induce vasculitis of large intracranial arteries. This means that additional circumstances, i.e. other contributing aetiologies, are required to promote vasculitis: for instance, a specific genetic background influencing the inflammatory response. In contrast, a risk factor is not sufficient on its own to cause a disease, but increases the likelihood of disease occurrence. It is measured by the relative risk, which allows the definition of the attributable fraction of a specific event in the genesis of a disease. There are distinct subtypes of risk factors. 'Predisposing risk factors' correspond to underlying conditions, such as age, sex, and diabetes. 'Favouring risk factors' are mainly genetic or environmental phenomenon such as infectious agents, diet or lifestyle. Thus, to establish an association, and to describe the type of link between an infectious event and a vascular disease, is a complex task, especially in the context of the relative rarity of strokes in childhood and the high frequency of infections in this age group. However, recent data from animal models and human infectious diseases have shed some light on the role of infection and immunoinflammatory reactions in the pathogenesis of childhood cerebral arteritis.

Animal models of cerebrovascular diseases associated with infections

Vascular disease, such as arteritis, has been demonstrated in natural and experimental viral infections in animals. Inflammation of the arterial wall was well recognized in animal diseases: for example, in horses infected with equine encephalitis virus, and fetal or neonatal infection of sheep with border disease virus (pestivirus). The arteritis of border disease virus involves preferentially the cerebral vessels. It appears 3 weeks after infection and has a protracted evolution over the following 6 months, leading to inflammatory and T-cell infiltration of arteriolar walls. A direct causal effect of border disease virus in arterial brain disease is implicated on the basis that viral antigens have been detected in vessel cells.

The mouse specific γ-herpes 68 virus (γHV) and β-herpes virus (murine cytomegalovirus) both infect multiple cell types, including endothelial cells.[14–16] γHV infection consistently results in vasculitis, which seems to especially affect young animals infected early in postnatal life (D7–D9). Interestingly, the γ-herpes vasculitis is a chronic disease involving specifically the walls of large arteries, leading to occlusion and death within a few weeks. Persistent γHV replication in the walls of the large elastic arteries is required for the maintenance of arteritis. The immune reaction, especially the interferon (IFN)-γ

pathway triggered by the virus, appears to influence, to some extent, the course of the vascular disease,[17,18] and the disruption of the IFN-γ pathway results in a significant worsening of the vasculitis. However, a major role for the virus is suggested by the dramatic improvement of the vascular lesions with antiviral therapy and the lack of immuno-inflammatory reaction detected in the vessels beyond the infected areas. Thus, murine herpes virus causes acute large-vessels arteritis, with some features in common with human vascular diseases. These models support the hypothesis that human cerebrovascular diseases could be associated with direct viral infection of cells from the vessel wall.

Cerebrovascular diseases and infections in human

BACTERIAL INFECTIONS AND VASCULITIS: A MODEL OF
CAUSAL LINK BETWEEN INFECTIOUS AGENTS AND
ISCHAEMIC STROKES

Cerebral infarction is not uncommon in meningitis (Fig. 5.1), particularly in those presenting under a year with *Streptococcus pneumoniae* (Fig. 5.1) and salmonella.[19] It is a particularly important cause of stroke in the developing world.[20] *Haemophilus influenzae* was also described as a cause of acute and delayed stroke in about 5% of patients in the era before vaccination (Fig. 5.1).[21,22] Frontal infarcts are typical[23] but basal ganglia strokes may appear in association with basal vasculopathy[24] and parieto-occipital involvement has been reported with blindness as the sequel.[25] In neonates, although vasculopathy may be seen on magnetic resonance angiography (MRA),[23] venous sinus thrombosis may be more common than arterial stroke in association with cerebral infarction[26] and this diagnosis may have been previously under-recognized in older children. Cavernous sinus thrombosis[27] and Lemierre syndrome (jugular venous thrombosis secondary to *Fusobacterium* infection)[28] are particularly serious complications of head and neck infection which may be associated with arterial[27,28] as well as venous sinus thrombosis[29] and meningitis. Around 20% of adults have arterial and 10% venous infarcts,[30] while a recent population-based study suggests that, in the era of vaccination, 40% of children with pneumococcal meningitis have a stroke during the course of the illness, with iron deficiency anaemia a possible risk factor.[31]

Most infarcts in tuberculous meningitis are in the anterior circulation (Fig. 5.1A),[32] although a few involve posterior territories and basilar embolus has been described.[33] There is evidence for a progressive vasculopathy in tuberculous meningitis with evidence of stenosis or spasm initially followed by progressive occlusion,[34] which may be accompanied by early recurrence of infarction.[35] Infarction in any brain region predicts poor outcome in tuberculous meningitis[36] but basal ganglia infarction, particularly if bilateral, is notably ominous.[37,36]

Many years after the introduction of antibiotics to treat bacterial infections, bacterial meningitis is still associated with a heavy burden of mortality and morbidity as, unfortunately, some physiopathological pathways remain, at least in part, out

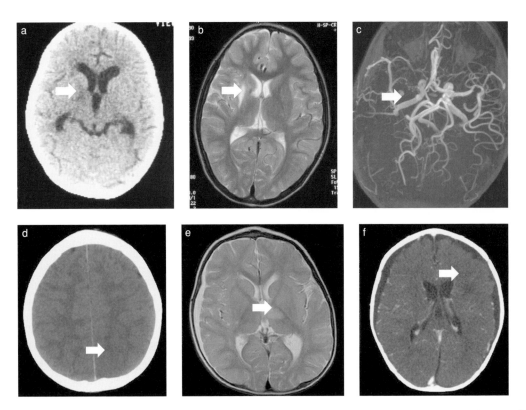

Fig. 5.1. Meningitis. (a) CT scan showing basal ganglia infarction (arrow) in a 1-year-old girl with tuberculous meningitis presenting with status epilepticus. (b) Basal ganglia infarct (arrow) in a child with *Haemophilus influenzae* meningitis. (c) Persistent middle cerebral artery disease (arrow) in the patient with *Haemophilus influenzae* meningitis whose infarct is depicted in B. (d) Venous infarction (arrow) in pneumococcal meningitis. (e) Thalamic infarction (arrow) in pneumococcal meningitis. (f) Lacunar infarction (arrow) and bilateral subdurals in pneumococcal meningitis.

of therapeutic control. Among them is the inflammatory reaction triggered by the infectious agent, which is one of the main mechanisms involved in vasculitis during infections involving the meninges and subarachnoidal spaces. The microvascular endothelium is a key component of the blood–brain barrier, which functions as a very specific filter. This endothelium has unique features, such as rare plasmalemmal vesicles and intercellular tight junctions. A bacterially induced breakdown of the blood–brain barrier is observed in animal models of the disease and this leads to separation of the intercellular tight junctions, increase of cytoplasmic vesicles and permeability to macromolecules such as proteins. In addition to the involvement of the microvasculature, large arterial segments are often invaded by immuno-inflammatory cells. The inflammatory molecular pathways involved in these vasculopathies are now more clearly understood. Diverse bacterial components, such as lipopolysaccharide, are among the most powerful inducers of proinflammatory cytokine (interleukin (IL)-1, tumour necrosis factor TNF-α) release. These cytokines are known to be produced by human blood and cerebral cells (microglia, endothelial cells, monocytes-macrophages)[38–40] inducing expression of cellular adhesion molecules on endothelial cells and triggering synthesis of chemokines, which stimulate neutrophil and monocyte-macrophage adherence to, and diapedesis through, the vascular wall. Within the vascular wall, activated monocytes and neutrophils release cytokines, prostaglandins, leukotrienes,

oxygen radicals and other harmful mediators. Bacterial infection is also known to induce a hypercoagulable state by increasing prothrombotic mediators such as fibrinogen, anti-cardiolipin antibodies and fibrin D-dimer.[6] This cascade may lead to multifocal vasculitis and thrombosis causing brain infarcts.[38]

These observations may have therapeutic implications, for example suggesting the use of adjunctive anti-inflammatory agents. Most studies support the use of corticosteroids in infants and children with tuberculous and other bacterial meningitis,[41,42] although there are few data on whether there is any beneficial effect in terms of the vasculopathy. More specifically targeted antiinflammatory agents, such as cytokine inhibitors or monoclonal antibodies against adhesion proteins, might be tested experimentally to protect the arterial wall.

OTHER AGENTS
In adulthood, a classical example of infectious vasculitis is that induced by *Treponema pallidum* spirochaetes in syphilis. Intima and adventitia are infiltrated by lymphocytes and macrophages. *Borrelia burgdorferi*, another spirochetal agent causing Lyme disease, can penetrate the blood–brain barrier and invade the brain parenchyma to induce neuroborreliosis. This infectious agent might also infiltrate the blood vessel wall to trigger a vasculitis. Some cases have been reported in children as well as in adults.[43–51] Idiopathic intracranial hypertension is also reported as a consequence of *Borrelia* infec-

tion[52–54] and may involve thrombosis or compression of the venous sinuses. Venous sinus thrombosis has been described in malaria[55] and might be the underlying pathophysiology for the subarachnoid haemorrhage[56] and cortical haemorrhagic infarcts[57,58] occasionally described. Much of the pathophysiology appears related to generalized cerebral oedema and reduced cerebral perfusion pressure[59,60] but as sequestration within the venules is the cardinal pathological finding, despite the difficulty of undertaking emergency CT or MR venography in the developing world, excluding venous sinus thrombosis as the underlying cause of the oedema, seizures and intracranial hypertension should be a priority in view of the possibility of anticoagulation treatment (see Chapters 7 and 16). Cystercercosis is an important cause of acute hemiparesis in endemic areas[61,62] and many cases have an associated arteritis.[61,63] It would be rare for the cardiomyopathy of American trypanosomias (Chagas' disease) to be sufficiently advanced for cardioembolic stroke to present in childhood.[64,65] Paragnomiasis has been reported as presenting with recurrent haemorrhagic stroke in China.[66]

Mycoplasma pneumoniae has been described in temporal association with childhood stroke,[67–74] and with acute demyelinating encephalopathy in sickle cell disease.[75] *Chlamydia pneumoniae* and *Helicobacter pylori* infections appear to be associated with strokes in adulthood[76–78] but the one study of *Chlamydia pneumoniae* in children with sickle cell disease showed no association.[79] Other agents, such as *Bartonella henselae* might also be involved.[80] However, it is still unknown whether the association between these infectious agents and stroke is consistent with a causal relationship in adults, or whether they are risk factors, perhaps triggering prothrombotic pathways or altering the balance of the lipid profile, or even whether the association is fortuitous. The majority of publications in children have been case reports and there have been few systematic studies.

ATHEROSCLEROSIS RECENTLY REVISITED BY IMMUNOLOGICAL AND INFECTIOUS APPROACHES: A PARADIGM FOR ARTERIAL WALL DISEASE IN CHILDHOOD?

Atherosclerosis, although multifactorial, is now considered as an inflammatory disease.[81,82] The lesions mainly occur in large and medium sized elastic and muscular arteries in some peculiar sites, such as arterial bifurcations and curvatures. These sites are characterized by modifications of the blood stream: increased turbulence and shear stress. Pathologically, in the first stage of these lesions, lipid-laden monocyte-macrophages are associated in the intimal part of the arterial wall with T lymphocytes and smooth muscle cells. Such lesions are frequently observed in pathological studies of fetuses and infants, suggesting that the disease has a much earlier start than previously thought.[83] Premature atherosclerosis might play a role in childhood cerebrovascular disease, raising the question of whether there are common physiopathological factors shared between atherogenesis and arterial wall diseases in childhood.

Endothelial dysfunction is likely to be one of the first steps of this process. Possible causes include hyper cholesterolaemia, free radical release induced by hypertension, diabetes or smoking, hyperhomocysteinaemia, and other genetic polymorphisms and/or infections.[84,85] The lesions are located, close to the endothelial epithelium, in the intima and are characterized by infiltration of immune cells: foamy macrophages and T lymphocytes mixed with ectopic proliferating smooth-muscle cells. A cascade of molecular synthesis is involved in cell recruitment (adhesion molecules, cytokines and chemokines, such as monocyte chemotactic protein (MCP)-1), cell proliferation (cytokine, such as fibroblast growth factor (FGF)-2 or transforming growth factor (TGF)-β for muscle cell), cell activation (interleukin (IL)-2 and IL-1 for T lymphocytes) and cell death (free radicals, proinflammatory cytokines and proteolytic enzymes such as metalloproteinases).[84] A heat shock protein, HSP-60, is implicated in atherosclerosis and titres are correlated with the degree of carotid atherosclerosis.[86] T-cell lines cultured from the atherosclerosis plaque proliferate when exposed to HSP-60.[81] Animal models provide other clues for the role of inflammatory reactions in the pathogenesis of the arterial diseases. For instance, IL-10, which inhibits metalloproteinase, proinflammatory cytokines and chemokines synthesis, has a protective role. Immunization of such models with HSP-60 leads to atherosclerotic plaque formation. The study of a xenotransplantation model – insertion of human arteries into the aorta of immunodeficient mice – showed that IFN-γ can induce arteriosclerotic changes by acting on vascular smooth muscle cells to potentiate growth factor induced mitogenesis.[87]

Some infectious agents seem to play a role in the pathophysiology of atherosclerosis. There is a close relationship between *Chlamydiae pneumoniae* infection, IgG and IgM titers, and increased evidence of atherosclerosis, including cerebrovascular lesions. *Chlamydia pneumoniae* and herpes virus antigens, such as CMV, are detected in atheromatous lesions.[81] Moreover, increased antibodies directed against these infectious agents have been correlated with progression of atheroma.[88] *Helicobacter pylori* and Epstein–Barr may also play a role and recent data have shown an association between atherosclerosis and chronic infection, such as bronchitis or periodontitis.[77,89,90] This suggests that any infectious agent, perhaps particularly those with multiple chronic manifestations, could accelerate atherosclerosis formation.[81] However, this remains a controversial area, in terms of which infectious agents might be involved and whether infection is an early trigger for endothelial dysfunction or an amplifier of an existing process.[91]

VIRAL INFECTION

Varicella zoster virus (VZV)

Cumulative evidence suggests that VZV can infect the walls of cerebral arteries and cause stroke in adult humans.[92] In adults, a causal relationship between herpes zoster ophthalmicus and delayed (days to months) infarction of the ipsilateral cerebral hemisphere is well established.[93,94] Zoster-related retinal arteritis has also been reported.[95,96] The course of the disease is usually uniphasic. Histopathological findings vary from thrombosis without vasculitic changes to a necrotizing granulomatous angiitis of uncertain aetiology.[97] Pathological studies showed patchy anomalies from one artery to another, as well as within a given artery: disruption of the internal elastic lamina, inflammatory response and fibrinoid necrosis.[98-100] From the pathophysiological point of view, there may be a viral induced auto immune process and/or a persistent infection of cerebral vessels. Viruses with the morphological aspect of herpes virus, VZV antigens and DNA have been detected in affected cerebral vessels in some cases,[93,97,101] but not all,[102] giving some support for the latter hypothesis.

Strokes following chickenpox in children have been reported as a number of single case reports and cases series.[103-105] However, this temporal link could have been fortuitous owing to the high frequency of this infection in this age group. In order to assess the relationship between *varicella* and idiopathic arterial ischaemic stroke in children, a case-control study was carried out demonstrating a significant statistical link between these strokes and *varicella* zoster virus infection.[106] The frequency of *varicella* with delayed hemiparesis was estimated to be 1:6500 *varicella* patients in Japan.[107] In retrospective studies of arterial ischaemic strokes, whatever the proportion of any underlying aetiology, about 15–20% of the children were reported to have had chickenpox during the 6–12 months preceding the infarct,[108-110] with an excess in the cryptogenic group in one series.[110] Prior *varicella* infection was not reported in a study from Montreal[12] but has been reported in the Toronto series.[105,111] These patients have a seemingly homogeneous presentation.[103-105,107,111-118] Typically the disease occurs in pre- and primary schoolchildren (mean age 4 years) with a delayed onset relative to the rash (mean 2 months; range 1 week to 12 months). Most of these children present with hemiparesis, aphasia or dysarthria, but not seizures or alteration of consciousness. The infarcts, mostly lacunar, are located in the basal ganglia and the internal capsule. The arterial lesions typically involve unilaterally the distal segment of the internal carotid artery and/or proximal portions of the anterior and middle cerebral arteries. Surprisingly, in view of the small size and deep location of parenchymal defects, arterial lesions often involve large vessels (supraclinoid portion and initial branches of carotid artery) (Fig. 5.2). Several hypotheses could account for this apparent discrepancy. The arteriopathy might be more extensive than suspected on the basis of the imaging results, since angiography does not enable visualization of small vessels such as lenticulostriate arteries, which might be associated with the lesions of large vessels. On the other hand, lesions of the large basal arteries detected by arteriography might be the visible manifestation of pathology arising at the origin of the lenticulostriate arteries. Finally, severe reduction of blood flow could be induced by vasculopathy affecting the large basal arteries with a more pronounced effect on deep areas than on cortex, where collateralization is better. One of the most striking features of this arteriopathy is the transient nature of the physiopathological process, which is typically monophasic.[111,119] This may be demonstrated arteriographically, by repeated examination showing regression or stabilization of arterial lesions often after an initial worsening, and/or by a long term clinical follow-up revealing some rare short-term recurrence of transient ischaemic attack or stroke, usually in the same arterial territory, in about one-third of the patients (Fig. 5.2),[111,120] but little evidence for long-term recurrence. An inflammatory and/or infectious process affecting the arterial wall seems to be the most likely physiopathological hypothesis. In favour are the detection of a protracted cerebrospinal fluid (CSF) inflammatory reaction (lymphocytes) in a significant number of the patients and IgG antibody synthesis against VZV in the CSF in some patients.[106,115] VZV DNA was only rarely detected by polymerase chain reaction in the CSF but very few patients have been studied.[106,121] Interestingly, some recent neuropathological observations from patients who died at the time of stroke detected VZV antigens by immunohistochemistry in the lesions of the arterial wall.[116] Some observations suggest a link between VZV infection and transient coagulopathies: deficiencies of protein S and protein C, synthesis of autoantibodies directed against cardiolipin or protein S. However it is not clear if these observations reflect only an epiphenomenon or could play a role in a physiopathological cascade.

Most children, around two thirds, had complete recovery or only mild deficiency. Life-threatening infarcts are very rare.[116] Rarely, patients have more severe arteriopathy, including moyamoya.[104]

We currently have an evidence-based association between chickenpox and brain infarcts in childhood. The precise position of this virus with regard to the physiopathology of the arteriopathy seems to be a direct infection of the arterial wall which might be associated with a local inflammatory reaction. In this context, some therapeutic intervention, for example antiviral and/or anti-inflammatory, might be tested. Of note is the global reduction of neurological complications, but without any specifically vascular analysis, obtained with a more systematic application of VZV vaccine in childhood.[122] However, stroke has been reported after *varicella* immunization[123] and the risk–benefit ratio may require requires further study.

Other viruses

Hepatitis B and C viruses have been associated with arteritis, some of them involving brain arteries. About 30% of patients with periarteritis nodosa have positive blood detection of hepatitis B surface antigen. Immunohistochemical studies of inflamed arteries detected this antigen. This arteriopathy had most often an acute course. Pathological studies in biopsy proven cases of hepatitis B-associated vasculitis showed intimal perforation, fibrinoid necrosis and periarterial infiltration of inflammatory cells.[124] Benefit from an antiviral agent (lamivudine) has been reported in the treatment of polyarteritis nodosa.[125,126] Stroke has also been reported in enteroviral,[127] parvovirus[128] and West Nile[129,130] viral infections in childhood.

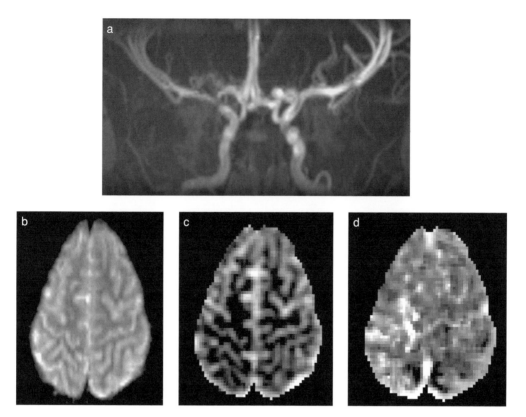

Fig. 5.2. Postvaricella angiopathy. (a) Magnetic resonance (MR) angiography in a 9-year-old boy who had nine clinical left-sided transient ischaemic attacks aged 18 months (9 months after chickenpox) and subsequently developed functionally disabling dystonia (b). MR imaging shows no infarct on this slice (there was a small infarct in the right lentiform nucleus). (c) Cerebral blood flow is reduced over a wide area in the right hemisphere which is more obvious on the mean transit time map (d).

Immunocompromised patients

Stroke has been described in several immunodeficiences,[110] but the best studied is human immunodeficiency virus (HIV), where there is some evidence for direct invasion of the vasculature by the virus.

Human immunodeficiency virus

Neurological dysfunction is a particularly distressing component of HIV infection in children. Reports from North America suggest that more than 50% of children with acquired immune deficiency syndrome (AIDS) have evidence of an encephalopathy, and in a prospective study from the European Collaborative Group,[131] neurological involvement was seen in 31% of children with HIV infection. In contrast with affected adults and children in the developing world,[132,133] opportunistic CNS infections are uncommon in children with AIDS in the developed world, and it seems likely that direct HIV infection of microglial and mononuclear cells is primarily responsible for the neurological manifestations of the disease. Two distinct encephalopathic syndromes have been described. The most common form is a progressive encephalopathy characterized initially by a subtle deterioration in cognitive, language and social skills, and later associated with arrest of head growth, and with pyramidal, extrapyramidal and cerebellar dysfunction. Serial CT may reveal progressive cerebral atrophy, white matter attenuation suggestive of demyelination and calcification of the basal ganglia. Although this condition may plateau, it is nevertheless thought to be clinically, radiologically and neurophysiologically distinct from the alternative form, a static encephalopathy seen in 25% of symptomatic children who present with developmental delay without regression. In both groups of children, the advent of focal neurological signs may indicate haemorrhagic or ischaemic infarction, a lymphoma, or an opportunistic infection. In the era before evidence-based treatment for HIV, the estimated clinical incidence of stroke in children with HIV was 1.3% per year but silent haemorrhagic and ischaemic stroke are also very common.[134]

Various types of cerebrovascular disease, including aneurysms (often multiple) and occlusive disease, have been reported in association with HIV1 infection, either at presentation or during the course of the disease (Fig. 5.3).[99,134–145] Large brain arterial involvement is characterized by a necrotizing vasculitis. The main histological anomalies are located within the adventitia: leukocytoclastic vasculitis of the vasa vasorum, angiogenesis, periadventitial vessels, chronic inflammation and fibrosis.[141] The aetiopathogenesis remains speculative but a multifactorial hypothesis is likely, combining several factors, such as opportunist infections, direct HIV infection, drug-induced toxic factors, prothrombotic factors (e.g. protein S deficiency) and inflammatory components which could act separately or in combination.[142–145] Evidence that vascular changes are provoked directly by the HIV infection include

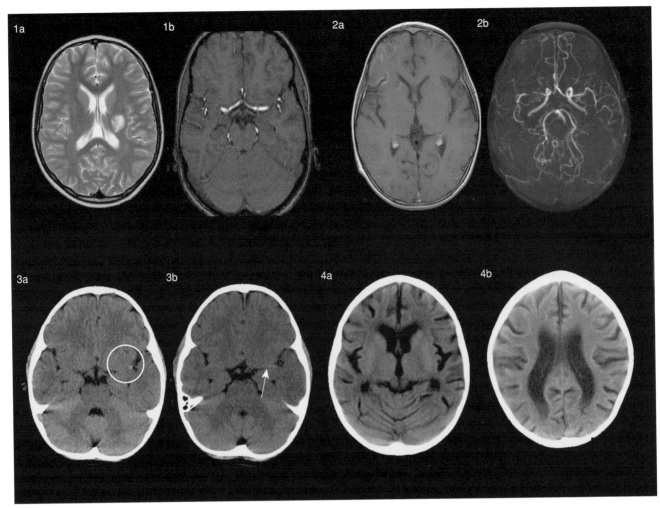

Fig. 5.3. Human immunodeficiency virus. (1a,1b) MRI showing a left basal ganglia infarct and left middle cerebral artery stenosis. (2a,2b) MRI showing attenuation of the middle cerebral artery with moyamoya-like collaterals. (3a,3b) CT scan showing a hyperdense left middle cerebral artery (circle, arrow) compatible with acute occlusion. (4a,4b) CT showing gross brain shrinkage. Courtesy of Dr Tracy Kilborn, Red Cross War Memorial Hospital, University of Cape Town, South Africa.

reports of cerebral vasculopathy with stenosis[142,143] and aneurysm formation[144] in children with HIV infection, and changes in vasomotor reactivity in patients with HIV infection without cerebrovascular symptoms.[145] The possibility that HIV-associated neuronal damage may be mediated by a metabolic dysregulation is supported by the virtual absence of HIV in neurones, astrocytes and oligodendrocytes in post-mortem tissue. There appears to be a similarity between the basal ganglia calcification and demyelination of HIV encephalopathy and lesions seen in children with defective folate metabolism. Surtees et al[146] reported low levels of the methyl group carriers (5H methyl-tetrahydrofolate, methionine and *S*-adenosylmethionine) and raised neopterins in the CSF of children with neurological complications of HIV infection. They postulated that neopterins, released from activated macrophages, may inhibit folate metabolism and suggested that treatment might be effective with methyl group donors such as methionine or betaine. Interestingly, brain tissues from several children with HIV encephalopathy have been studied with specific attention to the vessels. Angiocentric CD3 and CD8 positive T-cell infiltrates

were frequently observed. Rare perivascular macrophages were positive for viral proteins (p24) in a small proportion of the patients. There was no opportunistic viral infection. Based on these data, an autoimmune mechanism was suspected.[139,140] Antiretroviral treatment of paediatric AIDS prevents some but not all of the cognitive consequences;[147] there are few data on the effect on stroke risk in children despite concerns over atherogenesis in adults. Many patients with HIV also have a dyslipidaemia and other evidence of metabolic syndrome,[148] but although statins may reduce plasma lipids, they have little effect on CNS inflammation.[149]

FUNGAL VASCULITIS
Fungi are among the most common agents implicated in infectious complications associated with immunodeficiencies, but also occur in immunocompetent patients. Fungal emboli can be located in the intracranial arteries allowing the penetration of these agents in the vessel wall. The infectious/inflammatory invasion of large cerebral arteries can also result from fungal meningitis – sometimes eosinophilic – diffusing

to adjacent arteries. This results in a vasculitic process, seemingly due to fungal invasion of the arterial wall.[150] The most common fungi associated with ischaemic strokes are aspergillus, candida, coccioides and mucormycosis.[151,152] Aspergillus infection seems to involve large basal arterial wall and perforating arteries territories (basal nuclei).[153]

Conclusion

Research on childhood stroke has been limited by questionable classification of subtypes and by variations in coding. Understanding risk factors, such as infections, that predispose to stroke and influence its outcome will help in the design of therapeutic trials and prevention programmes. Decades of data collection on the epidemiology, aetiology and natural history of stroke have increased our knowledge of these diseases in childhood. However the role of numerous infectious agents still remains to be precisely defined.

The above mentioned infectious agents suspected to be associated with cerebrovascular disease and neurological symptoms should be sought in childhood ischaemic strokes with no obvious aetiologies provided by prior medical history. However, even in this situation we have to keep in mind that infectious agents can be combined with other factors or causes to produce the disease, as has been demonstrated for atherosclerosis. Thus, further extensive investigations are needed to define simultaneously the type of vascular anomalies, blood and CSF inflammatory markers, and infectious agents involved. Clearly, progress in this field requires controlled studies of well-characterized groups of patients allowing separate analysis of distinct conditions according to the clinicoradiological pattern as well as inflammatory and infectious markers of the diseases.

Acknowledgement
We are very grateful to Thomas Michiels, MD, PhD (Université catholique de Louvain, Belgium) for helpful discussion.

5.2 Thrombophilia and Childhood Stroke

Ulrike Nowak-Göttl and Ronald Sträter

Pathophysiology of vascular occlusion

The formation and growth of a thrombus are the result of local coagulation activation, combined with a disturbance in the balance between coagulation and fibrinolysis, leading to a prothrombotic state. Elevated thrombin generation with subsequent thrombus formation occurs in the context of a number of clinical and environmental conditions: the use of central lines, trauma or surgery, vessel abnormalities, malignant diseases, autoimmune diseases, cardiac malformations, polycythaemia, renal diseases, perinatal asphyxia, maternal diabetes, dehydration, septicaemia, obesity, acquired antiphospholipid

antibodies or the presence of lupus anticoagulants.[154–156] In addition, various genetic polymorphisms which affect levels of proteins regulating blood coagulation are well established as risk factors for thrombosis in adults.[157–161]

Owing to the special properties of the haemostatic system during infancy and childhood, symptomatic thrombotic manifestation occurs in 0.07/10 000 children overall, while 5.3/10 000 children and 2.4/1000 neonates admitted to intensive care units are affected.[154,155] Neonates are at greater risk of thromboembolic complications than older children,[162] perhaps due to the lower concentrations of antithrombin, heparin cofactor II and protein C, along with a reduced fibrinolytic capacity. The incidence of vascular accidents decreases significantly after the first year of life, with a second peak during puberty and adolescence, again associated with reduced fibrinolytic activity.[162,163]

Thromboembolic manifestations in children

Besides fetal wastage, preterm birth or intrauterine growth retardation due to placental infarction,[164–167] and peripartal thromboembolic stroke (see Chapter 9),[168–172] high rates of catheter-related thrombosis in neonates, infants and children have recently been demonstrated.[155,156,162] Other venous locations include cerebral,[173–176] renal, portal and mesenteric vein thrombosis.[155,156] Arterial vascular occlusions are usually associated with ischaemic stroke in neonates and older children.[110,168–172,177–186]

Established and putative prothrombotic risk factors

It is clear that there is a high risk of thrombosis in patients with homozygosity for the factor V G1691A mutation, protein C and protein S deficiency and cystathionine-β-synthase deficiency. Heterozygosity for antithrombin, protein C and protein S deficiency are also associated with increased risk, at least in the venous system. In contrast, a lower risk of developing early thromboembolism is observed in adult patients with the heterozygous FV G1691A mutation, the heterozygous prothrombin G20210A variant and heterozygous defects of the heparin-binding site of the antithrombin molecule. Moderate hyperhomocysteinaemia due to the homozygous methylenetetrahydrofolate reductase (MTHFR) polymorphism C677T appears to be a risk factor for thrombosis in large series.[157–161] Based on the great structural homology between lipoprotein(a) and plasminogen and on in vitro studies reporting that lipoprotein(a) inhibits fibrinolysis,[187] prospective and case-control studies have identified elevated lipoprotein(a) concentrations as a risk factor for premature myocardial infarction and stroke.[188,189]

Since the discovery of activated protein C resistance and the demonstration that it is a highly prevalent hereditary risk factor for thromboembolism,[158] evidence has been accumulating that thrombophilia is a multifactorial disorder. In addition, the association of multiple haemostatic prothrombotic defects[190] or the combination of established prothrombotic risk factors with acquired environmental or clinical conditions greatly increases the risk of thrombosis, not only in adults but also in infants and children.[175,182,191–195]

The role of prothrombotic disorders in ischaemic stroke in children

Conditions predisposing to cerebrovascular accidents in children include congenital heart malformations, haemolytic anaemias (e.g. haemoglobinopathy), single gene disorders (e.g. neurofibromatosis), chromosomal abnormalities (e.g. Down syndrome), infectious diseases (e.g. meningitis) and collagen tissue diseases as well as some rare inborn metabolic disorders.[196–198] One of the most important of the latter conditions to be clearly associated with thrombosis is homozygous cystathionine-β-synthase (CBS) deficiency leading to homocystinuria (see Chapter 14), which is established as a rare cause of symptomatic venous and arterial stroke in childhood.[199,200] As there are a few case reports of infants and older children presenting with stroke in the absence of other features of the condition,[199,201,202] it should always be excluded in cryptogenic cases.

In addition, as recently demonstrated, hypercoagulable states also represent a risk factor for stroke in childhood: The presence of the factor V G1691A mutation, the prothrombin G20210A variant, increased concentrations of lipoprotein(a), as well as deficiency states of natural anticoagulants such as antithrombin, protein C and protein S have been reported to be associated in single cases and in controlled studies of paediatric stroke populations, i.e. in neonates, infants and children.[169,171,177–183,185,186,203–214]

Tables 5.2 and 5.3 summarize results obtained from case-control studies in Caucasian paediatric patients recruited from different catchment areas in Germany, and suffering from ischaemic stroke with respect to prothrombotic risk factors.[182,185] The data presented here, however, may vary in different countries with respect to the ethnic population back-

ground,[186] the number of patient/controls investigated, the percentage with underlying disease, whether the study was population-based and perhaps most importantly, the proportion with venous and arterial mechanisms.[181,183,203,215–217] In a meta-analysis confined to stroke in an arterial territory, for which 18 publications fulfilled entry criteria, deficiency of antithrombin, protein C and protein S, activated protein C resistance, factor V G1691A, factor II G20210A, MTHFR C677T and homocysteine levels higher than the 95th centile for age were all more common in children with arterial ischaemic stroke (AIS) than controls and protein C deficiency and the MTHFR C677T polymorphism were significantly more common.[218] A full meta-analysis looking at cerebral venous sinus thrombosis (CVST) and perinatal stroke in addition to arterial ischaemic stroke found no evidence of heterogeneity or publication bias.[219] A statistically significant association with stroke onset was demonstrated for each thrombophilia trait evaluated, with no difference found between AIS and CSVT. Summary odds ratios/confidence intervals (ORs/CIs) (random-effects model) were as follows: antithrombin (6.95/1.93–24.95), protein C-deficiency (8.76/4.53–16.96), protein S (4.05/1.34–12.26), factor V G1691A (3.29/2.60–4.14), factor II G20210A (2.52/1.71–3.72), MTHFR C677T (AIS: 1.61/1.21–2.14), antiphospholipid antibodies (AIS: 5.84/3.05–11.17), elevated lipoprotein(a) (6.24/4.51–8.64) and combined thrombophilias (8.85/3.32–23.57). For perinatal AIS six studies were available. Summary odds ratios/confidence intervals were as follows: factor V G1691A (3.59/2.27–5.60) and factor II G20210A (2.05/1.04–4.04). Although these meta-analysis are very important in establishing that thrombophilias are risk factors for incident stroke, further studies are needed before the individual patient risk for primary and secondary stroke can be estimated; symptomatic patient groups should have arterial and venous imaging acutely and laboratory investigations at an appropriate

TABLE 5.2
Prothrombotic risk factors in Caucasian children (>6 months of age) suffering from spontaneous ischaemic stroke[182]

Risk factors	Controls (n=296)	Patients (n=148)	Odds ratio (95% CI)
Protein C deficiency	2 (0.7%)	9 (6.1%)	9.5 (2.0–44.6)
Factor V G1691A	12 (4.1%)	30 (20.3%)	6.0 (2.9–12.1)
Prothrombin G20210A	4 (1.4%)	9 (6.1%)	4.7 (1.4–15.6)
MTHFR C677TT	31 (10.5%)	35 (23.6%)	2.6 (1.5–4.5)
Lipoprotein(a) >30mg/dl	14 (4.7%)	39 (26.4%)	7.2 (3.8–13.8)

TABLE 5.3
Prothrombotic risk factors in Caucasian children suffering from neonatal ischaemic stroke[185]

Risk factors	Controls (n=182)	Patients (n=91)	Odds ratio (95% CI)
Protein C deficiency	–	6 (6.6%)	–
Factor V G1691A	10 (5.5%)	17 (18.7%)	3.9 (1.7–9.0)
Prothrombin G20210A	4 (2.2%)	4 (4.4%)	2.0 (0.5–8.3)
MTHFR C677TT	20 (11.0%)	15 (16.5%)	1.6 (0.8–3.3)
Lipoprotein(a) >30mg/dl	10 (5.5%)	20 (22.0%)	4.8 (2.2–10.9)

time after the stroke in comparison with age- and sex-matched healthy controls from the same geographiclal catchment areas, as well as comprehensive long-term follow-up.

Laboratory evaluation

Recurrent thromboembolic events and the duration of anticoagulant medication are possibly influenced by the presence of single or combined prothrombotic risk factors. Therefore the laboratory evaluation of genetic predisposition for vascular accidents is indicated. Based on the data obtained from case-control studies, at least the symptomatic propositus should be screened in a specialized coagulation unit for the following prothrombotic defects (Table 5.4). Besides a step-wise protein-based diagnostic procedure – the corresponding antigen concentration is not reduced when the activity of a protein is within its normal range – DNA-based assays are recommended. Protein-based assays, i.e. APC-resistance, protein C activity (first step) and antigen (second step), free and total protein S antigen, antithrombin activity (first step) and antigen (second step), lipoprotein(a) and fasting homocysteine concentrations should be investigated along with DNA-based assays, i.e. factor V G1691A mutation, prothrombin G20210A variant and MTHFR C677T genotype. However, potential variations are unavoidable due to different ethnic population backgrounds. In addition, rare prothrombotic defects, e.g. dysfibrinogenaemia, hypo-or dysplasminogenaemia, heparin

cofactor II deficiency, factor XII deficiency, increased levels of histidine-rich glycoprotein, protein Z or further genetic polymorphisms, should be kept in mind.[160] Besides testing for prothrombotic defects as stated above, all symptomatic children with thrombosis should be screened for antiphospholipid or anticardiolipin antibodies and the presence of lupus anticoagulants.[173,220] Family history is a poor screening tool for prothrombotic disorder in the child[221] and as abnormalities are common[222] and there may be longer-term management implications (see Chapter 17, Section 17.1), it is now difficult to argue against testing in the propositus, although as there may be insurance issues,[223] testing of other family members should be considered on an individual case basis.

INTERPRETATION OF LABORATORY RESULTS

To prevent results of protein-based assays from being affected by the acute thrombotic onset, blood samples should be obtained at least 3–6 months after the thrombotic episode. In contrast, since DNA-based assays are not influenced by the acute thrombotic onset, screening can be performed for factor V G1691A, prothrombin G20210A and MTHFR C677T and, in the future, potential further genetic polymorphisms immediately at the onset of the vascular accident.

For all plasma-based assays a clotting abnormality should be documented as a defect only if the plasma level of a protein is outside the limits of its normal range in at least two different samples.[224,225] A type I deficiency state can be diagnosed when the functional plasma activity and immunological antigen concentration of a protein are below the age-related limit (Table 5.5). A type II deficiency is present when repeatedly low functional activity levels are combined with normal antigen concentrations. The diagnosis of protein S deficiency is based on reduced free protein S antigen levels combined with decreased or normal total protein S antigen concentrations.[161] With respect to an antiphospholipid syndrome, repeated testing is necessary in paediatric patients with increased anticardiolipin/antiphospholipid or β2 glycoprotein I antibodies, or lupus anticoagulants.

Acknowledgement

The authors thank Susan Griesbach for help in editing this manuscript.

TABLE 5.4
Screening in symptomatic paediatric patients suffering from ischaemic stroke (may be modified with respect to different ethnic population backgrounds)[195,226]

Plasma/protein-based	DNA-based
APC-R (APC resistance)	Factor V G1691A
Protein C activity/antigen	Prothrombin G20210A
Free and total protein S antigen	MTHFR C677T
Antithrombin activity/antigen	
Lipoprotein(a)	Further potential polymorphisms
Fasting homocysteine	
Fibrinogen	
Plasminogen	
Factor VIIIC	
Factor XII	
Lupus anticoagulant/antiphospholipid antibodies	

TABLE 5.5
Age-dependent reference values (median, range) from 385 healthy Caucasian infants and children[225]

Parameter	Newborn (n=55)	3 months (n=50)	6 months (n=60)	1–5 years (n=60)	6–9 years (n=58)	10–18 years (n=52)
Protein C act. %	35 (14–55)	55 (25–82)	60 (38–95)	75 (45–102)	84 (64–125)	88 (62–128)
Protein C ag. %	30 (12–50)	50 (22–75)	55 (40–100)	70 (45–98)	80 (55–120)	82 (55–120)
Fr. prot. S ag. %	38 (15–55)	55 (35–92)	77 (45–115)	78 (62–120)	80 (62–130)	85 (60–140)
Antithrombin %	52 (30–85)	90 (55–120)	98 (65–126)	101 (85–140)	100 (85–136)	98 (84–139)
Plasminogen %	50 (35–70)	68 (45–95)	87 (65–100)	98 (63–123)	95 (68–120)	90 (70–115)
Lp(a) mg/dl	4.4 (0–125)					
kringle 4 repeats	>28					

act, activity; ag, antigen; Fr, free; Lp, lipoprotein(a); prot., protein.

5.3 Hypertension and Childhood Stroke

Juan C. Kupferman, Fenella J. Kirkham and Steven Pavlakis

Introduction

Normal ranges for blood pressure in childhood have been established for some time.[227,228] Paediatric hypertension is increasing in prevalence, probably secondary to the paediatric obesity epidemic.[229,230] Hypertension can cause end organ damage (i.e. left ventricular hypertrophy, vascular and retinal changes) in children similar to the damage seen in adults.[230–232] In adults, hypertension is the most consistent and powerful predictor of stroke, such that hypertension is causally involved in nearly 70% of all stroke cases.[233] Although hypertension has not been strongly identified as a risk factor in childhood stroke to date, there is literature that suggests that hypertension may, at least in part, be associated with stroke in children as well.[110,234]

Clinical data

The main problem with determining whether hypertension is a risk factor for paediatric stroke involves the fact that hypertension is not defined in children in ways that are accepted by all investigators. Many stroke studies do not specify how the blood pressure is obtained, defined or interpreted.[235,236] Furthermore, the evaluation of blood pressure in childhood stroke has not been emphasized. Hypertension and pre-hypertension are frequently undiagnosed in the paediatric population[237] and are just as likely undiagnosed in the paediatric stroke population as well. In contrast, the sickle cell disease literature has better assessed the role of hypertension in stroke and the literature in aggregate finds an association between hypertension and sickle cell-associated stroke.[230,238,239]

Paediatric stroke

Various stroke syndromes have been reported in children with hypertension and phaeochromocytoma, including border-zone infarction as a consequence of sudden reduction in blood pressure or cardiac failure,[240] haemorrhagic stroke[241] and embolism from a mural thrombus in the context of cardiomyopathy.[242] Pihko et al[243] reported transient ischaemic cerebral lesions during induction chemotherapy for acute lymphoblastic leukaemia in nine children with visual hallucinations progressing to confusion and seizure. The symptoms were often preceded by severe constipation and significantly elevated blood pressure. Neuroradiological examinations showed bilateral cortical or subcortical white matter lesions. The triangular shape and location of the lesions in the watershed areas between the major cerebral arteries suggested vascular ischaemia as the cause. There may have been overlap with posterior reversible encephalopathy syndrome (Fig. 5.4a) but the authors felt these cases might be distinct and instead represent borderzone ischaemia (Figs 5.4b and 5.5a). Reversible clinical and imaging manifestations has also been reported in association with hypertension in Cushing syndrome.[244]

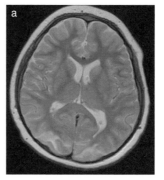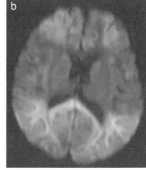

Fig. 5.4. (a) T2-weighted imaging from a child who became hypertensive on treatment with steroids for juvenile rheumatoid arthritis shows high signal posteriorly. (b) Diffusion-weighted imaging the following day shows more widespread ischaemia in the borderzones between the middle and anterior and middle and posterior arteries. From Sharma M, Kupferman JC, Brosgol Y, Paterno K, Goodman S, Prohovnik I, Kirkham FJ, Pavlakis SG. The effects of hypertension on the paediatric brain: a justifiable concern. Lancet Neurol. 2010; 9(9):933–40.

Left   Right

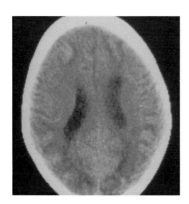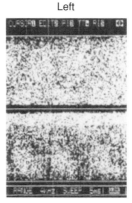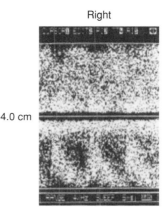

4.0 cm

Fig. 5.5. CT scan of patient with hypertensive encephalopathy and hypotension after treatment with hydralazine showing bilateral low density in the watershed region. Sonagrams recorded from left and right middle cerebral arteries (MCA) at a depth of 4.0cm from the temporal bone on admission. Time is on the abscissa, the ordinate represents the Doppler shift frequency and the intensity of the trace is proportional to the number of red blood cells travelling at that velocity. The Doppler shift was greater than twice the pulse repetition frequency of the beam so the peak of the signal appears at the bottom of the opposite channel (aliasing). Left: MCA velocity 190.6cm/s; right: MCA velocity 218.9cm/s.

The data on the role of hypertension in the remainder of the paediatric stroke population are scanty, however.[230] One study reported 36 children with infarctions in the basal ganglia and did not find hypertension to play a significant role.[114] There was no definition of hypertension nor comments about timing and methods of blood pressure analysis. Case series and review articles on paediatric stroke may not even mention hypertension as a potential risk factor.[204,232] In contrast, Ganesan et al[110] demonstrated a significant association between cerebral arterial abnormalities and systolic blood pressure greater than the 90th centile. They reported three patients with left ventricular hypertrophy, with systolic blood pressure greater than the 90th centile in two. However, a follow-up study showed that hypertension was not a significant factor in the risk of stroke recurrence in univariate analysis.[216] The same group reported a higher prevalence of hypertension in a series of 22 cases of posterior circulation stroke in children.[234] Nine children had hypertension, which was defined as a systolic blood pressure at discharge or on follow-up of >90th centile for height and age.[227]

Our group reported a case of ischaemic stroke in association with masked hypertension.[245] This patient had left ventricular hypertrophy as well as elevated blood pressure when measured for a 24-hour period, but not when measured at presentation in the emergency department. Masked hypertension is defined as a normal blood pressure in the surgery and elevated ambulatory blood pressures (obtained at regular intervals over a 24-hour period). Between 8% and 9% of children evaluated at two large hypertension centres were found to have masked hypertension.[246,247] In one of these studies, masked hypertension predisposed to the development of sustained hypertension and left ventricular hypertrophy, especially in children with parental history of hypertension.

Sickle cell disease, hypertension and stroke

Strouse et al[248] reported a series of primary haemorrhagic stroke in association with a history of hypertension and elevation of systolic blood pressure. The higher systolic blood pressure at presentation in patients with primary haemorrhagic stroke supported a contribution of elevated blood pressure to risk of haemorrhagic stroke. A history of hypertension was defined as previous treatment with an antihypertensive agent or a diagnosis of hypertension listed in the admission or clinic note. Other papers have found an association with hypertension and infarction or infarction recurrence.[238,249]

Haemorrhagic stroke and hypertension

The influence of elevated blood pressure may be even more significant in children with haemorrhagic rather than ischaemic stroke. Awada et al[250] reported 107 cases, including 12 children younger than 10 with haemorrhagic stroke. Systemic hypertension was found to be the cause in 20% of the cases in this series. The pooling of the causative data from this case and 253 others reported in the literature showed that even before 45 years of age systemic hypertension seems to be the leading risk factor for intracerebral haemorrhage. It accounted for approximately 30% of the cases. The pooled overall early mortality rate is approximately 20%, and only one-third of the patients returned to independent living.[250]

Transcranial Doppler

It has been shown in adults that hypertension increases the risks for stroke, coronary artery disease and heart failure. In hypertensive adults with end organ damage, abnormalities in cerebrovascular auto-regulation have been reported, which could be a precursor to stroke or subtle cognitive abnormalities.[230,251] As more children have been found to develop end organ damage secondary to uncontrolled hypertension, it is possible that subtle cerebrovascular changes are occurring as well. An abnormal transcranial Doppler (TCD) could be used as a clinical indicator (or pre-indicator) of end organ damage (brain). Very high velocities were demonstrated in one of our patients with hypertensive encephalopathy, subsequent hypotension and borderzone infarction (Fig. 5.5). If significant changes in vascular reactivity are found, it may suggest the need for starting or intensifying antihypertensive therapy to prevent further cerebrovascular complications.

In adults, hypertension affects cognitive function through abnormal cerebral perfusion and vascular insufficiency as well as stroke.[251] In addition, vascular reactivity of the brain as measured by TCD correlates directly with the severity of the hypertension and is a marker for disrupted cerebral perfusion. Adults with hypertension and end organ disease have a blunted response to hypercapnia and did not increase cerebral blood flow velocity with hypercapnia as seen in normotensive patients. This blunted response with significant hypertension is a potential biomarker for relative cerebrovascular insufficiency in the adult.[251] Hypercapnic reactivity is also abnormal in hypertensive children and improves after treatment.[230,252]

Abnormal brain vascular autoregulation is found in children with sickle cell and cyanotic heart disease, but has not been adequately tested in children with hypertension or indeed any other disorder. Children with hypertension and secondary cardiomyopathy have thickened aortic walls, which suggest a potential for abnormality in cerebral perfusion.[253] Abnormal autoregulation is a likely early marker for abnormal brain perfusion in childhood hypertension and if it is, TCD-derived abnormalities may prove to be an important biomarker for neurological involvement. TCD in children is becoming clinically appropriate and multiple laboratories are performing clinical studies.

Conclusion

Hypertension is the most important risk factor associated with stroke in the adult population. Although hypertension has not been strongly identified as a risk factor in childhood stroke to date, it is possible that hypertension plays an important role in its pathophysiology. Evaluation for possible hypertension should be undertaken thoroughly to identify children who may benefit from antihypertensive therapy and, therefore, prevent recurrences.

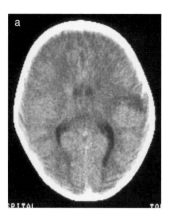
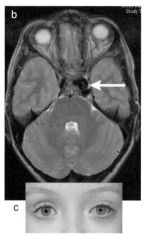

Fig. 5.6. (a) CT scan from a 3-year-old girl who banged her head on a table and lost consciousness about an hour later. She recovered fully within 6 hours but the following day developed a right hemiparesis and asymmetrical transcranial Doppler velocities consistent with vasospasm. The CT scan shows a small cortical infarct. (b) Carotid-cavernous fistula (arrow) in a boy with proptosis radiologically and (c) clinically after having his head trodden on during a football match.

5.4 Trauma

Fenella J. Kirkham

Stroke after apparent head injury, both major and minor, is well recognized (Fig. 5.6).[254–256] Some of these patients may have had a dissection of the carotid or vertebrobasilar arteries,[257] but others seem to have infarction in the territories of the small perforators supplying the basal ganglia.[254,258,259] Vasospasm[260] and venous sinus thrombosis[261–267] or congestion[268] are other mechanisms of injury. It is possible that these mechanisms play a role in brain injury after more serious head trauma with immediate loss of consciousness, although there are few data as vascular imaging is rarely performed in the acute phase.[257] Stroke may also occur from a variety of mechanisms, including dissection,[269,270] unilateral hypoxic-ischaemic injury[271] and venous sinus thrombosis[272] in the context of child abuse.[273] The vulnerability of children who sustain accidental or inflicted head injury to behavioural and cognitive problems may be, at least in part, determined pre-injury.

5.5 Iron Deficiency

Fenella J. Kirkham

As well as the evidence that the severity of the anaemia is a risk factor for stroke in sickle cell disease and that iron deficiency plays a role in stroke in children with congenital heart disease, it has recently been suggested that iron deficiency may also be aetiologically important in cryptogenic stroke in this age group.[110,274,275] In addition to an association of iron deficiency anaemias with sinovenous thrombosis,[176,275] nearly one-quarter of patients in a recent series of children with arterial stroke had evidence for iron deficiency;[110] currently there is no evidence for an effect on recurrence risk although numbers of patients are small and follow-up relatively short.[216] Some of these patients may have undiagnosed coeliac disease, which is associated with cerebrovascular disease in children and adults;[276] screening with antitransglutaminase antibodies is recommended in cryptogenic stroke as asymptomatic coeliac disease is common. Iron-deficiency anaemia per se has been identified as a risk factor for poor educational performance and nutritional intervention has been associated with higher scores on measures of numeracy, reading and vocabulary, so it worth excluding and/or treating iron deficiency.

5.6 Patent Foramen Ovale and Paradoxical Embolism

Vijeya Ganesan and Fenella J. Kirkham

Paradoxical emboli (from the systemic venous circulation or the right side of the heart to the brain) rely on the presence of a connection between the right and left sides of the heart. This can be a major structural anomaly such as a ventricular or atrial septal defect or more minor anomalies such as patent foramen ovale (PFO), often associated with atrial septal aneurysm or a pulmonary arteriovenous fistula. The source of embolic material is thought to be thrombosis within the venous circulation. A physiological left-to-right shunt through a PFO can be demonstrated on contrast echocardiography in 10–18% of otherwise healthy adults. However, post-mortem studies have found probe-patent PFO in up to 35% of individuals[277] with no difference with age in prevalence of echocardiographically determined shunts.[278] In the resting state when left atrial pressure exceeds right atrial pressure, there may be no inter-atrial shunting; however, increased right atrial pressure may enable right-to-left shunting of blood and therefore transmission of embolic material form the venous circulation to the cerebral arterial system.[279,280]

Lechat et al[281] reported that 40% of individuals who had had a stroke under the age of 55 had echocardiographic evidence of a PFO. This proportion rose to 54% in those patients in whom no other aetiology was identified. However, the mechanism of this association and its relative importance in the pathophysiology of cryptogenic stroke has been controversial. Although clinically evident or occult venous thrombosis is rarely demonstrated in these patients,[282] it is recognized that up to 30% of deep venous thromboses may be missed with currently available diagnostic techniques.[283] Furthermore, there is some evidence that affected individuals may have a propensity for transient atrial arrhythmias which could predispose to intra-cardiac thrombus formation.[284] A further difficulty is that several studies have found that Valsalva-provoking activities were not common at the onset of the stroke. However, although left atrial pressure is normally higher than right atrial pressure, this pressure gradient is transiently reversed in early systole. Reports of paradoxical embolus in cystic fibrosis[285] and of bubble microemboli on TCD during prolonged obstructive sleep apnoeas in adults[286] suggest that the shunt through a PFO may transiently reverse from the usual left-to-right to right-to-left under certain circumstances.

Many subsequent studies have found that the prevalence of PFO in young adults with otherwise unexplained stroke is in the order of 32–55%. A recent systematic review of the literature has shown that PFO (defined as a right-to-left shunt at atrial level) is significantly more common in patients aged <55 with ischaemic stroke and even more so in patients with cryptogenic stroke.[287] The presence of an atrial septal aneurysm may confer additional risk,[287–289] particularly of recurrent stroke.[290] However, prospective population-based studies have failed to confirm the association,[291,292] even with atrial septal aneurysm,[292] and an adequately powered study is now needed to confirm or exclude a link. Mitral valve prolapse is a commonly associated abnormality but is of uncertain aetiological significance.[288,293,294]

Echocardiographic evidence for a PFO comprises demonstration of the passage of contrast from the right to the left atrium, for example using bubble contrast transthoracic echocardiography (TTE). Provocative measures may be used to increase right atrial pressure, such as coughing, Valsalva manoeuvre or pressure on the liver. The potential for right-to-left shunting in an individual with a left-to-right shunt in the resting state cannot be excluded if a Valsalva manoeuvre or other measure which increases right atrial pressure is not incorporated into the study. This increases the detection rate of PFO by at least 25%.[293] The characteristics of the PFO, such as size of the defect and of the shunt, are also important considerations; larger defects and those with a larger right-to-left shunt appear to be more important, particularly in patients with cryptogenic stroke[277,295,296] Larger shunts are also more frequently associated with recurrent stroke or transient ischaemic attack (TIA).[297] Other factors which appear to be associated with a

higher risk of recurrent stroke include the presence of right-to left shunting at rest and high membrane mobility.[279] The risk of recurrent stroke or TIA in young adults with stroke due to paradoxical emboli appears to be around 3.5%/year;[283] however, most studies have included small numbers of patients followed for short periods. At present, there is little evidence that paradoxical embolism is a common mechanism of ischaemic stroke in children,[110,298] and atrial septal aneurysm, which is associated with a high risk of recurrent stroke,[290] is rare. However, well-documented case reports and series of PFO associated with stroke in neonates[299] and children[300,301] make the case for asking a paediatric cardiologist specifically to exclude a PFO in cryptogenic paediatric ischaemic stroke,[302] provided that resources are adequate to also exclude cerebrovascular disease.[110]

Transoesophageal echocardiography (TOE) has improved sensitivity compared with TTE in the detection of PFO in adults;[280] large shunts at atrial level should be detected but the need for general anaesthesia means that children cannot undertake the essential Valsava manoeuvre to exclude smaller PFOs. At Great Ormond Street Hospital, London, UK where between 1978 and 2001 TTE was conducted in 104 previously healthy children with arterial ischaemic stroke, unsuspected abnormalities were detected in 7 (7%).[110] One patient had an atrial septal defect without right to left shunt. However, he also had vasculitis. Three patients had left ventricular hypertrophy; systolic BP was greater than the 90th centile for height and age in two. Three other patients had poor ventricular function and posterior cerebral artery territory infarcts. In summary, none of these patients had evidence of large right-to-left shunts through these defects and all had other explanations for their stroke. A further important consideration in the paediatric age group is that thrombosis within the venous system is rare in the young.

An alternative method for demonstrating potential for paradoxical emboli is echocardiography (Fig. 5.7) or examination of the cerebral circulation with transcranial Doppler ultrasound (TCD) (Fig. 5.8. See also colour plate 3) during injection of microbubbles. A study is considered positive when

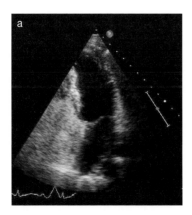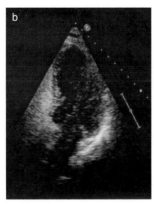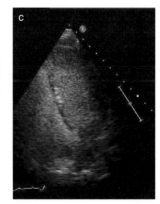

Fig. 5.7. Echocardiograms showing: (a) an intact interatrial septum; (b) a few microemboli crossing a patent foramen ovale; (c) many microemboli crossing a patent foramen ovale.

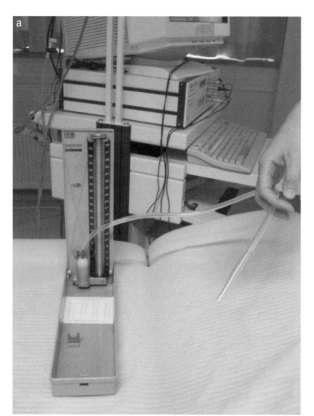

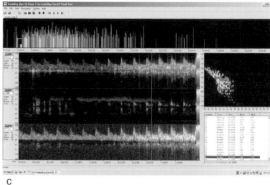

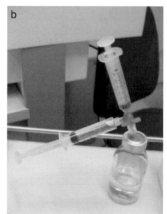

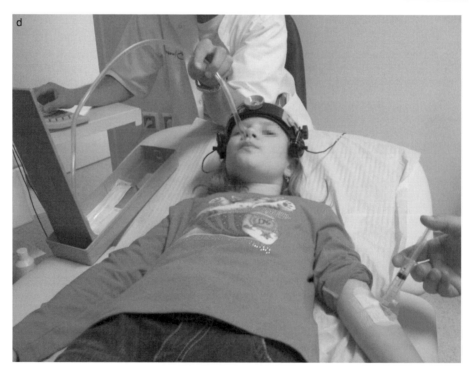

Fig. 5.8. (a) Apparatus used to exclude patent foramen ovale using bubble contrast transcranial Doppler during a Valsalva manouevre. Measurement of Valsalva pressure generated with transcranial Doppler equipment in the background. (b) Agitated saline. (c) Microemboli on transcranial Doppler. (d) Child undergoing the test. (See colour plate 3.)

high intensity transient signals are detected following injection of microbubbles.[300,303]

TCD is more sensitive than TTE with bubble contrast[304] and has a high sensitivity and specificity when compared with TOE as a criterion standard.[305] Moreover, it provides direct evidence of target organ involvement. In the Great Ormond Street study, nine children had injection of air bubbles with a Valsalva during TTE and none showed a right-to-left shunt.[110]

The publication of protocols for bubble echocardiography[302] and contrast TCD[300] for use in children is a big step forward as this will allow standardized investigation, although work on interobserver variation will be needed.[306] In the study reported by Benedik et al,[300] contrast TCD carried out with specially designed apparatus to enable children to perform the equivalent of a Valsalva manouevre by blowing into a glass tube (Fig. 5.8. See also colour plate 3) was positive in 4/6 children with cryptogenic ischaemic stroke and in 5/6 children with TIAs, but was not found in children with an alternative explanation for their strokes. The role of these small right-to-left shunts in the pathophysiology of initial and recurrent cryptogenic stroke requires further exploration.

PFOs can be surgically repaired or occluded by the transcatheter route. However, even surgical closure may not be effective in preventing recurrent stroke in patients with an otherwise cryptogenic first stroke.[307] Although Bogousslavsky et al[283] have argued that in the absence of definitive clinical evidence, both chronic anticoagulant therapy and surgery are low risk strategies with a risk which is outweighed by potential benefit, there is little evidence for benefit of anticoagulation over aspirin.[308] Transcatheter closure is feasible in children,[300,302,309] but it is not reasonable to argue in favour of a procedure with unknown long-term consequences in children where atrial septal aneurysm is rare and the association with PFO is unproven. Surgery and endovascular procedures may be associated with morbidity, including stroke, and neither surgery nor transcatheter occlusion is completely successful in abolishing the shunt.[307,310]

Transthoracic or transoesophageal echocardiography?

Transthroracic echocardiography is widely available and can be performed in most children without sedation. Transoesophageal echocardiography enables better visualization of basal cardiac structures such as the left atrium, left atrial appendage, atrial septum and mitral valve. However it has to be carried out under general anaesthetic in children. TOE is more sensitive than conventional echocardiography in the detection of atrial septal abnormalities (including PFO), thrombotic material in the atrial appendage, atrial myxoma and vegetations.[280,311,312]

TOE is recommended in the investigation of adults under 50 years of age who have a stroke.[293] There are few data in the paediatric age group. At Great Ormond Street Hospital, London, 36 children (of whom 33 were previously healthy) underwent TOE, which was abnormal in three cases, but in all cases the diagnosis had been made already.[110] Preliminary results from 10 patients enrolled in an ongoing study at Guys Hospital, London, comparing the yield of TOE and TTE in the acute phase of stroke found that TOE was abnormal in 1/6 patients with normal TTE; in 2/4 patients with abnormal TOE, TTE provided additional information. However, clinical management was not altered in any of these patients (K Lascelles, personal communication, 2009).

Clearly all children who have experienced ischaemic stroke should have TTE. Ideally this should include adminis-

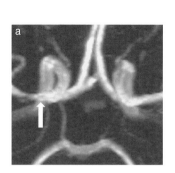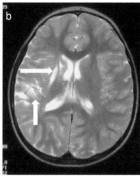

Fig. 5.9. (a) Magnetic resonance angiography showing embolic occlusion of the middle cerebral artery. (B) MRI showing a basal ganglia infarct (arrow) and subsequent silent infarction (arrow) in the same previously well child.

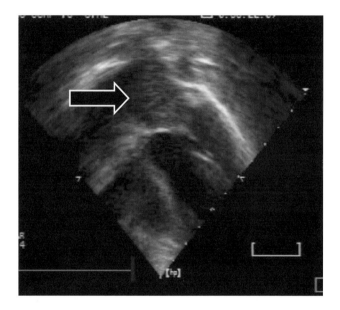

Fig. 5.10. Echocardiogram showing an atrial myxoma in a 9-year-old boy with a previous history of recurrent painful purpuric rash on his feet who became dizzy during football, and fell stiff to the ground with staring eyes and profuse sweating but no jerking movements. A CT scan (not shown) showed ventricular dilatation secondary to a cerebellar infarct; despite ventricular drainage he fulfilled the criteria for brain death.

tration of agitated saline as a contrast agent during a Valsava manoeuvre on a standardized protocol.[300–302] Particular attention should be paid to children likely to have had an embolic stroke (Figs 5.9 and 5.10) on clinical grounds, e.g. sudden onset,[313] no other cause found or rare clinical clues such as previous rash suggestive of left atrial myxoma.[314] It would be prudent to consider TOE in children known to have structural abnormalities of the heart (to look for intra-cardiac sources of embolism) and in children with unexplained stroke (to look for intracardiac thrombus, vegetations and rare but treatable conditions such as left atrial myxoma (Fig. 5.10)).[314] Again the TOE study should be carried out with contrast.

REFERENCES

1. Shillito J, Jr. Carotid arteritis: a cause of hemiplegia in childhood. J Neurosurg 1964; 21:540–551.

2. Aicardi J, Amsili J, Chevrie JJ. Acute hemiplegia in infancy and childhood. Dev Med Child Neurol 1969; 11(2):162–173.

3. Harwood-Nash DC, McDonald P, Argent W. Cerebral arterial disease in children. An angiographic study of 40 cases. Am J Roentgenol Radium Ther Nucl Med 1971; 111(4):672–686.

4. Raybaud CA, Livet MO, Jiddane M, Pinsard N. Radiology of ischemic strokes in children. Neuroradiology 1985; 27(6):567–578.

5. Satoh S, Shirane R, Yoshimoto T. Clinical survey of ischemic cerebrovascular disease in children in a district of Japan. Stroke 1991; 22(5):586–589.

6. Syrjanen J. Infection as a risk factor for cerebral infarction. Eur Heart J 1993; 14(Suppl K):17–19.

7. Kirkham FJ, Prengler M, Hewes DK, Ganesan V. Risk factors for arterial ischemic stroke in children. J Child Neurol 2000; 15(5):299–307.

8. Riou EM, Amlie-Lefond C, Echenne B, Farmer M, Sebire G. Cerebrospinal fluid analysis in the diagnosis and treatment of arterial ischemic stroke. Pediatr Neurol 2008; 38(1):1–9.

9. Riikonen R, Santavuori P. Hereditary and acquired risk factors for childhood stroke. Neuropediatrics 1994; 25(5):227–233.

10. Grau AJ, Brandt T, Forsting M, Winter R, Hacke W. Infection-associated cervical artery dissection. Three cases. Stroke 1997; 28(2):453–455.

11. Amlie-Lefond C, Barnard D, Sebire G, Friedman NR, Heyer GL, Lerner NB et al. Predictors of cerebral arteriopathy in children with arterial ischemic stroke: results of the international pediatric stroke study. Circulation 2009; 119(10):1417–1423.

12. Lanthier S, Carmant L, David M, Larbrisseau A, de VG. Stroke in children: the coexistence of multiple risk factors predicts poor outcome. Neurology 2000; 54(2):371–378.

13. Banker BQ. Cerebrovascular disease in infancy and childhood. 1. Occlusive Vascular Disease. J Neuropathol Exp Neurol 1961; 21:127–134.

14. Weck KE, Dal Canto AJ, Gould JD, O'Guin AK, Roth KA, Saffitz JE et al. Murine gamma-herpesvirus 68 causes severe large-vessel arteritis in mice lacking interferon-gamma responsiveness: a new model for virus-induced vascular disease. Nat Med 1997; 3(12):1346–1353.

15. Virgin HW, Speck SH. Unraveling immunity to gamma-herpesviruses: a new model for understanding the role of immunity in chronic virus infection. Curr Opin Immunol 1999; 11(4):371–379.

16. Dal Canto AJ, Virgin HW. Animal models of infection-mediated vasculitis: implications for human disease. Int J Cardiol 2000; 75(Suppl 1):S37–S45.

17. Presti RM, Pollock JL, Dal Canto AJ, O'Guin AK, Virgin HW. Interferon gamma regulates acute and latent murine cytomegalovirus infection and chronic disease of the great vessels. J Exp Med 1998; 188(3):577–588.

18. Dal Canto AJ, Swanson PE, O'Guin AK, Speck SH, Virgin HW. IFN-gamma action in the media of the great elastic arteries, a novel immunoprivileged site. J Clin Invest 2001; 107(2):R15–R22.

19. Chang CJ, Chang WN, Huang LT, Chang YC, Huang SC, Hung PL et al. Cerebral infarction in perinatal and childhood bacterial meningitis. QMJ 2003; 96(10):755–762.

20. Siddiqui TS, Rehman A, Ahmed B. Etiology of strokes and hemiplegia in children presenting at Ayub Teaching Hospital, Abbottabad. J Ayub Med Coll Abbottabad 2006; 18(2):60–63.

21. Kerr L, Filloux FM. Cerebral infarction as a remote complication of childhood *Haemophilus influenzae* meningitis. West J Med 1992; 157(2):179–182.

22. Taft TA, Chusid MJ, Sty JR. Cerebral infarction in *Haemophilus influenzae* type B meningitis. Clin Pediatr (Phila). 1986; 25(4):177–180.

23. Jan W, Zimmerman RA, Bilaniuk LT, Hunter JV, Simon EM, Haselgrove J. Diffusion-weighted imaging in acute bacterial meningitis in infancy. Neuroradiology 2003; 45(9):634–639.

24. Ramelli GP, Aebi C, Remonda L, Lovblad KO. Basal ganglia infarction complicating basilar meningitis: visualization by serial magnetic resonance imaging. Eur Neurol 2005; 54(4):227–229.

25. Mankhambo LA, Makwana NV, Carrol ED, Beare NA, Taylor T, Kampondeni S et al. Persistent visual loss as a complication of meningococcal meningitis. Pediatr Infect Dis J 2006; 25(6):566–567.

26. Fitzgerald KC, Golomb MR. Neonatal arterial ischemic stroke and sinovenous thrombosis associated with meningitis. J Child Neurol 2007; 22(7):818–822.

27. Rout D, Sharma A, Mohan PK, Rao VR. Bacterial aneurysms of the intracavernous carotid artery. J Neurosurg 1984; 60(6):1236–1242.

28. Bentham JR, Pollard AJ, Milford CA, Anslow P, Pike MG. Cerebral infarct and meningitis secondary to Lemierre's syndrome. Pediatr Neurol 2004; 30(4):281–283.

29. Bader-Meunier B, Pinto G, Tardieu M, Pariente D, Bobin S, Dommergues JP. Mastoiditis, meningitis and venous sinus thrombosis caused by *Fusobacterium necrophorum*. Eur J Pediatr 1994; 153(5):339–341.

30. Kastenbauer S, Pfister HW. Pneumococcal meningitis in adults: spectrum of complications and prognostic factors in a series of 87 cases. Brain 2003; 126(Pt 5):1015–1025.

31. Pryde K, Murugan V, Walker W, Wilson P, Faust S, Kirkham F. Stroke in paediatric pneumococcal meningitis – a case series of 8 patients. Eur J Paed Neurol 2009; 13(Suppl):S94.

32. Leiguarda R, Berthier M, Starkstein S, Nogues M, Lylyk P. Ischemic infarction in 25 children with tuberculous meningitis. Stroke 1988; 19(2):200–204.

33. Schoeman JF, Rutherfoord GS, Hewlett RH. Acute stroke in a child with miliary tuberculosis. Clin Neuropathol 1997; 16(6):303–308.

34. Kilic T, Elmaci I, Ozek MM, Pamir MN. Utility of transcranial Doppler ultrasonography in the diagnosis and follow-up of tuberculous meningitis-related vasculopathy. Childs Nerv Syst 2002; 18(3–4):142–146.

35. Andronikou S, Wieselthaler N, Smith B, Douis H, Fieggen AG, van TR et al. Value of early follow-up CT in paediatric tuberculous meningitis. Pediatr Radiol 2005; 35(11):1092–1099.

36. Andronikou S, Wilmshurst J, Hatherill M, VanToorn R. Distribution of brain infarction in children with tuberculous meningitis and correlation with outcome score at 6 months. Pediatr Radiol 2006; 36(12):1289–1294.

37. Schoeman JF, Van Zyl LE, Laubscher JA, Donald PR. Serial CT scanning in childhood tuberculous meningitis: prognostic features in 198 cases. J Child Neurol 1995; 10(4):320–329.

38. Quagliarello V, Scheld WM. Bacterial meningitis: pathogenesis, pathophysiology, and progress. N Engl J Med 1992; 327(12):864–872.

39. Lee SC, Liu W, Dickson DW, Brosnan CF, Berman JW. Cytokine production by human fetal microglia and astrocytes. Differential induction by lipopolysaccharide and IL-1 beta. J Immunol 1993; 150(7):2659–2667.

40. Sebire G, Emilie D, Wallon C, Hery C, Devergne O, Delfraissy JF et al. In vitro production of IL-6, IL-1 beta, and tumor necrosis factor-alpha by human embryonic microglial and neural cells. J Immunol 1993; 150(4):1517–1523.

41. Thwaites GE, Nguyen DB, Nguyen HD, Hoang TQ, Do TT, Nguyen TC et al. Dexamethasone for the treatment of tuberculous meningitis in adolescents and adults. N Engl J Med 2004; 351(17):1741–1751.

42. van de Beek D, de Gans J, McIntyre P, Prasad K. Corticosteroids in acute bacterial meningitis. Cochrane Review 2003; Version 3:CD004305.

43. Garcia-Monco JC, Villar BF, Alen JC, Benach JL. *Borrelia burgdorferi* in the central nervous system: experimental and clinical evidence for early invasion. J Infect Dis 1990; 161(6):1187–1193.

44. Defer G, Levy R, Brugieres P, Postic D, Degos JD. Lyme disease presenting as a stroke in the vertebrobasilar territory: MRI. Neuroradiology 1993; 35(7):529–531.

45. Hammers-Berggren S, Grondahl A, Karlsson M, von Arbin M, Carlsson A, Stiernstedt G. Screening for neuroborreliosis in patients with stroke. Stroke 1993; 24(9):1393–1396.

46. Laroche C, Lienhardt A, Boulesteix J. Ischemic stroke caused by neuroborreliosis. Arch Pediatr 1999; 6(12):1302–1305.

47. Wilke M, Eiffert H, Christen HJ, Hanefeld F. Primarily chronic and cerebrovascular course of Lyme neuroborreliosis: case reports and literature review. Arch Dis Child 2000; 83(1):67–71.

48. Klingebiel R, Benndorf G, Schmitt M, von Moers A, Lehmann R. Large cerebral vessel occlusive disease in Lyme neuroborreliosis. Neuropediatrics 2002; 33(1):37–40.

49. Cox MG, Wolfs TF, Lo TH, Kappelle LJ, Braun KP. Neuroborreliosis causing focal cerebral arteriopathy in a child. Neuropediatrics 2005; 36(2):104–107.

50. Renard C, Marignier S, Gillet Y, Roure-Sobas C, Guibaud L, Des P, V et al. Acute hemiparesis revealing a neuroborreliosis in a child. Arch Pediatr 2008; 15(1):41–44.

51. Topakian R, Stieglbauer K, Nussbaumer K, Aichner FT. Cerebral vasculitis and stroke in Lyme neuroborreliosis. Two case reports and review of current knowledge. Cerebrovasc Dis 2008; 26(5):455–461.

52. Raucher HS, Kaufman DM, Goldfarb J, Jacobson RI, Roseman B, Wolff RR. Pseudotumor cerebri and Lyme disease: a new association. J Pediatr 1985; 107(6):931–933.

53. Kan L, Sood SK, Maytal J. Pseudotumor cerebri in Lyme disease: a case report and literature review. Pediatr Neurol 1998; 18(5):439–441.

54. Hartel C, Schilling S, Neppert B, Tiemer B, Sperner J. Intracranial hypertension in neuroborreliosis. Dev Med Child Neurol 2002; 44(9):641–642.

55. Krishnan A, Karnad DR, Limaye U, Siddharth W. Cerebral venous and dural sinus thrombosis in severe falciparum malaria. J Infect 2004; 48(1):86–90.

56. Saraswat DK. Case of cerebral malaria presenting as subarachnoid haemorrhage. J Assoc Physicians India 1994; 42(9):756.

57. Millan JM, San Millan JM, Munoz M, Navas E, Lopez-Velez R. CNS complications in acute malaria: MR findings. AJNR Am J Neuroradiol 1993; 14(2):493–494.

58. Cordoliani YS, Sarrazin JL, Felten D, Caumes E, Leveque C, Fisch A. MR of cerebral malaria. AJNR Am J Neuroradiol 1998; 19(5):871–874.

59. Newton CR, Peshu N, Kendall B, Kirkham FJ, Sowunmi A, Waruiru C et al. Brain swelling and ischaemia in Kenyans with cerebral malaria. Arch Dis Child 1994; 70(4):281–287.

60. Idro R, Jenkins NE, Newton CR. Pathogenesis, clinical features, and neurological outcome of cerebral malaria. Lancet Neurol 2005; 4(12):827–840.

61. Jha S, Kumar V. Neurocysticercosis presenting as stroke. Neurol India 2000; 48(4):391–394.

62. Wraige E, Graham J, Robb SA, Jan W. Neurocysticercosis masquerading as a cerebral infarct. J Child Neurol 2003; 18(4):298–300.

63. Bouldin A, Pinter JD. Resolution of arterial stenosis in a patient with periarterial neurocysticercosis treated with oral prednisone. J Child Neurol 2006; 21(12):1064–1067.

64. Blum JA, Zellweger MJ, Burri C, Hatz C. Cardiac involvement in African and American trypanosomiasis. Lancet Infect Dis 2008; 8(10):631–641.

65. Nunes MC, Barbosa MM, Ribeiro AL, Barbosa FB, Rocha MO. Ischemic cerebrovascular events in patients with Chagas cardiomyopathy: a prospective follow-up study. J Neurol Sci 2009; 278(1–2):96–101.

66. Chen Z, Zhu G, Lin J, Wu N, Feng H. Acute cerebral paragonimiasis presenting as hemorrhagic stroke in a child. Pediatr Neurol 2008; 39(2):133–136.

67. Parker P, Puck J, Fernandez F. Cerebral infarction associated with *Mycoplasma pneumoniae*. Pediatrics 1981; 67(3):373–375.

68. Kirkham FJ, Calamante F, Bynevelt M, Gadian DG, Evans JP, Cox TC et al. Perfusion magnetic resonance abnormalities in patients with sickle cell disease. Ann Neurol 2001; 49(4):477–485.

69. Ovetchkine P, Brugieres P, Seradj A, Reinert P, Cohen R. An 8-year-old boy with acute stroke and radiological signs of cerebral vasculitis after recent *Mycoplasma pneumoniae* infection. Scand J Infect Dis 2002; 34(4):307–309.

70. Antachopoulos C, Liakopoulou T, Palamidou F, Papathanassiou D, Youroukos S. Posterior cerebral artery occlusion associated with *Mycoplasma pneumoniae* infection. J Child Neurol 2002; 17(1):55–57.

71. Leonardi S, Pavone P, Rotolo N, La RM. Stroke in two children with *Mycoplasma pneumoniae* infection. A causal or casual relationship? Pediatr Infect Dis J 2005; 24(9):843–845.

72. Greco F, Castellano CD, Sorge A, Perrini S, Sorge G. Multiple arterial ischemic strokes in a child with moyamoya disease and *Mycoplasma pneumoniae* infection. Minerva Pediatr 2006; 58(1): 63–68.

73. Tanir G, Aydemir C, Yilmaz D, Tuygun N. Internal carotid artery occlusion associated with *Mycoplasma pneumoniae* infection in a child. Turk J Pediatr 2006; 48(2):166–171.

74. Lee CY, Huang YY, Huang FL, Liu FC, Chen PY. *Mycoplasma pneumoniae – associated cerebral infarction in a child. J Trop Pediatr 2009; 55(4); 272–275.

75. Lee KH, McKie VC, Sekul EA, Adams RJ, Nichols FT. Unusual encephalopathy after acute chest syndrome in sickle cell disease: acute necrotizing encephalitis. J Pediatr Hematol Oncol 2002; 24(7):585–588.

76. Fryer RH, Schwobe EP, Woods ML, Rodgers GM. Chlamydia species infect human vascular endothelial cells and induce procoagulant activity. J Invest Med 1997; 45(4):168–174.

77. Markus HS, Mendall MA. *Helicobacter pylori* infection: a risk factor for ischaemic cerebrovascular disease and carotid atheroma. J Neurol Neurosurg Psychiatry 1998; 64(1):104–107.

78. Fagerberg B, Gnarpe J, Gnarpe H, Agewall S, Wikstrand J. *Chlamydia pneumoniae* but not cytomegalovirus antibodies are associated with future risk of stroke and cardiovascular disease: a prospective study in middle-aged to elderly men with treated hypertension. Stroke 1999; 30(2):299–305.

79. Goyal M, Miller ST, Hammerschlag MR, Gelling M, Gaydos CA, Hardick J et al. Is *Chlamydia pneumoniae* infection associated with stroke in children with sickle cell disease? Pediatrics 2004; 113(4):e318–e321.

80. Selby G, Walker GL. Cerebral arteritis in cat-scratch disease. Neurology 1979; 29(10):1413–1418.

81. Shoenfeld Y, Sherer Y, Harats D. Artherosclerosis as an infectious, inflammatory and autoimmune disease. Trends Immunol 2001; 22(6):293–295.

82. Paoletti R, Gotto AM, Jr, Hajjar DP. Inflammation in atherosclerosis and implications for therapy. Circulation 2004; 109(23 Suppl 1):III20–III26.

83. Nappoli C, D'Armiento FP, Mancini FP. Fatty streak formation occurs in human fetal aortas and is greatly enhanced by maternal hypercholesterolemia: intimal accumulation of low density lipoprotein and it's oxidation precede monocyte recruitment into early atherosclerotic lesions. J Clin Invest 1997; 100(2680):2690.

84. Ross R. Atherosclerosis – an inflammatory disease. N Engl J Med 1999; 340(2):115–126.

85. Jarvisalo MJ, Lehtimaki T, Raitakari OT. Determinants of arterial nitrate-mediated dilatation in children: role of oxidized lowdensity lipoprotein, endothelial function, and carotid intima-media thickness. Circulation 2004; 109(23):2885–2889.

86. Wick G, Schett G, Amberger A, Kleindienst R, Xu Q. Is atherosclerosis an immunologically mediated disease? Immunol Today 1995; 16(1):27–33.

87. Tellides G, Tereb DA, Kirkiles-Smith NC, Kim RW, Wilson JH, Schechner JS et al. Interferon-gamma elicits arteriosclerosis in the absence of leukocytes. Nature 2000; 403(6766):207–211.

88. Zhou YF, Leon MB, Waclawiw MA, Popma JJ, Yu ZX, Finkel T et al. Association between prior cytomegalovirus infection and the risk of restenosis after coronary atherectomy. N Engl J Med 1996; 335(9):624–630.

89. Ibrahim AI, Obeid MT, Jouma MJ, Moasis GA, Al-Richane WL, Kindermann I et al. Detection of herpes simplex virus, cytomegalovirus and Epstein–Barr virus DNA in atherosclerotic plaques and in unaffected bypass grafts. J Clin Virol 2005; 32(1):29–32.

90. Engebretson SP, Lamster IB, Elkind MS, Rundek T, Serman NJ, Demmer RT et al. Radiographic measures of chronic periodontitis and carotid artery plaque. Stroke 2005; 36(3):561–566.

91. Khairy P, Rinfret S, Tardif JC, Marchand R, Shapiro S, Brophy J et al. Absence of association between infectious agents and endothelial function in healthy young men. Circulation 2003; 107(15):1966–1971.

92. Martin JR, Mitchell WJ, Henken DB. Neurotropic herpesviruses, neural mechanisms and arteritis. Brain Pathol 1990; 1(1):6–10.

93. Hilt DC, Buchholz D, Krumholz A, Weiss H, Wolinsky JS. Herpes zoster ophthalmicus and delayed contralateral hemiparesis caused by cerebral angiitis: diagnosis and management approaches. Ann Neurol 1983; 14(5):543–553.

94. Amlie-Lefond C, Kleinschmidt-DeMasters BK, Mahalingam R, Davis LE, Gilden DH. The vasculopathy of varicella-zoster virus encephalitis. Ann Neurol 1995; 37(6):784–790.

95. Labetoulle M. Acute retinal necrosis syndrome. J Fr Ophtalmol 1995; 18(12):799–818.

96. Labetoulle M, Offret H, Haut J, Bloch-Michel E, Ullern M, Monin C. Acute retinal necrosis syndrome. Retrospective study apropos of 14 eyes in 11 patients. J Fr Ophtalmol 1995; 18(12):777–787.

97. Linnemann CC, Jr, Alvira MM. Pathogenesis of varicella-zoster angiitis in the CNS. Arch Neurol 1980; 37(4):239–240.

98. Ruppenthal M. Changes of the central nervous system in herpes zoster. Acta Neuropathol 1980; 52(1):59–68.

99. Chretien F, Gray F, Lescs MC, Geny C, Dubreuil-Lemaire ML, Ricolfi F et al. Acute varicella-zoster virus ventriculitis and meningo-myelo-radiculitis in acquired immunodeficiency syndrome. Acta Neuropathol 1993; 86(6):659–665.

100. Gilden DH, Kleinschmidt-DeMasters BK, Wellish M, Hedley-Whyte ET, Rentier B, Mahalingam R. Varicella zoster virus, a cause of waxing and waning vasculitis: the New England Journal of Medicine case 5 – 1995 revisited. Neurology 1996; 47(6):1441–1446.

101. Melanson M, Chalk C, Georgevich L, Fett K, Lapierre Y, Duong H et al. Varicella-zoster virus DNA in CSF and arteries in delayed contralateral hemiplegia: evidence for viral invasion of cerebral arteries. Neurology 1996; 47(2):569–570.

102. Hayman M, Hendson G, Poskitt KJ, Connolly MB. Postvaricella angiopathy: report of a case with pathologic correlation. Pediatr Neurol 2001; 24(5):387–389.

103. Eda I, Takashima S, Takeshita K. Acute hemiplegia with lacunar infarct after varicella infection in childhood. Brain Dev 1983; 5(5):494–499.

104. Ganesan V, Kirkham FJ. Mechanisms of ischaemic stroke after chickenpox. Arch Dis Child 1997; 76(6):522–525.

105. Askalan R, Laughlin S, Mayank S, Chan A, MacGregor D, Andrew M et al. Chickenpox and stroke in childhood: a study of frequency and causation. Stroke 2001; 32(6):1257–1262.

106. Sebire G, Meyer L, Chabrier S. Varicella as a risk factor for cerebral infarction in childhood: a case-control study. Ann Neurol 1999; 45(5):679–680.

107. Ichiyama T, Houdou S, Kisa T, Ohno K, Takeshita K. Varicella with delayed hemiplegia. Pediatr Neurol 1990; 6(4):279–281.

108. Sebire G, le Groupe d'Etude des AVC de l'Enfant de Bicetre. Accidents vasculaires cerebraux ischemiques d'origine arterielle. Paris: Flammarion, 1995.

109. Chabrier S, Husson B, Lasjaunias P, Landrieu P, Tardieu M. Stroke in childhood: outcome and recurrence risk by mechanism in 59 patients. J Child Neurol 2000; 15(5):290–294.

110. Ganesan V, Prengler M, McShane MA, Wade AM, Kirkham FJ. Investigation of risk factors in children with arterial ischemic stroke. Ann Neurol 2003; 53(2):167–173.

111. Lanthier S, Armstrong D, Domi T, deVeber G. Post-varicella arteriopathy of childhood: natural history of vascular stenosis. Neurology 2005; 64(4):660–663.

112. Caekebeke JF, Peters AC, Vandvik B, Brouwer OF, de Bakker HM. Cerebral vasculopathy associated with primary varicella infection. Arch Neurol 1990; 47(9):1033–1035.

113. Bodensteiner JB, Hille MR, Riggs JE. Clinical features of vascular thrombosis following varicella. Am J Dis Child 1992; 146(1):100–102.

114. Brower MC, Rollins N, Roach ES. Basal ganglia and thalamic infarction in children. Cause and clinical features. Arch Neurol 1996; 53(12):1252–1256.

115. Hausler MG, Ramaekers VT, Reul J, Meilicke R, Heimann G. Early and late onset manifestations of cerebral vasculitis related to varicella zoster. Neuropediatrics 1998; 29(4):202–207.

116. Berger TM, Caduff JH, Gebbers JO. Fatal varicella-zoster virus antigen-positive giant cell arteritis of the central nervous system. Pediatr Infect Dis J 2000; 19(7):653–656.

117. Moros-Pena M, Munoz-Albillos MS, Pena-Segura JL, Nagaraja D, Verma A, Taly AB. Cerebrovascular disease in children. Acta Neurol Scand 1994; 90:251–255.

118. Caruso JM, Tung GA, Brown WD. Central nervous system and renal vasculitis associated with primary varicella infection in a child. Pediatrics 2001; 107(1):E9.

119. Chabrier S, Rodesch G, Lasjaunias P, Tardieu M, Landrieu P, Sebire G. Transient cerebral arteriopathy: a disorder recognized by serial angiograms in children with stroke. J Child Neurol 1998; 13(1):27–32.

120. Husson B, Rodesch G, Lasjaunias P, Tardieu M, Sebire G. Magnetic resonance angiography in childhood arterial brain infarcts: a comparative study with contrast angiography. Stroke 2002; 33(5):1280–1285.

121. Hattori H, Higuchi Y, Tsuji M. Recurrent strokes after varicella. Ann Neurol 2000; 47(1):136.

122. Arvin AM. Varicella vaccine – the first six years. N Engl J Med 2001; 344(13):1007–1009.

123. Wirrell E, Hill MD, Jadavji T, Kirton A, Barlow K. Stroke after varicella vaccination. J Pediatr 2004; 145(6):845–847.

124. Sergent JS, Lockshin MD, Christian CL, Gocke DJ. Vasculitis with hepatitis B antigenemia: long-term observation in nine patients. Medicine (Baltimore) 1976; 55(1):1–18.

125. Guillevin L, Lhote F, Cohen P, Sauvaget F, Jarrousse B, Lortholary O et al. Polyarteritis nodosa related to hepatitis B virus. A prospective study with long-term observation of 41 patients. Medicine (Baltimore). 1995; 74(5):238–253.

126. Gupta S, Piraka C, Jaffe M. Lamivudine in the treatment of polyarteritis nodosa associated with acute hepatitis B. N Engl J Med 2001; 344(21):1645–1646.

127. Ribai P, Liesnard C, Rodesch G, Giurgea S, Verheulpen D, David P et al. Transient cerebral arteriopathy in infancy associated with enteroviral infection. Eur J Paediatr Neurol 2003; 7(2):73–75.

128. Guidi B, Bergonzini P, Crisi G, Frigieri G, Portolani M. Case of stroke in a 7-year-old male after parvovirus B19 infection. Pediatr Neurol 2003; 28(1):69–71.

129. Lowe LH, Morello FP, Jackson MA, Lasky A. Application of transcranial Doppler sonography in children with acute neurologic events due to primary cerebral and West Nile vasculitis. AJNR Am J Neuroradiol 2005; 26(7):1698–1701.

130. Alexander JJ, Lasky AS, Graf WD. Stroke associated with central nervous system vasculitis after West Nile virus infection. J Child Neurol 2006; 21(7):623–625.

131. Zahuranec DB, Brown DL, Lisabeth LD, Morgenstern LB. Is it time for a large, collaborative study of pediatric stroke? Stroke 2005; 36(9):1825–1829.

132. Madhi SA, Madhi A, Petersen K, Khoosal M, Klugman KP. Impact of human immunodeficiency virus type 1 infection on the epidemiology and outcome of bacterial meningitis in South African children. Int J Infect Dis 2001; 5(3):119–125.

133. Molyneux EM, Tembo M, Kayira K, Bwanaisa L, Mweneychanya J, Njobvu A et al. The effect of HIV infection on paediatric bacterial meningitis in Blantyre, Malawi. Arch Dis Child 2003; 88(12):1112–1118.

134. Park YD, Belman AL, Kim TS, Kure K, Llena JF, Lantos G et al. Stroke in pediatric acquired immunodeficiency syndrome. Ann Neurol 1990; 28(3):303–311.

135. Burns DK. The neuropathology of pediatric acquired immunodeficiency syndrome. J Child Neurol 1992; 7(4):332–346.

136. Katsetos CD, Fincke JE, Legido A, Lischner HW, de Chadarevian JP, Kaye EM et al. Angiocentric CD3(+) T-cell infiltrates in human immunodeficiency virus type 1-associated central nervous system disease in children. Clin Diagn Lab Immunol 1999; 6(1):105–114.

137. Gray F, Belec L, Lescs MC, Chretien F, Ciardi A, Hassine D et al. Varicella-zoster virus infection of the central nervous system in the acquired immune deficiency syndrome. Brain 1994; 117 (Pt 5):987–999.

138. Philippet P, Blanche S, Sebag G, Rodesch G, Griscelli C, Tardieu M. Stroke and cerebral infarcts in children infected with human immunodeficiency virus. Arch Pediatr Adolesc Med 1994; 148(9):965–970.

139. Legido A, Lischner HW, de Chadarevian JP, Katsetos CD. Stroke in pediatric HIV infection. Pediatr Neurol 1999; 21(2):588.

140. Visudtibhan A, Visudhiphan P, Chiemchanya S. Stroke and seizures as the presenting signs of pediatric HIV infection. Pediatr Neurol 1999; 20(1):53–56.

141. Ortiz G, Koch S, Romano JG, Forteza AM, Rabinstein AA. Mechanisms of ischemic stroke in HIV-infected patients. Neurology 2007; 68(16):1257–1261.

142. Leeuwis JW, Wolfs TF, Braun KP. A child with HIV-associated transient cerebral arteriopathy. AIDS 2007; 21(10):1383–1384.

143. Dlamini N, Wilmshurst J, Pohl K, Padayachee S, Eley B, Kirkham F. Transcranial Doppler and Stroke in South African Children with Human Immunodeficiency Virus. Arch Dis Child 2009; 94(Suppl I):A73–A79 (G185).

144. Bulsara KR, Raja A, Owen J. HIV and cerebral aneurysms. Neurosurg Rev. 2005;28(2):92–95.

145. Brilla R, Nabavi DG, Schulte-Altedorneburg G, Kemeny V, Reichelt D, Evers S et al. Cerebral vasculopathy in HIV infection revealed by transcranial Doppler: a pilot study. Stroke 1999; 30(4):811–813.

146. Surtees R, Hyland K, Smith I. Central-nervous-system methyl-group metabolism in children with neurological complications of HIV infection. Lancet 1990; 335(8690):619–621.

147. Van RA, Harrington PR, Dow A, Robertson K. Neurologic and neurodevelopmental manifestations of pediatric HIV/AIDS: a global perspective. Eur J Paediatr Neurol 2007; 11(1):1–9.

148. Oh J, Hegele RA. HIV-associated dyslipidaemia: pathogenesis and treatment. Lancet Infect Dis 2007; 7(12):787–796.

149. Probasco JC, Spudich SS, Critchfield J, Lee E, Lollo N, Deeks SG et al. Failure of atorvastatin to modulate CSF HIV-1 infection: results of a pilot study. Neurology 2008; 71(7):521–524.

150. Inamasu J, Uchida K, Mayanagi K, Suga S, Kawase T. Basilar artery occlusion due to mucormycotic emboli, preceded by acute hydrocephalus. Clin Neurol Neurosurg 2000; 102(1):18–22.

151. Somer T, Finegold SM. Vasculitides associated with infections, immunization, and antimicrobial drugs. Clin Infect Dis 1995; 20(4):1010–1036.

152. Nagashima T, Miyanoshita A, Sakiyama Y, Ozaki Y, Stan AC, Nagashima K. Cerebral vasculitis in chronic mucocutaneous candidiasis: autopsy case report. Neuropathology 2000; 20(4):309–314.

153. DeLone DR, Goldstein RA, Petermann G, Salamat MS, Miles JM, Knechtle SJ et al. Disseminated aspergillosis involving the brain: distribution and imaging characteristics. AJNR Am J Neuroradiol 1999; 20(9):1597–1604.

154. Andrew M, David M, Adams M, Ali K, Anderson R, Barnard D et al. Venous thromboembolic complications (VTE) in children: first analyses of the Canadian Registry of VTE. Blood 1994; 83(5):1251–1257.

155. Schmidt B, Andrew M. Neonatal thrombosis: report of a prospective Canadian and international registry. Pediatrics 1995; 96(5 Pt 1):939–943.

156. Nowak-Gottl U, von KR, Gobel U. Neonatal symptomatic thromboembolism in Germany: two year survey. Arch Dis Child Fetal Neonatal Ed 1997; 76(3):F163–F167.

157. Mudd SH, Skovby F, Levy HL, Pettigrew KD, Wilcken B, Pyeritz RE et al. The natural history of homocystinuria due to cystathionine beta-synthase deficiency. Am J Hum Genet 1985; 37(1):1–31.

158. Dahlback B, Carlsson M, Svensson PJ. Familial thrombophilia due to a previously unrecognized mechanism characterized by poor anticoagulant response to activated protein C: prediction of a cofactor to activated protein C. Proc Natl Acad Sci U S A 1993; 90(3):1004–1008.

159. Bertina RM, Koeleman BP, Koster T, Rosendaal FR, Dirven RJ, de RH et al. Mutation in blood coagulation factor V associated with resistance to activated protein C. Nature 1994; 369(6475):64–67.

160. Lane DA, Mannucci PM, Bauer KA, Bertina RM, Bochkov NP, Boulyjenkov V et al. Inherited thrombophilia: Part 1. Thromb Haemost 1996; 76(5):651–662.

161. Lane DA, Mannucci PM, Bauer KA, Bertina RM, Bochkov NP, Boulyjenkov V et al. Inherited thrombophilia: Part 2. Thromb Haemost 1996; 76(6):824–834.

162. Andrew M. Developmental hemostasis: relevance to thromboembolic complications in pediatric patients. Thromb Haemost 1995; 74(1):415–425.

163. Siegbahn A, Ruusuvaara L. Age dependence of blood fibrinolytic components and the effects of low-dose oral contraceptives on coagulation and fibrinolysis in teenagers. Thromb Haemost 1988; 60(3):361–364.

164. De Wolf F, Carreras LO, Moerman P, Vermylen J, Van AA, Renaer M. Decidual vasculopathy and extensive placental infarction in a patient with repeated thromboembolic accidents, recurrent fetal loss, and a lupus anticoagulant. Am J Obstet Gynecol 1982; 142(7):829–834.

165. Salafia CM, Vintzileos AM, Silberman L, Bantham KF, Vogel CA. Placental pathology of idiopathic intrauterine growth retardation at term. Am J Perinatol 1992; 9(3):179–184.

166. Berg K, Roald B, Sande H. High Lp(a) lipoprotein level in maternal serum may interfere with placental circulation and cause fetal growth retardation. Clin Genet 1994; 46(1 Spec No):52–56.

167. Dizon-Townson DS, Meline L, Nelson LM, Varner M, Ward K. Fetal carriers of the factor V Leiden mutation are prone to miscarriage and placental infarction. Am J Obstet Gynecol 1997; 177(2):402–405.

168. Ment LR, Duncan CC, Ehrenkranz RA. Perinatal cerebral infarction. Ann Neurol 1984; 16(5):559–568.

169. Debus O, Koch HG, Kurlemann G, Strater R, Vielhaber H, Weber P et al. Factor V Leiden and genetic defects of thrombophilia in childhood porencephaly. Arch Dis Child Fetal Neonatal Ed 1998; 78(2):F121–F124.

170. de Vries LS, Eken P, Groenendaal F, Rademaker KJ, Hoogervorst B, Bruinse HW. Antenatal onset of haemorrhagic and/or ischaemic lesions in preterm infants: prevalence and associated obstetric variables. Arch Dis Child Fetal Neonatal Ed 1998; 78(1):F51–F56.

171. Kraus FT, Acheen VI. Fetal thrombotic vasculopathy in the placenta: cerebral thrombi and infarcts, coagulopathies, and cerebral palsy. Hum Pathol 1999; 30(7):759–769.

172. Govaert P, Matthys E, Zecic A, Roelens F, Oostra A, Vanzieleghem B. Perinatal cortical infarction within middle cerebral artery trunks. Arch Dis Child Fetal Neonatal Ed 2000; 82(1):F59–F63.

173. deVeber G, Chan A, Monagle P, Marzinotto V, Armstrong D, Massicotte P et al. Anticoagulation therapy in pediatric patients with sinovenous thrombosis: a cohort study. Arch Neurol 1998; 55(12):1533–1537.

174. deVeber G, Andrew M, Adams C, Bjornson B, Booth F, Buckley DJ et al. Cerebral sinovenous thrombosis in children. N Engl J Med 2001; 345(6):417–423.

175. Heller C, Heinecke A, Junker R, Knofler R, Kosch A, Kurnik K et al. Cerebral venous thrombosis in children: a multifactorial origin. Circulation 2003; 108(11):1362–1367.

176. Sebire G, Tabarki B, Saunders DE, Leroy I, Liesner R, Saint-Martin C et al. Cerebral venous sinus thrombosis in children: risk factors, presentation, diagnosis and outcome. Brain 2005; 128(Pt 3):477–489.

177. Ganesan V, Kelsey H, Cookson J, Osborn A, Kirkham FJ. Activated protein C resistance in childhood stroke. Lancet 1996; 347(8996):260.

178. Riikonen RS, Vahtera EM, Kekomaki RM. Physiological anticoagulants and activated protein C resistance in childhood stroke. Acta Paediatr 1996; 85(2):242–244.

179. Becker S, Heller C, Gropp F, Scharrer I, Kreuz W. Thrombophilic disorders in children with cerebral infarction. Lancet 1998; 352(9142):1756–1757.

180. Heller C, Becker S, Scharrer I, Kreuz W. Prothrombotic risk factors in childhood stroke and venous thrombosis. Eur J Pediatr 1999; 158 Suppl 3:S117–S121.

181. McColl MD, Chalmers EA, Thomas A, Sproul A, Healey C, Rafferty I et al. Factor V Leiden, prothrombin 20210G→A and the MTHFR C677T mutations in childhood stroke. Thromb Haemost 1999; 81(5):690–694.

182. Nowak-Gottl U, Strater R, Heinecke A, Junker R, Koch HG, Schuierer G et al. Lipoprotein (a) and genetic polymorphisms of clotting factor V, prothrombin, and methylenetetrahydrofolate reductase are risk factors of spontaneous ischemic stroke in childhood. Blood 1999; 94(11):3678–3682.

183. Strater R, Vielhaber H, Kassenbohmer R, von KR, Gobel U, Nowak-Gottl U. Genetic risk factors of thrombophilia in ischaemic childhood stroke of cardiac origin. A prospective ESPED survey. Eur J Pediatr 1999; 158(Suppl 3):S122–S125.

184. Strater R, Becker S, von Eckardtstein A, Heinecke A, Gutsche S, Junker R et al. Prospective assessment of risk factors for recurrent stroke during childhood – a 5-year follow-up study. Lancet 2002; 360(9345):1540–1545.

185. Gunther G, Junker R, Strater R, Schobess R, Kurnik K, Heller C et al. Symptomatic ischemic stroke in full-term neonates: role of acquired and genetic prothrombotic risk factors. Stroke 2000; 31(10):2437–2441.

186. Kenet G, Sadetzki S, Murad H, Martinowitz U, Rosenberg N, Gitel S et al. Factor V Leiden and antiphospholipid antibodies are significant risk factors for ischemic stroke in children. Stroke 2000; 31(6):1283–1288.

187. Utermann G. The mysteries of lipoprotein(a). Science 1989; 246(4932):904–910.

188. Berg K, Dahlen G, Frick MH. Lp(a) lipoprotein and pre-beta₁-lipoprotein in patients with coronary heart disease. Clin Genet 1974; 6(3):230–235.

189. Jurgens G, Taddei-Peters WC, Koltringer P, Petek W, Chen Q, Greilberger J et al. Lipoprotein(a) serum concentration and apolipoprotein(a) phenotype correlate with severity and presence of ischemic cerebrovascular disease. Stroke 1995; 26(10):1841–1848.

190. Mandel H, Brenner B, Berant M, Rosenberg N, Lanir N, Jakobs C et al. Coexistence of hereditary homocystinuria and factor V Leiden – effect on thrombosis. N Engl J Med 1996; 334(12):763–768.

191. Formstone CJ, Hallam PJ, Tuddenham EG, Voke J, Layton M, Nicolaides K et al. Severe perinatal thrombosis in double and triple heterozygous offspring of a family segregating two independent protein S mutations and a protein C mutation. Blood 1996; 87(9):3731–3737.

192. Salomon O, Steinberg DM, Zivelin A, Gitel S, Dardik R, Rosenberg N et al. Single and combined prothrombotic factors in patients with idiopathic venous thromboembolism: prevalence and risk assessment. Arterioscler Thromb Vasc Biol 1999; 19(3):511–518.

193. Junker R, Koch HG, Auberger K, Munchow N, Ehrenforth S, Nowak-Gottl U. Prothrombin G20210A gene mutation and further prothrombotic risk factors in childhood thrombophilia. Arterioscler Thromb Vasc Biol 1999; 19(10):2568–2572.

194. Lawson SE, Butler D, Enayat MS, Williams MD. Congenital thrombophilia and thrombosis: a study in a single centre. Arch Dis Child 1999; 81(2):176–178.

195. Nowak-Gottl U, Junker R, Kreuz W, von Eckardstein A, Kosch A, Nohe N et al. Risk of recurrent venous thrombosis in children with combined prothrombotic risk factors. Blood 2001; 97(4):858–862.

196. Nicolaides P, Leonard J, Surtees R. Neurological outcome of methylmalonic acidaemia. Arch Dis Child 1998; 78(6):508–512.

197. Kirkham FJ. Stroke in childhood. Arch Dis Child 1999; 81(1):85–89.

198. Roach ES. Stroke in children. Curr Treat Options Neurol 2000; 2(4):295–304.

199. Cardo E, Campistol J, Caritg J, Ruiz S, Vilaseca MA, Kirkham F et al. Fatal haemorrhagic infarct in an infant with homocystinuria. Dev Med Child Neurol 1999; 41(2):132–135.

200. Buoni S, Molinelli M, Mariottini A, Rango C, Medaglini S, Pieri S et al. Homocystinuria with transverse sinus thrombosis. J Child Neurol 2001; 16(9):688–690.

201. Cochran FB, Packman S. Homocystinuria presenting as sagittal sinus thrombosis. Eur Neurol 1992; 32(1):1–3.

202. Lu CY, Hou JW, Wang PJ, Chiu HH, Wang TR. Homocystinuria presenting as fatal common carotid artery occlusion. Pediatr Neurol 1996; 15(2):159–162.

203. Ganesan V, McShane MA, Liesner R, Cookson J, Hann I, Kirkham FJ. Inherited prothrombotic states and ischaemic stroke in childhood. J Neurol Neurosurg Psychiatry 1998; 65(4):508–511.

204. Ganesan V, Savvy L, Chong WK, Kirkham FJ. Conventional cerebral angiography in children with ischemic stroke. Pediatr Neurol 1999; 20(1):38–42.

205. Ganesan V, Ng V, Chong WK, Kirkham FJ, Connelly A. Lesion volume, lesion location, and outcome after middle cerebral artery territory stroke. Arch Dis Child 1999; 81(4):295–300.

206. Nowak-Gottl U, Koch HG, Aschka I, Kohlhase B, Vielhaber H, Kurlemann G et al. Resistance to activated protein C (APCR) in children with venous or arterial thromboembolism. Br J Haematol 1996; 92(4):992–998.

207. Lynch JK, Han CJ. Pediatric stroke: what do we know and what do we need to know? Semin Neurol 2005; 25(4):410–423.

208. Bonduel M, Sciuccati G, Hepner M, Pieroni G, Torres AF, Frontroth JP et al. Arterial ischemic stroke and cerebral venous thrombosis in children: a 12-year Argentinean registry. Acta Haematol 2006; 115(3–4):180–185.

209. Johal SC, Garg BP, Heiny ME, Williams LS, Saha C, Walsh LE et al. Family history is a poor screen for prothrombotic genes in children with stroke. J Pediatr 2006; 148(1):68–71.

210. Salih MA, Abdel-Gader AG, Al-Jarallah AA, Kentab AY, Alorainy IA, Hassan HH et al. Perinatal stroke in Saudi children. Clinical features and risk factors. Saudi Med J 2006; 27(Suppl 1):S35–S40.

211. Salih MA, Abdel-Gader AG, Al-Jarallah AA, Kentab AY, Alorainy IA, Hassan HH et al. Stroke in Saudi children. Epidemiology, clinical features and risk factors. Saudi Med J 2006; 27(Suppl 1):S12–S20.

212. Gokben S, Tosun A, Bayram N, Serdaroglu G, Polat M, Kavakli K et al. Arterial ischemic stroke in childhood: risk factors and outcome in old versus new era. J Child Neurol 2007; 22(10):1204–1208.

213. Simma B, Martin G, Muller T, Huemer M. Risk factors for pediatric stroke: consequences for therapy and quality of life. Pediatr Neurol 2007; 37(2):121–126.

214. Lee YY, Lin KL, Wang HS, Chou ML, Hung PC, Hsieh MY et al. Risk factors and outcomes of childhood ischemic stroke in Taiwan. Brain Dev 2008; 30(1):14–19.

215. Kennedy CR, Warner G, Kai M, Chisholm M. Protein C deficiency and stroke in early life. Dev Med Child Neurol 1995; 37(8):723–730.

216. Ganesan V, Prengler M, Wade A, Kirkham FJ. Clinical and radiological recurrence after childhood arterial ischemic stroke. Circulation 2006; 114(20):2170–2177.

217. Kirkham FJ. Is there a genetic basis for pediatric stroke? Curr Opin Pediatr 2003; 15(6):547–558.

218. Haywood S, Liesner R, Pindora S, Ganesan V. Thrombophilia and first arterial ischaemic stroke: a systematic review. Arch Dis Child 2005; 90(4):402–405.

219. Kenet G & Lütkhoff LK (joint first authors), Albisetti M, Bernard T, Bonduel M, Brandao L et al. Impact of thrombophilia on arterial ischemic stroke or cerebral sinovenous thrombosis in children: a systematic review and meta-analysis of observational studies. Circulation 2010; 121(16):1838–1847.

220. Manco-Johnson MJ, Nuss R, Key N, Moertel C, Jacobson L, Meech S et al. Lupus anticoagulant and protein S deficiency in children with postvaricella purpura fulminans or thrombosis. J Pediatr 1996; 128(3):319–323.

221. Johal SC, Garg BP, Heiny ME, Williams LS, Saha C, Walsh LE et al. Family history is a poor screen for prothrombotic genes in children with stroke. J Pediatr 2006; 148(1):68–71.

222. Young G, Albisetti M, Bonduel M, Brandao L, Chan A, Friedrichs F et al. Impact of inherited thrombophilia on venous thromboembolism in children: a systematic review and meta-analysis of observational studies. Circulation 2008; 118(13):1373–1382.

223. Golomb MR, Garg BP, Walsh LE, Williams LS. Perinatal stroke in baby, prothrombotic gene in mom: does this affect maternal health insurance? Neurology 2005; 65(1):13–16.

224. Andrew M, Paes B, Johnston M. Development of the hemostatic system in the neonate and young infant. Am J Pediatr Hematol Oncol 1990; 12(1):95–104.

225. Ehrenforth S, Junker R, Koch HG, Kreuz W, Munchow N, Scharrer I et al. Multicentre evaluation of combined prothrombotic defects associated with thrombophilia in childhood. Childhood Thrombophilia Study Group. Eur J Pediatr 1999; 158(Suppl 3):S97–104.

226. Nowak-Gottl U, Kosch A, Schlegel N. Thromboembolism in newborns, infants and children. Thromb Haemost 2001; 86(1):464–474.

227. Update on the 1987 Task Force Report on High Blood Pressure in Children and Adolescents: a working group report from the National High Blood Pressure Education Program. National High Blood Pressure Education Program Working Group on Hypertension Control in Children and Adolescents. Pediatrics 1996; 98(4 Pt 1):649–658.

228. De Swiet M, Fayers P, Shinebourne EA. Blood pressure in first 10 years of life: the Brompton study. BMJ 1992; 304(6818):23–26.
229. Din-Dzietham R, Liu Y, Bielo MV, Shamsa F. High blood pressure trends in children and adolescents in national surveys, 1963 to 2002. Circulation 2007; 116(13):1488–1496.
230. Sharma M, Kupferman JC, Brosgol Y, Paterno K, Goodman S, Prohovnik I, Kirkham FJ, Parlakis SG. The impact of hypertension on the pediatric brain: a justifiable concern. Lancet Neurology 2010; 9:933–940.
231. Daniels SR. Hypertension-induced cardiac damage in children and adolescents. Blood Press Monit 1999; 4(3–4):165–170.
232. Mitchell P, Cheung N, de Haseth K, Taylor B, Rochtchina E, Islam FM et al. Blood pressure and retinal arteriolar narrowing in children. Hypertension 2007; 49(5):1156–1162.
233. Staessen JA, Kuznetsova T, Stolarz K. Hypertension prevalence and stroke mortality across populations. JAMA 2003; 289(18):2420–2422.
234. Ganesan V, Chong WK, Cox TC, Chawda SJ, Prengler M, Kirkham FJ. Posterior circulation stroke in childhood: risk factors and recurrence. Neurology 2002; 59(10):1552–1556.
235. Chung B, Wong V. Pediatric stroke among Hong Kong Chinese subjects. Pediatrics 2004; 114(2):e206–e212.
236. Lynch JK, Han CJ, Nee LE, Nelson KB. Prothrombotic factors in children with stroke or porencephaly. Pediatrics 2005; 116(2):447–453.
237. Hansen ML, Gunn PW, Kaelber DC. Underdiagnosis of hypertension in children and adolescents. JAMA 2007; 298(8):874–879.
238. Ohene-Frempong K, Weiner SJ, Sleeper LA, Miller ST, Embury S, Moohr JW et al. Cerebrovascular accidents in sickle cell disease: rates and risk factors. Blood 1998; 91(1):288–294.
239. Strouse JJ, Cox CS, Melhem ER, Lu H, Kraut MA, Razumovsky A et al. Inverse correlation between cerebral blood flow measured by continuous arterial spin-labeling (CASL) MRI and neurocognitive function in children with sickle cell anemia (SCA). Blood 2006; 108(1):379–381.
240. Rakototiana AF, Ramorasata AC, Rakoto-Ratsimba HN, Hunald FA, Rajaobelison T, Rantomalala HY. Pheochromocytoma revealed by stroke in a child. Arch Pediatr 2008; 15(10):1531–1534.
241. Van YH, Wang HS, Lai CH, Lin JN, Lo FS. Pheochromocytoma presenting as stroke in two Taiwanese children. J Pediatr Endocrinol Metab 2002; 15(9):1563–1567.
242. Dagartzikas MI, Sprague K, Carter G, Tobias JD. Cerebrovascular event, dilated cardiomyopathy, and pheochromocytoma. Pediatr Emerg Care 2002; 18(1):33–35.
243. Pihko H, Tyni T, Virkola K, Valanne L, Sainio K, Hovi L et al. Transient ischemic cerebral lesions during induction chemotherapy for acute lymphoblastic leukemia. J Pediatr 1993; 123(5):718–724.
244. Nguyen JH, Lodish MB, Patronas NJ, Ugrasbul F, Keil MF, Roberts MD et al. Extensive and largely reversible ischemic cerebral infarctions in a prepubertal child with hypertension and Cushing disease. J Clin Endocrinol Metab 2009; 94(1):1–2.
245. Kupferman JC, Singh A, Pavlakis SG. Lacunar stroke and masked hypertension in an adolescent male. Pediatr Neurol 2007; 36(2):125–127.
246. Lurbe E, Torro I, Alvarez V, Nawrot T, Paya R, Redon J et al. Prevalence, persistence, and clinical significance of masked hypertension in youth. Hypertension 2005; 45(4):493–498.
247. Stabouli S, Kotsis V, Toumanidis S, Papamichael C, Constantopoulos A, Zakopoulos N. White-coat and masked hypertension in children: association with target-organ damage. Pediatr Nephrol 2005; 20(8):1151–1155.
248. Strouse JJ, Hulbert ML, DeBaun MR, Jordan LC, Casella JF. Primary hemorrhagic stroke in children with sickle cell disease is associated with recent transfusion and use of corticosteroids. Pediatrics 2006; 118(5):1916–1924.
249. Pegelow CH, Colangelo L, Steinberg M, Wright EC, Smith J, Phillips G et al. Natural history of blood pressure in sickle cell disease: risks for stroke and death associated with relative hypertension in sickle cell anemia. Am J Med 1997; 102(2):171–177.
250. Awada A, Daif A, Obeid T, Al RS. Nontraumatic cerebral hemorrhage in the young: a study of 107 cases. J Stroke Cerebrovasc Dis 1998; 7(3):200–204.
251. Maeda H, Matsumoto M, Handa N, Hougaku H, Ogawa S, Itoh T et al. Reactivity of cerebral blood flow to carbon dioxide in hypertensive patients: evaluation by the transcranial Doppler method. J Hypertens 1994; 12(2):191–197.
252. Wong LJ, Kupferman JC, Prohovnik I, Kirkham FJ, Goodman S, Paterno K, Sharma M, Brosgol Y, Pavlakis SG. Hypertension impairs vascular reactivity in the pediatric brain. Stroke 2011; in press.
253. Sorof JM, Alexandrov AV, Cardwell G, Portman RJ. Carotid artery intimal-medial thickness and left ventricular hypertrophy in children with elevated blood pressure. Pediatrics 2003; 111(1):61–66.
254. Kieslich M, Fiedler A, Heller C, Kreuz W, Jacobi G. Minor head injury as cause and co-factor in the aetiology of stroke in childhood: a report of eight cases. J Neurol Neurosurg Psychiatry 2002; 73(1):13–16.
255. Shaffer L, Rich PM, Pohl KR, Ganesan V. Can mild head injury cause ischaemic stroke? Arch Dis Child 2003; 88(3):267–269.
256. Rana KS, Behera MK, Adhikari KM. Ischemic stroke following mild head injury: is it the cause. Indian Pediatr 2006; 43(11):994–997.
257. Chamoun RB, Mawad ME, Whitehead WE, Luerssen TG, Jea A. Extracranial traumatic carotid artery dissections in children: a review of current diagnosis and treatment options. J Neurosurg Pediatr 2008; 2(2):101–118.
258. Dharker SR, Mittal RS, Bhargava N. Ischemic lesions in basal ganglia in children after minor head injury. Neurosurgery 1993; 33(5):863–865.
259. Ahn JY, Han IB, Chung YS, Yoon PH, Kim SH. Posttraumatic infarction in the territory supplied by the lateral lenticulostriate artery after minor head injury. Childs Nerv Syst 2006; 22(11):1493–1496.
260. Aparicio JM, Tavares C, Teixeira-Pinto A, Almeida F, Silva ML, Vaz R et al. Cerebral vasospasm in pediatric head injuries: transcranial Doppler ultrasound findings. Cerebrovasc Dis 2002; 11:38.
261. Taha JM, Crone KR, Berger TS, Becket WW, Prenger EC. Sigmoid sinus thrombosis after closed head injury in children. Neurosurgery 1993; 32(4):541–545.
262. Meena AK, Naidu KS, Murthy JM. Cortical sinovenous thrombosis in a child with nephrotic syndrome and iron deficiency anaemia. Neurol India 2000; 48(3):292–294.
263. Satoh H, Kumano K, Ogami R, Nishi T, Onda J, Nishimura S et al. Sigmoid sinus thrombosis after mild closed head injury in an infant: diagnosis by magnetic resonance imaging in the acute phase – case report. Neurol Med Chir (Tokyo) 2000; 40(7):361–365.
264. Muthukumar N. Cerebral venous sinus thrombosis and thrombophilia presenting as pseudo-tumour syndrome following mild head injury. J Clin Neurosci 2004; 11(8):924–927.
265. Tamimi A, bu-Elrub M, Shudifat A, Saleh Q, Kharazi K, Tamimi I. Superior sagittal sinus thrombosis associated with raised intracranial pressure in closed head injury with depressed skull fracture. Pediatr Neurosurg 2005; 41(5):237–240.
266. Yuen HW, Gan BK, Seow WT, Tan HK. Dural sinus thrombosis after minor head injury in a child. Ann Acad Med Singapore 2005; 34(10):639–641.
267. Shigemori Y, Koshinaga M, Suma T, Nakamura S, Murata Y, Kawamata T et al. Jugular bulb venous thrombosis caused by mild head injury: a case report. Surg Neurol 2007; 68(6):660–664.
268. Matsushige T, Kiya K, Satoh H, Mizoue T, Kagawa K, Araki H. Cerebral venous congestion following closed head injury in a child. Pediatr Neurosurg 2004; 40(5):241–244.
269. Agner C, Weig SG. Arterial dissection and stroke following child abuse: case report and review of the literature. Childs Nerv Syst 2005; 21(5):416–420.
270. Nguyen PH, Burrowes DM, Ali S, Bowman RM, Shaibani A. Intracranial vertebral artery dissection with subarachnoid hemorrhage following child abuse. Pediatr Radiol 2007; 37(6):600–602.
271. McKinney AM, Thompson LR, Truwit CL, Velders S, Karagulle A, Kiragu A. Unilateral hypoxic-ischemic injury in young children from abusive head trauma, lacking craniocervical vascular dissection or cord injury. Pediatr Radiol 2008; 38(2):164–174.
272. Hoskote A, Richards P, Anslow P, McShane T. Subdural haematoma and non-accidental head injury in children. Childs Nerv Syst 2002; 18(6–7):311–317.
273. Fernandes AR, Pala AM, Ferreira M, Jasmin F. Shaken baby syndrome and stroke. Rev Neurol 2007; 45(11):701–702.

274. Hartfield DS, Lowry NJ, Keene DL, Yager JY. Iron deficiency: a cause of stroke in infants and children. Pediatr Neurol 1997; 16(1):50–53.

275. Maguire JL, deVeber G, Parkin PC. Association between iron-deficiency anemia and stroke in young children. Pediatrics 2007; 120(5):1053–1057.

276. Goodwin FC, Beattie RM, Millar J, Kirkham FJ. Celiac disease and childhood stroke. Pediatr Neurol 2004; 31(2):139–142.

277. Homma S, Di Tullio MR, Sacco RL, Mihalatos D, Li MG, Mohr JP. Characteristics of patent foramen ovale associated with cryptogenic stroke. A biplane transesophageal echocardiographic study. Stroke 1994; 25(3):582–586.

278. de Belder MA, Tourikis L, Leech G, Camm AJ. Risk of patent foramen ovale for thromboembolic events in all age groups. Am J Cardiol 1992; 69(16):1316–1320.

279. De Castro S, Cartoni D, Fiorelli M, Rasura M, Anzini A, Zanette EM et al. Morphological and functional characteristics of patent foramen ovale and their embolic implications. Stroke 2000; 31(10):2407–2413.

280. Manning WJ. Role of transesophageal echocardiography in the management of thromboembolic stroke. Am J Cardiol 1997; 80(4C):19D–28D.

281. Lechat P, Mas JL, Lascault G, Loron P, Theard M, Klimczac M et al. Prevalence of patent foramen ovale in patients with stroke. N Engl J Med 1988; 318(18):1148–1152.

282. Ranoux D, Cohen A, Cabanes L, Amarenco P, Bousser MG, Mas JL. Patent foramen ovale: is stroke due to paradoxical embolism? Stroke 1993; 24(1):31–34.

283. Bogousslavsky J, Devuyst G, Nendaz M, Yamamoto H, Sarasin F. Prevention of stroke recurrence with presumed paradoxical embolism. J Neurol 1997; 244(2):71–75.

284. Berthet K, Lavergne T, Cohen A, Guize L, Bousser MG, Le Heuzey JY et al. Significant association of atrial vulnerability with atrial septal abnormalities in young patients with ischemic stroke of unknown cause. Stroke 2000; 31(2):398–403.

285. Sritippayawan S, MacLaughlin EF, Woo MS. Acute neurological deficits in a young adult with cystic fibrosis. Pediatr Pulmonol 2003; 35(2):147–151.

286. Beelke M, Angeli S, Del SM, Gandolfo C, Cabano ME, Canovaro P et al. Prevalence of patent foramen ovale in subjects with obstructive sleep apnea: a transcranial Doppler ultrasound study. Sleep Med 2003; 4(3):219–223.

287. Overell JR, Bone I, Lees KR. Interatrial septal abnormalities and stroke: a meta-analysis of case-control studies. Neurology 2000; 55(8):1172–1179.

288. Cabanes L, Mas JL, Cohen A, Amarenco P, Cabanes PA, Oubary P et al. Atrial septal aneurysm and patent foramen ovale as risk factors for cryptogenic stroke in patients less than 55 years of age. A study using transesophageal echocardiography. Stroke 1993; 24(12):1865–1873.

289. Hanna JP, Sun JP, Furlan AJ, Stewart WJ, Sila CA, Tan M. Patent foramen ovale and brain infarct. Echocardiographic predictors, recurrence, and prevention. Stroke 1994; 25(4):782–786.

290. Mas JL. Patent foramen ovale, atrial septal aneurysm and ischaemic stroke in young adults. Eur Heart J 1994; 15(4):446–449.

291. Petty GW, Khandheria BK, Meissner I, Whisnant JP, Rocca WA, Christianson TJ et al. Population-based study of the relationship between patent foramen ovale and cerebrovascular ischemic events. Mayo Clin Proc 2006; 81(5):602–608.

292. Di Tullio MR, Sacco RL, Sciacca RR, Jin Z, Homma S. Patent foramen ovale and the risk of ischemic stroke in a multiethnic population. J Am Coll Cardiol 2007; 49(7):797–802.

293. Chambers JB, de Belder MA, Moore D. Echocardiography in stroke and transient ischaemic attack. Heart 1997; 78(Suppl 1):2–6.

294. Besson G, Bogousslavsky J, Hommel M, Stauffer JC, Siche JP. Patent foramen ovale in young stroke patients with mitral valve prolapse. Acta Neurol Scand 1994; 89(1):23–26.

295. Steiner MM, Di Tullio MR, Rundek T, Gan R, Chen X, Liguori C et al. Patent foramen ovale size and embolic brain imaging findings among patients with ischemic stroke. Stroke 1998; 29(5):944–948.

296. Serena J, Segura T, Perez-Ayuso MJ, Bassaganyas J, Molins A, Davalos A. The need to quantify right-to-left shunt in acute ischemic stroke: a case-control study. Stroke 1998; 29(7):1322–1328.

297. Stone DA, Godard J, Corretti MC, Kittner SJ, Sample C, Price TR et al. Patent foramen ovale: association between the degree of shunt by contrast transesophageal echocardiography and the risk of future ischemic neurologic events. Am Heart J 1996; 131(1):158–161.

298. Williams LS, Garg BP, Cohen ME, Fleck JD, Biller J. Subtypes of ischemic stroke in children and young adults. Neurology 1997; 49:1541–1545.

299. Filippi L, Palermo L, Pezzati M, Dani C, Matteini M, De Cristofaro MT et al. Paradoxical embolism in a preterm infant. Dev Med Child Neurol 2004; 46(10):713–716.

300. Benedik MP, Zaletel M, Meglic NP, Podnar T. Patent foramen ovale and unexplained ischemic cerebrovascular events in children. Catheter Cardiovasc Interv. 2007;70(7):999–1007.

301. Dowling MM, Lee N, Quinn CT, Rogers ZR, Boger D, Ahmad N et al. Prevalence of Intracardiac shunting in children with sickle cell disease and stroke. J Pediatr 2010;156(4):645–50.

302. Kenny D, Turner M, Martin R. When to close a patent foramen ovale. Arch Dis Child. 2008;93(3):255–259.

303. Itoh T, Matsumoto M, Handa N, Maeda H, Hougaku H, Tsukamoto Y et al. Paradoxical embolism as a cause of ischemic stroke of uncertain etiology. A transcranial Doppler sonographic study. Stroke 1994; 25(4):771–775.

304. Teague SM, Sharma MK. Detection of paradoxical cerebral echo contrast embolization by transcranial Doppler ultrasound. Stroke 1991; 22(6):740–745.

305. Klotzsch C, Janssen G, Berlit P. Transesophageal echocardiography and contrast-TCD in the detection of a patent foramen ovale: experiences with 111 patients. Neurology 1994; 44(9):1603–1606.

306. Cabanes L, Coste J, Derumeaux G, Jeanrenaud X, Lamy C, Zuber M et al. Interobserver and intraobserver variability in detection of patent foramen ovale and atrial septal aneurysm with transesophageal echocardiography. J Am Soc Echocardiogr 2002; 15(5):441–446.

307. Homma S, Di Tullio MR, Sacco RL, Sciacca RR, Smith C, Mohr JP. Surgical closure of patent foramen ovale in cryptogenic stroke patients. Stroke 1997; 28(12):2376–2381.

308. Homma S, Sacco RL, Di Tullio MR, Sciacca RR, Mohr JP. Effect of medical treatment in stroke patients with patent foramen ovale: patent foramen ovale in Cryptogenic Stroke Study. Circulation 2002; 105(22):2625–2631.

309. Bartz PJ, Cetta F, Cabalka AK, Reeder GS, Squarcia U, Agnetti A et al. Paradoxical emboli in children and young adults: role of atrial septal defect and patent foramen ovale device closure. Mayo Clin Proc 2006; 81(5):615–618.

310. Hung J, Landzberg MJ, Jenkins KJ, King ME, Lock JE, Palacios IF et al. Closure of patent foramen ovale for paradoxical emboli: intermediate-term risk of recurrent neurological events following transcatheter device placement. J Am Coll Cardiol 2000; 35(5):1311–1316.

311. Hart RG. Cardiogenic embolism to the brain. Lancet 1992; 339(8793):589–594.

312. Lee RJ, Bartzokis T, Yeoh TK, Grogin HR, Choi D, Schnittger I. Enhanced detection of intracardiac sources of cerebral emboli by transesophageal echocardiography. Stroke 1991; 22(6):734–739.

313. Braun KP, Rafay MF, Uiterwaal CS, Pontigon AM, DeVeber G. Mode of onset predicts etiological diagnosis of arterial ischemic stroke in children. Stroke 2007;38(2):298–302.

314. Al-Mateen M, Hood M, Trippel D, Insalaco SJ, Otto RK, Vitikainen KJ. Cerebral embolism from atrial myxoma in pediatric patients. Pediatrics. 2003;112(2):e162–e167.

6
ARTERIAL ISCHAEMIC STROKE AND VASCULAR DISEASE IN CHILDHOOD

6.1 Cervicocephalic Arterial Dissections in Childhood and Adolescence

Göran Darius Hildebrand and Stéphane Chabrier

Introduction

Dissection of the arteries of the neck and brain were not clearly described until the middle of the 20th century[1] but are now recognized to be an important cause of ischaemic stroke among children and young adults.[2–6] Since then more than 1000 adults and 150 children have been reported and there exist now a number of reviews regarding cervicocephalic arterial dissections in adults[7–9] and children.[10–12]

The role of cervicocephalic dissections in ischaemic stroke in children

Dissections of the arteries of the brain and neck account for ischaemic arterial accidents in a substantial proportion of young patients in all series: up to 15.5% of those 16–45 years,[13] 20.5% of those 9–45 years,[14] 22% of those under 30 years,[15] 13% of patients aged 18–44 years,[16] 33% with cerebellar and brainstem infarcts of those aged 18–44 years[17] and 40% of cerebellar infarction in patients younger than 40 years.[18] According to Williams et al[19] it is more common in young adults than in those under 15, although the children in this study were recruited retrospectively and the diagnosis may have been missed in them, while the young adults used for comparison were in a prospective stroke registry. Of the relatively small numbers of children reported so far, cervicocephalic dissections are reported in between 3% and 20% of any ischaemic arterial stroke[2,4,6,20–23] and up to 45% of children with posterior circulation ischaemic stroke.[24] Variation in prevalence in the published series reflects the lack of awareness of this diagnosis, particularly involving the intracranial circulation,[3] so that appropriate neuroimaging is not performed in the acute stage.

Epidemiology

The annual incidence of cervicocephalic dissections in childhood is unknown. In the general population, it is 1.7–2.9/100 000 for spontaneous internal carotid artery dissection (ICAD),[25–27] an estimated 0.5/100 000 for traumatic ICAD,[28,29] an estimated 1–1.5/100 000 for spontaneous vertebral artery dissection (VAD)[9,27] or approximately 4–5/100 000 for cervicocephalic dissections combined. However, the true incidence of cervicocephalic dissections is likely to be higher because of underrecognition, underinvestigation[12,30,31] and early healing.[27]

The age distribution of ICAD and VAD is unimodal with a peak in the fifth decade of life.[32–34] Children and adolescents accounted for 6.8% of patients with dissection in the Mayo Clinic series.[35]

The annual incidence of ischaemic strokes among children is thought to be between 1.2/100 000 and 7.91/100 000.[36–38] If 6.5–20% of paediatric ischaemic strokes are due to cervicocephalic dissection, the estimated annual incidence of strokes caused by dissections would be expected to be at least 0.078–0.24/100 000 children or 1–3 cases per week for the USA.

Pathology and aetiology (Table 6.1)

Cervicocephalic dissections are caused by arterial blood penetrating and splitting the wall of an artery supplying the brain. In both the adult and paediatric populations, the most frequently affected artery is the internal carotid artery (ICA) followed by the vertebral artery.[12,33,35] Dissections of the intracranial and basilar arteries are more common in children than in adults[12] but until the advent of computed tomography (CT)[39] and magnetic vesonance angiography (MRA), were rarely diagnosed as, in the absence of evidence-based treatment, the risks of conventional angiography were considered to outweigh the benefits of making a diagnosis. The common carotid and external carotid arteries are only rarely involved.[40–43] Occasionally, a dissection can extend from the ascending aorta.[44] Multiple dissections are common and seen in between 8% and 28% of children and adults.[12,33,35]

In adults, most cervicocephalic dissections are extracranial (up to 87%). The ICA is usually affected 2cm or more beyond its origin. In children, anterior circulation dissections are frequently intracranial (60%) affecting the distal internal carotid and middle cerebral arteries.[45,46] The vertebral artery can be affected anywhere between V1 and V4.[11,47] In children, 79% of all dissections of the posterior circulation are extracranial and 53% are located within the vertebral artery at the level of vertebral bodies C1 to C2. Intracranial dissections may be primary or due to intracranial extension of an extracranial dissection.

TABLE 6.1
Pre-existing conditions in which dissection has been described

Cardiac
Aortic coarctation
Bicuspid aortic valve
Pulmonary atresia
Pulmonary stenosis
Tricuspid atresia
Transposition of the great arteries
Truncus arteriosus

Renal
Adult polycystic kidneys

Skin
Multiple lentigines
Pseudoxanthoma elasticum

Connective tissue
Marfan
Ehlers–Danlos type IV
Osteogenesis imperfecta type I

Neck trauma
Athetoid cerebral palsy
Klippel–Feil anomaly ± Wildervanck syndrome (hearing loss, bilateral abducens palsy)

Other
Behçet's disease
Alpha-1 antitrypsin deficiency
Afibrinogenaemia
Homocystinuria

Intradural extension is more common in dissections of the vertebral artery than the ICA,[33] probably as compared with the foramen magnum, the tight carotid canal and its dural adhesions are a relatively effective barrier to ICAD extension.

The origin of the dissection probably is a small intimal tear or possibly a primary intramural haemorrhage of the vasa vasorum.[48] Despite extensive investigations, the exact aetiology remains unclear in most cases but is probably multifactorial, involving a variety of genetic and environmental factors whose exact roles are not understood at present.

TRAUMA

Severe head or neck trauma is a well-recognized cause of dissection.[49–51] However, any history of injury to the head or neck should be considered potentially significant[52] and if there is no history, non-accidental injury must be considered.[53,54] Dissection has been reported after trampolining,[55] surfing and riding on a roller coaster.[56] It is also worth remembering that intraoral injuries, for example from falling with a pencil or toothbrush in the mouth,[57–59] can cause contusion to and dissection of the carotid artery in the peritonsillar area. Anatomical variation probably plays a part in those dissections which follow minor trauma. Some children, particularly those with vertebrobasilar dissection, have anomalies of the cervical spine[24,60,61] and dissection has been reported in the Klippel–Feil syndrome with or without the additional hearing loss and abducens palsy described by Wildervanck.[61,62] Spinal manipulation appears to be a risk factor[63] and recurrent vertebral dissection

has been described in a child with dystonic cerebral palsy and frequent writhing movements of the neck.[24]

INFECTION, INFLAMMATION AND AUTOIMMUNITY

Infection appears to be a trigger in adults[64–66] and may be more important in children. The combination of trauma and infection may be synergistic, for example in *Pertussis* infection[67] and after adenotonsillectomy.[68,69] Infection may account, at least in part, for the higher incidence in winter.[70] Multiple simultaneous dissections are sometimes associated with infection.[71] Although there may be no obvious source of infection, C-reactive protein[72] and white cell count may be raised in the post-acute phase, particularly in spontaneous compared with traumatic dissections,[73] suggesting a role for acute or chronic inflammation. Homozygosity for the E variant of the E469K polymorphism of the *ICAM-1* proinflammatory gene appears to be associated with a high risk of spontaneous extracranial dissection.[74] Evidence of autoimmune thyroid disease is found in around one-third of patients with spontaneous carotid dissection, a significantly higher proportion than ischaemic stroke not due to dissection.[75]

CONGENITAL HEART DISEASE

Dissection has been reported in association with several forms of congenital heart disease,[76,77] particularly coarctation and congenitally bicuspid aortic valve.[77,78] Pulmonary atresia,[76] pulmonary stenosis, tricuspid atresia, transposition of the great arteries and truncus arteriosus have also been documented.[77] A wide aortic root[66,79] and hypertension[80] are risk factors in adults but there are no systematic studies in children.

UNDERLYING VASCULOPATHY AND GENETIC RISK FACTORS

Although an underlying arteriopathy has long been suspected, including a possibly unrecognized type, or *forme fruste*, and there is evidence for generalized endothelial dysfunction in terms of reduced endothelium-mediated vasodilatation,[81] no single factor has consistently been identified.[12,82] Some of these patients have been described as having fibromuscular dysplasia on digital subtraction arteriography,[81] although this term should be reserved for a pathological diagnosis. It is possible that there is an underlying connective tissue disorder in many cases of vascular dissection, particularly those occurring spontaneously. Ultrastructural abnormalities may be demonstrated in the skin[83,84] and a small proportion of patients have abnormalities of type III collagen with or without typical Ehlers–Danlos syndrome.[85] Although there is evidence for dominant inheritance,[86] studies looking at candidate genes, including those involved in pseudoxanthoma elasticum[87] and various disorders of collagen[66] as well as a genome-wide scan[86] have so far failed to identify a likely single gene, and it is clear that there is considerable heterogeneity between families.[86] It is also possible that factors such as anaemia play a role (see Chapter 15). Conditions such as α_1-antitrypsin deficiency may underly apparently spontaneous dissection, although there were no cases documented in a paediatric series[5] and a systematic review found no evidence.[66] Hyperhomocysteinaemia may be a risk factor,[88,89] although in adults the effect appears to be weak[66] and there are few data available in consecutive children. Ehlers–Danlos type IV and adult polycystic kidney might be responsible for a significant proportion of spontaneous arterial dissections[33,90] as well as aneurysm formation, although hereditary connective tissue disorders with a unique phenotype appear to be as common.[33]

It has been suggested that definite or probable[5,91] artery dissection should best be thought of as a sign, rather than a single disease, which is due to a variety of conditions predisposing that individual to a final pathway of single, multiple or recurrent dissections of the cervicocephalic vasculature and elsewhere in the circulation.[92]

Pathogenesis

Arterial dissection results in an intramural haematoma and its variable extension along the course of that artery. In the extracranial vessels, the media is involved while intracranial dissections are subintimal.[35] This primary pathological event may remain subclinical or produce clinical manifestations due to its secondary effects. These effects may be classified as local or distant.

LOCAL EFFECTS

The dissection may compress or stretch surrounding nerve structures and cause impairment of their nutrient blood supply. Subadventitial dissection deep into the arterial wall may lead to aneurysmal (or, of course, more precisely pseudo-aneurysmal) distention. These aneurysms may exert a direct local compressive effect or may sometimes give rise to thromboembolism from a nidus within the false lumen. As a rule, however, extracranial aneurysms associated with dissection do not rupture, unlike intracranial dissections, which carry a risk of subarachnoid haemorrhage because of their attenuated arterial wall architecture.[29,35] Subintimal dissection results in stenosis or occlusion of the arterial lumen. Abnormal flow, injury to the vessel wall and exposure of blood to tissue constitute potent thrombogenic stimuli (Virchow's triad) and result in subsequent local thrombosis.

DISTANT EFFECTS

Distant effects are ischaemic and are due to the direct haemodynamic effects of stenosis and thrombosis at the site of dissection and subsequent arterio-arterial embolism. Luminal stenosis may occasionally be associated with transient ischaemic attacks. Whilst haemodynamic mechanisms may be particularly important in intracranial dissections, artery-to-artery thromboembolism is probably the more important mechanism of stroke.[32,93,94] The evidence in support of the predominant role of artery-to-artery thromboembolism, especially among extracranial dissections, is based on a number of observations:

1. Arterial wall injury, exposure of tissue to blood and flow abnormalities result in the activation of Virchow's triad and thrombosis. The delay due to thrombus formation and

subsequent thromboembolism may be one explanation for the latency, usually ranging between minutes to days, usually observed between the presumed point of dissection and the onset of the first neurological ischaemic deficit.[33]

2. Angiographic features suggesting artery-to-artery embolization are reported in between 34% and 37% of young adults[94–96] and 50% of children[33] with dissection. Angiographic evidence of distal embolization may also be associated with the size of the infarction and poorer functional outcome.[95]

3. The pattern of stroke in ICAD supports an embolic mechanism in up to 92.2% and a haemodynamic mechanism in as few as 7.7%.[97,98]

4. Microemboli seen on transcranial Doppler in the middle cerebral artery downstream from an ICAD[99–102] correlate with the likelihood of developing stroke[98,99] and disappear with anticoagulation.[103]

5. Distant intracerebral thromboemboli are observed during surgery and at autopsy[95,98] and retinal emboli ipsilateral to the ICAD can be seen in occlusions of the ophthalmic artery.[104]

Presentation

The dissecting event is typically followed by a latent period which usually ranges from minutes to days, but which may on occasion last weeks or longer.[9,12,105] This latent period may either lead to spontaneous recovery or result in clinical manifestations, followed often by rapid step-wise deterioration. During the acute phase of dissection, the lesion is most unstable and evolving and the patient consequently at greatest risk of neurological injury. In children, an inaugural presentation with stroke is common,[3,23] whereas in most adult cases, stroke is preceded by either transient ischaemic attacks, amaurosis fugax or local clinical manifestations. However, in a recent series, one-third of children had had warning.[23] Seizures and coma are relatively common at presentation in children.[23] Local manifestations may include cranial nerve palsies, Horner syndrome, tinnitus or pain of the head, neck or face. There is frequently some history of minor trauma or physical exertion, although this often appears trivial in nature at the time.[3,23,106]

HISTORY

The child has usually been fit previously, may be of any age (including infancy),[76,107] and may or may not have sustained some form of trauma in the recent past. Unlike in adults in whom both sexes are equally represented, in children boys are affected more often (74% in anterior and 87% in posterior circulation dissection), even when traumatic dissections are excluded from analysis.[12] Not infrequently, children give a history of migraine[108] and may present with a concurrent history of respiratory tract infection. Adolescents sometimes present following alcohol or drug intoxication. There is rarely a personal or family history of connective tissue abnormality, previous dissection or early stroke in the family.[10,28,33,78,109–112]

PAIN

Pain affecting the head, neck or face is characteristic of cervicocephalic dissections and should raise suspicion. In adults, pain may be the only manifestation.[113] More typically, however, pain precedes the onset of cerebral ischaemia offering a potential window of opportunity for early intervention. In adults, headaches are seen in 68–75% of internal carotid and vertebral artery dissections and are inaugural in 33–59% of cases.[34,114] The location of pain can help with the localization of the lesion. Pain is usually ipsilateral to the site of ICAD (92%) and VAD (67%[34]). Frontal, facial or orbital pain were seen in 53–61% of ICAD, but less than 6% of VAD. Occipital pain was reported only in VAD.[33] Similarly, anterior neck pain was seen only in ICAD and posterior neck pain (with a few exceptions) only in VAD.

Among children, headache was reported in nine out of 11(82%) of cervical and seven out of seven (100%) of intracranial dissections in one series[35] but in a much smaller proportion in others[3,5,23] and not more commonly than in childhood stroke secondary to other pathologies.[5] In the large systematic review by Fullerton and coworkers, a history of headache was reported in only about half the cases of anterior (ACD) and posterior circulation dissection (PCD).[12] Moreover, neck pain was associated with PCD (11%) as opposed to ACD (1%). Similarly, neck stiffness was only seen in PCD (9%).

Though headaches among adults usually resolve within a median of 3–5 days, they may persist for months or even years in some cases.[34,113,114] Rarely, VAD can cause ipsilateral arm pain and weakness due to C5–C6 radiculopathy, cervical myelopathy or spinal epidural haematoma in adults.[115,116] It is important to remember, however, that arterial dissection can occur without pain in adults and especially in children, instead giving rise to neurological deficits.[3,12,13,23,114,117]

HORNER SYNDROME

Sudden onset of oculosympathetic paresis in a middle-aged or young person together with ischaemic manifestations, especially if painful or if following any degree of trauma, should be considered a cervicocephalic arterial dissection until proven otherwise.[118] Horner syndrome has been reported in 30–82% of cases of ICAD[32,118–120] and 27% of cases of VAD.[120,121] Although dissection may occasionally be associated with congenital Horner syndrome,[107,122] it appears that Horner syndrome is less common among children with cervicocephalic dissections for reasons that are unclear. Schievink et al reported oculosympathetic paresis in only two out of 19 (11%) cases.[35] Horner syndrome is thought to be central in VAD and due to brainstem ischaemia. In ICAD, Horner syndrome is a third-order lesion and probably due to mechanical or ischaemic injury to the periadventitial sympathetic plexus along the course of the ICA.[119] In ICAD, Horner syndrome is typically incomplete with ptosis and/or miosis, but usually no anhidrosis, because of the sparing of the vasoconstrictor and sudomotor sympathetic fibres that travel with the un-

affected external carotid artery. Oculosympathetic paresis often persists, but may be transient[123] or isolated.[119,124] The finding of oculosympathetic paresis is, therefore, always significant despite its rarity in children.[5] However, the absence of a Horner syndrome, like the absence of pain or trauma, does not rule out the possibility of dissection. Rarely, other pupillary disturbances have been reported in association with cervicocephalic dissections. They include ipsilateral mydriasis[125] due to ischaemia of the ciliary ganglion or iris[126] and third-nerve palsy[43] as well as pinpoint pupils due to brainstem infarction.[121]

CRANIAL NERVE INVOLVEMENT

Ocular motor misalignments are common in VAD and reported in 22% of VAD due to involvement of the VIth (14%), IIIrd (6%) and IVth (2%[121]) cranial nerves. Their significance in the acute setting has not historically been appreciated by paediatricians.

Cranial neuropathy is encountered in 2–16% of ICADs;[7,114,127,128] Mokri et al found cranial nerve palsies in 12% of 190 adult patients with spontaneous dissection of the extracranial ICA.[128] In decreasing order of frequency, these involved the XIIth (with or without IX, X and XI, 5.2%), Vth (3.7%), IIIrd, IVth or VIth (2.6%), IInd and VIIIth (less than 1% each) cranial nerves. Cranial nerve palsies occur ipsilateral to the side of ICAD and may be single[117,129–132] or multiple[128,133,134] and may present in isolation[133,134] or in conjunction with other manifestations of dissections.[121,127,128] Rarely patients with dissection present as unilateral palsy of the IXth to XIIth cranial nerves or Collet–Sicard syndrome.[135–137] It is worth remembering, therefore, that ipsilateral cranial nerve palsies or Horner syndrome in association with contralateral hemiparesis and headache can be false localizing signs resembling brainstem ischaemia and wrongly suggesting involvement of the posterior circulation when in fact the ICA is affected.[128,130] The mechanism of cranial neuropathy in ICAD is not well understood and may involve mechanical stretching or compression below the jugular foramen in the retrostyloid or posterior retroparotid spaces.[128] However, other mechanisms must exist, as aneurysms are not always seen in these cases and involvement of the IIIrd to VIth cranial nerves is well documented in dissections of the extracranial ICA. It is thought, therefore, that the nutrient vessels in the vasa nervorum of distant cranial nerves may be affected by mechanical, embolic or haemodynamic effects of proximal arterial dissection.[128] The lower cranial nerves appear to be particularly vulnerable in cervicocephalic dissections for reasons that are not clear.

CEREBRAL, CEREBELLAR AND BRAINSTEM ISCHAEMIA

Ischaemia may be transient or result in infarction and can affect any intracranial structure and rarely the spinal cord as well.[115,116,138] The majority of reported cases in children have had a stroke.[3,12,23,35,106] Schievink et al[35] reported cerebral or retinal ischaemia in all 18 children with cervical (11 patients) and intracranial arterial dissections (seven patients). Cervical dissections resulted in ischaemic stroke (9/11) or transient ischaemic attacks (2/11). Ischaemic stroke was also documented in all cases of intracranial dissection. One patient with intracranial dissection and coarctation of the aorta died. Seizures are relatively common at presentation in children with dissection,[23,35] as is seen with other causes of ischaemic stroke in childhood. The main clinical features reported in Schievink's series[35] were hemiparesis (94%), dysphasia (50%), seizures (33%), oculosympathetic paresis (11%), transient monocular blindness (11%), ataxia (11%), bruits (11%), pulsatile tinnitus (6%), vertigo (6%) and dysmetria (6%). A frequent presentation of VAD is the lateral medullary, or Wallenberg, syndrome, which should suggest the possibility of VAD in a young person, especially when preceded by posterior headache or neck pain.[48,139]

NEURO-OPHTHALMIC MANIFESTATIONS
Neuro-ophthalmic manifestations are very common in dissections of the internal carotid and vertebral arteries, affecting between 62% and 96% of patients.[118–121,140,141] Again, they may previously have been missed or misinterpreted in paediatric settings[23] and there is a good case for early consultation with an ophthalmologist.

Hicks et al[121] reported neuro-ophthalmic manifestations in 86% of VADs. In decreasing frequency, symptoms were diplopia (45%), blurred vision (14%), transient visual dimming (8%), oscillopsia (4%), photophobia (4%), upside-down vision (2%), positional transient visual obscurations (2%) and unilateral dry eye (2%). Neuro-ophthalmic signs reported were nystagmus (37%), ocular misalignment (33%) due to abducens nerve palsy (14%), oculomotor nerve palsy (6%), trochlear nerve palsy (2%) and skew deviation (12%), Horner syndrome (27%), decreased corneal sensation (22%), ptosis alone (16%), visual field defect (10%), abnormal pursuits/saccades (6%), ocular bobbing (4%), internuclear ophthalmoplegia (4%), anisocoria (4%) and pinpoint pupils (2%).[121]

Kerty reported neuro-ophthalmic findings in 27 out of 28 (96%) patients with ICAD,[120] but this may in part reflect referral bias in a neurophthalmology clinic. Biousse et al[119] reported 146 patients (age range 14–71 years) with extracranial ICADs who were asked about visual symptoms and, if present, referred to an ophthalmologist for formal assessment. Neuro-ophthalmic symptoms and signs were present in 62%. They included painful Horner syndrome (44.5%), transient monocular visual loss (28%) and permanent visual loss (2.5%).[142] Ocular motor nerve palsies are rarely reported in ICAD and range between 0.7% and 2.6%.[119,143,144] Visual loss may be transient or permanent and due to a number of mechanisms, including branch[145,146] and central retinal artery occlusion,[147–149] ophthalmic artery occlusion with loss of vision, ophthalmoparesis and orbital ischaemia,[104] anterior and posterior ischaemic optic neuropathy, which unlike other non-arteritic ischaemic optic neuropathies is painful and occurs in younger patients,[142,150,151] Terson syndrome,[152] ocular

ischaemic syndrome,[153] optic tract infarction,[154] occipital hemianopsia[155] and cortical blindness.[156]

NEURORADIOLOGY (Fig. 6.1)
Establishing the diagnosis of cervicocephalic dissection relies on urgent neurovascular imaging. The main aims of imaging are to establish the neuroradiological diagnosis of dissection, to look for evidence of neurological infarction and to corroborate the presence of factors that may affect early management (e.g. subarachnoid haemorrhage, size of infarction and mass effect). The principal investigations are conventional transfemoral digital subtraction angiography (DSA) and magnetic resonance imaging (MRI)/3D-phase contrast or time-of-flight angiography (MRI/A), but CT/angiography (CT/A) and various ultrasonographic techniques, including Doppler colour-flow and transcranial ultrasonography, have also been used to a lesser extent. Initial choice frequently is influenced by local expertise and availability.

Conventional angiography has helped define the vascular changes in cervicocephalic dissections (Fig. 6.1f,g).[157,158] Typical angiographic abnormalities of the ICA and vertebral artery (VA) are usually best seen extracranially and are similar in children and adults. They include luminal stenosis (irregular, elongated, tapered) and occlusion (often tapering with a flame-shape appearance) but aneurysmal pouch formation, intimal flaps and double lumina are more specific. Distal branch occlusions are common and indicate artery-to-artery embolization. In intracranial dissections, however, the smaller vessels have a much less characteristic radiological appearance (Fig. 6.1f) and may falsely raise the possibility of vasculitis or infection.[46]

The angiographic location and type of lesion affects the subsequent risk of subarachnoid haemorrhage. As a rule, intracranial involvement is much more prone to result in subarachnoid haemorrhage than extracranial dissections for both ICAD and VAD. Shin et al[47] reported the angiographic patterns of 24 VADs and grouped them as either aneurysmal or steno-occlusive. All 10 patients with the aneurysmal pattern dissected in V4 with a high proportion of subarachnoid haemorrhages (four cases). The 12 steno-occlusive dissections were more evenly distributed throughout V1 and V4 and presented with ischaemic deficits.[47] The propensity of aneurysms of the intradural V4 segment to cause subarachnoid haemorrhage may be due to a thicker internal lamina, an absent external elastic lamina, an attenuated adventitia and fewer elastic medial fibres.[47]

Conventional angiography is increasingly being supplanted by newer and non-invasive techniques, especially MRA. Combined MRI and MRA has been shown to have similar sensitivities and specificities to conventional angiography[9,11,159–161] and because of its non-invasive nature and ability to provide simultaneous neuroimaging, it is by many now considered the preferred choice of diagnosis and follow-up.[162,163] A further advantage of this combined protocol is the possibility to detect *in extracranial vessels* the pathognomonic intramural haematoma with T1-weighted fat-suppressed MRI

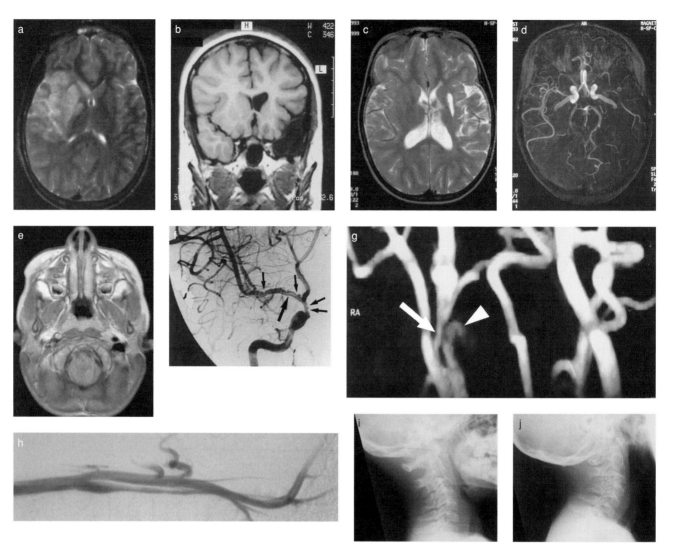

Fig. 6.1. Imaging in dissection. (a–c) Examples of infarcts on MRI. (d) magnetic resonance angiography (MRA) of the intracranial vessels in the child with the infarct shown in (c) showing less filling on the side of the infarct. (e) Fat-saturated T1 of the neck in a child with a XIIth nerve palsy after a peritonsilbr abcess (quincy) showing occlusion of the carotid secondary to dissection. (f) Double lumen (large arrow) diagnostic of intracranial dissection on digital subtraction arteriography in a 12-year-old girl who had banged her head whilst skiing. (g) MRA of the neck showing a tapering stenosis (arrow) and an aneurysmal pouch (arrowhead) diagnostic of dissection. (h) Digital subtraction arteriography of the common carotid artery showing a tapering occlusion with a flame-shape appearance highly suggestive of dissection. (i,j) X-ray of the neck in flexion and extension looking for bony abnormalities.

(Fig. 6.1e).[164,165] To detect the diagnostic intramural haematoma, it is important, therefore, to carry out an MRI of both the head and neck and not only of the head. MRA is also superior to conventional angiography in detecting aneurysmal dissections in which the vascular lumen is not compromised.

Whilst CT alone is an insensitive screening method,[166] the more recent advent of helical CTA is promising. However, experience with this new technique is still limited.[39] Various ultrasonographic techniques, especially a combination of Doppler colour-flow imaging and transcranial ultrasonography, have been tested. Their main limitation is that confirmatory MRI/MRA or conventional angiography is still required in many cases. However, they may have a role in routine follow-up.[29,127,167]

Whether MRA or conventional angiography is carried out, four-vessel angiography should always be attempted and should include the head and neck regions, as selective angio-

graphy may well miss a dissection and hence lead to diagnostic and therapeutic delay.[166] Interval MRA may be used to demonstrate healing.[168]

There are special considerations in children that influence the choice of investigation: difficulty and morbidity associated with obtaining vascular access and carrying out catheterization, the need for general anaesthesia in many cases as well as the greater cost of angiography compared with MRA should be considered.[169] Children will probably need longer follow-up and more overall examinations than adults. Follow-up examinations should, therefore, be by non-invasive means whenever possible. This usually involves combined MRI and MRA,[29,169] though ultrasound has been advocated by some as well.[127,162]

Combined MRI/MRA is frequently diagnostic on its own and is increasingly supplanting invasive conventional angiography as the preferred choice of initial neurovascular investigation. MR at 3 Tesla may increase sensitivity for the diagnosis of dissection.[170] Nonetheless, angiography still has a clear place in situations where the MRI/MRA has been inconclusive, particularly for intracranial dissection[35] and posterior circulation stroke.[171] Therefore, the different diagnostic modalities are complementary and should be selected depending on the individual findings. Even with a full protocol pursued exhaustively, pathognomic neuroimaging findings may only be suspected and the diagnosis of dissection in children often rests on a combination of clinical[5] and angiographic features.

Treatment

The aims of treatment are threefold: (1) to achieve early clinical stabilization; (2) to prevent recurrence in the short- and long-term; and (3) to provide rehabilitation. As clinical deterioration is most rapid during the acute stages of dissection and as long-term outcome is dependent on the extent of the neurological injury sustained, dissection should be considered a medical emergency and treatment initiated urgently. Because it is not possible to predict which dissection will result in stroke, all dissections should be treated unless there is a contraindication. Treatment is usually by immediate anticoagulation or by an antiplatelet agent (usually aspirin) though the effectiveness of this has never formally been tested in a prospective randomized controlled trial among either children or adults.[172] In the absence of a prospective randomized controlled trial, treatment should be based on our understanding of the pathophysiology and the natural history of cervicocephalic dissections, in particular the importance of artery-to-artery thromboembolism during the acute phase. In a few refractory cases, endovascular placement of stents or vascular surgery may be attempted if medical treatment fails to prevent recurrent symptoms.

ANTICOAGULATION AND ANTIPLATELET TREATMENT

Although haemodynamic mechanisms may be important in some cases, especially in intracranial dissections,[35,173] the main mechanism of cerebral and retinal ischaemia is probably artery-to-artery thromboembolism.[11,29,35,93,95–102,104] There have been no randomized controlled trials to prevent thromboembolic infarction, however most authors have advocated urgent anticoagulation or antiplatelet treatment for all patients with acute dissections in the absence of a contraindication.[20,29,31,35,48,120] As the prodromal phase is typically brief, anticoagulation or antiplatelet treatment should be started expeditiously, but judiciously. Although non-randomized studies have shown no clear difference in odds of survival or disability between aspirin and anticoagulation, immediate anticoagulation is preferred initially by many, aiming for a prothrombin time 1.5–2.5 times the normal control and a target international normalized ratio (INR) of 2.0–3.0.[29,48,172,174] Anticoagulation is absolutely contraindicated in the presence of subarachnoid haemorrhage, large brain infarction with mass effect and haemorrhagic transformation.[29]

Anticoagulation and antiplatelet treatment in intracranial dissections is controversial. Although, importantly, Chaves and coworkers reported no haemorrhagic complications among nine patients with spontaneous intracranial dissections of the ICA treated with either immediate anticoagulation (six patients) or antiplatelet agents (three patients),[173] haemorrhagic complications and fatal outcomes after treatment of intracranial dissections are well reported, especially when the dissection involves the posterior circulation. The use of anticoagulation and antiplatelet agents should, therefore, be embarked upon only with great caution.[7,8,21,29,175] Moreover, thromboembolism may be less and haemodynamic insufficiency relatively more important causes of ischaemia in intracranial dissections.[35,92,173] Some have recommended additional spinal fluid examination to exclude subarachnoid haemorrhage before initiating anticoagulation therapy in patients with intracranial dissection who have no evidence of haemorrhage on neuroimaging.

There is no evidence that anticoagulation causes extension of extracranial dissections or extracranial haemorrhage.[9,29,31,48] As there is no clear evidence from the available non-randomized studies for the superiority of anticoagulation over antiplatelet treatment, aspirin should be considered a valid alternative to anticoagulation.[172] With close supervision and judicious use in patients without contraindications, anticoagulation and aspirin treatment is generally safe and significant haemorrhagic complications relatively uncommon.[12,29,35]

OTHER MEDICAL THERAPY

Although there is no evidence of a detrimental effect of intravenous thrombolysis, e.g local or intracranial haemorrhage, in the published adult non-randomized series,[176] there is no evidence of benefit and this treatment cannot be recommended for children at present. Bedrest may reduce the haemodynamic effects of dissections.[119,120] There may be a case for immobilization of the neck, particularly if there is cervical instability.[24]

SURGERY VS ENDOVASCULAR TREATMENT

First-line medical treatment of cervicocephalic arterial dissection by either anticoagulation or antiplatelet therapy is adequate in the majority of cases in preventing further clinical deterioration. In adults, a number of surgical and more recently endovascular approaches have been attempted but there are no published data on the use of these invasive techniques in children. These interventions are technically demanding and associated with substantial risks of their own.[9,29] Techniques used include balloon angioplasty with placement of balloon-expandable or self-expanding stents, coil embolization, arterial ligation, resection with interposition vascular grafting or primary anastomosis and extracranial–intracranial bypass.[29,177–179] Consideration of endovascular or surgical intervention should be limited to patients in whom medical therapy fails to prevent recurrent symptoms or is contraindicated and in whom persistent ischaemic symptoms are due to surgically correctable and accessible lesions.[9,29] Indications include improvement of blood supply in patients with persistent haemodynamic symptoms and prevention of persistent shedding of thromboemboli from aneurysms despite adequate medical therapy.

Ligation is occasionally used for a post-traumatic pseudoaneurysm with ongoing thromboembolic events but the outcome for pseudoaneurysm is usually favourable[179,180] and the long-term risks of ligation include the development of cerebral ischaemia and intracranial aneurysms. Ligation may also further compromise cerebral blood supply in case of recurrence of a dissection in one of the other cervicocephalic arteries.[29] These patients and those who develop transient ischaemic attacks on a haemodynamic basis, which may be associated with the development of moyamoya collaterals after extracranial and intracranial dissection in children,[181,182] may benefit from extracranial–intracranial bypass.[182,183] Surgery for complications may also be required, for example decompression for intracranial hypertension or treatment of subarachnoid haemorrhage. Most patients are young and the long-term complications of many of these techniques are not well known.

Follow-up

The main aims of follow-up are to supervise the preventive and rehabilitative measures and to manage complications. Care for patients is multidisciplinary and should include the involvement of different subspecialties for further specialist assessment and care (see Chapter 17). The best long-term management of cervicocephalic dissections is unknown. Because of the risk of recurrent infarction, most patients are kept on medical treatment for varying lengths of time. Schievink has proposed the following protocol: (1) Patients are anticoagulated, or treated with antiplatelet agents if there are contraindications to anticoagulation. (2) At 3 months post-dissection, an MRI/MRA is performed. If the angiographic findings have normalized, treatment is discontinued. If they persist, treatment is continued. (3) At 6 months, MRI/MRA is repeated. If findings are still abnormal, life-long antiplatelet treatment is advised.[29] However, in the absences of randomized controlled trials, treatment and follow-up needs need to be individualized, taking into account individual clinical findings, response to treatment and presence of any predisposing risk factors. In the absence of contraindications, long-term treatment appears safe when closely monitored. Dissection can cause complications years later and it is not unreasonable therefore to give long-term antiplatelet prophylaxis for these reasons.

OUTCOME

Initial reports of outcome of cervicocephalic dissections were often based on post-mortem findings and hence associated with a high mortality. The introduction of non-invasive neuroimaging and greater clinical awareness of cervicocephalic dissection has led to the increasing detection of patients with earlier and less severe manifestations. More recent studies have therefore reported a more favourable outcome of cervicocephalic dissections in adults[27,96,184] and children.[3,12,23,35] In adults, outcome is related to the initial severity of the stroke,

underscoring the importance of early recognition and treatment[9,96] and thought to be better in extracranial than intracranial dissection.[11,12] Patients with spontaneous ICAD who developed Horner syndrome, cranial nerve palsy or who had normal internal carotid findings were much less likely to suffer ischaemic events in a recent large study.[185]

Of 105 adults with a cervical artery dissection, 73% remained fully independent, achieving a Barthel index of 100.[184] However, residual headache or cervical pain were frequent sequelae (20%). Vertebral artery dissection with posterior circulation ischaemia has a relatively good outcome, with only two deaths and 82% achieving Rankin scale of 0 or 1 at follow-up in a large series.[186] These hospital-based studies may be biased towards patients with poor outcome and a recent population-based study reported only one acute death, from intractable intracranial hypertension, and good outcome (Rankin scale 0 to 2) in 92% of adults with spontaneous cervical artery dissection.[27]

Schievink et al[35] described complete or good clinical recovery in 10 of 11 children with cervical arterial dissection. Similarly, Tabarki et al[187] reviewed 25 reports of vertebral artery dissection among children and reported complete recovery or mild remaining deficits in 22 of them. However, others have found less favourable outcomes. Patel et al[188] reviewed 10 children with extracranial carotid artery dissection and found hemiparesis or aphasia in seven (in two cases considered to be mild) and one death. Only two patients were left with no deficit.[188] The prognosis of intracranial arterial dissection in childhood and adolescence is generally thought more ominous. An early review by Manz et al revealed a mortality rate of 76% among 20 children with intracranial dissection in the first two months.[189] Schievink and coworkers described the only death in their series in a child with intracranial dissection and coarctation of the aorta.[35] In fact, four of the seven children with intracranial dissection in the same series had a complete or good recovery[35] and good outcomes in paediatric intracranial dissections have also been described by others.[59,181]

In their large systematic review, Fullerton and coworkers described the following outcome for 118 children with cervicocephalic dissections: dissection resulted in the death of 2% and 33% of patients in the PCD and ACD groups, respectively.[12] However, the mortality was much higher for cases reported before 1990 (ACD=45% and PCD=7%) than since 1990 (ACD=18% and PCD=0%) and higher among ACDs with intracranial (51%) than extracranial (11%) dissections. Although death from malignant middle cerebral infarction may occur[190] and the dissection may not be diagnosed in these very sick unconscious patients, survival does appear to be much better in recent single centre cohorts.[3,4,23,106]

In Fullerton's report,[12] among the survivors, the outcome was as follows: 37% with complete recovery, 33% with mild sequelae (subtle deficits not interfering with activities of daily living (ADL)), 8% with moderate sequelae (more readily apparent deficits or deficits that may be interfering with ADL), 6% with severe sequelae (deficits that significantly affect ADL or result in a low quality of life) and 15% with undefined residual deficits. In the recent prospective cohorts, between one- and two-thirds had significant neurological disability.[3,23]

Healing has been documented in around half of adults undergoing re-imaging.[27] Follow-up angiography of 39 children discussed in the systematic review showed complete resolution in 10 (26%), improvement in 16 (41%), no change in nine (23%) and progression in only four patients (10%[12]). In a cohort reported by Rafay et al,[23] follow-up angiography showed resolution of abnormalities in 60% of vessels but total occlusion often did not re-canalize.

RISK OF RECURRENCE

The cumulative rate of recurrent spontaneous cervical arterial dissection over a 10-year-period was 11.9% in the big Mayo clinic cohort.[191] However, a population-based study from the same centre found no recurrence over a mean follow-up period of 7.8 years[27] The exact recurrence risk in children is not known. Schievink described recurrent arterial dissection in three out of 17 paediatric patients with spontaneous dissections of cervicocephalic arteries who had been followed-up for between 1 and 21 years.[35]

The risk of recurrence among patients with spontaneous extracranial arterial dissections is highest during the first month following the initial dissection (2%) and then falls to 1% per year subsequently.[35] This risk remains increased for at least 10 years and probably longer.[29,35,191] Recurrent dissections may involve the original artery,[184,192,193] but more often occur in another cervicocephalic artery previously unaffected.[191] Importantly, they may also involve the aorta, renal, visceral and other extra-cervicocephalic arteries[9,191] and have been reported up to 40 years following the initial cervicocephalic dissection.[194] The risk of recurrent dissection is similar for internal carotid and vertebral artery dissection.[191,193]

Risk factors for recurrence include younger age[191] and the presence of a predisposing disorder, such as Ehlers–Danlos syndrome.[184] The cumulative 10-year-rate of recurrent dissection was 16.8% in those younger than 45 years of age compared with 6.1% in those 45 years and older.[35,191] Recurrent dissections have been reported following general anaesthesia years after the first dissection.[193] A family history is highly significant and should always be sought, as patients with a spontaneous cervical artery dissection and a family history of spontaneous arterial (cervicocephalic, renal or aortic) dissection have a much greater risk of recurrent arterial dissection (50%) than those without a family history (5.8%).[111] A multivariate analysis by Schievink et al showed no link between recurrent arterial dissection and the following: sex of the patient, site of dissection, multivessel dissection, hypertension, cigarette smoking, use of oral contraceptives or fibromuscular dysplasia.[111,191]

Patients, especially those in high-risk groups, should specifically be advised against contact sports and special care should be taken when undergoing a general anaesthetic procedure. The patient should understand the low but real risk of recurrence and be instructed to seek immediate medical attention should any symptoms recur.

Conclusions

Dissection of the cervicocephalic arteries is a leading cause of cerebrovascular accidents in the young, accounting for up to 20% of all ischaemic infarcts among children. Dissections of the anterior circulation are more common than dissections of the posterior circulation in children. Boys also appear to be more frequently affected than girls and multiple dissections are reported in at least 8% of children. Although arterial dissections are strongly linked with a history of trauma, most dissections occur in the absence of severe trauma and no clear cause can be found in the majority of cases. It has therefore been speculated that dissections are due to an as yet unknown underlying arteriopathy. Dissections cause neurological injury by a combination of local (compression, interference with nutrient vessels) and distant effects (thrombosis, haemodynamic compromise and artery-to-artery thromboembolism). Dissections typically lead to sudden, step-wise clinical deterioration. Manifestations include sudden onset of head, neck or facial pain, cranial nerve palsy, tinnitus, Horner syndrome, transient ischaemic attacks and stroke. A systematic review of published paediatric cases found that fatal outcomes were more common with ACD than PCD, particularly in association with intracranial dissection, with patients not receiving anticoagulation and with diagnosis before 1990. Recent data suggest better survival, although between one- and two-thirds of children have significant long-term disability. All affected children and young adults should have an urgent CT or MRI and vascular imaging (conventional or MRA-based four-vessel angiography) of the head and neck. Though no randomized controlled trial has been reported yet, for extracranial dissection, anticoagulation for up to 6 months, or aspirin, has been widely adopted because of the frequency of thromboembolic stroke. Caution is advised in intracranial dissections because they are more commonly associated with subarachnoid haemorrhage. Other interventions, for example ligation of a pseudoaneurysm or extracranial–intracranial bypass, are limited to cases in whom recurrent symptoms cannot be prevented medically.

6.2 Transient Cerebral Arteriopathy

Guillaume Sébire

Introduction

Ischaemic strokes in childhood arise from various mechanisms such as arteriopathy, thrombosis or embolism. Each of these processes results from different causes, many of which are relatively well recognized. Arterial wall injuries account for most of childhood arterial strokes[194] and account for 55–75% of all arterial strokes.[4,21,195–200] While some conditions

TABLE 6.2
Respective proportions of the different clinicoradiological patterns of arterial wall diseases among arterial brain infarcts in childhood[21,195–197,253]

Vascular wall disorders	%
Transient cerebral arteriopathy	35
Moyamoya syndrome	15
Dissections of cervical arteries	15
Emboli	15
Undetermined	15

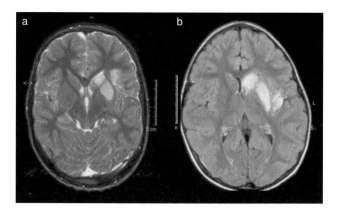

Fig. 6.2. Typical examples of infarct localization in transient cerebral arteriopathy (TCA), including the head of the caudate nucleus, the lentiform nucleus, some involvement but relative sparing of the internal capsule, and some extension in adjacent grey or white matter. (a) T2-weighted MRI in a 7-year-old boy. (b) Fiuid attenuation inversion recovery MRI in a 6-year-old girl.

can be attributed to well-defined aetiologies, others constitute less well-defined clinicoradiological patterns. The main causes are currently grouped within three categories, namely infectious, traumatic and genetic. Bacterial meningitis and varicella zoster virus (VZV) infection are the leading examples in the infectious group. The traumatic mechanism is principally illustrated by dissection of cervical arteries. Arterial wall injuries are also known to result from various genetic conditions. Moyamoya and sickle cell disease are the main examples. This genetic group includes other rarer pathologies, such as neurofibromatosis type 1 and metabolic disorders. Besides these direct aetiologies, many predisposing risk factors would also contribute in the pathogenesis of all these conditions. The main entities of childhood arterial wall injuries could be divided into three distinct clinicoradiological patterns: transient cerebral arteriopathy (TCA), moyamoya syndrome and cervical dissection (Table 6.2). One given cause can result in varying clinicoradiological patterns. A particular clinicoradiological pattern can, on the other hand, result from different causes. For instance TCA and moyamoya syndrome have been observed following the same cause, namely VZV infection.[201] Conversely, a single pattern such as moyamoya syndrome can result, for instance, from sickle cell disease, Down syndrome or neurofibromatosis type 1. Thus, correlations between aetiologies and the various clinicoradiological patterns remain complex.

General features
Repeated clinical evaluation and cerebral arteriography during the evolution of ischaemic strokes of idiopathic origin allowed us to characterize a non-progressive brain arterial wall disease named 'transient cerebral arteriopathy' (TCA).[200,202–204] This condition was characterized on the basis of the following specific clinical and angiographical features: (1) subcortical infarcts (basal ganglia or internal capsule; Fig. 6.2) associated with lesion(s) of the cerebral arterial wall (focal or segmental narrowing, tail-like occlusion) mostly located in the initial parts of basal arteries of the carotid system, and (2) clinical (lack of long-term recurrence of stroke more than 3 months after the initial event) and arteriographic follow-up disclosing regression or arrest of the evolution of the arteriopathy.[200,204,205] Several authors have previously pointed out the frequent occurrence

of acute strokes of idiopathic origin in childhood.[19,21,196–198,206] The analysis of the main series of strokes in childhood showed that many of these patients share clinical and paraclinical features with TCA (particularly a 'one shot' course and location of the disease, as noticed by some authors), making them very likely to be TCA patients;[181,207–225] however, in these studies, the lack of angiographic follow-up, except in a few reports,[216,226] failed to establish the specifically transitory action of the underlying pathophysiological process.

Epidemiology and physiopathology
TCA seems to represent a significant fraction of ischaemic strokes since it accounted for at least 26% of the whole group of ischaemic strokes we observed at the same time.[197] The lack of long-term recurrence of strokes and the improvement or stabilization of arterial lesions are in favour of a transient physiopathological process, such as arterial spasm, dissection or inflammatory/infectious angiitis. The vascular disease may involve an inflammatory response to infections such as meningitis, tonsillitis or *Varicella*.[203] Dissections affecting intracranial arteries are difficult to distinguish from stenosis or occlusion from other origins, even with the highest quality contrast angiography. However, some authors convincingly documented cases of intracranial dissections with clinical and paraclinical features close or similar to TCA,[3] occurring in traumatic circumstances or without any obvious precipitating event. It is noteworthy that, in our experience, 70% of the patients with TCA had had chickenpox at an average interval of 3 months (median, 6 weeks; range 9 days to 9 months) before stroke.[203] Some arterial wall injuries are already known, or suspected, to be associated with VZV. These include delayed onset arteriopathy following adult herpes zoster ophthalmicus, VZV vasculitis in patients with immunodeficiency, and anecdotal reports of temporal association between brain infarcts (TCA or moyamoya patterns) and chickenpox in childhood.[226–233] In order

to study the link between TCA and VZV we carried out a case-control study in which each of 11 patients with TCA was matched for age, sex and geographic residence, with four controls, to compare the frequency of VZV infection between both groups during the 9 months preceding the stroke.[203] Occurrence of chickenpox was significantly higher in the TCA group as compared with controls (64% versus 9%). These results were the first to provide a significant statistical link between idiopathic arterial ischaemic strokes in childhood, including TCA, and VZV infection. Whether this constitutes a direct aetiological link or a risk factor remains an open question. However, the following findings argue in favour of a causal relationship: (1) the presence of an acute or protracted VZV meningitis (intrathecal synthesis of VZV antibodies and/or VZV detection by polymerase chain reaction) observed concomitantly with the arteriopathy;[202,234,235] (2) the detection of VZV antigens and/or of an inflammatory reaction in the middle cerebral artery (MCA) wall from a patient presenting a fatal stroke;[236,237] (3) other 'models' of VZV-related vasculopathy in adulthood. So, recent virological, immunological and neuropathological data indicate that post-varicella angiopathy results, at least in some cases, from a focal viral invasion of the arterial wall inducing an acute vasculitis.[201,204] Similarly, we hypothesized that the aetiopathogenic mechanism involved in TCA not due to VZV infection could be either directly related to other infectious agents and/or the result of a secondary inflammatory reaction, or both. It might also implicate more specific immune pathways, such as anticardiolipin autoantibodies, which have been reported in close association with some VZV infections. Some other common infectious agents, such as parvovirus B19, cytomegalovirus (CMV), human immunodeficiency virus (HIV), *Mycoplasma pneumoniae*, *Borrelia burgdorferi*, enterovirus and *Helicobacter pylori*, are strongly suspected to generate an acute large vessel vasculitis, and might be responsible for TCAs not induced by varicella zoster virus;[20,238–243] (see Chapter 5.1). Immunological and infectious investigations, including repeated blood and cerebrospinal fluid (CSF) analysis for infectious culture, antibody titers, genome detection by PCR and study of the inflammatory reaction, should be undertaken more systematically in childhood stroke to further delineate the precise role of immune-inflammatory reactions and/or infectious agents in the pathogenesis of TCA.

Clinical and paraclinical features

The patients presenting with this condition display a particular pattern of clinicoradiological features.[202,216,226,244] All were previously healthy children. They ranged in age from 2 years to 13 years (mean age, 6 years). In children from 2 to 9 years of age, the stroke due to a transient arteriopathy occurred with a significantly higher frequency than strokes of other origin as compared with other pooled age groups, i.e. before 2 years old and 9 to 16 years old (89% vs 36%, $p<0.01$).[202] Motor symptoms prevailed with hemiplegia in all cases, most often proportional. This was associated with speech disorders in about half of the patients. Seizure or alteration of consciousness were rare. After the initial infarct, a single recurrence of the stroke may occur (within a maximum of 3 months) in one-third of the patients. Cerebral imaging showed small subcortical infarcts located in the territory of the lateral lenticulostriate arteries: i.e. the basal ganglia and internal capsule. Cortical strokes were only occasionally associated with these deep infarcts. Arteriography disclosed multifocal lesions of the arterial wall consisting of focal stenosis or segmental narrowing located in the large basal arteries of the brain, precisely at the distal parts of the internal carotids and at the initial segment of other cerebral arteries, namely anterior, middle or posterior cerebral arteries. Interestingly, serial arteriographic follow-ups showed initial worsening of the arterial lesions for a maximal duration of 7 months followed by complete regression, improvement or stabilization of the lesions. Recent studies showed the value of non-invasive tools, such as MRA (Figs 6.3–6.7) and transcranial Doppler, to diagnose TCA and to make the distinction between this condition and the other common arterial wall diseases such as moyamoya syndrome and dissection.[216,225,245,246] This technique makes the diagnosis possible with an excellent sensitivity and specificity. In fact, these various arterial wall disorders are located mainly at the bifurcation of

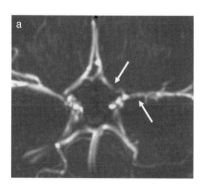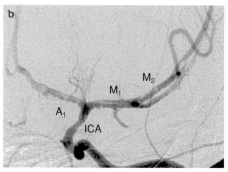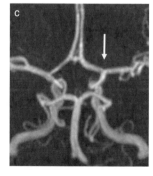

Fig. 6.3. Evolution of arterial abnormalities in a 6-year-old girl with typical transient cerebral arteriopathy. (a) Magnetic resonance angiography (MRA) at day 1 showing irregular stenosis of the A1 segment of the left anterior cerebral artery (ACA) (upper arrow) and M1 segment of the left middle cerebral artery (MCA) (lower arrow). (b) Conventional contrast angiography 4 days after stroke illustrating irregular stenoses with string-of-beads sign (beading) involving the distal segment of the internal carotid artery (ICA), and the A1 and M1 and M2 segments of the ACA and MCA respectively. (c) Complete resolution of arteriopathy (arrow) on MRA performed 15 months after stroke.

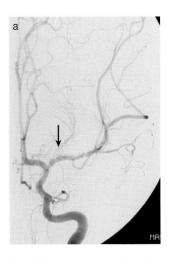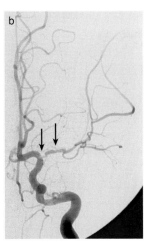

Fig. 6.4. Another example of the course of arteriopathy in transient cerebral arteriopathy (TCA). Conventional contrast angiography performed at 2 weeks (a) and 7 months (b) after stroke in a 7-year-old boy. (a) There is a long segmental irregular stenosis of the M1 of the middle cerebral artery (MCA) with beading at initial angiography. (b) Transient worsening of the disease with severe focal stenosis of the proximal M1 of the MCA (left arrow) and a long segmental stenosis of the M1 (right arrow). The beading, typical for the acute phase of TCA, is less prominent. Repeated angiography 22 months after stroke was identical, proving stabilization of arterial abnormalities (not shown).

the carotid artery, large segments of the arterial tree especially well studied by MR technique. Currently, digital subtraction arteriography remains the criterion standard for strict accurate anatomical investigation but indications for this method of

investigation are reduced to a relatively small fraction of cases in which MRA fails to establish the diagnosis.[225,247]

Diagnosis

Confirmation of the diagnosis of TCA requires MRA and/or CA showing *both* of two primary criteria.[205] *First is vascular imaging*, performed *within 3 months* following the infarct, displaying unilateral focal or segmental stenosis or occlusion which involve(s) the distal part of the internal carotid and initial segments and branches of anterior cerebral artery (ACA; A1 segment), MCA (M1 segment) or posterior cerebral artery (PCA; P1 segment). Note that in some cases initial vascular imaging can show no or minimal stenosis, which increases to maximum stenosis or occlusion within 3 months of the initial imaging, so an increase in vascular lesions detected on a second MRA performed only 1–3 months after the first one is often observed in TCA, sometimes associated with a second stroke. The lesions can be focal or multiple: additional distal lesions on medium sized cerebral arteries can occur. The *second primary criterion* is follow-up imaging showing non-progression of arterial lesions (no increase in stenosis and no new arterial lesions) 6 months after the initial stroke (Figs 6.3–6.7). Conversely, a worsening of arterial lesions detected on MRA at 6–12 months as compared with the 3–6 months MRA argues in favour of a chronic cerebral arteriopathy (Fig. 6.8). '*Post-varicella angiopathy*' *(PVA)* is defined by the same criteria as for TCA above *and* a clinical history of chicken pox infection in the 12 months preceding onset of stroke symptoms.

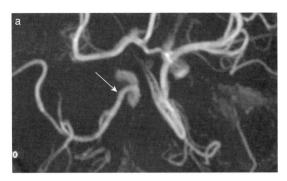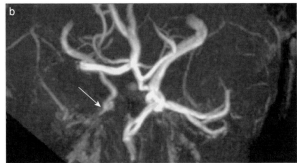

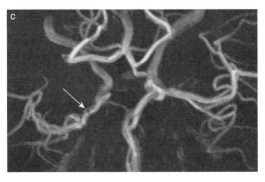

Fig. 6.5. Example of transient worsening in transient cerebral arteriopathy (TCA), leading to complete middle cerebral artery (MCA) occlusion but subsequent improvement in an 8-year-old boy. (a) Magnetic resonance angiography (MRA) shows a long segmental regular M1 stenosis (arrow) one day after stroke, and anterior cerebral artery (ACA) occlusion. (b) Three months later, there is complete occlusion of the origin of the MCA (arrow) and a tapered stenosis of the stroke distal interior carotid artery. (c) Twenty months after stroke, MRA has almost normalized, with a residual focal MCA stenosis (arrow) and patent (hypoplastic?) ACA.

118

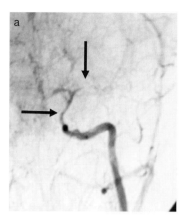
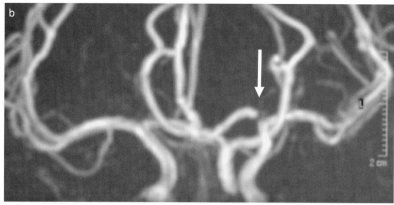

Fig. 6.6. Another example of occlusive transient cerebral arteriopathy with subsequent normalization. (a) Conventional angiography 2 weeks after basal ganglia stroke in a 7-year-old girl, showing a long tight distal internal carotid artery stenosis (horizontal arrow) and occlusion of the proximal middle cerebral artery (vertical arrow). (B) Eight years later, there is complete normalization of arteriopathic abnormalities (the arrow points at a flow artefact in the A1 of the anterior cerebral artery).

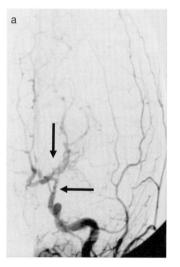
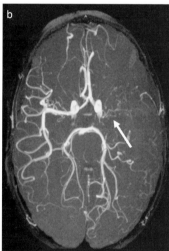
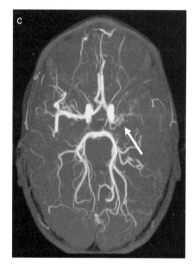

Fig. 6.7. Occlusive stabilizing unilateral transient cerebral arteriopathy in a 3-year-old boy who presented with three transient ischaemic attacks and a basal ganglia infarct on MRI. (a) Conventional angiography at 11 days after stroke shows an irregular distal internal carotid artery stenosis (horizontal arrow) and a proximal middle cerebral artery occlusion with the development of some abnormal moyamoya lenticulostriate collaterals (vertical arrow). Magnetic resonance angiography at 3 months (b) and 3 years (c) after stroke shows a persisting but unchanged MCA occlusion with some abnormal moyamoya collaterals (arrows). There is no contralateral involvement over time.

TCA is, therefore, a provisional diagnosis, likely to be further subclassified.

Treatment and outcome

Most of the patients had an antiplatelet treatment for at least 1 year, duration of treatment depending on the result of late arteriography.[202] No recurrence of stroke was observed in our patients after they received antiplatelet treatment.[203,234] Other authors observed a recurrence of stroke or transient ischaemic attack in one-third of their patients, mostly during the 2–3 months following the initial stroke.[245] The efficacy of anticoagulant treatment was not demonstrated in patients with TCA. Some of these patients might have strokes resulting from intracranial dissections in which anticoagulant treatment is not indicated owing to the risk of haemorrhaging. We have to keep in mind that some children with progressive arteriopathy, such as moyamoya syndrome, have initial angiographic findings

similar to those described here. That so many of these children recover, both clinically and radiographically, within such a short period of time, should discourage surgical treatment, at least until progression is certain. Frequent spontaneous improvement will also have to be considered when assessing the results of any treatment protocol. Longitudinal studies in large populations are required to define the natural history; this is important as recurrent stroke or transient ischamic attack (TIA) may be more common in those with progressive vasculopathy.[181] Studies are in progress to try to further delineate the early prognosis factors for progressive versus non-progressive cerebral arteriopathies. After a mean clinical follow-up of 3 years, one-third of the patients presented severe sequelae, hemiplegia and/or aphasia.[245]

Conclusion and perspectives

Other studies will be essential to better define the course of this disorder and to explore whether infectious, secondary

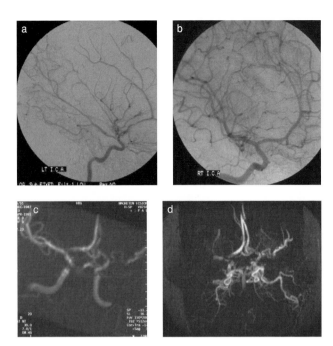

Fig. 6.8. Progressive arteriopathy in a girl who initially presented with an ischaemic stroke in the left basal ganglia and reduction of flow in the left internal carotid artery and proximal middle cerebral artery (MCA) on magnetic resonance angiography (MRA), 8 days after stroke. She was treated with aspirin and was left with a moderate right hemiparesis and some comprehension and word-finding difficulties. Conventional angiography at 3 months after stroke showed vasculopathy affecting the left side (a) but the right was normal (b). Further MRA 9 months later (c) suggested abnormality of the right proximal anterior cerebral artery, but the findings were interpreted cautiously in view of the image quality and it was not considered ethical to repeat the digital subtraction arteriography. Three months later, she had a contralateral infarct on MRI, involving the right basal ganglia and insular region (not shown). MRA (d), confirmed by conventional angiography, then showed bilateral arteriopathy with proximal stenosis of the right MCA and a more distal occlusion of the right M1 segment (arrowhead), as well as irregular stenosis of the left MCA.

inflammatory and/or thrombotic processes play a role. In relatively rare and heterogeneous conditions, such as TCA or other arterial brain diseases, there is an obvious need for multicentre studies in a sufficient number of patients to elucidate aetiopathogenic, therapeutic and prognostic questions. Such studies should take into account the biological specificities of, firstly, the vascular wall whose molecular and cellular components present important differences in venous versus arterial structures. In addition, the difference(s) in local perivascular environment between cerebral and extracerebral segments of a given vessel, has to be considered. Secondly, the specificity of the interactions between the haematological components and the various cellular elements of the vascular lining as well as with other possible factors should be also taken into account. These various vascular wall and haematological specifities are different according to the age group justifying separate studies in neonatal, infantile and juvenile strokes.[248]

Clarifying the physiological process in TCA should improve the therapeutic approach of the acute phase, defining the potential place of antiviral, anticoagulant or anti-inflammatory

drugs. The vaccine for varicella might prevent at least some cases of TCA, even if it is insufficient to determine whether neurological, and especially neurovascular, complications due to VZV infection will be reduced by this vaccination.[249] The well-demonstrated positive effect of vaccine in preventing severe varicella, associated bacterial complications and perhaps shingles seems to outweigh the rare danger of vaccinations.[250,251] This has led to the widespread use of the varicella vaccine in some countries (e.g., USA) but not in Europe, due to the more and more questionable reservations of some paediatricians.[249]

Finally, the risk of short-term recurrence of stroke in TCA opens the discussion about treatments targeted for secondary prevention. Large multicentre controlled treatment protocols comparing, for instance, antiplatelet versus anticoagulant, will be needed to try to improve morbidity due to recurrences.[252]

6.3 Moyamoya Syndrome in Childhood

Vijeya Ganesan and Brian G.R. Neville

Introduction

First described by Takeuchi and Shimizu,[254] moyamoya is a cerebral arteriopathy with bilateral severe stenosis or occlusion of the terminal ICAs, typically accompanied by basal collateral vessels. The name moyamoya derives from the Japanese word meaning 'something hazy like a puff of smoke drifting in the air' and describes the appearance of these collaterals. There may also be ethmoidal collaterals arising from the anterior and posterior ethmoidal arteries and external carotid system and vault collaterals, which are transdural vessels derived from the superficial temporal and middle meningeal arteries (Fig. 6.8).

Moyamoya is best considered an angiographically defined phenomenon rather than a pathological entity and may either be idiopathic or occur in the context of a wide range of other disorders. Most of the children have infarcts after presentation with stroke, transient ischaemic attacks or seizures (Fig. 6.9) but this is not essential for the diagnosis. Calcification is also well documented and haemorrhage occurs in childhood although it is more common in adults. The term moyamoya disease should be restricted to idiopathic Japanese cases. In order to promote consistency in the literature, the Japanese Research Committee on Spontaneous Occlusion of the Circle of Willis has proposed the following diagnostic criteria for moyamoya disease:[255]

- Stenosis or occlusion of the terminal internal carotid arteries on conventional cerebral angiography
- Moyamoya vessels observed at skull base or in the basal ganglia (if MRI is used for diagnosis, the criteria are that at least two flow voids are seen in one of the basal ganglia)[256]
- Bilateral changes
- Unknown aetiology.

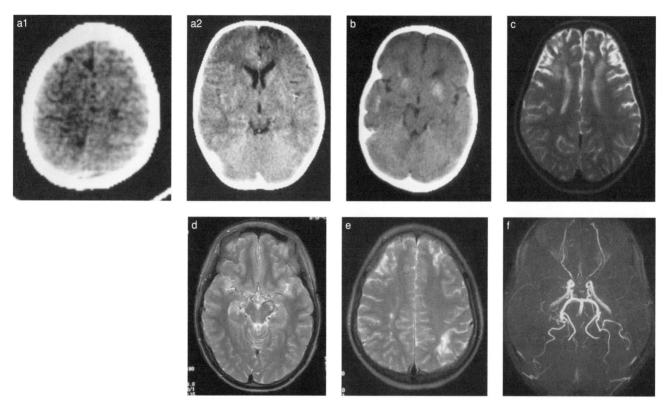

Fig. 6.9. Infarction in patients with moyamoya. (a) CT showing multiple infarcts from a child with Sneddon's syndrome. (b) CT showing bilateral basal ganglia calcification in a child with moyamoya after radiotherapy for optic glioma. (c) MRI showing bilateral frontal infarcts in a child with sickle cell disease. (d) MRI showing collaterals. (e) MRI showing infarct in the same patient as (d). (f) Magnetic resonance angiography (MRA) showing absent filling of the middle cerebral arteries in the same patient as (c); the collaterals were not obvious on MRA at this stage.

The Japanese define 'angiographic moyamoya' in cases where,

- There is unilateral involvement
- There is stenosis or occlusion of the proximal MCA
- There are other associated vascular malformations
- There is a recognized underlying cause.

The term '*moyamoya syndrome*' refers to non-Japanese patients with unilateral or bilateral terminal ICA stenosis or occlusion with basal collaterals, whether idiopathic or secondary. Symptomatic unilateral cases demonstrate the same pathophysiology and are amenable to similar diagnostic and therapeutic approaches; the majority of unilateral cases in childhood appear to progress to become bilateral,[256,257] although stabilization has been well-documented.[258]

Epidemiology

Moyamoya is not confined to the Japanese; although overall there is an increased incidence in people of Asian extraction, cases have been reported from all over the world, in all ethnic groups.[259,260] In Japan, the prevalence is 3/100 000 with an annual incidence of 0.35–0.54 per 100 000/year.[261,262] There is a female preponderance in the Japanese cases with a ratio of 1.8 to 1 and up to 12% of cases are familial.[262,263] In Europe, the incidence is about one-tenth that in Japan.[264] In the USA, the incidence has been estimated at 0.086/100 000

children[265] but the incidence in Asians was similar to that seen in Japan; compared with whites, the incidence was more than twice that in those of African extraction, while the relative rate in Hispanics was half. In contrast to the Japanese cases, where 80% are idiopathic, secondary cases are more common in other ethnic groups. Familial cases also appear to be less common in non-Japanese patients.[266] In Japan, there are two peaks in age of presentation, one in childhood (at around 5 years) and the other between 30 and 49 years of age.[261,267] The younger group usually presents with ischaemic symptoms, whereas the older patients tend to experience haemorrhagic complications. The ages and modes of presentation in other ethnic groups have been reported to be similar to those observed in the Japanese,[264] but a study of American patients[259,260] found that the peak age of presentation was in adulthood, and with ischaemic rather than haemorrhagic events in this age group.

Pathology

In primary moyamoya disease, there is a systemic vasculopathy in addition to the occlusion of the circle of Willis, which probably involves excessive amounts of elastin and collagen. Vascular histology in Japanese patients has shown that the stenosis or occlusion of the terminal ICA is due to eccentric intimal thickening, without disruption of the internal elastic laminae.[256,261,267,268] There is also fibrocellular intimal thickening and thinning of the media in other major branches of

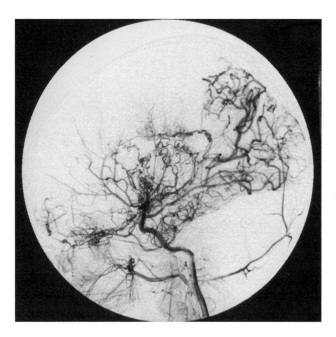

Fig. 6.10. Conventional angiography showing moyamoya.

the circle of Willis (i.e. anterior, middle and posterior cerebral arteries). Histological studies have also found evidence of intravascular thrombi in the intracranial and cervical arteries. These are most frequently found in association with intimal thickening and oedema.[269] Of note, none of the histological studies has shown evidence of inflammation in affected vessels. The collateral circulation is made up of dilatation of pre-existing channels rather than new vessels.[270] They show thinning of the vessel wall and obstruction due to mural thickening or thrombi (Fig. 6.10).[268]

Aetiology

Genetics

Familial moyamoya disease
There is considerable evidence that primary moyamoya disease has a genetic basis, probably polygenic. Approximately 7–12% of primary cases are familial[262] and 80% of monozygotic twins are concordant. Familial moyamoya disease (F-MMD) is inherited as an autosomal dominant trait with variable penetrance; affected females are more likely to have daughters who develop moyamoya later in life, suggesting a role for genomic imprinting.[271] In the Japanese F-MMD appears to be linked to markers on chromosome 3p[272] and a Greek family has also been reported;[273] interestingly the genes for Marfan disease and von Hippel–Lindau disease also map to 3p. Williams syndrome, which is associated with cerebrovascular[274,275] as well as cardiovascular disease, results from a mutation on chromosome 7q in a region which includes the elastin gene. In F-MMD, there is now evidence for involvement of a second gene on chromosome 17q25, close to the gene for neurofibromatosis type 1.[276,277] There may be

a third locus on chromosome 6 close to the HLA genes[278] and a fourth on chromosome 8.[279]

Growth factors and angiogenesis
Basic fibroblast (bFGF)[280] and hepatocyte growth factors[281] are increased in the CSF of Japanese patients with moyamoya disease. These growth factors are believed to have two effects, namely, proliferation of vascular endothelium and promotion of angiogenesis, and thus could lead to both ICA occlusion as well as collateralization.[282]

Infection, inflammation and autoimmunity
Moyamoya has been documented after infections[282] including *Varicella*,[233] although a case control study found no excess of head and neck infections such as tonsillitis or otitis media.[283] There appears to be an association with specific human leukocyte antigen (HLA) haplotypes (HLA B40 in patients younger than and HLA B52 antigen in those older than 10 years of age). Idiopathic cases in Japan have also been linked to HLA AW24, AW46, BW54[284] and B51-DR4.[285] Graves' disease is an occasional association in adults and children.[286] Although rapid progression and bilateral infarction has been described,[287] in one patient the vasculopathy reversed after plasmapheresis.[288]

Moyamoya syndrome
In the USA and Europe, most cases are of moyamoya syndrome secondary to other conditions with Mendelian inheritance, such as neurofibromatosis type 1,[289,290] Marfan syndrome, Noonan syndrome,[291] Robinow syndrome,[292] Seckel syndrome[293] and haemolytic anaemias such as hereditary spherocytosis, haemolytic-uraemic syndrome[294] and sickle cell disease[295,296] or chromosomal disorders such as Down and Williams syndromes (Table 6.3).[296,297] Moyamoya has also been described in the Alagille syndrome,[298] caused by mutations in the Jagged-1 gene (about half of which are inherited) responsible for signaling during embryonic development. Bicuspid aortic valve and coarctation of the aorta are also associated with moyamoya and other patients may have evidence of systemic vasculopathy involving the renal, abdominal, coronary and peripheral vessels. Other cerebrovascular pathologies, including aneurysms and arteriovenous malformations (Table 6.3), are seen on angiography in association with moyamoya, although they may not be more common in this group than in the general population.

Environmental Triggers
The relative importance of genetic and environmental factors remains controversial and although the radiological appearances are similar, there may be important differences in pathology. Environmental triggers, such as cranial irradiation for acute lymphoblastic leukaemia[299] or midline tumours, for example optic glioma,[300] are clearly important in some cases. There is also evidence for a role of prothrombotic disorders,[301] although some may be acquired, perhaps as a response to infection, and their aetiological role is not established. Some of the associated

TABLE 6.3
Conditions in which moyamoya has been described

Metabolic disease
Homocystinuria (homozygous and heterozygous)
Glycogen storage disease type Ia
Diabetes
Primary oxalosis
Hyperphosphatasia
Lactic acidosis, ptosis and impaired NADH-coenzyme Q reductase
　activity

Anaemias
Sickle cell disease
Hereditary spherocytosis
Hb Alesha
β-thalassaemia intermedia
Fanconi anaemia
Paroxysmal nocturnal haemoglobinuria
Haemolytic-uraemic syndrome

Disorders of thrombosis
Protein C deficiency
Protein S deficiency
Factor XII deficiency
Plasminogen deficiency
Lupus anticoagulant
Antiphospholipid antibodies
Factor V Leiden
Homozygosity for thermolabile variant of methylene tetrahydrofolate
　reductase
Thrombotic thrombocytopenic purpura
Haemophilia A

Neurocutaneous disorders
Neurofibromatosis type I
Hypomelanosis of Ito
Tuberous sclerosis
Elastosis perforans serpiginosa-like pseudoxanthoma elasticum
Microcephalic osteodysplastic primordial short stature type II with café-
　au-lait spots
Facial angioma and midline skin aplasia
Cutis marmorata telangiectatica congenita
Phakomatosis pigmentovascularis type IIIb
Aplasia cutis congenital
Harlequinism
Precocious puberty and pustular psoriasis
Livedo reticularis and Sneddon syndrome
Cardio-facial cutaneous syndrome

Tumours
Brain tumour – optic glioma, craniopharyngioma, cerebellar vermis,
　brainstem glioma, hypothalamic astrocytoma, pituitary adenoma,
　(with and without irradiation)
Wilm's tumour
Leukaemia

Autoimmune disease
Systemic lupus erythematosus (including neonatal lupus)
Sjögren syndrome
Juvenile rheumatoid arthritis
Graves thyrotoxicosis
Ulcerative colitis

Immunodeficiency
Schimke immuno-osseous dysplasia
Human immunodeficiency virus
IgA deficiency and Raynaud

Infection
Leptospirosis
Neurosyphilis in HIV

Tuberculous meningitis
Sarcoidosis
Epstein–Barr virus
Varicella zoster and herpes zoster opthalmicus
?Chronic upper airway infection

Miscellaneous chromosomal and single gene disorders
Down syndrome
Prader–Willi syndrome
Turner syndrome
Noonan syndrome
Marfan syndrome 2
Ehlers–Danlos syndrome VIIA1
Williams syndrome
Alagille syndrome
Marfan syndrome
Alport syndrome
Apert syndrome
Osteogenesis imperfecta
Robinow syndrome
Seckel syndrome
ACTA2 heterozygosity

Other conditions
Cranial irradiation
?Cranial trauma
Atherosclerosis
Cocaine dependency
Acute necrotizing encephalopathy
Synbrachydactylia, funnel chest, pes equinus, short stature
　(mesenchymal anomaly)
Grange syndrome
Morning glory optic discs, retinochoroidal coloboma and midline
　cranial defects
Meningoencephalocele
Pituitary gigantism
Schizophrenia
Central deafness
CREST syndrome
Hirschsprung disease
Polycystic kidneys and eosinophilic granuloma
Progressive myopathy
Behçet disease
Hemiplegic migraine

Vascular associations with moyamoya
Cerebral aneurysm
Cerebral arteriovenous malformation
Internal carotid artery dissection
Fibromuscular dysplasia
Persistent primitive trigeminal arteries
Persistent primitive hypoglossal artery
Sagittal sinus thrombosis
Renal artery stenosis
Renovascular hypertension
Primary pulmonary hypertension
Peripheral artery disease
Raynaud phenomenon

Cardiac disease
Patent ductus arteriosus, bilateral dolichoectatic internal carotid arteries
　in combination with iris hypoplasia with bilateral fixed dilated pupils
Aortic stenosis
Coronary artery disease
Dilated cardiomyopathy
Coarctation of the aorta

NADH, nicotinamide adenine dinucleotid, HIV, human immunodeficiency virus, ACTA2, atin, alpha 2, smooth muscle, aorta, CREST, Calcinosis Raynaud syndrome,
Esophagea; dismotility, Sclerodactyly, Telangiectasia.

disorders suggest possible aetiological mechanisms. In Down syndrome, for example, there may be a widespread vasculopathy affecting small and large vessels and the venous sinuses,[302] suggesting that moyamoya is part of a spectrum of vascular responses to environmental challenges experienced during development in a genetically predisposed individual. The association with Williams's syndrome,[274,275] a disorder which is associated with mutations in the elastin gene, suggests that abnormal vessel distensibility may lead to hypoperfusion and promote the development of collateral vessels. A vascular steal phenomenon in early life may lead to the development of moyamoya, as in patients with facial cavernous haemangioma (PHACES).[303] There is also an association with anaemias with unstable haemoglobin, haemolysis and oxygen desaturation, most commonly sickle cell disease (see Chapter 15). Although it has been observed that infection in the head and neck region frequently precedes the initial presentation,[267] a case–control study found no evidence of an excess of prior infection.[282,283] Fever may lead to systemic vasodilatation, which may in turn result in cerebral ischaemia due to reduced perfusion reserve.[303,304]

Clinical presentation

The clinical manifestations of moyamoya syndrome include arterial ischaemic stroke and transient ischaemic attacks (TIAs) (predominantly in children), intracranial haemorrhage, seizures (generalized tonic-clonic, absences[305] and partial), headache,[306,307] visual symptoms,[308] progressive cognitive dysfunction,[309] dementia,[310] psychosis[311] and movement disorders (e.g. chorea),[312,313] paroxysmal dyskinesia[314] and recurrent torticollis.[315] Some children have frequent recurrent TIAs, especially after hyperventilation, without developing cerebral infarction.[261]

Cerebral ischaemia is primarily due to cerebral perfusion failure. Embolic vascular occlusion due to artery to artery embolism may also play a part in the pathogenesis of focal ischaemia. The prevalence of ischaemic symptoms during childhood is thought to reflect increased cerebral metabolic requirements during childhood. There is then often a period of stabilization in young adulthood prior to the peak age of onset of haemorrhagic symptoms. Cerebral haemorrhage may occur in the subarachnoid, intracerebral or intraventricular spaces due to rupture of the fragile collateral vessels or of aneurysms.

Hypertension is a frequent clinical observation in patients with moyamoya syndrome. In some patients this is centrally driven and improves after surgical revascularization.[316] Around 5% of Japanese patients have renal artery stenosis.[317] Management of hypertension should be undertaken with extreme caution as the increased systemic blood pressure may be critical to maintaining cerebral perfusion.

Diagnosis

Catheter Cerebral Angiography
Prior to the availability of MRI, catheter cerebral angiography (CCA) was mandatory for the diagnosis of moyamoya.

Suzuki described an angiographic disease staging system[318] and in Japanese patients with idiopathic moyamoya disease there is progression through these stages. It is not clear whether this also occurs in secondary cases and disease staging is not especially helpful in clinical practice. In more advanced stages of the disease, the vertebrobasilar system is involved, with progressive occlusion of the posterior cerebral arteries. Cerebral infarction is more frequent in patients with more severe disease both in the ICA system and the posterior circulation.[319]

MRI
The availability of MRI has meant that CCA is no longer mandatory and criteria for MRI diagnosis have been defined (see above). MRA is able to demonstrate both the stenotic lesions and the collateral circulation.[319,320] Overall, MRA tends to overestimate the degree of stenosis and underestimate the amount of collateral. The collateral vessels may also be identified as flow voids in the basal ganglia on T1-weighted MRI (Fig. 6.9).

The newer MR techniques, in particular MR diffusion, perfusion and blood-oxygen imaging, have emerged as useful non-invasive techniques to explore cerebral perfusion and reactivity,[321,322] MR perfusion imaging using a bolus tracking method can demonstrate abnormal tissue perfusion in areas of cerebral tissue which appear normal in conventional and MR diffusion imaging[321,323–324] and therefore has potential to be used in the evaluation of patients for surgery.

Cerebral Haemodynamics
Cerebral autoregulation refers to the processes that maintain cerebral perfusion in response to changes in cerebral perfusion pressure. Stenosis or occlusion of major cerebral arteries reduces the arterial pressure in the distal circulation; distal perfusion is therefore dependent on collateral vessels. If these cannot maintain sufficient cerebral perfusion pressure, reflex vasodilatation occurs (stage 1 haemodynamic compromise).[325] Further reductions in perfusion pressure lead to an increase in the oxygen extracting capacity of the brain (the oxygen extraction fraction (OEF)) in order to maintain normal cerebral metabolic function (stage 2 haemodynamic compromise). This is described as 'misery perfusion'. Once OEF is maximal, further reductions in perfusion pressure lead to disruptions in tissue metabolism and ultimately to brain infarction.

In the resting state, patients with moyamoya may either have normal regional cerebral blood flow (rCBF) or focal reduction of rCBF, particularly in frontal regions:[326–328] i.e. resting rCBF is not adequate in the assessment of the haemodynamic state in these patients. It is useful to distinguish between areas where rCBF is inappropriately low for the metabolic demands of the tissue and areas where it is reduced because of reduced metabolic demand, as the areas showing the former pattern may potentially benefit from increased blood flow. Positron emission tomography (PET) studies in symptomatic patients may show areas of haemodynamic compromise with reduced rCBF, increased regional oxygen extraction fraction (rOEF) and regional cerebral blood volume (rCBV) and normal cerebral metabolic rate (CMRO$_2$).[329] Increased rCBV represents both compensatory vasodilatation related to the reduced rCBF as well as the blood contained with the collateral circulation. In patents with more advanced disease, there is a progressive fall in rCBF and eventually a decrease in rCMRO$_2$.

'Perfusion reserve' is the ability to maintain CBF following a vasodilatory stimulus, for example CO$_2$ or acetazolamide. A lack of increase in CBF following a vasodilatory stimulus implies that the cerebral circulation is already maximally vasodilated at rest (stage 1 haemodynamic compromise – see above). Perfusion reserve is reduced in patients with moyamoya and improves after revascularization surgery.[328–332] Taki et al[332,333] found that rCBV was increased but rCBF was relatively normal in symptomatic patients with moyamoya, suggesting that perfusion reserve (which is reduced in this instance as rCBV is increased) is more closely related to symptoms than resting rCBF. In this study reduced perfusion reserve correlated with increased rOEF on PET, i.e. areas of reduced perfusion reserve include areas with both stage 1 and stage 2 haemodynamic compromise.[334] Reduced perfusion reserve and increased rOEF and rCBV pre-operatively are more important predictors of postoperative collateral formation after indirect surgical revascularization than pre-operative rCBF.[335]

The relatively stable state of impaired cerebral perfusion, with full recruitment of the compensatory mechanisms of proliferation of collateral vessels, vasodilatation and hypertension, is a unique model of chronic cerebral ischaemia which has not been systematically explored in terms of its effects on cerebral function. Haemodynamic abnormalities improve but may still be outside the normal range after surgical revascularization.[329,332] Clinical improvement is not directly related to the improvement in haemodynamic studies.

ELECTROENCEPHALOGRAPHY (EEG)
Many patients have posterior slow wave activity at rest.[335,336] Hyperventilation results in generalized slow wave activity – which is referred to as 'build-up'. Between 20 and 60 seconds after cessation of hyperventilation a characteristic pattern termed 're-build-up' is seen. This consists of frontal polymorphous high voltage slow activity and is seen in 80% of children with moyamoya (Fig. 6.11). Re-build-up is caused by cerebral hypoxia due to both hypocapnic vasoconstriction ('ischaemic hypoxia') in areas of reduced perfusion reserve[328,337] as well as a delayed fall in pO$_2$ following hyperventilation ('hypoxic hypoxia').[338,339]

It is accepted practice that patients with moyamoya should not be asked to hyperventilate during routine EEG recordings as there is a risk of precipitating permanent ischaemic symptoms. We have seen a number of patients in whom the diagnosis was first suggested on the basis of the characteristic EEG pattern during the course of investigation for possible

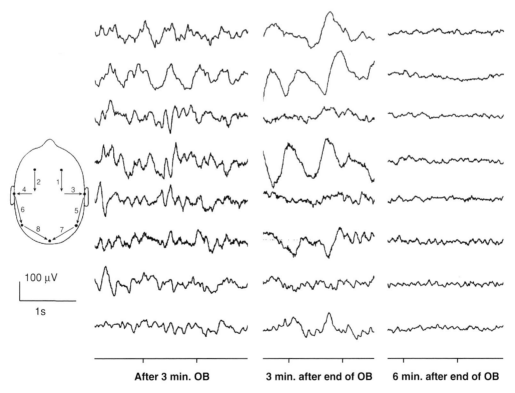

After 3 min. OB   **3 min. after end of OB**   **6 min. after end of OB**

100 μV

1s

Fig. 6.11. Electroencephalogram (EEG) features of moyamoya syndrome elicited in a previously undiagnosed child with intermittent right hemiparesis, referred as a possible case of epilepsy. At the end of a standard period of 3 minutes of overbreathing (OB), there is a limited amount of slowing, particularly over the left upper frontal region (left). However, this settled within a few seconds and was followed, 3 minutes after the end of overbreathing, by a 're-build-up' of much slower activity seen over a wider area of the left hemisphere and also the right frontal region (middle panel). This settled again and the EEG returned to its normal resting state 6 minutes after overbreathing ceased (right panel).

seizures. Many of the clinical attacks in these patients were in fact TIAs rather than partial seizures.

Treatment

Given that haemodynamic failure is responsible for cerebral ischaemia in the majority of patients, a variety of operations has been employed to improve cerebral perfusion in this group of children.[297,328,340–344] Those with moyamoya syndrome, for example secondary to sickle cell disease[344–347] or Down syndrome,[347] may also be considered for surgery.[297] Procedures can broadly be considered in two groups: direct extracranial-intracranial (EC-IC) bypass and indirect revascularization procedures.

Direct EC-IC bypass surgery usually involves anastomosis of a branch of the superficial temporal artery (STA) to a cortical branch of the MCA, bypassing the terminal ICA occlusion. Although direct anastomosis is technically challenging, in experienced hands microvascular anastomosis is possible in vessels with a calibre of at least 1mm.[348,349] STA–MCA anastomosis has been shown to be effective in immediately improving cerebral blood flow, which may be advantageous in patients who are clinically symptomatic at the time of surgery.

They are many techniques for indirect cerebral revascularization. Essentially these depend on promoting the formation of transdural collaterals. Encephalo-duro-arterio-synangiosis is a technique where the dura is cut and joined to a strip of galea containing a scalp artery. Pial synangiosis involves suturing the adventitia of the STA directly onto the pia. In Encephalo-myo-synangiosis, the dura is split and the temporalis muscle laid directly onto the temporoparietal brain surface. In EMAS (encephalo-myo-arterio-synangiosis), a flap of muscle with a strip of galea containing a branch of the STA is laid over the parasagittal frontal lobe. Other procedures include omental transplantation or creation of multiple burr holes.

Clinical stabilization and improvement in perfusion reserve appear to be related to the extent of new collateral formation.[350,351] Although collaterals may regress following surgical revascularization, the underlying vasculopathy may progress despite good collateralization. Collateralization appears to increase over the 6–12 months following surgery. Post-surgical collateralization is best in patients with the highest levels of CSF bFGF and the production of collaterals after surgery is much better in children with moyamoya than in adults with occlusive cerebrovascular disease.[329,335] The success of surgical revascularization in patients with moyamoya may have some mechanisms in common with the pathogenesis of the disorder.

The optimal surgical technique is controversial. Although the literature suggests that a combination of direct and indirect procedures appears to provide the greatest postoperative collateral formation[329,352,353] most likely to be associated with clinical stabilization,[327,353] indirect procedures are more technically straightforward and have been shown to be effective in providing a source of collaterals, improving clinical symptoms and cerebral haemodynamics.[351,354–356]

Normoxia, normocapnia, hydration and an adequate haematocrit should be maintained during general anaesthesia and in the postoperative period.[357] Adequate analgesia should be given as protracted crying because of pain has been associated with ischaemic events in the postoperative period.[354]

Although there are numerous case series reporting clinical stabilization (cessation of TIA and prevention of further ischaemic stroke), cognitive stabilization or improvement of haemodynamic parameters, the variability in natural history means that this in itself is not definitive evidence of the efficacy of surgery. Comparison of the long-term outcome in Japanese patients managed conservatively or treated surgically does not show clear differences between the two groups.[358] This may, of course, reflect selection bias as well the variability of the natural history. A review of the published English language literature concluded that surgery was of clinical benefit in terms of stroke prevention but commented that the literature was confounded by poor study design and reporting bias.[342] The timing of surgery is a further contentious issue. In Japan and Korea, surgery is offered to patients with repeated ischaemic symptoms and in whom cerebral perfusion studies have demonstrated reduced rCBF and perfusion reserve.[328,359] Even in Japan patients tend to be referred late[304] whereas the best improvements following surgery appear to be in young children who have not had repeated attacks.[328,354] However, the variability in natural history and the uncertainty about natural history in other ethnic groups has prompted debate about whether the Japanese criteria should also be applied to other patients. Whilst many centres would recommend revascularization at the point of diagnosis, given the variable natural history, our own practice is to offer surgery to patients with recurrent attacks or evidence of progressive ischaemic brain injury.

Revascularization surgery does not appear to be effective in preventing haemorrhagic events. Where haemorrhage has occurred from a ruptured aneurysm, surgical aneurysm repair appears to be effective in preventing further haemorrhage.[259]

Medical treatment (either aspirin or anticoagulation) is often used[256] but the efficacy of these in preventing further symptoms remains unproven. We routinely treat patients with low dose aspirin (1–2mg/kg/day) and only use anticoagulation in patients who continue to have TIA or stroke despite aspirin. Anticoagulation is generally contraindicated because of concern about rupture from collateral vessels but is occasionally used with caution in patients with intractable TIAs. The duration of medical therapy is contentious; our own practice is to continue antiplatelet agents through childhood and to stop at 18 years of age because of concerns about haemorrhage.

Outcome

Although some patients are prone to recurrent TIA and stroke, the functional sequelae of moyamoya are very variable. Olds reported that of 39 children reported in the literature followed up for at least 2 years, five died and 11 were 'normal' at follow-up.[358] Factors associated with poor outcome include an early age at presentation[350,360] and presentation with completed stroke. Cognitive function initially declines with longer duration of disease.[360,361] In a study with long follow-up of untreated patients, 16 out of 27 children with moyamoya disease had a lower Full Scale IQ at follow-up compared with baseline,[361] but there was evidence of stabilization around 10 years after the onset of symptoms.[361] Factors consistent with a poor outcome include early age at onset, TIAs followed by stroke, diffuse arteriographic occlusion, and bilateral or left hemisphere lesions.[362] Long-term functional outcome is good in between a third and a half of Japanese patients; between 20% and 30% have severe functional impairments.[360,363]

The natural history in non-Japanese patients is less clear. Chiu et al reported that of 31 American patients, four had died; all surviving patients had a modified Rankin score of 3 or less (corresponding to no or mild disability).[260] There was no significant difference in outcome or risk of further stroke between patients who had undergone surgery and those who had not. Decline in cognitive function appears to occur in moymoya syndrome as well. In a study of 15 children who developed moyamoya following a stroke (six with sickle cell disease [SCD]), and 19 controls (10 with SCD), there were significant reductions in IQ by the second assessment for the moyamoya patients compared with controls but IQ did not differ significantly between groups with and without SCA.[309] The pace and extent of decline in individual children may be unpredictable and intellectual status should be routinely documented longitudinally in individual patients.

6.4 Cerebral Vasculitis

Russell C. Dale

Introduction

Cerebral vasculitis is an inflammatory disorder of the central nervous system (CNS). By definition, the cerebral vessel walls are infiltrated by inflammatory cells, with consequent inflammatory neural damage and ischaemic injury. Cerebral vasculitis in children may occur as part of a systemic multi-organ vasculitis such as Henoch–Schönlein purpura, polyarteritis nodosa and Wegener's granulomatosis. In addition, cerebral vasculitis is a recognized complication of varicella infection. When CNS involvement occurs as part of a multi-system vasculitic disease, a diagnosis of cerebral vasculitis is usually possible. However, when the vasculitis is localized to the (primary angiitis of the CNS (PACNS)), diagnosis and consequent management is far more difficult.

PACNS is an uncommon disorder, although is frequently quoted as part of an acute neurology differential diagnosis. It is most frequently seen in the 5th to 7th decades, although it may occur at any age. A secure diagnosis requires relatively invasive procedures such as catheter cerebral angiography or cerebral biopsy, which should be reserved for cases with a high index of suspicion. However, definitive diagnosis is essential as immunosuppressive agents are effective, and have significantly reduced the mortality of this condition.

This chapter aims to review the clinical features of PACNS in both adults and children, followed by a review of the sensitivity and specificity of diagnostic investigations. Recent developments in the immunopathogenesis of vasculitis are not reviewed here, and readers are referred to literature dedicated to this subject.[364]

Clinical features

There is no classic or typical presentation of cerebral vasculitis. The tempo of clinical presentation of disease can be acute, subacute or chronic. A review of pathology proven cerebral vasculitis in childhood showed differences in the presentation tempo dependent upon the size of vessels involved.[365] Small vessel involvement presented subacutely with progressive multifocal neurological impairments. By contrast, large vessel involvement presented with acute ischaemic strokes or acute haemorrhages. Similarly, the mode of presentation is variable. Reviews of the adult literature have subdivided the mode of presentation as follows:[364]

Focal presentation

- Ischaemic 'stroke-like' events
- Rapidly increasing cerebral mass (often initially interpreted as malignant tumours)
- Intracerebral or subarachnoid haemorrhages
- Myelopathy.

Multiple/disseminated lesions

- Multiple lesion (two or more) sites. Cases are often initially interpreted as multiple sclerosis.

Diffuse (non-localizing) presentation

- Encephalitic presentation with encephalopathy and behavioural alteration
- Meningitic presentation
- Dementia or degenerative presentation (including progressive extrapyramidal disorder).

With such a diverse pattern of presentation, it is not surprising that a wide range of symptoms and signs may be present. The most common presenting features are headache, confusional state and hemiparesis.[366,367] Some children with haemorrhagic strokes have histological or arteriographic evidence of vasculitis in addition to an aneurysm[368] or arteriovenous malformation,[369] and venous infarcts have also been associated despite clear evidence of arteritis.[370] The clinical presentation of cerebral vasculitis is therefore not specific. However, the pattern of the disease is often progressive, fluctuant or recurrent. Therefore, there should be a low index of suspicion in acute isolated stroke in children.

The literature on PACNS in childhood was limited to case reports until several recent contributions from Benseler and colleagues in Toronto (Table 6.4). Of their series of 62 patients, common clinical features included hemiparesis, encephalopathy and headache. Twenty had a progressive clinical course; these patients were more likely to present with cognitive symptoms, multifocal MRI lesions and distal arterial disease.[371] Whilst this cohort is the largest described to date, it is worth noting that in the absence of histological diagnosis, there is likely to be a degree of overlap between the patients described in this study and those who have been categorized as having transient cerebral arteriopathy by other groups (see Chapter 6.2).

In general, cerebral angiography and/or brain biopsy have been the crucial diagnostic investigations in PACNS and it is worth noting that there have been histologically proven cases with negative catheter cerebral angiography.[372] Presentation with acute hemiparesis is not uncommon but subsequent disease course is usually complicated by further stroke-like events often with accompanying headache, encephalopathy and progressive disseminated disease. One child presented with an acute fatal subarachnoid haemorrhage. Subacute presentation with masslike lesions (three cerebral, one spinal and one carotid neck mass), often initially mistaken for tumour, is also well recognized. Another described clinical pattern is of multifocal presentation followed by a subsequent fluctuant or relapsing remitting course.

The outcome of the earlier cases must be placed in context, as before treatment was available cerebral vasculitis was universally fatal. In the earlier accounts of 12 patients who received adequate immunosuppressive treatment (reviewed later), five made a 'full' recovery, five patients had some residual disability and both patients who were not treated died. In contrast, more recent series report very good outcomes with modern immunosuppressive regimes.[373]

Investigation

PERIPHERAL BLOOD EXAMINATION

Investigation of the blood is usually unhelpful in providing a diagnosis of cerebral vasculitis, and is performed mainly to exclude differential diagnoses. From adult studies, the peripheral white cell count may be slightly elevated, although it is commonly normal.[364,367] The peripheral white cell count was normal in the majority of child PACNS cases. There may be slight elevation of the ethrocyte sedimentation rate, although significant elevation would be unusual,[3,364] but in Benseler's series, the ethrocyte sedimentation rate was elevated in 18 out of 35 and c-reactive protein in 14/19.[371] Antineutrophil cytoplasmic autoantibodies (ANCA) are usually normal, although exceptions are described.[374]

In conclusion, peripheral blood investigations are usually normal, in fact the absence of systemic inflammatory markers has been considered an important feature of PACNS in adults.[367] The normality of peripheral blood investigation in PACNS is in marked contrast to the systemic vasculitides.

CSF EXAMINATION

Laboratory examination of the CSF is a useful tool in the investigation of non-infectious inflammatory disorders of the CNS, although it rarely provides definitive diagnostic information.

From the adult literature, the CSF is usually abnormal in PACNS.[364] Most commonly, there is a steady elevation of CSF protein, or CSF lymphocytosis.[371]

Oligoclonal bands have not been routinely examined in PACNS patients; however intrathecal synthesis of oligoclonal bands has been occasionally described.[375] Interestingly, two biopsy-proven childhood PACNS cases had intrathecal synthesis of oligoclonal bands.[376,377] Both patients had a focal mass-like presentation with clear histological confirmation, and should therefore be considered definite PACNS. Although non-specific, examination of the CSF should be considered useful in the assessment of children with suspected PACNS.

NEUROIMAGING

MRI is more sensitive than CT in the management of cerebral vasculitis (Fig. 6.12). MRI frequently demonstrates the consequence of vascular inflammation such as haemorrhage, hyperintense lesions in the white matter, leptomeningeal enhancement and cerebral infarcts.[378,379] Frequently, the scan may provide evidence of a more widespread process than clinically suspected, and therefore lead clinicians to consider PACNS. However, the MRI changes are not specific to vascular inflammation. MRI is also not completely sensitive, as there has been one histologically defined case of PACNS where the MRI was normal.[380] Aviv et al[379] found that the most common pattern of abnormality on MRI was of multifocal unilateral parenchymal involvement in 42 of 45 children with PACNS. Isolated infratentorial lesions were not observed. MRI has other practical uses, namely to help select biopsy sites. When present, gadolinium enhancement of the leptomeninges is a useful diagnostic sign. Recently Kuker et al[381] have described vessel wall thickening and wall enhancement in patients with cerebral vasculitis, many of whom had a diagnosis of PACNS. Of note, 10 patients were aged 18 or under; vessel wall thickening/enhancement were identified in nine out of 10 but as only one had catheter cerebral angiography the relative sensitivities of the two investigations requires further investigation.

MRA does not reliably provide information about small vessels (which are most commonly affected in PACNS), and therefore may not be a sensitive tool in the diagnosis of PACNS. However, in patients with large vessel involvement, MRA may have comparable sensitivity to catheter angiography.[382] In a study of 42 children with PACNS, Aviv et al[379] reported that MRA was normal in 12; the majority of the rest had proximal vascular disease. Arterial disease was multifocal in two-thirds of those in whom it was identified. Patients with abnormal MRA always had abnormal MRI.

CATHETER CEREBRAL ANGIOGRAPHY

Catheter cerebral angiography (CCA) is the criterion standard technique for imaging the cerebral vessels. Angiographic features of cerebral vasculitis include arterial narrowing and dilatation, occlusion and alteration in circulation time of the affected vascular distributions. In addition, beading and aneurysm formation may be present.[383] However, CCA has significant diagnostic

TABLE 6.4

Primary angiitis of the central nervous system in childhood (where not stated N=1)

Author	Localization	Tempo	Clinical presentation	Course	Diagnostic investigation
LaMancusa and Steiman 1990[396]	Focal. 'Stroke-like'	Acute	Hemiplegia, aphasia	Recurrent hemiplegia	Angiography
Prengler et al 1997[391]	Focal. 'Stroke-like'	Acute	Hemiplegia, headaches, aphasia	Multiple stroke-like episodes	Angiography
Prengler et al 1997[391]	Focal. 'Stroke-like'	Acute	Hemiplegia, aphasia, dystonia, encephalopathy	Multiple stroke-like episodes	Angiography
Nishikawa et al 1998[397]	Focal. 'Stroke-like'	Acute	Headache, hemiplegia	Multiple stroke-like episodes and SAH	Angiography and autopsy
Gallagher et al 2001 (N=5)[392]	Focal. 'Stroke-like'	Acute	Headache, focal signs	Progressive	
Kamm et al 2008[398]	Focal. 'Stroke-like'	Acute	Hemiplegia, visual loss	Progressive	
Kumar et al 1997[399]	Focal. 'SAH'	Acute	Sudden death	Fatal	Autopsy
Derry et al 2002[377]	Focal. 'Mass-like'	Subacute	Hemiplegia, headache, seizures	Slowly progressive	Biopsy
Lanthier et al 2001[365]	Focal. 'Mass-like'	Subacute	Cerebellar lesion, headache	Full resolution	Biopsy
Katsicas et al 2000[400]	Focal. 'Mass-like'	Subacute			
Vella et al 1999[374]	Focal. 'Mass-like'	Subacute	Neck pain, cranial neuropathy	Full resolution	Angiography
Andrews et al 1990[376]	Focal. 'Mass-like'	Chronic	Hemiplegia, seizures	Slowly progressive	Biopsy
Giovanini et al 1994[401]	Focal. 'Mass-like'	Chronic	Myelopathy	Partial resolution	Biopsy
Barron et al 1993[402]	Multifocal	Subacute	Headache, hemiplegia	Fluctuant	Angiography
Lanthier et al 2001[365]	Multifocal	Subacute	Seizures, hemiplegia, headache	Partial resolution	Biopsy
Yaari et al 2004 (N=2)[403]	Multifocal	Subacute	Headache, hemiplegia	Partial resolution	
Matsell et al 1990[404]	Multifocal	Chronic	Headache, brainstem signs, seizures, quadriplegia	Relapsing remitting (died)	Autopsy
Calabrese and Mallek 1987[405]	Multifocal	Acute	Hemiplegia, hemianaesthesia, nystagmus	Full recovery	Angiography
Benseler et al 2005 (N=5)[372]	Mulifocal in 2, focal 'stroke-like' in 1, focal seizures in 1	Subacute	Hemiparesis, encephalopathy, seizures	Full recovery, no relapses	All angiogram negative, biopsy positive
Benseler et al 2006 (N=62)[371]	Variable	Variable	Focal neurological deficit, encephalopathy, headache	Progressive in 20	Clinical, MRI/A and angiography

SAH, subarachnoid haemorrhage.

129

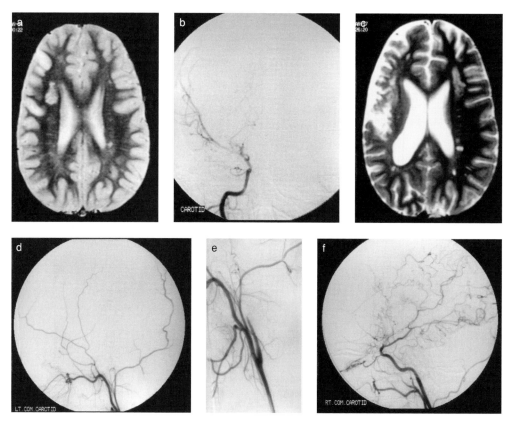

Fig. 6.12. Isolated cerebral angitis presenting with stroke in a 4-year old boy (a) T2-weighted brain MRI. Acute infarct in the right middle cerebral artery (MCA) territory. High T2 signal is seen in the right frontal cortex with further areas in both peritrigonal regions and centrum ovale on the right. (b) Carotid angiogram shows right MCA stenosis. (c) T2-weighted MRI brain demonstrates established infarction with associated atrophy in the right MCA territory. There is an additional patchy periventricular and deep white matter ischaemia on the right and left sides. (d–f) Four-vessel cerebral angiogram shows bilateral MCA stenosis. The right common carotid injection fills mainly the right posterior circulation with a combination of small collaterals, and retrograde filling of the ACA and MCA territories. (d). The new vessel formation is in the form of early moyamoya type change. The left common carotid is markedly stenosed near its origin (e,f). There is a progressive angiopathy with appearances consistent with a vasculitic process.

limitations. Firstly, the sensitivity of this investigation is limited. The majority of cerebral vessels involved in PACNS are smaller than 200 microns diameter, beyond angiographic resolution.[364] Therefore, CCA will only identify disease occurring in larger calibre vessels. The sensitivity is at best 85%,[384] although only 40% of histologically confirmed cases had abnormal angiograms.[372,385] The specificity of CCA is also problematical. There are a number of non-inflammatory angiopathies which can result in the 'typical' vasculitic angiographic features.[364] However, angiography continues to have an important role in PACNS although results should be carefully interpreted considering the clinical setting and laboratory findings.

In a study comparing CCA with MRA in children with PACNS, Aviv et al did not find significant differences between the two techniques in detection or characterization of lesions.[382] However, it should be noted that the majority of lesions in the 25 children who had contemporaneous MRA and CCA were unilateral and involved the anterior circulation and thus these finding cannot be extrapolated to patients with PACNS involving small vessels.

In conclusion, as with MRA, CCA is more likely to be diagnostic in cases suspected of having large or medium vessel disease and in those who present with recurrent ischaemic stroke.[366,365] Angiography in small vessel vasculitis presenting insidiously with mass lesions or multifocal lesions is likely to be normal, and biopsy should be considered the preferred diagnostic tool.

HISTOPATHOLOGY (CEREBRAL OR LEPTOMENINGEAL BIOPSY)
Examination of cerebral tissue remains the criterion standard method for diagnosing cerebral vasculitis. However, given its invasive nature it is only considered in a few patients. It should be noted that the morbidity of biopsy is quite low, and significantly lower than either delayed diagnosis or inappropriate therapy. The histopathological features of cerebral vasculitis are inflammatory infiltrate of the blood vessel wall. The inflammatory cells are predominantly lymphocytes, but also histiocytes, plasma cells and sometimes giant cells. There is often associated infarction and haemorrhage which may complicate the picture.[386] Cerebral vasculitis is often patchy in distribution, and, therefore, biopsy site selection is essential to maximize diagnostic yield. Authorities suggest a combined leptomeningeal/cortical biopsy (preferably stereotactic guided). If a 'blind' biopsy needs to be performed, it is recommended

to sample the leptomeninges and parenchyma from the non-dominant frontal or temporal lobe.[387] Given the patchy nature of the disease process, the sensitivity of biopsy is 65–75%.[367] In contrast, the specificity of biopsy in cerebral vasculitis is pleasingly high. Other than histopathology, more extensive examination of the tissue is recommended, in order to exclude causes of secondary vasculitis such as infection or neoplasm. The recommended tissue preparation and examination is reviewed by Parisi and Moore.[386]

Cerebral vasculitis as part of systemic disease

This chapter has predominantly discussed PACNS, although cerebral vasculitis can occur as part of systemic disease (secondary cerebral vasculitis). From the paediatric perspective the most common causes of secondary vasculitis are those associated with the systemic vasculitides or infection. Cerebral vasculitis is a recognized complication of various systemic conditions (Table 6.5).[385,388] The most important infectious precipitant of childhood cerebral vasculitis is *Varicella* (see Chapter 5, Section 5.1). Stroke after chickenpox is well described in immunocompetent children,[233] and intrathecal varicella antibodies should be measured in children with a recent history of chickenpox.[389] Co-existent retinal vasculitis may occur, and fundoscopy should be considered a routine investigation in suspected cerebral vasculitis. HIV and immunodeficiency states can lead to vasculitis secondary to multiple opportunistic infectious agents.[385] Finally, a drug history should be taken as drug-induced cerebral vasculitis has been described.[390]

Treatment

There have been no controlled studies in the treatment of cerebral vasculitis. However, conclusions have been made from the treatment of systemic vasculitis. Current authorities recommend the use of combined therapy with both steroids and cyclophosphamide.[364] Induction therapy with 2mg/kg/day prednisolone and 500–750mg/m^2 cyclophosphamide have been proposed, although dosage should be individualized to the clinical setting. Although the side effects associated with such therapies are significant, untreated cerebral vasculitis is often fatal. Treatment should therefore be aggressive. A recent landmark paper described a single centre open-label cohort study of 19 biopsy-proven patients with PACNS. The authors used induction therapy of 2 mg/kg prednisolone plus eleven pulses of 500–750mg/m cyclophosphamide every four weeks.

TABLE 6.5
Secondary cerebral vasculitis in childhood (also infections; see Chapter 5, Section 5.1)

Henoch–Schönlein purpura[406–408]
Polyarteritis nodosa[409]
Wegener granulomatosis[410]
Sjögren syndrome[411]
Scleroderma 'en coup de sabre'[412]
Goodpasture syndrome[413]
Dermatomyositis[414,415]
Wiskott–Aldrich syndrome[416]

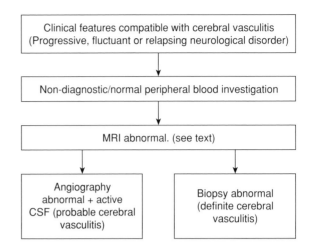

Fig. 6.13. Proposed diagnostic criteria for isolated cerebral vasculitis in children. CSF, cerebrospinal fluid.

Mycophenylate or azathloprine was used as maintenance therapy. Although 8 out of 19 patients experienced disease flares, 9 out of 19 had a good neurological outcome and four patients achieved remission off medication.[1] This author would recommend taking the advice of a paediatrician expert in the use of immunosuppressive agents when chosing a therapeutic regime as, for example, oral or intravenous agents may be effective in different patients.[391–393] Bypass procedures may relieve symptoms if there is chronic cerebral ischaemia.[391,394] Plasma exchange may be effective in improving CNS symptoms and signs in cerebral vasculitis secondary to Henoch–Schönlein purpura or polyarteritis nodosa.[391,395]

Conclusion

Although PACNS is rare in children and diagnosis is sometimes difficult, treatment is available which can reduce morbidity and mortality. As diagnostic investigations are invasive, they should be reserved for those patients with a high index of suspicion. A diagnostic protocol is suggested in Fig. 6.13, although caution should be applied as no diagnostic protocols have been clinically tested.

6.5 Vasospasm

Fenella J. Kirkham

In adults, vasospasm is most commonly detected after subarachnoid haemorrhage (SAH) as patients are screened with transcranial Doppler (TCD) as well as MRA and conventional angiography. There are few systematic studies in children but vasospasm was detected in eight out of 50 (16%) in one series of aneurysmal SAH, only in children over 9 years of age,[417] although it has been described in toddlers.[418,419] Ischaemic stroke has occasionally been described[420] but vasospasm does not necessarily predict poor outcome.[417] Non-aneurysmal intracerebral haemorrhage may also be associated with vasospasm, with case reports in children with congenital heart disease[420] and post-varicella angiopathy.[421] Children with infection or head injury may also have evidence of vasospasm on vascular imaging or TCD, not necessarily associated with haemorrhage on CT;[422-425] again there are few data but no evidence for an association with poor outcome.[425] Vasospasm has occasionally been described after surgery or chemotherapy in children with cancer[426,427] but the prevalence, and any association with neurological sequelae, is currently unknown. Children with migraine may have high velocities on TCD interictally[428,429] and reversible vasospasm has been reported in association with thunderclap headache in this age group, as well as in adults.[430,431] It is possible that some other vasculopathies common in children, for example in those with sickle cell disease, begin as potentially reversible vasospasm, but longitudinal studies are needed.

6.6 Tortuosity and Dolichoectasia

Katharine M.L. Forrest

Arterial tortuosity of the large vessels is not an uncommon finding on digital subtraction arteriography[432] and is rarely associated with symptoms of cerebrovascular insufficiency in adults.[433] It has been described in Menkes disease[434] and velocardiofacial syndrome[435] and at least two genetic syndromes have recently been described: Loeys–Dietz syndrome types 1 and 2 which may be associated with hypertelorism, dissection and aneurysms and are secondary to mutations in transforming growth factor[436,437] and the arterial tortuoisity syndrome which is secondary to mutations in the *SLC2A10* gene encoding a facilitating glucose transporter, GLUT10.[438] One case series found tortuosity on digital subtraction arteriography in nine children with epilepsy and TIAs,[439] Although criteria for diagnosis are not robust and there are no population-based or case-control data, children have been described with stroke in the context of extracranial cerebral vessel tortuosity.[69,440–442] One case with an anomalous vertebrobasilar circulation in addition had iron deficiency anaemia, and tortuosity has also been reported in sickle cell anaemia and trait,[443,444] although there is currently no evidence of a link to stroke.[445] It is important to distinguish between tortuosity of the large and small vessels and ectasia as there is evidence that the former is congenital[446] while the latter may be acquired, perhaps alongside widening of the arterial lumen in patients with chronic anaemia or hypoxia.[443,444,447]

The ectasia, elongation and tortuosity defining dolichoectasia (Fig. 6.14) affects intracranial and basilar arteries more commonly than the carotid system[448] and rarely both.[449–451] Wolfe et al. have found that while African-American ethnicity, diabetes mellitus, peripheral vascular disease and smoking were risk factors predictive of morbidity in adults with vertebrobasilar dolichoectasia (VBD), hypertension was predictive of mortality.[452] However, Passero's multivariate analysis revealed that the presence of superimposed atherosclerotic changes of the posterior circulation was not significantly associated with the occurrence of ischaemic stroke, suggesting that mechanisms

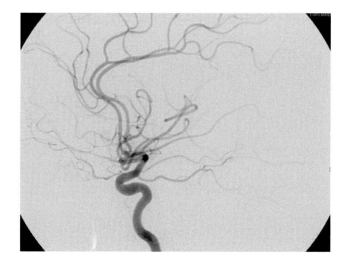

Fig. 6.14. Arterial tortuosity in an 8-year-old girl with recurrent strokes.

other than atherosclerosis are involved.[453] Pathological studies have demonstrated defects in the elastic lamina and deficiency of the reticular fibre in the muscular layer, features that are also common to berry aneurysms, and independendent of atherosclerosis.[454] A peri-embryogenesis event involving several cephalic neural crest segments of the dorsal aorta has been proposed to underly the spectrum of angiogenic dysfunction seen in two paediatric cases of PHACES syndrome.[455] Dolichoectasia has also been found in lysosomal disease, specifically Pompe disease,[450,451] and in around a quarter of people with Fabry disease,[456,457] as well as in a child with dysmorphism and developmental delay due to chromosomal aberrations.[458] Infection may also play a role. Association of dolichoectasia with acquired immune deficiency syndrome (AIDS) carries a grave prognosis[459] (see Chapter 5.1).

Presenting features relate to the complications of dolichoectasia. Brain ischaemia and infarction have recently been reported in children.[460] Potential mechanisms for ischaemia include thrombus formation and micro-embolization secondary to haemodynamic changes in the dilated vessel or stretching and distortion of the orifices of the paramedian perforators.[461] Compression of nerves causing diploplia due to trochlear nerve palsy, orbital pain due to trigeminal neuralgia, abducens nerve palsy, hemifacial spasm and hypoglossal nerve palsy have occurred.[462] Medullary compression leading to tinnitus, headache, vertigo and limb weakness,[463] and ventricular compression resulting in hydrocephalus is recognized. Haemorrhage is associated with the degree of ectasia and elongation of the basilar artery and may be favoured by hypertension and use of antiplatelet or anticoagulant agents.[464]

The place for antiplatelet agents or anticoagulants in prevention of ischaemic stroke in association with dolichoectasia is unclear and there is currently a lack of evidence to guide such intervention. Follow-up of 93 patients with VBD over an average of 11.7 years suggested that such therapy had little if any impact on the likelihood of recurrent stroke,[453] but a beneficial role for antiplatelet or anticoagulant treatment should not be completely discounted.[465]

6.7 Developmental venous anomalies

Mara Prengler and Fenella J. Kirkham

Developmental venous anomalies (DVAs),[466] previously known as cerebral venous angiomas, are the most common cerebral vascular malformations, as they are found in 2.6% of autopsies, but are considered extreme anatomical variants draining normal territories. This entity consists of a collection of fine medullary veins which lack smooth muscle or elastic fibres, and are interspersed in normal neuronal tissue.[467] The medullary veins converge on a large and dilated central vein which drains to the cortical veins and less frequently to the deep venous system (20%) or dural sinuses. On angiography, DVAs appear in the early venous phase, with typically a characteristic 'caput medusae-like' appearance, and persist into the late venous phase. Arterial and capillary times are normal. DVAs may be the result of cerebrovascular accidents, such as occlusion, or maldevelopment of medullary veins or tributaries during embryogenesis when cerebral veins are formed (Padget's fourth to seventh stage), in order to compensate the cerebral venous drainage. These lesions have been associated with cavernous haemangiomas, arteriovenous malforma-

tions, developmental defects of the cranial base, and head and neck venous malformations. DVAs have been reported predominantly in the frontal (36–56%) and parietal (12–24%) lobes and the cerebellum (14–29%), less frequently in occipital and temporal lobes, deep cerebrum and brainstem. Complex DVAs, which combine superficial and deep venous angiomas, occur in 10%, of cases and are found in supra- and infratentorial regions, uni- or bilaterally. They have been encountered with facial lymphatic malformations and anomalies of sinus pericranii.

DVAs are usually asymptomatic incidental findings on neuroimaging but can be associated with haemorrhagic stroke, usually if there is also a cavernous malformation, and occasionally with infarction, probably secondary to venous thrombosis.[467] They are typically found in middle aged patients with neurological symptoms such as headaches, dizziness, seizures or focal deficits and in those cases are usually considered incidental unless corresponding to an anatomical site which explains the symptoms. Cortical dysplasia has been described but is probably not secondary to the DVA.[467] These venous anomalies were considered an uncommon diagnosis in childhood, suggesting that either DVAs or complex DVAs are well tolerated without CSF circulatory disorders and cerebral dysfunction, but children have been reported[468–470] (Figs 6.15 and 6.16) and formed a substantial proportion of

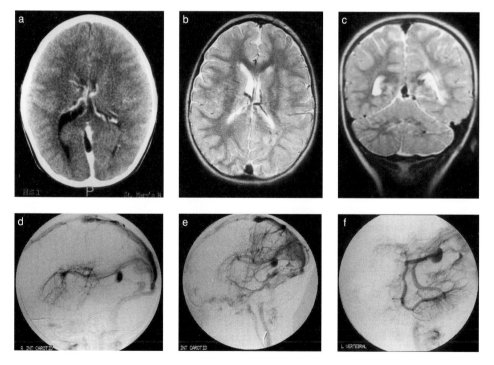

Fig. 6.15. Images from a 3-year-old girl with a pre-existing left orbital varix, ipsilateral enlarged pupil, abnormal vessels, failure of the iris to develop and decreased vision. Motor and speech development were mildly delayed. At 2 years and 7 months she had a short episode of looking pale without focusing, which lasted for a few minutes. Two months later, she developed diarrhoea and vomiting and collapsed with left-sided weakness, preceded by pain in the left eye which showed remarkable prominence of the orbital varices. (a) Axial CT scan shows multiple developmental venous anomalies in deep cerebrum. Axial (b) and coronal (c) T2-weighted MRI show high signal changes in periventricular areas of the brain related to the location of the developmental venous anomalies. (d–f) A four-vessel cerebral angiogram shows an anomalous deep venous drainage with the internal cerebral vein draining into a persistent falcine sinus on the right (d). On the left, there is a relative paucity of cortical veins in this region and the internal cerebral vein is draining to a persistent falcine sinus which appears dysplastic. Prominent medullary veins are present in the medullary white matter (e). Vertebral veins show a similar pattern with striking delay in the passage of the contrast in the left cerebellar hemisphere (f).

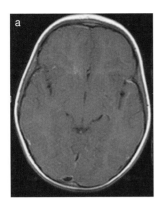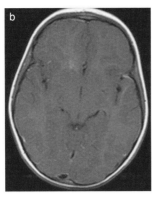

Fig. 6.16. (a,b) Right frontal and left temporal developmental venous anomalies in a 4-year-old girl who presented unconscious with seizures in the context of dehydration secondary to severe acute diarrhoea and vomiting. Although they may be incidental and an MR venogram was normal, transient venous sinus thrombosis may account for the clinical presentation.

cases in a large series with review of the literature,[470] supporting that these lesions are congenital.

Clinically symptomatic events in DVAs may be related to venous hypertension in weak and less flexible veins draining the brain parenchyma. In addition, there may be focal stenosis in the DVA at the point that the vein penetrates the dural sinus or venous thrombosis, while anomalous blood flow through abnormal venous vessels may play a role. Furthermore, there may be additional factors, such as hypercoagulabilty, dehydration in association with diarrhoea and vomiting (Figs 6.15 and 6.16), or cyanotic heart disease, which increase the risk of thrombosis and/or haemorrhage.

The management of DVAs is controversial. Surgical resection, neuroradiological embolization and gamma knife surgery may be appropriate in individual cases.[467] As these venous anomalies are related to the drainage for a portion of the brain parenchyma, potentially fatal venous infarctions may occur in adjacent brain after resection; this can be avoided if the collecting vein is preserved. The management of thrombosis within a DVA is that of cerebral venous sinus thrombosis (see Chapter 7); if symptoms do not improve with supportive measures such as rehydration, anticoagulation may be required.

REFERENCES

1. Hutchinson C, Elbers J, Halliday W, Branson H, Laughlins S, Armstrong D, et al. Treatment of small vessel primary CNS vasculitis in children: an open-label cohort study. Lancet Neurol 2010; 9(11):1078–1084.
2. de Bray JM, Baumgartner RW. History of spontaneous dissection of the cervical carotid artery. Arch Neurol 2005; 62(7):1168–1170.
3. Giroud M, Lemesle M, Madinier G, Manceau E, Osseby GV, Dumas R. Stroke in children under 16 years of age. Clinical and etiological difference with adults. Acta Neurol Scand 1997; 96(6):401–406.
4. Chabrier S, Lasjaunias P, Husson B, Landrieu P, Tardieu M. Ischaemic stroke from dissection of the craniocervical arteries in childhood: report of 12 patients. Eur J Paediatr Neurol 2003; 7(1):39–42.
5. Ganesan V, Prengler M, McShane MA, Wade AM, Kirkham FJ. Investigation of risk factors in children with arterial ischemic stroke. Ann Neurol 2003; 53(2):167–173.
6. Hildebrand D, Prengler M, Chawda SJ, Chong WK, Cox TC, Wade A et al. Clinical predictors of dissection in a stroke cohort. Ann Neurol 2003; 54(S7):137.
7. Bowen MD, Burak CR, Barron TF. Childhood ischemic stroke in a nonurban population. J Child Neurol 2005; 20(3):194–197.
8. Stapf C, Elkind MS, Mohr JP. Carotid artery dissection. Annu Rev Med 2000; 51:329–347.
9. Mokri B. Cervicocephalic arterial dissections. In: Uncommon Cause of Stroke (eds J Bogousslavsky, L Caplan L). Cambridge: Cambridge University Press, 2001; 211–229.
10. Schievink WI. Spontaneous dissection of the carotid and vertebral arteries. N Engl J Med 2001; 344:898–906.
11. Schievink WI, Mokri B, Michels VV, Piepgras DG. Familial association of intracranial aneurysms and cervical artery dissections. Stroke 1991; 22(11):1426–1430.
12. Silverboard G, Tart R. Cerebrovascular arterial dissection in children and young adults. Semin Pediatr Neurol 2000; 7(4):289–300.
13. Fullerton HJ, Johnston SC, Smith WS. Arterial dissection and stroke in children. Neurology 2001; 57(7):1155–1160.
14. Ducrocq X, Lacour JC, Debouverie M, Bracard S, Girard F, Weber M. Cerebral ischemic accidents in young subjects. A prospective study of 296 patients aged 16 to 45 years. Rev Neurol (Paris) 1999; 155(8):575–582.
15. Gautier JC, Pradat-Diehl P, Loron P, Lechat P, Lascault G, Juillard JB et al. Cerebral vascular accidents in young subjects. A study of 133 patients 9 to 45 years of age. Rev Neurol (Paris) 1989; 145(6–7):437–442.
16. Bogousslavsky J, Despland PA, Regli F. Spontaneous carotid dissection with acute stroke. Arch Neurol 1987; 44(2):137–140.
17. Kristensen B, Malm J, Carlberg B, Stegmayr B, Backman C, Fagerlund M et al. Epidemiology and etiology of ischemic stroke in young adults aged 18 to 44 years in northern Sweden. Stroke 1997; 28(9):1702–1709.
18. Malm J, Kristensen B, Carlberg B, Fagerlund M, Olsson T. Clinical features and prognosis in young adults with infratentorial infarcts. Cerebrovasc Dis 1999; 9(5):282–289.
19. Barinagarrementeria F, Amaya LE, Cantu C. Causes and mechanisms of cerebellar infarction in young patients. Stroke 1997; 28(12):2400–2404.
20. Williams LS, Garg BP, Cohen ME, Fleck JD, Biller J. Subtypes of ischemic stroke in children and young adults. Neurology 1997; 49:1541–1545.
21. Kirkham FJ, Prengler M, Hewes DK, Ganesan V. Risk factors for arterial ischemic stroke in children. J Child Neurol 2000; 15(5):299–307.
22. Chabrier S, Husson B, Lasjaunias P, Landrieu P, Tardieu M. Stroke in childhood: outcome and recurrence risk by mechanism in 59 patients. J Child Neurol 2000; 15(5):290–294.
23. Salih MA, Al-Jarallah AA, Al-Salman MM, Alorainy IA, Hassan HH. Stroke from cervicocephalic arterial dissection in Saudi children. Saudi Med J 2006; 27(Suppl 1):S103–S107.
24. Rafay MF, Armstrong D, deVeber G, Domi T, Chan A, MacGregor DL. Craniocervical arterial dissection in children: clinical and radiographic presentation and outcome. J Child Neurol 2006; 21(1):8–16.
25. Ganesan V, Chong WK, Cox TC, Chawda SJ, Prengler M, Kirkham FJ. Posterior circulation stroke in childhood: risk factors and recurrence. Neurology 2002; 59(10):1552–1556.
26. Schievink WI, Mokri B, Whisnant JP. Internal carotid artery dissection in a community. Rochester, Minnesota, 1987–1992. Stroke 1993; 24(11):1678–1680.
27. Giroud M, Fayolle H, Andre N, Dumas R, Becker F, Martin D et al. Incidence of internal carotid artery dissection in the community of Dijon. J Neurol Neurosurg Psychiatry 1994; 57(11):1443.
28. Lee VH, Brown RD, Jr, Mandrekar JN, Mokri B. Incidence and outcome of cervical artery dissection: a population-based study. Neurology 2006; 67(10):1809–1812.
29. Schievink WI, Wijdicks EF, Michels VV, Vockley J, Godfrey M. Heritable connective tissue disorders in cervical artery dissections: a propective study. Neurology 1998; 50:1166–1169.

30. Schievink WI. The treatment of spontaneous carotid and vertebral artery dissections. Curr Opin Cardiol 2000; 15:316–321.

31. Chan MT, Nadareishvili ZG, Norris JW. Diagnostic strategies in young patients with ischemic stroke in Canada. Can J Neurol Sci 2000; 27(2):120–124.

32. Neau JP, Petit E, Gil R. Dissection of cervical arteries. Presse Med 2001; 30(38):1882–1889.

33. Hart RG, Easton JD. Dissections of cervical and cerebral arteries. Neurol Clin 1983; 1(1):155–182.

34. Schievink WI, Michels VV, Piepgras DG. Neurovascular manifestations of heritable connective tissue disorders. A review. Stroke 1994; 25(4):889–903.

35. Silbert PL, Mokri B, Schievink WI. Headache and neck pain in spontaneous internal carotid and vertebral artery dissections. Neurology 1995; 45(8):1517–1522.

36. Schievink WI, Mokri B, Piepgras DG. Spontaneous dissections of cervicophalic arteries in childhood and adolescence. Neurology 1994; 44:1607–1612.

37. Broderick J, Talbot GT, Prenger E, Leach A, Brott T. Stroke in children within a major metropolitan area: the surprising importance of intracerebral hemorrhage. J Child Neurol 1993; 8(3):250–255.

38. deVeber G. Cerebrovascular disease in children. In: Pediatric Neurology – Principles and Practice (eds KF Swaiman, S Ashwal). St Louis: Mosby, 1999; 1099–1125.

39. Giroud M, Lemesle M, Gouyon JB, Nivelon JL, Milan C, Dumas R. Cerebrovascular disease in children under 16 years of age in the city of Dijon, France: a study of incidence and clinical features from 1985 to 1993. J Clin Epidemiol 1995; 48(11):1343–1348.

40. Robertson WC, Jr, Given CA. Spontaneous intracranial arterial dissection in the young: diagnosis by CT angiography. BMC Neurol 2006; 6:16.

41. Burklund CW. Spontaneous dissecting aneurysm of the cervical carotid artery: a report of surgical treatment in two patients. Johns Hopkins Med J 1970; 126(3):154–159.

42. O'Dwyer JA, Moscow N, Trevor R, Ehrenfeld WK, Newton TH. Spontaneous dissection of the carotid artery. Radiology 1980; 137(2):379–385.

43. Graham JM, Miller T, Stinnett DM. Spontaneous dissection of the common carotid artery. Case report and review of the literature. J Vasc Surg 1988; 7(6):811–813.

44. Koennecke H, Seyfert S. Mydriatic pupil as the presenting sign of common carotid artery dissection. Stroke 1998; 29(12):2653–2655.

45. Schievink WI, Bjornsson J, Piepgras DG. Coexistence of fibromuscular dysplasia and cystic medial necrosis in a patient with Marfan's syndrome and bilateral carotid artery dissection. Stroke 1994; 25:2492–2496.

46. Chabrier S, Lasjaunias P, Tardieu M. Specifics in pediatric arterial cerebral infarctions. Arch Pediatr 2001; 8(3):299–307.

47. Dlamini N, Mackay M, Fullerton H, Freeman J, deVeber G. Intracranial dissection mimicking transient cerebral arteriography in childhood arterial ischemic stroke. Stroke 2010; 41:e18.

48. Shin JH, Suh DC, Choi CG, Leei HK. Vertebral artery dissection: spectrum of imaging findings with emphasis on angiography and correlation with clinical presentation. Radiographics 2000; 20(6):1687–1696.

49. Leys D, Lucas C, Gobert M, Deklunder G, Pruvo JP. Cervical artery dissections. Eur Neurol 1997; 37(1):3–12.

50. Chuvhin MI, Naumenko LL. Posttraumatic ischemic stroke in childhood. Zh Nevrol Psikhiatr Im S S Korsakova 2004; (Suppl 12):3–13.

51. de Borst GJ, Slieker MG, Monteiro LM, Moll FL, Braun KP. Bilateral traumatic carotid artery dissection in a child. Pediatr Neurol 2006; 34(5):408–411.

52. Lin JJ, Lin KL, Chou ML, Wong AM, Wang HS. Cerebellar infarction in the territory of the superior cerebellar artery in children. Pediatr Neurol 2007; 37(6):435–437.

53. Dittrich R, Rohsbach D, Heidbreder A, Heuschmann P, Nassenstein I, Bachmann R et al. Mild mechanical traumas are possible risk factors for cervical artery dissection. Cerebrovasc Dis 2007; 23(4):275–281.

54. Agner C, Weig SG. Arterial dissection and stroke following child abuse: case report and review of the literature. Childs Nerv Syst 2005; 21(5):416–420.

55. Nguyen PH, Burrowes DM, Ali S, Bowman RM, Shaibani A. Intracranial vertebral artery dissection with subarachnoid hemorrhage following child abuse. Pediatr Radiol 2007; 37(6):600–602.

56. Wechsler B, Kim H, Hunter J. Trampolines, children, and strokes. Am J Phys Med Rehabil 2001; 80(8):608–613.

57. Lascelles K, Hewes D, Ganesan V. An unexpected consequence of a roller coaster ride. J Neurol Neurosurg Psychiatry 2001; 71(5):704–705.

58. Woodhurst WB, Robertson WD, Thompson GB. Carotid injury due to intraoral trauma: case report and review of the literature. Neurosurgery 1980; 6(5):559–563.

59. Pierrot S, Bernardeschi D, Morrisseau-Durand MP, Manach Y, Couloigner V. Dissection of the internal carotid artery following trauma of the soft palate in children. Ann Otol Rhinol Laryngol 2006; 115(5):323–329.

60. Lubarsky M, Helmer R, Knight C, Mullins ME. Internal carotid artery dissection following wooden arrow injury to the posterior pharynx. Case report. J Neurosurg Pediatr 2008; 1(4):334–336.

61. Cushing KE, Ramesh V, Gardner-Medwin D, Todd NV, Gholkar A, Baxter P et al. Tethering of the vertebral artery in the congenital arcuate foramen of the atlas vertebra: a possible cause of vertebral artery dissection in children. Dev Med Child Neurol 2001; 43(7):491–496.

62. Hasan I, Wapnick S, Kutscher ML, Couldwell WT. Vertebral arterial dissection associated with Klippel–Feil syndrome in a child. Childs Nerv Syst 2002; 18(1–2):67–70.

63. Dirik E, Yis U, Dirik MA, Cakmakci H, Men S. Vertebral artery dissection in a patient with Wildervanck syndrome. Pediatr Neurol 2008; 39(3):218–220.

64. Smith WS, Johnston SC, Skalabrin EJ, Weaver M, Azari P, Albers GW et al. Spinal manipulative therapy is an independent risk factor for vertebral artery dissection. Neurology 2003; 60(9):1424–1428.

65. Grau AJ, Buggle F, Ziegler C, Schwarz W, Meuser J, Tasman AJ et al. Association between acute cerebrovascular ischemia and chronic and recurrent infection. Stroke 1997; 28(9):1724–1729.

66. Grau AJ, Brandt T, Buggle F, Orberk E, Mytilineos J, Werle E et al. Association of cervical artery dissection with recent infection. Arch Neurol 1999; 56(7):851–856.

67. Rubinstein SM, Peerdeman SM, van Tulder MW, Riphagen I, Haldeman S. A systematic review of the risk factors for cervical artery dissection. Stroke 2005; 36(7):1575–1580.

68. Skowronski DM, Buxton JA, Hestrin M, Keyes RD, Lynch K, Halperin SA. Carotid artery dissection as a possible severe complication of pertussis in an adult: clinical case report and review. Clin Infect Dis 2003; 36(1):e1–e4.

69. Wraige E, Ganesan V, Pohl KR. Arterial dissection complicating tonsillectomy. Dev Med Child Neurol 2003; 45(9):638–639.

70. Carvalho KS, Edwards-Brown M, Golomb MR. Carotid dissection and stroke after tonsillectomy and adenoidectomy. Pediatr Neurol 2007; 37(2):127–129.

71. Paciaroni M, Georgiadis D, Arnold M, Gandjour J, Keseru B, Fahrni G et al. Seasonal variability in spontaneous cervical artery dissection. J Neurol Neurosurg Psychiatry 2006; 77(5):677–679.

72. Dziewas R, Konrad C, Drager B, Evers S, Besselmann M, Ludemann P et al. Cervical artery dissection – clinical features, risk factors, therapy and outcome in 126 patients. J Neurol 2003; 250(10):1179–1184.

73. Genius J, Dong-Si T, Grau AP, Lichy C. Postacute C-reactive protein levels are elevated in cervical artery dissection. Stroke 2005; 36(4):e42–e44.

74. Forster K, Poppert H, Conrad B, Sander D. Elevated inflammatory laboratory parameters in spontaneous cervical artery dissection as compared to traumatic dissection: a retrospective case-control study. J Neurol 2006; 253(6):741–745.

75. Longoni M, Grond-Ginsbach C, Grau AJ, Genius J, Debette S, Schwaninger M et al. The ICAM-1 E469K gene polymorphism is a risk factor for spontaneous cervical artery dissection. Neurology 2006; 66(8):1273–1275.

76. Pezzini A, Del ZE, Mazziotti G, Ruggeri G, Franco F, Giossi A et al. Thyroid autoimmunity and spontaneous cervical artery dissection. Stroke 2006; 37(9):2375–2377.

77. Ganesan V, Kirkham FJ. Stroke due to arterial disease in congenital heart disease. Arch Dis Child 1997; 76(2):175.

78. Schievink WI, Mokri B, Piepgras DG, Gittenberger-de Groot AC. Intracranial aneurisms and cervicophalic arterial dissections associated with congenital heart disease. Neurosurgery 1996; 39:685–690.

79. Schievink WI, Mokri B. Familial aorto-cervicocephalic arterial dissections and congenitally bicuspid aortic valve. Stroke 1995; 26:1935–1940.

80. Tzourio C, Cohen A, Lamisse N, Biousse V, Bousser MG. Aortic root dilatation in patients with spontaneous cervical artery dissection. Circulation 1997; 95(10):2351–2353.

81. Pezzini A, Caso V, Zanferrari C, Del ZE, Paciaroni M, Bertolino C et al. Arterial hypertension as risk factor for spontaneous cervical artery dissection. A case-control study. J Neurol Neurosurg Psychiatry 2006; 77(1):95–97.

82. Lucas C, Lecroart JL, Gautier C, Leclerc X, Dauzat M, Leys D et al. Impairment of endothelial function in patients with spontaneous cervical artery dissection: evidence for a general arterial wall disease. Cerebrovasc Dis 2004; 17(2–3):170–174.

83. Guillon B, Tzourio C, Biousse V, Adrai V, Bousser MG, Touboul PJ. Arterial wall properties in carotid artery dissection: an ultrasound study. Neurology 2000; 55(5):663–666.

84. Brandt T, Hausser I, Orberk E, Grau A, Hartschuh W, Anton-Lamprecht I et al. Ultrastructural connective tissue abnormalities in patients with spontaneous cervicocerebral artery dissections. Ann Neurol 1998; 44(2):281–285.

85. Brandt T, Orberk E, Weber R, Werner I, Busse O, Muller BT et al. Pathogenesis of cervical artery dissections: association with connective tissue abnormalities. Neurology 2001; 57(1):24–30.

86. van den Berg JS, Limburg M, Kappelle LJ, Pals G, Arwert F, Westerveld A. The role of type III collagen in spontaneous cervical arterial dissections. Ann Neurol 1998; 43(4):494–498.

87. Wiest T, Hyrenbach S, Bambul P, Erker B, Pezzini A, Hausser I et al. Genetic analysis of familial connective tissue alterations associated with cervical artery dissections suggests locus heterogeneity. Stroke 2006; 37(7):1697–1702.

88. Morcher M, Hausser I, Brandt T, Grond-Ginsbach C. Heterozygous carriers of pseudoxanthoma elasticum were not found among patients with cervical artery dissections. J Neurol 2003; 250(8):983–986.

89. Pezzini A, Del ZE, Archetti S, Negrini R, Bani P, Albertini A et al. Plasma homocysteine concentration, C677T MTHFR genotype, and 844ins68bp CBS genotype in young adults with spontaneous cervical artery dissection and atherothrombotic stroke. Stroke 2002; 33(3):664–669.

90. Kloss M, Wiest T, Hyrenbach S, Werner I, Arnold ML, Lichy C et al. MTHFR 677TT genotype increases the risk for cervical artery dissections. J Neurol Neurosurg Psychiatry 2006; 77(8):951–952.

91. Schievink WI. Cerebrovascular involvement in Ehlers–Danlos syndrome. Curr Treat Options Cardiovasc Med 2004; 6(3):231–236.

92. Ganesan V, Cox TC, Gunny R. Abnormalities of cervical arteries in children with arterial ischemic stroke. Neurology. 2011;76(2):166–71.

93. Guillon B, Brunereau L, Biousse V, Djouhri H, Levy C, Bousser MG. Long-term follow-up of aneurysms developed during extracranial internal carotid artery dissection. Neurology 1999; 53(1):117–122.

94. Schievink WI, Mokri B, Piepgras DG. Spontaneous dissections of cervicophalic arteries in childhood and adolescence. Neurology 1994; 44:1607–1612.

95. Cronqvist SE, Norrving B, Nilsson B. Young stroke patients. An angiographic study. Acta Radiol Suppl 1986; 369:34–37.

96. Bogousslavsky J, Regli F. Ischemic stroke in adults younger than 30 years of age. Cause and prognosis. Arch Neurol 1987; 44(5):479–482.

97. Desfontaines P, Despland PA. Dissection of the internal carotid artery: aetiology, symptomatology, clinical and neurosonological follow-up, and treatment in 60 consecutive cases. Acta Neurol Belg 1995; 95(4):226–234.

98. Lucas C, Moulin T, Deplanque D, Tatu L, Chavot D. Stroke patterns of internal carotid artery dissection in 40 patients. Stroke 1998; 29(12):2646–2648.

99. Steinke W, Schwartz A, Hennerici M. Topography of cerebral infarction associated with carotid artery dissection. J Neurol 1996; 243(4):323–328.

100. Srinivasan J, Newell DW, Sturzenegger M, Mayberg MR, Winn HR. Transcranial Doppler in the evaluation of internal carotid artery dissection. Stroke 1996; 27(7):1226–1230.

101. Babikian VL, Forteza AM, Gavrilescu T, Samaraweera R. Cerebral microembolism and extracranial internal carotid artery dissection. J Ultrasound Med 1996; 15(12):863–866.

102. Koennecke HC, Trocio SH, Jr, Mast H, Mohr JP. Microemboli on transcranial Doppler in patients with spontaneous carotid artery dissection. J Neuroimaging 1997; 7(4):217–220.

103. Droste DW, Ritter M, Kemeny V, Schulte-Altedorneburg G, Ringelstein EB. Microembolus detections at follow-up in 19 patients with acute stroke: correlation with stroke etiology and antithrombotic treatment. Cerebrovasc Dis 2000; 10(4):272–277.

104. Koch S, Romano JG, Bustillo IC, Concha M, Forteza AM. Anticoagulation and microembolus detection in a case of internal carotid artery dissection. J Neuroimaging 2001; 11(1):63–66.

105. Galetta SL, Leahey A, Nichols CW, Raps EC. Orbital ischemia, ophthalmoparesis, and carotid dissection. J Clin Neuroophthalmol 1991; 11(4):284–287.

106. Biousse V, Anglejan-Chatillon J, Touboul PJ, Amarenco P, Bousser MG. Time course of symptoms in extracranial carotid artery dissections. A series of 80 patients. Stroke 1995; 26(2):235–239.

107. Camacho A, Villarejo A, de Aragon AM, Simon R, Mateos F. Spontaneous carotid and vertebral artery dissection in children. Pediatr Neurol 2001; 25(3):250–253.

108. Robertson WC, Pettigrew LC. 'Congenital' Horner's syndrome and carotid dissection. J Neuroimaging 2003; 13(4):367–370.

109. Pezzini A, Granella F, Grassi M, Bertolino C, Del ZE, Immovilli P et al. History of migraine and the risk of spontaneous cervical artery dissection. Cephalalgia 2005; 25(8):575–580.

110. Mokri B, Stanson AW, Houser OW. Spontaneous dissections of the renal arteries in a patient with previous spontaneous dissections of the internal carotid arteries. Stroke 1985; 16(6):959–963.

111. Mokri B, Piepgras DG, Wiebers DO, Houser OW. Familial occurrence of spontaneous dissection of the internal carotid artery. Stroke 1987; 18(1):246–251.

112. Schievink WI, Mokri B, Piepgras DG, Kuiper JD. Recurrent spontaneous arterial dissections: risk in familial versus non-familial disease. Stroke 1996; 27:622–624.

113. Perez EF, Gil PA, Garzon FJ, Salinas E, Franco E. Familial internal carotid dissection. Neurologia 1998; 13(5):247–249.

114. Biousse V, Woimant F, Amarenco P, Touboul PJ, Bousser MG. Pain as the only manifestation of internal carotid artery dissection. Cephalalgia 1992; 12(5):314–317.

115. Biousse V, D'Anglejan-Chatillon J, Massiou H, Bousser MG. Head pain in non-traumatic carotid artery dissection: a series of 65 patients. Cephalalgia 1994; 14(1):33–36.

116. de Bray JM, Penisson-Besnier I, Giroud M, Klein J, Tanguy JY, Pasco A et al. Cervical deficit radiculopathy in 3 cases of vertebral artery dissection. Rev Neurol (Paris) 1998; 154(11):762–766.

117. Crum B, Mokri B, Fulgham J. Spinal manifestations of vertebral artery dissection. Neurology 2000; 55(2):304–306.

118. Davies L. A case of vagal palsy due to dissecting aneurysm of the carotid artery. Med J Aust 1987; 147(7):352–353.

119. Andre-Sereys P, Petit E, Benrabah R, Abanouh A, Rancurel G, Haut J. Spontaneous dissection of the internal carotid artery in ophthalmological milieu. Apropos of 10 cases. J Fr Ophtalmol 1996; 19(4):259–264.

120. Biousse V, Touboul PJ, D'Anglejan-Chatillon J, Levy C, Schaison M, Bousser MG. Ophthalmologic manifestations of internal carotid artery dissection. Am J Ophthalmol 1998; 126(4):565–577.

121. Kerty E. The ophthalmology of internal carotid artery dissection. Acta Ophthalmol Scand 1999; 77(4):418–421.

122. Hicks PA, Leavitt JA, Mokri B. Ophthalmic manifestations of vertebral artery dissection. Patients seen at the Mayo Clinic from 1976 to 1992. Ophthalmology 1994; 101(11):1786–1792.

123. Ganesan V, Kirkham FJ. Stroke due to arterial disease in congenital heart disease. Arch Dis Child 1997; 76(2):175.

124. Leira EC, Bendixen BH, Kardon RH, Adams HP, Jr. Brief, transient Horner's syndrome can be the hallmark of a carotid artery dissection. Neurology 1998; 50(1):289–290.

125. Bilbao R, Amoros S, Murube J. Horner syndrome as an isolated manifestation of an intrapetrous internal carotid artery dissection. Am J Ophthalmol 1997; 123(4):562–564.

126. Inzelberg R, Nisipeanu P, Blumen SC, Kovach I, Groisman GM, Carasso RL. Transient unilateral mydriasis as the presenting sign of aortic and carotid dissection. Neurology 2000; 55(12):1934–1935.

127. Newman NJ, Kline LB, Leifer D, Lessell S. Ocular stroke and carotid artery dissection. Neurology 1989; 39(11):1462–1464.

128. Sturzenegger M. Spontaneous internal carotid artery dissection: early diagnosis and management in 44 patients. J Neurol 1995; 242(4):231–238.

129. Mokri B, Silbert PL, Schievink WI, Piepgras DG. Cranial nerve palsy in spontaneous dissection of the extracranial internal carotid artery. Neurology 1996; 46(2):356–359.

130. Maitland CG, Black JL, Smith WA. Abducens nerve palsy due to spontaneous dissection of the internal carotid artery. Arch Neurol 1983; 40(7):448–449.

131. Lieschke GJ, Davis S, Tress BM, Ebeling P. Spontaneous internal carotid artery dissection presenting as hypoglossal nerve palsy. Stroke 1988; 19(9):1151–1155.

132. Moussouttas M, Tuhrim S. Spontaneous internal carotid artery dissection with isolated vagus nerve deficit. Neurology 1998; 51(1):317–318.

133. Mizumaki Y, Endo S, Yamatani K, Takaku A, Tsukamoto E. Hypoglossal nerve paresis caused by spontaneous dissection of kinked internal carotid artery – case report. Neurol Med Chir (Tokyo) 1998; 38(3):165–167.

134. Panisset M, Eidelman BH. Multiple cranial neuropathy as a feature of internal carotid artery dissection. Stroke 1990; 21(1):141–147.

135. Fink JN, Anderson TJ. Lower cranial nerve palsies due to carotid artery dissection. N Z Med J 1998; 111(1065):166–168.

136. Rees JH, Valentine AR, Llewelyn JG. Spontaneous bilateral carotid and vertebral artery dissection presenting as a Collet–Sicard syndrome. Br J Radiol 1997; 70(836):856–858.

137. Schmidt F, Dihne M, Steinbach J, Buhring U, Kuker W. Raeder- and Collet–Siccard–Syndrome. Acute pareses of cranial nerves symptomatic of a dissection of internal carotid artery. Nervenarzt 2000; 71(6):502–505.

138. Heckmann JG, Tomandl B, Duhm C, Stefan H, Neundorfer B. Collet–Sicard syndrome due to coiling and dissection of the internal carotid artery. Cerebrovasc Dis 2000; 10(6):487–488.

139. Labouret P, Tranchant C, Jesel M, Dietemann JL, Warter JM. Cervical myelopathy disclosing dissection of the extracranial vertebral artery. Rev Neurol (Paris) 1993; 149(10):559–561.

140. Mokri B. Dissections of cervical and cephalic arteries. In: Sundt's Occlusive Cerebrovascular Disease, 2nd edn (ed FB Meyer). Philadelphia: WB Saunders, 1994; 45–70.

141. Kline LB. The neuro-opthalmologic manifestations of spontaneous dissection of the internal carotid artery. Semin Opthalmol 1992; 7:30–37.

142. Biousse V. Carotid disease and the eye. Curr Opin Ophthalmol 1997; 8(6):16–26.

143. Biousse V, Schaison M, Touboul PJ, D'Anglejan-Chatillon J, Bousser MG. Ischemic optic neuropathy associated with internal carotid artery dissection. Arch Neurol 1998; 55(5):715–719.

144. Vargas ME, Desrouleaux JR, Kupersmith MJ. Ophthalmoplegia as a presenting manifestation of internal carotid artery dissection. J Clin Neuroophthalmol 1992; 12(4):268–271.

145. Schievink WI, Mokri B, Garrity JA, Nichols DA, Piepgras DG. Ocular motor nerve palsies in spontaneous dissections of the cervical internal carotid artery. Neurology 1993; 43(10):1938–1941.

146. McDonough RL, Forteza AM, Flynn HW, Jr. Internal carotid artery dissection causing a branch retinal artery occlusion in a young adult. Am J Ophthalmol 1998; 125(5):706–708.

147. Godfrey DG, Biousse V, Newman NJ. Delayed branch retinal artery occlusion following presumed blunt common carotid dissection. Arch Ophthalmol 1998; 116(8):1120–1121.

148. Rao TH, Schneider LB, Patel M, Libman RB. Central retinal artery occlusion from carotid dissection diagnosed by cervical computed tomography. Stroke 1994; 25(6):1271–1272.

149. Wurm G, Loffler W, Wegenschimmel W, Fischer J. Traumatic injury of the internal carotid artery in the extracranial segment.

Description of a severe late complication. Chirurg 1995; 66(9):916–919.

150. Mokhtari F, Massin P, Paques M, Biousse V, Houdart E, Blain P et al. Central retinal artery occlusion associated with head or neck pain revealing spontaneous internal carotid artery dissection. Am J Ophthalmol 2000; 129(1):108–109.

151. Rivkin MJ, Hedges TR, III, Logigian EL. Carotid dissection presenting as posterior ischemic optic neuropathy. Neurology 1990; 40(9):1469.

152. Tsai RK, Sun CY. Spontaneous dissection of internal carotid artery presenting as isolated posterior ischaemic optic neuropathy. Br J Ophthalmol 1997; 81(6):513.

153. Yamaura A, Watanabe Y, Saeki N. Dissecting aneurysms of the intracranial vertebral artery. J Neurosurg 1990; 72(2):183–188.

154. Duker JS, Belmont JB. Ocular ischemic syndrome secondary to carotid artery dissection. Am J Ophthalmol 1988; 106(6):750–752.

155. Archer JS, Gracies JM, Tohver E, Crimmins DS, O'Leary BJ, Milder DG. Bilateral optic disk pallor after unilateral internal carotid artery occlusion. Neurology 1998; 50(3):809–811.

156. Bourcier-Bareil F, Hommet C, Cottier JP, Arsene S, Rossazza C. Hemianopsia related to dissection of the internal carotid artery. J Neuroophthalmol 1999; 19(2):136–139.

157. Greselle JF, Zenteno M, Kien P, Castel JP, Caille JM. Spontaneous dissection of the vertebro-basilar system. A study of 18 cases (15 patients). J Neuroradiol 1987; 14(2):115–123.

158. Miller Fisher C, Ojemann RG, Roberson GH. Spontaneous dissection of cervico-cerebral arteries. J Canad Sci Neurol 1978; 5:9–19.

159. Houser OW, Mokri B, Sundt TM, Jr, Baker HL, Jr, Reese DF. Spontaneous cervical cephalic arterial dissection and its residuum: angiographic spectrum. AJNR Am J Neuroradiol 1984; 5(1):27–34.

160. Gelbert F, Assouline E, Hodes JE, Reizine D, Woimant F, George B et al. MRI in spontaneous dissection of vertebral and carotid arteries. 15 cases studied at 0.5 tesla. Neuroradiology 1991; 33(2):111–113.

161. Stringaris K, Liberopoulos K, Giaka E, Kokkinis K, Bastounis E, Klonaris EC et al. Three-dimensional time-of-flight MR angiography and MR imaging versus conventional angiography in carotid artery dissections. Int Angiol 1996; 15(1):20–25.

162. Kirsch E, Kaim A, Engelter S, Lyrer P, Stock KW, Bongartz G et al. MR angiography in internal carotid artery dissection: improvement of diagnosis by selective demonstration of the intramural haematoma. Neuroradiology 1998; 40(11):704–709.

163. Bakke SJ, Smith HJ, Kerty E, Dahl A. Cervicocranial artery dissection. Detection by Doppler ultrasound and MR angiography. Acta Radiol 1996; 37(4):529–534.

164. Oelerich M, Stogbauer F, Kurlemann G, Schul C, Schuierer G. Craniocervical artery dissection: MR imaging and MR angiographic findings. Eur Radiol 1999; 9(7):1385–1391.

165. Ozdoba C, Sturzenegger M, Schroth G. Internal carotid artery dissection: MR imaging features and clinical-radiologic correlation. Radiology 1996; 199(1):191–198.

166. Keller E, Flacke S, Gieseke J, Sommer T, Brechtelsbauer D, Gass S et al. Craniocervical dissections: study strategies in MR imaging and MR angiography. Rofo 1997; 167(6):565–571.

167. Provenzale JM, Barboriak DP, Taveras JM. Exercise-related dissection of craniocervical arteries: CT, MR, and angiographic findings. J Comput Assist Tomogr 1995; 19(2):268–276.

168. Steinke W, Rautenberg W, Schwartz A, Hennerici M. Noninvasive monitoring of internal carotid artery dissection. Stroke 1994; 25(5):998–1005.

169. Kasner SE, Hankins LL, Bratina P, Morgenstern LB. Magnetic resonance angiography demonstrates vascular healing of carotid and vertebral artery dissections. Stroke 1997; 28(10):1993–1997.

170. James CA, Glasier CM, Angtuaco EE. Altered vertebrobasilar flow in children: angiographic, MR, and MR angiographic findings. AJNR Am J Neuroradiol 1995; 16(8):1689–1695.

171. Bachmann R, Nassenstein I, Kooijman H, Dittrich R, Kugel H, Niederstadt T et al. Spontaneous acute dissection of the internal carotid artery: high-resolution magnetic resonance imaging at 3.0 tesla with a dedicated surface coil. Invest Radiol 2006; 41(2):105–111.

172. Ganesan V, Savvy L, Chong WK, Kirkham FJ. Conventional cerebral angiography in children with ischemic stroke. Pediatr Neurol 1999; 20(1):38–42.

173. Lyrer P, Engelter S. Antithrombotic drugs for carotid artery dissection. Cochrane Database Syst Rev 2003; (3):CD000255.

174. Chaves C, Estol C, Esnaola MM, Gorson K, O'Donoghue M, De Witt LD et al. Spontaneous intracranial internal carotid artery dissection: report of 10 patients. Arch Neurol 2002; 59(6):977–981.

175. Engelter ST, Lyrer PA, Kirsch EC, Steck AJ. Long-term follow-up after extracranial internal carotid artery dissection. Eur Neurol 2000; 44(4):199–204.

176. Zetterling M, Carlstrom C, Konrad P. Review Article: Internal carotid artery dissection. Acta Neurol Scand 2000; 101:1–7.

177. Georgiadis D, Lanczik O, Schwab S, Engelter S, Sztajzel R, Arnold M et al. IV thrombolysis in patients with acute stroke due to spontaneous carotid dissection. Neurology 2005; 64(9):1612–1614.

178. Schievink WI, Piepgras DG, McCaffrey TV, Mokri B. Surgical treatment of extracranial internal carotid artery dissecting aneurisms. Neurosurgery 1994; 35:809–815.

179. Vishteh AG, Marciano FF, David CA, Schievink WI, Zabramski JM, Spetzler RF. Long-term graft patency rates and clinical outcomes after revascularization for symptomatic traumatic internal carotid artery dissection. Neurosurgery 1998; 43(4):761–767.

180. Muller BT, Luther B, Hort W, Neumann-Haefelin T, Aulich A, Sandmann W. Surgical treatment of 50 carotid dissections: indications and results. J Vasc Surg 2000; 31(5):980–988.

181. Touze E, Randoux B, Meary E, Arquizan C, Meder JF, Mas JL. Aneurysmal forms of cervical artery dissection: associated factors and outcome. Stroke 2001; 32(2):418–423.

182. Pozzati E, Galassi E, Godano U, Cordella L. Regressing intracranial carotid occlusions in childhood. Pediatr Neurosurg 1994; 21(4):243–247.

183. Danchaivijitr N, Cox TC, Saunders DE, Ganesan V. Evolution of cerebral arteriopathies in childhood arterial ischemic stroke. Ann Neurol 2006; 59(4):620–626.

184. Nussbaum ES, Erickson DL. Extracranial-intracranial bypass for ischemic cerebrovascular disease refractory to maximal medical therapy. Neurosurgery 2000; 46(1):37–42.

185. Leys D, Moulin T, Stojkovic T, Begey S, Chavot D, Donald Investigators. Follow-up of patients with history of cervical artery dissection. Cerebrovasc Dis 1995; 5:43–49.

186. Baumgartner RW, Arnold M, Baumgartner I, Mosso M, Gonner F, Studer A et al. Carotid dissection with and without ischemic events: local symptoms and cerebral artery findings. Neurology 2001; 57(5):827–832.

187. Arnold M, Bousser MG, Fahrni G, Fischer U, Georgiadis D, Gandjour J et al. Vertebral artery dissection: presenting findings and predictors of outcome. Stroke 2006; 37(10):2499–2503.

188. Tabarki B, el Madani A, Alvarez H, Husson B, Lasjaunias P, Landrieu P et al. Ischemic cerebral vascular accident caused by vertebral artery dissection. Arch Pediatr 1997; 4(8):763–766.

189. Patel H, Smith RR, Garg BP. Spontaneous extracranial carotid artery dissection in children. Pediatr Neurol 1995; 13(1):55–60.

190. Manz HJ, Vester J, Lavenstein B. Dissecting aneurysm of cerebral arteries in childhood and adolescence. Case report and literature review of 20 cases. Virchows Arch A Pathol Anat Histol 1979; 384(3):325–335.

191. Smith SE, Kirkham FJ, Deveber G, Millman G, Dirks PB, Wirrell E, Telfeian AE, Sykes K, Barlow K, Ichord R. Outcome following decompressive craniectomy for malignant middle cerebral artery infarction in children. Dev Med Child Neurol. 2011;53(1):29–33.

192. Schievink WI, Mokri B, O'Fallon WM. Recurrent spontaneous cervical-artery dissection. N Engl J Med 1994; 330(6):393–397.

193. Goldstein LB, Gray L, Hulette CM. Stroke due to recurrent ipsilateral carotid artery dissection in a young adult. Stroke 1995; 26(3):480–483.

194. Bassetti C, Carruzzo A, Sturzenegger M, Tuncdogan E. Recurrence of cervical artery dissection. A prospective study of 81 patients. Stroke 1996; 27(10):1804–1807.

195. Schievink WI, Mokri B. Aortic dissection decades following internal carotid artery dissection – report of two cases. Angiology 1997; 48:985–988.

196. Dusser A, Goutieres F, Aicardi J. Ischemic strokes in children. J Child Neurol 1986; 1(2):131–136.

197. Satoh S, Shirane R, Yoshimoto T. Clinical survey of ischemic cerebrovascular disease in children in a district of Japan. Stroke 1991; 22(5):586–589.

198. Sebire G, le Groupe d'Etude des AVC de l'Enfant de Bicetre. Accidents vasculaires cerebraux ischemiques d'origine arterielle. Paris: Flammarion, 1995.

199. Kirkham FJ. Stroke in childhood. Arch Dis Child 1999; 81(1):85–89.

200. Fullerton HJ, Wu YW, Sidney S, Johnston SC. Risk of recurrent childhood arterial ischemic stroke in a population-based cohort: the importance of cerebrovascular imaging. Pediatrics 2007; 119(3):495–501.

201. Braun KP, Bulder MM, Chabrier S, Kirkham FJ, Uiterwaal CS, Tardieu M et al. The course and outcome of unilateral intracranial arteriopathy in 79 children with ischaemic stroke. Brain 2009; 132(Pt 2):544–557.

202. Miravet E, Danchaivijitr N, Basu H, Saunders DE, Ganesan V. Clinical and radiological features of childhood cerebral infarction following varicella zoster virus infection. Dev Med Child Neurol 2007; 49(6):417–422.

203. Chabrier S, Rodesch G, Lasjaunias P, Tardieu M, Landrieu P, Sebire G. Transient cerebral arteriopathy: a disorder recognized by serial angiograms in children with stroke. J Child Neurol 1998; 13(1):27–32.

204. Sebire G, Meyer L, Chabrier S. Varicella as a risk factor for cerebral infarction in childhood: a case-control study. Ann Neurol 1999; 45(5):679–680.

205. Sebire G. Transient cerebral arteriopathy in childhood. Lancet 2006; 368(9529):8–10.

206. Sebire G, Fullerton H, Riou E, deVeber G. Toward the definition of cerebral arteriopathies of childhood. Curr Opin Pediatr 2004; 16(6):617–622.

207. Kirkham FJ, Hogan AM. Risk factors for arterial ischemic stroke in childhood. CNS Spectr 2004; 9(6):451–464.

208. Banker BQ. Cerebrovascular disease in infancy and childhood. 1. Occlusive vascular disease. J Neuropathol Exp Neurol 1961; 21:127–134.

209. Shillito J, Jr. Carotid arteritis: a cause of hemiplegia in childhood. J Neurosurg 1964; 21:540–551.

210. Hilal SK, Solomon GE, Gold AP, Carter S. Primary cerebral arterial occlusive disease in children. I. Acute acquired hemiplegia. Radiology 1971; 99(1):71–86.

211. Harwood-Nash DC, McDonald P, Argent W. Cerebral arterial disease in children. An angiographic study of 40 cases. Am J Roentgenol Radium Ther Nucl Med 1971; 111(4):672–686.

212. Demierre B, Rondot P. Dystonia caused by putamino-capsulo-caudate vascular lesions. J Neurol Neurosurg Psychiatry 1983; 46(5):404–409.

213. Zimmerman RA, Bilaniuk LT, Packer RJ, Goldberg HI, Grossman RI. Computed tomographic-arteriographic correlates in acute basal ganglionic infarction of childhood. Neuroradiology 1983; 24(5): 241–248.

214. Bladin PF, Berkovic SF. Striatocapsular infarction: large infarcts in the lenticulostriate arterial territory. Neurology 1984; 34(11):1423–1430.

215. Raybaud CA, Livet MO, Jiddane M, Pinsard N. Radiology of ischemic strokes in children. Neuroradiology 1985; 27(6):567–578.

216. Wanifuchi H, Kagawa M, Takeshita M, Izawa M, Kitamura K. Ischemic stroke in infancy, childhood, and adolescence. Childs Nerv Syst 1988; 4(6):361–364.

217. Bode H, Harders A. Transient stenoses and occlusions of main cerebral arteries in children – diagnosis and control of therapy by transcranial Doppler sonography. Eur J Pediatr 1989; 148(5):406–411.

218. Kappelle LJ, Willemse J, Ramos LM, van der Grond J. Ischaemic stroke in the basal ganglia and internal capsule in childhood. Brain Dev 1989; 11(5):283–292.

219. Shirane R, Sato S, Yoshimoto T. Angiographic findings of ischemic stroke in children. Childs Nerv Syst 1992; 8(8):432–436.

220. Trescher WH. Ischemic stroke syndromes in childhood. Pediatr Ann 1992; 21(6):374–383.

221. Zimmerman RA, Bogdan AR, Gusnard DA. Pediatric magnetic resonance angiography: assessment of stroke. Cardiovasc Intervent Radiol 1992; 15(1):60–64.

222. Godefroy O, Rousseaux M, Pruvo JP, Cabaret M, Leys D. Neuropsychological changes related to unilateral lenticulostriate infarcts. J Neurol Neurosurg Psychiatry 1994; 57(4):480–485.

223. Nagaraja D, Verma A, Taly AB, Kumar MV, Jayakumar PN. Cerebrovascular disease in children. Acta Neurol Scand 1994; 90(4):251–255.

224. Powell FC, Hanigan WC, McCluney KW. Subcortical infarction in children. Stroke 1994; 25(1):117–121.

225. Brower MC, Rollins N, Roach ES. Basal ganglia and thalamic infarction in children. Cause and clinical features. Arch Neurol 1996; 53(12):1252–1256.

226. Rollins N, Dowling M, Booth T, Purdy P. Idiopathic ischemic cerebral infarction in childhood: depiction of arterial abnormalities by MR angiography and catheter angiography. AJNR Am J Neuroradiol 2000; 21(3):549–556.

227. Caekebeke JF, Peters AC, Vandvik B, Brouwer OF, de Bakker HM. Cerebral vasculopathy associated with primary varicella infection. Arch Neurol 1990; 47(9):1033–1035.

228. Linnemann CC, Jr, Alvira MM. Pathogenesis of varicella-zoster angiitis in the CNS. Arch Neurol 1980; 37(4):239–240.

229. Ichiyama T, Houdou S, Kisa T, Ohno K, Takeshita K. Varicella with delayed hemiplegia. Pediatr Neurol 1990; 6(4):279–281.

230. Schwid S, Ketonen L, Betts R, Richfield E, Kieburtz K. Cerebrovascular complications after primary varicella-zoster infection. Lancet 1992; 340(8820):669.

231. Amlie-Lefond C, Kleinschmidt-DeMasters BK, Mahalingam R, Davis LE, Gilden DH. The vasculopathy of varicella-zoster virus encephalitis. Ann Neurol 1995; 37(6):784–790.

232. Gilden DH, Kleinschmidt-DeMasters BK, Wellish M, Hedley-Whyte ET, Rentier B, Mahalingam R. Varicella zoster virus, a cause of waxing and waning vasculitis: the New England Journal of Medicine case 5 – 1995 revisited. Neurology 1996; 47(6):1441–1446.

233. Melanson M, Chalk C, Georgevich L, Fett K, Lapierre Y, Duong H et al. Varicella-zoster virus DNA in CSF and arteries in delayed contralateral hemiplegia: evidence for viral invasion of cerebral arteries. Neurology 1996; 47(2):569–570.

234. Ganesan V, Kirkham FJ. Mechanisms of ischaemic stroke after chickenpox. Arch Dis Child 1997; 76(6):522–525.

235. Sebire G, Chabrier S. Reply. Ann Neurol 1999; 46:934.

236. Hattori H, Higuchi Y, Tsuji M. Recurrent strokes after varicella. Ann Neurol 2000; 47(1):136.

237. Berger TM, Caduff JH, Gebbers JO. Fatal varicella-zoster virus antigen-positive giant cell arteritis of the central nervous system. Pediatr Infect Dis J 2000; 19(7):653–656.

238. Singhal AB, Singhal BS, Ursekar MA, Koroshetz WJ. Serial MR angiography and contrast-enhanced MRI in chickenpox-associated stroke. Neurology 2001; 56(6):815–817.

239. Cox MG, Wolfs TF, Lo TH, Kappelle LJ, Braun KP. Neuroborreliosis causing focal cerebral arteriopathy in a child. Neuropediatrics 2005; 36(2):104–107.

240. Craze JL, Salisbury AJ, Pike MG. Prenatal stroke associated with maternal parvovirus infection. Dev Med Child Neurol 1996; 38(1):84–85.

241. Guidi B, Bergonzini P, Crisi G, Frigieri G, Portolani M. Case of stroke in a 7-year-old male after parvovirus B19 infection. Pediatr Neurol 2003; 28(1):69–71.

242. Mandrioli J, Portolani M, Cortelli P, Sola P. Middle cerebral artery thrombosis in course of parvovirus B19 infection in a young adult: A new risk factor for stroke? J Neurovirol 2004; 10(1):71–74.

243. Ribai P, Liesnard C, Rodesch G, Giurgea S, Verheulpen D, David P et al. Transient cerebral arteriopathy in infancy associated with enteroviral infection. Eur J Paediatr Neurol 2003; 7(2):73–75.

244. Leeuwis JW, Wolfs TF, Braun KP. A child with HIV-associated transient cerebral arteriopathy. AIDS 2007; 21(10):1383–1384.

245. Lanthier S, Armstrong D, Domi T, deVeber G. Post-varicella arteriopathy of childhood: natural history of vascular stenosis. Neurology 2005; 64(4):660–663.

246. Husson B, Rodesch G, Lasjaunias P, Tardieu M, Sebire G. Magnetic resonance angiography in childhood arterial brain infarcts: a comparative study with contrast angiography. Stroke 2002; 33(5):1280–1285.

247. Imamura A, Matsuo N, Ariki M, Horikoshi H, Hattori T. MR imaging and [1]H-MR spectroscopy in a case of cerebral infarction with transient cerebral arteriopathy. Brain Dev 2004; 26(8):535–538.

248. Gout A, Seibel N, Rouviere C, Husson B, Hermans B, Laporte N et al. Aphasia owing to subcortical brain infarcts in childhood. J Child Neurol 2005; 20(12):1003–1008.

249. Sebire G. Factor V Leiden as a cause of hemiplegic cerebral palsy, neonatal stroke, and placental thrombosis? Ann Neurol 1998; 44(3):426–427.

250. Vazquez M, LaRussa PS, Gershon AA, Steinberg SP, Freudigman K, Shapiro ED. The effectiveness of the varicella vaccine in clinical practice. N Engl J Med 2001; 344(13):955–960.

251. Wirrell E, Hill MD, Jadavji T, Kirton A, Barlow K. Stroke after varicella vaccination. J Pediatr 2004; 145(6):845–847.

252. Donahue JG, Kieke BA, Yih WK, Berger NR, McCauley JS, Baggs J et al. Varicella vaccination and ischemic stroke in children: is there an association? Pediatrics 2009; 123(2):e228–e234.

253. Roach ES. Stroke in children. Curr Treat Options Neurol 2000; 2(4):295–304.

254. Lanthier S, Carmant L, David M, Larbrisseau A, de Veber G. Stroke in children: the coexistence of multiple risk factors predicts poor outcome. Neurology 2000; 54(2):371–378.

255. Takeuchi K, Shimizu H. Hypogenesis of bilateral internal carotid arteries. No to Shinkei. Brain Nerve 1957; 9(37):43.

256. Natori Y, Ikezaki K, Matsushima T, Fukui M. 'Angiographic moyamoya' its definition, classification, and therapy. Clin Neurol Neurosurg 1997; 99(Suppl 2):S168–S172.

257. Fukui M. Guidelines for the diagnosis and treatment of spontaneous occlusion of the circle of Willis ('moyamoya' disease). Research Committee on Spontaneous Occlusion of the Circle of Willis (Moyamoya Disease) of the Ministry of Health and Welfare, Japan. Clin Neurol Neurosurg 1997; 99(Suppl 2):S238–S240.

258. Hirotsune N, Meguro T, Kawada S, Nakashima H, Ohmoto T. Long-term follow-up study of patients with unilateral moyamoya disease. Clin Neurol Neurosurg 1997; 99(Suppl 2):S178–S181.

259. Seol HJ, Wang KC, Kim SK, Lee CS, Lee DS, Kim IO et al. Unilateral (probable) moyamoya disease: long-term follow-up of seven cases. Childs Nerv Syst 2006; 22(2):145–150.

260. Peerless SJ. Risk factors of moyamoya disease in Canada and the USA. Clin Neurol Neurosurg 1997; 99(Suppl 2):S45–S48.

261. Chiu D, Shedden P, Bratina P, Grotta JC. Clinical features of moyamoya disease in the United States. Stroke 1998; 29(7):1347–1351.

262. Fukui M. Current state of study on moyamoya disease in Japan. Surg Neurol 1997; 47(2):138–143.

263. Kuriyama S, Kusaka Y, Fujimura M, Wakai K, Tamakoshi A, Hashimoto S et al. Prevalence and clinicoepidemiological features of moyamoya disease in Japan: findings from a nationwide epidemiological survey. Stroke 2008; 39(1):42–47.

264. Kitahara T, Ariga N, Yamaura A, Makino H, Maki Y. Familial occurrence of moyamoya disease: report of three Japanese families. J Neurol Neurosurg Psychiatry 1979; 42(3):208–214.

265. Yonekawa Y, Ogata N, Kaku Y, Taub E, Imhof HG. Moyamoya disease in Europe, past and present status. Clin Neurol Neurosurg 1997; 99(Suppl 2):S58–S60.

266. Uchino K, Johnston SC, Becker KJ, Tirschwell DL. Moyamoya disease in Washington State and California. Neurology 2005; 65(6):956–958.

267. Numaguchi Y, Gonzalez CF, Davis PC. Moyamoya disease in the United States. Clin Neurol Neurosurg 1997; 99:26–30.

268. Suzuki J, Kodama N. Moyamoya disease – a review. Stroke 1983; 14(1):104–109.

269. Hosoda Y, Ikeda E, Hirose S. Histopathological studies on spontaneous occlusion of the circle of Willis (cerebrovascular moyamoya disease). Clin Neurol Neurosurg 1997; 99(Suppl 2):S203–S208.

270. Yamashita M, Oka K, Tanaka K. Cervico-cephalic arterial thrombi and thromboemboli in moyamoya disease – possible correlation with progressive intimal thickening in the intracranial major arteries. Stroke 1984; 15(2):264–270.

271. Kono S, Oka K, Sueishi K, Sonobe M. Histopathological studies on spontaneous vault moyamoya and revascularized collaterals formed by encephalomyosynangiosis. Clin Neurol Neurosurg 1997; 99(Suppl 2):S209–S212.

272. Mineharu Y, Takenaka K, Yamakawa H, Inoue K, Ikeda H, Kikuta KI et al. Inheritance pattern of familial moyamoya disease: autosomal dominant mode and genomic imprinting. J Neurol Neurosurg Psychiatry 2006; 77(9):1025–1029.

273. Ikeda H, Sasaki T, Yoshimoto T, Fukui M, Arinami T. Mapping of a familial moyamoya disease gene to chromosome 3p24.2-p26. Am J Hum Genet 1999; 64(2):533–537.

274. Zafeiriou DI, Ikeda H, Anastasiou A, Vargiami E, Vougiouklis N, Katzos G et al. Familial moyamoya disease in a Greek family. Brain Dev 2003; 25(4):288–290.

275. Kawai M, Nishikawa T, Tanaka M, Ando A, Kasajima T, Higa T et al. An autopsied case of Williams syndrome complicated by moyamoya disease. Acta Paediatr Jpn 1993; 35(1):63–67.

276. Kaplan P, Levinson M, Kaplan BS. Cerebral artery stenoses in Williams syndrome cause strokes in childhood. J Pediatr 1995; 126(6):943–945.

277. Yamauchi T, Tada M, Houkin K, Tanaka T, Nakamura Y, Kuroda S et al. Linkage of familial moyamoya disease (spontaneous occlusion of the circle of Willis) to chromosome 17q25. Stroke 2000; 31(4):930–935.

278. Mineharu Y, Liu W, Inoue K, Matsuura N, Inoue S, Takenaka K et al. Autosomal dominant moyamoya disease maps to chromosome 17q25.3. Neurology 2008; 70(24 Pt 2):2357–2363.

279. Inoue TK, Ikezaki K, Sasazuki T, Matsushima T, Fukui M. Linkage analysis of moyamoya disease on chromosome 6. J Child Neurol 2000; 15(3):179–182.

280. Sakurai K, Horiuchi Y, Ikeda H, Ikezaki K, Yoshimoto T, Fukui M et al. A novel susceptibility locus for moyamoya disease on chromosome 8q23. J Hum Genet 2004; 49(5):278–281.

281. Yoshimoto T, Houkin K, Takahashi A, Abe H. Angiogenic factors in moyamoya disease. Stroke 1996; 27(12):2160–2165.

282. Nanba R, Kuroda S, Ishikawa T, Houkin K, Iwasaki Y. Increased expression of hepatocyte growth factor in cerebrospinal fluid and intracranial artery in moyamoya disease. Stroke 2004; 35(12):2837–2842.

283. Czartoski T, Hallam D, Lacy JM, Chun MR, Becker K. Postinfectious vasculopathy with evolution to moyamoya syndrome. J Neurol Neurosurg Psychiatry 2005; 76(2):256–259.

284. Yamaguchi T, Matsushima Y, Takada Y, Niimi Y, Umezu R, Fukuyama Y et al. Case-control study of moyamoya disease. No To Shinkei 1989; 41(5):485–491.

285. Kitahara T, Okumura K, Semba A, Yamaura A, Makino H. Genetic and immunologic analysis on moyamoya. J Neurol Neurosurg Psychiatry 1982; 45(11):1048–1052.

286. Aoyagi M, Ogami K, Matsushima Y, Shikata M, Yamamoto M, Yamamoto K. Human leukocyte antigen in patients with moyamoya disease. Stroke 1995; 26(3):415–417.

287. Golomb MR, Biller J, Smith JL, Edwards-Brown M, Sanchez JC, Nebesio TD et al. A 10-year-old girl with coexistent moyamoya disease and Graves' disease. J Child Neurol 2005; 20(7):620–624.

288. Hsu SW, Chaloupka JC, Fattal D. Rapidly progressive fatal bihemispheric infarction secondary to moyamoya syndrome in association with Graves thyrotoxicosis. AJNR Am J Neuroradiol 2006; 27(3):643–647.

289. Utku U, Asil T, Celik Y, Tucer D. Reversible MR angiographic findings in a patient with autoimmune Graves disease. AJNR Am J Neuroradiol 2004; 25(9):1541–1543.

290. Tomsick TA, Lukin RR, Chambers AA, Benton C. Neurofibromatosis and intracranial arterial occlusive disease. Neuroradiology 1976; 11(5):229–234.

291. Erickson RP, Woolliscroft J, Allen RJ. Familial occurrence of intracranial arterial occlusive disease (moyamoya) in neurofibromatosis. Clin Genet 1980; 18(3):191–196.

292. Schuster JM, Roberts TS. Symptomatic moyamoya disease and aortic coarctation in a patient with Noonan's syndrome: strategies for management. Pediatr Neurosurg 1999; 30(4):206–210.

293. Qaiser R, Scott RM, Smith ER. Identification of an association between Robinow syndrome and moyamoya. Pediatr Neurosurg 2009; 45(1):69–72.

294. Codd PJ, Scott RM, Smith ER. Seckel syndrome and moyamoya. J Neurosurg Pediatr 2009; 3(4):320–324.

295. Singla M, John E, Hidalgo G, Grewal D, Macmillan C. Moyamoya vasculopathy in a child after hemolytic uremic syndrome: a possible etiopathogenesis. Neuropediatrics 2008; 39(2):128–130.

296. Dobson SR, Holden KR, Nietert PJ, Cure JK, Laver JH, Disco D et al. Moyamoya syndrome in childhood sickle cell disease: a predictive factor for recurrent cerebrovascular events. Blood 2002; 99(9):3144–3150.

297. Scott RM, Smith ER. Moyamoya disease and moyamoya syndrome. N Engl J Med 2009; 360(12):1226–1237.

298. Roach ES, Riela AR. Vasculopathies of the nervous system. In: Pediatric Cerebrovascular Disorders, 2nd edn (eds RS Roach, AR Riela). Aronk, New York: Futura Publishing Company, 1995; 163–180.

299. Connor SE, Hewes D, Ball C, Jarosz JM. Alagille syndrome associated with angiographic moyamoya. Childs Nerv Syst 2002; 18(3–4):186–190.

300. Beyer RA, Paden P, Sobel DF, Flynn FG. Moyamoya pattern of vascular occlusion after radiotherapy for glioma of the optic chiasm. Neurology 1986; 36(9):1173–1178.

301. Kondoh T, Morishita A, Kamei M, Okamura Y, Tamaki M, Kohmura E. Moyamoya syndrome after prophylactic cranial irradiation for acute lymphocytic leukemia. Pediatr Neurosurg 2003; 39(5):264–269.

302. Bonduel M, Hepner M, Sciuccati G, Torres AF, Tenembaum S. Prothrombotic disorders in children with moyamoya syndrome. Stroke 2001; 32(8):1786–1792.

303. Worley G, Shbarou R, Heffner AN, Belsito KM, Capone GT, Kishnani PS. New onset focal weakness in children with Down syndrome. Am J Med Genet A 2004; 128A(1):15–18.

304. Hsia TY, Kirkham F, Waldman A, Tsang V. The implications of extensive cerebral vascular dysplasia in surgical repair of coarctation of the aorta and ventricular septal defect. J Thorac Cardiovasc Surg 2001; 121(5):998–1001.

305. Matsushima Y, Aoyagi M, Niimi Y, Masaoka H, Ohno K. Symptoms and their pattern of progression in childhood moyamoya disease. Brain Dev 1990; 12(6):784–789.

306. Kikuta K, Takagi Y, Arakawa Y, Miyamoto S, Hashimoto N. Absence epilepsy associated with moyamoya disease. Case report. J Neurosurg 2006; 104(4 Suppl):265–268.

307. Aydin K, Okuyaz C, Gucuyener K, Serdaroglu A, Akpek S. Moyamoya disease presented with migrainelike headache in a 4-year-old girl. J Child Neurol 2003; 18(5):361–363.

308. Seol HJ, Wang KC, Kim SK, Hwang YS, Kim KJ, Cho BK. Headache in pediatric moyamoya disease: review of 204 consecutive cases. J Neurosurg 2005; 103(5 Suppl):439–442.

309. Barrall JL, Summers CG. Ocular ischemic syndrome in a child with moyamoya disease and neurofibromatosis. Surv Ophthalmol 1996; 40(6):500–504.

310. Hogan AM, Kirkham FJ, Isaacs EB, Wade AM, Vargha-Khadem F. Intellectual decline in children with moyamoya and sickle cell anaemia. Dev Med Child Neurol 2005; 47(12):824–829.

311. Levin SD, Hoare RD, Robinson RO. Childhood moyamoya presenting as dementia: report of a case. Dev Med Child Neurol 1983; 25(6):794–797.

312. Klasen H, Britton J, Newman M. Moyamoya disease in a 12-year-old Caucasian boy presenting with acute transient psychosis. Eur Child Adolesc Psychiatry 1999; 8(2):149–153.

313. Pavlakis SG, Schneider S, Black K, Gould RJ. Steroid-responsive chorea in moyamoya disease. Mov Disord 1991; 6(4):347–349.

314. Zheng W, Wanibuchi M, Onda T, Liu H, Koyanagi I, Fujimori K et al. A case of moyamoya disease presenting with chorea. Childs Nerv Syst 2006; 22(3):274–278.

315. Gonzalez-Alegre P, Ammache Z, Davis PH, Rodnitzky RL. Moyamoya-induced paroxysmal dyskinesia. Mov Disord 2003; 18(9):1051–1056.

316. Yasutomo K, Hashimoto T, Miyazaki M, Kuroda Y. Recurrent torticollis as a presentation of moyamoya disease. J Child Neurol 1993; 8(2):187–188.

317. Yamada I, Himeno Y, Matsushima Y, Shibuya H. Renal artery lesions in patients with moyamoya disease: angiographic findings. Stroke 2000; 31(3):733–737.

318. Togao O, Mihara F, Yoshiura T, Tanaka A, Kuwabara Y, Morioka T et al. Prevalence of stenoocclusive lesions in the renal and abdominal arteries in moyamoya disease. AJR Am J Roentgenol 2004; 183(1):119–122.

319. Suzuki J, Takaku A. Cerebrovascular 'moyamoya' disease. Disease showing abnormal net-like vessels in base of brain. Arch Neurol 1969; 20(3):288–299.

320. Mugikura S, Takahashi S, Higano S, Shirane R, Kurihara N, Furuta S et al. The relationship between cerebral infarction and angiographic characteristics in childhood moyamoya disease. AJNR Am J Neuroradiol 1999; 20(2):336–343.

321. Yamada I, Matsushima Y, Suzuki S. Moyamoya disease: diagnosis with three-dimensional time-of-flight MR angiography. Radiology 1992; 184(3):773–778.

322. Calamante F, Ganesan V, Kirkham FJ, Jan W, Chong WK, Gadian DG et al. MR perfusion imaging in moyamoya syndrome: potential implications for clinical evaluation of occlusive cerebrovascular disease. Stroke 2001; 32(12):2810–2816.

323. Mikulis DJ, Krolczyk G, Desal H, Logan W, deVeber G, Dirks P et al. Preoperative and postoperative mapping of cerebrovascular reactivity in moyamoya disease by using blood oxygen level-dependent magnetic resonance imaging. J Neurosurg 2005; 103(2):347–355.

324. Togao O, Mihara F, Yoshiura T, Tanaka A, Noguchi T, Kuwabara Y et al. Cerebral hemodynamics in moyamoya disease: correlation between perfusion-weighted MR imaging and cerebral angiography. AJNR Am J Neuroradiol 2006; 27(2):391–397.

325. Tanaka Y, Nariai T, Nagaoka T, Akimoto H, Ishiwata K, Ishii K et al. Quantitative evaluation of cerebral hemodynamics in patients with moyamoya disease by dynamic susceptibility contrast magnetic resonance imaging – comparison with positron emission tomography. J Cereb Blood Flow Metab 2006; 26(2):291–300.

326. Derdeyn CP, Grubb RL, Jr, Powers WJ. Cerebral hemodynamic impairment: methods of measurement and association with stroke risk. Neurology 1999; 53(2):251–259.

327. Ishikawa T, Houkin K, Kamiyama H, Abe H. Effects of surgical revascularization on outcome of patients with pediatric moyamoya disease. Stroke 1997; 28(6):1170–1173.

328. Kuroda S, Houkin K, Kamiyama H, Abe H, Mitsumori K. Regional cerebral hemodynamics in childhood moyamoya disease. Childs Nerv Syst 1995; 11(10):584–590.

329. Kim SK, Cho BK, Phi JH, Lee JY, Chae JH, Kim KJ, Hwang YS, Kim IO, Lee DS, Lee J, Wang KC. Pediatric moyamoya disease: An analysis of 410 consecutive cases. Ann Neurol. 2010;68(1):92–101.

330. Ikezaki K, Matsushima T, Kuwabara Y, Suzuki SO, Nomura T, Fukui M. Cerebral circulation and oxygen metabolism in childhood moyamoya disease: a perioperative positron emission tomography study. J Neurosurg 1994; 81(6):843–850.

331. Tatemichi TK, Prohovnik I, Mohr JP, Correll JW, Quest DO, Jarvis L. Reduced hypercapnic vasoreactivity in moyamoya disease. Neurology 1988; 38(10):1575–1581.

332. Kuwabara Y, Ichiya Y, Sasaki M, Yoshida T, Masuda K, Ikezaki K et al. Cerebral hemodynamics and metabolism in moyamoya disease – a positron emission tomography study. Clin Neurol Neurosurg 1997; 99(Suppl 2):S74–S78.

333. Nakagawara J, Takeda R, Suematsu K, Nakamura J. Quantification of regional cerebral blood flow and vascular reserve in childhood moyamoya disease using [123I]IMP-ARG method. Clin Neurol Neurosurg 1997; 99(Suppl 2):S96–S99.

334. Taki W, Yonekawa Y, Kobayashi A, Ishikawa M, Kikuchi H, Nishizawa S et al. Cerebral circulation and oxygen metabolism in moyamoya disease of ischemic type in children. Childs Nerv Syst 1988; 4(5):259–262.

335. Nariai T, Suzuki R, Hirakawa K, Maehara T, Ishii K, Senda M. Vascular reserve in chronic cerebral ischemia measured by the acetazolamide challenge test: comparison with positron emission tomography. AJNR Am J Neuroradiol 1995; 16(3):563–570.

336. Nariai T, Suzuki R, Matsushima Y, Ichimura K, Hirakawa K, Ishii K et al. Surgically induced angiogenesis to compensate for hemodynamic cerebral ischemia. Stroke 1994; 25(5):1014–1021.

337. Kodama N, Aoki Y, Hiraga H, Wada T, Suzuki J. Electroencephalographic findings in children with moyamoya disease. Arch Neurol 1979; 36(1):16–19.

338. Kazumata K, Kuroda S, Houkin K, Abe H, Mitumori K. Regional cerebral hemodynamics during re-build-up phenomenon in childhood moyamoya disease. An analysis using ^{99m}Tc-HMPAO SPECT. Childs Nerv Syst 1996; 12(3):161–165.

339. Kuroda S, Houkin K, Hoshi Y, Tamura M, Kazumata K, Abe H. Cerebral hypoxia after hyperventilation causes 're-build-up' phenomenon and TIA in childhood moyamoya disease. A near-infrared spectroscopy study. Childs Nerv Syst 1996; 12(8):448–452.

340. Lin Y, Yoshiko K, Negoro T, Watanabe K, Negoro M. Cerebral oxygenation state in childhood moyamoya disease: a near-infrared spectroscopy study. Pediatr Neurol 2000; 22(5):365–369.

341. Ikezaki K, Loftus CM, Iloeje SO, American Association of Neurological Surgeons. psychiatric morbidity among children with sickle cell disease. Dev Med Chld Neurol 2001; 33(12):1087–1094.

342. Moyamoya Disease. Rolling Meadows III: American Association of Neurological Surgeons, 2001.

343. Fung LW, Thompson D, Ganesan V. Revascularization surgery for paediatric moyamoya: a review of the literature. Childs Nerv Syst 2005; 21(5):358–364.

344. Guzman R, Lee M, Achrol A, Bell-Stephens T, Kelly M, Do HM et al. Clinical outcome after 450 revascularization procedures for moyamoya disease. J Neurosurg 2009; 111(5):927–935.

345. Czabanka M, Vajkoczy P, Schmiedek P, Horn P. Age-dependent revascularization patterns in the treatment of moyamoya disease in a European patient population. Neurosurg Focus 2009; 26(4):E9.

346. Fryer RH, Anderson RC, Chiriboga CA, Feldstein NA. Sickle cell anemia with moyamoya disease: outcomes after EDAS procedure. Pediatr Neurol 2003; 29(2):124–130.

347. Ganesan V, Lumley JSP, Toolis C, Thompson DNP. Surgical revascularization in children with sickle cell disease. Dev Med Child Neurol 2007; 49(S1):3.

348. Jea A, Smith ER, Robertson R, Scott RM. Moyamoya syndrome associated with Down syndrome: outcome after surgical revascularization. Pediatrics 2005; 116(5):e694–e701.

349. George BD, Neville BG, Lumley JS. Transcranial revascularization in childhood and adolescence. Dev Med Child Neurol 1993; 35(8):675–682.

350. Golby AJ, Marks MP, Thompson RC, Steinberg GK. Direct and combined revascularization in pediatric moyamoya disease. Neurosurgery 1999; 45(1):50–58.

351. Nakashima H, Meguro T, Kawada S, Hirotsune N, Ohmoto T. Long-term results of surgically treated moyamoya disease. Clin Neurol Neurosurg 1997; 99(Suppl 2):S156–S161.

352. Robertson RL, Burrows PE, Barnes PD, Robson CD, Poussaint TY, Scott RM. Angiographic changes after pial synangiosis in childhood moyamoya disease. AJNR Am J Neuroradiol 1997; 18(5):837–845.

353. Kim DS, Kye DK, Cho KS, Song JU, Kang JK. Combined direct and indirect reconstructive vascular surgery on the frontoparietooccipital region in moyamoya disease. Clin Neurol Neurosurg 1997; 99(Suppl 2):S137–S141.

354. Takikawa S, Kamiyama H, Abe H, Mitsumori K, Tsuru M. Hemodynamic evaluation of vascular reconstructive surgery for childhood moyamoya disease using single photon emission computed tomography. Neurol Med Chir (Tokyo) 1990; 30(6):389–395.

355. Choi JU, Kim DS, Kim EY, Lee KC. Natural history of moyamoya disease: comparison of activity of daily living in surgery and non surgery groups. Clin Neurol Neurosurg 1997; 99(Suppl 2):S11–S18.

356. Matsushima Y, Aoyagi M, Koumo Y, Takasato Y, Yamaguchi T, Masaoka H et al. Effects of encephalo-duro-arterio-synangiosis on childhood moyamoya patients – swift disappearance of ischemic attacks and maintenance of mental capacity. Neurol Med Chir (Tokyo) 1991; 31(11):708–714.

357. Scott RM, Smith JL, Robertson RL, Madsen JR, Soriano SG, Rockoff MA. Long-term outcome in children with moyamoya syndrome after cranial revascularization by pial synangiosis. J Neurosurg 2004; 100(2 Suppl Pediatrics):142–149.

358. Sato K, Shirane R, Yoshimoto T. Perioperative factors related to the development of ischemic complications in patients with moyamoya disease. Childs Nerv Syst 1997; 13(2):68–72.

359. Olds MV, Griebel RW, Hoffman HJ, Craven M, Chuang S, Schutz H. The surgical treatment of childhood moyamoya disease. J Neurosurg 1987; 66(5):675–680.

360. Ikezaki K. Rational approach to treatment of moyamoya disease in childhood. J Child Neurol 2000; 15(5):350–356.

361. Kurokawa T, Tomita S, Ueda K, Narazaki O, Hanai T, Hasuo K et al. Prognosis of occlusive disease of the circle of Willis (moya-moya disease) in children. Pediatr Neurol 1985; 1(5):274–277.

362. Imaizumi C, Imaizumi T, Osawa M, Fukuyama Y, Takeshita M. Serial intelligence test scores in pediatric moyamoya disease. Neuropediatrics 1999; 30(6):294–299.

363. Maki Y, Nakada Y, Nose T, Yoshii Y. Clinical and radioisotopic follow-up study of 'Moyamoya'. Childs Brain 1976; 2(4):257–271.

364. Imaizumi T, Hayashi K, Saito K, Osawa M, Fukuyama Y. Long-term outcomes of pediatric moyamoya disease monitored to adulthood. Pediatr Neurol 1998; 18(4):321–325.

365. Schmidley JW. Isolated CNS angiitis: Clinical Aspects. Central Nervous System Angiitis. London: Butterworth-Heinemann, 2000; 1–22.

366. Lanthier S, Lortie A, Michaud J, Laxer R, Jay V, deVeber G. Isolated angiitis of the CNS in children. Neurology 2001; 56(7):837–842.

367. Zivkovic S, Moore PM. Systemic and central nervous system vasculitides. Curr Treat Options Neurol 2000; 2(5):459–472.

368. Moore PM. Vasculitis of the central nervous system. Curr Rheumatol Rep 2000; 2(5):376–382.

369. Love S, Renowden S, Carter M. Ruptured vertebrobasilar aneurysm associated with giant cell arteritis in a young boy. Clin Neurol Neurosurg 2008; 110(1):92–96.

370. Abe T, Maruyama T, Nagai Y, Kamida T, Wakabayashi Y, Ishii K et al. Severe postoperative vasculitis of the central nervous system in a child with arteriovenous malformation: case report. Surg Neurol 2007; 68(3):317–321.

371. Kava MP, Tullu MS, Kamat JR, Vaswani RK. Primary angiitis of the central nervous system. Indian Pediatr 2002; 39(7):684–689.

372. Benseler SM, Silverman E, Aviv RI, Schneider R, Armstrong D, Tyrrell PN et al. Primary central nervous system vasculitis in children. Arthritis Rheum 2006; 54(4):1291–1297.

373. Benseler SM, deVeber G, Hawkins C, Schneider R, Tyrrell PN, Aviv RI et al. Angiography-negative primary central nervous system vasculitis in children: a newly recognized inflammatory central nervous system disease. Arthritis Rheum 2005; 52(7):2159–2167.

374. Elbers J, Benseler SM. Central nervous system vasculitis in children. Curr Opin Rheumatol 2008; 20(1):47–54.

375. Vella S, Ramelli GP, Schroth G, Bianchetti MG. Circulating antineutrophil autoantibodies in a child with isolated central nervous system vasculitis. Neuropediatrics 1999; 30(5):268–269.

376. Petrasek JG, Panitch H, Woofsy D. IgA-associated granulomas angiitis (GA) of brain: successful therapy with cyclophosphamide. Neurology 1980; 30:442.

377. Andrews JM, Thompson JA, Pysher TJ, Walker ML, Hammond ME. Chronic encephalitis, epilepsy, and cerebrovascular immune complex deposits. Ann Neurol 1990; 28(1):88–90.

378. Derry C, Dale RC, Thom M, Miller DH, Giovannoni G. Unihemispheric cerebral vasculitis mimicking Rasmussen's encephalitis. Neurology 2002; 58(2):327–328.

379. Harris KG, Tran DD, Sickels WJ, Cornell SH, Yuh WT. Diagnosing intracranial vasculitis: the roles of MR and angiography. AJNR Am J Neuroradiol 1994; 15(2):317–330.

380. Aviv RI, Benseler SM, Silverman ED, Tyrrell PN, deVeber G, Tsang LM et al. MR imaging and angiography of primary CNS vasculitis of childhood. AJNR Am J Neuroradiol 2006; 27(1):192–199.

381. Imbesi SG. Diffuse cerebral vasculitis with normal results on brain MR imaging. AJR Am J Roentgenol 1999; 173(6):1494–1496.

382. Kuker W, Gaertner S, Nagele T, Dopfer C, Schoning M, Fiehler J et al. Vessel wall contrast enhancement: a diagnostic sign of cerebral vasculitis. Cerebrovasc Dis 2008; 26(1):23–29.

383. Aviv RI, Benseler SM, deVeber G, Silverman ED, Tyrrell PN, Tsang LM et al. Angiography of primary central nervous system angiitis of childhood: conventional angiography versus magnetic resonance angiography at presentation. AJNR Am J Neuroradiol 2007; 28(1):9–15.

384. Hurst RW, Grossman RI. Neuroradiology of central nervous system vasculitis. Semin Neurol 1994; 14(4):320–340.

385. Lie JT. Primary (granulomatous) angiitis of the central nervous system: a clinicopathologic analysis of 15 new cases and a review of the literature. Hum Pathol 1992; 23(2):164–171.

386. Fieschi C, Rasura M, Anzini A, Beccia M. Central nervous system vasculitis. J Neurol Sci 1998; 153(2):159–171.

387. Parisi JE, Moore PM. The role of biopsy in vasculitis of the central nervous system. Semin Neurol 1994; 14(4):341–348.

388. Moore PM. Diagnosis and management of isolated angiitis of the central nervous system. Neurology 1989; 39(2 Pt 1):167–173.

389. Duzova A, Bakkaloglu A. Central nervous system involvement in pediatric rheumatic diseases: current concepts in treatment. Curr Pharm Des 2008; 14(13):1295–1301.

390. Hausler MG, Ramaekers VT, Reul J, Meilicke R, Heimann G. Early and late onset manifestations of cerebral vasculitis related to vari-cella zoster. Neuropediatrics 1998; 29(4):202–207.

391. Nagaratnam N, James WE. Isolated angiitis of the brain in a young female on the contraceptive pill. Postgrad Med J 1987; 63(746):1085–1086.

392. Prengler M, McShane MA, Ganesan V, Kirkham FJ. Isolated angi-itis of the central nervous system in childhood and immunosuppressive therapy with cyclophosphamide. Dev Med Child Neurol 1997; 39(Suppl 77):30.

393. Gallagher KT, Shaham B, Reiff A, Tournay A, Villablanca JP, Curran J et al. Primary angiitis of the central nervous system in chil-dren: 5 cases. J Rheumatol 2001; 28(3):616–623.

394. Bitter KJ, Epstein LG, Melin-Aldana H, Curran JG, Miller ML. Cyclophosphamide treatment of primary angiitis of the central nervous system in children: report of 2 cases. J Rheumatol 2006; 33(10):2078–2080.

395. Sanai N, Fullerton H, Karl TR, Lawton MT. Aortocarotid bypass for hemispheric hypoperfusion in a child. J Neurosurg Pediatr 2008; 1(4):343–347.

396. Wright E, Dillon MJ, Tullus K. Childhood vasculitis and plasma exchange. Eur J Pediatr 2007; 166(2):145–151.

397. LaMancusa J, Steiman G. Suspected isolated angiitis causing stroke in a child. Stroke 1990; 21(9):1380.

398. Nishikawa M, Sakamoto H, Katsuyama J, Hakuba A, Nishimura S. Multiple appearing and vanishing aneurysms: primary angiitis of the central nervous system. Case report. J Neurosurg 1998; 88(1):133–137.

399. Kamm C, Nagele T, Mittelbronn M, Schoning M, Melms A, Gasser T et al. Primary central nervous system vasculitis in a child mimi-cking parasitosis. J Neurol 2008; 255(1):130–132.

400. Kumar R, Wijdicks EF, Brown RD, Jr, Parisi JE, Hammond CA. Isolated angiitis of the CNS presenting as subarachnoid haemorrhage. J Neurol Neurosurg Psychiatry 1997; 62(6):649–651.

401. Katsicas MM, Russo R, Taratuto A, Pociecha J, Zelazko M. Primary angiitis of the central nervous system presenting as a mass lesion in a child. J Rheumatol 2000; 27(5):1297–1298.

402. Giovanini MA, Eskin TA, Mukherji SK, Mickle JP. Granulomatous angiitis of the spinal cord: a case report. Neurosurgery 1994; 34(3):540–543.

403. Barron TF, Ostrov BE, Zimmerman RA, Packer RJ. Isolated angi-itis of CNS: treatment with pulse cyclophosphamide. Pediatr Neurol 1993; 9(1):73–75.

404. Yaari R, Anselm IA, Szer IS, Malicki DM, Nespeca MP, Gleeson JG. Childhood primary angiitis of the central nervous system: two biopsy-proven cases. J Pediatr 2004; 145(5):693–697.

405. Matsell DG, Keene DL, Jimenez C, Humphreys P. Isolated angiitis of the central nervous system in childhood. Can J Neurol Sci 1990; 17(2):151–154.

406. Calabrese LH, Mallek JA. Primary angiitis of the central nervous system. Report of 8 new cases, review of the literature, and pro-posal for diagnostic criteria. Medicine (Baltimore) 1988; 67(1):20–39.

407. Chiaretti A, Caresta E, Piastra M, Pulitano S, Di RC. Cerebral hem-orrhage in Henoch–Schöenlein syndrome. Childs Nerv Syst 2002; 18(8):365–367.

408. Eun SH, Kim SJ, Cho DS, Chung GH, Lee DY, Hwang PH. Cerebral vasculitis in Henoch–Schönlein purpura: MRI and MRA findings, treated with plasmapheresis alone. Pediatr Int 2003; 45(4):484–487.

409. Ozkaya O, Bek K, Alaca N, Ceyhan M, Acikgoz Y, Tasdemir HA. Cerebral vasculitis in a child with Henoch–Schönlein purpura and familial Mediterranean fever. Clin Rheumatol 2007; 26(10):1729–1732.

410. Paula De Carvalho Panzeri Carlotti, Paes LF, V, Tanuri CC, Celia CM, Pileggi G, Carvalho C et al. Polyarteritis nodosa with central nervous system involvement mimicking meningoencephalitis. Pediatr Crit Care Med 2004; 5(3):286–288.

411. Haas JP, Metzler M, Ruder H, Waldherr R, Boswald M, Rupprecht T. An unusual manifestation of Wegener's granulomatosis in a 4-year-old girl. Pediatr Neurol 2002; 27(1):71–74.

412. Berman JL, Kashii S, Trachtman MS, Burde RM. Optic neuropathy and central nervous system disease secondary to Sjögren's syndrome in a child. Ophthalmology 1990; 97(12):1606–1609.

413. Holl-Wieden A, Klink T, Klink J, Warmuth-Metz M, Girschick HJ. Linear scleroderma 'en coup de sabre' associated with cerebral and ocular vasculitis. Scand J Rheumatol 2006; 35(5):402–404.

414. Gittins N, Basu A, Eyre J, Gholkar A, Moghal N. Cerebral vasculitis in a teenager with Goodpasture's syndrome. Nephrol Dial Transplant 2004; 19(12):3168–3171.

415. Ramanan AV, Sawhney S, Murray KJ. Central nervous system complications in two cases of juvenile onset dermatomyositis. Rheumatology (Oxford) 2001; 40(11):1293–1298.

416. Elst EF, Kamphuis SS, Prakken BJ, Wulffraat NM, van der Net JJ, Peters AC et al. Case report: severe central nervous system involvement in juvenile dermatomyositis. J Rheumatol 2003; 30(9):2059–2063.

417. Dupuis-Girod S, Medioni J, Haddad E, Quartier P, Cavazzana-Calvo M, Le Deist F et al. Autoimmunity in Wiskott–Aldrich syndrome: risk factors, clinical features, and outcome in a single-center cohort of 55 patients. Pediatrics 2003; 111(5 Pt 1):e622–e627.

418. Aryan HE, Giannotta SL, Fukushima T, Park MS, Ozgur BM, Levy ML. Aneurysms in children: review of 15 years experience. J Clin Neurosci 2006; 13(2):188–192.

419. Sert A, Aydin K, Pirgon O, Emlik D, Ustun ME. Arterial spasm following perimesencephalic nonaneurysmal subarachnoid hemorrhage in a pediatric patient. Pediatr Neurol 2005; 32(4):275–277.

420. Nahed BV, Ferreira M, Naunheim MR, Kahle KT, Proctor MR, Smith ER. Intracranial vasospasm with subsequent stroke after traumatic subarachnoid hemorrhage in a 22-month-old child. J Neurosurg Pediatr 2009; 3(4):311–315.

421. Rojiani AM, Poskitt KJ, Cochrane DD, Macnab AJ, Norman MG. Ruptured intracranial aneurysm presenting as cerebral infarction in a young child. Pediatr Neurosurg 1990; 16(6):326–330.

422. Carpenter J, Keating R, Weinstein S, Vezina G, Berger J, Bell MJ. Cerebral hemorrhage and vasospasm in a child with congenital heart disease. Neurocrit Care 2008; 8(2):276–279.

423. Danchaivijitr N, Miravet E, Saunders DE, Cox T, Ganesan V. Post-varicella intracranial haemorrhage in a child. Dev Med Child Neurol 2006; 48(2):139–142.

424. Nabika S, Kiya K, Satoh H, Mizoue T, Oshita J, Kondo H. Ischemia of the internal capsule due to mild head injury in a child. Pediatr Neurosurg 2007; 43(4):312–315.

425. Ojha BK, Jha DK, Kale SS, Mehta VS. Trans-cranial Doppler in severe head injury: evaluation of pattern of changes in cerebral blood flow velocity and its impact on outcome. Surg Neurol 2005; 64(2):174–179.

426. Aparicio JM, Tavares C, Teixeira-Pinto A, Almeida F, Silva ML, Vaz R et al. Cerebral vasospasm in pediatric head injuries: transcranial Doppler ultrasound findings. Cerebrovasc Dis 2002; 11:38.

427. Lee TT, Ragheb J, Bruce JC, Altman N, Morrison G. Diffuse cerebral vasospasm with ischemia after resection of a cerebellopontine angle primitive neuroectodermal tumor in a child. Pediatr Neurosurg 1998; 29(6):300–303.

428. Pound CM, Keene DL, Udjus K, Humphreys P, Johnston DL. Acute encephalopathy and cerebral vasospasm after multiagent chemotherapy including PEG-asparaginase and intrathecal cytarabine for the treatment of acute lymphoblastic leukemia. J Pediatr Hematol Oncol 2007; 29(3):183–186.

429. Boasso LE, Fischer AQ. Cerebral vasospasm in childhood migraine during the intermigrainous period. J Neuroimaging 2004; 14:158–161.

430. Prodan CI, Holland NR, Lenaerts ME, Parke JT. Magnetic resonance angiogram evidence of vasospasm in familial hemiplegic migraine. J Child Neurol 2002; 17(6):470–472.

431. Kirton A, Diggle J, Hu W, Wirrell E. A pediatric case of reversible segmental cerebral vasoconstriction. Can J Neurol Sci 2006; 33(2):250–253.

432. Liu HY, Fuh JL, Lirng JF, Chen SP, Wang SJ. Three paediatric patients with reversible cerebral vasoconstriction syndromes. Cephalalgia 2009; 17 July 17 (epub ahead of print).

433. Weibel J, Fields WS. Tortuosity, coiling, and kinking of the internal carotid artery. I. Etiology and radiographic anatomy. Neurology 1965; 15:7–18.

434. Weibel J, Fields WS. Tortuosity, coiling, and kinking of the internal carotid artery. II. Relationship of morphological variation to cerebrovascular insufficiency. Neurology 1965; 15:462–468.

435. Takahashi S, Ishii K, Matsumoto K, Higano S, Ishibashi T, Zuguchi M et al. Cranial MRI and MR angiography in Menkes' syndrome. Neuroradiology 1993; 35(7):556–558.

436. Kenzie-Stepner K, Witzel MA, Stringer DA, Lindsay WK, Munro IR, Hughes H. Abnormal carotid arteries in the velocardiofacial syndrome: a report of three cases. Plast Reconstr Surg 1987; 80(3):347–351.

437. Loeys BL, Schwarze U, Holm T, Callewaert BL, Thomas GH, Pannu H et al. Aneurysm syndromes caused by mutations in the TGF-beta receptor. N Engl J Med 2006; 355(8):788–798.

438. Rodrigues VJ, Elsayed S, Loeys BL, Dietz HC, Yousem DM. Neuroradiologic manifestations of Loeys–Dietz syndrome type 1. AJNR Am J Neuroradiol 2009; 30(8):1614–1619.

439. Coucke PJ, Willaert A, Wessels MW, Callewaert B, Zoppi N, De Backer J et al. Mutations in the facilitative glucose transporter GLUT10 alter angiogenesis and cause arterial tortuosity syndrome. Nat Genet 2006; 38(4):452–457.

440. Sarkari NB, Holmes JM, Bickerstaff ER. Neurological manifestations associated with internal carotid loops and kinks in children. J Neurol Neurosurg Psychiatry 1970; 33(2):194–200.

441. Cartwright MS, Hickling WH, Roach ES. Ischemic stroke in an adolescent with arterial tortuosity syndrome. Neurology 2006; 67(2):360–361.

442. Drera B, Barlati S, Colombi M. Ischemic stroke in an adolescent with arterial tortuosity syndrome. Neurology 2007; 68(19):1637.

443. Golomb MR, Fullerton HJ. Kinky vessels and double joints: useful clues for childhood stroke? Neurology 2006; 67(2):199–200.

444. Steen RG, Hankins GM, Xiong X, Wang WC, Beil K, Langston JW et al. Prospective brain imaging evaluation of children with sickle cell trait: initial observations. Radiology 2003; 228(1):208–215.

445. Steen RG, Emudianughe T, Hankins GM, Wynn LW, Wang WC, Xiong X et al. Brain imaging findings in pediatric patients with sickle cell disease. Radiology 2003; 228(1):216–225.

446. Deane CR, Goss D, Bartram J, Pohl KR, Height SE, Sibtain N et al. Extracranial internal carotid arterial disease in children with sickle cell anemia. Haematologica 2010; 95(8):1287–1292.

447. Beigelman R, Izaguirre AM, Robles M, Grana DR, Ambrosio G, Milei J. Are kinking and coiling of carotid artery congenital or acquired? Angiology 2010; 61(1):107–112.

448. Thore CR, Anstrom JA, Moody DM, Challa VR, Marion MC, Brown WR. Morphometric analysis of arteriolar tortuosity in human cerebral white matter of preterm, young, and aged subjects. J Neuropathol Exp Neurol 2007; 66(5):337–345.

449. Lou M, Caplan LR. Vertebrobasilar dilatative arteriopathy. Ann N Y Acad Sci 2010; 1184:121–133.

450. Takeuchi S, Takasato Y, Masaoka H, Hayakawa T, Otani N, Yoshino Y et al. Dolichoectasia involving the vertebrobasilar and carotid artery systems. J Clin Neurosci. 2009; 16(10):1344–1346.

451. Makos MM, McComb RD, Hart MN, Bennett DR. Alpha-glucosidase deficiency and basilar artery aneurysm: report of a sibship. Ann Neurol 1987; 22:629–633.

452. Braunsdorf WE. Fusiform aneurysm of basilar artery and ectatic internal carotid arteries associated with glycogenosis type 2 (Pompe's disease). Neurosurgery 1987; 21:748–749.

453. Wolfe T, Ubogu EE, Fernandes-Filho JA, Zaidat OO. Predictors of clinical outcome and mortality in vertebrobasilar dolichoectasia diagnosed by magnetic resonance angiography. J Stroke Cerebrovasc Dis. 2008; 17(6):388–393.

454. Passero SG. Natural history of vertebrobasilar dolichoectasia. Neurology 2008; 71:1460.

455. Hyung-Min Kwon, Ji-hoon Kim, Jae-Sung Lim, Jong-Ho Park, Sang-Hyung Lee, Yong-Seok Lee. Basilar artery dolichoectasia is associated with paramedian pontine infarction. Cerebrovasc Dis 2009; 27(2):114–118.

456. Baccin CE, Krings T, Alvarez H, Ozanne A, Lasjaunias PL. A report of two cases with dolichosegmental intracranial arteries as a new feature of PHACES syndrome. Childs Nerv Syst. 2007; 23(5):559–567.

457. Garzuly F, Marodi L, Erdos M et al. Megadolichobasilaranomaly with thrombosis in a family with Fabry's disease and a novel mutation in the alpha-galactosidase A gene. Brain 2005; 128(Pt 9):2078–2083.

458. Gavazzi C, Borsini W, Guerrini L, Della Nave R, Rocca MA, Tessa C et al. Subcortical damage and cortical functional changes in men and women with Fabry disease: a multifaceted MR study. Radiology 2006; 241(2):492–500.

459. Su PH, Chen JY, Chen SJ, Yang MS, Liu YL. Basilar artery dolichoectasia in a boy with a combination of partial monosomy 18p and partial trisomy 20q. Clin Dysmorphol. 2006; 15(4):225–228.

460. Mahadevan A, Tagore R, Siddappa NB, Santosh V, Yasha TC, Ranga U et al. Giant serpentine aneurysm of vertebrobasilar artery mimicking dolichoectasia – an unusual complication of pediatric AIDS. Report of a case with review of the literature. Clin Neuropathol 2008; 27(1):37–52.

461. Forrest KM, Siddiqui A, Lim M, Wraige E. Basilar artery dolichoectasia in childhood: evidence of vascular compromise. Childs Nerv Syst. 2011; 27(1):193–6.

462. Hegedüs K. Ectasia of the basilar artery with special reference to possible pathogenesis. Surg Neurol 1985; 24:463–469.

463. Toldo I, Manara R, Sartori S, Suppiej A, Drigo P. Unilateral hypoglossal nerve palsy due to neurovascular conflict in a child. Brain Dev 2009; 31(6):461–464.

464. Savitz SI, Ronthal M, Caplan LR. Vertebral artery compression of the medulla. Arch Neurol 2006; 63(2):234–241.

465. Stefano G, Passero MD, Calchetti B, Bartalini S. Intracranial bleeding in patients with vertebrobasilar dolichoectasia. Stroke 2005; 36:1421–1425.

466. Sarikaya S, Sarikaya B. Natural history of vertebrobasilar dolichoectasia. Neurology 2008; 71(18):1460; author reply 1460.

467. Lasjaunias P, Burrows P, Planet C. Developmental venous anomalies (DVA): the so-called venous angioma. Neurosurg Rev 1986; 9:233–244.

468. Ruíz DS, Yilmaz H, Gailloud P. Cerebral developmental venous anomalies: current concepts. Ann Neurol 2009; 66(3):271–283.

469. Kim P, Castellani R, Tresser N. Cerebral venous malformation complicated by spontaneous thrombosis. Child's Nerv Syst 1996; 12:172–175.

470. Prengler M, Taylor W, Kirkham FJ. Risk of venous thrombosis in complex developmental venous anomalies associated with orbital varices in childhood. Dev Med Child Neurol 1998; 40(Suppl 79):29.

471. Pereira VM, Geibprasert S, Krings T, Aurboonyawat T, Ozanne A, Toulgoat F et al. Pathomechanisms of symptomatic developmental venous anomalies. Stroke 2008; 39(12):3201–3215.

7
CEREBAL SINOVENOUS (VENOUS SINUS) THROMBOSIS

Gabrielle deVeber

Introduction

Stroke in childhood can be secondary to vascular occlusion in the venous drainage of the brain, termed cerebal sinovenous (venous sinus) thrombosis (CSVT). Venous infarction is a frequent sequel of CSVT and may be 'haemorrhagic' if there is visible haemorrhage into the area of infarction.[1] The diagnosis and treatment of children with CSVT differs from adults in important ways. First, CSVT may be more difficult to recognize in children compared with adults. As a result, the diagnosis of this disorder is frequently missed and delayed, especially in neonates. Second, CSVT in adults is frequently secondary to puerperal thrombosis or malignancy, in contrast to children in whom CSVT is secondary to a multitude of diseases (Table 7.1).[2–8] Third, there are several well-designed studies investigating prophylactic and therapeutic options for adults with CSVT.[9–11] There are no randomized controlled trials in children. Fourth, the neonatal period is the time in which 43% of childhood CSVT occurs. The presence of developmental differences in the haemostatic, cerebrovascular and neurological systems of the young negate the simple extrapolation of guidelines from adults to children with stroke.

Epidemiology

The incidence of childhood CSVT is 0.67 per 100 000 children per year aged term birth to 18 years.[3] Neonates comprise 43% of patients (Fig. 7.1). In a study excluding neonates, the incidence was 0.34 per 100 000 children per year. No prior estimates are available but the incidence may be increasing for two reasons. First, increased detection of CSVT in children has been enabled by the development of diagnostic tests such as power Doppler, computerized tomography (CT) with venography (CTV) and magnetic resonance imaging (MRI) with venography (MRV).[12,13] Second, the number of children at risk for CSVT is increasing as a result of more aggressive therapies and increased survival in previously lethal childhood disease including preterm birth, haemolytic anaemia, leukaemia and congenital heart disease. Thrombotic complications of these illnesses and treatments include CSVT. Thrombotic strokes in the venous system are still under-diagnosed because of subtle clinical signs and lack of use of appropriate radiographic tests including dedicated venous imaging.[14] The increasing incidence of CSVT in children has contributed to a growing awareness and has resulted in research focussed on this problem.[15]

The economic impact of childhood stroke including CSVT has not been assessed. However, given the special needs of developing children and since many decades of disability result over a full lifespan in children with neurological damage from CSVT, the burden of illness per individual will inevitably be greater than for an adult.

Anatomy and physiology

The venous drainage of the brain occurs through the 'superficial' or 'deep' cerebral sinovenous systems, which consist of a network of cerebral sinuses and veins (Fig. 7.2). Cerebral sinuses are external to the brain and are enclosed between two layers of fibrous dura mater, with the outermost layer being attached to bone along bony suture lines. The rigid attachment of sinuses and lack of venous valves results in a passive drainage of blood flow in the cerebral venous system.[16] As a result of these anatomical factors, the flow in the dural sinuses is highly responsive to changes in the systemic blood pressure. Reductions in systemic blood pressure can result in stasis or reversal of blood flow within the dural sinuses. A relative reduction of thrombomodulin in the lining of cerebral sinuses may further increase the tendency to thrombosis.[17]

The 'superficial' venous system begins with cortical veins, which drain the cerebral hemispheres into the superior sagittal sinus. In most humans, the superior sagittal sinus drains predominantly into the right lateral sinus (which is composed of both a transverse and sigmoid portion) and jugular vein. The 'deep venous system' includes the inferior sagittal sinus and the paired internal cerebral veins, which join to form the vein of Galen and the straight sinus. This deep system drains predominantly into the smaller calibre left lateral sinus and jugular vein.[18] Anteriorly, the paired cavernous sinuses communicate with the jugular system via the petrosal sinuses, although these structures are only rarely involved in childhood CSVT.

In addition to the major role played by the superior sagittal sinus in venous drainage of the brain, the sinus plays a major role in the absorption of cerebrospinal fluid (CSF). The CSF is normally absorbed from the subarachnoid space into the venous blood circulation through 'arachnoid granulations', which line the superior sagittal sinus. Thrombotic occlusion of the superior sagittal sinus or the right lateral sinus can result in reduced or absent function of the arachnoid granulations resulting in communicating hydrocephalus.[19,20]

TABLE 7.1
Conditions in which cerebral sinovenous thrombosis (venous sinus thrombosis) has been described in childhood

General
Dehydration
Hypoxia, e.g. poststrangulation
Post lumbar puncture

Inflammatory bowel disease
Ulcerative colitis
Crohn disease

Systemic diseases
Systemic lupus erythematosus
Thyrotoxicosis
Cushing syndrome
Behçet disease

Anaemias
Iron deficiency
Sickle cell disease
Thalassaemia
Autoimmune haemolytic anaemia
Paroxysmal nocturnal haemoglobinuria

Malignancies and their treatment
Leukaemia (asparaginase, steroids)
Lymphoma

Cardiac disease
Cyanotic congenital heart disease
Post-operative
Post-catheterization

Renal disease
Nephrotic syndrome

Chromosomal disorders
Down syndrome

Head and neck infections, e.g. *Pneumococcus, Fusobacterium necrophorum*
Meningitis
Mastoiditis
Ear infections
Tonsillitis
Sinusitis

Other head and neck disorders
Head injury
Brain tumour
Multiple sclerosis
Hydrocephalus (+/− shunt)

Metabolic conditions
Homocystinuria

Drugs
L-Asparaginase
Oral contraceptives
Corticosteroids
Epoetin-alfa

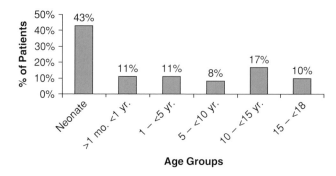

Fig. 7.1. Age distribution of children with sinovenous thrombosis in the Canadian Paediatric Ischaemic Stroke Registry: *N*=160.

trauma, impingement by other intracranial pathologies, for example brain tumours, or direct spread of infection from adjacent soft tissue infections. The latter scenario results in a septic thrombophlebitis, which accounts for the traditional classification of CSVT as either 'septic' or 'non-septic'. The aetiological head and neck infections in 'septic' CSVT usually arise from the inner ear, mastoid or air sinuses. The advent of antibiotics has resulted in a reduced frequency of 'septic' sinus thrombosis; however in young children in whom otitis media, mastoiditis and meningitis are still relatively common, or inadequately treated, 'septic' CSVT is still frequently encountered. In a recent series, for example, 3% of children with acute mastoiditis had lateral sinus thrombosis.[22]

Intravascular risk factors for CSVT promote thrombosis from within the structures, although they may overlap with vascular risk factors. At all ages, dehydration is a major risk factor for CSVT, with haemoconcentration contributing to thrombus formation. Anaemia and iron deficiency have been well-documented in childhood CSVT[6,23] and congenital or acquired prothrombotic disorders are frequently associated;[4,6,24,25] both affect endothelial function as well as promoting thrombosis. Finally, alterations in blood flow dynamics within the sino-venous system can contribute to the formation of thrombus. In the postnatal period, the rate of blood flow within the venous sinuses is significantly dependent on head positioning. In young infants with vein of Galen malformations or older children with arteriovenous malformations, thrombosis of the sinovenous system may be associated.

VENOUS INFARCTION
Cerebral infarction results when perfusion to the affected area of the brain is reduced to critical levels. In contrast to arterial ischaemic stroke in which there is 'inflow' obstruction, in sino-venous thrombosis the mechanism for venous infarction is related to venous 'outflow' obstruction with increasing regional venous pressure in the affected region of the brain. The venous congestion results in significant extravasation of fluid into the brain, producing focal cerebral oedema. The resultant oedema may be transient, if venous flow is re-established, or associated with permanent infarction. With infarction, the increased regional tissue pressure due to lack of venous drainage

Pathophysiology of cerebal sinovenous thrombosis
The mechanisms of thrombosis in CSVT are either vascular or intravascular. The primary vascular factor for neonates is the mechanical distortion of the cranial bones during the birth process with damage and thrombosis of the underlying venous sinuses.[21] Vascular factors in older children include mechanical distortion or damage with the sinuses with head

Fig. 7.2. Vascular stuctures most frequently involved in childhoood sinovenous thrombosis.

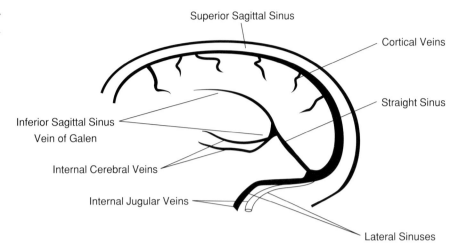

eventually exceeds the incoming arterial blood pressure resulting in insufficient delivery of arterial blood and regional ischaemic infarction in non-arterial vascular territories. Diffusion-weighted imaging has demonstrated that venous infarcts have restricted diffusion (cytotoxic oedema) in the early stages,[26,27] supporting the proposed theory that retrograde venous pressure decreases cerebral blood flow causing tissue damage, akin to arterial infarction. Haemorrhage accompanies venous infarction more frequently than arterial infarction, because of the extravasation of blood from the congested cerebral venous system. Subdural effusion or haematoma,[28,29] subarachnoid haemorrhage[30,31] and intracerebral haemorrhage, particularly in the parietal or occipital regions,[6,32,33] have all been reported. The risk for venous infarction is increased with rapid rates of sinovenous occlusion, with total occlusion of the lumen, and with thrombosis located at the entry points of cerebral veins into the sagittal sinus.[20,32] A further consequence of venous obstruction is the potential for propagation of existing thrombosis due to venous stasis within the vascular channels, with the potential for further infarction. Relief of the venous obstruction, even if delayed, may relieve the circulatory congestion with clinical benefit.

In addition to the intracerebral and intravascular events in CSVT, the disruption of CSF absorption within the superior sagittal sinus results in a communicating hydrocephalus,[19,33] and in diffuse cerebral swelling, both of which further increase intracranial pressure which may lead to cerebral herniation[34] and death.[35] Pressure on the optic nerves secondary to raised intracranial pressure initially causes papilloedema,[6] which if unrelieved over time can progress to permanent visual loss.

Clinical setting (Table 7.2)

Risk factors are identifiable in more than 95% of children with CSVT,[3,4,6] many of which are clinical and deserve a higher profile, as increased awareness is likely to be a cost-effective way of increasing diagnosis and therefore improving management and outcome. In the Canadian Registry, idiopathic CSVT, with no clinical or laboratory associations, occurred in only 3% of children compared with an estimated 10–25% of

TABLE 7.2
Symptoms and signs of cerebral sinovenous thrombosis in older children

Lethargy
Nausea
Vomiting
Headache
Seizures (focal, generalized)
Confusion
Acute psychiatric symptoms
Depressed level of consciousness (drowsiness, coma)
Respiratory failure
Hemiparesis
Ataxia
Jittery movements
Hemisensory loss
Speech impairment, mutism
Visual impairment (transient obscurations, reduced acuity, blindness)
Cranial nerve palsies (VI)
Papilloedema

adults.[20] Risk factors are different for the neonatal and older age groups, and individual patients frequently have multiple risk factors. Common risk factors for CSVT in adults, such as malignancy,[36,37] pregnancy[38] and oral contraceptive use,[39] are relatively rare in children.

In neonates, risk factors consist of normal physiological factors including a relatively increased haematocrit and the forced overlapping of cranial sutures during the birth process, acute neonatal illnesses and prothrombotic disorders. Pre-eclampsia in the mother may be a risk factor.[40] In neonates studied in the Canadian Registry, acute systemic insults or illnesses were present in 84% and frequently overlapped in individual neonates. The most frequent risk factors were perinatal complications including asphyxia or hypoxic-ischaemic encephalopathy (HIE), which were reported in 51%[3] and may be under-diagnosed.[41] Of note, HIE is likely to be over-diagnosed in neonates with CSVT since both asphyxia and CSVT present with seizures and lethargy, but CSVT has also been frequently found on cerebral angiography or MR venography performed in neonates with established asphyxia.[41,42]

Dehydration accounted for 30% of cases in the Canadian Registry and can be associated with hypernatraemia.[43,44] The other neonatal illnesses were systemic bacterial sepsis (16%) and head or neck disorders (16%) including meningitis, vascular malformations and other pathologies including a variety of perinatal complications in addition to birth asphyxia.

In older infants and children, clinical risk factors (pre-existing diagnoses and/or infection and/or dehydration; Table 7.1) are found in the majority of patients. CSVT occurs in various everyday clinical settings, including infection, dehydration, renal failure, trauma, cancer, cardiac disease and haematological disorder,[2–4,6,45–47] but as there is often difficulty in making the diagnosis, data for incidence remain a minimum estimate.[3] Postoperative (e.g. adenotonsillectomy, cardiopulmonary bypass, neurosurgery) CSVT has almost certainly been under-recognized.[6,48,49] A wide variety of chronic diseases, usually diagnosed prior to presentation (Table 7.1), are found in around 60% of patients, many of whom have multiple clinical and laboratory risk factors[4,6]. Although the diagnosis is rarely recognized in those undergoing surgery or catherization,[49] structural cardiac disease is found in up to 10% of children[3,4,6], and up to 25% of neonates.[50] Acute systemic insults or illnesses make up a further third. Hypoxic-ischaemic insults and acute hypoxia may be an under-recognized cause.[51–53] The most frequent is dehydration (around 20%), which in many cases develops in the setting of a viral gastroenteritis with vomiting and diarrhoea.

Common infections, including ear infections,[54] sinusitis[55] and meningitis,[56] may be complicated by CSVT. Head and neck infections resulting in 'septic' CSVT are present in 23% of older infants and children and are particularly common in preschool children.[3] Although the frequency of septic thombosis is decreasing, because of antibiotic development, recent studies have shown that it is still responsible for a substantial proportion of thrombosis in older children.[2–4,6,47] Human immunodeficiency virus[57] and other infections more commonly seen in tropical countries, e.g. neurocystercercosis,[58] may also be associated with CSVT.

Certain chronic illnesses such as inflammatory bowel disease,[59,60] systemic lupus erythematosus,[61,62] Behçet disease,[63] Cushing syndrome,[64] and thyrotoxicosis[65,66] appear to predispose to CVST, which may present in unusual ways, including psychiatric manifestations,[67] particularly if the deep venous system is involved.[68,69] Other conditions, such as nephrotic syndrome[6,70–76] or gastroenteritis,[3,6] may be associated with CVST in the context of dehydration. CSVT has also been reported in Down syndrome[77] and homocystinuria.[78,79]

Underlying haematological disorders (Table 7.3) account for around 20% of childhood CSVT.[3] The use of steroids, as well as L-asparaginase, appears to be important in leukaemia.[80,81] CSVT occurs in the context of chronic haemolytic anaemia including Evans' syndrome,[82] beta-thalassaemia major,[83] paroxysmal nocturnal haemoglobinuria[84,85] and sickle cell disease.[6,86–89] Iron deficiency anaemia and microcytosis are associated with childhood CSVT,[6,23,70,90–94] sometimes in association with thrombocytosis. Lead poisoning and sideroblastic anaemia may also be associated with dural sinus thrombosis[95,96] which may cause acute encephalopathy in children.[97] Anaemia may be obscured by relative haemo-concentration in children who are dehydrated and ferritin may be an acute phase protein, so the diagnosis of iron deficiency should be comprehensively excluded or treated.

Although occasionally recognized, there are few data on the prevalence of CSVT in convulsive and non-convulsive seizures and status epilepticus[98] and otherwise unexplained hydrocephalus.[6,19,33] CSVT may also be an important determinant of outcome in coma of traumatic[99–101] and non-traumatic origin, including diabetic ketoacidosis[93] and cerebral malaria.[102] Minor head injury may be associated with CSVT,[99,103–109] as may extradural[110] and subdural[111–113] haematoma. CSVT is certainly an important differential but the question of whether this is an important component of the pathophysiology of non-accidental injury has received little attention.[113]

Clinical features (Table 7.2)
The clinical features of CSVT are subtle, diffuse, frequently associated with seizures (Table 7.2), and typically develop gradually over hours, days or even weeks. Variables influencing the clinical presentation include the age of the child, the extent and location of the thrombus, and the presence or absence of venous infarction. Concomitant underlying diseases involving the nervous system (including asphyxia or meningitis) can cause additional neurological signs.

In neonates, in spite of the presence of venous infarcts in over one third of cases, seizures and lethargy are frequent and focal neurological deficits are rare.[47,50,114,115] In the Canadian Paediatric Ischaemic Stroke Registry, a population-based prospective registry composed of 160 consecutive paediatric patients with CSVT, only 6% of neonates with CSVT had hemiparesis. In contrast, the majority of neonates presented with seizures (72%) and diffuse signs including jitteriness and lethargy (59%).[3,14,24] Physical findings of a tense fontanelle, splaying of cranial sutures, dilated scalp veins and swelling of the eyelids, are found in infants with extensive CSVT.[116]

In older infants and children, seizures are present in nearly half of cases. Even more frequent symptoms are headache, papilloedema and decreased level of consciousness resulting from raised intracranial pressure.[3,4,6] Presentation with pseudotumour cerebri[117,118] and isolated headache[119] have been well-documented, although this is a very rare presentation in children compared with the number of children with migraine and tension headache.[120] The headache and papilloedema secondary to CSVT are indistinguishable from pseudotumour cerebri.[6] Sinus thrombosis has been found in 25% of patients with pseudotumour cerebri undergoing angiography[121] and there is increasing evidence for an association between lateral sinus stenosis, perhaps related to CSVT, and pseudotumour cerebri.[122,123] Visual disturbances are present in around one-fifth of children, in most cases related to papilloedema or sixth nerve palsy.

TABLE 7.3
Laboratory investigations in cryptogenic cerebral venous sinus thrombosis

Essential
Blood culture
Full blood count
Iron studies
Thyroid function
Antinuclear antibody or DNA binding

Potentially useful
Homocysteine
Vitamin status, i.e. folate, B_6, B_{12}
Full prothrombotic screen (DNA and citrated samples)

TABLE 7.4
Diagnosis of sinovenous thrombosis

High index of suspicion in children with associated pre-existing disorder
High index of suspicion in children presenting with headache, seizures, coma
Plain CT insufficient to rule out CSVT
MRI (T1-, T2-weighted, T2*, FLAIR)
MRI with contrast
Diffusion-weighted MRI
CT venography
MR venography
Contrast MR venography
Transcranial Doppler
Conventional angiography

FLAIR, fluid attenuated inversion recovery.

LABORATORY INVESTIGATION (Table 7.3)
High D-dimer levels are associated with the diagnosis of CSVT, while low levels make the diagnosis very unlikely.[124] It is important to exclude treatable underlying conditions including infection, iron deficiency anaemia, thyrotoxicosis and systemic lupus erythematosus (Table 7.3). Prothrombotic testing is more controversial, as it is expensive, but the yield is high, although finding an abnormality may not alter management.

Prothrombotic risk factors (Table 7.3) (see also Chapter 5, Section 5.2)
Prothrombotic abnormalities (Table 7.3) have been described in 15–20% of neonates with CSVT.[3,24,115,125] The presence of anticardiolipin antibodies (ACLA) is the most frequent finding. The persistence and contribution of these abnormalities to the causation of neonatal CSVT have not been defined.[4,6,24] The presence of congenital or acquired prothrombotic disorders has been reported in 33 to 96% of children with CSVT, with the latter figure representing children with otherwise idiopathic CSVT.[4–6,24,61,125–130] Although the yield for investigating idiopathic CSVT is higher,[5] prothrombotic disorders probably play a role in septic CSVT[54] and perhaps in other symptomatic cases. These figures exceed the estimates in adults with CSVT, in whom the incidence of prothrombotic disorders is 15–21%.[131,132] Congenital disorders that have been reported include activated protein C resistance and Factor V Leiden, Prothrombin gene G20210A, dysfibrinogenaemia, deficiencies of protein C, protein S, antithrombin, plasminogen, and factor XII and high factor VIII levels.[6,115,133,134]

Acquired prothrombotic states are more frequent than congenital prothrombotic disorders, and include ACLA, lupus anticoagulant, acquired activated protein C resistance, and acquired protein C, protein S and antithrombin deficiencies, which may co-exist in individual patients.[129,135,136] Hyperhomocysteinaemia may be an important risk factor for genetic and acquired origin.[6,137] The presence of ACLA is the single most common prothrombotic disorder in children with CSVT. However, ACLAs are frequently transient and may be merely associations with CSVT or with underlying diseases and their role in the causation of CSVT is not known. Heterozygosity

for prothrombin G20210A appears to be associated with recurrence.[138]

Radiographic diagnosis and features (Table 7.4)
In order to confirm the diagnosis of CSVT it is necessary to either image the thrombus within sinovenous channels, or image a reduction or obliteration of venous flow within the affected venous sinus. The following section presents a summary of the various diagnostic studies for CSVT and a description of the radiographic features including location of thrombosis and frequency and location of venous infarcts.

A number of radiographic techniques are used for the diagnosis of CSVT.[139]

CT
CT is still the initial test used in children with suspected CSVT however, plain CT misses the diagnosis in most children. On a non-contrast CT, signs of CSVT include the 'filled triangle' or 'dense triangle' sign, and the 'cord sign' which reflect the presence of a thrombus in sinovenous channels (Fig. 7.3). On a contrast enhanced CT, an empty triangle or 'delta sign' represents bright contrast enhancement of the dura surrounding a clot in the sinovenous system (Fig. 7.4). CT will usually also show any associated intraparenchymal, subarachnoid or intraventricular[30,140–142] haemorrhage (Fig. 7.5). However, CT has significant limitations in the diagnosis of CSVT. First, CT misses the presence of CSVT in 16–40% of children and adults and underestimate both the extent of sinus involvement and the presence of infarcts.[3,20,47,121,143] The lack of sensitivity of CT is likely to be related in part to the location of the sinuses adjacent to the bony skull, since CT is subject to significant interference by 'bone artifact'. Second, CT can yield falsely positive results.[144] This is particularly true for neonates, in whom increased haematocrit,[145] decreased unmyelinated brain density and slower venous flow can combine to produce a high-density triangle in the torcular area mimicking the 'dense triangle' sign.[146] CT venography is superior to conventional CT because of increased resolution and intravascular contrast, but the sensitivity of this technique remains to be proven.[12,147] In neonates in whom slow flow and smaller transverse sinus channels can cause flow alterations in

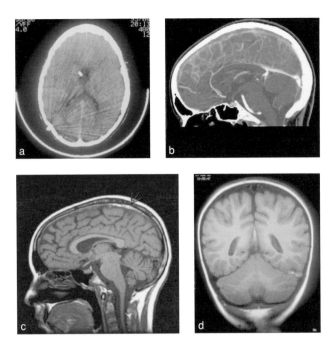

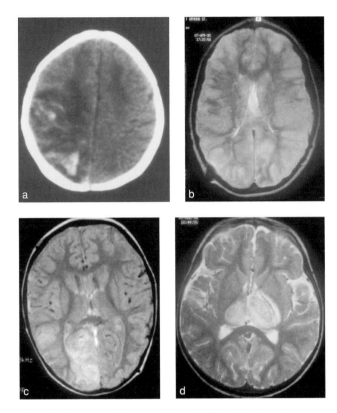

Fig. 7.3. Examples of thrombosis in the straight sinus on CT (a,b), and in the sagittal (c) and transverse (d) sinus on MRI.

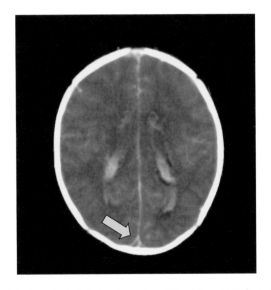

Fig. 7.4. 'Empty delta' sign (arrow) on CT with contrast in a child with sinovenous thrombosis.

the sinuses, CT venography may be superior to MRV because the administration of contrast clarifies the actual anatomy within the sinuses rather than simply the flow signal.

MRI and MRV

MRI is the currently the diagnostic study of choice in CSVT. The increased sensitivity and specificity of MRI/MRV compared with CT reflect the capacity of MRI to visualize flow, the presence of thrombus (Fig. 7.3), clot progression and resolution over time and associated parenchymal lesions (Fig. 7.7).[121,138,143,148–151] On MRI, thrombus appears as an increased signal on T1-weighted, proton density and T2-weighted images in a cerebral vein or dural sinus (Fig. 7.3).

Fig. 7.5. Examples of venous ischaemia/infarction throughout one hemisphere – with haemorrhage on CT (a), or on MRI in the parieto-occipital region bilaterally (b), the occipital lobe (c) and bilaterally in the thalami (d).

The signal characteristics of the thrombus change over time and permit approximate ageing of acute, subacute or chronic thrombus.[148] The rate and extent of recanalization after CSVT has not been established; however in adults partial or full recanalization is seen in at least 25% of cases and occurs as early as 2 weeks after symptom onset.[148,151] Recanalization may not occur in those with a subacute onset.[6] Recent modifications to the MRI technique include the 'single-slice thick slab phase-contrast angiography' (SSPCA) technique which takes less than 30 seconds to acquire, and provides a reliable and rapid technique for the diagnosis of CSVT.[152] MRV may show lack of flow in the sinuses (Fig. 7.6), although artefacts and anatomical variation may make interpretation difficult. MRV techniques utilizing gadolinium enhancement (e.g. ATECO techniques) show great promise and may be the best non-invasive method, with the added benefit of avoiding the significant contrast load and radiation dose associated with CT venography.

Ultrasound

In young infants in the presence of an open fontanelle, Doppler flow ultrasound provides an inexpensive non-invasive means of screening for and monitoring the course of CSVT[153,154] and there is now some experience with venous transcranial duplex sonography to monitor venous flow patterns in CSVT in older patients.[155] Doppler ultrasound is most successful at defining total obstruction of the sinus, since residual flow through areas of partial sinus occlusion may appear normal. Regular cranial

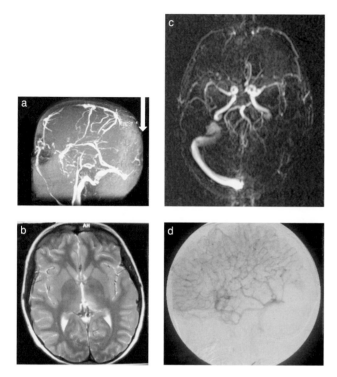

Fig. 7.6. Vascular imaging in venous sinus thrombosis. (a,b) Images from a child with a chronic haemolytic anaemia and recent onset of a butterfly rash over the face. She presented with confusion and was thought to have cerebral systemic lupus erythematosus with 'cerebral lupus' but an magnetic resonance venogram (MRV) demonstrated lack of flow in the posterior part of the superior sagittal sinus (a; arrow) with normal parenchymal imaging (b) and she recovered after treatment with intravenous heparin (c). MRV in a child with sickle cell disease who presented with seizures and coma after 2 weeks of headache and vomiting. The right sigmoid and lateral (transverse) sinus can be clearly seen, while the straight sinus and left sigmoid and transverse sinuses have been obliterated. (d) Digital subtraction arteriography 5 months after presentation in the 3-year-old boy with iron deficiency and occipital abnormality in Fig. 7.5c showing chronically poor filling in the sagittal sinus.

ultrasound is useful for monitoring the presence and severity of centrally located cerebral haemorrhage associated with CSVT, for example intraventricular haemorrhage which in term infants has been found to be associated with CSVT in approximately one-third[50] and may be demonstrated in preterm infants.[142]

Conventional angiography
Conventional angiography (Fig. 7.6D) remains the reference test if CSVT cannot be confirmed by CTV or MRI/MRV. Partial or complete lack of filling of cerebral veins or sinuses is the usual finding in CSVT, although anatomical variants including hypoplastic left transverse sinus can be difficult to differentiate from partial thrombosis. The other angiographic features of CSVT include enlarged collateral veins, delayed venous emptying, reversal of normal venous flow direction, abnormal cortical veins (broken or corkscrew-like), and regional or global delayed venous flow.[121,156] Since angiography is an invasive procedure, which may cause local thrombosis at the site of catheter entry, particularly in small infants with small

vessels, conventional angiography is rarely performed when CTV or MRI/MRV are available. In the Canadian Registry fewer than 10% of children underwent conventional angiography.[3]

LOCATION OF THROMBOSIS
CSVT in children most commonly involves multiple sinovenous channels. The 'superficial sinovenous system', including the sagittal sinus and related lateral sinus (typically right sided), is involved in 61% of patients and the remainder have thrombosis in the 'deep system' including internal cerebral veins, vein of Galen, straight sinus or related lateral sinus (typically left). The cavernous sinus and inferior sagittal sinus are rarely involved. In the Canadian Registry, the superior sagittal sinus was involved in 58% of patients, the lateral sinus(es) in 54% and the straight sinus in 25%.[3] Cortical vein thrombosis is difficult to diagnose,[156] and was found in only 10%, similar to the involvement of the internal cerebral veins (10%).

VENOUS INFARCTS
The frequency of venous infarction associated with CSVT is similar for children across various age groups, however neonates are more likely to have haemorrhagic components to their infarcts. In the Canadian Registry, 58% of neonates had no infarcts, 35% had haemorrhagic infarcts and 7% had bland infarcts. In older infants and children, 59% had no infarcts, 23% had haemorrhagic infarcts and 18% had bland infarcts.[3] Venous infarcts related to the thrombosis within the superficial system are located in the hemispheric cortex and white matter and can be unilateral or bilateral. With thrombosis of the 'deep' system, the infarcts are usually located in one or both thalami or the cerebellum.

Acute treatment (Tables 7.5 and 7.6)

GENERAL TREATMENT
Acute supportive therapy includes maintenance of hydration, antibiotics, adequate blood pressure, normoglycaemia and aggressive therapy for seizures[98] (Fig. 7.7), as well as appropriate treatment of the underlying cause. These are important to minimize the risk of propagation of the thrombus, and the extent of cerebral damage (Tables 7.5 and 7.6). For unconscious patients measures aimed at monitoring and managing intracranial pressure and preventing cerebral herniation, including surgical decompression,[157,158] may be life-saving (Tables 7.5 and 7.6). Antibiotic treatment should be discussed with the local microbiologist. Anaerobic cover such as metronidazole and clindamycin or vancomycin may be required to cover organisms such as *Fusobacterium necrophorum* in Lemierre syndrome (jugular venous thrombosis associated with anaerobic infection of the head and neck)[159] or aspergillosis.[160] For otitis media with or without mastoiditis, high dose antibiotic therapy can assist in promoting recanalization of the lateral sinus. The role of mastoidectomy is controversial[161] but some patients develop otitic hydrocephalus and may require shunting.

TABLE 7.5
Acute management of sinovenous thrombosis

Supportive treatment
Rehydration
Treat infection, e.g. antibiotics for meningitis/mastoiditis/pharyngitis
Treat cause, e.g. mastoidectomy, steroids for systemic lupus
   erythematosus, inflammatory bowel
Treat seizures
Treat iron deficiency

**Anticoagulate/monitor for 3–6 months whether or not there is
haemorrhage**
Intravenous heparin/activated partial thromboplastin time (APPT)
Subcutaneous LMWH/anti-factor Xa
Warfarin/international normalised ratio

**Possible management for seriously ill patients not improving with
anticoagulation**
Thrombolysis
Thrombectomy
Surgical decompression

TABLE 7.6
Monitoring of patient with acute sinovenous thrombosis

Clinical seizures (duration, semiology)
Level of consciousness (Glasgow Coma Scale adapted for children)
Focal neurological signs, e.g. hemiparesis
Visual acuity and fields

For those on intravenous heparin:
   4-hourly APPT
For those on subcutaneous low molecular weight heparin:
   Daily anti-factor Xa

For those who are not anticoagulated:
   Repeat venous neuroimaging at 5 days to check for further
      propagation of thrombus

For those who are unconscious and/or ventilated:
   Continuous EEG monitoring to detect seizures (Fig. 7.7)
   Intracranial pressure monitoring
   Repeat neuroimaging

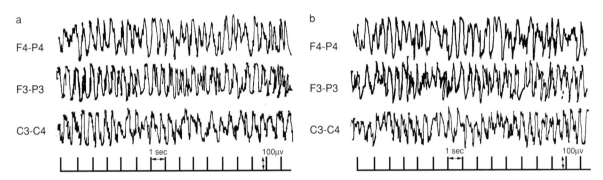

Fig. 7.7. (a,b) Oxford Medilog continuous electroencephalogram (EEG) trace from a 4-year-old girl with cavernous sinus thrombosis showing a very prolonged electrographic seizure, which commenced at 01:30. The discharges continued unrecognized by the nursing staff until 05:00. Subsequently the EEG became isoelectric and the child died a brain death.

ANTICOAGULANT TREATMENT
Anticoagulant therapy for childhood CSVT is controversial and non-standardized, reflecting the lack of clinical trials for this condition. In the absence of intracranial haemorrhage treatment of children and neonates with CSVT with either heparin or low molecular weight heparin is justified.[3,115] In the past decade, in the Canadian Registry, 37% of neonates and 67% of older infants and children with CSVT received anticoagulant medications without major haemorrhagic complications. The medications used were low molecular weight heparin in 32%, unfractionated heparin in 22% and warfarin in 39%.[3]

The increasing tendency to treat childhood CSVT with anticoagulants is based on several lines of evidence including the established risk of propagation or recurrence of the thrombosis in childhood CSVT, the compelling data on the efficacy and safety of heparin in adults with clinical trials,[11] and the evidence for safety of anticoagulants in children.[6,138,162,163] The efficacy and safety of heparin in adults with CSVT include four randomized controlled trials.[10,164–166] The one randomized placebo controlled trial of intravenous heparin in adults[164] was stopped early because there was clear evidence of benefit, in terms of mortality. A randomized placebo controlled trial

of subcutaneous low molecular weight heparin in adults[10] showed a trend for better outcome in the treated group, but the mortality was lower in this series and there were more patients with milder presentations in the placebo arm. There are currently no randomized data in the paediatric age group. Single-centre and small multi-centre series in children[6,24,138,167,168] have shown that intravenous and subcutaneous low molecular weight heparin (LMWH) can be used safely in children, provided that there is close attention to detail, particularly in terms of monitoring APPT for intravenous heparin or anti-Xa levels for subcutaneous heparin. However, case reports and cohort studies in which anticoagulant treatment is non-standardized, such as the Canadian Registry, cannot establish the efficacy of anticoagulants in children with CSVT since treatment is highly selected and likely to be biased. Cohort studies in which consecutive children with CSVT are treated with anticoagulants using standardized protocols are now becoming available, therefore the safety of anticoagulants in this population can be established. One large prospective consecutive cohort study has assessed the safety of anticoagulants for a variety of childhood thrombotic events. In that study 146 children (33% neonates) including 15 with CSVT and 29 with arterial ischaemic stroke were treated, in the absence of contraindications, with therapeutic doses of LMWH. The study showed a 5% rate of major haemorrhages, which occured predominantly in neonates.[162]

One cohort study has reported on anticoagulant therapy used in consecutive children with CSVT.[163] In 30 children, eight were ineligible for anticoagulation because of significant intracranial haemorrhage at diagnosis. However 10 children received initial unfractionated heparin (UFH) and 12 initial LMWH. The majority of children (18) then received warfarin for 3 months. There were no extensions of the CSVT, although two children had recurrent CSVT during the chronic phase of anticoagulation and only one child who received UFH had a clinically silent intracranial haemorrhage during therapy. Mortality was three out of eight of those ineligible for treatment, mainly because of haemorrhage, compared with none of the 22 who were anticoagulated. The same group has recently shown that propagation of thrombus is more common in those who were not anticoagulated and that, although there was haemorrhages in those who were anticoagulated, none was fatal and while outcome was not worsened by haemorrhage, one of the predictors of poor outcome was propagation.[169] Another series suggested that cognitive outcome might be better in the anticoagulated group[6] (see below). However, death is uncommon in this age group and many children have apparently made a full recovery without anticoagulation, although long term follow-up data are scanty.

Concerns about anticoagulant treatment in CSVT include a potential for intracerebral haemorrhage, given the frequency of haemorrhagic venous infarction, and a perception that treatment is not needed because the outcome is uniformly good in childhood CSVT. In the published adult trials the authors have emphasized that patients with initial haemorrhagic infarction who were treated benefited from heparin therapy.[121,164] The outcome for CSVT in childhood is not necessarily benign; in the Canadian Registry, between 40% and 50% of children in all age groups died or had neurological deficits resulting from the CSVT, and 13% experienced propogation or recurrence of thrombosis.

The results from the adult trials and childhood consecutive cohort studies suggest that anticoagulant therapy should be considered in children with CSVT and that clinical trials assessing the potential benefit of anticoagulants are urgently needed, particularly in neonates where the risk–benefit ratio of anticoagulants is likely to differ from adults. Large multicentre randomized controlled trials will be necessary to establish efficacy. Whether older children could ethically be randomized to placebo in light of the strong evidence for efficacy in adult studies is questionable. However, since neonates differ markedly from older age groups, a randomized controlled trial, assessing anticoagulants for neonatal CSVT, would be justifiable.

Several factors will influence the decision to treat individual patients, and the duration of treatment.[8,169] The extent of the thrombus, presence and extent of associated haemorrhage, transiency of risk factors of the CSVT, and the ability to monitor anticoagulant therapy are all factors to consider. While awaiting more definitive evidence on which to base therapy, one approach is to treat neonates with UFH or LMWH for 10 to 14 days and reassess[170] (see Chapter 16). The current treatment regimen for neonates by the author consists initially of 6 weeks of anticoagulation in the absence of contraindications followed by an additional 6 weeks only if persistent thrombus is seen on MRV or CTV at 6 weeks. During the treatment of neonates with anticoagulants, ultrasound can be used to monitor for haemorrhage and in some patients, with Doppler added, for extension of the thrombus. For older infants and children, UFH or LMWH for 7–10 days followed by warfarin or LMWH for 3 to 6 months should be considered (see Chapter 16), as given to most adults with CSVT. After anticoagulant therapy is discontinued, a repeat radiographic assessment confirming the absence of extension of the thrombus is suggested.

THROMBOLYTIC THERAPY

There are no randomized data on thrombolysis[171–173] or thrombectomy[174] in CVST even in adults, but each has been used with apparent success in isolated cases or small series of seriously ill patients, usually in coma and with extensive thrombosis of superficial and deep venous structures.[172,173] A non-randomized study comparing urokinase thrombolysis with heparin in adults suggested better functional outcome for the thrombolysed patients but higher risk of haemorrhage.[175] In situations where there is progression of the CSVT in spite of maximal systemic anticoagulation, local intra-clot thrombolytic treatment has been used in adults and children with CSVT.[169,171,175–178] Failure of local thrombolytic therapy has also been reported.[179] Since the risk–benefit ratio of thrombolytic therapy is not known in adults or children, and the haemorrhagic risks of thrombolytic therapy may be considerable in children outside of controlled trials, the use of thrombolytic therapy should, in general, be discouraged.

Long-term management

'BENIGN' INTRACRANIAL HYPERTENSION (PSEUDOTUMOUR CEREBRI)

In the chronic phase, measures to relieve the diffuse cerebral swelling, which can persist for many weeks or months, include repeated lumbar puncture with the removal of CSF, treatment with acetazolamide, and in intractable cases, lumbo-peritoneal shunt.[180,181] It is important to monitor both the severity of papilloedema and visual field defects during these prolonged periods of raised intracranial pressure.[182] Rarely, when visual loss is progressing in spite of maximal therapy aimed at reducing intracranial pressure, optic nerve sheath fenestration is performed.

PREVENTION OF RECURRENCE

Between 10% and 20% of children who have a cerebral venous sinus thrombosis will experience a recurrent symptomatic venous event, at least half of which are systemic rather than

TABLE 7.7
Management of risk factors to prevent recurrence

Improve diet, e.g. 5 portions of fruit and/or vegetables per day
Reduce cows' milk intake and increase solids in infants and toddlers
Treat cause, e.g. steroids for sytemic lupus erythematosus, inflammatory bowel
Suggest alternative contraception
Treat iron deficiency
Treat hyperhomocysteinaemia/frank vitamin deficiency, e.g. folate, B_6 or B_{12}
Consider prolonged oral anticoagulation after recurrence

cerebral.[138] In one study, non-administration of anticoagulant before relapse (hazard ratio [HR] 11.2, 95% CI 3.4–37.0; $p<0.0001$), persistent occlusion on repeat venous imaging (4.1, 1.1–14.8; $p=0.032$) and heterozygosity for the G20210A mutation in factor II (4.3, 1.1–16.2; $p=0.034$) were independently associated with recurrent venous thrombosis.[138] There are, however, few robust predictors of recurrence and there have been no trials of preventative strategies in children or adults. There is a little evidence that stopping the use of oral contraceptives reduces the risk. There are several low risk strategies, such as improving the quality of the diet, which can be recommended (Table 7.7). It would be difficult to recommend a higher risk strategy, such as prolonged oral anticoagulation, unless significant risks for recurrence are present.

Mortality
Large cohort studies in adults with CSVT report mortality rates ranging from 14% to 36%.[121,143] The overall death rate in the two major adult randomized controlled trials of anticoagulation was 11%, and was 14–30% in control patients compared with 0–7% in patients treated with heparin or LMWH. Of note, both trials randomized patients with haemorrhagic venous infarction[10,164].

There is some evidence that mortality with CSVT is less in children compared with adults. In the historical cohort of 150 children with CSVT derived from pooled literature analysis, 9% received anticoagulants and the mortality was 9%.[163] However, historical or literature derived controls could over- or under-estimate mortality because of publication and time bias. In the Canadian Registry 53% of 160 children were treated with anticoagulants and the mortality rate was 8%.[3] Of 17 children in the Dutch study,[183] five died, one of CSVT. The three (18%) who died acutely were not anticoagulated. Of 396 children enrolled in the European Collaborative Paediatric Database, 12 (3%) died, 12 children died within 2 weeks of presentation with a first episode of CSVT, only one of whom had received anticoagulation. Causes of death were severe infection in three, intracranial haemorrhaging in two and brain herniation after severe brain oedema in seven cases. In a multicentre cohort study from the USA reported by Wasays et al,[8] overall mortality was 13% (9/70) but 25% (6/25) of neonates died. One patient who underwent thrombolysis died, one died in the anticoagulation treatment group and seven children in the antibiotic/hydration group died.[8]

Neurological outcome
The long-term outcome of CSVT in children is difficult to assess for several reasons, including the relatively small numbers of children with CSVT at any one institution, non-standardized outcome assessment and insufficient duration of follow-up. It is difficult to adjust for the potential influence of anticoagulants on outcomes given their inconsistent use. Multicentre studies and long-term follow-up of consecutive children with CSVT, combined with a standardized approach to using anticoagulants, will be needed to fully define outcome. Factors that may influence outcome include the age at the time of the event, rapidity of diagnosis, extent of the thrombosis, associated neurological disorders and the use of anticoagulants.

The outcome following CSVT is likely to be influenced by the age of the child at the time of the event, with younger ages traditionally being expected to have a better outcome. However, recent evidence shows that in rats, the neonatal brain is more susceptible to hypoxic-ischaemic injury.[184] Clinical manifestations of damage sustained in the neonatal period from CSVT will likely be delayed as has been shown for other forms of cerebral ischaemia in neonates because of ongoing acquisition during childhood of developmental milestones.[185] The delay in clinical neurological signs is related to the relatively immature brain in the neonate, and the maturational changes in the nervous system during the first year of life when myelination, neuronal pruning and synapse modelling are occurring. The practical implication is that prognostication in individual neonates and very young infants is difficult, and probably unreliable.

In neonates with CSVT, 37 of 63 (59%) in a large recent study had neurological deficitor death.[169] Previous case series have reported conflicting outcomes, with some reporting disability or death in 38–50%[47,115] and others reporting a normal outcome in over 90% of neonates with CSVT.[114] However, the study reporting a normal outcome in most infants used only CT without confirmatory MRI or CT or MR venography, and the follow-up interval was less than 1 year in half of the patients.

DeVeber et al[163] reviewed the previously available literature and found 150 patients with CVT reported, 136 of whom had not been anticoagulated. Mortality was 16% and poor neurological outcome was documented in 22% of the untreated. Thirty additional patients were reported, including eight who were not anticoagulated; three of this group died. Holzmann[186] and Lancon[187] reported mainly good outcome in patients with lateral sinus thrombosis who were not anticoagulated, although details were scanty in these neurosurgical series. In Carvalho's[2] series of 12 non-neonates from Indianapolis, none of whom were treated, two died, neither of CSVT (one brain tumour, one leukaemia) and of 10 survivors followed up, six (60%) had normal outcome; no data were reported on recurrent CVT or peripheral venous thrombosis. Interestingly, in this series of non-anticoagulated patients, five out of 19 neonates had haemorrhage on initial imaging and one out of 12 of the older children had haemorrhagic conversion of an infarct. Anticoagulation is often withheld in children with

VST and intracranial haemorrhage, although there is no evidence for an enhanced risk of extension of haemorrhage.

There are several recent studies that provide insight into the long-term outcome of CSVT in children.[3,6,8,169,188,189] First, in a consecutive cohort study of 68 children, 43 (63%) were normal and the remainder had neurological deficits at long-term follow-up.[169] Previously in a single centre consecutive cohort study 38 infants and children who survived CSVT were assessed using a standard outcome measure and protocol.[189] In the study, 26% of patents received anticoagulants. The mean follow-up was 2.1 years with a range of 0.8–6.6 years. Two-thirds of the children were neurologically normal, including 14 of 18 neonates and 10 of 19 older infants and children, and one-third had neurological deficits. The neurological deficits were mild in seven and moderate or severe with functional consequences in the other seven. Additional outcomes included seizures in 16%, headaches in 24%, and recurrent thromboembolism in two patients. In the latter study the EuroQuol outcome measure[190,191] was modified and assessed in a subset of children. The parental impression was of complete recovery in two-thirds including seven of 10 neonates and seven out of 11 older infants and children. In the same study, one-third of the neonates with arterial ischaemic stroke showed an increasing number and severity of neurological deficits over time, emphasizing the importance of longitudinal study in neonatal cerebrovascular injury.[189]

Second in is the Canadian Registry, 160 children with CSVT were followed for a mean of 1.13 years and mortality data were included.[3] In this study nearly 50% of neonates had either neurological impairments or had died 1 year following the event. Overall, 55% of all children were normal, 35% had a neurological deficit and 8% died. Age was not a predictor of outcome. The neurological deficits were motor (80%), cognitive (10%), developmental delay (9%), speech deficits (6%), visual deficits (6%) and other (26%). Of the 12 (8%) deaths, six were attributable to CSVT. There were seizures at follow-up in 15% and recurrent events in 13%.[3] Predictors of adverse neurological outcomes included seizures in non-neonates at presentation and the presence of infarcts (bland or haemorrhagic) in all patients.

In De Schryver's[183] series, 12 survivors returned for follow-up. Five survivors who were not anticoagulated had normal IQ but one had cognitive difficulties and behavioural problems. Two received heparin and four oral anticoagulation. One had impairment of fine movement but none of the others had neurological sequelae and IQ was normal in 10 tested (two were excluded as their command of Dutch was insufficient), although two who had had lateral sinus thrombosis after mastoiditis had mild cognitive difficulties. Decreased physical well-being was described on the Child Health Questionnaire in three of the 12 for whom this was completed.

In Sébire's study,[6] five patients died, three acutely and two later; one during a recurrent episode of CSVT and one with severe neurological sequelae, respectively 3 and 6 months after the initial event. For the 37 survivors, follow-up ranged from 6 months to 10 years (median 1 year). Eleven children had no neurological or cognitive difficulties at follow-up. Twelve had symptoms and signs compatible with chronic pseudotumour cerebri and 14 had cognitive difficulties (of whom two had a permanent hemiparesis, three had reduced visual acuity and two developed epilepsy). None of the patients with cognitive difficulties was diagnosed with pseudotumour cerebri. Anticoagulated patients were more likely to have good cognitive outcome, with a statistical trend of borderline significance, and a reduction in mortality which was not statistically significant. There was no association between persistent thrombosis visible at follow-up venography (*N*=19) and death, cognitive sequelae or pseudotumour cerebri, but two of the three patients with epilepsy as an outcome had persistent occlusion. The only statistically significant association with death was an admission Glasgow Coma Score <12. Chronic pseudotumour cerebri was more common in those with lateral and/or sigmoid sinus involvement. In multiple logistic regression, older age, involvement of the lateral and/or sigmoid sinus, lack of parenchymal abnormality and anticoagulation were all independent predictors of good cognitive outcome.

In a cohort reported by Wasay et al[8] from the USA, 29 of 70 children, including neonates (41%) were normal, whereas 32 patients (46%) had a neurological deficit at discharge.

Conclusion

CSVT in children is a serious event with long-term ramifications. Neonates are at significant risk compared with older children, and aetiology can be established in the majority of children if adequate investigations are performed. The outcome even with current treatments is death or neurological deficit in nearly 50% of neonates and children. Information on the epidemiology of childhood CSVT has recently become available. These data contribute to the feasibility of developing clinical trials to provide evidence-based treatments, which will decrease the adverse outcomes. An international multicentre approach will be necessary in order to make these trials a reality.

REFERENCES

1. Teksam M, Moharir M, deVeber G, Shroff M. Frequency and topographic distribution of brain lesions in pediatric cerebral venous thrombosis. AJNR Am J Neuroradiol 2008; 29(10):1961–1965.
2. Carvalho KS, Bodensteiner JB, Connolly PJ, Garg BP. Cerebral venous thrombosis in children. J Child Neurol 2001; 16(8):574–580.
3. deVeber G, Andrew M, Adams C, Bjornson B, Booth F, Buckley DJ et al. Cerebral sinovenous thrombosis in children. N Engl J Med 2001; 345(6):417–423.
4. Heller C, Heinecke A, Junker R, Knofler R, Kosch A, Kurnik K et al. Cerebral venous thrombosis in children: a multifactorial origin. Circulation 2003; 108(11):1362–1367.
5. Kenet G, Waldman D, Lubetsky A, Kornbrut N, Khalil A, Koren A et al. Paediatric cerebral sinus vein thrombosis. A multicenter, case-controlled study. Thromb Haemost 2004; 92(4):713–718.
6. Sebire G, Tabarki B, Saunders DE, Leroy I, Liesner R, Saint-Martin C et al. Cerebral venous sinus thrombosis in children: risk factors, presentation, diagnosis and outcome. Brain 2005; 128(Pt 3): 477–489.

7. Fitzgerald KC, Williams LS, Garg BP, Carvalho KS, Golomb MR. Cerebral sinovenous thrombosis in the neonate. Arch Neurol 2006; 63(3):405–409.

8. Wasay M, Dai AI, Ansari M, Shaikh Z, Roach ES. Cerebral venous sinus thrombosis in children: a multicenter cohort from the United States. J Child Neurol 2008; 23(1):26–31.

9. Einhäupl K, Kempski O, Baethmann A (eds). Cerebral Sinus Thrombosis. New York: Plenum Press, 1991.

10. de Bruijn SF, Stam J. Randomized, placebo-controlled trial of anti-coagulant treatment with low-molecular-weight heparin for cerebral sinus thrombosis. Stroke 1999; 30(3):484–488.

11. Stam J, de Bruijn SF, deVeber G. Anticoagulation for cerebral sinus thrombosis. Cochrane Database Syst Rev 2002; (4): CD002005.

12. Casey SO, Alberico RA, Patel M, Jimenez JM, Ozsvath RR, Maguire WM et al. Cerebral CT venography. Radiology 1996; 198:163–170.

13. Hunerbein R, Reuter P, Meyer W, Kuhn FP. CT angiography of cerebral venous circulation: anatomical visualization and diagnostic pitfalls in interpretation. Rofo 1997; 167(6):612–618.

14. Rivkin MJ, Anderson ML, Kaye EM. Neonatal idiopathic cerebral venous thrombosis: an unrecognized cause of transient seizures or lethargy. Ann Neurol 1992; 32(1):51–56.

15. Lynch JK, Nelson KB, Curry CJ, Grether JK. Cerebrovascular disorders in children with the factor V Leiden mutation. J Child Neurol 2001; 16(10):735–744.

16. Capra N, Anderson K. Anatomy of the cerebral venous system. In: Knapp JP, Schmidek HH (eds). The Cerebral Venous System and it's Disorders. Orlando, USA: Grune and Stratton Inc; 1984.

17. Maroney SA, Cooley BC, Sood R, Weiler H, Mast AE. Combined tissue factor pathway inhibitor and thrombomodulin deficiency produces an augmented hypercoagulable state with tissue-specific fibrin deposition. J Thromb Haemost. 2008; 6(1):111–117.

18. Woodhall B. Variations of the cranial venous sinuses in the region of the torcular heophili. Arch Surg 1936; 33:297.

19. Norrell H, Wilson C, Howieson J, Megison L, Bertan V. Venous factors in infantile hydrocephalus. J Neurosurg 1969; 31(5): 561–569.

20. Bousser MG, Ross-Russell R. Cerebral Venous Thrombosis. Vol 1: Major J Problems in Neurology, 1st edn. London: WB Saunders; 1997.

21. Newton TH, Gooding CA. Compression of superior sagittal sinus by neonatal calvarial molding. Radiology 1975; 115(3):635–640.

22. Niv A, Nash M, Slovik Y, Fliss DM, Kaplan D, Leibovitz E et al. Acute mastoiditis in infancy: the Soroka experience:1990–2000. Int J Pediatr Otorhinolaryngol 2004; 68(11):1435–1439.

23. Maguire JL, deVeber G, Parkin PC. Association between iron-deficiency anemia and stroke in young children. Pediatrics 2007; 120(5):1053–1057.

24. deVeber G, Monagle P, Chan A, MacGregor D, Curtis R, Lee S et al. Prothrombotic disorders in infants and children with cerebral thromboembolism. Arch Neurol 1998; 55(12):1539–1543.

25. Bonduel M, Sciuccati G, Hepner M, Pieroni G, Torres AF, Frontroth JP et al. Arterial ischemic stroke and cerebral venous thrombosis in children: a 12-year Argentinean registry. Acta Haematol 2006; 115(3–4):180–185.

26. Forbes KP, Pipe JG, Heiserman JE. Evidence for cytotoxic edema in the pathogenesis of cerebral venous infarction. AJNR Am J Neuroradiol 2001; 22(3):450–455.

27. Mullins ME, Grant PE, Wang B, Gonzalez RG, Schaefer PW. Parenchymal abnormalities associated with cerebral venous sinus thrombosis: assessment with diffusion-weighted MR imaging. AJNR Am J Neuroradiol 2004; 25(10):1666–1675.

28. Marquardt G, Weidauer S, Lanfermann H, Seifert V. Cerebral venous sinus thrombosis manifesting as bilateral subdural effusion. Acta Neurol Scand 2004; 109(6):425–428.

29. Singh S, Kumar S, Joseph M, Gnanamuthu C, Alexander M. Cerebral venous sinus thrombosis presenting as subdural haematoma. Australas Radiol 2005; 49(2):101–103.

30. Sztajzel R, Coeytaux A, Dehdashti AR, Delavelle J, Sinnreich M. Subarachnoid hemorrhage: a rare presentation of cerebral venous thrombosis. Headache 2001; 41(9):889–892.

31. Adaletli I, Sirikci A, Kara B, Kurugoglu S, Ozer H, Bayram M. Cerebral venous sinus thrombosis presenting with excessive sub-arachnoid hemorrhage in a 14-year-old boy. Emerg Radiol 2005; 12(1–2):57–59.

32. Ungersbock K, Heimann A, Kempski O. Cerebral blood flow alterations in a rat model of cerebral sinus thrombosis. Stroke 1993; 24(4):563–569.

33. Weidauer S, Marquardt G, Seifert V, Zanella FE. Hydrocephalus due to superior sagittal sinus thrombosis. Acta Neurochir (Wien) 2005; 147(4):427–430.

34. Petzold A, Smith M. High intracranial pressure, brain herniation and death in cerebral venous thrombosis. Stroke 2006; 37(2):331–332.

35. Canhao P, Ferro JM, Lindgren AG, Bousser MG, Stam J, Barinagarrementeria F. Causes and predictors of death in cerebral venous thrombosis. Stroke 2005; 36(8):1720–1725.

36. Brown MT, Friedman HS, Oakes WJ, Boyko OB, Schold SC, Jr. Sagittal sinus thrombosis and leptomeningeal medulloblastoma. Neurology 1991; 41(3):455–456.

37. Hickey WF, Garnick MB, Henderson IC, Dawson DM. Primary cerebral venous thrombosis in patients with cancer – a rarely diagnosed paraneoplastic syndrome. Report of three cases and review of the literature. Am J Med 1982; 73(5):740–750.

38. Cantu C, Barinagarrementeria F. Cerebral venous thrombosis associated with pregnancy and puerperium. Review of 67 cases. Stroke 1993; 24(12):1880–1884.

39. Dindar F, Platts ME. Intracranial venous thrombosis complicating oral contraception. Can Med Assoc J 1974; 111(6):545–548.

40. Hunt RW, Badawi N, Laing S, Lam A. Pre-eclampsia: a predisposing factor for neonatal venous sinus thrombosis? Pediatr Neurol 2001; 25(3):242–246.

41. Battin MR, Teele RL. Abnormal sagittal sinus blood flow in term infants following a perinatal hypoxic ischaemic insult. Pediatr Radiol 2003; 33(8):559–562.

42. Lee BC, Voorhies TM, Ehrlich ME, Lipper E, Auld PA, Vannucci RC. Digital intravenous cerebral angiography in neonates. AJNR Am J Neuroradiol 1984; 5(3):281–286.

43. van Amerongen RH, Moretta AC, Gaeta TJ. Severe hypernatremic dehydration and death in a breast-fed infant. Pediatr Emerg Care 2001; 17(3):175–180.

44. Gebara BM, Everett KO. Dural sinus thrombosis complicating hypernatremic dehydration in a breastfed neonate. Clin Pediatr (Phila) 2001; 40(1):45–48.

45. Cottrill CM, Kaplan S. Cerebral vascular accidents in cyanotic congenital heart disease. Am J Dis Child 1973; 125(4):484–487.

46. Phornphutkul C, Rosenthal A, Nadas AS, Berenberg W. Cerebrovascular accidents in infants and children with cyanotic congenital heart disease. Am J Cardiol 1973; 32(3):329–334.

47. Barron TF, Gusnard DA, Zimmerman RA, Clancy RR. Cerebral venous thrombosis in neonates and children. Pediatr Neurol 1992; 8(2):112–116.

48. Reilly MJ, Milmoe G, Pena M. Three extraordinary complications of adenotonsillectomy. Int J Pediatr Otorhinolaryngol 2006; 70(5): 941–946.

49. Emir M, Ozisik K, Cagli K, Bakuy V, Ozisik P, Sener E. Dural sinus thrombosis after cardiopulmonary bypass. Perfusion 2004; 19(2): 133–135.

50. Wu YW, Miller SP, Chin K, Collins AE, Lomeli SC, Chuang NA et al. Multiple risk factors in neonatal sinovenous thrombosis. Neurology 2002; 59(3):438–440.

51. Saito S, Tanaka SK. A case of cerebral sinus thrombosis developed during a high-altitude expedition to Gasherbrum I. Wilderness Environ Med 2003; 14(4):226–230.

52. Torgovicky R, Azaria B, Grossman A, Eliyahu U, Goldstein L. Sinus vein thrombosis following exposure to simulated high altitude. Aviat Space Environ Med 2005; 76(2):144–146.

53. Yamamoto K, Yanagawa Y, Iwamoto S, Kaneko N, Sakamoto T, Okada Y. Case of suicide by hanging complicated by cerebral sinus thrombosis. No Shinkei Geka 2005; 33(3):251–254.

54. Oestreicher-Kedem Y, Raveh E, Kornreich L, Yaniv I, Tamary H. Prothrombotic factors in children with otitis media and sinus thrombosis. Laryngoscope 2004; 114(1):90–95.

55. Cannon ML, Antonio BL, McCloskey JJ, Hines MH, Tobin JR, Shetty AK. Cavernous sinus thrombosis complicating sinusitis. Pediatr Crit Care Med 2004; 5(1):86–88.

56. Kastenbauer S, Pfister HW. Pneumococcal meningitis in adults: spectrum of complications and prognostic factors in a series of 87 cases. Brain 2003; 126(Pt 5):1015–1025.

57. Karim MS, Athar MK, Ghobrial MW. Superior sagittal sinus thrombosis and HIV. Ann Intern Med 2002; 137(5 Pt 1):375.

58. Prasad R, Singh R, Joshi B. Lateral sinus thrombosis in neurocysticercosis. Trop Doct 2005; 35(3):182–183.

59. Kao A, Dlugos D, Hunter JV, Mamula P, Thorarensen O. Anticoagulation therapy in cerebral sinovenous thrombosis and ulcerative colitis in children. J Child Neurol 2002; 17(7):479–482.

60. Standridge S, de los RE. Inflammatory bowel disease and cerebrovascular arterial and venous thromboembolic events in 4 pediatric patients: a case series and review of the literature. J Child Neurol 2008; 23(1):59–66.

61. Uziel Y, Laxer RM, Blaser S, Andrew M, Schneider R, Silverman ED. Cerebral vein thrombosis in childhood systemic lupus erythematosus. J Pediatr 1995; 126(5 Pt 1):722–727.

62. Chan YL, Roebuck DJ, Yuen MP, Yeung KW, Lau KY, Li CK et al. Long-term cerebral metabolite changes on proton magnetic resonance spectroscopy in patients cured of acute lymphoblastic leukemia with previous intrathecal methotrexate and cranial irradiation prophylaxis. Int J Radiat Oncol Biol Phys 2001; 50(3):759–763.

63. Alper G, Yilmaz Y, Ekinci G, Kose O. Cerebral vein thrombosis in Behçet's disease. Pediatr Neurol 2001; 25(4):332–335.

64. Yoshimura S, Ago T, Kitazono T, Yonekura T, Kumai Y, Kuroda J et al. Cerebral sinus thrombosis in a patient with Cushing's syndrome. J Neurol Neurosurg Psychiatry 2005; 76(8):1182–1183.

65. Siegel MJ, Luker GD, Glauser TA, DeBaun MR. Cerebral infarction in sickle cell disease: transcranial Doppler US versus neurologic examination. Radiology 1995; 197(1):191–194.

66. Ra CS, Lui CC, Liang CL, Chen HJ, Kuo YL, Chen WF. Superior sagittal sinus thrombosis induced by thyrotoxicosis. Case report. J Neurosurg 2001; 94(1):130–132.

67. McQueen A. "I think she's just crazy". Lancet 2005; 365(9469):1513.

68. Kothare SV, Ebb DH, Rosenberger PB, Buonanno F, Schaefer PW, Krishnamoorthy KS. Acute confusion and mutism as a presentation of thalamic strokes secondary to deep cerebral venous thrombosis. J Child Neurol 1998; 13(6):300–303.

69. von MM, Stiefel M, Brockmann K, Nau R. Deep cerebral venous sinus thrombosis often presents with neuropsychologic symptoms. J Clin Neurosci 2003; 10(3):310–312.

70. Meena AK, Naidu KS, Murthy JM. Cortical sinovenous thrombosis in a child with nephrotic syndrome and iron deficiency anaemia. Neurol India 2000; 48(3):292–294.

71. Lin CC, Lui CC, Tain YL. Thalamic stroke secondary to straight sinus thrombosis in a nephrotic child. Pediatr Nephrol 2002; 17(3):184–186.

72. Rodrigues MM, Zardini LR, de Andrade MC, Mangia CM, Carvalhaes JT, Vilanova LC. Cerebral sinovenous thrombosis in a nephrotic child. Arq Neuropsiquiatr 2003; 61(4):1026–1029.

73. Gangakhedkar A, Wong W, Pitcher LA. Cerebral thrombosis in childhood nephrosis. J Paediatr Child Health 2005; 41(4):221–224.

74. Papachristou FT, Petridou SH, Printza NG, Zafeiriou DI, Gompakis NP. Superior sagittal sinus thrombosis in steroid-resistant nephrotic syndrome. Pediatr Neurol 2005; 32(4):282–284.

75. Fluss J, Geary D, deVeber G. Cerebral sinovenous thrombosis and idiopathic nephrotic syndrome in childhood: report of four new cases and review of the literature. Eur J Pediatr 2006; 165(10):709–716.

76. Balci YI, Tavil B, Fidan G, Ozaltin F. Cerebral sinovenous thrombosis in a child with steroid sensitive nephrotic syndrome. Eur J Pediatr 2007; 166(7):757–758.

77. del-Rio CG, Orozco AL, Perez-Higueras A, Camino LM, Al-Assir I, Ruiz-Moreno M. Moyamoya disease and sagittal sinus thrombosis in a child with Down's syndrome. Pediatr Radiol 2001; 31(2):125–128.

78. Buoni S, Molinelli M, Mariottini A, Rango C, Medaglini S, Pieri S et al. Homocystinuria with transverse sinus thrombosis. J Child Neurol 2001; 16(9):688–690.

79. Vorstman E, Keeling D, Leonard J, Pike M. Sagittal sinus thrombosis in a teenager: homocystinuria associated with reversible antithrombin deficiency. Dev Med Child Neurol 2002; 44(7):498.

80. Kieslich M, Porto L, Lanfermann H, Jacobi G, Schwabe D, Bohles H. Cerebrovascular complications of L-asparaginase in the therapy of acute lymphoblastic leukemia. J Pediatr Hematol Oncol 2003; 25(6):484–487.

81. Nowak-Gottl U, Ahlke E, Fleischhack G, Schwabe D, Schobess R, Schumann C et al. Thromboembolic events in children with acute lymphoblastic leukemia (BFM protocols): prednisone versus dexamethasone administration. Blood 2003; 101(7):2529–2533.

82. Shiozawa Z, Ueda R, Mano T, Tsugane R, Kageyama N. Superior sagittal sinus thrombosis associated with Evans' syndrome of haemolytic anaemia. J Neurol 1985; 232(5):280–282.

83. Incorpora G, Di GF, Romeo MA, Pavone P, Trifiletti RR, Parano E. Focal neurological deficits in children with beta-thalassemia major. Neuropediatrics 1999; 30(1):45–48.

84. Hassan KM, Varadarajulu R, Sharma SK, Motwani H, Mishra DK, Dhall A et al. Cerebral venous thrombosis in a patient of paroxysmal nocturnal haemoglobinuria following aplastic anaemia. J Assoc Physicians India 2001; 49:753–755.

85. Naithani R, Mahapatra M, Dutta P, Kumar R, Pati HP, Choudhry VP. Paroxysmal nocturnal hemoglobinuria in childhood and adolescence – a retrospective analysis of 18 cases. Indian J Pediatr 2008; 75(6):575–578.

86. Garcia JH. Thrombosis of cranial veins and sinuses: brain parenchymal effects. In: Einhaupl KM, Kempski O, Baethmann A (eds). Cerebral Sinus Thrombosis: Experimental and Clinical Aspects. New York: Plenum Press, 1990.

87. Oguz M, Aksungur EH, Soyupak SK, Yildirim AU. Vein of Galen and sinus thrombosis with bilateral thalamic infarcts in sickle cell anaemia: CT follow-up and angiographic demonstration. Neuroradiology 1994; 36(2):155–156.

88. Di RC, Jourdan C, Yilmaz H, Artru F. Cerebral deep vein thrombosis: three cases. Rev Neurol (Paris) 1999; 155(8):583–587.

89. van Mierlo TD, van den Berg HM, Nievelstein RA, Braun KP. An unconscious girl with sickle-cell disease. Lancet 2003; 361(9352):136.

90. Belman AL, Roque CT, Ancona R, Anand AK, Davis RP. Cerebral venous thrombosis in a child with iron deficiency anemia and thrombocytosis. Stroke 1990; 21(3):488–493.

91. Hartfield DS, Lowry NJ, Keene DL, Yager JY. Iron deficiency: a cause of stroke in infants and children. Pediatr Neurol 1997; 16(1):50–53.

92. Swann IL, Kendra JR. Severe iron deficiency anaemia and stroke. Clin Lab Haematol 2000; 22(4):221–223.

93. Keane S, Gallagher A, Ackroyd S, McShane MA, Edge JA. Cerebral venous thrombosis during diabetic ketoacidosis. Arch Dis Child 2002; 86(3):204–205.

94. Benedict SL, Bonkowsky JL, Thompson JA, Van Orman CB, Boyer RS, Bale JF, Jr et al. Cerebral sinovenous thrombosis in children: another reason to treat iron deficiency anemia. J Child Neurol 2004; 19(7):526–531.

95. Viader F, Bakchine S, Gaudin H, Dhermy D, Masson M, Carbon C. Lead encephalopathy with thrombosis of the superior longitudinal sinus. Ann Med Interne (Paris) 1985; 136(5):401–404.

96. Domingo-Claros A, Alonso E, Banda Ed EL. Schizophrenia and refractory anaemia with ring sideroblasts. Br J Haematol 2004; 125(5):543.

97. McLaurin RL, Nichols JB, Jr. Extensive cranial decompression in the treatment of severe lead encephalopathy. Pediatrics 1957; 20(4):653–667.

98. Ferro JM, Correia M, Rosas MJ, Pinto AN, Neves G. Seizures in cerebral vein and dural sinus thrombosis. Cerebrovasc Dis 2003; 15(1–2):78–83.

99. Stiefel D, Eich G, Sacher P. Posttraumatic dural sinus thrombosis in children. Eur J Pediatr Surg 2000; 10(1):41–44.

100. Huisman TA, Holzmann D, Martin E, Willi UV. Cerebral venous thrombosis in childhood. Eur Radiol 2001; 11(9):1760–1765.

101. Yuen HW, Gan BK, Seow WT, Tan HK. Dural sinus thrombosis after minor head injury in a child. Ann Acad Med Singapore 2005; 34(10):639–641.

102. Krishnan A, Karnad DR, Limaye U, Siddharth W. Cerebral venous and dural sinus thrombosis in severe falciparum malaria. J Infect 2004; 48(1):86–90.

103. Brors D, Schafers M, Schick B, Dazert S, Draf W, Kahle G. Sigmoid and transverse sinus thrombosis after closed head injury presenting with unilateral hearing loss. Neuroradiology 2001; 43(2): 144–146.

104. Liang CL, Yang LC, Lui CC, Hsiao M, Hung KS. Parietal contusion and transient superior sagittal sinus occlusion presenting with cortical blindness. J Trauma 2002; 53(5):1006–1009.

105. Barbati G, Dalla MG, Coletta R, Blasetti AG. Post-traumatic superior sagittal sinus thrombosis. Case report and analysis of the international literature. Minerva Anestesiol 2003; 69(12):919–925.

106. Muthukumar N. Cerebral venous sinus thrombosis and thrombophilia presenting as pseudo-tumour syndrome following mild head injury. J Clin Neurosci 2004; 11(8):924–927.

107. Sousa J, O'Brien D, Bartlett R, Vaz J. Sigmoid sinus thrombosis in a child after closed head injury. Br J Neurosurg 2004; 18(2):187–188.

108. Quinones-Hinojosa A, Binder DK, Hemphill JC, III, Manley GT. Diagnosis of posttraumatic transverse sinus thrombosis with magnetic resonance imaging/magnetic resonance venography: report of two cases. J Trauma 2004; 56(1):201–204.

109. Siegel LJ, Gerigk L, Tuettenberg J, Dempfle CE, Scharf J, Fiedler F. Cerebral sinus thrombosis in a trauma patient after recombinant activated factor VII infusion. Anesthesiology 2004; 100(2):441–443.

110. Owler BK, Besser M. Extradural hematoma causing venous sinus obstruction and pseudotumor cerebri syndrome. Childs Nerv Syst 2005; 21(3):262–264.

111. Hoskote A, Richards P, Anslow P, McShane T. Subdural haematoma and non-accidental head injury in children. Childs Nerv Syst 2002; 18(6–7):311–317.

112. Takitani K, Nishino A, Tanabe T, Tanaka H, Harada K, Mimaki T et al. White matter lesion due to dural sinus thrombosis in an infant with subdural hematoma. Pediatr Int 2002; 44(6):680–682.

113. Erdogan B, Caner H, Aydin MV, Yildirim T, Kahveci S, Sen O. Hemispheric cerebrovascular venous thrombosis due to closed head injury. Childs Nerv Syst 2004; 20(4):239–242.

114. Shevell MI, Silver K, O'Gorman AM, Watters GV, Montes JL. Neonatal dural sinus thrombosis. Pediatr Neurol 1989; 5(3):161–165.

115. Berfelo FJ, Kersbergen KJ, van Ommen CH, Govaert P, van Straaten HL, Poll-The BT, van Wezel-Meijler G, Vermeulen RJ, Groenendaal F, de Vries LS, de Haan TR. Neonatal cerebral sinovenous thrombosis from symptom to outcome. Stroke. 2010;41(7): 1382–1388.

116. Hartmann A, Wappenschmidt J, Solymosi L. Clinical findings and differential diagnosis of cerebral vein thrombosis. In: Einhaupl KM (ed). Cerebral Sinus Thrombosis. Experimental and Clinical Aspects. New York: Plenum Press, 1987; 171.

117. Biousse V, Ameri A, Bousser MG. Isolated intracranial hypertension as the only sign of cerebral venous thrombosis. Neurology 1999; 53(7):1537–1542.

118. Ansari I, Crichlow B, Gunton KB, Diamond GR, Melvin J. A child with venous sinus thrombosis with initial examination findings of pseudotumor syndrome. Arch Ophthalmol 2002; 120(6):867–869.

119. Cumurciuc R, Crassard I, Sarov M, Valade D, Bousser MG. Headache as the only neurological sign of cerebral venous thrombosis: a series of 17 cases. J Neurol Neurosurg Psychiatry 2005; 76(8):1084–1087.

120. Abu-Arafeh I, Macleod S. Serious neurological disorders in children with chronic headache. Arch Dis Child 2005; 90(9):937–940.

121. Ameri A, Bousser MG. Cerebral venous thrombosis. Neurol Clin 1992; 10(1):87–111.

122. Farb RI, Vanek I, Scott JN, Mikulis DJ, Willinsky RA, Tomlinson G et al. Idiopathic intracranial hypertension: the prevalence and morphology of sinovenous stenosis. Neurology 2003; 60(9):1418–1424.

123. Higgins JN, Gillard JH, Owler BK, Harkness K, Pickard JD. MR venography in idiopathic intracranial hypertension: unappreciated and misunderstood. J Neurol Neurosurg Psychiatry 2004; 75(4):621–625.

124. Kosinski CM, Mull M, Schwarz M, Koch B, Biniek R, Schlafer J et al. Do normal D-dimer levels reliably exclude cerebral sinus thrombosis? Stroke 2004; 35(12):2820–2825.

125. Bonduel M, Sciuccati G, Hepner M, Torres AF, Pieroni G, Frontroth JP. Prethrombotic disorders in children with arterial ischemic stroke and sinovenous thrombosis. Arch Neurol 1999; 56(8):967–971.

126. Prats JM, Garaizar C, Zuazo E, Lopez J, Pinan MA, Aragues P. Superior sagittal sinus thrombosis in a child with protein S deficiency. Neurology 1992; 42(12):2303–2305.

127. Rich C, Gill JC, Wernick S, Konkol RJ. An unusual cause of cerebral venous thrombosis in a four-year-old child. Stroke 1993; 24(4):603–605.

128. van Kuijck MA, Rotteveel JJ, van Oostrom CG, Novakova I. Neurological complications in children with protein C deficiency. Neuropediatrics 1994; 25(1):16–19.

129. Ganesan V, Kelsey H, Cookson J, Osborn A, Kirkham FJ. Activated protein C resistance in childhood stroke. Lancet 1996; 347(8996):260.

130. von SE, Athreya BH, Rose CD, Goldsmith DP, Morton L. Clinical characteristics of antiphospholipid antibody syndrome in children. J Pediatr 1996; 129(3):339–345.

131. Deschiens MA, Conard J, Horellou MH, Ameri A, Preter M, Chedru F et al. Coagulation studies, factor V Leiden, and anticardiolipin antibodies in 40 cases of cerebral venous thrombosis. Stroke 1996; 27(10):1724–1730.

132. Zuber M, Toulon P, Marnet L, Mas JL. Factor V Leiden mutation in cerebral venous thrombosis. Stroke 1996; 27(10):1721–1723.

133. Cakmak S, Derex L, Berruyer M, Nighoghossian N, Philippeau F, Adeleine P et al. Cerebral venous thrombosis: clinical outcome and systematic screening of prothrombotic factors. Neurology 2003; 60(7):1175–1178.

134. Kurekci AE, Gokce H, Akar N. Factor VIII levels in children with thrombosis. Pediatr Int 2003; 45(2):159–162.

135. Gouault-Heilman M, Quentin P, Dreyfus M, Gandrille S, Emmerich J, Leroy-Matherson C et al. Massive thrombosis of venous cerebral sinuses in a 2 year old boy with a combined inherited deficiency of antithrombin III and protein C. Thromb Haemost 1994; 72:782.

136. Martinelli I, Landi G, Merati G, Cella R, Tosetto A, Mannucci PM. Factor V gene mutation is a risk factor for cerebral venous thrombosis. Thromb Haemost 1996; 75(3):393–394.

137. Martinelli I, Battaglioli T, Pedotti P, Cattaneo M, Mannucci PM. Hyperhomocysteinemia in cerebral vein thrombosis. Blood 2003; 102(4):1363–1366.

138. Kenet G, Kirkham F, Niederstadt T, Heinecke A, Saunders D, Stoll M et al. Risk factors for recurrent venous thromboembolism in the European collaborative paediatric database on cerebral venous thrombosis: a multicentre cohort study. Lancet Neurol 2007; 6(7): 595–603.

139. Connor SE, Jarosz JM. Magnetic resonance imaging of cerebral venous sinus thrombosis. Clin Radiol 2002; 57(6):449–461.

140. Lietz K, Kuehling SE, Parkhurst JB. Hemorrhagic stroke in a child with protein S and factor VII deficiencies. Pediatr Neurol 2005; 32(3):208–210.

141. Wu O, Ostergaard L, Weisskoff RM, Benner T, Rosen BR, Sorensen AG. Tracer arrival timing-insensitive technique for estimating flow in MR perfusion-weighted imaging using singular value decomposition with a block-circulant deconvolution matrix. Magn Reson Med 2003; 50(1):164–174.

142. Ramenghi LA, Gill BJ, Tanner SF, Martinez D, Arthur R, Levene MI. Cerebral venous thrombosis, intraventricular haemorrhage and white matter lesions in a preterm newborn with factor V (Leiden) mutation. Neuropediatrics 2002; 33(2):97–99.

143. Jacewicz M, Plum F. Aseptic cerebral venous thrombosis. In: Einhaupl KM (ed). Cerebral Sinus Thrombosis. New York: Plenum Press, 1990; 157–170.

144. Hamburger C, Villringer A, Bauer M, Lorz T. Delta (empty triangle) sign in patients without thrombosis of the superior sagittal sinus. In: Einhaupl KM, Kempski O, Baethmann A (eds). Cerebral Sinus Thrombosis: Experimental and Clinical Apects. New York: Plenum Press, 1990; 211–219.

145. Healy JF, Nichols C. Polycythemia mimicking venous sinus thrombosis. AJNR Am J Neuroradiol 2002; 23(8):1402–1403.

146. Ludwig B, Brand M, Brockerhoff P. Postpartum CT examination of the heads of full term infants. Neuroradiology 1980; 20(3): 145–154.

147. Kirchhof K, Jansen O, Sartor K. CT angiography of the cerebral veins. Rofo 1996; 165(3):232–237.

148. Macchi PJ, Grossman RI, Gomori JM, Goldberg HI, Zimmerman RA, Bilaniuk LT. High field MR imaging of cerebral venous thrombosis. J Comput Assist Tomogr 1986; 10(1):10–15.

149. Medlock MD, Olivero WC, Hanigan WC, Wright RM, Winek SJ. Children with cerebral venous thrombosis diagnosed with magnetic resonance imaging and magnetic resonance angiography. Neurosurgery 1992; 31(5):870–876.

150. Zimmerman RA, Bogdan AR, Gusnard DA. Pediatric magnetic resonance angiography: assessment of stroke. Cardiovasc Intervent Radiol 1992; 15(1):60–64.

151. Dormont D, Anxionnat R, Evrard S, Louaille C, Chiras J, Marsault C. MRI in cerebral venous thrombosis. J Neuroradiol 1994; 21(2):81–99.

152. Adams WM, Laitt RD, Beards SC, Kassner A, Jackson A. Use of single-slice thick slab phase-contrast angiography for the diagnosis of dural venous sinus thrombosis. Eur Radiol 1999; 9(8):1614–1619.

153. Govaert P, Voet D, Achten E, Vanhaesebrouck P, van RH, van GD et al. Noninvasive diagnosis of superior sagittal sinus thrombosis in a neonate. Am J Perinatol 1992; 9(3):201–204.

154. Bezinque SL, Slovis TL, Touchette AS, Schave DM, Jarski RW, Bedard MP et al. Characterization of superior sagittal sinus blood flow velocity using color flow Doppler in neonates and infants. Pediatr Radiol 1995; 25(3):175–179.

155. Stolz E, Gerriets T, Bodeker RH, Hugens-Penzel M, Kaps M. Intracranial venous hemodynamics is a factor related to a favorable outcome in cerebral venous thrombosis. Stroke 2002; 33(6): 1645–1650.

156. Jacobs K, Moulin T, Bogousslavsky J, Woimant F, Dehaene I, Tatu L et al. The stroke syndrome of cortical vein thrombosis. Neurology 1996; 47(2):376–382.

157. Stefini R, Latronico N, Cornali C, Rasulo F, Bollati A. Emergent decompressive craniectomy in patients with fixed dilated pupils due to cerebral venous and dural sinus thrombosis: report of three cases. Neurosurgery 1999; 45(3):626–629.

158. Keller E, Pangalu A, Fandino J, Konu D, Yonekawa Y. Decompressive craniectomy in severe cerebral venous and dural sinus thrombosis. Acta Neurochir Suppl 2005; 94:177–183.

159. Goldenberg NA, Knapp-Clevenger R, Hays T, Manco-Johnson MJ. Lemierre's and Lemierre's-like syndromes in children: survival and thromboembolic outcomes. Pediatrics 2005; 116(4):e543–e548.

160. Deveze A, Facon F, Latil G, Moulin G, Payan-Cassin H, Dessi P. Cavernous sinus thrombosis secondary to non-invasive sphenoid aspergillosis. Rhinology 2005; 43(2):152–155.

161. Wong I, Kozak FK, Poskitt K, Ludemann JP, Harriman M. Pediatric lateral sinus thrombosis: retrospective case series and literature review. J Otolaryngol 2005; 34(2):79–85.

162. Dix D, Andrew M, Marzinotto V, Charpentier K, Bridge S, Monagle P et al. The use of low molecular weight heparin in pediatric patients: a prospective cohort study. J Pediatr 2000; 136(4): 439–445.

163. deVeber G, Chan A, Monagle P, Marzinotto V, Armstrong D, Massicotte P et al. Anticoagulation therapy in pediatric patients with sinovenous thrombosis: a cohort study. Arch Neurol 1998; 55(12): 1533–1537.

164. Einhaupl KM, Villringer A, Meister W, Mehraein S, Garner C, Pellkofer M et al. Heparin treatment in sinus venous thrombosis. Lancet 1991; 338(8767):597–600.

165. Nagarajat D, Rao BS, Taly AB, Subhash MN. Randomised controlled trial of heparin in puerpal cerebral venous/sinus thrombosis. Nimhans J 1995; 13:111–115.

166. Chakrabarti I, Maiti B. Study on cerebral venous thrombosis with special references to efficacy of heparin. J Neurol Sciences 1997; 150:147.

167. Johnson MC, Parkerson N, Ward S, de Alarcon PA. Pediatric sinovenous thrombosis. J Pediatr Hematol Oncol 2003; 25(4): 312–315.

168. Barnes C, Newall F, Furmedge J, Mackay M, Monagle P. Cerebral sinus venous thrombosis in children. J Paediatr Child Health 2004; 40(1–2):53–55.

169. Moharir MD, Shroff M, Stephens D, Pontigon A-M, Chan A, MacGregor D et al. Anticoagulants in pediatric cerebral sinovenous thrombosis: a safety and outcome study. Ann Neurol 2010; 67(5):590–599.

170. Mallick AA, Sharples PM, Calvert SE, Jones RW, Leary M, Lux AL et al. Cerebral venous sinus thrombosis: a case series including thrombolysis. Arch Dis Child 2009; 94(10):790–794.

171. Griesemer DA, Theodorou AA, Berg RA, Spera TD. Local fibrinolysis in cerebral venous thrombosis. Pediatr Neurol 1994; 10(1): 78–80.

172. Soleau SW, Schmidt R, Stevens S, Osborn A, MacDonald JD. Extensive experience with dural sinus thrombosis. Neurosurgery 2003; 52(3):534–544.

173. Liebetrau M, Mayer TE, Bruning R, Opherk C, Hamann GF. Intra-arterial thrombolysis of complete deep cerebral venous thrombosis. Neurology 2004; 63(12):2444–2445.

174. Chahlavi A, Steinmetz MP, Masaryk TJ, Rasmussen PA. A transcranial approach for direct mechanical thrombectomy of dural sinus thrombosis. Report of two cases. J Neurosurg 2004; 101(2):347–351.

175. Wasay M, Bakshi R, Kojan S, Bobustuc G, Dubey N, Unwin DH. Nonrandomized comparison of local urokinase thrombolysis versus systemic heparin anticoagulation for superior sagittal sinus thrombosis. Stroke 2001; 32(10):2310–2317.

176. Wong VK, LeMesurier J, Franceschini R, Heikali M, Hanson R. Cerebral venous thrombosis as a cause of neonatal seizures. Pediatr Neurol 1987; 3(4):235–237.

177. Higashida RT, Helmer E, Halbach VV, Hieshima GB. Direct thrombolytic therapy for superior sagittal sinus thrombosis. AJNR Am J Neuroradiol 1989; 10(5 Suppl):S4–S6.

178. Wasay M, Bakshi R, Dai A, Roach S. Local thrombolytic treatment of cerebral venous thrombosis in three paediatric patients. J Pak Med Assoc 2006; 56(11):555–556.

179. Monagle P, Phelan E, Downie P, Andrew M. Local thrombolytic therapy in childen. Thromb Haemost 1997; 78:504.

180. Salman MS, Kirkham FJ, MacGregor DL. Idiopathic 'benign' intracranial hypertension: case series and review. J Child Neurol 2001; 16(7):465–470.

181. Erdem H, Dinc A, Pay S, Simsek I, Uysal Y. A neuro-Behçet's case complicated with intracranial hypertension successfully treated by a lumboperitoneal shunt. Joint Bone Spine 2006; 73(2):200–201.

182. Gout A, Seibel N, Rouviere C, Husson B, Hermans B, Laporte N et al. Aphasia owing to subcortical brain infarcts in childhood. J Child Neurol 2005; 20(12):1003–1008.

183. De Schryver EL, Blom I, Braun KP, Kappelle LJ, Rinkel GJ, Peters AC et al. Long-term prognosis of cerebral venous sinus thrombosis in childhood. Dev Med Child Neurol 2004; 46(8):514–519.

184. Yager JY, Thornhill JA. The effect of age on susceptibility to hypoxic-ischemic brain damage. Neurosci Biobehav Rev 1997; 21(2):167–174.

185. Bouza H, Rutherford M, Acolet D, Pennock JM, Dubowitz LM. Evolution of early hemiplegic signs in full-term infants with unilateral brain lesions in the neonatal period: a prospective study. Neuropediatrics 1994; 25(4):201–207.

186. Holzmann D, Huisman TA, Linder TE. Lateral dural sinus thrombosis in childhood. Laryngoscope 1999; 109(4):645–651.

187. Lancon JA, Killough KR, Tibbs RE, Lewis AI, Parent AD. Spontaneous dural sinus thrombosis in children. Pediatr Neurosurg 1999; 30(1):23–29.

188. De Schryver EL, Blom I, Braun KP, Kappelle LJ, Rinkel GJ, Peters AC et al. Long-term prognosis of cerebral venous sinus thrombosis in childhood. Dev Med Child Neurol 2004; 46(8):514–519.

189. deVeber GA, MacGregor D, Curtis R, Mayank S. Neurologic outcome in survivors of childhood arterial ischemic stroke and sinovenous thrombosis. J Child Neurol 2000; 15(5):316–324.

190. Lindley WF, Livingstone M, Warlow C. 'Can simple questions assess outcome after stroke?'. Cerebrovasc Dis 1994; 4:314–324.

191. Dorman PJ, Waddell F, Slattery J, Dennis M, Sandercock P. Is the EuroQol a valid measure of health-related quality of life after stroke? Stroke 1997; 28(10):1876–1882.

HAEMORRHAGIC STROKE

8.1 Non-traumatic Intracranial Haemorrhage in Children

Vijeya Ganesan and Dawn E. Saunders

The term intracranial haemorrhage (ICH) encompasses intra-ventricular (IVH), intra-parenchymal (IPH) and subarachnoid (SAH) haemorrhage. IVH alone is a subarachnoid haemorrhage, but can also result from extension of IPH into the ventricles. For the purposes of this chapter, we will use the term ICH to include all of these (Fig. 8.1) and will confine our discussion to non-traumatic ICH. The term haemorrhagic stroke is ambiguous and although often used in the literature, we will use the term primary IPH to differentiate this from haemorrhagic transformation in patients with arterial ischaemia. Primary IPH and ICH are synonymous. ICH in the neonatal age group is covered in Section 8.2. In this section we will firstly discuss clinical aspects of ICH, then cerebrovascular and systemic aetiologies and, finally, radiological investigation.

Clinical aspects of intracranial haemorrhage in children

EPIDEMIOLOGY

ICH is at least as common as arterial ischaemic stroke (AIS) in childhood.[1] However, as cases may present to a variety of departments (emergency, neurosurgery, radiology, neurology, paediatrics), few groups have been able to undertake systematic studies of this subject. Schoenberg et al reported the incidence of 'haemorrhagic stroke' in children in Rochester, Minnesota between 1965 and 1974 to be 1.9 per 100 000 per year.[2] A study in Dijon (1985–1993) found the incidence to be 5 per 100 000 per year.[3] Analysing California hospital discharge data for a 10-year interval for children aged 1 month to 19 years of age, Fullerton[4] estimated the haemorrhagic stroke incidence in children to be 1.1 per 100 000 per year. In her more detailed Kaiser-Permanate study,[5] the average annual incidence rate of haemorrhagic stroke was 1.7 per 100 000 person-years (95% binomial exact CI, 1.5–2.0), 62% were male with a mean age at the time of stroke of 10.9 years (SD 6.9). Half were pure ICH, whereas 22% were pure SAH/

IVH, and 37% were a combination of ICH and SAH/IVH. In a study of Chinese children in Hong Kong, Chung and Wong[6] found a similar overall stroke rate to previous studies, but only 28% of those children had haemorrhagic strokes. In the United Kingdom Birmingham Children's Hospital[7] and British Paediatric Surveillance Unit[8] studies, the proportion of those with ICH was also lower than those with ischaemic stroke or normal imaging. The peak age for ICH is the first year of life, with around one-third of cases presenting in this age group, while SAH, often aneurysmal, is more common among adolescents.[4,9]

RISK OF RECURRENT HAEMORRHAGE

In the study of Blom et al,[10] recurrence occurred in nine out of 56 (16%) patients with initial ICH, ICH or SAH during a mean of 10.3 years of follow-up; three were fatal and four children had more than one recurrence. Four had anteriovenous malformations (AVM) and two arterial aneurysms (AA) (for these six, three before planned surgery and three inoperable), and there was an inoperable intracerebral tumour and an intracranial infection, while one was idiopathic. In Meyer-Heim's[11] study, three out of 34 (9%) children had a recurrent haemorrhage, all within the first year, one idiopathic and two with vascular disease (one just before a planned embolization). The likelihood and timing of recurrent haemorrhage depends on the underlying aetiology, i.e. whether the initial ICH has an underlying structural aetiology (and if so whether it is extirpated in a timely fashion), occurs in the context of a medical illness or trauma or is idiopathic.[5] Recurrence after traumatic or idiopathic ICH is unusual, although cases have been reported[5,11] and most recurrences in the context of medical aetiologies (e.g. hypertension, thrombocytopenia) occur in the first week. However, the majority of those who suffer reccurence have untreated or partially treated structural vascular lesions[5] (see below).

OUTCOME

Mortality is higher in children with ICH compared with AIS;[8,12,13] see Chapter 15, Section 15.1). For example, Al Jarallah et al[14] reported a mortality of around 10% in their series; this is similar to the rate in other series.[15] Half the patients regained normal neurological function and the rest had a variety of

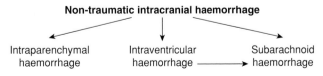

Non-traumatic intracranial haemorrhage

| Intraparenchymal haemorrhage | Intraventricular haemorrhage | Subarachnoid haemorrhage |

Fig. 8.1. Definition of intracranial haemorrhage.

residual sequelae.[14] Around 10% of children experience post-treatment seizures,[10] compared with over 20% of adults.[16] In a series from Switzerland, a quarter died and morbidity was considerable, particularly in infratentorial haemorrhages, in aneurysms, in children younger than 3 years and in those with underlying haematological disorders.[11] Although motor disability may be less frequent and functional outcome is often good,[10] only a quarter have no cognitive or physical sequelae and the majority of survivors have low self-esteem.[10] The cognitive difficulties are often subtle; in five children undergoing detailed neuropsychological testing after surgery for AVM, mild to moderate weaknesses in executive functions were suggested regardless of AVM location.[17]

Intraparenchymal haemorrhage

The clinical presentation of IPH may be very similar to that of AIS and it is not possible to confidently distinguish between these diagnoses on clinical grounds. However, children with primary IPH more frequently present with symptoms and signs of raised intracranial pressure, such as headache and vomiting.[14] Seizures occur in around a third of cases. Focal neurological signs may even be absent, depending on the site of the lesion. The clinical presentation may be very non-specific in infants, even with large haematomas. A depressed conscious level is a poor prognostic sign.[14]

An underlying cause is identified in more than 90% of children with IPH.[14] This is most commonly a vascular abnormality, and in contrast to adults, arteriovenous malformations (AVM) are a much more common cause in children than arterial aneurysms (AA).[11,14,18,19] Benign and malignant vascular tumours can also present with IPH[20] and can be difficult to identify on imaging in the presence of a large haematoma (e.g. see Fig. 8.2). Reperfusion of ischaemic tissue may result in haemorrhagic transformation of an infarct which may mimic IPH. Haemorrhagic transformation is particularly common in patients with large embolic infarcts and in areas of venous ischaemia.

SUBARACHNOID HAEMORRHAGE
Children with SAH present with symptoms and signs of meningeal irritation, including neck stiffness and photophobia. However, these may not be apparent in young infants, in whom signs of raised intracranial pressure or meningeal irritation are much less specific. Autonomic dysfunction may be a feature. Seizures occur in around 20% of cases at presentation. The risk of rebleeding following SAH is 10% in the early period and 30% within 4 weeks. Overall, around 75% of survivors of SAH have another haemorrhage.

In a study of 56 Thai children with SAH, Visudhiphan et al[21] made a diagnosis in 54 (96%): underlying haemorrhagic disorder in 22, AVM or AA in 18, gnathostomiasis (a helminthic infestation) in nine, bleeding tumours in four and hypernatraemia in one. Hourihan et al[22] reported that of 167 children presenting with SAH, 52% were due to AA and 26% were due to

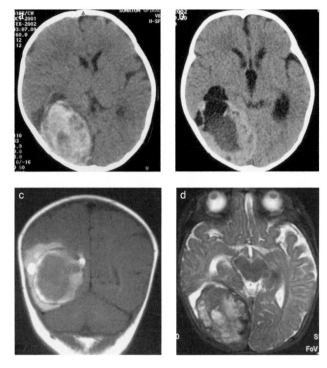

Fig. 8.2. Imaging of a 3-month-old child who presented with seizures and was found to have a large posterior haematoma on the presenting unenhanced CT scan (a) with no definite underlying tumour. (b) Six weeks later the CT scan shows an area of rim enhancement with a central low density area typical of a tumour. The (c) coronal T1- and (d) axial T2-weighted images 1 week after presentation demonstrate early subacute haemorrhage in the rim of the tumour (high on T1- and very dark on T2-weighted images). The central area of low signal on T1- and high signal on T2-weighted images is not compatible with the signal characteristics of haematoma and represents tumour. The child was found to have a malignant glioma at surgery.

AVM. This is in contrast to adults where over three-quarters of SAH are secondary to AA. In 15–30% of children with SAH an underlying vascular lesion may not be identified even with catheter angiography. However, in Hourihan's series, four of the 26 patients with no underlying lesion initially identified had a recurrent SAH; of these two were then found to have AVMs and one an AA. Over half of those with pure SAH had aneurysms in the Kaiser Permanante series.[9] SAH may occur in patients with moyamoya, the cerebral vasculopathy associated with sickle cell disease[23] and in association with venous sinus thrombosis.[24]

Computed tomography is positive in 95% of patients with SAH within the first 24 hours; however, this falls to 50% after a week. Cerebrospinal fluid (CSF) should be examined for the presence of xanthochromia, as negative visual inspection does not exclude the presence of blood breakdown products.

INTRAVENTRICULAR HAEMORRHAGE
IVH is most commonly seen in the neonatal age group (see Section 8.2). In older children IVH can be secondary to AVM, cavernous malformation, AA or extension of IPH.[25]

Vascular causes of non-traumatic intracranial haemorrhage

VASCULAR MALFORMATIONS

Arteriovenous malformations (AVMs)

AVMs are defined by the presence of high flow arteriovenous shunts through a nidus of abnormal thin walled, coiled and tortuous connections between feeding arteries and draining veins, without an intervening capillary network. The vascular channels are separated by glial tissue. Histologically, cells found within the nidus show reactive changes and are thought to be non-functioning. Current views suggest that they represent abnormalities of developmental vascular remodelling, rather than structural abnormalities per se,[26] and may be acquired as well as congenital.[27,28]

Estimation of the prevalence of AVMs had varied widely[26] but recent studies provide a firm basis for planning services. In a Swedish population-based study of adults and children,[29] there were 12.4 de novo diagnosed AVMs per 1 000 000 population per year (135 AVMs) and of these, 4.4 per 1 000 000 had haematomas needing expedient surgical evacuation. In the New York islands population-based study across all ages from 2000, the annual AVM detection rate was 1.34 per 100 000 person-years (95% CI, 1.18 to 1.49).[30] The incidence of first-ever AVM haemorrhage was 0.51 per 100 000 person-years and the estimated prevalence of AVM haemorrhage among detected cases was 0.68 per 100 000 (95% CI, 0.57–0.79). In the Western Australian population-based study, the first haemorrhage was fatal in 4.6% of patients.[31] Around 20% of cerebral AVMs are diagnosed during infancy and childhood.[32]

Pial AVMs account for 30–50% of ICH in the paediatric age group. They usually cause IPH, but this may extend to the subarachnoid space or the ventricular system. Compared with adults, AVMs more commonly present with haemorrhage in children under the age of 10,[30,33,34] probably, at least in part, because they less often undergo neuroimaging for seizures and headaches. Size is larger in younger patients[33] and a site in eloquent or deep areas of the brain (particularly basal ganglia and thalamus)[15,33,35] and in the posterior fossa is also more frequent than in adults[18,33] (although 80% are supratentorial). Aneurysms presenting in the same patient as an AVM is more common in adults.[33] AVMs are multiple in 17% of children and may occasionally be familial. In these cases, inherited underlying conditions, such as hereditary haemorrhagic telangiectasia, hypomelanosis of Ito, neurofibromatosis, Wyburn–Mason syndrome and cancer-predisposing overgrowth syndromes such as Beckwith–Wiedemann and those caused by PTEN mutations (see Chapter 15) should be excluded clinically or with genetic testing.

Clinical presentation of AVM in childhood is most commonly with haemorrhage (in 80–85% of cases),[32,34,35] but also may be with seizures, headache (including benign intracranial hypertension[36]) and focal neurological deficits. The high risk of recurrence (see below) justifies an aggressive approach to the treatment of AVMs presenting in childhood.

The Spetzler–Martin system for classifying AVMs takes three factors into consideration: (1) size of the AVM (small = maximum diameter <3cm, medium = maximum diameter 3–6cm, large = maximum diameter of >6cm); (2) eloquence of adjacent brain area (eloquent areas = sensorimotor, language and visual cortex, hypothalamus and thalamus, internal capsule, brainstem, cerebellar peduncles, deep cerebellar nuclei); and (3) presence of deep venous drainage.[37] Interobserver agreement is good overall, but variability, typically between neuroradiologists and neurosurgeons presumably related to different approaches, can affect reporting of results, surgical risk assessment and patient selection.[38] This classification is used mainly in the context of evaluating cases for surgical treatment (see Chapter 8, Section 8.2) Features associated with a higher risk of haemorrhage include the presence of flow-related or intranidal aneurysm, small nidus size (<3cm), deep venous drainage, deep location, high pressure in the feeding artery, slow arterial filling and venous stenosis.[26] In the Swedish population-based study, Grades 1–3 lesions represented 85% of the caseload.[29] In addition to the 4.4 per 1 000 000 presenting with life-threatening haemorrhage, there were 5.8 cases per 1 000 000 population per year of Grade 1 or 2 and larger non-critically located Grade 3 malformations, potentially amenable to surgery. Small, critically located Grades 3 and 4 lesions, potentially requiring radiosurgery, amounted to 1.6 cases per 1 000 000 population per year. There were 0.5 cases per 1 000 000 population per year of Grade 5 AVMs, which are difficult to treat with any modality.

The risk of rebleeding from an AVM after an initial haemorrhage is around 2–3% per year in series combining adults and children but is reported as being much higher, around 25% after 5 years, in paediatric series.[39] In series reporting only children with known AVMs, the annual risk of haemorrhage is also 2–4%; in around 25% of patients the haemorrhage is fatal.[18,35] The annual risk of haemorrhage for patients presenting in childhood is actually lower than for those presenting as adults, once adjusted for mode of presentation, as haemorrhage accounts for the majority of children whose AVM or AA comes to light and those who present with haemorrhage have a higher risk of subsequent haemorrhage.[34,40] However, they have a substantial cumulative risk. The overall lifetime risk of haemorrhage can be approximated by the formula (105 minus the age of the patient)[41] and therefore is substantial for patients presenting in childhood. Recurrence after apparently complete obliteration has been reported, especially in children,[42] supporting the need for ongoing follow-up.[26]

Cavernomas

Cavernomas are well circumscribed vascular malformations comprising thin-walled sinusoidal spaces lined with endothelial tissue and containing intra- or intervascular calcifications, without any intervening parenchymal tissue. These contain clotted and flowing blood. As the blood is slow flowing, the feeding arteries and draining veins are of normal calibre and there is no arteriovenous shunting. Both sporadic and genetic forms have been identified and where familial, the mode of inheritance is usually autosomal dominant. Familial cases are particularly frequent in Hispanics (accounting for up to 50% of cases) and tend to be associated with multiple lesions.[43,44] Retinal and cutaneous cavernomas are an infrequent but well-recognized association with familial cases. Three cerebral cavernous malformation (CCM) genes have been identified (*CCM1*, *CCM2* and *CCM3*); the sensitivity of genetic screening is >95% in patients with an affected relative and 57% in sporadic cases, but the role of screening should be carefully considered as genetic diagnosis may enable counseling but may not alter the affected individuals' clinical management.[44]

Cavernomas most commonly occur in the cortical and subcortical areas in the Rolandic area and basal ganglia, pons and cerebellar hemispheres. Although congenital, they may increase in size over time. This is thought to be due to repeated episodes of haemorrhage with subsequent tissue fibrosis and calcification.[45] De novo lesions may arise in familial cases. Developmental venous malformations are often found in association with cavernomas and it is thought that venous hypertension resulting from obstructed outflow results in the formation of the cavernoma.[46] Clinical presentation may be with haemorrhage, seizures or focal neurological deficits. The risk of recurrent haemorrhage is in the region of 4.5% per year.

Developmental venous anomalies

Developmental venous anomalies (DVA) are thin-walled venous channels with normal intervening neural tissue and should not be considered true vascular malformations. The channels are morphologically normal and drain the brain normally, though venous outflow may be somewhat slower than normal. DVA are generally asymptomatic and are most commonly identified incidentally. The risk of ICH associated with DVA is extremely low and other potential causes should be considered and excluded. ICH may, for example, arise from an adjacent cavernoma as the two are commonly co-located.

Capillary telangiectasias

These are collections of dilated ectatic capillaries with normal intervening neural tissue, without smooth muscle or elastic fibres. They are rarely associated with ICH or SAH.

ARTERIAL ANEURYSMS

Arterial aneurysms are acquired lesions which are rare in children, who account for less than 5% of all cases. They are multiple in 2–5% of children. The apparent male preponderance in childhood persisting until early adulthood was not borne out in a recent series.[47] The age of presentation during childhood and adolescence is biphasic, with symptom onset most often before age 2 or after age 10;[48] rupture in the neonatal period has been documented.[49,50] The most common are dissecting and saccular[47] aneurysms which, in children, have a predilection for the posterior circulation and the bifurcation of the ICA respectively. Haemorrhage in patients below 2 years of age is

usually due to dissecting aneurysms, while saccular aneurysms were responsible in patients above 5 years of age. Compared with adults, children are more likely to have giant aneurysms (Fig. 8.3) and lesions in the posterior circulation and less likely to develop an aneurysm of the anterior and posterior communicating arteries.[47,51–56] In Lasjaunias'[52] series of 59 children with 75 aneurysms, 33 children had dissecting, two had chronic post-traumatic, eight had infectious and 16 had saccular lesions. Five children had familial disease and nine presented with multiple aneurysms. Half to three-quarters of patients with AA present with ICH[52] but younger children are particularly likely to present with other symptoms. Infectious aneurysms are especially likely to cause IPH. The risk of recurrent haemorrhage from a saccular aneurysm is around 50% in the first 6 months which subsequently decreases to around 3% per year. Lasjaunias reports that AA are more likely than AVM to cause ICH in Caucasians whereas AVM are implicated more frequently in Asian patients.[53]

Typically around 10–20% of AAs are post-traumatic; a similar proportion are mycotic and are associated with infection with, for example, *Staphylococcus*, *Streptococcus*, gram negative organisms or human immunodeficiency virus.[47] Mycotic aneurysms may also arise secondary to embolization of infective thrombi into the intracranial circulation in

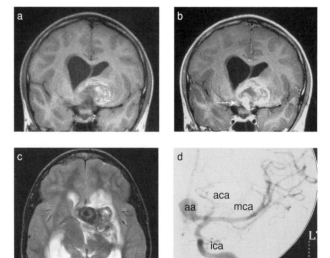

Fig. 8.3. (a) Pre- and (b) post-contrast coronal T1-weighted images at the level of the frontal horns show the presence of an aneurysm – signal void surrounded by haematoma which enhances following the administration of contrast. The signal characteristics of the haematoma on T1-weighted (a,b) and T2-weighted (c) images indicate the presence of blood of different ages. The haematoma immediately surrounding the aneurysm is of low signal on both sequences (acute, deoxyhaemoglobin) and more peripherally is an area of high signal on T1-weighted (a,b) and low signal on T2-weighted (c) images (early acute, intracellular haematoma). The concentric rings of the aneurysm indicate the presence of recurrent haemorrhaging typical of giant aneurysm. (d) A conventional angiogram confirms the presence of a giant aneurysm (aa) arising from the left terminal carotid artery. aa, arterial aneurysm; aca, anterior cerebral artery; ica, internal carotid artery; mca, middle cerebral artery.

patients with subacute bacterial endocarditis (SBE); rupture of the aneurysm may be the presenting sign of SBE. Mycotic aneurysms also result from invasion of intracranial vessels by adjacent infections such as middle ear or sinus infection, meningitis, osteomyelitis of the skull, and septic cavernous sinus thrombosis. Traumatic aneurysms may be intra- or extracranial. The latter are typically associated with injuries to the neck, for example after road traffic accidents or penetrating injuries to the skull base. Other associations with AA in children are sickle cell disease, polycystic kidney disease, coarctation of the aorta, tuberous sclerosis, neurofibromatosis, incontinentia pigmenti, Sneddon syndrome, Alagille syndrome, hereditary haemorrhagic telangiectasia, Marfan syndrome, Ehlers Danlos syndrome type IV, pseudoxanthoma elasticum, hypertension and human immunodeficiency virus. However, no underlying systemic disorder is found in the majority of children.[47]

Systemic causes of intracranial haemorrhage

These are collectively rarer than the vascular causes of ICH.[14] A systemic cause should be considered particularly in children with known medical diagnoses, for example sepsis or malignancy. Haemorrhagic disease of the newborn should be considered in neonates with ICH (see Chapter 9). Haematological evaluation of patients with ICH should include a platelet count, clotting screen as well as measurement of clotting factor levels (factors VII, VIII, IX, X, XI, XIII). Intracranial haemorrhage occurs in 0.5–1.0% of children with idiopathic thrombocyopenic purpura, and half are fatal.[57] Patients with severe haemophilia are still at risk, particularly if they are not on prophylaxis, for example because they have an inhibitor, and should undergo neuroimaging if they have any alteration of consciousness.[58] Children with leukaemia and other cancers are at risk of both IPH and SAH;[59] in addition to direct effects (e.g. haemorrhaging into tumours or decreased platelet count), certain chemotherapy drugs (e.g. asparaginase) may promote hypercoagulability, resulting in cerebral venous thrombosis and secondary haemorrhagic infarction (Fig. 8.4). Recent transfusion and the use of steroids are risk factors for intracranial haemorrhage in sickle cell disease;[23] AA are more commonly found in adults (see Chapter 15). Recreational drug use should also be considered as a cause of ICH (IPH and SAH) in the young. For example, amphetamine may be associated with a necrotizing angiitis, cocaine causes a surge of hypertension followed by vasospasm and ecstasy causes acute sympathetic surge. Affected individuals may additionally have an underlying vascular lesion and should therefore be comprehensively evaluated.[60]

Radiological investigations and appearances

CT

Because of the ease of use and availability, CT is the first radiological examination performed in the vast majority of children with ICH. On the initial scan the size of the haematoma, shown as high density on CT within the first 7–10 days, the degree

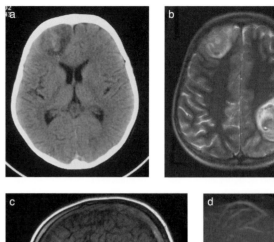
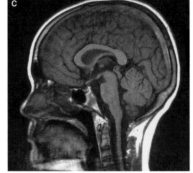
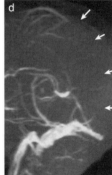

Fig. 8.4. Venous sinus thrombosis in a child with acute lymphoblastic leukaemia (ALL) on asparginase. (a) A large right frontal haematoma and clot within the superior sagittal sinus (SSS) is seen on the axial CT at presentation. (b) Two days later the child deteriorated and a left parietal haematoma is visible with layering of blood within it (long arrow). Midline sagittal T1-weighted image (c) confirms the presence of clot (high signal) in the posterior SSS and absence of flow is seen on the magnetic resonance venogram (d).

of mass effect, and the presence of intraventricular blood and hydrocephalus are important observations to be made. The presence of subarachnoid and intraventricular blood contribute to hydrocephalus either by blocking CSF resorption or by obstructing ventricular outflow. Calcification or a large deep draining vein may indicate the presence of an AVM (Fig. 8.5). High density within the venous sinuses, indicating clot, should be looked for, particularly in children with multiple haematomas which do not conform to a vascular territory (e.g. see Fig. 8.4). An important caveat is that in neonates the blood within the venous sinuses can appear bright because of the raised haematocrit. Multiple haematomas may also be seen in children with septic emboli (e.g. Fig. 8.6) and haemorrhagic diatheses.

More recently CT angiography (CTA; Fig. 8.7), which now has an established role in the evaluation of adults with AA,[61] was been shown to be useful in the initial evaluation of children with non-traumatic ICH due to a variety of vascular pathologies.[62] CTA is more rapid and accessible than MRI/MRA, especially in a sick child. Although incurring an additional radiation burden, early identification of the vascular lesion using CTA may enable deferment of digital substraction angiogram (DSA) to a time when it may be combined with endovascular treatment.

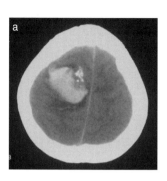
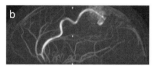
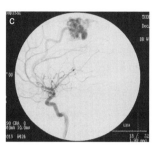
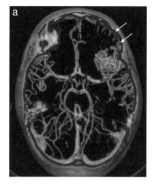
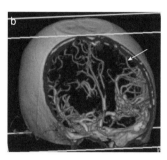

Fig. 8.7. Axial (a) and oblique (b) coronal 3D CT images of an DSA with feeders from the insular branches of the left middle cerebral artery.

Fig. 8.5. (a) CT of a patient presenting with intra-parenchymal haemorrhage. The presence of punctate calcification seen on CT is suggestive of an arterial venous malformation (AVM) which is confirmed on MRI and magnetic resonance angiography (MRA). MRA (b) and catheter angiography (c) demonstrate that the nidus is small, the arterial feeder is a large pericallosal branch and venous drainage is into the superior sagittal sinus.

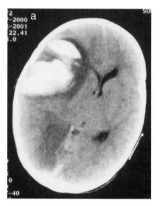
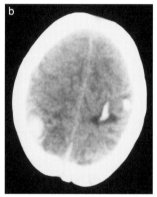

Fig. 8.6. CT scan at the level of the basal ganglia (a) and the level of the cerebral convexities (b). Multiple cerebral haematomas with significant mass effect are compressing the ventricles. A right posterior cerebral artery territory infarct has resulted from tentorial herniation. Vegetations were found on the mitral valve and despite treatment for subacute bacterial endocarditis, the child did not survive.

MRI

Conventional MRI techniques are sensitive to deoxy-haemoglobin, methaemoglobin and haemosiderin, the paramagnetic breakdown products of haemoglobin found in subacute and chronic haemorrhage, but are not sensitive to oxyhaemoglobin present in acute haemorrhage.[63,64] Small amounts of paramagnetic breakdown products found in acute haemorrhage can be detected by more sensitive gradient echo imaging.[63] The appearance of cerebral haemorrhage on MRI is complex and depends on a number of factors such as the age and location of the haemorrhage, the strength of the magnet and the presence of an underlying lesion.[65]

The breakdown products of haemoglobin[63] are paramagnetic and result in a disruption of the local magnetic field and an alteration in the relaxation properties of the water molecules that produce the MRI. At 1.5T, the evolution of the breakdown products are summarized in Table 8.1. In the hyperacute stage (within several hours) when there is minimal deoxyhaemoglobin, conventional MR sequences are less sensitive than CT to the detection of haematoma (Fig. 8.8). However, the addition of newer gradient echo images, which are highly sensitive to magnetic field inhomogeneity, have been shown to be as reliable as CT in the assessment of hyperacute intracranial haemorrhage.[63,65,66] MRI is less sensitive than CT in the detection of SAH and is not recommended in the hyperacute stages of SAH, despite reports of improved sensitivity of fluid attenuated inversion recovery images in the detection of acute SAH.

In a study of 50 children with either SAH or primary IPH, MRI and MRA alone contributed to the identification of the cause in 25 out of 38 children with IPH; 18 had a vascular aetiology and five had underlying tumours. MRA was shown to be of value in three patients in which standard MRI was normal.[67] There were three false negatives. Neurosurgeons may operate on the basis of MRI/MRA in cases where the anatomy of the underlying vascular lesion is well demonstrated, thereby

TABLE 8.1
Appearance of blood and blood breakdown products over time on MRI

Time scale	Stage	T1 change	T2 change	Product
0–2 days	Acute	Dark	Dark	Deoxyhaemoglobin
3–7 days	Early subacute	Bright	Dark	Intracellular methaemoglobin
8–14 days	Late subacute	Bright	Bright	Extracellular methaemoglobin
>14 days	Chronic	Dark	Dark	Haemosiderin

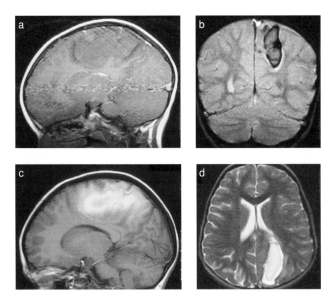

Fig. 8.8. (a,b) Acute haematoma. Images acquired within 36 hours of presentation; isointense signal of the haematoma shown on the sagittal T1-weighted image and dark on the T2-weighted image as the oxyhaemoglobin changes to deoxyhaemoglobin. (c,d) Late subacute haematoma. Images acquired 2 weeks later; the high signal on both T1- and T2-weighted images resulting from the presence of extracellular methaemoglobin.

eliminating or deferring the need for DSA. Although the use of MRI and MRA as first line non-invasive vascular evaluation techniques in patients with IPH may be obviated by increasing availability of and experience of CTA, there is likely to be an ongoing role for MRI in evaluation of patients with negative CTA, to exclude pathologies such as an underlying tumour.

Prior to the widespread use of CTA to characterize AA, MRI and MRA were shown to have a complementary role to DSA in these patients. In a series of adults with SAH, 3D MRA detected five aneurysms not seen on DSA and DSA detected five aneurysms not seen on MRA.[68] In two series of adult patients with aneurysms, 50%[69] and 40%[70] were operated on following 3D MRA alone. There are no reports comparing aneurysm detection using MRA and conventional angiography in children. The majority of aneurysms are small and peripherally sited, but may still be demonstrated by MRA (Fig. 8.9). Giant aneurysms (diameter >2.5cm) arise from major intracranial vessels and are often detected by CT and MRI.

CONVENTIONAL CEREBRAL ANGIOGRAPHY

Despite the increasing use of non-invasive methods for cerebrovascular imaging, digital substraction angiogram (DSA) has a continuing role in the evaluation of children with IPH. However, increasingly DSA is a relatively elective investigation following identification of an underlying vascular lesion on CTA or MRI/MRA. This has the advantage of combining the investigation with potential endovascular treatment. The anatomical detail provided by DSA is unparalleled (Fig. 8.10) and is of use in planning and delivering endovascular, surgical or radiosurgical treatments. In addition, DSA provides dynamic evaluation of vascular lesion such as the degree of AV shunting.

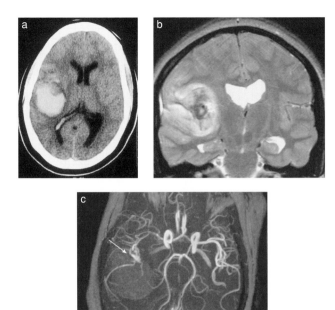

Fig. 8.9. An 11-year-old girl presented with a sudden onset of a left hemiparesis. (a) Axial CT scan demonstrates a hyperdense haematoma with an area of lower hyperdensity thought to represent an aneurysm. (b) The MRI was acquired within 24 hours of onset. A coronal T2-weighted image shows that the haematoma is centred in the Sylvian fissure with the aneurysm in the centre and a rim of more acute low signal representing extracellular haemoglobin. (c) Three-dimensional time-of-flight magnetic resonance angiography confirms the presence of an aneurysm (long arrow) arising from a branch of the middle cerebral artery. The patient underwent emergency evacuation of the clot and clipping of the aneurysm. Histology revealed inflammation within the wall in keeping with a mycotic aneurysm.

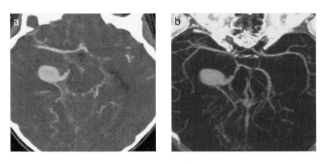

Fig. 8.10. A 12-year-old girl presented with headache, neck stiffness and loss of consciousness. (a) Axial CT (not shown) demonstrated the presence of subarachnoid blood and the CT angiography showed an aneurysm. (b) An amergency angiogram confirmed the presence of a posterior cerebral artery territory aneurysm.

The timing of DSA depends on the patient's clinical condition and the urgency of surgery. The risk of rebleeding in children with AA means that DSA is usually undertaken relatively early in the clinical course in cases with negative CTA/MRA or in those where endovascular treatment of AA is proposed. If clinically acceptable, patients with IPH thought to be due to an AVM (indicated by calcification on CT, the presence of a nidus of vessels or large draining vein, or the position of the haematoma, e.g. within the thalamus, or identified on MRI/CTA) should have DSA delayed for 4–6 weeks.

This allows resolution of the haematoma and the resulting mass effect, which in the acute phase may compress the abnormal vessels and prohibit visualization of the underlying AVM. DSA is particularly valuable in detecting small peripheral AVMs which may not be seen on conventional MRI or MRA (Fig. 8.11). In a small proportion of patients, DSA in the acute phase will not identify a vascular lesion subsequently demonstrated.

MR IMAGING FEATURES OF VASCULAR LESIONS

The cardinal features of an AVM seen on MRI are a nidus of abnormal vessels and a large draining vein, visualized as signal voids due to fast flowing blood on the conventional images or as abnormal vessels on the MRA (Fig. 8.12). The nidus of vessels and both deep and superficial draining veins can also be identified by MRA. Flow aneurysms and intranidal aneurysms may be associated with AVMs.

On MRI, the characteristic appearance of a cavernoma is of a sharply marginated, lobulated mass with heterogeneous signal characteristics and without surrounding oedema. Classically, a haemosiderin rim (low signal on both T1- and T2-weighted) is seen. Gradient echo imaging is of particular value in the detection of additional and often small lesions (Fig. 8.13).

Developmental venous anomalies (Fig. 8.14) are radially orientated dilated veins, separated by brain parenchyma, that drain into a single, dilated venous structure and have a very typical 'caput medusa' appearance on MRI. They most commonly occur in the frontal lobe (40%), the posterior fossa (20%) and the parietal lobe (15%).[71]

Capillary telangiectasia are seen on gradient echo imaging or as an area of enhancement following contrast.[72] They

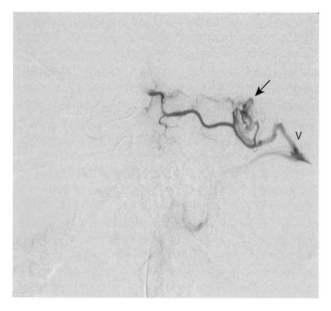

Fig. 8.11. A 9-year-old boy presented with a small peripheral haematoma. MRI/MRA did not reveal a vascular cause. Conventional angiography shows an arteriovenous malformation (arrow) fed from branches of the posterior cerebral artery and draining early into an enlarged vein (v).

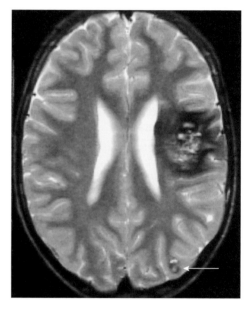

Fig. 8.13. A large area of low signal on the T2-weighted sequence indicates the presence of haemosiderin in a large cavernoma. A second smaller cavernoma with a typical haemosiderin rim is also seen (arrow).

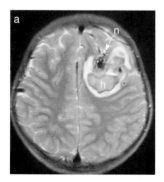
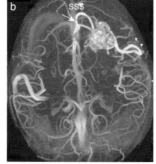

Fig. 8.12. (a) An arteriovenous malformation is well visualized on the axial T2-weighted images as signal voids from the nidus of vessels surrounded by a haematoma and odema. (b) A three-dimensional time of flight angiogram demonstrates the nidus of abnormal vessels with superficial draining veins to the superior saggital sinus (arrow) and peripheral cortical veins (arrowheads). h, haematoma; n, nidus.

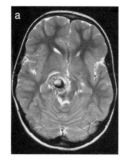
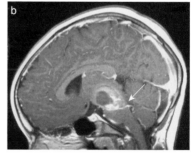

Fig. 8.14. A haematoma is seen within the midbrain on the left on the axial T2-weighted (a) and sagittal post-contrast T1-weighted (b) images. A large pontomesencephalic vein (arrow) lies inferior to the haematoma indicating the presence of an underlying developmental venous anomaly.

are most commonly found in the pons, rarely bleed and are usually found at autopsy.

The presence of a haematoma or subarachnoid blood detected by CT or MRI will help to localize the site of an *arterial aneurysm*. Associated cerebritis, abscess, oedema or infarction may also be visualized. Saccular aneurysms are dilatations which in children arise more distal to the circle of Willis than those seen on adults. One-third to one-half arise from the posterior circulation[39,72] although they are commonly found in the anterior circulation in children.[52] Giant aneurysms are seen on CT and MRI as blood-filled saccular dilatations arising from major vessels (e.g. see Fig. 8.3). Mycotic aneurysms are fusiform dilatations and are often small and peripherally sited. Even though MRA is currently less reliable than DSA for the diagnosis of aneurysms in people at risk, it is preferred in most asymptomatic individuals.

MR features of tumours

Although CT may suggest the presence of an underlying tumour, MRI is a much more sensitive imaging modality to the presence of a tumour. In the majority of cases, the signal characteristics of tumour (low signal on T1-weighted images and high signal on T2-weighted images) can be distinguished from those of the haematoma (Fig. 8.2). Gadolinium enhancement may be demonstrated in the presence of tumour but can also be seen in the periphery of haematomas.

RECOMMENDATIONS FOR IMAGING IN CHILDREN WITH INTRACRANIAL HAEMORRHAGE (Fig. 8.15)

Once acute ICH is identified, we recommend initial evaluation with CTA in order to identify a potential underlying vascular lesion. If this is positive, subsequent imaging is planned based on the clinical state of the patient, proposed treatment modality

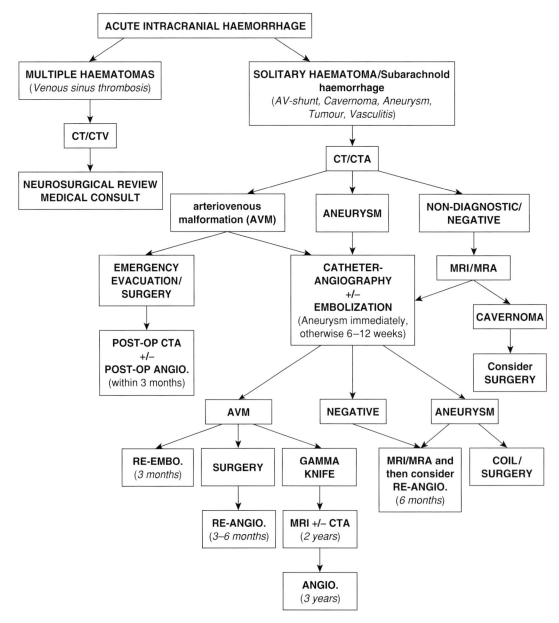

Fig. 8.15. Recommendations for imaging other children with intracranial haemorrhage.

and characteristics of the lesion. If CTA is negative we recommended MRI with gadolinium as a contrast agent and intracranial MRA to identify both vascular and non-vascular causes of IPH. Early MRI (within 48 hours) is ideal to avoid contamination of the MRA by T1 changes arising from the haematoma (e.g. see Fig. 8.8). We recommend using a time of flight sequence to maximize the resolution of the MRA sequence. Children found to have a systemic cause for ICH do not usually require further imaging unless venous sinus thrombosis is suspected when this can be confirmed on MRA and MR venography (Fig. 8.4). If no structural or systemic cause is found in the acute period, we recommend repeating the MRI examination after an interval of 2–3 months. If this remains negative, DSA is recommended.

Children with SAH or IVH should have an early CTA and if this is negative we recommend early DSA, proceeding to MRI with contrast enhancement and MRA if there is still no diagnosis. In a small study of 30 adult patients with angiogram negative SAH, MRI was positive in two studies; one demonstrated an aneurysm and another demonstrated a brainstem lesion of unknown aetiology.[73] In adult studies of angiogram negative SAH who had not had MRI, repeat DSA revealed an aneurysm in 5% and 6% of patients respectively.[74,75] However the aetiology of SAH differs in children from adults and as there are currently no data available in children, we recommend that if DSA and MRI are negative, a repeat DSA should be considered. This should be determined on a case by case basis and only after review of all the imaging together by the multidisciplinary team.

8.2 Surgical Treatment of Haemorrhagic Stroke in Children

Joan P. Grieve and Neil D. Kitchen

Introduction
The principles of surgical treatment of haemorrhagic stroke differ little between adult and paediatric populations, although this problem is less commonly encountered in children. However, the spectrum of disease causing ICH is very different and is often due to developmental or genetic causes. Thorough investigation is required to elucidate the problem fully before considering surgery, both to identify the cause and elucidate the extent of the pathology. A team approach in dealing with these children is of utmost importance. Input is often required from several specialities, including paediatricians, neurosurgeons, neurologists, neuroradiologists and radiotherapists, in order to decide the most appropriate treatment for each specific case.

Haemorrhage due to structural lesions
Vascular anomalies are the most common cause of primary ICH in infants and children (see Chapter 8, Section 8.1). Thus any spontaneous haemorrhage in a child should be presumed to be due to an underlying structural abnormality until proven otherwise. In the acute setting of raised intracranial pressure and coma as a result of a haematoma, immediate consideration has to be given to surgical treatment of the haematoma. Adequate investigation preoperatively should be undertaken, if time allows, including four-vessel angiography to delineate any structural lesion, in particular AVMs or aneurysms. Angiography should demonstrate the type, size and orientation of any lesion, the relationship between AVM or aneurysm and parent vessels, collateral flow through the circle of Willis, the presence of adjacent perforators and the state of the cerebral vasculature, including other associated AVMs or aneurysms. MRI can also add useful information, particularly demonstrating the site and surrounding anatomy of the lesion, as well as identifying angiographically occult lesions. It should be borne in mind that the mass effect caused by the haematoma can totally obscure or prevent complete demonstration of a vascular lesion on angiography.

There is no compelling evidence that surgical evacuation of a supratentorial intraparenchymal haematoma is beneficial at any age. Mendelow and colleagues[76] found no benefit from early (less than 24 hours) haematoma evacuation in a randomized trial of individuals with non-traumatic supratentorial haemorrhage. A smaller study investigating earlier (less than 4 hours) surgery was halted after rebleeding occurred in 4 of 11 individuals who underwent early haematoma evacuation.[77] Haematoma evacuation may occasionally alleviate impending brain herniation in selected individuals with a cerebellar lesion or a large haemorrhage in the cerebral hemisphere. There is currently no evidence base for the use of Factor VII in children with ICH.

ARTERIOVENOUS MALFORMATIONS
AVMs (Figs 8.5, 8.7 and 8.12) are the most common structural lesion to present with haemorrhage in the paediatric population. Intracranial haemorrhage is the most common initial manifestation and is seen in as many as 80% of symptomatic AVMs. The haemorrhage is generally parenchymal but blood may dissect into the subarachnoid space and ventricular system. As a consequence of haemorrhage, the patient may develop signs and symptoms of raised intracranial pressure, focal neurological signs or coma. As AVM surgery can be protracted, it is desirable, whenever possible, to plan the malformation excision as an elective procedure after adequate investigation. Consideration of treatment of these lesions is undertaken as a team approach including neurosurgeons, interventional radiologists and radiotherapists. Although surgical excision of a brain AVM is considered by most to be the ideal treatment, not all lesions are amenable to surgery. In particular, galenic AVMs are the domain of the interventional radiologist (see Chapter 13). All treatment options should be considered with combined approaches (e.g. preoperative embolization followed by definitive surgery with complete resection of the AVM) being increasingly used.

If only subarachnoid haemorrhage has occurred, or if the intracerebral haemorrhage is small and the patient's condition stable, interval surgery may be staged after a wait of a few days to weeks. During that time, the child is monitored appropriately. This may include observation on the intensive care unit, monitoring of intracranial pressure and control of cerebral perfusion pressure. The advantages of delay include a relaxed brain and liquefying haematoma. In the acute setting of coma and raised intracranial pressure, delayed surgery is not always an option. In this situation, some surgeons prefer to remove only the haematoma initially, avoiding any possible underlying vascular lesion, to relieve the mass effect and alleviate the acutely raised intracranial pressure. However other individuals feel that both the haematoma and underlying AVM can be dealt with at the same time. Decisions such as these are often dependent on the clinical condition of the patient as well as the site and size of the lesion concerned. Surgical principles generally suggest that removal of the lesion should only be undertaken acutely if a total resection is possible. Straying into a vascular malformation, with subsequent partial removal of the lesion, increases the postoperative rehaemorrhage risk. It can also be extremely difficult to gain adequate haemostasis prior to closure.

There is not the same urgency in the group of children who present with symptoms other than raised intracranial pressure as a result of haemorrhage. In these situations the objective of surgery for AVMs is to eliminate the risk of ICH and, where possible, to halt neurological deterioration. The decision to offer treatment to a child with an AVM must be supported by an understanding of the risks related to treatment of that particular AVM. The Spetzler–Martin[37] grading system for AVMs (see Chapter 8, Section 8.1) attempts to deal with the complexity surrounding surgical decision-making. Although this grading system was based on surgical results in an adult population, it remains a useful guide as to the resectability of any AVM. Children with intracranial AVMs pose special challenges because of their unacceptable life-long risk of haemorrhage, neurological deficits or death when treated conservatively. The younger the child is, the greater the indication for attempted resection, because of the longer vulnerable period for rupture or worsening symptomatology.

Perioperative management of a child with an AVM requires all of the major neuro-anaesthetic and pharmacological techniques currently available. A craniotomy is performed in a routine fashion depending on the precise location of the lesion. When haemorrhage does occur, it usually represents transgression into the malformation itself, rather than from the original site of haemorrhage. This haemorrhage can be controlled with general packing while the dissection proceeds at a remote site. A parenchymal clot, if present, can create considerable 'autodissection' of the AVM. After the haematoma has been removed, the surgeon will recognize the AVM hanging from the wall or roof of the cavity. The dissection proceeds with microinstruments in an organized circumferential fashion around the malformation, preserving until the end the

majority of major draining veins. Total excision of the lesion can only be confirmed on postoperative angiography. If there is residual malformation, further intervention becomes necessary to occlude the remnant. Thereafter, the child's convalescence depends only on rehabilitation needs. The degree of their motor, speech and cerebellar recovery can be remarkable.

The reported mortality rate following surgery ranges between 0 and 8%.[18,32,78–80] Between 50% and 75% have no neurological deficit at follow-up, with severe complications after surgery being reported in about 10% of patients.[81] Humphreys et al[78] reported on a series of 160 children over a 45-year period, of whom 129 (82%) underwent surgical treatment. Complete AVM resection was possible in 88 children. Fifty-six (64%) of those had a normal neurological outcome, 21 had persistent deficits, eight developed seizures and one had cognitive difficulties. One patient died on the day following surgery and another died of causes unrelated to the AVM. Surgical resection provided complete relief from seizures (off anticonvulsant medication) in 13 of 22 (59%) children. Complete removal of an AVM is currently achieved in 70–90% of children.[32,78] Surgery allows a definitive cure for these lesions. However, there have been cases where recanalization has occurred despite documented evidence that the AVMs have been completely obliterated.[18]

Patients presenting with haemorrhage tend to have improvement in neurological function on the modified Rankin scale whereas those with non-haemorrhagic presentations are more likely to experience deterioration, albeit usually slight.[82] Several groups have had excellent results by offering surgery to patients with Spetzler–Martin grades I–III lesions.[83–85] Grade 3 lesions are heterogeneous and have variable outcomes after surgery: small AVMs having a better prognosis than medium/deep AVMs which have a better prognosis than medium/eloquent AVMs; large grade 3 lesions are very rare.[82] There appears to be a higher chance of neurological deficit if embolization is undertaken before surgery.[86] In a recent statistical model looking at prediction of outcome for surgery, diffuseness, white matter configuration, arterial perforator supply and associated aneurysms were added to the Spetzler–Martin criteria and brain eloquence, diffuse nidus and deep venous drainage were significant predictors of early disabling neurological deficits.[87] Allowing for differences in clinical presentation, anatomical location and surgical technique, children undergoing microsurgical resection of AVMs do better than adults, with greater improvement on the modified Rankin scale.[88] This is likely to be related to neural plasticity as well as better general health and should be taken into account when deciding between surgery, interventional neuroradiology and stereotactic radiotherapy.

CEREBRAL ANEURYSMS

Cerebral aneurysms present less commonly than AVMs in the paediatric population. The reason for this is that, unlike AVMs, the vast majority of aneurysms are thought not to be congenital, but rather acquired during life. The principles of aneurysmal management are similar in both the adult and paediatric populations. The primary aim is to exclude the aneurysm from the cerebral circulation. This is most commonly performed by craniotomy and placing a clip across the neck of the aneurysm. The adult population is increasingly being treated using Guglielmi Detachable Coils (GDC),[89] particularly for those lesions found arising from the vertebrobasilar system. However the indications for coiling and results of long-term follow-up need to be examined further before their role in the management of paediatric SAH patients can be fully delineated. It is an attractive minimally invasive alternative to surgical clipping that can be carried out at the same time as diagnostic angiography and the International Subarachnoid Aneurysm Trial (ISAT) showed better outcome in terms of death and dependency on the modified Rankin scale.[90] One particular problem with coiled aneurysms is that the limited long-term studies available suggest that neck remnants can lead to recurrent aneurysms. Recurrence rates of 16–32% within 2–3 years have been seen.[91,92] This is clearly not acceptable in the paediatric population and, in addition, the rate of initial obliteration appears to be higher for surgical treatment in the paediatric population so aneurysmal clipping via craniotomy remains a good option in children.[55]

Aneurysms in children are often found at unusual sites.[93] They are more often giant, with only one-quarter of them being small and saccular, typical features of adult aneurysms.[94] There is a higher proportion of mycotic lesions that are often small and peripherally located[95] (Fig. 8.9). Mycotic aneurysms are typically treated by craniotomy and excision of the aneurysm, the vessels often being too friable and small to tolerate isolation of the aneurysm alone, leaving the parent vessel intact. These children commonly have predisposing factors such as congenital heart disease. Traumatic aneurysms or those associated with connective tissue disorders, such as polycystic kidney disease or Marfan or Ehlers–Danlos syndrome, are also more commonly encountered.[96] Incidental lesions found on imaging are generally treated more aggressively than those found in the adult population because of the life-long risk of rupture.

Aneurysmal rupture is primarily associated with SAH, although intraventricular and intracerebral haematoma can occur. Surgery for evacuation of intracerebral haematomas associated with aneurysmal rupture is only occasionally needed. Adult data suggest that if unprotected, 15–20% of patients will rebleed in the first 2 weeks,[97,98] carrying with it a significant mortality and morbidity. In most studies there is an initial peak in the first 48 hours of rehaemorrhage of approximately 4% per day, which rapidly steadies at 1–2% per day until 40 days posthaemorrhage.[99] After 6 months there is a long-term risk of further haemorrhage of 3% per year. Because of this, individuals suffering a spontaneous SAH require prompt investigation to determine the cause of haemorrhage. Surgery is often also needed in these children to treat hydrocephalus, acutely in the form of an external ventricular drain, or in the long term with a ventriculo-peritoneal shunt once the blood has resolved.

Neurological deficits following aneurysmal rupture are commonly caused by the initial haemorrhage, but may develop subsequently as a result of vasospasm. Symptomatic vasospasm occurs in 20–30% of patients following SAH and is clinically at its worst 3–14 days after the haemorrhage.[99] The mechanism by which vasospasm occurs is poorly understood. Although not treated surgically, this is a problem commonly encountered by the neurosurgeon in these children. All patients suffering an aneurysmal SAH are treated with both volume expansion and nimodipine, a calcium channel antagonist, in an effort to counteract the effects of spasm, which if severe can result in ischaemic stroke.

Results of surgery are dependent upon the clinical condition of the child prior to surgery, as is indeed the case in adults. Aneurysms are more commonly giant in children with a corresponding increase in surgical mortality and morbidity. Surgery to aneurysms in the paediatric population has an associated 5–20% mortality and 10% morbidity.[94,95,100]

ANGIOMATOUS MALFORMATIONS

These lesions are increasingly being identified with the advent of modern neuroimaging. The number, size and anatomical location should be evaluated carefully with regard to relevance to the patient's symptoms. The most commonly identified are cavernous angiomas and developmental venous anomalies.

Cavernous angiomas appear as a dark blue or purple lobulated lesions which, although unencapsulated, are well circumscribed. The surrounding brain is frequently stained with haemosiderin. The natural history of these lesions remains unclear. A small percentage do appear to develop progressive symptoms with haemorrhage, seizures or progressive neurological deficit. With the exception of those lesions in the brainstem, most episodes of haemorrhage from cavernous angiomas are minor, and indeed some may be undetected. Fatal haemorrhage has been reported, but usually from a posterior fossa lesion. MRI is now the investigation of choice, where a central core of mixed signal intensity surrounded by a rim of hypointense signal produced by haemosiderin is seen (Fig. 8.13).

For children who have suffered a haemorrhage, the angioma is best excised early, when the haematoma bed can facilitate the surgical definition and the malformation can be completely excised. If presenting with seizures, the focal lesion and surrounding haemosiderin-stained brain should be considered the epileptogenic focus and should be excised. Small cavernous angiomas may be difficult to localize at operation, especially if it does not present at the cortex. Some form of intra-operative image guidance in this situation will allow the surgeon to make a safe, judicious entry thorough the cortex to the malformation. At that point, the lesion is easily dissected free, and haemorrhaging from disrupted vessels is seldom a problem. Other lesions however may not be surgically accessible, particularly those found within the brainstem. These are commonly treated conservatively, though the role of stereotactic radiosurgery has yet to be defined fully. There is preliminary evidence in the adult population that radiosurgery may reduce the risk of further haemorrhage.[101]

In a series of 24 children, 13 presented with epilepsy, nine presented with haemorrhage, whilst the remaining two were asymptomatic with the diagnosis made as an incidental finding.[102] Only nine children had a persistence of the presurgical neurological signs, although improved with surgery; no patient showed a progression of preoperative neurological signs; one child died, but his clinical condition was critical prior to surgery. Removal of the cavernoma allowed control of the seizures in all epilepsy cases.

Developmental venous anomalies, although the most common intracranial vascular lesion, are the least likely structural abnormality to cause symptoms. Indeed, many regard them simply as a variant of normal. This type of lesion is composed of enlarged medullary veins converging into a central draining channel, separated by normal-appearing parenchyma (Fig. 8.14). It is generally believed that they are frequently associated with other more symptomatic conditions, such as cavernous angiomas, and are often wrongly identified as the source of symptoms. When haemorrhage does occur, it more commonly affects the posterior fossa. Occasionally it may be necessary to evacuate the haematoma created by a developmental venous anomaly, when only clot removal should be attempted. Obliteration of any of the major draining veins should be avoided.

Haemorrhage due to non-structural causes

The operative technique used in the treatment of non-structural ICH does not differ from that for ICH from a structural cause. However, it is important that any underlying haematological predisposition that the child has to spontaneous ICH is detected and that it is a true primary haemorrhage that has occurred. Haemophilia, vitamin K deficiency, disseminated intravascular coagulation and idiopathic thrombocytopenia purpura may all be complicated by intracerebral haemorrhage. Intracerebral haematomas may also be due to haemorrhage into tumours. The underlying primary cause may have already been diagnosed, but rarely haemorrhage into a secondary deposit may be the initial presentation.

Any coagulopathy will predispose the child to ICH and it is therefore of vital importance that this has been reversed prior to surgery and that clotting remains normal both perioperatively and in the postoperative period, to prevent major life-threatening haemorrhage at the time of surgery or recurrent postoperative haemorrhage.

Summary

Any child suffering ICH requires adequate imaging and investigation to identify possible causes or predisposing factors. Each child requires assessment on an individual basis, when frequently a multidisciplinary approach is required to ensure that the child undergoes the most appropriate form of treatment, safely and effectively.

8.3 Interventional Neuroradiology in the Management of Aneurysms and Arteriovenous Shunts in Children

Chao Bao Luo, Marina Sachet Ferreira, Hortensia Alvarez, Georges Rodesch, Pierre L. Lasjuanias and Stefan K. Brew

Introduction

Cerebral arteriovenous shunts (CAVS) and aneurysms are uncommon lesions[52,103,104] although children form an important proportion of patients[105,106] and their needs must be met appropriately.

Aneurysms

The aetiology, pathology, epidemiology and natural history of aneurysm is children is poorly understood, but is likely to be different to adults. The aneurysms have different angiographic morphology, and are found in different locations, particularly commonly in the posterior circulation. Treatment of children whose aneurysms do not thrombose spontaneously is similar to that used in adult aneurysm patients. Overall, complete or partial spontaneous thrombosis occurs in 10–20%.[52] A large randomized trial in adults showed a benefit in terms of reduced death or dependency for detachable Gugliemi coils over surgical clipping in the treatment of ruptured aneurysms, although late recurrence was greater in the endovascularly treated group.[90,107] Obliteration with onyx is now widely used (Fig. 8.16). Both microsurgical and endovascular techniques have been used effectively in children with intracranial aneurysms.[52,55,108] Posterior circulation aneurysms seem to be more prevalent in children, and are usually better tackled endovascularly. There is some concern that an endovascular aneurysm occlusion might not provide the same long-lasting protection from rupture as surgery, but most endovascular procedures are effective in permanently obliterating the aneurysm and parents often prefer the non-surgical approach.[55] Infectious aneurysms can occasionally be treated medically if the patient is systemically ill, but both endovascular and conventional surgical treatments should be considered.

Of 59 patients referred to Le Kremlin-Bicêtre,[52] 32 underwent surgical (22%), endovascular (63%) or combined (9%) treatment. Eleven patients were treated conservatively and in five patients the aneurysms had spontaneously thrombosed at admission. Presumed dissecting aneurysms were frequent in children of all ages with either associated thrombosis or arterial tear with repeated acute haemorrhage and poor outcome. Two types of dissection seem identifiable despite the small number of cases collected: (1) acute segmental arterial tear without thrombosis, acute SAH and recurrence before 5 years; and

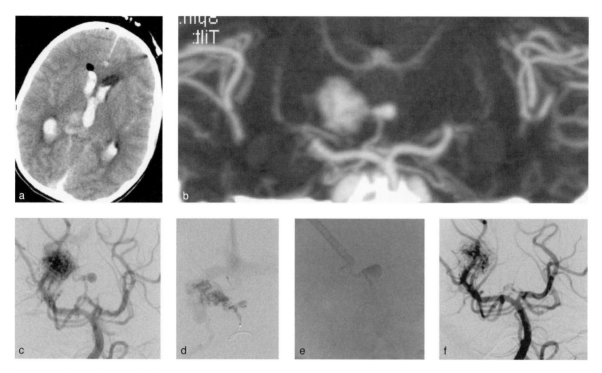

Fig. 8.16. Images from a 10-year-old girl who collapsed unconscious suddenly and had intraventricular haemorrhage on CT (a). The CT angiogram (b) showed an arteriovenous malformation and an aneurysm confirmed on the formal arteriogram (c). As she had bled from the aneurysm, this was embolized with onyx (d,e) and occlusion of the aneurysm was confirmed on the post-procedure arteriogram (f). The arteriovenous malformation was subsequently treated with stereotactic radiosurgery. (Images courtesy of Dr John Millar, Consultant Neuroradiologist, Southampton University Hospitals NHS Trust, UK.)

(2) subacute focal dissection with partial thrombosis (or mural haematoma), rare SAH and no early recurrence. The former would require aggressive management whereas the latter often do not require interventional approaches.

In contrast, conventionally located saccular aneurysms are relatively rare in children. When found, usually in the context of recent SAH, they are managed in an analogous way to those found in adults.

The posterior cerebral artery is a particularly common site for aneurysms in childhood. Treatment of these aneurysms is difficult, as it is seldom possible to spare the parent artery. Children often, but not always, tolerate occlusion of the aneurysm sac and parent artery without stroke.

Arteriovenous shunts

Intracranial arterio-venous shunts can be divided into pure pial AV fistula, pial arteriovenous malformation (PAVM), vein of Galen malformation (VGAM) and other rare conditions such as dural sinus malformation. VGAM will be addressed separately. It should be noted that even experienced practitioners may have difficulty classifying some cases; a high flow pial fistula of the medial surface of the parietal lobe can look very much like a VGAM. This lack of diagnostic clarity contaminates all the literature in this field and makes any effort to predict natural history difficult.

In most surgical series, children represent 20% of the overall pial AV shunt cases. The age at the time of diagnosis varies in the literature.[109,110] In over 600 cases, the following incidences were noted: before 5 years, 10–20%; 6–10 years, 25–30%; 11–15 years, 42–60%. These figures are significantly different from our personal statistics, as more than 50% of our patients were diagnosed before 2 years of age. Considering the PAVM, only 27.6% of them were diagnosed in neonates or infants. From this difference we conclude that most of the literature relates to the management of AVM in children over 5 years of age, and it indirectly suggests that some of the earlier diagnosed AVMs were VGAMs (see Chapter 13). There is, however, almost certainly an element of referral bias in our cohort.

Embolization is one of the treatment options for AVMs (Fig. 8.17). For a population of 1 000 000 adults and children, figures for embolization as well as radiosurgery procedures range from two to seven per year, depending on the strategy at hand.[29] This means that published experience with embolization as one of the modalities for managing children with PAVMs has mainly been accrued in a handful of centres.[111,112] Although embolization is an option in many children with PAVMs,[111] the results of surgery for Grades 1–3 lesions in this group are good (see Chapter 8, Section 8.2). There are no randomized controlled trials and very few data comparing techniques in children but in adults undergoing non-surgical approaches to Grades 1–3 lesions, the number of patients requiring treatment with more than one method for obliteration increases drastically, as does the potential risk for procedure-related complications.[29] However, it is clear that some patients benefit from embolization. This chapter reviews the experience with embolization

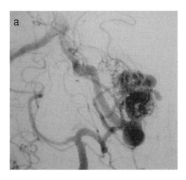
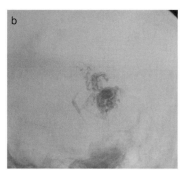
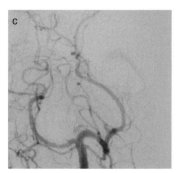

Fig. 8.17. Embolization of an arteriovenous malformation (AVM) with onyx. Digital subtraction arteriography before (a), and after (b) showing the cast of onyx in the AVM and occlusion confirmed on the delayed angiogram (c). (Images courtesy of Dr John Millar, Consultant Neuroradiologist, Southampton University Hospitals NHS Trust, UK.)

for pial AVMs at Le Kremlin-Bicêtre and Great Ormond Street Hospital for Children.

Clinical manifestations and natural history of cerebral arteriovenous shunts

PAVMs usually present with ICH.[106] Only 7–29% of PAVM patients present with epilepsy, which may represent a recent haemorrhage event in any case. The severity of such episodes is different from those in adults, both with regards to diagnostic imaging and clinical symptoms. The revealing symptoms in a series of 93 children were as follows: cerebral haemorrhage, seizure from haemorrhage, seizure without haemorrhage, subarachnoid haemorrhage, progressive deficit, headache, learning disability, failure to thrive and facial collateral circulation. A convulsion in a neonate or a seizure in a child suggests a different type of cerebral insult. Successful medical management of seizure activity in the child is important, as it has an impact on the child's ability to be independent as well as on psychological development. Contrary to previous reports in the literature, there is no sex dominance in true PAVM; the few reports in which male dominance has been noted included patients with VGAM, though even in this group there may be confounding variables. In the Great Ormond Street Hospital experience, there is no clear-cut sex difference in either group.

Although the numbers are small, in our early experience we saw several cases of early rebleed in children, without specific angio-architectural features that had predicted this. We are therefore increasingly prepared to intervene early in PAVM presenting with haemorrhage in children.

Pathophysiology and anatomical predictors of risk

Knowledge and understanding of the natural history of the disease and its symptomatology have allowed guidelines to be developed in treatment planning. Abnormalities of the venous system are common in paediatric PAVM. Venous high flow angiopathy is very commonly encountered in paediatric PAVM. It represents the most active part of an AVM and it is probable that many symptoms in young children are related to the venous system.[39,113] We have divided the venous angiopathy into three main groups: dural sinus high flow, venous

thrombosis and venous stenosis. In infancy, venous high flow angiopathy and venous hypertension can lead to learning disability, neurological deficit, haemorrhage and seizure. Arterial angiopathies are mainly observed in children and rarely in neonates or infants;[39] this can be an isolated or diffuse stenotic response or arterial enlargement as well as mural impairment with aneurysmal formation. These can induce clinical symptoms such as headache, neurological deficits, seizure and ICH.

CAVSs are different in children and adults. Fistulas are more frequent in children and are always superficial and cortical. They may present with heart failure, and those on the medial surface of the hemisphere are often misdiagnosed as VGAM. They are most often diagnosed in the first 5 years of life. They can be seen arising from any one artery of the brain, including those of the posterior fossa, and are consistently associated with large venous pouches. Depending on the age of discovery, their tolerance in young children is amazing when one considers their size and flow. They are probably a completely different entity to PAVM, though PAVM in children often contain fistulous components. The second feature of interest to note in children is the existence of multifocal AVM or arteriovenous fistulas (AVF). Series and case reports of multifocal lesions and unusual associations have been published.[114,115] In our experience, twice as many children have multifocal lesions. The lesions are randomly distributed, both supra- and infratentorially.

Pure AVF are more often encountered in neonates, whereas lesions detected in infants are more often nidus-type AVM. Unfortunately, most children that present in the neonatal period with a convulsion or mild congestive cardiac failure are wrongly diagnosed and managed as a well-tolerated VGAM patient and are later referred with a significant neurological deficit. During the weeks between the clinical onset of symptoms and referral, a significant proportion of infants develop 'melting-brain' syndrome.

In comparison, intracranial arteriovenous shunts diagnosed in infancy with mild manifestations are more readily considered for treatment before hydrodynamic disorders or haemorrhage, as the subsequent brain damage does not develop rapidly. Thus we recommend urgent and sometimes emergency management of PAVM in the neonatal and early infancy age group. The angioarchitecture analysis of these patients shows no apparent arterial weakness, but anomalies of venous drainage were noted in many cases.

In summary, paediatric patients more frequently present with multifocal lesions, induced remote arteriovenous shunts,[116] venous thromboses and systemic phenomena,[117–119] large venous ectasia and high-flow lesions, as well as rapid atrophy. Conversely, high-flow angiopathic changes are not seen with the same frequency and flow-related arterial aneurysms are seen only exceptionally[120] whereas proximal occlusive arteriopathy is more frequent. The Spetzler–Martin grading system may need to be applied cautiously in young children, in whom: (1) cerebral eloquence is difficult to assess, particularly in the infant and toddler; (2) many lesions are fistulas or multifocal; (3) because of their flow the lesions usually involve the entire venous system; and (4) the possibilities of recovery in children are different from adults. The decision-making process in children includes, in addition to the conventional objectives, various peculiar factors such as anatomic analysis of veins and the myelination process. Thereafter, progressive deficits related to congested cerebral veins; poorly controlled seizures, haemorrhages with or without specific arterial or venous changes upstream and downstream of the AVMs, or headaches in children without hydrocephalus or macrocrania can become immediate objectives for staged or partial treatment. The relative radiosensitivity of the immature brain must also be taken into account, making radiosurgery relatively unappealing.

Objective of treatment

Ever since AV shunts were first recognized, obliteration of the lesion has been the only acceptable goal. However, rapidly obtaining complete exclusion is not always appropriate if it occurs at the expense of neurological deterioration.

In most instances, the morphological goal can be superimposed on the clinical one. In infants, however, as seen in VGAM (see Chapter 13), these objectives can be separate in time or even contradictory if the attempt to obtain a cure compromises neurological outcome. Staged treatment is the organization of steps to reach a more favourable situation and to achieve a complete exclusion with lower morbidity than if it was accomplished in a single session. Partial treatment is an incomplete exclusion motivated by a clinical concern and targeted to a specific portion of the lesion when complete exclusion cannot be offered with an acceptable level of risk. This means that we aim to obtain – by endovascular or other technique – total exclusion only if a good neurological outcome can be anticipated.

Technical management

Endovascular embolization is performed according to modern principles of AVM embolization.[121] Briefly, transarterial embolizations are accomplished via a transfemoral route with the placement of an arterial sheath. All embolizations are performed with the patient under general anaesthesia. When possible, techniques of superselective angiography are used in pre-embolization planning. Modern flow-assisted wire-guided microcatheters of various sizes are used to inject histocryl or onyx (Fig. 8.17) into the intended vessels. The target vessels are determined depending on the aim of the embolization procedure. Patients may be kept asleep after closure of the shunt in the intensive care unit for 24 hours with normotensive blood pressure. To achieve complete occlusion of fistula,[122,123] usually only one session is needed, whereas the endovascular approach is usually completed in several sessions for the nidus type of AVM.

When discussing partial or complete endovascular exclusion in CAVS patients, we are referring to transarterial embolization with glue or, more recently, onyx (Fig. 8.17). Other embolic agents such as coils, particles, balloons, threads, collagen mixture and other methods have not shown any reliable and predictable results. In our experience, they have never constituted a better embolic agent to reach our therapeutic goal, nor do they represent a satisfactory alternative as a primary embolic agent. Some have been associated with specific complications, such as contrast leakage[124] and hypoglycaemia[125] with ethanol. The transvenous approach to PAVM is currently still an anecdotal method. The basic technique consists of occluding the arterial part of the nidus with the immediate portion of the draining vein. The entire nidus demonstrated may not have to be occluded, as secondary regression of another supply can sometimes be seen in young children. The dangers related to the venous passage of glue and possible subsequent haemorrhage depend on the converging or diverging position of the venous outlets. Multiplicity of the nidus veins and the length of the course in the subpial compartment indicate the distal point of possible venous occlusion.

PAVMs at Hôpital Bicêtre

In the years from 1982 to 2001 Pierre Lasjaunias and his group were actively involved actively involved in the management of 476 CAVSs in children and infants. Of these 258 were true VGAMs and 218 were PAVMs. Haemorrhage occurred as the first symptoms in the children with PAVMs (Tables 8.2–8.4), but none of the VGAM cases. In the PAVM group, 23 children were found to be unsuitable for endovascular treatment, and in 159 cases embolization was indicated as the primary treatment, but 23 children were treated in other institutions. Seventeen children underwent a direct surgical approach (none in the VGAM group). The morphological results after embolization are shown in Table 8.5. In our experience, no child

TABLE 8.2
Clinical presentation of brain arteriovenous malformation in neonates (N=8)

Clinical presentation	Patients	
	Number	**%**
Cardiac failure	4	50
Haemorrhage	3	37.5
Incidental	1	12

TABLE 8.3
Clinical presentation of PAVM in infants (*N*=30)

Clinical presentation	Patients	
	Number	%
Haemorrhage	9	30
Macrocrania	8	26.6
Cardiac failure	7	23.3
Neurological deficit	2	6.6
Seizures	2	6.6
Incidental	2	6.6

AVM, arteriovenous malformation.

TABLE 8.4
Clinical presentation of PAVM in children >2 years old (*N*=180)

Clinical presentation	Patients	
	Number	%
Haemorrhage	90	50
Seizures	30	16.6
Neurological deficit	27	15
Headache	14	7.7
Incidental	6	3.3
Cardiac failure	4	2.2
Psychomotor development retardation	3	1.6
Macrocrania	2	1.1
Other	4	2.2

AVM, arteriovenous malformation.

TABLE 8.5
Morphological results in 136 patients with PAVM

Occlusion	Patients	
	Number	%
100%	28	20.5
80–95%	35	25.7
50–80%	36	26.4
<50%	37	.2

considered completely cured at follow-up showed any recurrent arteriovenous shunting or any new symptom at later clinical or angiographic follow-up.

OUTCOME FOR PAVM UNDERGOING EMBOLIZATION
Normal maturation is an important follow-up criterion in neonates and infants. Even without deficit, haemorrhage or seizure, it helps in assessing treatment quality and success. Failure to obtain a normal brain maturation process may constitute a therapeutic failure if the optimum moment for intervention has been missed. This points to the difference between early irreversible damage and damage by persistent disorder and secondary destruction. Brain calcification, which can be observed in both instances, indicates failure to restore normal haemo- and hydrodynamic conditions in the maturing brain.

In the paediatric series from Le Kremlin-Bicêtre, half of the treated children had a normal neurological examination at final follow-up, and 34.5% had minimal neurological deficit compatible with normal life (Table 8.6). In 6.6% of treated children there were permanent neurological symptoms, 3.6% presented with a temporary neurological symptom and the mortality rate was 1.4% (Table 8.7).

In a population-based study, when using non-surgical approaches to Grades 1–3 lesions, the number of patients requiring treatment with more than one method for obliteration increased drastically as did the potential risk for procedure-related complications.[29] Endovascular treatment carries a procedural risk related to AVM grade (worse in Spetzler–Martin grades III–V particularly related to location in an eloquent part of the brain), presence of a fistula, number of branches treated, venous deposition of glue and periprocedural haemorrhage.[126-128] Haemorrhage as a complication is more common in older patients and in those undergoing partial AVM reduction of >60%.[129] This, together with the poorer outcome with a larger number of branches treated, argues for staged endovascular procedures when these are indicated for AVMs which cannot be obliterated by microsurgery or radiosurgery alone. The stages may be all embolization or a combination of embolization with either microsurgery or

TABLE 8.6
Clinical results in embolized PAVM patients (*N*=136)

Clinical results	Patients	
	Number	%
Asymptomatic	48	35
Non-treated minimal neurological symptom	14	10
Non-treated temporary neurological symptom (including seizures)	4	2.9
Permanent neurological symptom, psychomotor development within 20% of normal school level with support	47	34.5
Severe neurological symptoms, psychomotor development retardation greater than 20% compared with normal education in special school	13	9.5
Death	10	7.3

TABLE 8.7
Complications of embolization for PAVM

Complication	Patients	
	Number	**%**
Permanent neurological symptom	9	6.6
Temporary neurological symptom	5	3.6
Death	2	1.4

radiosurgery, with comparable results for small lesions. For example, in a series of 50 patients treated with embolization followed by radiosurgery (see Chapter 8, Section 8.4), actuarial complete obliteration rate was 67% after 3 years and 78% after 4 years.[130] The complete obliteration rate was significantly higher in AVM <3cm (92% vs 60%) and in AVM Spetzler–Martin Grade I/II (90% vs 59%). Intracranial haemorrhage after radiosurgery was seen in 12% after a median of 8.5 months. Annual haemorrhage risk was 7.9% after 1 year and 2.2% after 2 years. However, in a recent paediatric study, one of the main predictive factors for obliteration was no previous embolization as well as low AVM volume.[131]

Treatment in children should aim to preserve normal neurocognitive maturation as well long-term protection from acute episodes. Staged treatment is the organization of steps to reach a more favourable situation. The decision to stage a procedure carries some significant advantages; particularly in children, where the length of the procedure is limited by puncture time or fluid volumes. In addition, with the haemodynamic triggers being modified, the correction of some disorders induces a normal, although delayed maturation. The remaining patients cannot be cured with the current treatment modalities, either because the lesion cannot be reached or because the disease is multifocal. In this subgroup, treatment is partial and is repeated in time with large intervals between sessions. Palliative treatment is an incomplete exclusion of a lesion in order to stabilize a critical situation. Partial targeted treatment is an incomplete exclusion motivated by a clinical concern requiring improvement and directed towards a specific portion of the lesion. The aim of partial targeted treatment is to eliminate dangerous portions of the AVM progressively or its effects on the adjacent brain or to reduce the seizure activity, progressive deficits or migrainous headaches. In our experience, partial targeted embolization is an acceptable therapeutic objective only if a complete cure cannot be obtained at a satisfactory level of risk, and if the procedure is performed with a permanent agent, such as histocryl. This means that we aim to obtain – by endovascular or other technique – total exclusion if a good neurological outcome can be anticipated. The fact that most lesions in patients referred to us are large or multifocal explains the small number of complete cures in our series. Complete exclusion is frequently obtained, but not as frequently as in VGAM. Even if endovascular management is the primary choice, complementary treatment is usually planned.

Conclusion

When writing this chapter, Pierre Lasjaunias and his group had more than 20 years of experience in the management of CAVSs in children. The adult-based grading should be used with caution in the management of CAVSs in the first few years of life when the anatomy and physiology are different, and because of the specificity of the angioarchitecture. An understanding of the inter-relationship between the lesion to be treated and the other structures has shown its value and permits better patient selection. In the Bicêtre experience, endovascular management of CAVSs in children offers the largest range of possibilities and results. Prediction of the risks of CAVSs in children is different, depending on the anatomophysiological status of the child. Before 2 years of age, the lesions are mainly VGAMs causing systemic and hydrodynamic disorders for which the best therapeutic option is the endovascular approach. Non-Galenic lesions at the same age have a very poor prognosis. After 5–7 years of age, the physiology, type and architecture of these lesions are closer to those in adults and prompt a similar type of management, which in our group is primarily endovascular, followed by surgery if anatomical exclusion cannot be obtained by embolization. Between these ages, management will still be mainly endovascular but, because of late referral, it will often be applied to children who already have cognitive impairment with unpredictable outcomes. Management of children with these lesions requires a large multidisciplinary team, which is the only way of offering the most suitable and effective treatment, the sole guarantee of a good result.

8.4 Stereotactic Radiosurgery in the Management of Arteriovenous Malformations in Children

M.W.R. Radatz and A.A. Kemeny

Introduction

The vast majority of cerebral arteriovenous malformations (AVMs) are congenital lesions. Inheritance is only shown in very rare scenarios in association with neurocutaneous syndromes. They are non-neoplastic anomalies and occur after abnormal development of embryonic vascular channels.[132] The incidence of new symptomatic AVMs presented for neurosurgical intervention is about 12 patients per million population per annum.[133] Additionally there are about seven patients per million per year found to have an AVM on imaging incidentally. AVMs have a 2–4% annual haemorrhage risk and account for 1–2% of all strokes with a mortality rate of about 30% per haemorrhage. About 20% of AVMs present in childhood and they are one of the most frequent causes of haemorrhagic stroke in the paediatric population. Other presentations include headaches, seizures and neurological deficit as result of haemorrhage or steal phenomena.[81,134,135] Spontaneous obliteration is very rare and is described in only 1.3% of PAVMs,[136] usually in post-haemorrhagic lesions with few arterial feeding arteries.

For those considered operable with minimal risk of morbidity and mortality, an immediate removal of the lesion is the ideal treatment. The same applies in the emergency setting where surgical intervention may be life saving. However, surgery for arteriovenous malformations places great demand on the surgeon. The anatomy of the lesion is of vital importance, particularly the size and location of the nidus and its feeding and draining vessels. Spetzler and Martin's[37] classification correlates with surgical morbidity and mortality and is a useful tool in the evaluation of surgical suitability. The surgeon is faced with a high variability of lesions and it is an important task to consider different treatment options such as surgery, embolization and stereotactic radiosurgery and combinations of these options to tailor them to the most appropriate treatment for each individual. This selection process usually involves a multi-disciplinary approach and decision-making process which combines the opinions of neurosurgeons, radiosurgeons and interventional radiologists. Stereotactic radiosurgery using the Leksell Gamma Knife is playing an important part in the treatment of AVMs since it was established in clinical practice at the Karolinska Institute in Stockholm, Sweden.

Leksell gamma knife radiosurgery for arteriovenous malformation

The aim of the treatment in AVMs is prophylaxis of haemorrhages. Therefore, morbidity and mortality of the treatment must be well below the risks of the lesions' natural history. Stereotactic radiosurgery is delivering these standards with its ability to ensure a highly conformal application of single dose radiation to the target. Since the early reports[137] describing radiosurgical AVM obliteration, radiosurgery has become a well-established treatment modality with a good long-term outcome, although surgical excision has advantages for lesions in non-eloquent territories, as the risk of recurrent haemorrhage is reduced immediately. It was shown that the mechanism of action of radiation is a combination of endothelial change[138] and activation of myofibroblasts[139] leading to stenosis and obliteration of the nidus. Protection from future haemorrhage can only be achieved by complete obliteration.[80,140] Complete obliteration in this context is defined as total occlusion of the nidus without any early venous drainage.

Treatment

The treatment involves hospital admission for 1 or 2 days, depending on the suitability of the child for the procedure being carried out under local anaesthetic. Under the age of 14 usually a general anaesthetic is required. After induction the stereotactic frame is applied and the patient undergoes DSA and MRI. The latter helps to improve the 3D appreciation of the nidus and thus it enables a more precise conformation to the shape of the lesion and a reduction in the volume of brain exposed to radiation. This helps to minimize the adverse

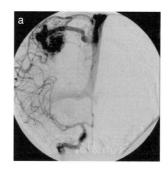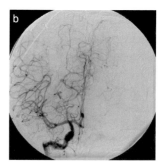

Fig. 8.18. (a,b) Pre- and 3 years post-radiosurgery cerebral arteriography in a teenage girl with an arteriovenous malformation successfully treated with radiosurgery.

effects of radiosurgery. The target definition is followed by dose planning. The dose is prescribed to the margin of the lesion, usually to the 50% isodose, which represents the steepest portion of radiation fall-off curve.[141,142] The dose depends on the location and volume of the lesion as well as the age of the patient and possible previous irradiation. It is a trade-off between the maximal wanted effect and the attempt to minimize radiation-induced side-effects. Therefore the maximum dose (100% isodose) does not exceed 50Gy and may be as little as 24Gy. Once the treatment is finished, the frame is removed, and the patient transferred back to the ward to be discharged the next morning.

Follow-up

To evaluate the treatment results, patients require a series of follow-up examinations, which involve repeat MRI/MRA[140,143–145] and DSA (Fig. 8.18). In the early stages MRI has proven to be a sensitive technique to evaluate cerebral radiation injury and nidus regression by avoiding the more invasive cerebral angiography. The latter remains, however, the criterion-standard in the evaluation of outcome and it is performed when MRI/MRA suggests obliteration. Once complete obliteration has been achieved further follow-up is only required if late symptomatic side-effects occur.

Results

Since the early successes of stereotactic radiosurgery in the treatment of AVMs reported by Steiner et al,[137] many more series have been published. Obliteration rates range from 100% in very small lesions (<1cm^3) to 50% in lesions with a much larger volume (8–10cm^3) and an average obliteration rate of ~80% is reproduced worldwide using the Leksell Gamma Knife.[146–148] The radiation response is significantly better in younger patients, often achieving complete obliteration within the first year.[149,150] In recent paediatric series, complete obliteration of the AVM was documented in 35–92% of patients using either the gamma knife or linear accelerators (LINAC) systems.[130,131,151–154]

With longer follow-up times, better imaging and better dose planning available, the understanding of dose–volume effects and side-effects of stereotactic radiosurgery are much better understood[155] and have allowed clinicians to make treatment safer. Multidisciplinary teams are evaluating now the suitability of each individual and treatment plans are tailored to maximize cure rates. Combinations of embolization and microsurgery with stereotactic radiosurgery are routine in supraregional centres of excellence, allowing for otherwise inoperable or untreatable lesions to be cured.[156–158] In some cases, obliteration of the nidus may require repeated stereotactic irradiation, which offers as good obliteration rates as after the primary treatment with some increase in side-effects.[159] Excellent results may be seen in seizure outcome in children, with 85% becoming seizure free and off medication already 1 year after stereotactic radiosurgery.[160] In addition, stereotactic radiosurgery was shown to improve headaches in ~75% in a series of 247 consecutive patients reported by Steiner et al.[148]

Complications

Post-radiosurgical serial MRI shows radiation-induced changes in about 30% of patients, of which only ~10% are symptomatic.[161] Symptomatic radionecrosis is reported in about 3–4% of cases[153] and is highly dependant on dose to and volume of the treated target; it appears on neuroimaging as focal oedema. Neurological sequelae are seen in 5–15%.[131,152] Rebleeding before total obliteration occurred within 4 years in only 4%.[153,162] The haemorrhage risk is already significantly reduced in the first two years after stereotactic radiosurgery if compared with the natural course of these lesions. Symptomatology is highly dependent on eloquence of the irradiated tissue and is highest within the brainstem. A few cases of meningioma have been reported at least 10 years after radiosurgery.[163]

Conclusions

Gamma knife or LINAC stereotactic radiosurgery offers an excellent treatment option in inaccessible, deep or eloquently placed paediatric AVM presenting with haemorrhage, epilepsy or headaches. The combination with interventional and microsurgical techniques brings some previously inoperable lesions into the realm of curable abnormalities.

REFERENCES

1. Broderick J, Talbot GT, Prenger E, Leach A, Brott T. Stroke in children within a major metropolitan area: the surprising importance of intracerebral hemorrhage. J Child Neurol 1993; 8(3):250–255.
2. Schoenberg BS, Mellinger JF, Schoenberg DG. Cerebrovascular disease in infants and children: a study of incidence, clinical features, and survival. Neurology 1978; 28(8):763–768.
3. Giroud M, Lemesle M, Gouyon JB, Nivelon JL, Milan C, Dumas R. Cerebrovascular disease in children under 16 years of age in the city of Dijon, France: a study of incidence and clinical features from 1985 to 1993. J Clin Epidemiol 1995; 48(11):1343–1348.
4. Fullerton HJ, Wu YW, Zhao S, Johnston SC. Risk of stroke in children: ethnic and gender disparities. Neurology 2003; 61(2): 189–194.
5. Fullerton HJ, Wu YW, Sidney S, Johnston SC. Recurrent hemorrhagic stroke in children: a population-based cohort study. Stroke 2007; 38(10):2658–2662.
6. Chung B, Wong V. Pediatric stroke among Hong Kong Chinese subjects. Pediatrics 2004; 114(2):e206–e212.
7. Williams AN, Davies P, Eunson PD, Kirkham FJ, Green SH. Stroke and cerebrovascular disease: Brimingham Children's Hospital 1993–1998. Dev Med Child Neurol 2002; 45(suppl):10.
8. Williams AN, Kirkham FJ. Childhood stroke, stroke-like illness and cerebrovascular disease. Stroke 2004; 35(Suppl):311.
9. Jordan LC, Johnston SC, Wu YW, Sidney S, Fullerton HJ. The importance of cerebral aneurysms in childhood hemorrhagic stroke: a population-based study. Stroke 2009; 40(2):400–405.
10. Blom I, De Schryver EL, Kappelle LJ, Rinkel GJ, Jennekens-Schinkel A, Peters AC. Prognosis of haemorrhagic stroke in childhood: a long-term follow-up study. Dev Med Child Neurol 2003; 45(4):233–239.
11. Meyer-Heim AD, Boltshauser E. Spontaneous intracranial haemorrhage in children: aetiology, presentation and outcome. Brain Dev 2003; 25(6):416–421.
12. Higgins JJ, Kammerman LA, Fitz CR. Predictors of survival and characteristics of childhood stroke. Neuropediatrics 1991; 22(4): 190–193.
13. Keidan I, Shahar E, Barzilay Z, Passwell J, Brand N. Predictors of outcome of stroke in infants and children based on clinical data and radiologic correlates. Acta Paediatr 1994; 83(7):762–765.
14. Al-Jarallah A, Al-Rifai MT, Riela AR, Roach ES. Nontraumatic brain hemorrhage in children: etiology and presentation. J Child Neurol 2000; 15(5):284–289.
15. Celli P, Ferrante L, Palma L, Cavedon G. Cerebral arteriovenous malformations in children. Clinical features and outcome of treatment in children and in adults. Surg Neurol 1984; 22(1):43–49.
16. Thorpe ML, Cordato DJ, Morgan MK, Herkes GK. Postoperative seizure outcome in a series of 114 patients with supratentorial arteriovenous malformations. J Clin Neurosci 2000; 7(2):107–111.
17. Whigham KB, O'Toole K. Understanding the neuropsychologic outcome of pediatric AVM within a neurodevelopmental framework. Cogn Behav Neurol 2007; 20(4):244–257.
18. Kondziolka D, Humphreys RP, Hoffman HJ, Hendrick EB, Drake JM. Arteriovenous malformations of the brain in children: a forty year experience. Can J Neurol Sci 1992; 19(1):40–45.
19. Papadias A, Taha A, Sgouros S, Walsh AR, Hockley AD. Incidence of vascular malformations in spontaneous intra-cerebral haemorrhage in children. Childs Nerv Syst 2007; 23(8):881–886.
20. Licata B, Turazzi S. Bleeding cerebral neoplasms with symptomatic hematoma. J Neurosurg Sci 2003; 47(4):201–210.
21. Visudhiphan P, Chiemchanya S, Somburanasin R, Dheandhanoo D. Causes of spontaneous subarachnoid hemorrhage in Thai infants and children. A study of 56 patients. J Neurosurg 1980; 53(2):185–187.
22. Hourihan MD, Gates PC, McAllister VL. Subarachnoid hemorrhage in childhood and adolescence. J Neurosurg 1984; 60(6):1163–1166.
23. Strouse JJ, Hulbert ML, DeBaun MR, Jordan LC, Casella JF. Primary hemorrhagic stroke in children with sickle cell disease is associated with recent transfusion and use of corticosteroids. Pediatrics 2006; 118(5):1916–1924.
24. Sebire G, Tabarki B, Saunders DE, Leroy I, Liesner R, Saint-Martin C et al. Cerebral venous sinus thrombosis in children: risk factors, presentation, diagnosis and outcome. Brain 2005; 128(Pt 3):477–489.
25. Parmar RC, Bavdekar SB, Goel A, Limaye U, Muranjan MN. Primary intraventricular haemorrhage: a rare presenting feature of arteriovenous malformation in children. J Indian Med Assoc 2002; 100(4):254–256.
26. Fleetwood IG, Steinberg GK. Arteriovenous malformations. Lancet 2002; 359(9309):863–873.
27. Gonzalez LF, Bristol RE, Porter RW, Spetzler RF. De novo presentation of an arteriovenous malformation. Case report and review of the literature. J Neurosurg 2005; 102(4):726–729.
28. O'Shaughnessy BA, DiPatri AJ, Jr, Parkinson RJ, Batjer HH. Development of a de novo cerebral arteriovenous malformation in a child with sickle cell disease and moyamoya arteriopathy. Case report. J Neurosurg 2005; 102(2 Suppl):238–243.
29. Hillman J. Population-based analysis of arteriovenous malformation treatment. J Neurosurg 2001; 95(4):633–637.
30. Stapf C, Mast H, Sciacca RR, Berenstein A, Nelson PK, Gobin YP et al. The New York Islands AVM Study: design, study progress, and initial results. Stroke 2003; 34(5):e29–e33.

31. Apsimon HT, Reef H, Phadke RV, Popovic EA. A population-based study of brain arteriovenous malformation: long-term treatment outcomes. Stroke 2002; 33(12):2794–2800.

32. Di Rocco C, Tamburrini G, Rollo M. Cerebral arteriovenous malformations in children. Acta Neurochir (Wien). 2000; 142(2):145–156.

33. Stapf C, Khaw AV, Sciacca RR, Hofmeister C, Schumacher HC, Pile-Spellman J et al. Effect of age on clinical and morphological characteristics in patients with brain arteriovenous malformation. Stroke 2003; 34(11):2664–2669.

34. Fullerton HJ, Achrol AS, Johnston SC, McCulloch CE, Higashida RT, Lawton MT et al. Long-term hemorrhage risk in children versus adults with brain arteriovenous malformations. Stroke 2005; 36(10):2099–2104.

35. Smith ER, Butler WE, Ogilvy CS. Surgical approaches to vascular anomalies of the child's brain. Curr Opin Neurol 2002; 15(2): 165–171.

36. Vorstman EB, Niemann DB, Molyneux AJ, Pike MG. Benign intracranial hypertension associated with arteriovenous malformation. Dev Med Child Neurol 2002; 44(2):133–135.

37. Spetzler RF, Martin NA. A proposed grading system for arteriovenous malformations. J Neurosurg 1986; 65(4):476–483.

38. Du R, Dowd CF, Johnston SC, Young WL, Lawton MT. Interobserver variability in grading of brain arteriovenous malformations using the Spetzler–Martin system. Neurosurgery 2005; 57(4):668–675.

39. Lasjaunias P. Pial arteriovenous malformations. In: Lasjaunias P (ed.) Vascular diseases in neonates, infants and children. Berlin, Heidelberg, Springer-Verlag 1997; 203–309.

40. Mast H, Young WL, Koennecke HC, Sciacca RR, Osipov A, Pile-Spellman J et al. Risk of spontaneous haemorrhage after diagnosis of cerebral arteriovenous malformation. Lancet 1997; 350(9084): 1065–1068.

41. Brown RD, Jr. Simple risk predictions for arteriovenous malformation hemorrhage. Neurosurgery 2000; 46(4):1024.

42. Hoh BL, Ogilvy CS, Butler WE, Loeffler JS, Putman CM, Chapman PH. Multimodality treatment of nongalenic arteriovenous malformations in pediatric patients. Neurosurgery 2000; 47(2): 346–357.

43. Rigamonti D, Hadley MN, Drayer BP, Johnson PC, Hoenig-Rigamonti K, Knight JT et al. Cerebral cavernous malformations. Incidence and familial occurrence. N Engl J Med 1988; 319(6): 343–347.

44. Labauge P, Denier C, Bergametti F, Tournier-Lasserve E. Genetics of cavernous angiomas. Lancet Neurol 2007; 6(3):237–244.

45. Frima-Verhoeven PA, Op de Coul AA, Tijssen CC, Maat B. Intracranial cavernous angiomas: diagnosis and therapy. Eur Neurol 1989; 29(1):56–60.

46. Dillon WP. Cryptic vascular malformations: controversies in terminology, diagnosis, pathophysiology, and treatment. AJNR Am J Neuroradiol 1997; 18(10):1839–1846.

47. Hetts SW, Narvid J, Sanai N, Lawton MT, Gupta N, Fullerton HJ, Dowd CF, Higashida RT, Halbach VV. Intracranial aneurysms in childhood: 27-year single-institution experience. AJNR Am J Neuroradiol. 2009; 30(7):1315–24.

48. Orozco M, Trigueros F, Quintana F, Dierssen G. Intracranial aneurysms in early childhood. Surg Neurol 1978; 9(4):247–252.

49. Newcomb AL, Munns GF. Rupture of aneurysm of the circle of Willis in the newborn. Pediatrics 1949; 3(6):769–772.

50. Lee YJ, Kandall SR, Ghali VS. Intracerebral arterial aneurysm in a newborn. Arch Neurol 1978; 35(3):171–172.

51. Proust F, Toussaint P, Garnieri J, Hannequin D, Legars D, Houtteville JP et al. Pediatric cerebral aneurysms. J Neurosurg 2001; 94(5):733–739.

52. Lasjaunias P, Wuppalapati S, Alvarez H, Rodesch G, Ozanne A. Intracranial aneurysms in children aged under 15 years: review of 59 consecutive children with 75 aneurysms. Childs Nerv Syst 2005; 21(6):437–450.

53. Lasjaunias PL, Campi A, Rodesch G. Aneurysmal disease in children: review of 20 cases with intracranial arterial localizations. Intervent Neuroradiol 1997; 3:215–229.

54. Huang J, McGirt MJ, Gailloud P, Tamargo RJ. Intracranial aneurysms in the pediatric population: case series and literature review. Surg Neurol 2005; 63(5):424–432.

55. Buis DR, van Ouwerkerk WJ, Takahata H, Vandertop WP. Intracranial aneurysms in children under 1 year of age: a systematic review of the literature. Childs Nerv Syst 2006; 22(11):1395–1409.

56. Sanai N, Quinones-Hinojosa A, Gupta NM, Perry V, Sun PP, Wilson CB et al. Pediatric intracranial aneurysms: durability of treatment following microsurgical and endovascular management. J Neurosurg 2006; 104(2 Suppl):82–89.

57. Fogarty PF, Segal JB. The epidemiology of immune thrombocytopenic purpura. Curr Opin Hematol 2007; 14(5):515–519.

58. Traivaree C, Blanchette V, Armstrong D, Floros G, Stain AM, Carcao MD. Intracranial bleeding in haemophilia beyond the neonatal period – the role of CT imaging in suspected intracranial bleeding. Haemophilia 2007; 13(5):552–559.

59. Kyrnetskiy EE, Kun LE, Boop FA, Sanford RA, Khan RB. Types, causes, and outcome of intracranial hemorrhage in children with cancer. J Neurosurg 2005; 102(1 Suppl):31–35.

60. McEvoy AW, Kitchen ND, Thomas DG. Intracerebral haemorrhage caused by drug abuse. Lancet 1998; 351(9108):1029.

61. Wallace RC, Karis JP, Partovi S, Fiorella D. Noninvasive imaging of treated cerebral aneurysms, Part II: CT angiographic follow-up of surgically clipped aneurysms. AJNR Am J Neuroradiol 2007; 28(7):1207–1212.

62. Gatscher S, Brew S, Banks T, Simcock C, Sullivan Y, Crockett J. Multislice spiral computed tomography for pediatric intracranial vascular pathophysiologies. J Neurosurg 2007; 107(3 Suppl): 203–208.

63. Atlas SW, Mark AS, Grossman RI, Gomori JM. Intracranial hemorrhage: gradient-echo MR imaging at 1.5T. Comparison with spin-echo imaging and clinical applications. Radiology 1988; 168(3): 803–807.

64. Hayman LA, McArdle CB, Taber KH, Saleem A, Baskin D, Lee HS et al. MR imaging of hyperacute intracranial hemorrhage in the cat. AJNR Am J Neuroradiol 1989; 10(4):681–686.

65. Patel MR, Edelman RR, Warach S. Detection of hyperacute primary intraparenchymal hemorrhage by magnetic resonance imaging. Stroke 1996; 27(12):2321–2324.

66. Schellinger PD, Jansen O, Fiebach JB, Hacke W, Sartor K. A standardized MRI stroke protocol: comparison with CT in hyperacute intracerebral hemorrhage. Stroke 1999; 30(4):765–768.

67. Liu AC, Segaren N, Cox TS, Hayward RD, Chong WK, Ganesan V et al. Is there a role for magnetic resonance imaging in the evaluation of non-traumatic intraparenchymal haemorrhage in children? Pediatr Radiol 2006; 36(9):940–946.

68. Jaeger HR, Mansmann U, Hausmann O, Partszch U, Moseley IF, Taylor WJ. MRA versus digital subtraction angiography in actue subarachnoid haemorrhage: a blinded multireader study of prospectively recruited patients. Neuroradiology 2000; 42:313–326.

69. Watanabe Z, Kikuchi Y, Izaki K, Hanyu N, Lim FS, Gotou H et al. The usefulness of 3D MR angiography in surgery for ruptured cerebral aneurysms. Surg Neurol 2001; 55(6):359–364.

70. Sankhla SK, Gunawardena WJ, Coutinho CM, Jones AP, Keogh AJ. Magnetic resonance angiography in the management of aneurysmal subarachnoid haemorrhage: a study of 51 cases. Neuroradiology 1996; 38(8):724–729.

71. Lee C, Pennington MA, Kenney CM, III. MR evaluation of developmental venous anomalies: medullary venous anatomy of venous angiomas. AJNR Am J Neuroradiol 1996; 17(1):61–70.

72. Lee RR, Becher MW, Benson ML, Rigamonti D. Brain capillary telangiectasia: MR imaging appearance and clinicohistopathologic findings. Radiology 1997; 205(3):797–805.

73. Renowden SA, Molyneux AJ, Anslow P, Byrne JV. The value of MRI in angiogram-negative intracranial haemorrhage. Neuroradiology 1994; 36(6):422–425.

74. Duong H, Melancon D, Tampieri D, Ethier R. The negative angiogram in subarachnoid haemorrhage. Neuroradiology 1996; 38(1):15–19.

75. Urbach H, Zentner J, Solymosi L. The need for repeat angiography in subarachnoid haemorrhage. Neuroradiology 1998; 40(1):6–10.

76. Mendelow AD, Gregson BA, Fernandes HM, Murray GD, Teasdale GM, Hope DT et al. Early surgery versus initial conservative treatment in patients with spontaneous supratentorial intracerebral haematomas in the International Surgical Trial in Intracerebral Haemorrhage (STICH): a randomized trial. Lancet 2005; 365(9457):387–397.

77. Morgenstern LB, Demchuk AM, Kim DH, Frankowski RF, Grotta JC. Rebleeding leads to poor outcome in ultra-early craniotomy for intracerebral hemorrhage. Neurology 2001; 56(10):1294–1299.

78. Humphreys RP, Hoffman HJ, Drake JM, Rutka JT. Choices in the 1990s for the management of pediatric cerebral arteriovenous malformations. Pediatr Neurosurg 1996; 25(6):277–285.

79. Malik GM, Sadasivan B, Knighton RS, Ausman JI. The management of arteriovenous malformations in children. Childs Nerv Syst 1991; 7(1):43–47.

80. Ventureyra EC, Herder S. Arteriovenous malformations of the brain in children. Childs Nerv Syst 1987; 3(1):12–18.

81. Gerosa MA, Cappellotto P, Licata C, Iraci G, Pardatscher K, Fiore DL. Cerebral arteriovenous malformations in children (56 cases). Childs Brain 1981; 8(5):356–371.

82. Lawton MT. Spetzler–Martin Grade III arteriovenous malformations: surgical results and a modification of the grading scale. Neurosurgery 2003; 52(4):740–748.

83. Kiris T, Sencer A, Sahinbas M, Sencer S, Imer M, Izgi N. Surgical results in pediatric Spetzler–Martin grades I–III intracranial arteriovenous malformations. Childs Nerv Syst 2005; 21(1):69–74.

84. Bristol RE, Albuquerque FC, Spetzler RF, Rekate HL, McDougall CG, Zabramski JM. Surgical management of arteriovenous malformations in children. J Neurosurg 2006; 105(2 Suppl):88–93.

85. Klimo P, Jr, Rao G, Brockmeyer D. Pediatric arteriovenous malformations: a 15-year experience with an emphasis on residual and recurrent lesions. Childs Nerv Syst 2007; 23(1):31–37.

86. Hartmann A, Mast H, Mohr JP, Pile-Spellman J, Connolly ES, Sciacca RR et al. Determinants of staged endovascular and surgical treatment outcome of brain arteriovenous malformations. Stroke 2005; 36(11):2431–2435.

87. Spears J, Terbrugge KG, Moosavian M, Montanera W, Willinsky RA, Wallace MC et al. A discriminative prediction model of neurological outcome for patients undergoing surgery of brain arteriovenous malformations. Stroke 2006; 37(6):1457–1464.

88. Sanchez-Mejia RO, Chennupati SK, Gupta N, Fullerton H, Young WL, Lawton MT. Superior outcomes in children compared with adults after microsurgical resection of brain arteriovenous malformations. J Neurosurg 2006; 105(2 Suppl):82–87.

89. Guglielmi G, Vinuela F, Sepetka I, Macellari V. Electrothrombosis of saccular aneurysms via endovascular approach. Part 1: Electrochemical basis, technique, and experimental results. J Neurosurg 1991; 75(1):1–7.

90. Molyneux AJ, Kerr RS, Yu LM, Clarke M, Sneade M, Yarnold JA et al. International subarachnoid aneurysm trial (ISAT) of neurosurgical clipping versus endovascular coiling in 2143 patients with ruptured intracranial aneurysms: a randomized comparison of effects on survival, dependency, seizures, rebleeding, subgroups, and aneurysm occlusion. Lancet 2005; 366(9488):809–817.

91. Raymond J, Roy D, Bojanowski M, Moumdjian R, L'Esperance G. Endovascular treatment of acutely ruptured and unruptured aneurysms of the basilar bifurcation. J Neurosurg 1997; 86(2):211–219.

92. McDougall CG, Halbach VV, Dowd CF, Higashida RT, Larsen DW, Hieshima GB. Endovascular treatment of basilar tip aneurysms using electrolytically detachable coils. J Neurosurg 1996; 84(3): 393–399.

93. Ito M, Yoshihara M, Ishii M, Wachi A, Sato K. Cerebral aneurysms in children. Brain Dev 1992; 14(4):263–268.

94. Gerosa M, Licata C, Fiore DL, Iraci G. Intracranial aneurysms of childhood. Childs Brain 1980; 6(6):295–302.

95. Pasqualin A, Mazza C, Cavazzani P, Scienza R, DaPian R. Intracranial aneurysms and subarachnoid hemorrhage in children and adolescents. Childs Nerv Syst 1986; 2(4):185–190.

96. Ventureyra EC, Higgins MJ. Traumatic intracranial aneurysms in childhood and adolescence. Case reports and review of the literature. Childs Nerv Syst 1994; 10(6):361–379.

97. Longstreth WT, Jr, Nelson LM, Koepsell TD, van Belle G. Clinical course of spontaneous subarachnoid hemorrhage: a population-based study in King County, Washington. Neurology 1993; 43(4):712–718.

98. Kassell NF, Torner JC. Aneurysmal rebleeding: a preliminary report from the Cooperative Aneurysm Study. Neurosurgery 1983; 13(5):479–481.

99. Kassell NF, Sasaki T, Colohan AR, Nazar G. Cerebral vasospasm following aneurysmal subarachnoid hemorrhage. Stroke 1985; 16(4):562–572.

100. Amacher AL, Drake CG. The results of operating upon cerebral aneurysms and angiomas in children and adolescents. I. Cerebral aneurysms. Childs Brain 1979; 5(3):151–165.

101. Regis J, Bartolomei F, Hayashi M, Roberts D, Chauvel P, Peragut JC. The role of gamma knife surgery in the treatment of severe epilepsies. Epileptic Disord 2000; 2(2):113–122.

102. Di Rocco C, Iannelli A, Tamburrini G. Surgical management of paediatric cerebral cavernomas. J Neurosurg Sci 1997; 41(4):343–347.

103. Miller LJ, Roid GH. Toddler and Infant Motor Evaluation (TIME). San Antonio, TX: Therapy Skill Builders, 1994.

104. Partington MD, Davis DH, Kelly PJ. Stereotactic resection of pediatric vascular malformations. Pediatr Neurosci 1989; 15(5): 217–222.

105. Garza-Mercado R, Cavazos E, Tamez-Montes D. Cerebral arteriovenous malformations in children and adolescents. Surg Neurol 1987; 27(2):131–140.

106. Hladky JP, Lejeune JP, Blond S, Pruvo JP, Dhellemmes P. Cerebral arteriovenous malformations in children: report on 62 cases. Childs Nerv Syst 1994; 10(5):328–333.

107. van der Schaaf I, Algra A, Wermer M, Molyneux A, Clarke M, van Gijn J et al. Endovascular coiling versus neurosurgical clipping for patients with aneurysmal subarachnoid haemorrhage. Cochrane Database Syst Rev 2005;(4):CD003085.

108. Agid R, Jonas KT, Lee SK, Ter Brugge KG. Diagnostic characteristics and management of intracranial aneurysms in children. Neuroimaging Clin N Am 2007; 17(2):153–163.

109. Tamaki N, Ehara K, Lin TK, Kuwamura K, Obora Y, Kanazawa Y et al. Cerebral arteriovenous malformations: factors influencing the surgical difficulty and outcome. Neurosurgery 1991; 29(6): 856–861.

110. Fong D, Chan ST. Arteriovenous malformation in children. Childs Nerv Syst 1988; 4(4):199–203.

111. Lasjaunias P, Hui F, Zerah M, Garcia-Monaco R, Malherbe V, Rodesch G et al. Cerebral arteriovenous malformations in children. Management of 179 consecutive cases and review of the literature. Childs Nerv Syst 1995; 11(2):66–79.

112. Terbrugge KG. Neurointerventional procedures in the pediatric age group. Childs Nerv Syst 1999; 15(11–12):751–754.

113. Suh DC, Alvarez H, Bhattacharya JJ, Rodesch G, Lasjaunias PL. Intracranial haemorrhage within the first two years of life. Acta Neurochir (Wien). 2001; 143(10):997–1004.

114. Rodesch G, Lasjaunias P, Ter Brugge KG, Burrows P. Lesions vasculaires arteriovenouses intra craniennes de l'enfants. Place des techniques endovasculaires a propos de 44 cas. Neurochirurgie 1988; 34:243–251.

115. Tada T, Sugita K, Kobayashi S, Watanabe N. Supra- and infratentorial arteriovenous malformations with an aneurysmal dilatation: a case report. Neurosurgery 1986; 19(5):831–834.

116. Garcia-Monaco R, Rodesch G, Terbrugge K, Burrows P, Lasjaunias P. Multifocal dural arteriovenous shunts in children. Childs Nerv Syst 1991; 7(8):425–431.

117. Cronqvist S, Granholm L, Lundstrom NR. Hydrocephalus and congestive heart failure caused by intracranial arteriovenous malformations in infants. J Neurosurg 1972; 36(3):249–254.

118. Cumming GR. Circulation in neonates with intracranial arteriovenous fistula and cardiac failure. Am J Cardiol 1980; 45(5): 1019–1024.

119. Willinsky R, Lasjaunias P, Terbrugge K, Burrows P. Multiple cerebral arteriovenous malformation: review of our experience from 203 patients with cerebral vascular lesions. Neuroradiology 1991; 32:207–210.

120. Lasjaunias P, Piske R, Terbrugge K, Willinsky R. Cerebral arteriovenous malformations (C. AVM). and associated arterial aneurysms (AA). Analysis of 101 C. AVM cases, with 37 AA in 23 patients. Acta Neurochir (Wien) 1988; 91(1–2):29–36.

121. Berenstein A, Lasjaunias P. Endovascular treatment of cerebral intracranial lesions. In: Surgical Neuroangiography, Vol. 4 (eds P Lasjaunias, A Berenstein, KG ter Brugge). New York: Berlin Heidelberg, 1992; 189–266.

122. Weon YC, Yoshida Y, Sachet M, Mahadevan J, Alvarez H, Rodesch G et al. Supratentorial cerebral arteriovenous fistulas (AVFs) in children: review of 41 cases with 63 non choroidal single-hole AVFs. Acta Neurochir (Wien) 2005;147(1):17–31; discussion 31.

123. Yoshida Y, Weon YC, Sachet M, Mahadevan J, Alvarez H, Rodesch G et al. Posterior cranial fossa single-hole arteriovenous fistulae in children: 14 consecutive cases. Neuroradiology 2004;46(6):474–481.

124. Phatouros CC, Halbach VV, Malek AM, Meyers PM, Dowd CF, Higashida RT. Intraventricular contrast medium leakage during ethanol embolization of an arteriovenous malformation. AJNR Am J Neuroradiol 1999; 20(7):1329–1332.

125. Joffe D, Bank WO. Morbidity in a pediatric patient having alcohol ablation of an arteriovenous malformation. Can J Anaesth 2006; 53(5):527–528.

126. Kim LJ, Albuquerque FC, Spetzler RF, McDougall CG. Postembolization neurological deficits in cerebral arteriovenous malformations: stratification by arteriovenous malformation grade. Neurosurgery 2006; 59(1):53–59.

127. Ledezma CJ, Hoh BL, Carter BS, Pryor JC, Putman CM, Ogilvy CS. Complications of cerebral arteriovenous malformation embolization: multivariate analysis of predictive factors. Neurosurgery 2006; 58(4):602–611.

128. Haw CS, Terbrugge K, Willinsky R, Tomlinson G. Complications of embolization of arteriovenous malformations of the brain. J Neurosurg 2006; 104(2):226–232.

129. Heidenreich JO, Hartlieb S, Stendel R, Pietila TA, Schlattmann P, Wolf KJ et al. Bleeding complications after endovascular therapy of cerebral arteriovenous malformations. AJNR Am J Neuroradiol 2006; 27(2):313–316.

130. Zabel-du BA, Milker-Zabel S, Huber P, Schlegel W, Debus J. Pediatric cerebral arteriovenous malformations: the role of stereotactic linac-based radiosurgery. Int J Radiat Oncol Biol Phys 2006; 65(4):1206–1211.

131. Reyns N, Blond S, Gauvrit JY, Touzet G, Coche B, Pruvo JP et al. Role of radiosurgery in the management of cerebral arteriovenous malformations in the pediatric age group: data from a 100-patient series. Neurosurgery 2007; 60(2):268–276.

132. Padget DH. The cranial venous system in man in reference to development, adult configuration, and relation to the arteries. Am J Anat 1956; 98(3):307–355.

133. Brown RD Jr, Wiebers DO, Torner JC, O'Fallon WM. Frequency of intracranial hemorrhage as a presenting symptom and subtype analysis: a population-based study of intracranial vascular malformations in Olmsted Country, Minnesota. J Neurosurg 1996; 85(1):29–32.

134. Crawford PM, West CR, Chadwick DW, Shaw MD. Arteriovenous malformations of the brain: natural history in unoperated patients. J Neurol Neurosurg Psychiatry 1986; 49(1):1–10.

135. So SC. Cerebral arteriovenous malformations in children. Childs Brain 1978; 4(4):242–250.

136. Patel MC, Hodgson TJ, Kemeny AA, Forster DM. Spontaneous obliteration of pial arteriovenous malformations: a review of 27 cases. AJNR Am J Neuroradiol 2001; 22(3):531–536.

137. Steiner L, Leksell L, Forster DM, Greitz T, Backlund EO. Stereotactic radiosurgery in intracranial arterio-venous malformations. Acta Neurochir (Wien) 1974; Suppl 21:195–209.

138. Schneider BF, Eberhard DA, Steiner LE. Histopathology of arteriovenous malformations after gamma knife radiosurgery. J Neurosurg 1997; 87(3):352–357.

139. Szeifert GT, Kemeny AA, Timperley WR, Forster DM. The potential role of myofibroblasts in the obliteration of arteriovenous malformations after radiosurgery. Neurosurgery 1997; 40(1):61–65.

140. Guo WY, Karlsson B, Ericson K, Lindqvist M. Even the smallest remnant of an AVM constitutes a risk of further bleeding. Case report. Acta Neurochir (Wien) 1993; 121(3–4):212–215.

141. Larsson B, Liden K, Sarby B. Irradiation of small structures through the intact skull. Acta Radiol Ther Phys Biol 1974; 13(6):512–534.

142. Steiner L, Lindquist C, Steiner M. Cerebrovascular disease in children and adolescents: radiosurgery with focused gamma-beam irradiation in children. In: Cerebral Vascular Disease in Children and Adolescents (eds MS Edwards, HJ Hoffman). Baltimore: Williams and Wilkins, 1989; 367–388.

143. Abe T, Matsumoto K, Horichi Y, Hayashi T, Ikeda H, Iwata T. Magnetic resonance angiography of cerebral arteriovenous malformations. Neurol Med Chir (Tokyo) 1995; 35(8):580–583.

144. Flickinger JC, Lunsford LD, Kondziolka D, Maitz AH, Epstein AH, Simons SR et al. Radiosurgery and brain tolerance: an analysis of neurodiagnostic imaging changes after gamma knife radiosurgery for arteriovenous malformations. Int J Radiat Oncol Biol Phys 1992; 23(1):19–26.

145. Warren DJ, Hoggard N, Walton L, Radatz MW, Kemeny AA, Forster DM et al. Cerebral arteriovenous malformations: comparison of novel magnetic resonance angiographic techniques and conventional catheter angiography. Neurosurgery 2001; 48(5):973–982.

146. Pollock BE, Lunsford LD, Kondziolka D, Maitz A, Flickinger JC. Patient outcomes after stereotactic radiosurgery for "operable" arteriovenous malformations. Neurosurgery 1994; 35(1):1–7; discussion 7–8.

147. Lunsford LD, Kondziolka D, Flickinger JC, Bissonette DJ, Jungreis CA, Maitz AH et al. Stereotactic radiosurgery for arteriovenous malformations of the brain. J Neurosurg 1991; 75(4):512–524.

148. Steiner L, Lindquist C, Adler JR, Torner JC, Alves W, Steiner M. Clinical outcome of radiosurgery for cerebral arteriovenous malformations. J Neurosurg 1992; 77(1):1–8.

149. Altschuler EM, Lunsford LD, Coffey RJ, Bissonette DJ, Flickinger JC. Gamma knife radiosurgery for intracranial arteriovenous malformations in childhood and adolescence. Pediatr Neurosci 1989; 15(2):53–61.

150. Kemeny AA, Dias PS, Forster DM. Results of stereotactic radiosurgery of arteriovenous malformations: an analysis of 52 cases. J Neurol Neurosurg Psychiatry 1989; 52(5):554–558.

151. Cohen-Gadol AA, Pollock BE. Radiosurgery for arteriovenous malformations in children. J Neurosurg 2006; 104(6 Suppl):388–391.

152. Zadeh G, Andrade-Souza YM, Tsao MN, Scora D, Armstrong D, Humphreys R et al. Pediatric arteriovenous malformation: University of Toronto experience using stereotactic radiosurgery. Childs Nerv Syst 2007; 23(2):195–199.

153. Kiran NA, Kale SS, Vaishya S, Kasliwal MK, Gupta A, Sharma MS et al. Gamma knife surgery for intracranial arteriovenous malformations in children: a retrospective study in 103 patients. J Neurosurg 2007; 107(6 Suppl):479–484.

154. Buis DR, Dirven CM, Lagerwaard FJ, Mandl ES, Lycklama ANG, Eshghi DS et al. Radiosurgery of brain arteriovenous malformations in children. J Neurol 2008; 255(4):551–560.

155. Flickinger JC, Kondziolka D, Pollock BE, Maitz AH, Lunsford LD. Complications from arteriovenous malformation radiosurgery: multivariate analysis and risk modeling. Int J Radiat Oncol Biol Phys 1997; 38(3):485–490.

156. Dion JE, Mathis JM. Cranial arteriovenous malformations. The role of embolization and stereotactic surgery. Neurosurg Clin N Am 1994; 5(3):459–474.

157. Gobin YP, Laurent A, Merienne L, Schlienger M, Aymard A, Houdart E et al. Treatment of brain arteriovenous malformations by embolization and radiosurgery. J Neurosurg 1996; 85(1):19–28.

158. Steiner L, Lindquist C, Cail W, Karlsson B, Steiner M. Microsurgery and radiosurgery in brain arteriovenous malformations. J Neurosurg 1993; 79(5):647–652.

159. Karlsson B, Kihlstrom L, Lindquist C, Steiner L. Gamma knife surgery for previously irradiated arteriovenous malformations. Neurosurgery 1998; 42(1):1–5.

160. Gerszten PC, Adelson PD, Kondziolka D, Flickinger JC, Lunsford LD. Seizure outcome in children treated for arteriovenous malformations using gamma knife radiosurgery. Pediatr Neurosurg 1996; 24(3):139–144.

161. Flickinger JC, Kondziolka D, Maitz AH, Lunsford LD. Analysis of neurological sequelae from radiosurgery of arteriovenous malformations: how location affects outcome. Int J Radiat Oncol Biol Phys 1998; 40(2):273–278.

162. Sutcliffe JC, Forster DM, Walton L, Dias PS, Kemeny AA. Untoward clinical effects after stereotactic radiosurgery for intracranial arteriovenous malformations. Br J Neurosurg 1992; 6(3):177–185.

163. Sheehan J, Yen CP, Steiner L. Gamma knife surgery-induced meningioma. Report of two cases and review of the literature. J Neurosurg 2006; 105(2):325–329.

9
NEONATAL STROKE

9.1 Perinatal Arterial Stroke

Frances Cowan and Eugenio Mercuri

Introduction

There has been increasing interest in the clinical aspects of perinatal stroke,[1-3] as well as in the parallel development of experimental perinatal stroke models.[4] The term perinatal stroke is used mainly to describe focal ischaemic brain injury in an arterial territory or perinatal arterial stroke (PAS); the term perinatal ischemic stroke or PIS[3] has also been coined. This lesion occurs most frequently within the left middle cerebral artery territory in term infants and commonly presents with seizures in the first few days after birth. Some infants present beyond the neonatal period with hemiplegia, seizures or developmental delay and are found to have lesions consistent with a perinatally occurring arterial territory stroke – these lesions have been called "presumed perinatal stroke" or PPERI.[5] Most neonatally presenting strokes appear to occur in the later intrapartum or early postnatal period rather than earlier, but the timing of PPERI is less clear and may be in the late third trimester. Maternal and intrapartum risk factors appear to be important.[6,7] PAS also occurs in preterm infants. The vascular territory of the lesion in preterm infants tends to be more central than in later gestation and aetiologies may be different from stroke in term-born infants.[8] PAS may also occur in the fetus, with the characteristics of strokes occurring in either term or preterm infants, depending on the gestational age at which the injury is sustained; however many lesions recorded as fetal stroke are probably primarily haemorrhagic rather than ischaemic lesions.[9]

The term perinatal stroke has been more loosely used to cover other pathologies that lead to focal and unilateral or asymmetrical forms of brain injury. The most common of these other lesions occur at the junction of arterial territories and is referred to as borderzone, watershed or parasagittal infarction[10] often associated with sub-acute hypoxia-ischaemia or hypoglycaemia.[11] Other focal lesions include isolated large focal haematomas or infarction/haemorrhage associated with venous thrombosis,[12-15] which may occur following intrapartum fetal distress, acidosis and low Apgar scores at birth or with infection or electrolyte disturbance, although most often evidence for such problems is lacking (see Chapter 7). Children with early neurodevelopmental delay or hemiplegia may be found to have evidence of an established venous or haemorrhagic parenchymal infarction (HPI) typically occurring neonatally in preterm infants but which may occur antenatally and go undetected until symptoms in infancy lead to investigation.[16,17] In this chapter we will focus on strokes occurring in arterial territories or PAS defining aetiology, presentation and outcome.

PAS is primarily ischaemic but may have haemorrhagic elements especially in the subcortical and cortical grey matter. They most commonly involve white matter and cortical grey matter but not always subcortical grey matter. However lesions can be solely in the subcortical grey matter. They occur most commonly in territory of the middle cerebral artery (MCA) but may also occur in the anterior (ACA) or posterior (PCA) arterial territories and they may be in multiple sites.

Occurrence

The incidence of PAS in term infants has varied between studies, at least in part because of variability in definition. Estan and Hope[18] found it to be 1/4000 or 0.025% in a population-based study of symptomatic infants in Oxford, UK. Stroke ascertainment was dependent on investigating infants with neonatal symptoms of sufficient severity to warrant brain imaging, which was performed with cranial ultrasound and computerized tomography (CT) but not magnetic resonance imaging (MRI). It is likely that smaller strokes were not detected either because the symptoms were not thought sufficient to warrant investigation or they were not detected using ultrasound or CT. Wang and colleagues[19] found, using ultrasound, that focal areas of echogenicity were not uncommon on screening asymptomatic term infants in the first postnatal three days although only one infant of 2309 had definite evidence of infarction. Schulzke et al[20] found using a 1.0 Tesla MRI system in symptomatic infants an incidence of 1 in 2300 with only one-third of the infarcts being detected with ultrasound. Other studies have also found MRI to be superior to ultrasound[21] though our own experience was that ultrasound was abnormal in 67% of infants scanned in the first three postnatal days and 87% when scanned between days 4 and 10.[22] There has been no formal comparison of ultrasound or MRI with CT but we have seen cases where strokes have been diagnosed with CT but not seen with MRI and vice versa.

Uvebrant[23] found, in the term born population around Göteborg, Sweden, 44/100 000 children (~1 per 2300 infants) with congenital hemiplegia. However this dataset is not very useful for estimating the population incidence of PAS as it will include children with developmental abnormalities and asymmetrical periventricular lesions resulting in hemiplegia[24] and will not include those with PAS in territories away from motor pathways. Data for white infants in Germany from Günther et al[25] give a low incidence of 1.35/100 000 live births.

Studies using the Kaiser Permanante system in California from 1997 to 2002 found a prevalence of PAS (excluding watershed, venous infarction and primary haemorrhage) of 20/100 000[26] but importantly this study of 40 infants included six preterm infants: additionally 14 of the 34 term infants presented beyond the neonatal period. The 20 infants born at term and presenting neonatally give an incidence of 10/100 000 or 1/10 000, far less than the Oxford data.[18] In an earlier study of infants with motor impairment due to PAS (1991–1998), the prevalence was 17/100 000 live births[6] but this study also included those presenting with hemiparesis or seizures beyond the neonatal period (26/38 cases, 68%). The incidence reported by Laugesaar et al[27] using CT and MRI and including both PAS and PPERI from Estonia was 63/100 000 or ~1/1600; 12 infants presented neonatally giving an incidence of 1/5000.

Govaert et al[28] report on 17 strokes in 1729 term infants admitted to a tertiary neonatal unit, i.e. 1%, similar to the data from Ment et al.[29] Barmada's autopsy data[30] gives an occurrence of 5.4% in term newborns but the vast majority of neonates with stroke do not die and the relevance of this data in terms of lesion incidence is unclear.

It is now generally agreed that stroke is the second most common cause for neonatal seizures after hypoxic-ischaemic encephalopathy.[31] We have described 350 full-term infants (excluding infants with major congenital malformations and chromosomal abnormalities) presenting with neonatal encephalopathy (NE) and/or seizures alone, all of whom had early brain MRI.[32] Of the 90 presenting with seizures but not encephalopathy, 40% had a focal infarction (~two-thirds arterial territory and one-third borderzone) and 25% focal haemorrhagic lesions (large focal haematoma or scattered white matter haemorrhage). Only eight of the 260 infants with NE had focal infarction.

Stroke in the preterm population has been well described by de Vries et al[33] and Bender et al[8] in data from a large population of infants <34 weeks' gestational age. They found an incidence of 1%, and as most infants born who are this preterm will be admitted to a neonatal unit this incidence is likely to be correct. The site of lesion is more likely to be in the basal ganglia in the preterm infant than in the term infant.

Classification

PAS is usually classified according to the arterial territory involved.[33] The territory supplied by the MCA is most commonly affected, and lesions are subclassified into the main branch, the cortical branches and the lenticulostraite branches.

A different classification system takes into account the following sites of tissue involvement:[34]

Cerebral hemispheres
Basal ganglia and thalami
Internal capsule
Mesencephalon and brainstem
Cerebellum.

MCA territory infarction is most common in the term infant but also occurs in the preterm infant and may occur antenatally. These lesions are three to four times more common in the left than the right hemisphere. Main branch MCA PAS is the lesion most likely to be detected if cranial ultrasound is the only imaging modality, as infarctions in the anterior and posterior regions and smaller branch MCA infarcts are more difficult to visualize.[28,35]

In the term infant cortical branch involvement of the MCA may not result in severe perinatal symptoms, there may be no motor sequelae and it is likely that many such lesions are not diagnosed (Fig. 9.1) and may not be recognized as infarcts if imaged later (Fig. 9.2). Arterial territory infarctions also occur in preterm infants often without specific symptomatology, they will be detected by careful and sequential ultrasound.[28,33] Lesions in the subcortical grey matter are more common in the preterm than the term infant.

Background and aetiology of perinatal arterial stroke

Normal physiological circumstances render the newborn term infant susceptible to embolus and thrombosis. The fetus and newborn have a high circulating haemoglobin and packed cell volume and blood flow is relatively slow. Feeding may be slow to establish and accentuate the normal postnatal fluid loss, leaving the infant relatively dehydrated. During pregnancy and delivery the hypercoagulable state in the mother may

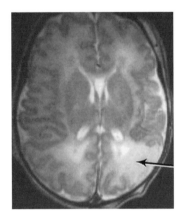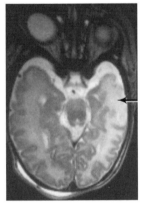

Fig. 9.1. 1 Left cortical branch middle cerebral artery territory stroke in a 38-week gestation 2.9-kg infant considered normal at birth. The Apgar scores were 9 at 1 and 10 at 5 minutes: the cord pH was not measured. He was recruited as a 'normal control' and first scanned on day 2–3 after birth. He was however born by Caesarean section after a failed ventouse and forceps for failure to progress. He did not develop seizures. Note the loss of cortical differentiation and clear infarct margins on the T2-weighted images seen on these axial images taken on day 5. There was no involvement of the basal ganglia or internal capsule and motor and cognitive outcomes were normal at early school age.

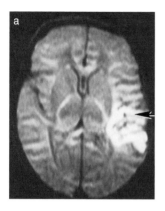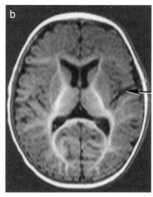

Fig. 9.2. An acute left middle cerebral artery branch artery infarction (a) seen on diffusion weighted imaging in a term infant presenting with early neonatal seizures. Imaging later in the first year (b) shows the region of infarction to appear much smaller than seen originally, now with the appearance of a cleft.

contribute to placental infarction.[36–38] The natural clotting and thrombophilic status of the term infant is also hypercoagulable relative to later in the neonatal period.[39,40] Specific abnormalities of thrombophilic activity are increasingly described in infants with neonatal stroke (see below for text and references).

CIRCULATORY FACTORS

The patent foramen ovale may allow emboli from the placenta, umbilical vessels, portal veins or caval veins to bypass the lungs and enter the cerebral circulation both before, during and just after delivery.[41,42] A similar mechanism may account for the occasional case of perinatal stroke associated with subclavian steal syndrome.[43] Occasionally, perinatal stroke may be the presentation of an atrial septal defect.[44] It is thought that the ageing placenta may release thrombi into the fetal circulation.[37,38] In infants with some fetal distress and acidosis causing pulmonary hypertension and persisting fetal circulation, the foramen ovale may remain patent postnatally leaving the cerebral circulation vulnerable to emboli. The anatomy of the aortic arch and carotid arteries may predispose such emboli to enter the left rather than the right carotid artery, explaining the predilection for left-sided stroke.

Blood flows through the still patent ductus arteriosus after birth in a left to right direction for some time. This may allow backflow from the carotid arteries in diastole. Very low end-diastolic blood flow velocities can be seen in cerebral arterial vessels in the first few hours after birth.[45] It is suggested that this backflow may create turbulence near to the origin of the left carotid artery, which may contribute to the left-sided preponderance for stroke in term neonates.

The cerebral venous circulation is very vulnerable to interruption as the head is moulded during delivery in both normal and instrumental deliveries and flow in the sinuses may vary hugely with inevitable swings in venous pressure.[46] Changes in cranial venous pressure may alter inflow, especially if the infant is hypotensive. The role of blood pressure and its control around the time of birth in the aetiology of neonatal stroke is unknown.

OTHER FACTORS

Sepsis, disseminated intravascular coagulation, polycythaemia,[47] congenital heart disease,[48] and the need for vascular cannulation (all frequent occurrences in sick newborns), as well as extracorporeal membrane oxygenation and endocarditis, have definite associations with stroke, although these problems are more commonly seen in the preterm infant or in specialist units and we have rarely seen them in our own term patients. Stroke is more common in fetuses and neonates following twin-to-twin transfusion syndrome[49] and fetomaternal haemorrhage.[50] It is also reported following maternal cocaine abuse[51] though this is not universally accepted.[52] Stroke has been associated with birth trauma[53] and difficult instrumental delivery[54] with a well-recognized association between skull fracture and contralateral stroke.[55] This may account for the occasional documentation of carotid thrombosis[56] and dissection[57] in neonates. The incidence of maternal trauma and shock associated with neonatal stroke is not known[58] but we have one possible case.

Maternal factors

In our own studies[59,60] most term infants with focal infarction are born to primigravidas and this was also a risk factor in the study reported by Lee et al[7]. The pregnancies are often recorded as normal but in our experience on detailed questioning many mothers have had some abdominal pain or haemorrhage, raised blood pressure, infections, traumas, some systemic disease (11 of 24 infants in the 1999 series of Mercuri et al[60]) and some infants are growth restricted.[61] These problems together occur more often than in the normal population[60] but individually none is specifically related to the occurrence or severity of the lesion.

Two recent studies from the Kaiser Permanante healthcare system in Northern California have looked at risk factors for PAS (excluding those in a watershed or venous distribution as well as pure haemorrhage). In a study of PAS presenting with motor impairment reported by Wu et al[6], prepartum risk factors significantly associated with PAS multivariate analysis were pre-eclampsia and intrauterine growth restriction. In Lee et al's[7] nested case control study of risk factors for PAS where they included both term-born and preterm infants and infants with PPERI, univariate analysis identified primiparity, pre-eclampsia, prolonged rupture of membranes, chorioamnionitis and oligohydramnios. On multivariate analysis, risk factors independently associated with PAS were entirely maternal: history of infertility and/or ovarian stimulation (not significant in univariate analysis as they were associated with lower risk of pre-eclampsia and oligohydramnios), pre-eclampsia, prolonged rupture of membranes and chorioamnionitis. Primiparity and oligohydramnios were of borderline significance. The presence of multiple risk factors substantially increased the risk of PAS.

Labour and delivery
Labour is often prolonged and the delivery complicated (14 of 24 infants in the 1999 series of Mercuri et al) in infants with PAS. In the study reported by Wu et al[6], neonates with PAS were at higher risk of delivery complications, such as emergency Caesarean section, 5-minute Apgar <7 and resuscitation at birth. Prolonged second stage of labour, emergency Caesarean section and vacuum extraction were all predictors on univariate analysis in the study reported by Lee et al[7]. A mild to moderate degree of fetal distress is common (15/23 infants in the series of Mercuri et al[60]). However, despite fetal heart rate abnormality being a predictor of PAS in the study of Lee et al,[7] significant acidosis or low Apgar scores are rare. The infants may need some resuscitation but usually not intubation and most are thought initially well enough to stay with their mothers on the postnatal wards.

An association with hypoxic-ischaemic encephalopathy undoubtedly exists[63] though in our experience it is uncommon. In our study of infants with NE and early MRI, only eight of the 260 infants with NE had PAS (3%), whereas focal infarction was found in 40% of the 90 infants presenting with seizures alone.[32] An association between acute subdural haematoma and perinatal stroke has also been reported[64] though the mechanism of the association is unclear.

Familial and congenital factors
Consanguinity or significant family history are very uncommon. Most studies have found that boys are more commonly affected[65] though Günther et al[25] reported a slight preponderance of females (1.1:1) in their series of 91 term infants with PAS. Hemiplegia is reported to be more common in boys (1.4:1) but this is not based on an accurate ascertainment of neonatal stroke. A few reports of genetic disorders associated with early stroke exist but almost all are outside the neonatal period. These include fibromuscular dysplasia,[66] mitochondrial disorders,[67] homocystinuria,[68,69] carbamyl-phosphate synthetase deficiency[70] and the carbohydrate deficient glycoprotein group.[71] The one exception is a syndrome associating infantile hemiparesis with retinal artery tortuosity and leukoencephalopathy.[72] All are rare and we have not seen an example of any of these. We have seen four children with relatively small strokes without motor consequences. Three were mildly dysmorphic neonatally with more hypotonia than usually seen following neonatal stroke and had later developmental delay; one developed mild autistic spectrum behaviour, one had transient hyperhomocysteinaemia in the first 3 months[73] but was later diagnosed with Soto syndrome. One had a haemorrhagic infarct in the caudate nucleus and continued systemic haemorrhagic tendencies that have not been possible to categorize, two had a small MCA branch artery infarction and one a PCA. We have also seen one child with a mesencephalic haemorrhagic infarct and multiple small infarct lesions in the cerebellum who was unable to open her eyes (related to the mesencephalic lesion), who developed severe dystonia and gained an unusual amount of weight. She eventually died without a unifying diagnosis. Her father required coronary artery bypass surgery in his thirties.

Prothrombotic abnormalities
There is an increasing body of evidence showing a significant association between neonatal stroke and thromboembolic disorders[5,25,74–77] as well as some data to suggest that such abnormalities are important in the aetiology of all types of spastic cerebral palsy.[76,78]

Our own data show that 10 of 24 (42%) neonates with stroke of perinatal origin confirmed on early brain MRI had at least one prothrombotic risk factor. Five were heterozygous for the factor V Leiden (G1691A) mutation (FVL) and six had high levels of factor VIIIc.[75] There was no significant abnormality in the coagulation profile (prothrombin time, activated partial thromboplastin time, thrombin time, platelet count, fibrinogen and von Willebrand factor antigen), and no children had protein C, S or antithrombin deficiency, lupus anticoagulant or the prothrombin gene (G20210A mutation of the prothrombin gene). Lipoprotein (a) (Lp(a)), plasminogen (PAI), homocysteine and anticardiolipin antibodies (ACLA) were not measured, nor was the genotype for methylene tetrahydrofolate reductase (MTHFR) consistently ascertained.

There was an association between the occurrence of these abnormalities and the presence of haemorrhage on MRI and poor neurological outcome. Eight of eleven patients (73%) with hemiplegia or global delay had one prothrombotic abnormality, whereas only one of thirteen (8%) with a normal outcome had any prothrombotic risk factors. In addition, all five children with the FVL mutation developed a hemiplegia.

Günther et al[25] found that 68% of 91 term neonates with PAS had at least one prothrombotic factor compared with 24% of 182 controls. The most common finding was an increase in the level of Lp(a) in 20 patients (22%) versus 10 controls (5.5%). The FVL mutation was found in 17 patients (18.7%, findings very similar to our data) compared with 10 controls (5.5%). The PT gene was found in four patients (4.4%) and four controls (2.2%) and the MTHFR TT677 genotype in 15 patients (16.5%) and 20 controls (10.9%), neither significantly raised in the patients. Protein C deficiency was found in six patients (6.6%) and none of the controls. Acquired ACLA IgG was found in three patients but not IgM. No case of protein C or antithrombin deficiency was found. Levels of factor VIIIc were not recorded. Forty-nine (54%) of these patients has additional triggering factors, e.g. asphyxia, sepsis, patent foramen ovale, and two-thirds of these had at least one prothrombotic abnormality. Thus this study suggests a significant role for Lp(a), FVL, the PT gene and protein C in neonatal stroke in combination with other perinatal risk factors. The low incidence of ACLAs may be related to the late sampling.

Golomb et al[5] studied 22 infants who were thought to be asymptomatic at birth and presented either with early hand preference or seizures between 2 and 6 months when they were found to have an established lesion on MRI suggestive of PAS.

ACLAs were found in 12 of 17 patients, which persisted in two patients. Two patients had the FVL mutation and one was homozygous for MTHFR. It is not possible to know whether these children had a stroke around the time of birth or before but the apparent absence of symptoms at birth suggests that the infarcts were already established at that time. The high incidence of ACLAs and low incidence of FVL and other prothrombotic disorders in this group of children leads one to speculate that antenatally and perinatally occurring stroke may be aetiologically different.

There remains much scope for research into prothrombotic abnormalities in neonatal stroke and thrombosis in the newborn infant. Genetically regulated prothrombotic factors vary greatly between populations; cultures where consanguinity is accepted are at particularly higher risk of homozygous states.[79–81] Prothrombotic abnormalities may be transiently related to altered cytokines and sepsis. We do not know how alterations in cytokines and inflammatory processes affect thrombotic processes but it is highly likely they are interdependent. The correct timing of investigation in relation to the onset of lesions and symptoms and birth is not defined. Prothrombotic disorders have been reported with intraventricular haemorrhage in the preterm infant.[82] The role of other factors, e.g. factors II, V, VII, protein Z and various glycoproteins, remains largely unexplored. Hogeveen et al[73] found homocysteine levels to be higher in neonates with stroke, compared with healthy age-matched controls. However, in a recent study, there was no evidence for an excess of any candidate gene polymorphisms.[83] The prevalence of other mutations, such as those regulating collagen IV, remains to be determined.[84]

In summary there is a multiplicity of aetiological factors and it is likely that it is a combination of factors that leads to the insult. It is of great interest that familial occurrences of neonatal AIS and recurrence of stroke within the index case are very rare. The question of health insurance should be discussed with families before testing.[85]

Placenta

There is a dearth of placental data from children with neonatal stroke. Kraus and Acheen[37] in a review of 84 placentas found evidence of thrombosis in 16 (19%) and three of the fetuses appeared to have cerebral thrombi. However all these infants were <36 weeks' gestation and no clear association with neonatal stroke was apparent. Placental thrombi have been associated with cerebral lesions on ultrasound in growth-restricted infants but this was a preterm population and the lesions were not typical of stroke.[38] Chorioamnionitis has also been implicated in stroke.[7]

Clinical presentation

Seizures, which may be quite subtle in the first 24–72 hours after birth, are the most common first clinical sign of perinatal stroke in infants who were thought well enough to go to the postnatal wards with their mothers. On questioning, however, the infants have often been rather quiet or irritable and not interested in feeding. First time parents may not consider this unusual and the staff may have given reassurance. After the seizures have been identified many parents say that they have seen similar movements in the preceding hours. Infants may also present with apnoea, cyanosis, poor feeding and lethargy, and signs that suggest sepsis. Some infants are undoubtedly asymptomatic and we have found an acutely evolving infarction in an infant scanned as a normal control (Fig. 9.1). This infant was born by Caesarean section to a primigravida for failure to progress and failed instrumental delivery but he had normal Apgar scores and was considered normal by the clinical team.

Neurological examination between seizures may be normal, but generalized hypotonia is common though few infants have this recorded before they have been given anticonvulsants. A proportion of infants with AIS show some asymmetry of tone pattern in the first days/weeks after birth, which is usually transient. Abnormal patterns of movements can also be observed.[86] Many infants with cerebral infarction do not show other signs of encephalopathy and they are responsive to visual and auditory stimuli unless sedated by anticonvulsants. A few infants will require early respiratory support and these are usually the ones with signs of encephalopathy and/or ongoing seizures that are difficult to treat.[63]

Infants with focal infarction rarely have specific dysmorphic features or cutaneous markers of neurological problems; occasionally limb ischaemia is associated. This is usually present at birth suggesting that, at least in these infants, the PAS is initiated before delivery.[87] We have seen two infants with PAS and Erb's palsy but this does not seem a common association.

Diagnosis

Cranial ultrasound generally provides the first evidence of a focal hemispheric lesion. If the scan is performed soon after the onset of symptoms it may not be abnormal or not sufficiently so to provide a diagnosis.[18,32,88,89] In contrast, scans performed at the end of the first week usually provide evidence of focal changes suggestive of infarction. In a study of 40 infants who had early (day 1–3) and later (day 4–7) ultrasound, all eight lesions with a haemorrhagic component were diagnosable on early ultrasound scan. Major lesions with midline shift (*n*=3) were also easily detected. In the remaining 29 infants 13 had normal early scans but only six had normal later scans. These six were all smaller cortical branch lesions not associated with motor sequelae. Identifying brainstem and cerebellar involvement and posterior and small convexity lesions can be difficult[28,35] though modern scanners and the use of additional acoustic windows allow better insonation of these areas. Whilst cranial ultrasound almost always gives some indication of the problem (~90%), specific site and lesion diagnosis and identifying additional smaller peripheral lesions is better done with MRI (Fig. 9.3). However ultrasound is very useful and if lesions are well seen on early ultrasound this suggests that their onset predated labour.

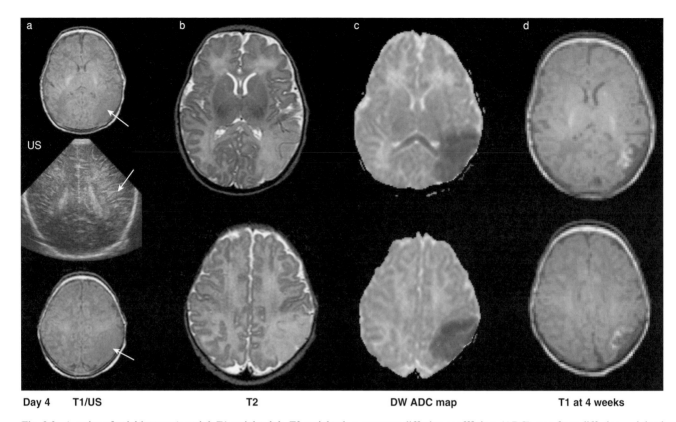

| Day 4 T1/US | T2 | DW ADC map | T1 at 4 weeks |

Fig. 9.3. A series of axial images (a and d, T1-weighted; b, T2-weighted; c, apparent diffusion coeffficient (ADC) map from diffusion weighted sequences) and one coronal ultrasound image. (a–c) were obtained on day 4 after birth and (d) at 4 weeks from an infant born at 39 weeks' gestation who presented with seizures. The ultrasound image shows increased echogenicity on the left suggestive but not absolutely diagnostic of infarction. A left-sided posterior branch MCA infarction is clearly seen on all images but most easily on the ADC map (c), then the T2 images (b) and least on the T1 (arrows, a). There is no cortical highlighting to be seen yet. By 4 weeks the infarction has evolved with tissue loss well seen. Cortical highlighting is still seen at this age. The lesion appears smaller than the size of the infarct as determined from the earlier imaging. The ADC image indicated involvement of the posterior limb of the internal capsule (PLIC) and the corpus callosum: however the PLIC did not seem involved on the conventional images and, although slightly smaller than on the contralateral side, was well myelinated on the follow-up scan. The corpus callosum was slightly thinner adjacent to the infarction on follow-up scans. This child has not developed a hemiplegia.

CT has been the definitive mode of imaging in many studies. However, we have seen the diagnosis of PAS made on CT when there has been no evidence for it on MRI and vice versa. No large comparative study has been performed between CT and MRI and it would probably now not be judged ethical. In a study by Krishnamoorthy et al,[90] three of eight patients had a normal CT followed by an abnormal MRI within 24 hours. It is difficult to make valid comparisons from observational studies as inevitably CT is performed before MRI and differences in the time interval from the onset of symptoms to scan may account for some of the increased accuracy of MRI. Most infants that are referred for MRI after CT are those with ongoing symptomatology and not necessarily typical of all infants with AIS.

Care should therefore be taken in not underdiagnosing PAS on early CT and, in the face of a normal CT, if no other explanation for the symptoms is forthcoming, MRI is indicated. Prognosis for motor function after neonatal stroke is dependent on which regions of the brain are affected, particularly the internal capsule[60,91] and brainstem[92,93] (Fig. 9.4), and this is difficult to determine from CT, which therefore cannot continue to be recommended.

MRI is the preferred method of diagnosis. Conventional T1- and T2-weighted images allow the identification of the vascular distribution of the lesion and the extent of involvement of cortical and subcortical structures, such as the internal capsule, basal ganglia and also secondary changes in the brainstem and thalami. It gives optimal imaging of the whole brain so that small additional lesions in, for example, the contralateral hemisphere, the brainstem and posterior fossa or evidence of small longstanding lesions are not missed. In addition it allows for diffusion and perfusion weighted imaging and non-invasive MR angiography.

Initially on T1-weighted images the cortex is of low signal intensity (long T1) and the white matter of intermediate signal (Fig. 9.4) though lower than on T2 where both cortex and white matter are of high signal intensity (long T2) (Fig. 9.1 and 9.3) – by 5–7 days the cortical signal becomes high on T1 and low on T2 giving the typical appearance of 'cortical highlighting' (Fig. 9.4). This is probably due to capillary proliferation or infiltration by lipid-laden macrophages. Sometimes within the infarction there is obvious haemorrhage. Within a few days the white matter becomes of low signal on T1. During these early periods of signal change a

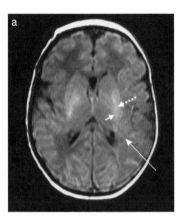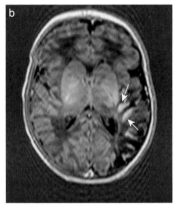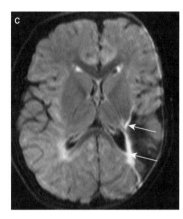

Fig. 9.4. Axial T1-weighted day 2 (a), Inversion recovery day 7 (b) and later fluid attenuated inversion recovery (FLAIR) scan (c) images from a term infant with early neonatal seizures. The early images (a) show the region of infarction on the left (arrow) with relative loss of grey-white matter differentiation and the white and cortical grey matter are almost isointense. The left posterior limb of the internal capsule (PLIC) is not clearly seen (short arrow) and there is abnormal high signal intensity (SI) in the left putamen (dotted arrow). A few days later (b) the signal in the white matter is lower and cortical highlighting is seen (arrows). Some high signal in the PLIC is seen but it is not normal and there is an abnormal line of low SI adjacent to it. Again there is abnormal high SI in the posterior putamen. A FLAIR image (c) at 10 months shows a porencephalic cyst and gliosis (arrows) around the margins of the infarct and along the posterior PLIC. As expected this child developed a hemiplegia. He is cognitively normal in early secondary school and has not had seizures.

loss of grey/white matter differentiation is seen. Swelling is a feature of larger lesions, sometimes with mid-line shift. Secondary signal changes in the brainstem tracts and thalami can be seen as early as the first week (Fig. 9.5).

The very early signal changes are seen more clearly on T2- than on T1-weighted images (Figs 9.3 and 9.5) but in our experience, most lesions can be detected on both within 24–48 hours from seizure onset. We have seen two patients where the infarction was only visualized on T2-weighted scans in the first week. Using diffusion weighted imaging (DWI), all lesions were clearly evident on the first scan.[94–96] The DWI "pseudonormalizes" or becomes less abnormal after days 5–7 from birth,[97,98] losing the characteristic signal in the region of the infarction 1–2 weeks after birth. Diffusion restriction in the corticospinal tracts is also well seen and appears to represent pre-Wallerian degeneration and can be used to predict outcome.[92,93,99,100]

In addition to acutely evolving lesions, we have found evidence of longer standing lesions in two of our patients. Whilst this is a very small proportion it does lend weight to the view that antenatal factors may play a role in increasing susceptibility to perinatal insults.

In a series of 12 infants who had serial conventional MRI and DWI from the first week, the early DWIs were most abnormal on the first scan in eight infants.[95] In the other four infants the lesion was seen to evolve over days 2–4, showing more tissue involvement with time although the change was not clinically significant. The extent of tissue involvement was usually the same on conventional T2-weighted and DWI and both sometimes overestimated the size of the infarction determined from scans at 6–8 weeks (Figs 9.2 and 9.4) though not always (Fig. 9.5). The time course of DWI changes is similar to that described in the adult human literature.[101] In contrast to adults and animal experimental data, it is not known when neonates incur their lesions. We have not seen infants with infarction where the initial DWI was normal but the earliest we have imaged an in-patient infant is 2.5 hours after seizures started and in our cohort the median time from seizure onset to scan was 33 hours and 55 hours from birth (most infants having to be transferred in). Because of this practical difficulty there are limitations in using DWI alone to time the onset of the lesion, and a combination of very early and sequential ultrasound, and conventional and diffusion weighted MRI in the first few days after symptom onset is the most helpful.

Electroencephalography (EEG) performed soon after onset of seizures may be normal or only show some asymmetry in the background activity. Epileptic features, such as recurrent sharp waves and/or multiple spikes, are often found and these are not always associated with abnormal background activity. It is the persistence of abnormal background activity rather than the occurrence of seizures that is associated with a poor motor prognosis.[102,126] The occurrence of periodic lateralized epileptiform discharges (PLEDs) suggests a diagnosis of stroke.[103] In our experience, status epilepticus with PAS is not common, occurring more often with bilateral parasagittal type of lesions.

Blood flow studies Decreased blood velocities are reported on the side of the stroke,[104] with reduced pulsation within the first 6–12 hours of presentation as compared with the contralateral side. This may be followed by an increase in velocities in ipsilateral vessels. On MRA we have seen absence of signal in ipsilateral vessels on early imaging with restoration of signal a few days later. However we do not know of a systematic study, with repeated MRA in the first few days, to know how common this is with PAS.

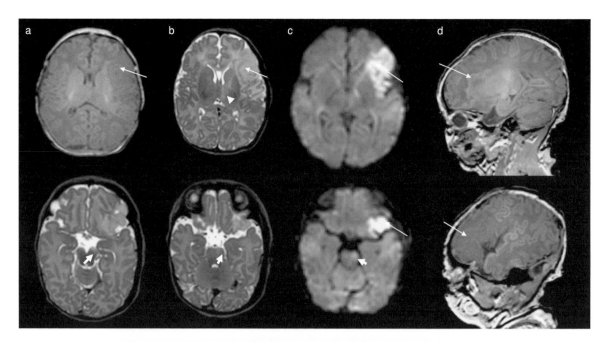

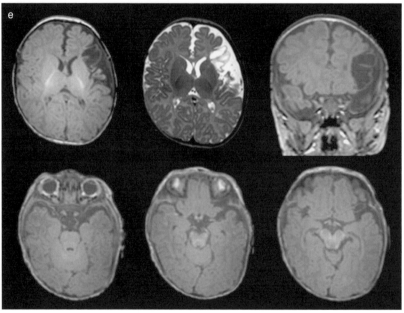

Fig. 9.5. Axial T1 and T2 (a), axial T2 (b), diffusion (c) and sagittal T1 (d) weighted images from a term born infant who developed seizures at 30 hours after birth. He was born by forceps delivery: Apgar scores and cord gases were normal. His ultrasound showed increased echogenicity on the left. His MRI done on day 4 (a–d), 60 hours after the onset of seizures, shows an acute left fronto-parietal infarction (thin arrows). There is a clear highlighted rim to the infarct seen best on the upper sagittal image. Additionally there is abnormal high signal in the anterior limb of the internal capsule (ALIC) and the anterior part of the posterior limb of the internal capsule (PLIC) on the T2 and diffusion weight images, as well as the medial left thalamus and left brainstem on T2-weighted images remote from the infarct (short thick arrows). The posterior part of the PLIC appears normally myelinated both at term and on a follow up scan at 8 weeks (e), though on the later scan the ALIC is not as well myelinated on the left. However on the later scan his brainstem appears normal and symmetrical. He has developed some plagiocephaly. Note cortical highlighting is not seen at 2 months but a cortical rim around the atrophic infarct remains clearly visible and the volume of the region of the infarct is still well seen. From our data we would not expect him to develop a hemiplegia because his basal ganglia and PLIC do not seem involved in the infarct on his early scan[60] but the changes in the brainstem are of concern.[92,93] From our own data we might expect him to have some minor right-sided neurological signs at early school age.[113] Follow up at 15 months shows no clinical or functional asymmetry and normal development in all domains.

Summary of early diagnostic investigations:

- The clinical presentation of an apparently well term infant who develops seizures in the first 1–3 days should give a high index of suspicion for the diagnosis.
- Cranial ultrasound performed soon after the onset of the convulsions may not detect the lesion.
- Rarely will the lesion not be seen on a conventional MRI and it is always seen on DWI.
- The presence of focal asymmetrical changes on ultrasound scans after a few days and the presence of asymmetries of background and/or seizure activity or the presence of periodic lateralized epileptiform discharges on EEG provide additional evidence of the presence of the lesion.
- Brain MRI is the most reliable diagnostic tool to establish the type and extent of the lesion together with very early ultrasound in timing lesion onset.

LATER EVOLUTION OF LESIONS

Atrophy starts to set in after 3 weeks (Fig. 9.3) and is maximally obvious by 6–8 weeks. In infarction of a main or branch artery a porencephalic cyst is obvious at this time though there is almost always some tissue within the region (Fig. 9.4) and interestingly it rarely looks completely cystic on ultrasound. In contrast, borderzone infarctions, which cross arterial territories, rarely become cystic on MRI.

After 2 months, in some but not all infants, the infarcted region decreases in size and there appears to be regeneration of tissue at the infarct margins over the next 6–8 months. Using a computer program designed to match and subtract accurately serially acquired volume acquisions images, we have shown that there is excessive growth in and around the infarct during this time.[105,106] This tissue has the MRI appearances of white matter and its growth may account for the virtual disappearance of smaller infarcts. Regeneration of tissue has been described in animal experiments[107] but not in adult humans or older children.

After several months tissue adjacent to the infarct will show evidence of gliosis (Fig. 9.4) but the amount of gliosis around an infarct is variable and not predictable and is often small. In infants with smaller peripheral lesions, the site of infarction may develop the appearance of a schizencephalic cleft (Fig. 9.2)[108] and very little gliosis. For all infants the affected hemisphere as a whole remains smaller than the unaffected side (Figs 9.3 and 9.6) and myelination is reduced, most obviously around the site of the infarction.

Wallerian degeneration

In the acute stages of MCA infarction there may be abnormal signal (long T1 and long T2) within the brainstem (Fig. 9.5), probably resulting from metabolic change within tissue distant from but connected to the primary lesion. This phenomenon is known as diaschisis and may be temporary. However with larger lesions, mainly those affecting the central motor pathway, Wallerian degeneration in the brainstem can be seen as persisting abnormal signal intensity occurring within a few days with atrophy appearing over 5–8 weeks.[109] Similar signal changes and later thalamic atrophy ipsilateral to an infarct are often seen where there has not been any primary involvement (Figs 9.4 and 9.6). Cerebellar atrophy, both ipsilateral and contralateral, is reported after large focal hemispheric infarction though we have not seen this in our patients in the first year after birth.[110]

Recurrence after perinatal stroke

We have not yet seen evidence of a recurrence of stroke either within the child or within the family. However none of these children has cardiovascular risk factors or sickle cell disease. A few cases have been reported by others[111] but recurrence is rare and reassurance can generally be given that will not occur. This is unlike the situation in older children where recurrence is not uncommon.[112]

Neurodevelopmental outcome

Reported outcome data of perinatal stroke depends on study population and it is difficult to compare different datasets unless there is consistent data relating to lesion site and type. Different cohorts may not only consist of neonatally symptomatic term-born infants but may include preterm infants, those who present late with symptoms and those whose lesions are acquired antenatally, further complicating valid comparisons.

Hemiplegia is the most frequently reported sequela for infants with focal infarction.[113] The incidence of hemiplegia in different series is very variable[114–124] for the reasons given above. Our experience, which is not population based and is obtained from term-born infants mainly presenting with early seizures, is that about one-third develop a hemiplegia.[34,61,113] The first signs of hemiplegia can be detected between 3 and 6 months and consist of mild asymmetry or abnormal patterns of movements[86,125] and become more evident between 6 and 12 months.[109]

Not all PAS is associated with abnormal motor outcome; it is therefore important to identify early signs which predict outcome. In our experience early MRI and early EEG can reliably be used to do this. We found that the concomitant involvement of hemispheric tissue, the PLIC and the basal ganglia in the primary lesion as seen on conventional T1 and T2-weighted MRI was associated with an abnormal motor outcome (Fig. 9.4), whilst the involvement of only one or two of the three regions was associated with a mater normal outcome.[126,127] However, we had few children in our cohort with isolated posterior basal ganglia and PLIC involvement and this combination, which perhaps occurs more often in preterm infants, does increase the risk of hemiplegia. The motor outcome did not appear to depend on the vascular distribution of the lesion. In the more recent studies by de Vries et al[92] and Kirton et al[93] early acute DWI changes in the corticospinal tracts also predict hemiplegia, though we have seen acute changes in the brainstem without subsequent atrophy (Fig. 9.5).

Not surprisingly the population-based studies of PAS, which included children with PPERI who presented with neurological problems beyond the neonatal period, found that hemiplegia was common[6,26] (Fig. 9.6). In addition in the study of

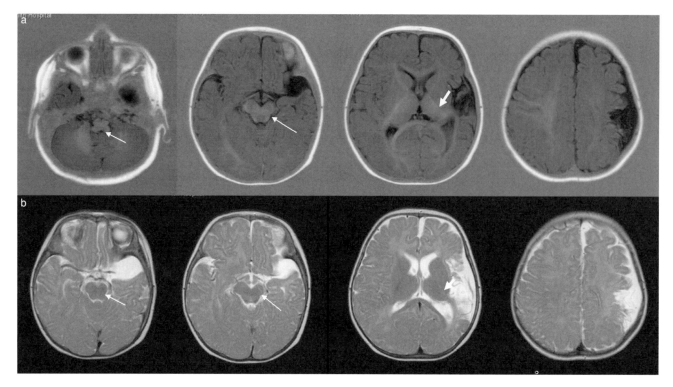

Fig. 9.6. Presumed perinatal stroke in a 4-kg infant born at term by emergency Caesarean section for fetal distress, meconium-stained liquor and a prolonged second stage. He had Apgar scores of 9 at 1 minute and 10 at 5 minutes. He developed respiratory distress thought secondary to mild meconium aspiration but did not require ventilation and was discharged home by day 4. There were no neonatal neurological concerns. He had one ultrasound scan on day 1 reported as normal which on review showed some mild left-sided echogenicity. He presented with poor right upper limb function at 4 months. A left-sided middle cerebral artery territory infarction is seen on his T1 (a) and T2 (b) weighted MRI done at 5 months. The left posterior limb of the internal capsule (short fat arrows) is involved, the left thalamus is small, as are the left corticospinal tracts seen at the level of the mesencephalon and in the brainstem (thin white arrows). He has a moderate right-sided hemiplegia with some independent finger movements and good cognitive skills at 18 months. He started to walk at 12 months and has appropriate language development. He has not had any seizures.

Lee et al[26], 85% of whom were born at term, large stroke size and involvement of Broca's area, Wernicke's area, the internal capsule or the basal ganglia were predictors of hemiplegic cerebral palsy.

We have also found that abnormal background EEG activity in the neonatal period was associated with abnormal motor outcome whilst a normal background, with or without seizure activity, was related to normal outcome.[126] In contrast, neither the neonatal clinical examination nor the neonatal cranial ultrasound was helpful in prognosis. We have found an association between heterozygosity for FVL and the development of hemiplegia.[75]

The pattern of hemiplegia following PAS in the term-born infant is usually such that the upper limb appears more affected than the lower limb[125]. Almost all infants with PAS and hemiplegia will walk, although the age at which they do this may be delayed to 2 years.[21] We have found good consistency between neurological findings at 2 and 5.5 years with only one child being classified as having a mild hemiplegia later that was not identified at 2 years. Some children with involvement of the ALIC but the PLIC had some minor neurological signs or suboptimal scores on the Movement ABC detected at 5.5 years but not a hemiplegia. Hand function in the non-hemiplegic hand is normal, regardless of the severity

of the hemiplegia, if the contralateral hemisphere is normal on MRI.[34] However, hand function in the non-hemiplegic hand is not normal when there are bilateral brain lesions even though the lesion in the hemisphere ipsilateral to the hemiplegia is small, suggesting that the larger lesion limits plasticity.

Seizures have been reported to be common in children who suffered neonatal infarction[118,120,128] and developed hemiplegia. Rarely, children with larger lesions may develop hypsarrhythmia and infantile spasms.[129] A few children require surgical removal of epileptogenic tissue. The incidence of later seizures in those who do not develop hemiplegia is low but in most studies follow-up is relatively short term.[18,34,61,88,130] Timing may be particularly important in relation to the generation of hippocampal sclerosis, which appears to be a sequel of focal injury relatively late in gestation.[131] In the series of Golomb,[132] 67% of those with perinatal stroke developed seizures; time to presentation was shorter in those with prenatal ultrasound abnormality and in those with a family history of epilepsy. Golomb et al[130] also found that for children with hemiplegic cerebral palsy, 47% had epilepsy, and this was more likely to occur in children who had both a neonatal presentation and delivery by Caesarean section. Only eight of 40 children in our cohort with neonatal stroke have had later seizures and only four so far have required long-term anticonvulsant therapy; however relatively few children in the cohort had very large lesions and the follow up is relatively short even though 31 have reached early school age.[61] There is a strong correlation between seizures and low IQ[128] and the presence of seizures has a deleterious effect on cognitive functioning.[133,134]

In general, children with neonatal stroke are thought to have a good *cognitive outcome* though importantly there are no large long-term follow-up studies of infants with stroke without hemiplegia. Data from children with hemiplegia of different aetiologies shows that two-thirds have intelligence considered in the normal range though those with major motor impairment have a lower mean IQ. In the series of Golomb et al,[130] children with cerebral palsy after perinatal stroke who had neonatal presentation were more likely to have severe cognitive impairment than children with delayed presentation. In our own studies, all but six of 31 children of school age are in a mainstream school setting with an IQ in the normal range.[61] Six of these children have a mild to moderate hemiplegia. Two of the children with lower IQs have small lesions and do not have a hemiplegia but are slightly dysmorphic; the other children with low IQs have other unusual features. Several groups have reported a fall in IQ over time and relate this to the occurrence of seizures.[128,134]

Speech and language development in infants and children with focal lesions is still a subject of controversy. Speech delay has been observed in children, more commonly with left hemisphere infarcts,[128,134,135] but it has been recently suggested that these early abnormalities tend to recover in the course of development.[136] These authors did not find an effect of lesion size on language development. They suggest that the effect of left hemisphere lesions on language is more on early grammar and expression and that the effects of right hemisphere lesions may not be noted until there is a demand for more complex contextual and pragmatic use of language. Deficits in prosodic aspects of language have been shown for lesions in either hemisphere, although affective comprehension was only impaired with right hemisphere lesions.[137] Differences in reading and spelling skills have been shown in boys but not girls in association with left hemisphere lesions.[138]

Visual development Visual field abnormalities are unusual in the absence of hemiplegia. Acuity is generally normal but narrow visual fields and other aspects of abnormal visual processing (fixation shifts, orientation-reversal VEP) can be found in two-thirds of term children with focal infarction when assessed in the first years after birth,[139–141] although less than a third were abnormal by school age[113] confirming other observations that there may be recovery in some.[142] These abnormalities are not always related to the involvement of optic radiation and primary visual cortex on MRI but probably reflect the involvement of other cortical and subcortical structures that are also involved in a wider network responsible for different aspects of visual function. We would suggest that all

children with focal lesions should have a detailed assessment of visual function regardless of the site of their lesion.

A variety of visuospatial difficulties have been reported in children with strokes of pre- and perinatal origin. Ballantyne and Trauner[143] found that these children performed poorly on tests of facial recognition, particularly when there was parietal lobe involvement of either side. This observation could not be accounted for by differences in IQ or lesion severity. Processing differences have been noted between left and right hemisphere lesions in block design tasks, suggesting that the right hemisphere is responsible for more global aspects of visual processing and the left hemisphere more detailed local function.[144] Right hemisphere lesions may lead to difficulties with spatial integrative functions that may improve with time. Stiles et al[145] have shown that this improvement is more likely to be the result of the development of compensatory strategies rather than a true recovery of function. Our own cohort of term children with lesions that have been very clearly defined on MRI in the neonatal period are now entering the age when these sort of studies can be performed and we hope that this will help to clarify some of these issues.

Psychological and behavioural problems have been extensively studied by Goodman,[146] who found problems with behaviour, emotions and relationships in 50% of children with hemiplegia; these are sufficient to cause considerable difficulties for the children and their families. Temper tantrums are common and reluctance to comply with parental requests. Anxiety is also common, with marked shyness and some specific phobias. Severely antisocial behaviour is rare. Many of these problems are compounded by a lack of understanding of the complex issues that may accompany hemiplegia, particularly in the school setting and in peer relationships. Goodman's studies however are not limited to children with PAS. Trauner at al[147] found in 39 children with focal unilateral brain lesions of perinatal onset, not all of whom had hemiplegia, that when the effects of IQ were allowed for, there was no increase in clinically significant behavioural or emotional problems over controls or in relation to the site of the lesions. Our experience is that there are more behavioural difficulties at a preschool age than one might expect but numbers are small. We have found that many parents feel their children are emotionally labile and prone to outbursts of temper and that discussing these issues has been very helpful.

Compensatory abilities The remarkably good outcome in many infants with neonatal stroke is likely to relate to cortical and subcortical plasticity. Cortical reorganization to two sites has been demonstrated using magnetic encephalography in an adult in response to median nerve stimulation following neonatal MCA infarction.[148] Villabranca and Hovda[149] found abundant evidence for long-term remodelling of the brain following extensive unilateral brain damage. This ability occurred preferentially during a distinct period in early life that includes the perinatal period, suggesting that injury at this time may be followed by considerable functional recovery as compared with injury in other age periods. Functional MRI studies have demonstrated the anatomical basis in a few infants.[150] Eyre et al[151] have shown that, following early onset unilateral brain lesions, evoked responses elicited using transcranial magnetic stimulation of the undamaged cortex have onsets, thresholds and amplitudes within the normal range for contralateral responses. This observation was not seen in adult onset stroke. They argue that dense ipsilateral projections from the unaffected hemisphere must persist and they suggest that the process by which they would normally withdraw in the immediate postnatal period is governed by a competitive activity dependent process that does not take place because of the loss of cortical control.

These studies, together with the observations of good motor, language, intellectual and visual development in these children, all provide evidence for considerable plasticity and functional recovery in the neonatal brain injured at term. A consequence of this plasticity may be crowding that may explain difficulites with skills and behaviours that develop later in childhood.

Treatment – neonatal

At present there is no specific acute therapy for neonatal stroke. A few infants require intensive care, with ventilation, volume expansion and inotropic support. Care should be taken not to hyperventilate and cause cerebral vasoconstriction from hypocapnia, thereby decreasing blood flow to unaffected areas of the brain. Hyperthermia should be avoided.[152]

We treat clinical seizures if they last longer than 5 minutes and occur on two occasions. We also treat subclinical seizures if there are runs of half an hour or more seen on EEG or cerebral function monitor. We use phenobarbitone as a first line medication – most children are transferred into us and are already on this therapy. Second line anticonvulsant drugs are midazolam and lidocaine although the use of, in particular, the benzodiazepine drugs may necessitate ventilation. Levetiracetam is a promising drug. We rarely continue anticonvulsants longer than 10–14 days.

We do not anticoagulate infants. There is no strong evidence to support this at present.[153] Most infants are not diagnosed before their infarction is well established. There are considerable concerns about haemorrhaging into infarcted tissue, worsening the prognosis for a condition that may have a normal outcome. However, there may be a case for anticoagulation in infants where the diagnosis has been made very early and the lesion is extending and involves regions of the brain that will lead to hemiplegia or where there are other problems, for example cardiac abnormality or thrombi that might lead to further stroke. All infants should have coagulation and thrombophilic studies.

Hypothermia is now a standard therapeutic tool in the treatment of acute perinatal asphyxia.[154] At present this therapy is not being applied to neonatal stroke, partly because of the late diagnosis and also because of the relatively good outcome.

However Taylor et al[155] suggest that hypothermia delayed a few hours after onset of the lesion may be protective. As MRI becomes increasingly available, and it becomes possible to identify sites of tissue involvement and predict outcome very early, it may be possible to target this therapy at those likely to have long-term morbidity. The use of Xenon is also being trialled for global perinatal hypoxia-ischaemia and may also be promising in neonatal stroke.[156]

Longer term management and rehabilitation are discussed in Chapter 17.

A useful self help group run by parents in co-operation with many professionals is HemiHelp (www.hemihelp.org.uk).

9.2 Intracranial Haemorrhage in the Newborn

Fenella J. Kirkham and Frances Cowan

Introduction

Intracranial haemorrhage is an important management problem in the neonate, particularly those born preterm, although it is also well recognized in term infants, the main focus of this chapter. With improvements in perinatal care, the relative importance of birth trauma has fallen considerably, but it continues to cause perinatal death in approximately 1 in 2000 deliveries[157] and is a relatively rare cause of cerebral palsy. In parallel with this decline, however, there has probably been an increase in intracranial haemorrhage in 'high-risk' neonates, e.g. those requiring extracorporeal membrane oxygenation (ECMO) for severe lung disease due to meconium aspiration[158] or cardiopulmonary bypass for the repair of a congenital heart defect.[159,160] Vitamin K deficiency continues to cause intracranial haemorrhage in infants who do not receive adequate prophylaxis, through parental choice as well as prematurity and biliary atresia.[161] In the US Nationwide Inpatient Sample for haemophilia for for 1988 to 2001, the overall incidence of intracranial haemorrhage, including those born preterm, was 0.11%.[162] The incidence of intracranial, including extradural and subdural haemorrhage, in term infants has been estimated to be 0.027% of live births.[163] In a recent population-based survey in Estonia, seven of 12 of those of gestational age >32 weeks presenting in the neonatal period with symptomatic stroke had haemorrhage on neuroimaging (one subarachnoid, four intraventricular and two intraparenchymal) and the incidence of haemorrhagic perinatal stroke was 0.0117% or 11.7 per 100 000.[27] In the Kaiser Permanante system, the incidence was 6.2 per 100 000.[164] These are less than Hanigan's figure, at least in part because subdural and extradural haemorrhages were excluded, but it is almost certainly an underestimate of the incidence of perinatal haemorrhagic stroke, as those who died acutely and those undergoing cardiac surgery or ECMO may not have been reported. Intracranial haemorrhage remains common among some groups. In addition to the high prevalence in infants with congenital heart disease undergoing MRI,[160] the incidence was 1.9% between 1988 and 2001 in term neonates with haemophilia A, B or C or von Willibrand's disease, but without comorbidities such as sepsis or respiratory or cardiac disease.[162] Fetal intracranial haemorrhage has also been documented[165] and is probably a cause of otherwise unexplained cerebral palsy.

There are a number of different intracranial sites at which haemorrhage may occur, and the aetiology in an individual case may be deduced at least in part from this information, although the gestation of the infant and the circumstances surrounding the delivery may also be important. Intraventricular haemorrhage, usually due to rupture of the germinal matrix, is much more common in those born before 32 weeks, although it may also occur in the term neonate. Haemorrhagic transformation of spontaneous cerebral infarction (see Chapter 8, Section 8.1), due to either arterial or venous[166] thrombosis, may occur at any gestation. Subdural and subarachnoid haemorrhages may be asymptomatic and are not necessarily related to traumatic delivery.[167,195]

The timing of the presentation may be important in determining aetiology, although caution is advised if there are potential legal issues regarding breach of duty or child protection. Many children with severe birth trauma present with reduced level of consciousness or seizures within 24 hours of birth, although others, usually, but not always, with lesser degrees of injury may not present until after discharge from hospital. There may then be difficulty in distinguishing birth trauma from postnatal causes of intracerebral haemorrhage, such as minor trauma in the context of vitamin K deficiency and venous sinus thrombosis associated with dehydration (Fig. 9.7). It is also well recognized that intracranial haemorrhage may occur antenatally.[167,168]

In Jhawar's[169] study, 66 term infants with intracranial haemorrhage were identified, and 104 control infants were matched. The following were independently associated with increased risk of intracranial haemorrhage: forceps assistance compared with spontaneous vaginal delivery; 1-minute Apgar scores of 1 through 4 and 5 through 8, compared with scores of 9 or 10 (corresponding 5-minute Apgar scores were also statistically significant); and requirements for resuscitation, compared with no resuscitation requirements. Interestingly, of the 52 case patients for whom platelet counts were recorded within 48 hours after birth, 31% had counts of less than $70 \times 10(9)/L$ and those with platelets of $<50 \times 10(9)/L$ were more likely

to have intraparenchymal haemorrhage and a more severe radiological grade. Forceps-associated haemorrhage was more frequently subarachnoid and subdural and less frequently intraparenchymal and was more caudal in location.

It is very important to exclude disorders of coagulation,[161,162,164] such as haemophilia (Fig. 9.8) and other congenital[170,171] and acquired[172] factor deficiencies, liver disease, disseminated intravascular coagulation or vitamin K deficiency. The latter may be a particular risk in infants born to mothers on anticonvulsants or certain antibiotics, and some sources recommend prophylactic vitamin K in the latter stages of pregnancy in these groups, although this remains controversial.[173] Oral or intramuscular vitamin K prophylaxis immediately after birth has been associated with a reduction in the incidence of early and late haemorrhagic disease of the newborn in healthy term infants,[161,174] although there is continuing work on regimens for 'high-risk' infants, such as those born preterm and breastfed[175] and those with undiagnosed biliary atresia.[176] Thrombocytopenia may also be the major risk factor for neonatal intracranial haemorrhage, and may be either auto- or iso-immune or secondary to congenital or postnatal infection, congenital bone marrow aplasias or metabolic disease, such as methylmalonic, propionic, isovaleric and alpha-aminoadipic acidaemias[177,178] (see Chapter 9). The risk of neonatal intracerebral haemorrhage if the mother has auto-immune thrombocytopenia is now very small and does not appear to be related to the mode of delivery.[54,179] Other metabolic condition associated with intracranial haemorrhage in newborn infants

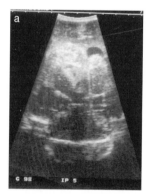
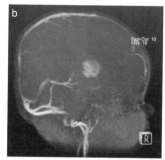

Fig. 9.7. (a) Cranial ultrasound showing intraventricular haemorrhage in a term infant. (b) Magnetic resonance venogram showing poor flow in the sagittal sinus posteriorly.

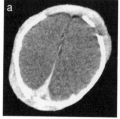
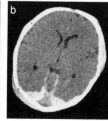
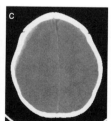
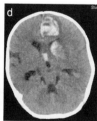
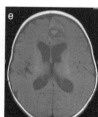
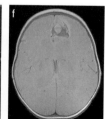

Fig. 9.8. (a–f) CT scans showing subarachnoid and subdural haemorrhage as well as cephalhaematoma in a boy who was diagnosed with haemophilia.

include the disorders of glycosylation[180] in addition to the subdural effusions seen in glutaric aciduria type I. Lactic acidosis, with or without coagulopathy, appears to be a risk factor for intracranial haemorrhage in those undergoing ECMO.[181,182] Infants with coarctation of the aorta are at particular risk of intracranial haemorrhage,[183] either secondary to systemic hypertension or occasionally due to associated intracranial aneurysms. Maternal cocaine,[184] alcohol[185] and salicylate[186] ingestion and smoking[187] may also be associated with intracranial haemorrhage in the fetus and neonate, particularly in those born preterm.

Structural abnormalities of the brain, including tumours,[188] and vascular anomalies such as aneurysms[189] and arteriovenous malformations[190,191] are rare causes of intracranial haemorrhage. Although head ultrasound is very useful in diagnosing and monitoring preterm infants with intraventricular haemorrhage, this technique may miss these structural lesions and other forms of neonatal intracranial haemorrhage in the posterior fossa[192] or in the supratentorial subdural space and urgent CT or MRI (see Chapter 4 Section 4.2) is mandatory, particularly in term infants whose neurological condition is deteriorating, and to exclude potentially treatable conditions such as venous sinus thrombosis.[166] Very careful review of the clinical presentation and the available neuroimaging and haematological investigations will usually lead to the correct diagnosis.

Extradural haemorrhage

This is a comparatively unusual site of haemorrhage in the newborn, probably because the dura is relatively thick and is closely applied to the inner periosteum of the skull in this age group. The haemorrhage usually originates from the middle meningeal artery, or occasionally from the venous sinuses. Skull fracture and cephalhaematoma in the same region are common accompanying features. The infant usually presents within a few hours of a traumatic delivery with signs of intracranial hypertension, such as a bulging fontanelle, together with focal signs suggestive of uncal herniation, for example a fixed dilated pupil and ptosis and sometimes seizures. The lesion is easily seen as a lens-shaped hyperdensity on CT[193] and may be detected on ultrasound.[194] Rapid neurosurgical decompression is essential as the haemorrhage usually continues inexorably, with deterioration in the level of consciousness and signs of brainstem compression eventually. The outcome is related to the depth of coma at the time of surgery, and may be excellent in those who are treated early.

Subdural haemorrhage

Subdural haemorrhage remains slightly more common in term infants, although the proportion of preterm born infants has risen. The aetiology of subdural haemorrhage was traditionally always considered to be trauma but self-resolving lesions are not uncommon in asymptomatic infants after routine normal and uncomplicated forceps and Ventouse extractions.[167,195,196] These usually disappear by 1 month, usually allowing a distinction from subdural haemorrhages or effusions secondary to non-accidental injury; serial head circumference measurements, including that taken at birth, are often very useful in making the correct deduction. For neonatal subdural haemorrhage, the obstetric risk factors are those which predispose to extreme moulding of the head, for example birthweight >4.5kg, face or brow presentation, very prolonged labour, or to rotational and stretching forces. Forceps delivery and vacuum extraction were implicated in the pathogenesis of subdural haemorrhage, particularly with high rotation for persistent occipto-posterior, but it appears that the risk factor is abnormal labour.[197–199] Birth asphyxia was considered to be an association but there is little supporting evidence.[200] Infants with a haemorrhagic diathesis, for example secondary to isoimmune thrombocytopenia, are at particular risk and prothrombotic abnormalities have also been reported,[201] perhaps related to venous sinus thrombosis, which can be difficult to diagnose.[166] Although there remains a significant associated mortality and morbidity, the incidence of this potentially serious lesion is falling. Improved prediction of cephalo-pelvic dysproportion and management with elective Caesarean section has made this the least common cause of neonatal intracranial haemorrhage.

There are several common origins for subdural haemorrhage in neonates, each with a typical location. Rupture of the superficial bridging veins produces subdural haematoma over the lateral aspect of the cerebrum. The typical presentation is with seizures, with or without focal neurological signs such as an ipsilateral third nerve palsy, with ptosis of the eyelid and an enlarged pupil. Other infants may present with symptoms and signs of raised intracranial pressure, such as irritability, lethargy and a full fontanelle. The haematoma may resolve or evolve into a chronic subdural, with or without hydrocephalus. If there is a tentorial tear, the straight and/or transverse sinus and the vein of Galen may be ruptured and the haemorrhage is infratentorial, with the risk if the haemorrhage is large of brainstem compression and death. These infants may present with apnoea and a reduction in conscious level. Laceration of the falx cerebri is associated with rupture of the inferior sagittal sinus, with haemorrhage in the longitudinal cerebral fissure above the corpus callosum. These infants are very ill, with a depressed level of consciousness, opisthotonus, abnormal pupillary signs and bradycardia; fortunately this is very rare. Infants born by the breech are at risk of occipital osteodiastasis, with separation of the squamous and lateral parts of the occipital bone and associated occipital sinus rupture.[202]

Ischaemic infarcts are sometimes seen in association with subdural haemorrhage.[195] It is possible that basal subdural haemorrhage causes vasospasm and infarction in the middle cerebral artery territory,[54] although this is controversial[203] and it is also possible that the subdural haematoma is secondary to the infarct.[64]

Ultrasound may miss subdural haemorrhage, as the convexity may not be visualized in the window available through the fontanelle. CT is usually adequate for diagnosis, but MRI may be required for the demonstration of any associated ischaemic lesions and for determining the timing of the haemorrhage. Lumbar puncture should be considered with care because of the risk of herniation of the temporal lobes through the tentorium or of the cerebellum through the foramen magnum.

Large supratentorial subdural haematomas over the convexities of the cerebral hemispheres may occasionally require drainage, which may be performed through the fontanelle using a subdural needle.[204] Neurosurgical intervention, i.e. longer term drainage, is rarely required in this situation, but may be life saving in infratentorial subdural haemorrhages.[205,206] The majority of these patients do well at long-term follow up particularly if the motor pathways were not involved.[207] If the lesion is diagnosed incidentally, or in an infant without signs of brainstem compression, the prognosis may be equally good with conservative management. Communicating hydrocephalus may require medical or surgical intervention either acutely or at a later stage.

The prognosis for subdural haemorrhage is variable and depends on the site of the lesion. While normal outcome has been reported for infants surviving infratentorial haemorrhage, the majority of those with large haemorrhages die rapidly or have significant disability. The prognosis for supratentorial haemorrhage is variable and probably depends on the degree of associated focal[208] and global ischaemia, although the majority of those with haemorrhage over the convexity do well and there is no evidence for sequelae in those with asymptomatic subdurals.[195] Occipital osteodiasthesis is usually a post-mortem diagnosis.

Subarachnoid haemorrhage

Subarachnoid haemorrhage can occur in both preterm infants and those born at term, but is more common in the former, usually as an incidental finding. The haemorrhage is presumed to originate from the anastomosis between the leptomeningeal arteries which are present during development, but gradually involute. The haemorrhaging may be either supratentorial, usually posteriorly, or infratentorial. The common associations with subarachnoid haemorrhage are haemorrhagic diatheses and exchange transfusion; there is little evidence for an association with birth trauma.[209] Infants with subarachnoid haemorrhage are usually less ill than those with subdural haemorrhage, and are commonly asymptomatic. Some present with seizures without other clinical signs; in these the prognosis is usually good. Others may present with a catastrophic deterioration, often associated with acute hydrocephalus; outcome is much worse in this group. The diagnosis may be made at lumbar puncture, if an atraumatic tap yields uniformly blood-stained CSF in the later bottles, or on CT.[209] In contrast to adults, the prognosis is usually good, unless there is associated birth asphyxia or CT evidence of cerebral atrophy.[209] Occasionally, medical or surgical intervention for communicating hydrocephalus may be required.

Intraparenchymal haemorrhage

Primary intraparenchymal haemorrhage is rare in the neonatal period and most intracerebral haemorrhages are secondary to ischaemic infarction.[210] It is important to exclude haemorrhagic

diathesis. There are case reports of arteriovenous malformations and aneurysms presenting in the neonatal period[189,190] and arteriography is sometimes indicated, particularly if the haemorrhage is located in a site suggestive of a vascular lesion or if there are associated features such as cardiac failure. Interventional neuroradiology or surgery may be beneficial in some cases.[191] It has been argued that birth trauma may cause arterial aneurysm, particularly at the tentorial incisura,[211] but it may be impossible to distinguish a traumatic from a congenital lesion.

Haemorrhage into a previous infarction is more likely, and although birth trauma may sometimes play a role,[210,211] predisposing factors should be actively excluded as many of these infants have no obstetric risk factors.[163] These include infection, either pre- or postnatal, and prothrombotic disorders, such as the Factor V Leiden mutation. Ischaemic infarction may occur in the anterior or posterior circulations. Traumatic carotid or vertebral dissection may play a role, although the diagnosis may often be missed unless the appropriate MR sequences are requested. Again, arteriography is rarely justified to exclude this possibility.

Thalamic Haemorrhage

The common presentation is with seizures, often associated with 'sunsetting' of the eyes, secondary to vertical gaze impairment. Many of these infants have predisposing factors for cerebral venous thrombosis such as sepsis, cyanotic congenital heart disease, and coagulopathy.[213] Recent studies have shown the presence of venous sinus thrombosis in a substantial proportion (see Chapter 7).[15,214] The prognosis is usually relatively good, although cerebral palsy is more common than in other causes of intraventricular haemorrhage and there is commonly some evidence of a hemiparesis.[212]

Intracerebellar Haemorrhage

This is more common in preterm infants[215,216] and may be primary or secondary to venous infarction or to extension of an intraventricular haemorrhage. Birth trauma, particularly during breech or forceps delivery, and asphyxia may play a role, as may postnatal events including hypoxia and fluid balance abnormalities. Limeropoulos et al[217] found emergency caesarean section, patent ductus arteriosus and lower 5-day minimum pH to be risk factors in preterm infants. Haemorrhagic diatheses, including abnormalities of the coagulation cascade, such as vitamin K deficiency or thrombocytopenia, may be important. Fixation of tubing across the occiput may be associated with intracerebellar haemorrhage because of obstruction of the venous sinuses and should be avoided.

Infants usually present with signs of brainstem compression or of intracranial hypertension or both. Although intracerebellar haemorrhage may be diagnosed by ultrasound,[217] a CT is usually required for confirmation, to distinguish this lesion from subdural haemorrhage and to define the extent of the haemorrhage. The prognosis in preterm infants is uniformly poor, but the majority of term infants survive, with or without neurosurgical intervention, usually but not always with some degree of language, cognitive and social-behavioural problems[218] as well as motor disability.[218,219] Surgical drainage may occasionally be life saving in deteriorating infants,[220] but is not usually indicated in those who remain clinically stable. Venticulostomy and eventually lumbo-peritoneal shunt may be required for the associated obstructive hydrocephalus.

Intraventricular haemorrhage

Intraventricular haemorrhage is much more common in infants born preterm than in those born at term, and is usually due to rupture of the germinal matrix in this group. The diagnosis is usually made by head ultrasound, which is undertaken routinely in most infants at risk. Some of these infants remain asymptomatic, but others present with a catastrophic collapse or a more gradual deterioration in level of consciousness with hypotonia and abnormal eye signs. The incidence in infants born before 32 weeks' gestation is as high as 35–45% and there is a significant associated morbidity whatever the grade of the haemorrhage.[221,223] The haemorrhage may be confined to the region of the germinal matrix (Grade I) or may spread into the ventricular system (Grade II). There may be associated ventricular dilatation in the early stages (Grade III) with a high risk of both obstructive and communicating hydrocephalus in the long term, which often requires medical and/or surgical intervention. In some infants, there may be intraparenchymal extension (Grade IV), which is associated with a poorer long-term prognosis.

Risk factors and strategies for prevention of intraventricular haemorrhage in the preterm infant have been the subject of intensive research.[222,223] For early intraventricular haemorrhage, risk factors include vaginal delivery and low Apgar scores, while those presenting later often have low flow in the superior vena cava in relation to high mean airway pressure.[223] The evidence suggests that up to one-third of germinal matrix and intraventricular haemorrhages are of antenatal or immediate postnatal origin.[224] Present efforts focus on antenatal management, specifically the use of steroids for mothers in preterm labour,[225] antimicrobial therapy after preterm premature rupture of the membranes[226] and indomethacin to close the patent ductus arteriosus.[29,227] Antenatal vitamin K and phenobarbitone and neonatal ethamsylate have not been shown to be of benefit. Excessive heparin use, for example in flushing arterial lines, should be avoided in neonates.[228] It may be more difficult in an individual case to ensure the prevention of preterm labour or of manouevres which cause swings in cerebral blood flow in preterm infants, and the role of elective caesarean section remains controversial.[229]

The germinal matrix usually involutes at around 36 weeks' gestation, but subependymal haemorrhage is seen in approximately 4% of term infants who are scanned with ultrasound,[230] and intraventricular haemorrhage occurs, either secondary to choroid plexus or germinal matrix haemorrhage or as an extension from a parenchymal bleed. Birth trauma and asphyxia may be aetiological in some with intraventricular haemorrhage,[210] although prospective studies have failed to identify this as a risk factor[230] in the group with isolated germinal matrix haemorrhage; the majority of this group appear to be associated with low birth weight and the prognosis is usually good. Outcome is more variable in those with intraventricular haemorrhage, particularly if there has been birth trauma and/or asphyxia.[210]

Outcome

In the surviving preterm infant, the outcome for intracranial haemorrhage is variable,[231] except that cerebellar haemorrhage is associated with poor motor and congnitive outcome.[218,231] In Jhawar's[232] study of term infants with intracranial haemorrhage, death occurred most frequently among those with primarily subarachnoid haemorrhage (19%) and the most favorable outcomes occurred among those with subdural haemorrhage (80% had no disability). In univariate models the following increased risk for poor outcome: thrombocytopenia with a platelet count of <70 000, increasing overall haemorrhage severity, frontal location and spontaneous vaginal delivery as opposed to forceps-assisted delivery. In multivariate models, only thrombocytopenia remained significant for physical disability and was of borderline significance for cognitive disability.

Conclusions

There are a number of different types of intracranial haemorrhage in preterm and term neonates. Some are potentially preventable, but trauma is relatively rarely the cause nowadays and the majority of the disabling lesions occur in very sick, 'high-risk' infants. Venous sinus thrombosis may play a more important role than previously recognized but this may be very difficult to prove as it is reversible.

REFERENCES

1. Nelson KB, Lynch JK. Stroke in newborn infants. Lancet Neurol 2004; 3(3):150–158.
2. Nelson KB. Perinatal ischemic stroke. Stroke 2007; 38(2 Suppl):742–745.
3. Raju TN, Nelson KB, Ferriero D, Lynch JK. Ischemic perinatal stroke: summary of a workshop sponsored by the National Institute of Child Health and Human Development and the National Institute of Neurological Disorders and Stroke. Pediatrics 2007; 120(3):609–616.
4. Vexler ZS, Sharp FR, Feuerstein GZ, Ashwal S, Thoresen M, Yager JY et al. Translational stroke research in the developing brain. Pediatr Neurol 2006; 34(6):459–463.
5. Golomb MR, MacGregor DL, Domi T, Armstrong DC, McCrindle BW, Mayank S et al. Presumed pre- or perinatal arterial ischemic stroke: risk factors and outcomes. Ann Neurol 2001; 50(2):163–168.
6. Wu YW, March WM, Croen LA, Grether JK, Escobar GJ, Newman TB. Perinatal stroke in children with motor impairment: a population-based study. Pediatrics 2004; 114(3):612–619.
7. Lee J, Croen LA, Backstrand KH, Yoshida CK, Henning LH, Lindan C et al. Maternal and infant characteristics associated with perinatal arterial stroke in the infant. JAMA 2005; 293(6):723–729.
8. Benders MJ, Groenendaal F, Uiterwaal CS, Nikkels PG, Bruinse HW, Nievelstein RA et al. Maternal and infant characteristics associated with perinatal arterial stroke in the preterm infant. Stroke 2007; 38(6):1759–1765.
9. Ozduman K, Pober BR, Barnes P, Copel JA, Ogle EA, Duncan CC et al. Fetal stroke. Pediatr Neurol 2004; 30(3):151–162.

10. Groenendaal F, de Vries LS. Watershed infarcts in the full term neonatal brain. Arch Dis Child Fetal Neonatal Ed 2005; 90(6):F488.

11. Burns CM, Rutherford MA, Boardman JP, Cowan FM. Patterns of cerebral injury and neurodevelopmental outcomes after symptomatic neonatal hypoglycemia. Pediatrics 2008; 122(1):65–74.

12. deVeber G, Andrew M, Adams C, Bjornson B, Booth F, Buckley DJ et al. Cerebral sinovenous thrombosis in children. N Engl J Med 2001; 345(6):417–423.

13. Carvalho KS, Bodensteiner JB, Connolly PJ, Garg BP. Cerebral venous thrombosis in children. J Child Neurol 2001; 16(8):574–580.

14. Wu YW, Miller SP, Chin K, Collins AE, Lomeli SC, Chuang NA et al. Multiple risk factors in neonatal sinovenous thrombosis. Neurology 2002; 59(3):438–440.

15. Wu, YW, Hamrick, SE, Miller, SP, Haward, MF, Lai, MC, Callen, PW, Barkovich, AJ, Ferriero, DM (2003 'Intraventricular hemorrhage in term neonates caused by sinovenous thrombosis.' Ann Neurol 54:123–126.

16. Takanashi J, Barkovich AJ, Ferriero DM, Suzuki H, Kohno Y. Widening spectrum of congenital hemiplegia: periventricular venous infarction in term neonates. Neurology 2003; 61(4):531–533.

17. Kirton A, deVeber G, Pontigon AM, MacGregor D, Shroff M. Presumed perinatal ischemic stroke: vascular classification predicts outcomes. Ann Neurol 2008; 63(4):436–443.

18. Estan J, Hope P. Unilateral neonatal cerebral infarction in full term infants. Arch Dis Child Fetal Neonatal Ed 1997; 76(2):F88–F93.

19. Wang LW, Huang CC, Yeh TF. Major brain lesions detected on sonographic screening of apparently normal term neonates. Neuroradiology 2004; 46(5):368–373.

20. Schulzke S, Weber P, Luetschg J, Fahnenstich H. Incidence and diagnosis of unilateral arterial cerebral infarction in newborn infants. J Perinat Med 2005; 33(2):170–175.

21. Golomb MR, deVeber GA, MacGregor DL, Domi T, Whyte H, Stephens D et al. Independent walking after neonatal arterial ischemic stroke and sinovenous thrombosis. J Child Neurol 2003; 18(8):530–536.

22. Cowan F, Mercuri E, Groenendaal F, Bassi L, Ricci D, Rutherford M et al. Does cranial ultrasound imaging identify arterial cerebral infarction in term neonates? Arch Dis Child Fetal Neonatal Ed 2005; 90(3):F252–F256.

23. Uvebrant P. Hemiplegic cerebral palsy. Aetiology and outcome. Acta Paediatr Scand Suppl 1988; 345:1–100.

24. Wiklund LM, Uvebrant P, Flodmark O. Computed tomography as an adjunct in etiological analysis of hemiplegic cerebral palsy; II: Children born at term. Neuropediatrics 1991; 22(3):121–128.

25. Gunther G, Junker R, Strater R, Schobess R, Kurnik K, Heller C et al. Symptomatic ischemic stroke in full-term neonates: role of acquired and genetic prothrombotic risk factors. Stroke 2000; 31(10):2437–2441.

26. Lee J, Croen LA, Lindan C, Nash KB, Yoshida CK, Ferriero DM et al. Predictors of outcome in perinatal arterial stroke: a population-based study. Ann Neurol 2005; 58(2):303–308.

27. Laugesaar R, Kolk A, Tomberg T, Metsvaht T, Lintrop M, Varendi H et al. Acutely and retrospectively diagnosed perinatal stroke: a population-based study. Stroke 2007; 38(8):2234–2240.

28. Govaert P, Matthys E, Zecic A, Roelens F, Oostra A, Vanzieleghem B. Perinatal cortical infarction within middle cerebral artery trunks. Arch Dis Child Fetal Neonatal Ed 2000; 82(1):F59–F63.

29. Ment LR, Duncan CC, Ehrenkranz RA. Perinatal cerebral infarction. Ann Neurol 1984; 16(5):559–568.

30. Barmada MA, Moossy J, Shuman RM. Cerebral infarcts with arterial occlusion in neonates. Ann Neurol 1979; 6(6):495–502.

31. Tekgul H, Gauvreau K, Soul J, Murphy L, Robertson R, Stewart J et al. The current etiologic profile and neurodevelopmental outcome of seizures in term newborn infants. Pediatrics 2006; 117(4):1270–1280.

32. Cowan F, Rutherford M, Groenendaal F, Eken P, Mercuri E, Bydder GM et al. Origin and timing of brain lesions in term infants with neonatal encephalopathy. Lancet 2003; 361(9359):736–742.

33. de Vries LS, Groenendaal F, Eken P, van H, I, Rademaker KJ, Meiners LC. Infarcts in the vascular distribution of the middle cerebral artery in preterm and fullterm infants. Neuropediatrics 1997; 28(2):88–96.

34. Mercuri E, Jongmans M, Bouza H, Haataja L, Rutherford M, Henderson S et al. Congenital hemiplegia in children at school age: assessment of hand function in the non-hemiplegic hand and correlation with MRI. Neuropediatrics 1999; 30(1):8–13.

35. Dudink J, Mercuri E, Al-Nakib L, Govaert P, Counsell SJ, Rutherford MA, Cowan FM Evolution of Unilateral Perinatal Arterial Ischemic Stroke on Conventional and Diffusion-Weighted MR Imaging. AJNR Am J Neuroradiol 30:998–1004.

36. Greer IA. Thrombosis in pregnancy: maternal and fetal issues. Lancet 1999; 353(9160):1258–1265.

37. Kraus FT, Acheen VI. Fetal thrombotic vasculopathy in the placenta: cerebral thrombi and infarcts, coagulopathies, and cerebral palsy. Hum Pathol 1999; 30(7):759–769.

38. Viscardi RM, Sun CC. Placental lesion multiplicity: risk factor for IUGR and neonatal cranial ultrasound abnormalities. Early Hum Dev 2001; 62(1):1–10.

39. Andrew M, Paes B, Milner R, Johnston M, Mitchell L, Tollefsen DM et al. Development of the human coagulation system in the full-term infant. Blood 1987; 70(1):165–172.

40. Reverdiau-Moalic P, Delahousse B, Body G, Bardos P, Leroy J, Gruel Y. Evolution of blood coagulation activators and inhibitors in the healthy human fetus. Blood 1996; 88(3):900–906.

41. Parker MJ, Joubert GI, Levin SD. Portal vein thrombosis causing neonatal cerebral infarction. Arch Dis Child Fetal Neonatal Ed 2002; 87(2):F125–F127.

42. Filippi L, Palermo L, Pezzati M, Dani C, Matteini M, De Cristofaro MT et al. Paradoxical embolism in a preterm infant. Dev Med Child Neurol 2004; 46(10):713–716.

43. Beattie LM, Butler SJ, Goudie DE. Pathways of neonatal stroke and subclavian steal syndrome. Arch Dis Child Fetal Neonatal Ed 2006; 91(3):F204–F207.

44. Christensen DD, Vincent RN, Campbell RM. Presentation of atrial septal defect in the pediatric population. Pediatr Cardiol 2005; 26(6):812–814.

45. Weir FJ, Ohlsson A, Myhr TL, Fong K, Ryan ML. A patent ductus arteriosus is associated with reduced middle cerebral artery blood flow velocity. Eur J Pediatr 1999; 158(6):484–487.

46. Cowan F, Thoresen M. Changes in superior sagittal sinus blood velocities due to postural alterations and pressure on the head of the newborn infant. Pediatrics 1985; 75(6):1038–1047.

47. Amit M, Camfield PR. Neonatal polycythemia causing multiple cerebral infarcts. Arch Neurol 1980; 37(2):109–110.

48. McQuillen PS, Hamrick SE, Perez MJ, Barkovich AJ, Glidden DV, Karl TR et al. Balloon atrial septostomy is associated with preoperative stroke in neonates with transposition of the great arteries. Circulation 2006; 113(2):280–285.

49. Denbow ML, Battin MR, Cowan F, Azzopardi D, Edwards AD, Fisk NM. Neonatal cranial ultrasonographic findings in preterm twins complicated by severe fetofetal transfusion syndrome. Am J Obstet Gynecol 1998; 178(3):479–483.

50. Boyce LH, Khandji AG, DeKlerk AM, Nordli DR. Fetomaternal hemorrhage as an etiology of neonatal stroke. Pediatr Neurol 1994; 11(3):255–257.

51. Heier LA, Carpanzano CR, Mast J, Brill PW, Winchester P, Deck MD. Maternal cocaine abuse: the spectrum of radiologic abnormalities in the neonatal CNS. AJNR Am J Neuroradiol 1991; 12(5):951–956.

52. King TA, Perlman JM, Laptook AR, Rollins N, Jackson G, Little B. Neurologic manifestations of in utero cocaine exposure in near-term and term infants. Pediatrics 1995; 96(2 Pt 1):259–264.

53. Mannino FL, Trauner DA. Stroke in neonates. J Pediatr 1983; 102(4):605–610.

54. Govaert P, Vanhaesebrouck P, de Praeter C. Traumatic neonatal intracranial bleeding and stroke. Arch Dis Child 1992; 67(7 Spec No):840–845.

55. Choy CM, Tam WH, Ng PC. Skull fracture and contralateral cerebral infarction after ventouse extraction. BJOG 2001; 108(12):1298–1299.

56. Alfonso I, Prieto G, Vasconcellos E, Aref K, Pacheco E, Yelin K. Internal carotid artery thrombus: an underdiagnosed source of brain emboli in neonates? J Child Neurol 2001; 16(6):446–447.

57. Lequin MH, Peeters EA, Holscher HC, de KR, Govaert P. Arterial infarction caused by carotid artery dissection in the neonate. Eur J Paediatr Neurol 2004; 8(3):155–160.

58. Gilles MT, Blair E, Watson L, Badawi N, Alessandri L, Dawes V et al. Trauma in pregnancy and cerebral palsy: is there a link? Med J Aust 1996; 164(8):500–501.

59. Mercuri E, Cowan F, Rutherford M, Acolet D, Pennock J, Dubowitz L. Ischaemic and haemorrhagic brain lesions in newborns with seizures and normal Apgar scores. Arch Dis Child Fetal Neonatal Ed 1995; 73(2):F67–74.

60. Mercuri E, Cowan F. Cerebral infarction in the newborn infant: review of the literature and personal experience. Eur J Paediatr Neurol 1999; 3(6):255–263.

61. Ricci D, Mercuri E, Barnett A, Rathbone R, Cota F, Haataja L et al. Cognitive outcome at early school age in term-born children with perinatally acquired middle cerebral artery territory infarction. Stroke 2008; 39(2):403–410.

62. Rutherford M, Ramenghi LA, Edwards AD, Brocklehurst P, Halliday H, Levene M, et al. Assessment of brain tissue injury after moderate hypothermia in neonates with hypoxic-ischaemic encephalopathy: a nested substudy of a randomised controlled trial. Lancet Neurol. 2010;9(1):39–45.

63. Ramaswamy V, Miller SP, Barkovich AJ, Partridge JC, Ferriero DM. Perinatal stroke in term infants with neonatal encephalopathy. Neurology 2004; 62(11):2088–2091.

64. Steinbok P, Haw CS, Cochrane DD, Kestle JR. Acute subdural hematoma associated with cerebral infarction in the full-term neonate. Pediatr Neurosurg 1995; 23(4):206–215.

65. Golomb MR, Dick PT, MacGregor DL, Curtis R, Sofronas M, deVeber GA. Neonatal arterial ischemic stroke and cerebral sinovenous thrombosis are more commonly diagnosed in boys. J Child Neurol 2004; 19(7):493–497.

66. Currie AD, Bentley CR, Bloom PA. Retinal haemorrhage and fatal stroke in an infant with fibromuscular dysplasia. Arch Dis Child 2001; 84(3):263–264.

67. Pavlakis SG, Kingsley PB, Bialer MG. Stroke in children: genetic and metabolic issues. J Child Neurol 2000; 15(5):308–315.

68. Cardo E, Campistol J, Caritg J, Ruiz S, Vilaseca MA, Kirkham F et al. Fatal haemorrhagic infarct in an infant with homocystinuria. Dev Med Child Neurol 1999; 41(2):132–135.

69. Prengler M, Sturt N, Krywawych S, Surtees R, Liesner R, Kirkham F. Homozygous thermolabile variant of the methylenetetrahydrofolate reductase gene: a potential risk factor for hyperhomocysteinaemia, CVD, and stroke in childhood. Dev Med Child Neurol 2001; 43(4):220–225.

70. Sperl W, Felber S, Skladal D, Wermuth B. Metabolic stroke in carbamyl phosphate synthetase deficiency. Neuropediatrics 1997; 28(4):229–234.

71. Kjaergaard S, Schwartz M, Skovby F. Congenital disorder of glycosylation type Ia (CDG-Ia): phenotypic spectrum of the R141H/F119L genotype. Arch Dis Child 2001; 85(3):236–239.

72. Vahedi K, Massin P, Guichard JP, Miocque S, Polivka M, Goutieres F et al. Hereditary infantile hemiparesis, retinal arteriolar tortuosity, and leukoencephalopathy. Neurology 2003; 60(1):57–63.

73. Hogeveen M, Blom HJ, Van AM, Boogmans B, van Beynum IM, I, Van De Bur M. Hyperhomocysteinemia as risk factor for ischemic and hemorrhagic stroke in newborn infants. J Pediatr 2002; 141(3):429–431.

74. Thorarensen O, Ryan S, Hunter J, Younkin DP. Factor V Leiden mutation: an unrecognized cause of hemiplegic cerebral palsy, neonatal stroke, and placental thrombosis. Ann Neurol 1997; 42(3):372–375.

75. Mercuri E, Cowan F, Gupte G, Manning R, Laffan M, Rutherford M et al. Prothrombotic disorders and abnormal neurodevelopmental outcome in infants with neonatal cerebral infarction. Pediatrics 2001; 107(6):1400–1404.

76. Lynch JK, Nelson KB, Curry CJ, Grether JK. Cerebrovascular disorders in children with the factor V Leiden mutation. J Child Neurol 2001; 16(10):735–744.

77. Lynch JK, Han CJ, Nee LE, Nelson KB. Prothrombotic factors in children with stroke or porencephaly. Pediatrics 2005; 116(2):447–453.

78. Nelson KB, Dambrosia JM, Grether JK, Phillips TM. Neonatal cytokines and coagulation factors in children with cerebral palsy. Ann Neurol 1998; 44(4):665–675.

79. Brouwer DA, Mulder H, Fokkens B, Ramsewak S, Muskiet FA, Ramdath DD. Cord blood apolipoprotein-E genotype distribution and plasma lipid indices in newborns of different ethnicity. Ann Hum Biol 2000; 27(4):367–375.

80. Mahonty D, Das KC, al-Hussain H, Naglen P. Thrombophilia in ethnic Arabs in Kuwait. Ann Hematol 1996; 73:283–290.

81. Chan DK, Hu G, Tao H, Owens D, Vun CM, Woo J et al. A comparison of polymorphism in the 3′-untranslated region of the prothrombin gene between Chinese and Caucasians in Australia. Br J Haematol 2000; 111(4):1253–1255.

82. Petaja J, Hiltunen L, Fellman V. Increased risk of intraventricular hemorrhage in preterm infants with thrombophilia. Pediatr Res 2001; 49(5):643–646.

83. Miller SP, Wu YW, Lee J, Lammer EJ, Iovannisci DM, Glidden DV et al. Candidate gene polymorphisms do not differ between newborns with stroke and normal controls. Stroke 2006; 37(11):2678–2683.

84. Van der Knaap MS, Smit LM, Barkhof F, Pijnenburg YA, Zweegman S, Niessen HW et al. Neonatal porencephaly and adult stroke related to mutations in collagen IV A1. Ann Neurol 2006; 59(3):504–511.

85. Golomb MR, Garg BP, Walsh LE, Williams LS. Perinatal stroke in baby, prothrombotic gene in mom: does this affect maternal health insurance? Neurology 2005; 65(1):13–16.

86. Guzzetta A, Mercuri E, Rapisardi G, Ferrari F, Roversi MF, Cowan F et al. General movements detect early signs of hemiplegia in term infants with neonatal cerebral infarction. Neuropediatrics 2003; 34(2):61–66.

87. Raine J, Davies H, Gamsu HR. Multiple idiopathic emboli in a full term neonate. Acta Paediatr Scand 1989; 78(4):644–646.

88. Clancy R, Malin S, Laraque D, Baumgart S, Younkin D. Focal motor seizures heralding stroke in full-term neonates. Am J Dis Child 1985; 139(6):601–606.

89. Stillger A, Kumar RK. Neonatal cerebral infarction: USS or CT for imaging? Indian J Pediatr 1999; 66(1):141–143.

90. Krishnamoorthy KS, Soman TB, Takeoka M, Schaefer PW. Diffusion-weighted imaging in neonatal cerebral infarction: clinical utility and follow-up. J Child Neurol 2000; 15(9):592–602.

91. Cowan FM, de Vries LS. The internal capsule in neonatal imaging. Semin Fetal Neonatal Med 2005; 10(5):461–474.

92. de Vries LS, van der Grond J, van Hasteert I, Groenendaal F. Prediction of outcome in new-born infants with arterial ischaemic stroke using diffusion-weighted magnetic resonance imaging. Neuropediatrics 2005; 36(1):12–20.

93. Kirton A, Shroff M, Visvanathan T, deVeber G. Quantified corticospinal tract diffusion restriction predicts neonatal stroke outcome. Stroke. 2007; 38(3):974–980.

94. Cowan FM, Pennock JM, Hanrahan JD, Manji KP, Edwards AD. Early detection of cerebral infarction and hypoxic ischemic encephalopathy in neonates using diffusion-weighted magnetic resonance imaging. Neuropediatrics 1994; 25(4):172–175.

95. Al-Nakib LA, Pennock J, Bydder G, Cowan F. Diffusion weighted (DW). MR imaging in neonatal stroke – timing of lesions, prediction of lesion size. Eur J Paediatr Neurol 1999; 199(29):124–125.

96. Robertson RL, Ben-Sira L, Barnes PD, Mulkern RV, Robson CD, Maier SE et al. MR line-scan diffusion-weighted imaging of term neonates with perinatal brain ischemia. AJNR Am J Neuroradiol 1999; 20(9):1658–1670.

97. Mader I, Schoning M, Klose U, Kuker W. Neonatal cerebral infarction diagnosed by diffusion-weighted MRI: pseudonormalization occurs early. Stroke 2002; 33(4):1142–1145.

98. Kuker W, Mohrle S, Mader I, Schoning M, Nagele T. MRI for the management of neonatal cerebral infarctions: importance of timing. Childs Nerv Syst 2004; 20(10):742–748.

99. Mazumdar A, Mukherjee P, Miller JH, Malde H, McKinstry RC. Diffusion-weighted imaging of acute corticospinal tract injury preceding Wallerian degeneration in the maturing human brain. AJNR Am J Neuroradiol 2003; 24(6):1057–1066.

100. Groenendaal F, Benders MJ, de Vries LS. Pre-Wallerian degeneration in the neonatal brain following perinatal cerebral

hypoxia-ischemia demonstrated with MRI. Semin Perinatol 2006; 30(3):146–150.

101. Schlaug G, Siewert B, Benfield A, Edelman RR, Warach S. Time course of the apparent diffusion coefficient (ADC) abnormality in human stroke. Neurology 1997; 49(1):113–119.

102. van Rooij LG, de Vries LS, Handryastuti S, Hawani D, Groenendaal F, van Huffelen AC et al. Neurodevelopmental outcome in term infants with status epilepticus detected with amplitude-integrated electroencephalography. Pediatrics 2007; 120(2):e354–e363.

103. Rando T, Ricci D, Mercuri E, Frisone MF, Luciano R, Tortorolo G et al. Periodic lateralized epileptiform discharges (PLEDs) as early indicator of stroke in full-term newborns. Neuropediatrics 2000; 31(4):202–205.

104. Perlman JM, Rollins NK, Evans D. Neonatal stroke: clinical characteristics and cerebral blood flow velocity measurements. Pediatr Neurol 1994; 11(4):281–284.

105. Rutherford MA, Pennock JM, Cowan FM, Dubowitz LM, Hajnal JV, Bydder GM. Does the brain regenerate after perinatal infarction? Eur J Paediatr Neurol 1997; 1(1):13–17.

106. Rutherford MA, Pennock JM, Cowan FM, Saeed N, Hajnal JV, Bydder GM. Detection of subtle changes in the brains of infants and children via subvoxel registration and subtraction of serial MR images. AJNR Am J Neuroradiol 1997; 18(5):829–835.

107. Goldman PS, Galkin TW. Prenatal removal of frontal association cortex in the fetal rhesus monkey: anatomical and functional consequences in postnatal life. Brain Res 1978; 152(3):451–485.

108. Fernandez-Bouzas A, Harmony T, Santiago-Rodriguez E, Ricardo-Garcell J, Fernandez T, vila-Acosta D. Schizencephaly with occlusion or absence of middle cerebral artery. Neuroradiology 2006; 48(3):171–175.

109. Bouza H, Dubowitz LM, Rutherford M, Cowan F, Pennock JM. Late magnetic resonance imaging and clinical findings in neonates with unilateral lesions on cranial ultrasound. Dev Med Child Neurol 1994; 36(11):951–964.

110. Le SE, Saeed N, Cowan FM, Edwards AD, Rutherford MA. MR imaging quantification of cerebellar growth following hypoxic-ischemic injury to the neonatal brain. AJNR Am J Neuroradiol 2004; 25(3):463–468.

111. Kurnik K, Kosch A, Strater R, Schobess R, Heller C, Nowak-Gottl U. Recurrent thromboembolism in infants and children suffering from symptomatic neonatal arterial stroke: a prospective follow-up study. Stroke 2003; 34(12):2887–2892.

112. Fullerton HJ, Wu YW, Sidney S, Johnston SC. Risk of recurrent childhood arterial ischemic stroke in a population-based cohort: the importance of cerebrovascular imaging. Pediatrics 2007; 119(3):495–501.

113. Mercuri E, Anker S, Guzzetta A, Barnett A, Haataja L, Rutherford M et al. Neonatal cerebral infarction and visual function at school age. Arch Dis Child Fetal Neonatal Ed 2003; 88(6):F487–F491.

114. Trauner DA, Mannino FL. Neurodevelopmental outcome after neonatal cerebrovascular accident. J Pediatr 1986; 108(3):459–461.

115. Sran SK, Baumann RJ. Outcome of neonatal strokes. Am J Dis Child 1988; 142(10):1086–1088.

116. Allan WC, Riviello JJ Jr. Perinatal cerebrovascular disease in the neonate. Parenchymal ischemic lesions in term and preterm infants. Pediatr Clin North Am 1992; 39(4):621–650.

117. Rollins NK, Morriss MC, Evans D, Perlman JM. The role of early MR in the evaluation of the term infant with seizures. AJNR Am J Neuroradiol 1994; 15(2):239–248.

118. Koelfen W, Freund M, Varnholt V. Neonatal stroke involving the middle cerebral artery in term infants: clinical presentation, EEG and imaging studies, and outcome. Dev Med Child Neurol 1995; 37(3):204–212.

119. Jan MM, Camfield PR. Outcome of neonatal stroke in full-term infants without significant birth asphyxia. Eur J Pediatr 1998; 157(10):846–848.

120. Sreenan C, Bhargava R, Robertson CM. Cerebral infarction in the term newborn: clinical presentation and long-term outcome. J Pediatr 2000; 137(3):351–355.

121. Marret S, Lardennois C, Mercier A, Radi S, Michel C, Vanhulle C et al. Fetal and neonatal cerebral infarcts. Biol Neonate 2001; 79(3–4):236–240.

122. Miller V. Neonatal cerebral infarction. Semin Pediatr Neurol 2000; 7(4):278–288.

123. Mercuri E, Barnett A, Rutherford M, Guzzetta A, Haataja, L, Cioni G, et al. Neonatal cerebral infarction and neuromotor outcome at school age. Pediatrics 2004;113:95–100.

124. Golomb MR, Garg BP, Saha C, Azzouz F, Williams LS. Cerebral palsy after perinatal arterial ischemic stroke. J Child Neurol 2008; 23(3):279–286.

125. Bouza H, Rutherford M, Acolet D, Pennock JM, Dubowitz LM. Evolution of early hemiplegic signs in full-term infants with unilateral brain lesions in the neonatal period: a prospective study. Neuropediatrics 1994; 25(4):201–207.

126. Mercuri E, Rutherford M, Cowan F, Pennock J, Counsell S, Papadimitriou M et al. Early prognostic indicators of outcome in infants with neonatal cerebral infarction: a clinical, electroencephalogram, and magnetic resonance imaging study. Pediatrics 1999; 103(1):39–46.

127. Boardman JP, Ganesan V, Rutherford MA, Saunders DE, Mercuri E, Cowan F. Magnetic resonance image correlates of hemiparesis after neonatal and childhood middle cerebral artery stroke. Pediatrics 2005; 115(2):321–326.

128. Cioni G, Sales B, Paolicelli PB, Petacchi E, Scusa MF, Canapicchi R. MRI and clinical characteristics of children with hemiplegic cerebral palsy. Neuropediatrics 1999; 30(5):249–255.

129. Golomb MR, Garg BP, Williams LS. Outcomes of children with infantile spasms after perinatal stroke. Pediatr Neurol 2006; 34(4):291–295.

130. Golomb MR, Saha C, Garg BP, Azzouz F, Williams LS. Association of cerebral palsy with other disabilities in children with perinatal arterial ischemic stroke. Pediatr Neurol 2007; 37(4):245–249.

131. Squier W, Salisbury H, Sisodiya S. Stroke in the developing brain and intractable epilepsy: effect of timing on hippocampal sclerosis. Dev Med Child Neurol 2003; 45(9):580–585.

132. Golomb MR, Garg BP, Carvalho KS, Johnson CS, Williams LS. Perinatal stroke and the risk of developing childhood epilepsy. J Pediatr 2007; 151(4):409–413.

133. Chilosi AM, Cipriani PP, Bertuccelli B, Pfanner PL, Cioni PG. Early cognitive and communication development in children with focal brain lesions. J Child Neurol 2001; 16(5):309–316.

134. Muter V, Taylor S, Vargha-Khadem F. A longitudinal study of early intellectual development in hemiplegic children. Neuropsychologia 1997; 35(3):289–298.

135. Thal DJ, Marchman V, Stiles J, Aram D, Trauner D, Nass R et al. Early lexical development in children with focal brain injury. Brain Lang 1991; 40(4):491–527.

136. Vicari S, Albertoni A, Chilosi AM, Cipriani P, Cioni G, Bates E. Plasticity and reorganization during language development in children with early brain injury. Cortex 2000; 36(1):31–46.

137. Trauner DA, Ballantyne A, Friedland S, Chase C. Disorders of affective and linguistic prosody in children after early unilateral brain damage. Ann Neurol 1996; 39(3):361–367.

138. Frith U, Vargha-Khadem F. Are there sex differences in the brain basis of literacy related skills? Evidence from reading and spelling impairments after early unilateral brain damage. Neuropsychologia 2001; 39(13):1485–1488.

139. Mercuri E, Atkinson J, Braddick O, Anker S, Nokes L, Cowan F et al. Visual function and perinatal focal cerebral infarction. Arch Dis Child Fetal Neonatal Ed 1996; 75(2):F76–F81.

140. Mercuri E, Spano M, Bruccini F. Visual outcome in childen with congenital hemiplegia: correlation with MRI findings. Neuropediatrics 1996; 27:184–188.

141. Mercuri E, Atkinson J, Braddick O, Anker S, Cowan F, Pennock J et al. The aetiology of delayed visual maturation: short review and personal findings in relation to magnetic resonance imaging. Eur J Paediatr Neurol 1997; 1(1):31–34.

142. Seghier ML, Lazeyras F, Zimine S, Saudan-Frei S, Safran AB, Huppi PS. Visual recovery after perinatal stroke evidenced by functional and diffusion MRI: case report. BMC Neurol 2005; 5:17.

143. Ballantyne AO, Trauner DA. Facial recognition in children after perinatal stroke. Neuropsychiatry Neuropsychol Behav Neurol 1999; 12(2):82–87.

144. Schatz AM, Ballantyne AO, Trauner DA. A hierarchical analysis of block design errors in children with early focal brain damage. Dev Neuropsychol 2000; 17(1):75–83.

145. Stiles J, Trauner D, Engel M, Nass R. The development of drawing in children with congenital focal brain injury: evidence for limited functional recovery. Neuropsychologia 1997; 35(3):299–312.

146. Goodman R. Psychological aspects of hemiplegia. Arch Dis Child 1997; 76(3):177–178.

147. Trauner DA, Nass R, Ballantyne A. Behavioural profiles of children and adolescents after pre- or perinatal unilateral brain damage. Brain 2001; 124(Pt 5):995–1002.

148. Lewine JD, Astur RS, Davis LE, Knight JE, Maclin EL, Orrison WW Jr. Cortical organization in adulthood is modified by neonatal infarct: a case study. Radiology 1994; 190(1):93–96.

149. Villablanca JR, Hovda DA. Developmental neuroplasticity in a model of cerebral hemispherectomy and stroke. Neuroscience 2000; 95(3):625–637.

150. Fair DA, Brown TT, Petersen SE, Schlaggar BL. fMRI reveals novel functional neuroanatomy in a child with perinatal stroke. Neurology 2006; 67(12):2246–2249.

151. Eyre JA, Taylor JP, Villagra F, Smith M, Miller S. Evidence of activity-dependent withdrawal of corticospinal projections during human development. Neurology 2001; 57(9):1543–1554.

152. Yager JY, Armstrong EA, Jaharus C, Saucier DM, Wirrell EC. Preventing hyperthermia decreases brain damage following neonatal hypoxic-ischemic seizures. Brain Res 2004; 1011(1):48–57.

153. Andrew ME, Monagle P, deVeber G, Chan AK. Thromboembolic disease and antithrombotic therapy in newborns. Hematology Am Soc Hematol Educ Program 2001; 358–374.

154. Azzopardi DV, Strohm B, Edwards AD, Dyet L, Halliday HL, Juszczak E, et al; TOBY Study Group. Moderate hypothermia to treat perinatal asphyxial encephalopathy. N Engl J Med. 2009 Oct 1;361(14):1349–58.

155. Taylor DL, Mehmet H, Cady EB, Edwards AD. Improved neuroprotection with hypothermia delayed by 6 hours following cerebral hypoxia-ischemia in the 14-day-old rat. Pediatr Res 2002; 51(1):13–19.

156. Hobbs C, Thoresen M, Tucker A, Aquilina K, Chakkarapani E, Dingley J. Xenon and hypothermia combine additively, offering long-term functional and histopathologic neuroprotection after neonatal hypoxia/ischemia. Stroke 2008; 39(4):1307–1313.

157. Geirsson RT. Birth trauma and brain damage. Baillieres Clin Obstet Gynaecol 1988; 2(1):195–212.

158. Jarjour IT, hdab-Barmada M. Cerebrovascular lesions in infants and children dying after extracorporeal membrane oxygenation. Pediatr Neurol 1994; 10(1):13–19.

159. Krull F, Latta K, Hoyer PF, Ziemer G, Kallfelz HC. Cerebral ultrasonography before and after cardiac surgery in infants. Pediatr Cardiol 1994; 15(4):159–162.

160. Tavani F, Zimmerman RA, Clancy RR, Licht DJ, Mahle WT. Incidental intracranial hemorrhage after uncomplicated birth: MRI before and after neonatal heart surgery. Neuroradiology 2003; 45(4):253–258.

161. McNinch A, Busfield A, Tripp J. Vitamin K deficiency bleeding in Great Britain and Ireland: British Paediatric Surveillance Unit Surveys, 1993–94 and 2001–02. Arch Dis Child 2007; 92(9):759–766.

162. Tarantino MD, Gupta SL, Brusky RM. The incidence and outcome of intracranial haemorrhage in newborns with haemophilia: analysis of the Nationwide Inpatient Sample database. Haemophilia 2007; 13(4):380–382.

163. Hanigan WC, Powell FC, Miller TC, Wright RM. Symptomatic intracranial hemorrhage in full-term infants. Childs Nerv Syst 1995; 11(12):698–707.

164. Armstrong-Wells J, Johnston SC, Wu YW, Sidney S, Fullerton HJ. Prevalence and predictors of perinatal hemorrhagic stroke: results from the Kaiser pediatric stroke study. Pediatrics 2009; 123(3):823–828.

165. Morioka T, Hashiguchi K, Nagata S, Miyagi Y, Mihara F, Hikino S et al. Fetal germinal matrix and intraventricular hemorrhage. Pediatr Neurosurg 2006; 42(6):354–361.

166. Eichler F, Krishnamoorthy K, Grant PE. Magnetic resonance imaging evaluation of possible neonatal sinovenous thrombosis. Pediatr Neurol 2007; 37(5):317–323.

167. Rooks VJ, Eaton JP, Ruess L, Petermann GW, Keck-Wherley J, Pedersen RC. Prevalence and evolution of intracranial hemorrhage in asymptomatic term infants. AJNR Am J Neuroradiol. 2008 Jun;29(6):1082–9.

168. Vergani P, Strobelt N, Locatelli A, Paterlini G, Tagliabue P, Parravicini E et al. Clinical significance of fetal intracranial hemorrhage. Am J Obstet Gynecol 1996; 175(3 Pt 1):536–543.

169. Sohda S, Hamada H, Takanami Y, Kubo T. Prenatal diagnosis of fetal subdural haematomas. Br J Obstet Gynaecol 1996; 103(1):89–90.

170. Jhawar BS, Ranger A, Steven D, Del Maestro RF. Risk factors for intracranial hemorrhage among full-term infants: a case-control study. Neurosurgery 2003; 52(3):581–590.

171. Ucsel R, Savasan S, Coban A, Metin F, Can G. Fatal intracranial hemorrhage in a newborn with factor VII deficiency. Turk J Pediatr 1996; 38(2):257–260.

172. El Kalla S, Menon NS. Neonatal congenital Factor X deficiency. Pediatr Hematol Oncol 1991; 8(4):347–354.

173. Ries M, Wolfel D, Maier-Brandt B. Severe intracranial hemorrhage in a newborn infant with transplacental transfer of an acquired factor VII:C inhibitor. J Pediatr 1995; 127(4):649–650.

174. Thorp JA, Gaston L, Caspers DR, Pal ML. Current concepts and controversies in the use of vitamin K. Drugs 1995; 49(3):376–387.

175. Clark FI, James EJ. Twenty-seven years of experience with oral vitamin K1 therapy in neonates. J Pediatr 1995; 127(2):301–304.

176. Clarke P, Mitchell SJ, Wynn R, Sundaram S, Speed V, Gardener E et al. Vitamin K prophylaxis for preterm infants: a randomized, controlled trial of 3 regimens. Pediatrics 2006; 118(6):e1657–e1666.

177. van Hasselt PM, de Koning TJ, Kvist N, de VE, Lundin CR, Berger R et al. Prevention of vitamin K deficiency bleeding in breastfed infants: lessons from the Dutch and Danish biliary atresia registries. Pediatrics 2008; 121(4):e857–e863.

178. Ozand PT, Rashed M, Gascon GG, Youssef NG, Harfi H, Rahbeeni Z et al. Unusual presentations of propionic acidemia. Brain Dev 1994; 16 (Suppl):46–57.

179. Candito M, Richelme C, Parvy P, Dageville C, Appert A, Bekri S et al. Abnormal alpha-aminoadipic acid excretion in a newborn with a defect in platelet aggregation and antenatal cerebral haemorrhage. J Inherit Metab Dis 1995; 18(1):56–60.

180. Suri V, Aggarwal N, Saxena S, Malhotra P, Varma S. Maternal and perinatal outcome in idiopathic thrombocytopenic purpura (ITP) with pregnancy. Acta Obstet Gynecol Scand 2006; 85(12):1430–1435.

181. Cohn RD, Eklund E, Bergner AL, Casella JF, Woods SL, Althaus J et al. Intracranial hemorrhage as the initial manifestation of a congenital disorder of glycosylation. Pediatrics 2006; 118(2):e514–e521.

182. Grayck EN, Meliones JN, Kern FH, Hansell DR, Ungerleider RM, Greeley WJ. Elevated serum lactate correlates with intracranial hemorrhage in neonates treated with extracorporeal life support. Pediatrics 1995; 96(5 Pt 1):914–917.

183. la Cruz TV, Stewart DL, Winston SJ, Weatherman KS, Phelps JL, Mendoza JC. Risk factors for intracranial hemorrhage in the extracorporeal membrane oxygenation patient. J Perinatol 1997; 17(1):18–23.

184. Young RS, Liberthson RR, Zalneraitis EL. Cerebral hemorrhage in neonates with coarctation of the aorta. Stroke 1982; 13(4):491–494.

185. Singer LT, Yamashita TS, Hawkins S, Cairns D, Baley J, Kliegman R. Increased incidence of intraventricular hemorrhage and developmental delay in cocaine-exposed, very low birth weight infants. J Pediatr 1994; 124(5 Pt 1):765–771.

186. Holzman C, Paneth N, Little R, Pinto-Martin J. Perinatal brain injury in premature infants born to mothers using alcohol in pregnancy. Neonatal Brain Hemorrhage Study Team. Pediatrics 1995; 95(1):66–73.

187. Karlowicz MG, White LE. Severe intracranial hemorrhage in a term neonate associated with maternal acetylsalicylic acid ingestion. Clin Pediatr (Phila)1993; 32(12):740–743.

188. Spinillo A, Ometto A, Stronati M, Piazzi G, Iasci A, Rondini G. Epidemiologic association between maternal smoking during pregnancy and intracranial hemorrhage in preterm infants. J Pediatr 1995; 127(3):472–478.

189. Hamada H, Kuwayama N, Hirashima Y, Hayashi N, Endo S, Takaku A. Intracranial hemorrhage associated with congenital

organic disease in neonates. Report of two cases and review of literature. Childs Nerv Syst 2001; 17(7):423–426.

190. Buis DR, van Ouwerkerk WJ, Takahata H, Vandertop WP. Intracranial aneurysms in children under 1 year of age: a systematic review of the literature. Childs Nerv Syst 2006; 22(11):1395–1409.

191. Rodesch G, Malherbe V, Alvarez H, Zerah M, Devictor D, Lasjaunias P. Nongalenic cerebral arteriovenous malformations in neonates and infants. Review of 26 consecutive cases (1982–1992). Childs Nerv Syst 1995; 11(4):231–241.

192. Ozek E, Ozek M, Bilgen H, Kilic T, Pamir N. Neonatal intracranial hemorrhage due to rupture of arteriovenous malformation. Pediatr Neurol 1996; 15(1):53–56.

193. de Campo M. Neonatal posterior fossa haemorrhage: a difficult ultrasound diagnosis. Australas Radiol 1989; 33(2):150–153.

194. Gama CH, Fenichel GM. Epidural hematoma of the newborn due to birth trauma. Pediatr Neurol 1985; 1(1):52–53.

195. Lam A, Cruz GB, Johnson I. Extradural hematoma in neonates. J Ultrasound Med 1991; 10(4):205–209.

196. Whitby EH, Griffiths PD, Rutter S, Smith MF, Sprigg A, Ohadike P et al. Frequency and natural history of subdural haemorrhages in babies and relation to obstetric factors. Lancet 2004; 363(9412):846–851.

197. Rooks VJ, Eaton JP, Ruess L, Petermann GW, Keck-Wherley J, Pedersen RC. Prevalence and evolution of intracranial hemorrhage in asymptomatic term infants. AJNR Am J Neuroradiol. 2008;29(6):1082–9.

198. Cardozo LD, Gibb DM, Studd JW, Cooper DJ. Should we abandon Kielland's forceps? Br Med J (Clin Res Ed) 1983; 287(6388):315–317.

199. Castillo M, Fordham LA. MR of neurologically symptomatic newborns after vacuum extraction delivery. AJNR Am J Neuroradiol 1995; 16(4 Suppl):816–818.

200. Towner D, Castro MA, Eby-Wilkens E, Gilbert WM. Effect of mode of delivery in nulliparous women on neonatal intracranial injury. N Engl J Med 1999; 341(23):1709–1714.

201. Byard RW, Blumbergs P, Rutty G, Sperhake J, Banner J, Krous HF. Lack of evidence for a causal relationship between hypo-xicischemic encephalopathy and subdural hemorrhage in fetal life, infancy, and early childhood. Pediatr Dev Pathol 2007; 10(5):348–350.

202. Cheung PY, Obaid L, Rajani H. Spontaneous subdural haemorrhage in newborn babies. Lancet 2004; 363(9425):2001–2002.

203. Wigglesworth JS, Husemeyer RP. Intracranial birth trauma in vaginal breech delivery: the continued importance of injury to the occipital bone. Br J Obstet Gynaecol 1977; 84(9):684–691.

204. Hanigan WC, Olivero WC, Miller TC. Traumatic neonatal intracranial bleeding and stroke. Arch Dis Child 1993; 68(3 Spec No):339–340.

205. Macdonald RL, Hoffman HJ, Kestle JR, Rutka JT, Weinstein G. Needle aspiration of acute subdural hematomas in infancy. Pediatr Neurosurg 1994; 20(1):73–76.

206. Takagi T, Fukuoka H, Wakabayashi S, Nagai H, Shibata T. Posterior fossa subdural hemorrhage in the newborn as a result of birth trauma. Childs Brain 1982; 9(2):102–113.

207. Romodanov AP, Brodsky Y. Subdural hematomas in the newborn. Surgical treatment and results. Surg Neurol 1987; 28(4):253–258.

208. Brouwer AJ, Groenendaal F, Koopman C, Nievelstein RJ, Han SK, de Vries LS. Intracranial hemorrhage in full-term newborns: a hospital-based cohort study. Neuroradiology. 2010 Jun;52(6):567–76.

209. Duhaime AC, Durham S. Traumatic brain injury in infants: the phenomenon of subdural hemorrhage with hemispheric hypodensity ("Big Black Brain"). Prog Brain Res 2007; 161:293–302.

210. Avrahami E, Amzel S, Katz R, Frishman E, Osviatzov I. CT demonstration of intracranial bleeding in term newborns with mild clinical symptoms. Clin Radiol 1996; 51(1):31–34.

211. Bergman I, Bauer RE, Barmada MA, Latchaw RE, Taylor HG, David R et al. Intracerebral hemorrhage in the full-term neonatal infant. Pediatrics 1985; 75(3):488–496.

212. Piatt JH Jr, Clunie DA. Intracranial arterial aneurysm due to birth trauma. Case report. J Neurosurg 1992; 77(5):799–803.

213. Roessmann U, Miller RT. Thrombosis of the middle cerebral artery associated with birth trauma. Neurology 1980; 30(8):889–892.

214. Roland EH, Flodmark O, Hill A. Thalamic hemorrhage with intraventricular hemorrhage in the full-term newborn. Pediatrics 1990; 85(5):737–742.

215. Puig J, Pedraza S, Mendez J, Trujillo A. [Neonatal cerebral venous thrombosis: diagnosis by magnetic resonance angiography.] Radiologia 2006; 48(3):169–171.

216. Merrill JD, Piecuch RE, Fell SC, Barkovich AJ, Goldstein RB. A new pattern of cerebellar hemorrhages in preterm infants. Pediatrics 1998; 102(6):E62.

217. Miall LS, Cornette LG, Tanner SF, Arthur RJ, Levene MI. Posterior fossa abnormalities seen on magnetic resonance brain imaging in a cohort of newborn infants. J Perinatol 2003; 23(5):396–403.

218. Limperopoulos C, Benson CB, Bassan H, DiSalvo DN, Kinnamon DD, Moore M et al. Cerebellar hemorrhage in the preterm infant: ultrasonographic findings and risk factors. Pediatrics 2005; 116(3):717–724.

219. Limperopoulos C, Bassan H, Gauvreau K, Robertson RL, Jr., Sullivan NR, Benson CB et al. Does cerebellar injury in premature infants contribute to the high prevalence of long-term cognitive, learning, and behavioral disability in survivors? Pediatrics 2007; 120(3):584–593.

220. Rijhsinghani A, Belsare TJ. Neonatal intracerebellar hemorrhage after forceps delivery. Report of a case without neurologic damage. J Reprod Med 1997; 42(2):127–130.

221. Perrin RG, Rutka JT, Drake JM, Meltzer H, Hellman J, Jay V et al. Management and outcomes of posterior fossa subdural hematomas in neonates. Neurosurgery 1997; 40(6):1190–1199; discussion 1199–1200.

222. Van De Bor M, Ens-Dokkum M, Schreuder AM, Veen S, Brand R, Verloove-Vanhorick SP. Outcome of periventricular-intraventricular haemorrhage at five years of age. Dev Med Child Neurol 1993; 35(1):33–41.

223. Wells JT, Ment LR. Prevention of intraventricular hemorrhage in preterm infants. Early Hum Dev 1995; 42(3):209–233.

224. Osborn DA, Evans N, Kluckow M. Hemodynamic and antecedent risk factors of early and late periventricular/intraventricular hemorrhage in premature infants. Pediatrics 2003; 112(1 Pt 1):33–39.

225. Paneth N, Pinto-Martin J, Gardiner J, Wallenstein S, Katsikiotis V, Hegyi T et al. Incidence and timing of germinal matrix/intraventricular hemorrhage in low birth weight infants. Am J Epidemiol 1993; 137(11):1167–1176.

226. Garland JS, Buck R, Leviton A. Effect of maternal glucocorticoid exposure on risk of severe intraventricular hemorrhage in surfactant-treated preterm infants. J Pediatr 1995; 126(2):272–279.

227. Mercer BM, Arheart KL. Antimicrobial therapy in expectant management of preterm premature rupture of the membranes. Lancet 1995; 346(8985):1271–1279.

228. Fowlie PW. Prophylactic indomethacin: systematic review and meta-analysis. Arch Dis Child Fetal Neonatal Ed 1996; 74(2):F81–F87.

229. Malloy MH, Cutter GR. The association of heparin exposure with intraventricular hemorrhage among very low birth weight infants. J Perinatol 1995; 15(3):185–191.

230. Ment LR, Oh W, Ehrenkranz RA, Philip AG, Duncan CC, Makuch RW. Antenatal steroids, delivery mode, and intraventricular hemorrhage in preterm infants. Am J Obstet Gynecol 1995; 172(3):795–800.

231. Hayden CK Jr, Shattuck KE, Richardson CJ, Ahrendt DK, House R, Swischuk LE. Subependymal germinal matrix hemorrhage in full-term neonates. Pediatrics 1985; 75(4):714–718.

232. Dyet LE, Kennea N, Counsell SJ, Maalouf EF, jayi-Obe M, Duggan PJ et al. Natural history of brain lesions in extremely preterm infants studied with serial magnetic resonance imaging from birth and neurodevelopmental assessment. Pediatrics 2006; 118(2):536–548.

233. Jhawar BS, Ranger A, Steven DA, Del Maestro RF. A follow-up study of infants with intracranial hemorrhage at full-term. Can J Neurol Sci 2005; 32(3):332–339.

10
VEIN OF GALEN ANEURYSMAL MALFORMATION

Chao Bao Luo, Marina Sachet Ferreira, Hortensia Alvarez, Georges Rodesch, Pierre L. Lasjaunias and Stefan K. Brew

Introduction

The first description of a possible vein of Galen aneurysmal malformation (VGAM) in 1895 was a cerebral arteriovenous malformation of the diencephalon draining into a dilated vein of Galen (Steinhel cited by Dandy).[1] In 1946 Jeager reported bilateral arteriovenous communications draining into an aneurysmally dilated vein of Galen,[2] and Boldrey treated two similar patients with arterial ligation.[3] Authors have subsequently used the same generic name of 'vein of Galen arteriovenous malformation' for very different entities. Subsequent surgical[4-6] and endovascular[7-9] series attempted to deal with this rare, and still poorly understood, disease entity and its natural history, often emphasizing the technical challenge related to the treatment. In the British Paediatric Surveillance Unit study,[10] the incidence for vein of Galen malformation was 0.11 per 100 000.

The link between the lesion and cardiac failure in neonates was noted by Pollock and Laslett in 1958.[11] Since that time the relationship between intracranial arteriovenous lesions, and, for instance, hydrodynamic disorders with ventricular enlargement, facial venous collateral circulation in infants and epistaxis has been accepted. Gold et al[12] reviewed 34 cases and described three consecutive clinical stages: (1) neonates with cardiac insufficiency; (2) infants and young children with hydrocephalus and convulsions; and (3) older children or adults with headaches[13] and subarachnoid haemorrhage.[14] Johnston[15] analysed in an exhaustive fashion the clinical presentations of VGAM. In 82 infants he found the following percentages of symptoms: cerebrospinal fluid disorders (70%), neurological deficits (31%) and neurocognitive delay (12%). In children between 1 and 5 years of age these symptoms occurred in 61%, 33% and 5%. For comparison in our series of the same age group, more than 50% had neurocognitive delay and almost none had neurological manifestations unless they had been previously shunted. This apparent discrepancy in the clinical profile of our material emphasizes the variability in the way symptoms have been documented by various specialists.

Morphology of the vein of Galen aneurysmal malformation

Padget[16] first explicitly dealt with the embryology of this condition, a fact that has seldom been acknowledged by the few of those who have written subsequent accounts. She explicitly refers to the possibility of an early embryonic arteriovenous shunt developing in the telea choroidea of the third ventricle, and speculates as to its consequences. Charles and his colleagues explicitly stated that the ectatic vein in VGAM was the embryonic precursor of the median vein of the prosencephalon, and not the vein of Galen itself.[2] We appreciated the dural sinus abnormalities[17] and persistent alternative embryonic routes of the deep venous drainage in this condition.[18] From then on the VGAM was recognized as the first embryonic vascular malformation. It is an arteriovenous malformation. The potential for antenatal diagnosis of the VGAM has already been documented using non-invasive tools such as ultrasound including colour flow Doppler and magnetic resonance imaging (MRI). It is puzzling that it has never been demonstrated on a 20-week antenatal ultrasound scan, when the embryology suggests it must be present at this stage.

The arterial supply is usually by all choroidal arteries including subfornical and anterior choroidal contributions[19] (Fig. 10.1); it may also receive a significant contribution from the subependymal network originating from the posterior circle of Willis through the thalamus. In fact, subependymal contributions can sometimes be used for the purpose of an endovascular approach, but most of the time they will disappear following the proper occlusion of the most prominent shunts. Finally, the limbic arterial arch, which bridges the cortical branch of

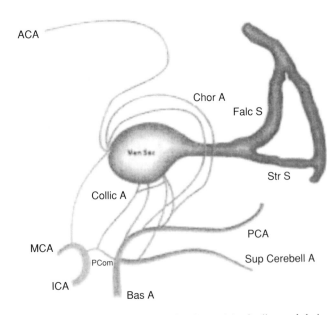

Fig. 10.1. Anatomy of the vein of Galen and its feeding and draining vessels. ACA, anterior cerebral artery; Bas A, basilar artery; Chor A, choroidal artery; Collic A, collicular artery; Falc S, falcine sinus; ICA, internal carotid artery; MCA, middle cerebral artery; PCA, posterior cerebral artery; PCom, posterior communicating artery; Sup Cerebell A, superior cerebellar artery; Str S, straight sinus.

the posterior cerebral artery with the pericallosal artery, is often seen.

Grossly two types of angioarchitecture are encountered: choroidal and mural. The former corresponds to a very primitive disposition, with the contribution of all the choroidal arteries and an interposed network before opening into the large venous pouch. The latter corresponds to direct arteriovenous fistulae within the wall of the median vein of the prosencephalon. In reality, there is a spectrum ranging from a single arteriovenous shunt to innumerable arterial feeders from every conceivable course.

The venous drainage by definition is towards the dilated median vein of the prosencephalon and usually no communication exists with the deep venous system of the brain (Fig. 10.1), although there are reports of thalamic haemorrhage after embolization, and we have seen at least two cases where thalamic veins were retrogradely catheterized off the sac. Thalamostriate veins will open into the posterior and inferior thalamic (diencephalic) veins as occurs normally during the 3rd month in utero. They secondarily join either the anterior confluence or more often a subtemporal vein demonstrating a typical epsilon shape on the lateral angiogram. The remainder of the venous drainage is variable, with the straight sinus being absent in almost all cases. Falcine dural channels drain the pouch towards the posterior third of the superior sagittal sinus. There is presently no convincing evidence to suggest a hereditary or genetic influence on the development of VGAM.

Natural history of the vein of Galen aneurysmal malformations

Cardiac Manifestations

Congestive cardiac failure (CCF) is usually present during the neonatal period in VGAM. What is the prognosis of an antenatally diagnosed VGAM? Currently around one-fifth of the babies will have evidence of cerebral damage at birth and often die; the remainder (and more controversially those who survive despite severe problems at birth) should undergo embolization at various times depending on their individual response to medical treatment, and their late neurological outcome is excellent at 2–6 years follow up. Therapeutic interruption of the pregnancy should only be discussed in cases where there is evidence of in utero parenchymal damage to the brain. While in utero heart failure probably indicates a relatively poor prognosis, this is not yet clear, though work is currently being conducted to try and find predictors of outcome in utero, perhaps even enabling in utero intervention to be offered to those with poor prognosis. Macrocrania in utero is not a negative prognostic sign in our experience.

After a brief period of stabilization most CCF will worsen during the first three days of life, and then stabilize again and improve with appropriate medical management. In only two of the babies referred to us (Bicêtre and Great Ormond Street) with the diagnosis of VGAM did the cardiac failure developed de novo after the 2nd week of life. However, it can decompensate at 3 weeks or recur later following lung infec-

tions or other concurrent disease. The degree of failure is variable from one child to the other. We have no reliable predictors of severity of heart failure, as yet. Renal and hepatic damage may further aggravate the CCF and their function can be transiently impaired (oliguria, increase of enzymes) or become rapidly unstable despite intensive medical care.

After the diagnosis of VGAM is suspected by clinical examination, a pre-therapeutic evaluation should be obtained and include the following information: (1) clinical evaluation of the infant as well as the documentation of all the possible events that occurred since birth (convulsions, for example, do not occur in VGAM at that age unless brain damage has already taken place); (2) evaluation of the renal and liver function; (3) head ultrasound (Fig. 10.2a) or computed tomography (CT) (Fig. 10.2b) for diagnosis and to initially evaluate for possible encephalomalacia; (4) cardiac ultrasound to assess the cardiac tolerance and to diagnose any associated cardiac malformation that might require specific treatment; (5) good-quality MRI (Fig. 10.3)

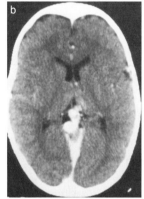
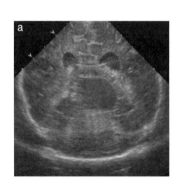

Fig. 10.2. Initial imaging. (a) Head ultrasound of an infant in heart failure showing dilated lateral ventricles and a midline abnormality consistent with a vein of Galen malformation. (b) CT scan of an 8-year-old boy with proptosis and prominent cranial veins showing contrast enhancement of a vein of Galen malformation.

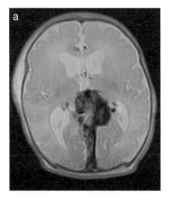
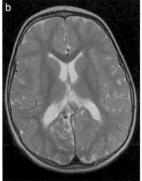

Fig. 10.3. (a,b) Magnetic resonance images before and after embolization in an infant in whom the diagnosis of vein of Galen aneurysmal malformation was made antenatally and confirmed on head ultrasound at birth (Fig. 10.2a). He was very sick with renal and hepatic failure as well as heart failure requiring maximal inotropes but his brain was normal on imaging and his parents wanted treatment. After embolization his heart failure and systemic complications improved and at the age of 6 years he is neurologically intact.

to provide all the necessary morphological information regarding the lesion (the diagnosis of a pial arteriovenous malformation (AVM) at that age would have completely different therapeutic consequences) and the status of myelination; and (6) Electroencephalography, ideally once the baby is in an intensive care unit, intubated and sedated. Angiography in the neonatal workup is not indicated and not recommended. Only when an embolization is contemplated will the angiographic procedure be performed at the same time.

The Bicêtre group led by Lasjauniais, the pioneers in this field, designed a specific neonatal score[20] (Table 10.1) which documents the significant non-neurological manifestations in that age group in addition to assessing the gross neurological status. A score of less than 8/21 resulted in a decision not to treat; a score between 8/21 and 12/21 entailed emergency endovascular intervention; while a score of over 12/21 led to the decision to manage with medical treatment until the child was at least 5 months of age providing there was no failure to thrive. At that time a decision was made to proceed with endovascular treatment no matter what the symptoms. The scoring system was a useful prognostic tool in the series from the Hospital for Sick Children, Toronto.[21] However, at Great

Ormand Street Hospital, after several early experiences of treating children too sick to treat by the Bicêtre criteria (<8) with excellent outcomes, we have abandoned rigid criteria in the decision-making process of whom to offer treatment We now use a multi-disciplicary approach akin to that in other life-threatening paediatric conditions, and will generally offer treatment to any child without evidence of diffuse parenchymal damage. Paediatric follow-up criteria include monthly head circumference, infant's weight and MRI at 3-month intervals. Obviously, alteration in any of these parameters will prompt endovascular management. A decrease in the head circumference is probably the most ominous finding to be noted since it indicates the loss of brain substance and early suture fusion.

MACROCRANIA AND HYDROCEPHALUS

The next phase in the evolution of the disorder is marked by the hydrovenous disorders (Figs 10.4 and 10.5). As opposed to CCF, hydrodynamic disorders can manifest themselves in fetuses, neonates and infants. They constitute the primary revealing factor in infancy when the diagnosis has not been made previously. They result from the abnormal haemodynamic conditions present in the torcular venous sinus confluence,

TABLE 10.1
Bicêtre neonatal score

Points	Cardiac	Cerebral	Respiratory	Renal	Hepatic
5	Normal	Normal	Normal	–	–
4	Overload, no treatment	EEG abnormal, Nll clinical signs	Tachypnoea, Finishes bottle	–	–
3	Failure, stable with drugs	Isolated neurological signs	Tachypnoea, Cannot drink	Normal	Normal
2	Failure, not stable	Single seizure	Ventilated, FiO$_2$<25%	Transient anuria	Hepatomegaly
1	Ventilation necessary	Seizures	Ventilated, FiO$_2$>25%	Unstable	Hepatic failure
0	Resistant to therapy	Permanent neurological signs	Ventilated, Desaturated	Anuric	Coagulopathy

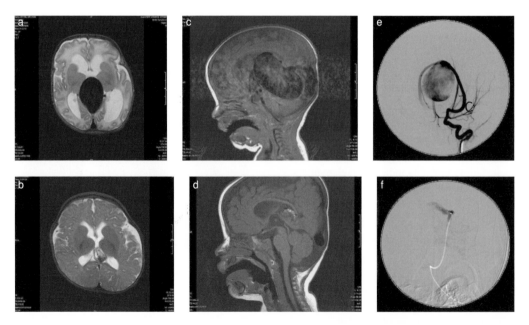

Fig. 10.4. Axial MR images (a,b), sagittal MR images (c,d) and arteriograms (e,f) before and after embolization in an infant born at 30 weeks' gestation with vein of Galen malformation in whom the diagnosis was made on antenatal ultrasound. Although his heart failure was mild, his head circumference increased from the 50th to the 98th centile between birth and 4 weeks of age and he was referred for embolization at 5 weeks. After embolization, his head circumference stabilized and he has made good developmental progress.

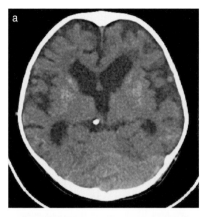

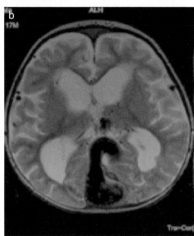

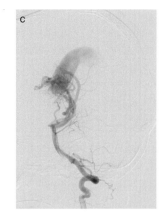

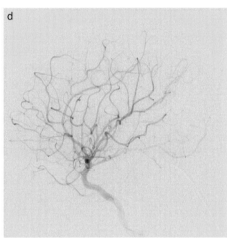

Fig. 10.5. CT (a) and MRI (b) from a 17-month-old infant with VGAM who was irritable with macrocephaly, developmental regression and 'blank spells'. On examination, she was pale and floppy, lying immobile in bed, severely delayed and with poor eye contact. There was a dilemma as to whether to offer embolization because of the child's clinical state and imaging appearances, but parents were adamant treatment should be offered and it was eventually agreed. After four procedures (arteriograms: c,d) the malformation was cured (d). Six months after presentation the child's head growth had normalized and she was alert with an acceleration in development so that she was approximately 6 months behind.

the posterior convergence of the venous drainage of the brain and the immaturity of the granulation system. If the sutures quickly stop growing or if the medullary vein resorption decreases (or the pial vein pressure increases), or if for any other unknown reason the compliance of the venous system fails, the patient will develop hydrocephalus and intracranial hypertension. Spontaneous stabilization of the enlarging head can occur with the cavernous sinus capture of the sylvian veins. A new low-pressure venous system will offer an alternate pathway for water resorption, and therefore improves the subsequent cerebral venous congestion. Evolution from macrocrania to hydrocephalus is therefore not inevitable. Although not clear-cut, we increasingly suspect stenosis of the jugular bulbs to be a common precipitant of this pathway of evolution.

Ventricular shunting in VGAM carries high morbidity. Johnston,[15] in a literature review, noted that of 11 shunted infants, 7/11 died and only 1/11 had no deficit. In an additional group of 6 shunted children, only 2/6 had 'no deficit'. In Zerah's[22] series, only 1/17 infants had an uneventful shunting procedure. The others had enlargement of the VGAM (7/16), persistent seizures (3/16), subdural haematomas (6/16), mechanical problems (3/16) or slit ventricles (1/16), although there was no mortality. The deficits, seizures or haemorrhages seen following ventricular shunting have been so well accepted that they have even been considered as part of the natural history of the VGAM. Endovascular management in similar situations today has shown that, even with a partial treatment of the arteriovenous

shunt, these secondary symptoms do not occur unless additional factors intervene to change the angioarchitecture of the lesion.

Development delay is part of the natural history of untreated VGAMs. Careful evaluation of neurocognitive performances shows that most macrocranic children present with some degree of learning disability. In view of the poor prognosis of the disease, specialists and parents tend to accept as normal a child with a mild learning disability (<20% of the chronological age). To measure the neurocognitive dimension during follow up, we recommend the Denver[23] and Brunet-Lezine tests, which are easy to administer and reproducible.

LONG-TERM EVOLUTION OF VEIN OF GALEN ANEURYSMAL MALFORMATION WITH PATENT SINUSES
Seizures and learning disability will be the main symptoms seen if the correction of the arteriovenous shunt was not done in time. They often occur in children referred late in the evolution of their disease or after ventricular shunting. Therefore, convulsions are not a necessary phase through which all children with VGAM will pass, but rather indicate a failure in the timing of treatment. They often reflect increased intracranial venous pressure due to an imbalance between the high flow of the arteriovenous shunt, and limited pathways of outflow (jugular bulb stenoses for instance).

Calcifications are usually bilateral and symmetrically located preferentially in the frontal region. They can be asymmetrically located mostly in unilaterally shunted children and often on the side opposite of the shunt. Focal evidence of iatrogenic haemorrhage or acute hydrocephalus is infrequent, and their occurrence should further diminish with the increased use of early endovascular management of macrocrania. Cerebral angiography may provide crucial information as it demonstrates that in the absence of pial reflux and in the absence of late venous thrombosis, haemorrhage will not occur. It is important to realize the comparatively good clinical outcome of children with patent sinuses compared with those with secondarily occluded sinuses. At Great Ormand Street Hospital we now consider stenting stenotic sinuses to relieve venous hypertension, if there is no alternative. We have seen good clinical outcomes in patients even in the presence of parenchymal calcification, which may even be reversible.[24]

Dural sinus occlusion and supratentorial pial congestion and reflux
The cause of the occlusion is unknown. In the presence of moderate jugular bulb stenosis and capture of the cerebral veins by the cavernous sinus outlets, macrocrania and developmental delay may be stabilized, as long as the stenosis does not progress further. This evolution will facilitate collateralization of the facial veins in infants; they are not present in the neonatal period as the redistribution and capture of veins has not occurred yet. Under these circumstances, the VGAM and the prominent facial veins are good indicators of relief of cerebral venous hypertension. Epistaxis related to nasal vein congestion can occur, indicating increased flow through the ophthalmic vein. The long-term result is likely to be chronic venous ischaemia with delayed calcifications and a peculiar appearance of the cortical veins. Conversely, if the superior to inferior petrosal sinus collateral patency is inadequate, a longer collateral circuit for the VGAM drainage will be necessary. Pial venous reflux is then demonstrated, the macrocrania may progress to hydrocephalus and acute focal damage may occur: seizures, deficit and haemorrhage.

If the stenosis is complete and bilateral, even if it has been present for a few years, its clinical tolerance is exclusively dependent on the capacity of the alternative outlets to drain the VGAM and the brain. These pathways always exist in infancy or early childhood; otherwise the condition would be rapidly fatal as it is often but not always the case in neonatal dural sinus malformations, although even in this condition with a formerly grave prognosis we have seen neonates cured by embolization. The risk of haemorrhage and venous infarction is high when there is significant pial reflux and the VGAM has become an AVM draining into the pial venous system.

Failure to thrive, proptosis, bone hypertrophy, learning disability, cerebral calcifications and some psychiatric syndromes can be noted in older children or young adults, who may present with haemorrhage (Fig. 10.6) as well as symptoms of ischaemia. Once the optimal therapeutic window has been missed, these symptoms are less likely to be reversed even if the lesion is obliterated.

Dural sinus occlusion and infratentorial pial reflux
The infratentorial consequence of the sinus occlusion is the tonsilar prolapse phenomenon, which is secondary to the pial congestion and only appears in its presence. It subsequently disappears with correction of the arteriovenous shunt provided that the prolapse has not existed for a long time. It does not create any specific symptoms at that age.

SPONTANEOUS THROMBOSIS
Spontaneous thrombosis of the VGAM, although often referred to by those who oppose interventional treatment, is in fact rare.[25,26] In our series, 5 out of 120 patients (4%) developed spontaneous thrombosis, but only 2 are neurologically normal, i.e. a lower proportion than those treated actively. In cases in which angiography was available, mural forms were demonstrated, easily curable by embolization. Spontaneous thrombosis should not be considered as a favourable outcome, and waiting for it does not represent a therapeutic strategy and constitutes today an unacceptable choice.

Objectives and methods of treatment

GENERAL REMARKS
Our aim is to preserve a child who will develop normally without neurological deficit. To achieve this normal cerebral

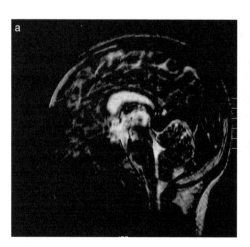
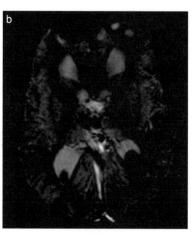

Fig. 10.6. Sagittal (a) and axial (b) MR images from an adult with VGAM presenting with haemorrhage.

development does not require a rapid morphological disappearance of the arteriovenous shunt or a rapid shrinkage of the ectasia. To reach these objectives we have chosen transarterial embolization using the femoral approach with glue (Histocryl) as the embolic agent (Figs 10.4 and 10.5). This method has proven to offer reliable and predictable results.

Our choice has been not to use coils, balloons or particles because they are, in our opinion, inappropriate materials for the treatment of these lesions, as they produce proximal occlusion preventing access for definitive embolization, without reliably reducing the arteriovenous shunt. We will not comment on the transvenous approach other than to say that it may be effective, and may be the only option in some instances.

Neonates

We do not perform an embolization on a neonate with diffuse parenchymal damage. Patients with severe cerebral damage or severe multiorgan failure (score <8), where embolization would only be a technical challenge with little hope of good outcome, represent 10% of our referral in VGAM. Mortality rate is high. It is self-evident that the very sick children with low scores will tend to have worse outcomes, but at Great Ormand Street Hospital we will offer treatment to even very sick children provided there is no evidence of diffuse parenchymal damage. We have seen cure, and normal children, even in these circumstances.

In neonates the immediate goal is to restore a satisfactory systemic physiology and to gain time. Failure to observe a response to the intensive care unit management will lead to early embolization in the neonatal period. The end point of partial embolization is usually the reduction of one-third of the shunt in order to obtain a significant change. Lack of response to drugs must lead to a careful search for an associated cardiac malformation or a patent ductus arteriosus with a large shunt. The aim of symptomatic therapy is to improve oxygen delivery to the tissues and decrease tissue oxygen consumption. If cardiac failure cannot be controlled by these measures, embolization of the arteriovenous shunt should be considered. We are beginning to quantify shunt reduction, in the hope of identifying predictors of how aggressive embolization needs to be to relieve heart failure. Pulmonary arterial hypertension seems to be a common finding in those with persistent heart failure.

Infants and Children

Our concern at this age is to anticipate the natural history to avoid ventricular shunting.[15] Premature attempts to exclude an asymptomatic lesion or taking significant technical risks to exclude in one session a VGAM that presents no immediate risks and can be eradicated in two or three sessions, should not be promoted. Conversely, to decide not to treat on the assumption that an asymptomatic lesion is a well tolerated lesion is certainly naive and dangerous. Paediatric neurologists will provide all the necessary information on the progression of the child and the need to improve the capacity for normal development. Although the volume of the ectatic vein does not seem

to be mechanically responsible for brainstem compression, shrinkage of the pouch is always a welcome reward for an efficient transarterial embolization.

Technical management

General Technical Remarks

We use the transarterial femoral approach to deliver glue in situ as the first treatment modality in every case. No cut down has been necessary in our experience. In our series of 258 cases and more than 400 embolizations, the venous route was used in only four when it became impossible to achieve effective embolization from the arterial route.[27]

The microcatheters we use are a combination of flow guided and over the wire type of devices (mini torquer sensor, CathNet-Science, Paris, France, and custom-made short Magic 1.8, Balt, Montmorency, France); these are used directly through the 4F sheath, without guiding catheter; therefore no coaxial system is used in 90% of cases. Catheters which are too soft are often unstable during fast injection of pure glue while most of the over-the-wire microcatheters tend to kink in these looping vessels.

The neonatal and infant group of children, whenever the occlusion of the malformation of the vein of Galen is complete or almost complete, are kept under general anaesthesia for the next 24 hours in the intensive care unit. They are subsequently woken up the following day. Endovascular treatment sessions are arranged every 3–6 months depending on the clinical status and response to the embolization.

Follow Up

During follow up, all children are clinically evaluated by the referring physicians or the paediatric neurologists. Clinical assessment is based on neurocognitive examination using the Denver and Brunet–Lezine test. After treatment is completed, children are followed up with a clinical examination every year, and MRI every 2 years since we have created a population of children that did not exist 20 years ago. This ongoing clinical follow-up is mandatory in the paediatric population since therapeutic success can only be truly evaluated when brain maturation is complete and functionally evaluated over time.

Total exclusion of a VGAM is a clear and simple observation as demonstrated by a repeat angiogram, most often 1 year after the final session of embolization. Total obliteration of the lesion has already been obtained in 50.6% of the children that were embolized. In 97% of the cases where the treatment of the lesion was considered complete, total exclusion of the shunt has been obtained and confirmed.

Overall Mortality and Morbidity

At Bicêtre, following our selection criteria, in some children treatment was withheld. Of 216 treated patients, 23 died despite or because of the embolization (10.6%).[28] In Fullerton's[29] series, of 16 patients with CCF all presented either prenatally or neonatally and 4 died acutely, while none of those presenting later died. By angiographic classification, outcome was worse for those with choroidal VGAM (3/13 died) than for those with mural VGAM (none died).

Complications: morbidity

In our series,[28] 20 out of the 193 (10.4%) surviving patients had severe learning disability, 30 (15.6%) had moderate learning disability and 143 (74%) were neurologically normal on follow up. In Fullerton's[29] series assessed with a modification of the Denver Developmental Screening Test, of those presenting in the perinatal period with heart failure, six had significant delay and six had no or minor developmental delay. Of those presenting in the neonatal period without heart failure, two of five were significantly delayed, and three of five had no delay. Of those presenting after the neonatal period, only one of six was delayed. Overall, 14 of 27 children who received treatment for VGAM had a favourable outcome, which was predicted by presentation after the neonatal period, absence of heart failure and choroidal angioarchitecture.[29]

In our recent series from Great Ormand Street Hospital,[30] there have been 4% non-neurological complications related to the embolization procedure and the technical difficulty of injecting pure Bucrylate glue. We have had few venous passages of glue (<3%) into the sinuses, or further distally despite the fact that we are not using hypotension or flow arrest. However, in case of a converging venous drainage of the VGAM and the brain any glue passage into the venous outlet may produce a post-embolization venous infarction. If the glue remains in the sinuses further occlusion of the shunt must be obtained to avoid the effect of rerouting of the VGAM flow into the pial venous system. Heparin in these cases will be needed to preserve the remaining lumen if the iatrogenic occlusion is incomplete. In this same group of treated patients, 5% developed permanent neurological disability. Two children treated by the transvenous route after failure to achieve further embolization by transarterial approach sustained an intracerebral haemorrhage within a few hours after embolization. In both cases the occlusion of the venous outlet to the pouch was complete and the remaining flow into the VGAM insufficiently reduced. A third case developed a hemianopsia when the microcatheter became inadvertently glued in the vessel during embolization. Recent results are a substantial improvement as in the initial series of 11 patients managed at Great Ormand Street Hospital during the 1980s and early 1990s, only three survived and only one was intact.[31]

Overall mortality and morbidity at Great Ormand Street Hospital

The multidisciplinary team at Great Ormand Street Hospital have taken a more liberal approach than the Bicêtre group in offering treatment to any child without evidence of diffuse parenchymal damage. Of 33 children (26 neonates, seven infants) referred to our team for management of VGAM over the last six years, 28 underwent endovascular treatment. Four patients were not offered treatment as they had evidence of severe diffuse brain injury at presentation; treatment was deferred in one other who subsequently died. In total seven children died (two who had endovascular treatment and five who did not). Of the survivors (all treated) 13 are neurodevelopmentally intact, seven have mild neurodevelopmental impairment and the remaining six have significant neurological impairment. Of note, two children with low Bicêtre scores were neurologically intact after successful treatment. Our overall outcomes and complication rates and those of others[29-36] are broadly similar to the Bicêtre experience, although we may well have been aided by advances in equipment and intensive care. There is clearly still much progress to be made.

The place of other techniques

THE PLACE OF SURGERY

The majority of surgical treatments reported are only partial, with ligature often far from the point of the fistula, while others were excisions of already thrombosed lesions.[33] It is above all ventricular shunting that must be viewed with suspicion; while it alleviates acute hydrocephalus it carries a high morbidity and may worsen the neurological outcome. If one takes as a reference Johnston's[15] review, then the results of surgery in VGAM management are very poor with a 38–91% mortality in the overall group and 33–77% mortality in the operated group. Normal children represented 4–32% of overall group depending on the age group. These results are certainly quite different from the results we published in over 177 cases managed by transarterial embolization with a 18.4% overall mortality and 80% of the children having normal neurological examination on follow-up.

Today, with proper embolization, we have demonstrated that there is no indication for the primary surgical approach to VGAM, either to ligate feeders or to attack the pouch itself. In addition, ventricular shunting should be avoided, and instead a well-planned embolization be performed at the stage of macrocrania, although ventricular drainage may still be necessary. Third ventriculostomy appears a promising alternative.

THE PLACE OF RADIOSURGERY

In our series, four children had radiotherapy, three before they had been referred to us. In each of the three cases a linear accelerator had been used with no effect on the lesion; these three were subsequently cured by embolization. The last case completed treatment with a combination of multifocused radiotherapy following embolization of 80% of the lesion. The search for minimally invasive techniques to cure difficult or unreachable vascular malformations of the brain has made radiosurgery a therapeutic alternative, even in the paediatric population. The main problem in applying this technique in VGAMs is the vulnerability of the child's brain and necessary time needed for the progressing 'endarteritis' to be completed. During this delay the haemodynamic and hydrodynamic effects, either on the supratentorial or infratentorial spaces created by the VGAM with concurrent maturing and developing brain, will induce irreversible damage and neurocognitive delay. This retardation is one of the most challenging problems, often overlooked and rarely reported in the literature. It was present in nearly all the infants who were referred to us, despite the fact that they were considered 'neurologically normal'. To avoid irreversible delay, we believe that in none of these cases can one actually wait 2 years to obtain occlusion of the shunt. Although theoretically efficient, we believe that there is no indication for radiosurgery as the first modality in the treatment of VGAMs.

REFERENCES

1. Dandy WE. Experimental hydrocephalus. Ann Surg 1919; 70(2): 129–142.
2. Lasjaunias P. Vascular Diseases in Neonates, Infants and Children, 1 edn. Berlin: Springer-Verlag, 1997.
3. Boldrey E, Miller ER. Arteriovenous fistula (aneurysm) of the great cerebral vein (of Galen) and the circle of Willis; report on two patients treated by ligation. Arch Neurol Psychiatry 1949; 62(6):778–783.
4. Yasargil MG, Antic J, Laciga R, Jain KK, Boone SC. Arteriovenous malformations of vein of Galen: microsurgical treatment. Surg Neurol 1976; 6(3):195–200.
5. Menezes AH, Graf CJ, Jacoby CG, Cornell SH. Management of vein of Galen aneurysms. Report of two cases. J Neurosurg 1981; 55(3):457–462.
6. Hoffman HJ, Chuang S, Hendrick EB, Humphreys RP. Aneurysms of the vein of Galen. Experience at The Hospital for Sick Children, Toronto. J Neurosurg 1982; 57(3):316–322.
7. Ciricillo SF, Edwards MS, Schmidt KG, Hieshima GB, Silverman NH, Higashida RT et al. Interventional neuroradiological management of vein of Galen malformations in the neonate. Neurosurgery 1990; 27(1):22–27.
8. Dowd CF, Halbach VV, Barnwell SL, Higashida RT, Edwards MS, Hieshima GB. Transfemoral venous embolization of vein of Galen malformations. AJNR Am J Neuroradiol 1990; 11(4):643–648.
9. Casasco A, Lylyk P, Hodes JE, Kohan G, Aymard A, Merland JJ. Percutaneous transvenous catheterization and embolization of vein of Galen aneurysms. Neurosurgery 1991; 28(2):260–266.
10. Williams AN, Kirkham FJ. Childhood stroke, stroke-like illness and cerebrovascular disease. Stroke 2004; 35:311.
11. Pollock AQ, Laslett PA. Cerebral arteriovenous fistula producing cardiac failure in the newborn infant. J Pediatr 1958; 53(6):731–736.
12. Gold AP, Ransohoff J, Carter S. Vein of Galen Malformation. Acta Neurol Scand 1964; 11(40):5–31.
13. Gupta R, Connolly ES, Mayer S, Elkind MS. Hemicraniectomy for massive middle cerebral artery territory infarction: a systematic review. Stroke 2004; 35(2):539–543.
14. Abend NS, Ichord R, Aijun Z, Hurst R. Vein of Galen aneurysmal malformation with deep venous communication and subarachnoid hemorrhage. J Child Neurol 2008; 23(4):441–446.
15. Johnston IH, Whittle IR, Besser M, Morgan MK. Vein of Galen malformation: diagnosis and management. Neurosurgery 1987; 20(5):747–758.
16. Padget DH. The cranial venous system in man in reference to development, adult configuration, and relation to the arteries. Am J Anat 1956; 98(3):307–355.
17. Lasjaunias P, Ter Brugge, Lopez IL, Chiu M, Flodmark O, Chuang S et al. The role of dural anomalies in vein of Galen aneurysms: report of six cases and review of the literature. AJNR Am J Neuroradiol 1987; 8(2):185–192.
18. Lasjaunias P, Garcia-Monaco R, Rodesch G, Terbrugge K. Deep venous drainage in great cerebral vein (vein of Galen) absence and malformations. Neuroradiology 1991; 33(3):234–238.
19. Lasjaunias PL, Campi A, Rodesch G. Aneurysmal disease in children: review of 20 cases with intracranial arterial localizations. Intervent Neuroradiol 1997; 3:215–229.
20. Foran A, Donohue V, McParland P, Lynch B, Lasjaunias P, Rodesch G et al. Vein of Galen aneurysm malformation (VGAM): closing the management loop. Ir Med J 2004; 97(1):8–10.
21. Geibprasert S, Krings T, Armstrong D, Terbrugge KG, Raybaud CA. Predicting factors for the follow-up, outcome and management decisions in vein of Galen aneurysmal malformations. Childs Nerv Syst 2010, 26(1):35–46.
22. Zerah M, Garcia-Monaco R, Rodesch G, Terbrugge K, Tardieu M, de Victor D et al. Hydrodynamics in vein of Galen malformations. Childs Nerv Syst 1992; 8(3):111–117.
23. Frankenburg WK, Dodds J, Archer P, Shapiro H, Bresnick B. The Denver II: a major revision and restandardization of the Denver Developmental Screening Test. Pediatrics 1992; 89(1):91–97.
24. Bansal A, Gailloud P, Jordan L, Ruiz DS. Regression of cerebral calcifications after endovascular treatment in a case of vein of Galen arteriovenous malformation. J Neurosurg Pediatr 2009; 4(1):17–20.
25. Irfan M, Lohman B, McKinney AM. Confirmation of T1-bright vein of Galen aneurysm spontaneous thrombosis by subtraction magnetic resonance venography: a case report. Acta Radiol 2009; 50(7):812–815.
26. Shah QA, Qureshi AI. Spontaneous thrombosis of a large vein of Galen malformation. J Neuroimaging 2011, 21:87–8.
27. Lasjaunias P, Hui F, Zerah M, Garcia-Monaco R, Malherbe V, Rodesch G et al. Cerebral arteriovenous malformations in children. Management of 179 consecutive cases and review of the literature. Childs Nerv Syst 1995; 11(2):66–79.
28. Lasjaunias PL, Chng SM, Sachet M, Alvarez H, Rodesch G, Garcia-Monaco R. The management of vein of Galen aneurysmal malformations. Neurosurgery 2006; 59(5 Suppl 3):S184–S194.
29. Fullerton HJ, Aminoff AR, Ferriero DM, Gupta N, Dowd CF. Neurodevelopmental outcome after endovascular treatment of vein of Galen malformations. Neurology. 2003;61(10):1386–90.
30. McSweeney N, Brew S, Bhate S, Cox T, Roebuck DJ, Ganesan V. Management and outcome of vein of Galen malformation. Arch Dis Child. 2010;95(11):903–9.
31. Parker A, Taylor W, Kirkham FJ. Vein of Galen malformations presenting in early infancy. In: Proceedings of the British Paediatric Association 1996; 58: G78.
32. Heuer GG, Gabel B, Beslow LA, Stiefel MF, Schwartz ES, Storm PB, Ichord RN, Hurst RW. Diagnosis and treatment of vein of Galen aneurysmal malformations. Childs Nerv Syst. 2010;26(7): 879–87.
33. Li AH, Armstrong D, terBrugge KG. Endovascular treatment of vein of Galen aneurysmal malformation: management strategy and 21-year experience in Toronto. J Neurosurg Pediatr. 2011;7(1):3–10.
34. Heuer GG, Gabel B, Beslow LA, Stiefel MF, Schwartz ES, Storm PB, Ichord RN, Hurst RW. Diagnosis and treatment of vein of Galen aneurysmal malformations. Childs Nerv Syst. 2010;26(7): 879–87.
35. Pongpech S, Aurboonyawat T, Visudibhan A, Jiarakongmun P. Endovascular management in children with vein of Galen aneurysmal malformation. Minim Invasive Neurosurg. 2010;53(4):169–74.
36. Beltramello A, Perini S, Mazza C. Spontaneously healed vein of Galen aneurysms. Clinical radiological features. Childs Nerv Syst 1991; 7(3):129–134.

11
STURGE–WEBER SYNDROME

Sarah Aylett

Background

Sturge–Weber syndrome (SWS) is a sporadic condition in which an ischaemic mechanism results in epilepsy, hemiplegia and learning disability. SWS is characterized by a facial capillary haemangioma involving the periorbital area, forehead or scalp, a venous angioma of the leptomeninges and a choroidal angioma. The leptomeningeal angioma involves the pia mater, most commonly in the occipito-parietal region, and is more commonly unilateral. The angioma is bilateral in 15% of cases.[1] Rarely, the pial angioma may be present without a facial naevus.[2] However, in these cases occipital calcification in association with epilepsy and coeliac disease requires consideration.[3] It is thought that failure of regression of a vascular plexus around the cephalic portion of the neural tube between 6 and 9 weeks' gestation results in the facial, choroidal and cerebral angioma. The range of severity of SWS with regard to epilepsy, physical disability and learning disability is variable.

Pathological studies

The leptomeningeal angioma involves the pia mater, most commonly in the occipito-parietal region, but may involve the entire cerebral hemisphere. Pathological studies in adults and children with SWS are described by Alexander and Norman.[4] The layer of blood vessels within the subarachnoid space includes blood vessels of arteriolar or arterial type in addition to vessels with thin angiomatous walls. Calcification both within superficial and deeper layers of the cortex, subcortical white matter and in a perivascular distribution occurs beneath the areas involved with the angioma. In areas where gyri are heavily calcified, loss of myelinated fibres is also observed. Micropolygyria and heterotopias may be found in the cerebrum and cerebellum. It is postulated that this is secondary to chronic ischaemia occurring after cortical migration.

Neuroimaging

In addition to the presence of the angioma, there is an abnormality of the venous circulation in SWS, with a decrease in the numbers of superficial cortical veins, and enlargement of the deep medullary veins and choroid plexus. In young children the degree of enlargement is related to the extent of the pial angioma.[5] Angiography has shown stasis and slowing of the venous circulation.[6] Typical neuroimaging findings are demonstrated in the majority, although there is a wide range of alternative pathologies associated with facial capillary haemangiomas.[7]

Progressive gliosis and atrophy seen in SWS are consistent with an ischaemic process involving the cortical and subcortical regions of the brain underlying the venous angioma.[8] On presentation with seizures in infancy there is little atrophy, but beyond the age of 2 years there is evolving atrophy and calcification, both within the angioma and the underlying cerebral cortex, which become more extensive with increasing age. Calcification is likely to be the end result of cell necrosis secondary to chronic ischaemia. Calcification and focal or generalized atrophy are well demonstrated by computed tomography (CT) (Fig. 11.1). However, gadolinium-enhanced magnetic resonance imaging (MRI) is a superior technique both for detection of the pial angioma (Figs 11.2 and 11.3) and the associated vascular anomalies.[9] MRI is more sensitive than CT in demonstrating the extent of the pial angioma at an early, and often presymptomatic, stage.[5,10] Involvement of the infratentorial structures is common.[7]

Since the arterial tree is anatomically normal in the majority of cases, and there is a major venous abnormality, it seems likely that the pathophysiological mechanism involves either poor venous drainage and/or venous hypertension.[11,12] Sagittal venous thrombosis has been observed and is presumed to be secondary to the venous stasis.[9]

Cortical enhancement is seen in relation to acute seizures, suggestive of an increase in permeability of the blood–brain barrier occurring in relation to these acute episodes.[13] In infants with SWS an accentuation of T2 shortening in the white matter underlying the angioma may be seen. Although it has been suggested that this finding is secondary to an acceleration in myelination,[14–16] there is no associated accentuation of T1 shortening or evidence from pathological studies to

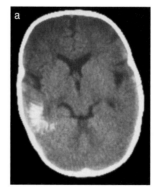
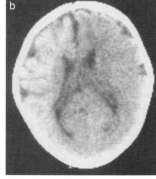

Fig. 11.1. (a,b) CT scans from patients with Sturge–Weber syndrome.

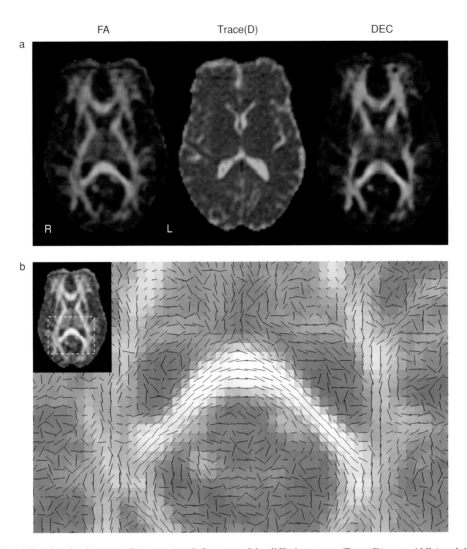

Plate 1. (Figure 4.25) (a) Fractional anisotropy (FA) map (top left), trace of the diffusion tensor (Trace(D), top middle) and directionally encoded colour (DEC) map (top right) calculated from diffusion tensor imaging in a normal volunteer. The contrast of the FA and Trace(D) maps is very different. While the FA map has very high grey/white matter contrast, that is not the case for the Trace(D). Three different diffusion properties can be identified in the brain: (1) high anisotropy and moderate average diffusivity (white matter); (2) low anisotropy and moderate average diffusivity (grey matter); (3) low anisotropy and high average diffusivity cerebrospinal fluid). The DEC map is created by colouring each voxel in the FA map according to the direction of the eigenvector associated with the largest eigenvalue of the diffusion tensor ((λ_1) (red, left–right; green, anterior–posterior; blue, inferior–superior). (b) Expansion of a portion of the FA map (see dotted white insert in left inset image) showing in each voxel the projection of the eigenvector associated with the largest eigenvalue. As can be seen, the direction of the eigenvector is a good representation of the white matter fibre direction.

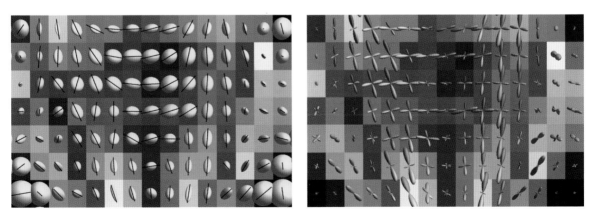

Plate 2. (Figure 4.26) Diffusion tensor (left) and constrained spherical deconvolution (right) results displayed as a coronal slice through the pons, in a region known to contain crossing fibres. The principal direction of diffusion (i.e. the eigenvector with the largest eigenvalue) is shown overlaid on the diffusion tensor ellipsoid to aid visualization of the estimated white matter orientations. It can readily be appreciated that the diffusion tensor model fails to adequately characterize the complex arrangement of the fibre tracts in this region. These erroneous orientations have obvious deleterious consequences for fibre tractography results. Constrained spherical deconvolution, on the other hand, is robust to crossing fibre effects, and provides a much more adequate estimate of the fibre orientations present in this region. In particular, the corticospinal tracts and transverse pontine fibres can easily be identified.

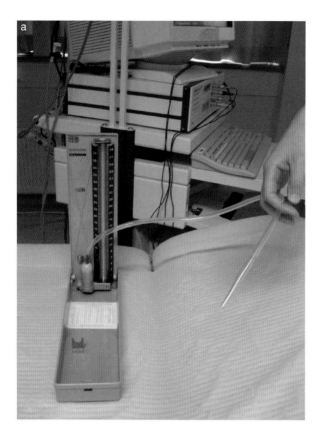

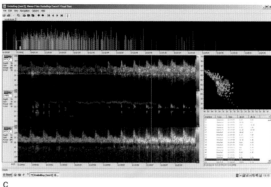

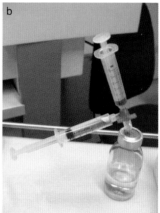

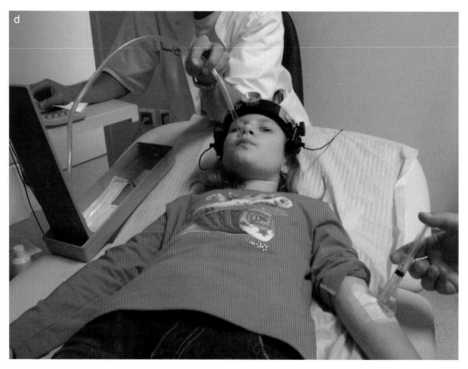

Plate 3. (Figure 5.8) (a) Apparatus used to exclude patent foramen ovale using bubble contrast transcranial Doppler during a Valsalva manouevre. Measurement of Valsalva pressure generated with transcranial Doppler equipment in the background. (b) Agitated saline. (c) Microemboli on transcranial Doppler. (d) Child undergoing the test.

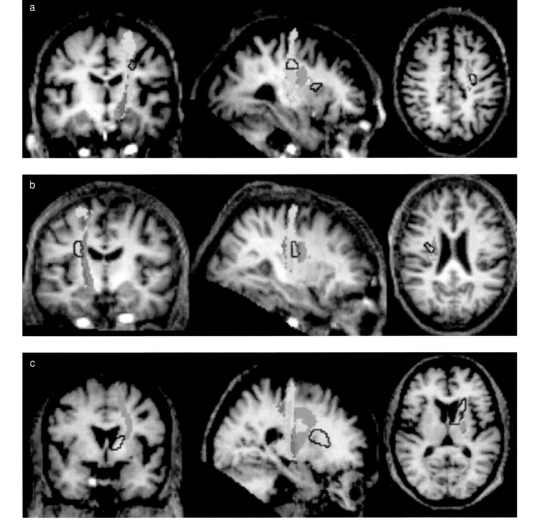

Plate 4. (Figure 4.35) An example of the application of fibre tractography to stroke recovery, showing the location of the lesion in three stroke patients (as identified by the area of low diffusion anisotropy) in relation to the path of different corticofugal pathways, identified in a group of healthy controls using fibre tractography. The inferred disconnections were found to explain enhanced hand-grip-related responses as assessed using functional MRI. (From a figure previously published in Newton JM, Ward NS, Parker GJ, Deichmann R, Alexander DC, Friston KJ et al. Non-invasive mapping of corticofugal fibres from multiple motor areas – relevance to stroke recovery. Brain 2006; 129(Pt 7):1844–1858. Copyright © 2006, Jennifer M Newton, published by Oxford University Press).

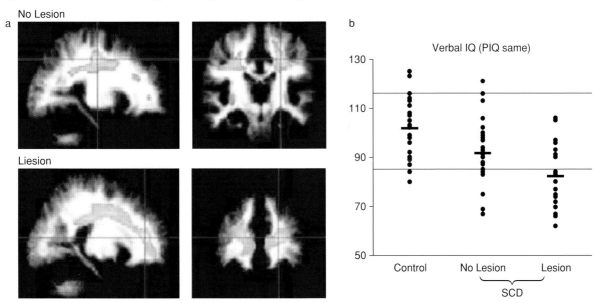

Plate 5. (Figure 15.28) (a,b) Voxel-based morphometry comparison of white matter density between controls and patients with SCA with and without covert infarction. Regions of reduced white matter density in those with SCA and covert infarction are displayed on the mean white matter segment. The white matter abnormality distribution is similar to that in the patient with overt stroke shown in Fig. 15.18C and in the patient with apparently reversible ischaemia in Fig. 15.17C. The patients with covert lesions have lower verbal (and performance; not shown) IQ than those with no covert lesion, who have lower verbal (and performance; not shown) IQ than sibling controls; part of the explanation for which the voxel-based morphometry data provides evidence, is that there is tissue damage not visible on T2-weighted MRI.

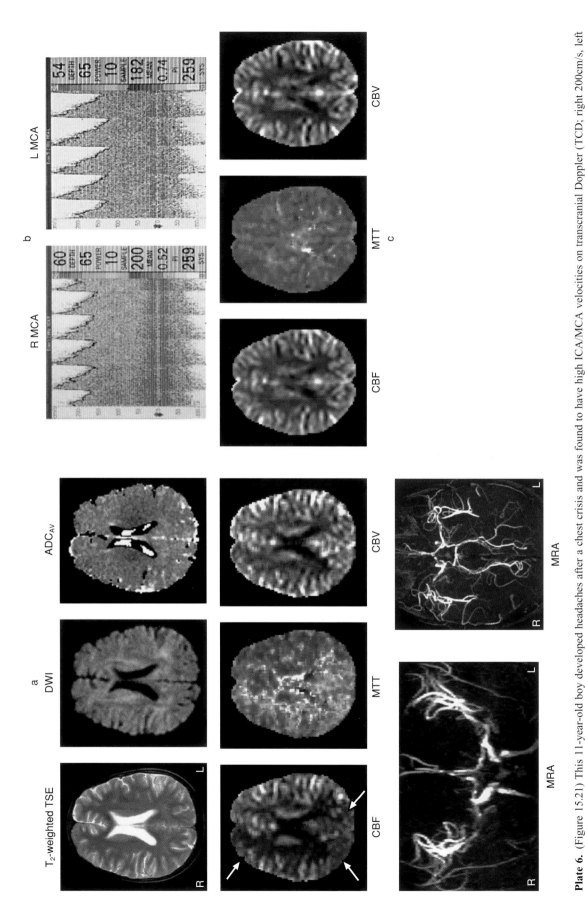

Plate 6. (Figure 15.21) This 11-year-old boy developed headaches after a chest crisis and was found to have high ICA/MCA velocities on transcranial Doppler (TCD; right 200cm/s, left 182cm/s) (b). (a) MR results obtained at the time of initial presentation. MRA showed turbulence in the M2 segments bilaterally (grade 2 on the right and 1 on the left) and in the P1 segment on the right (grade 2; a, bottom row). T2-weighted and diffusion-weighted imaging were normal (a, top row) but perfusion imaging showed reduced cerebral blood flow (CBF), high mean transit time (MTT) and decreased cerebral blood volume (CBV) throughout the right hemisphere and posteriorly on the left (arrows, a, middle row). The patient was transfused on the basis of the TCD and severely abnormal perfusion imaging findings; his headaches improved and he has not had a subsequent event. (b,c) MR perfusion data obtained after 1 year of monthly transfusions, when his MRA and TCD had returned to normal. There are no abnormalities of CBF, CBV or MTT; 6 months after discontinuation of the transfusion regimen, his TCD, MRA and perfusion imaging remained normal.

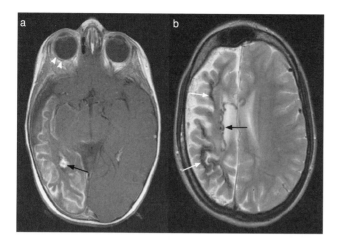

Fig. 11.2. (a) Axial T1-weighted MRI with gadolinium showing right pial angioma, cortical and subcortical atrophy, enlargement of the choroid plexus (black arrow) and right choroidal angioma (white arrowheads). (b) Axial T2-weighted MRI showing hypointensity of the subcortical white matter (white arrows) and developmental venous anomaly (black arrow).

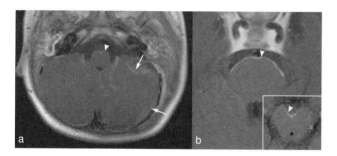

Fig. 11.3. (a,b) Axial T1-weighted MRI with gadolinium showing enhancement of midbrain (a, b and inset) and cerebellum (a).

support this. Alternatively, the T2 shortening may be related to an increase in deoxyhaemoglobin within the venous system.

Diffusion weighted imaging (DWI) has been used in patients with acute stroke to distinguish between tissue which is inevitably destined to infarct and that which is underperfused but not irreversibly damaged. The diffusion changes may be quantified by calculating the apparent diffusion coefficient (ADC), which allows for errors inherent in collecting the data in three planes. In animal experiments using echo-planar imaging within minutes of vessel occlusion, the ADC in the territory perfused by the vessel reduces to about half the normal value and unless there is reperfusion within about 3 hours, T2-weighted changes compatible with infarction begin to appear. The ADC returns to normal over the next few days (pseudonormalization) and then becomes permanently high in the infarcted region. The same phenomenon, with a similar time course, has been demonstrated in adults and children with acute stroke.[17] There is evidence of restricted diffusion in infants with SWS, with associated T2 hypointensity. In one infant this persisted over several months. The T2 hypointensity was consistent with an increase in local deoxyhaemoglobin, with

the findings suggesting compromised tissue with an increased oxygen extraction[18,19] (Fig. 11.4). DWI abnormality has also been demonstrated in the cerebellum.[20] The possible relationship of these changes with long-term prognosis and developmental outcome requires further study.

CEREBRAL BLOOD FLOW AND GLUCOSE UTILIZATION STUDIES

Studies of cerebral blood flow[21] using single photo emission CT (SPECT) have shown a reduction in regional cerebral blood flow within the cortex and subcortical regions of the affected hemisphere. There is evidence of a reduction in glucose utilization extending beyond the area of the radiological abnormality; in two infants in this series a paradoxical increase in cerebral glucose utilization was observed.[22] More recently it has been suggested that a marked asymmetry of cortical glucose utilization is associated with a more favourable cognitive and seizure outcome.[23] It is postulated that marked asymmetry may be associated with a greater potential for relocation of function.

Hemiplegia and migraine

Transient hemiparesis associated with headache, vomiting and migraine-like phenomena, but without evidence of ictal activity is well described in SWS and is considered to be related to an abnormal vasomotor response.[24] Riela et al[25] demonstrated a reduction in the cerebral blood flow response to carbon dioxide in SWS, suggesting that the cerebral circulation can mount only a limited vasodilator response. Okudaira et al[26] reported a reduction in vasoactivity to acetazolamide in eight patients, which was more marked in the affected and contralateral cortex in those showing progressive neurological symptoms.

Epilepsy

The majority of children with SWS appear to develop seizures in the first 2 years of life,[27] with the onset of seizures below the age of 6 months being associated with intractability and a poor outcome. The onset of seizures was with a febrile episode in one-third of one series.[28] In this retrospective review of 30 patients with SWS, the mean age of onset of seizures was 6 months. Resistance to treatment is variably reported in between 40% and 83%.[24,27,28] In one reported series,[28] all patients with the onset of seizures in the first year of life had poor control and subsequent cognitive impairment. High seizure intensity in young patients appeared to predict poorer cognitive outcome, but in this series the presence of a hemiplegia was not associated with a poorer prognosis.[29] However, Arzimanoglou and Aicardi[24] found that an associated hemiplegia increased the likelihood of cognitive problems. A relatively high incidence of epileptic status is reported in SWS, with this occurring in over 50% of one series.[24] Frequently, the onset of seizures in SWS is followed by the appearance for the first time of a hemiplegia and a homonymous hemianopia. Clinically, acute episodes of encephalopathy occur with altered consciousness associated with recurrent

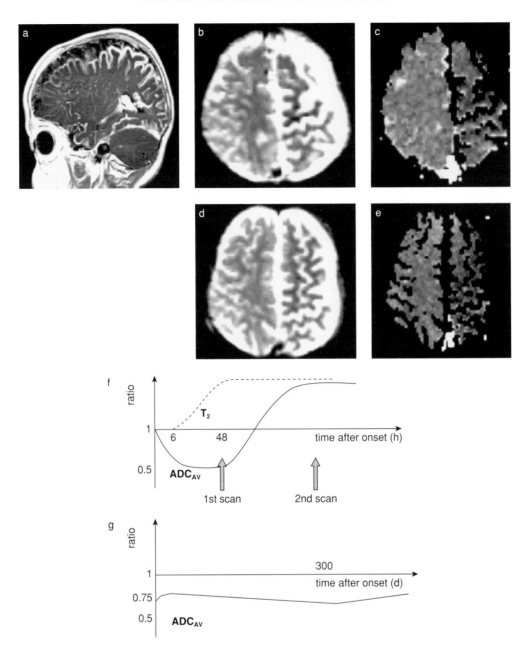

Fig. 11.4. This patient was born with a left capillary haemangioma in the V1–2 distribution. She presented at age 4 months with right-sided twitching lasting 40 minutes, treated with diazepam. Despite treatment with sodium valproate and further boluses of diazepam, she continued to have further seizures over a period of 6 days, including one of 2 hours and one of 30 minutes. The child was loaded with phenytoin, and no further clinical seizures or abnormal EEG discharges were observed. Sagittal (a) and axial (b–e) T2-weighted imaging and diffusion imaging were performed 6, 12, and 25 days after initial presentation (b,d). Diffusion-weighted imaging has been used within 48 hours of acute stroke to demonstrate areas of tissue which are ischaemic and at high risk of infarction, while there is pseudonormalization thereafter (f) but in this patient, the apparent diffusion coefficient (ADC) maps obtained at 6 days after initial onset of the seizures showed evidence of ongoing restricted diffusion throughout a substantial part of the abnormal left hemisphere (d). Representative regions showed an ipsi/contralateral ADC ratio of 0.79 (shown graphically in g, compared with values of the order of 0.5 in the first 48 hours after stroke and 1.0 in controls, shown graphically in f). The ADC remained low in the affected areas at 12 and 25 days after presentation (shown graphically in g, ipsi/contralateral ADC ratio 0.81 and 0.84 respectively). Throughout this period, the T2-weighted images showed hypointensity in corresponding regions. The patient developed a right hemiparesis and continued to have daily single clonic jerks of this side with secondary generalized seizures once or twice a month despite treatment with phenytoin, sodium valproate and aspirin. A follow-up scan was performed at the age of 14 months (c,e); the ADC remained low with an ipsi/contralateral ADC ratio of 0.79 (shown graphically in g). At the age of 15 months, her development was delayed to the 10-month level. Two months later, she had an episode of intractable status epilepticus for 2 weeks despite aggressive anticonvulsant therapy. She underwent a further magnetic resonance scan to determine whether she had bilateral damage at the ages of 16 and 30 month and persistently low ADC was again demonstrated (shown graphically in g), suggesting ongoing ischaemia. The patient underwent a hemispherectomy for intractable epilepsy at the age of 33 months and has remained seizure-free postoperatively (from Kirkham FJ, Datta AK. Hypoxic adaptation during development: relation to pattern of neurological presentation and cognitive disability. Dev Sci. 2006;9(4):411–27).

seizures, with neurological deficits often becoming more severe after each episode of encephalopathy. There is evidence of an impairment of the haemodynamic response to seizures in infants with SWS,[30] which could contribute to a lack of oxygen and substrate delivery to the affected cortex.

Although simple partial seizures are most frequently seen at onset, multiple seizure types may occur, including complex partial seizures, generalized tonic clonic seizures, my conic-astatic epilepsy[31] and infantile spasms.[32] Sporadic severe and prolonged seizures and status epilepticus are common presentations, although epilepsy may not continue between these bouts.[33]

Electroencephalographic (EEG) abnormalities may be both non-epileptiform, with asymmetry of the background amplitude, or frankly epileptic with focal or generalized discharges.[34] The striking features of the EEG in SWS are the attenuation and the excess of slow activities; bilateral polymorphic delta activity, which is often an EEG marker for ischaemia, appears to be related to severe mental retardation, even if the lesion is unilateral.[35] The absence of interictal spiking and the occurrence of EEG seizure discharges only in the periphery of the lesion are compatible with focal ischaemia underlying the pial angioma itself.[35] Quantitative EEG may allow diagnosis of an underlying pial angioma in a child with a facial haemangioma.[36]

Neurodevelopmental and cognitive outcome

Following normal early development, children with SWS often experience catastrophic neurological deterioration in association with the evolution of epilepsy, and consequently suffer a high rate of disability.[1,27,37] Children with SWS also frequently develop glaucoma and a homonymous hemianopia. Although a bihemispheric angioma appears to be associated with a poor outcome,[27] it is noteworthy that in cases with unilateral leptomeningeal involvement, global cognitive impairment is common.[1,27,28,37,38]

Retrospective studies suggest that there is a spectrum of neurological and cognitive disability in children with unihemispheric SWS. In one series 30% were found to fall within the normal ability range, whilst 60% showed cognitive impairment which varied from mild (12.5%) to severe (32.5%).[27] It is noteworthy that in cases with unilateral leptomeningeal involvement, global cognitive impairment is common. In a small prospective series, Barling et al[39] found that language skills were at a comparable level to cognitive ability in a group of infants with SWS. There was, however, evidence of fluctuation in both expressive and receptive language. Whether the abnormalities in language development are of the same severity as an epileptic aphasia, and related to the extent of the underlying vascular abnormality, requires further study. It is possible that a high rate of discharges from the abnormal hemisphere in SWS interferes with the function of the normal hemisphere. Another possibility is that an impairment of contralateral vascular control renders the hemisphere incapable of reorganization of function. Whilst the onset of epilepsy in the first year of life is associated with a high rate of developmental delay,[24,40] global delay is seen in infants with

no, or relatively well controlled seizures (personal observation). Bilateral cerebral glucose hypometabolism appears to be associated with learning disability even with a unilateral pial nevus[22] and the extent of white matter abnormality demonstrable on MRI also seems to be predictive.[41–43]

Management

Although there are no controlled studies, there is a theoretical rationale for the use of aspirin prophylaxis in symptomatic cases of SWS. Maria et al[44] observed fewer stroke-like episodes in those treated with aspirin. However, there is controversy over whether aspirin has benefit[45] and intracranial haemorrhage has been reported.[46] Anticoagulation with warfarin has been used acutely, and should be considered if there is evidence of venous sinus thrombosis or if there is an associated prothrombotic abnormality.

There are no studies comparing efficacy of different antiepileptic drugs in SWS. The modified Atkins diet may be of benefit.[47] In view of the associated neurological deficits which may occur in association with seizures in SWS, prompt and aggressive treatment of seizures is indicated.

The rationale behind surgical treatment of SWS has been removal or disconnection of the epileptogenic tissue. In most cases this requires hemispherectomy[48–51] although peri-insular hemispherotomy has been used successfully by some groups.[52] Progressive cognitive decline may be halted or show some recovery.[53] Acquired motor deficits in infants or children with an established hemiplegia following hemispherectomy are often minimal.[49,53] The timing of such surgery appears to be crucial, although this is controversial.[45,50,51] Treatment very early in life, often before 1 year, appears to be more successful in abolishing seizures and ensuring more normal development.[49] Lobar resection can however be successful in appropriately selected children.[54,55] Where the angioma is unilateral and resection can be complete, this may be associated with a positive outcome.[56] In this series of 20 patients, five underwent hemispherectomy and 14 cortical resection; Of these 13 were seizure free at follow up.

Epilepsy surgery should be considered where there is resistance to medical treatment or signs of progression in SWS. The latter includes increasing duration of seizures and postictal deficits, and an increase in atrophy or calcified lesions or both.[56]

REFERENCES

1. Bebin EM, Gomez MR. Prognosis in Sturge–Weber disease: comparison of unihemispheric and bihemispheric involvement. J Child Neurol 1988; 3(3):181–184.
2. Ambrosetto P, Ambrosetto G, Michelucci R, Bacci A. Sturge–Weber syndrome without port-wine facial nevus. Report of 2 cases studied by CT. Childs Brain 1983; 10(6):387–392.
3. Gobbi G, Bouquet F, Greco L, Lambertini A, Tassinari CA, Ventura A et al. Coeliac disease, epilepsiy and cerebral calcifications. Lancet 1992; 340:439–443.
4. Alexander GL, Norman RM. The Sturge–Weber Syndrome, 1st edn. Bristol: John Wright & Sons, 1960.
5. Griffiths PD. Sturge–Weber syndrome revisited: the role of neuroradiology. Neuropediatrics 1996; 27(6):284–294.

6. Probst FP. Vascular morphology and angiographic flow patterns in Sturge–Weber angiomatosis: facts, thoughts and suggestions. Neuroradiology 1980; 20(2):73–78.

7. Adams ME, Aylett SE, Squier W, Chong W. A spectrum of unusual neuroimaging findings in patients with suspected Sturge–Weber syndrome. AJNR Am J Neuroradiol 2009; 30(2):276–281.

8. Marti-Bonmati L, Menor F, Mulas F. The Sturge–Weber syndrome: correlation between the clinical status and radiological CT and MRI findings. Childs Nerv Syst 1993; 9(2):107–109.

9. Benedikt RA, Brown DC, Walker R, Ghaed VN, Mitchell M, Geyer CA. Sturge–Weber syndrome: cranial MR imaging with Gd-DTPA. AJNR Am J Neuroradiol 1993; 14(2):409–415.

10. Griffiths PD, Boodram MB, Blaser S, Armstrong D, Gilday DL, Harwood-Nash D. ^{99m}Technetium HMPAO imaging in children with the Sturge–Weber syndrome: a study of nine cases with CT and MRI correlation. Neuroradiology 1997; 39(3):219–224.

11. Coley SC, Britton J, Clarke A. Status epilepticus and venous infarction in Sturge–Weber syndrome. Childs Nerv Syst 1998; 14(12):693–696.

12. Parsa CF. Sturge–Weber syndrome: a unified pathophysiologic mechanism. Curr Treat Options Neurol 2008; 10(1):47–54.

13. Terdjman P, Aicardi J, Sainte-Rose C, Brunelle F. Neuroradiological findings in Sturge–Weber syndrome (SWS) and isolated pial angiomatosis. Neuropediatrics 1991; 22(3):115–120.

14. Jacoby CG, Yuh WT, Afifi AK, Bell WE, Schelper RL, Sato Y. Accelerated myelination in early Sturge–Weber syndrome demonstrated by MR imaging. J Comput Assist Tomogr 1987; 11(2):226–231.

15. Porto L, Kieslich M, Yan B, Zanella FE, Lanfermann H. Accelerated myelination associated with venous congestion. Eur Radiol 2006; 16(4):922–926.

16. Moritani T, Kim J, Sato Y, Bonthius D, Smoker WR. Abnormal hypermyelination in a neonate with Sturge–Weber syndrome demonstrated on diffusion-tensor imaging. J Magn Reson Imaging 2008; 27(3):617–620.

17. Connelly A, Chong WK, Johnson CL, Ganesan V, Gadian DG, Kirkham FJ. Diffusion weighted magnetic resonance imaging of compromised tissue in stroke. Arch Dis Child 1997; 77(1):38–41.

18. Calamante F, Kirkham FJ, Connelly A. Persistent reduced apparent diffusion coefficient in SWS: possible relationship to increased tissue oxygen extraction. In: Proceedings of the International Society of Magnetic Resonance in Medicine, 8th Annual Meeting; Denver, 2000.

19. Kirkham FJ, Datta AK. Hypoxic adaptation during development: relation to pattern of neurological presentation and cognitive disability. Dev Sci. 2006;9(4):411–27.

20. Arulrajah S, Ertan G, Comi M, Tekes A, Lin L, Huisman GM. MRI with diffusion-weighted imaging in children and young adults with simultaneous supra- and infratentorial manifestations of Sturge–Weber syndrome. J Neuroradiol 2010; 37(1):51–59.

21. Chiron C, Raynaud C, Tzourio N, Diebler C, Dulac O, Zilbovicius M et al. Regional cerebral blood flow by SPECT imaging in Sturge–Weber disease: an aid for diagnosis. J Neurol Neurosurg Psychiatry 1989; 52(12):1402–1409.

22. Chugani HT, Mazziotta JC, Phelps ME. Sturge–Weber syndrome: a study of cerebral glucose utilization with positron emission tomography. J Pediatr 1989; 114(2):244–253.

23. Lee JS, Asano E, Muzik O, Chugani DC, Juhasz C, Pfund Z et al. Sturge–Weber syndrome: correlation between clinical course and FDG PET findings. Neurology 2001; 57(2):189–195.

24. Arzimanoglou A, Aicardi J. The epilepsy of Sturge–Weber syndrome: clinical features and treatment in 23 patients. Acta Neurol Scand Suppl 1992; 140:18–22.

25. Riela AR, Stump DA, Roach ES, McLean WT, Jr, Garcia JC. Regional cerebral blood flow characteristics of the Sturge–Weber syndrome. Pediatr Neurol 1985; 1(2):85–90.

26. Okudaira Y, Arai H, Sato K. Hemodynamic compromise as a factor in clinical progression of Sturge–Weber syndrome. Childs Nerv Syst 1997; 13(4):214–219.

27. Pascual-Castroviejo I, Diaz-Gonzalez C, Garcia-Melian RM, Gonzalez-Casado I, Munoz-Hiraldo E. Sturge–Weber syndrome: study of 40 patients. Pediatr Neurol 1993; 9(4):283–288.

28. Oakes WJ. The natural history of patients with the Sturge–Weber syndrome. Pediatr Neurosurg 1992; 18(5–6):287–290.

29. Kramer U, Kahana E, Shorer Z, Ben-Zeev B. Outcome of infants with unilateral Sturge–Weber syndrome and early onset seizures. Dev Med Child Neurol 2000; 42(11):756–759.

30. Aylett SE, Neville BG, Cross JH, Boyd S, Chong WK, Kirkham FJ.

31. Ewen JB, Comi AM, Kossoff EH. Myoclonic-astatic epilepsy in a child with Sturge–Weber syndrome. Pediatr Neurol 2007; 36(2):115–117.

32. Barbagallo M, Ruggieri M, Incorpora G, Pavone P, Nucifora C, Spalice A et al. Infantile spasms in the setting of Sturge–Weber syndrome. Childs Nerv Syst 2009; 25(1):111–118.

33. Kossoff EH, Ferenc L, Comi AM. An infantile-onset, severe, yet sporadic seizure pattern is common in Sturge–Weber syndrome. Epilepsia 2009; 50(9):2154–2157.

34. Brenner RP, Sharbrough FW. Electroencephalographic evaluation in Sturge–Weber syndrome. Neurology 1976; 26(7):629–632.

35. Sassower K, Duchowny M, Jayakar P, Resnick T, Levin B, Alvarez L et al. EEG evaluation in children with Sturge–Weber syndrome and epilepsy. Epilepsia 1994; 7:286–289.

36. Ewen JB, Kossoff EH, Crone NE, Lin DD, Lakshmanan BM, Ferenc LM et al. Use of quantitative EEG in infants with port-wine birthmark to assess for Sturge–Weber brain involvement. Clin Neurophysiol 2009; 120(8):1433–1440.

37. Uram M, Zubillaga C. The cutaneous manifestations of Sturge–Weber syndrome. J Clin Neuroophthalmol 1982; 2(4):245–248.

38. Enjolras O, Riche MC, Merland JJ. Facial port-wine stains and Sturge–Weber syndrome. Pediatrics 1985; 76(1):48–51.

39. Barling E, Aylett SE, Sonksen P, Stackhouse J, Lees J. Early speech and language development in Sturge–Weber syndrome – is it related to seizure activity? Eur J Paediatr Neurol 1997; 1(A):102.

40. Sujansky E, Conradi S. Outcome of Sturge–Weber syndrome in 52 adults. Am J Med Genet 1995; 57(1):35–45.

41. Juhasz C, Lai C, Behen ME, Muzik O, Helder EJ, Chugani DC et al. White matter volume as a major predictor of cognitive function in Sturge–Weber syndrome. Arch Neurol 2007; 64(8):1169–1174.

42. Juhasz C, Batista CE, Chugani DC, Muzik O, Chugani HT. Evolution of cortical metabolic abnormalities and their clinical correlates in Sturge–Weber syndrome. Eur J Paediatr Neurol 2007; 11(5):277–284.

43. Alkonyi B, Govindan RM, Chugani HT, Behen ME, Jeong JW, Juhász C. Focal white matter abnormalities related to neurocognitive dysfunction: an objective diffusion tensor imaging study of children with sturge-weber syndrome. Pediatr Res. 2011;69(1):74–9.

44. Maria BL, Neufeld JA, Rosainz LC, Drane WE, Quisling RG, Ben-David K et al. Central nervous system structure and function in Sturge–Weber syndrome: evidence of neurologic and radiologic progression. J Child Neurol 1998; 13(12):606–618.

45. Comi AM. Update on Sturge–Weber syndrome: diagnosis, treatment, quantitative measures, and controversies. Lymphat Res Biol 2007; 5(4):257–264.

46. Greco F, Fiumara A, Sorge G, Pavone L. Subgaleal hematoma in a child with Sturge–Weber syndrome: to prevent stroke-like episodes, is treatment with aspirin advisable? Childs Nerv Syst 2008; 24(12):1479–1481.

47. Kossoff EH, Borsage JL, Comi AM. A pilot study of the modified Atkins diet for Sturge–Weber syndrome. Epilepsy Res. 2010 Dec;92(2–3):240–3.

48. Falconer MA, Rushworth RG. Treatment of encephalotrigeminal angiomatosis (Sturge–Weber disease) by hemispherectomy. Arch Dis Child 1960; 35:433–447.

49. Hoffman HJ, Hendrick EB, Dennis M, Armstrong D. Hemispherectomy for Sturge–Weber syndrome. Childs Brain 1979; 5(3):233–248.

50. Kossoff EH, Buck C, Freeman JM. Outcomes of 32 hemispherectomies for Sturge–Weber syndrome worldwide. Neurology. 2002;59(11): 1735–8.

51. Bourgeois M, Crimmins DW, de Oliveira RS, Arzimanoglou A, Garnett M, Roujeau T et al. Surgical treatment of epilepsy in Sturge–Weber syndrome in children. J Neurosurg 2007; 106(1 Suppl):20–28.

52. Schropp C, Sorensen N, Krauss J. Early periinsular hemispherotomy in children with Sturge–Weber syndrome and intractable epilepsy – outcome in eight patients. Neuropediatrics 2006; 37(1):26–31.

53. Vargha-Khadem F, Carr LJ, Isaacs E, Brett E, Adams C, Mishkin M. Onset of speech after left hemispherectomy in a nine-year-old boy. Brain 1997; 120(Pt 1):159–182.

54. Bye AM, Matheson JM, MacKenzie RA. Epilepsy surgery in Sturge–Weber syndrome. Aust Paediatr J 1989; 25(2):103–105.

55. Ito M, Sato K, Ohnuki A, Uto A. Sturge–Weber disease: operative indications and surgical results. Brain Dev 1990; 12(5):473–477.

56. Arzimanoglou AA, Andermann F, Aicardi J, Sainte-Rose C, Beaulieu MA, Villemure JG et al. Sturge–Weber syndrome: indications and results of surgery in 20 patients. Neurology 2000; 55(10):1472–1479.

12
HEMIPLEGIC MIGRAINE

Sarah Benton, Michel D. Ferrari, Fenella J. Kirkham and Peter J. Goadsby

Introduction

Hemiplegic migraine is not a form of cerebrovascular disease but is occasionally associated with stroke. It is also an important condition for the way in which its genetics, pathophysiology, clinical features and management illustrate the broader understanding of childhood primary headache, particularly migraine. The International Headache Society recognizes 96 pages worth of headache types (Headache Classification Committee 1988) and detailed accounts of headache in general and paediatric headache in particular are available.[1,2]

Migraine is in essence an episodic disorder of sensory modulation: headache with features of sensory disturbance, to distinguish it from tension-type headache, which is, in turn, headache that is otherwise featureless. Migraine is a disorder of brain function involving midbrain[3–5] and pontine structures.[3–6] We will not deal in any detail with the broader aspects of migraine that have been reviewed in detail[7,8] but will focus on the pathophysiology of migraine aura, which is a crucial component of hemiplegic migraine. There is no reason, in principle, or as far as it has been studied, to suppose that the other aspects of a migraine attack are particularly different for patients with hemiplegic migraine. We will deal with the classification, clinical features and genetics of hemiplegic migraine, the pathophysiology of aura and then management of the condition.

Classification, clinical features and genetics of hemiplegic migraine

Classification of Hemiplegic Migraine

A number of subtypes of migraine aura are recognized. The current diagnostic criteria for migraine with aura[9] have been revised.[10] This has not altered the basic description of migraine with aura but will bring some order to the various subtypes of aura. Two forms of hemiplegic migraine are now recognized, a familial and a sporadic type (Table 12.1). The essential characteristics of hemiplegic migraine are:

- Fully reversible motor weakness in association with at least one of visual, sensory or speech disturbance.
- Aura symptoms that develop gradually, over more than 5 minutes, and last less than 24 hours.
- A first- or second-degree relative with migraine with aura that includes motor weakness.

Headache associated with aura has features of migraine.[9] It must be immediately recognized that the description is of hemiparetic aura, not just hemiplegic aura, in the strict use of the term, but the word hemiplegic has historical currency that will preserve it.

TABLE 12.1
Proposed International Headache Society classification for hemiplegic migraine

Familial hemiplegic migraine	
Description	Migraine with aura including motor weakness and where at least one first- or second-degree relative has migraine aura including motor weakness
Diagnostic criteria	1. At least two attacks
	2. Fully reversible motor weakness and at least one of the following:
	(a) Visual, sensory or speech disturbance
	(b) At least two of the following:
	(i) At least one aura symptom develops gradually over 5 minutes and/or different symptoms occur in succession
	(ii) Each aura symptom lasts less than 24 hours
	(iii) Headache that meets criteria for migraine without aura, begins during the aura or follows aura within 60 minutes
	3. At least one first- or second-degree relative has attacks with aura including motor weakness (fulfilling current migraine with aura criteria)
	4. Not attributed to another disorder
Sporadic hemiplegic migraine	
Description	Migraine with aura including motor weakness but no first- or second-degree relative has aura including motor weakness
Diagnostic criteria	Fulfils diagnostic criteria 1, 2, 4. Familial hemiplegic migraine except criterion 3

CLINICAL, NEUROPHYSIOLOGICAL AND NEURORADIOLOGICAL FEATURES AND GENOTYPE–PHENOTYPE CORRELATIONS

Familial hemiplegic migraine (FHM) is a rare autosomal dominantly inherited subtype of migraine with aura.[9,11] Patients with FHM have attacks of migraine with aura, which, in addition to the typical migraine aura and headache symptoms, are associated with hemiparesis, contralateral slowing on electroencephalogram (EEG) (Fig. 12.1) and sometimes in the acute phase with neuroimaging evidence of focal cytotoxic oedema in the contralateral hemisphere (Figs 12.2a and 12.3). In some FHM families there may be, in addition, associated progressive cerebellar ataxia with neuroimaging evidence of cerebellar atrophy (Fig. 12.2b). If there is frank infarction, other conditions such as cerebral autosomal dominant arteriopathy with subcortical infarcts and leukoencephalopathy (CADASIL; Fig. 12.2c, see also Chapter 15) should be considered, although stroke secondary to dissection has been documented (Fig. 12.2d,e). As well as having hemiplegic attacks, patients may also have attacks of typical migraine with or without aura; in families with FHM, both individuals with FHM and with 'non-hemiplegic' typical migraine are to be found. FHM is part of the migraine spectrum, and genes involved in FHM are candidates for sporadic HM as well as 'non-hemiplegic' typical migraine with and without aura, although there is currently more evidence for the former.[12,13]

In approximately 50% of the reported families (but only 7% of families in a population-based study), FHM is associated with the FHM1 gene, *CACNA1A*, on chromosome 19p13 (Fig. 12.2).[13,14] Two groups also found linkage to chromosome 1;[13–16] the French group showed linkage to chromosome 1q21-q23 in three FHM families and this has subsequently been identified as *ATP1A* or *FHM2*, which was found in 7% of families in the population-based study. A third gene involved in FHM as well as in epilepsy is *SCN1A* on chromosome 2 or *FMF3*,[14,16] and it is likely that there are several other genes involved on chromosomes including 1 and 14.

Few clinical differences have been found between FHM families with mutations in these three genes.[14] The most striking exception is cerebellar ataxia and atrophy (Fig. 12.2b), which occurs in approximately 50% of those with *CACNA1A*[13,14,17–19] and the association of *CACNA1A* with attacks which can be triggered by minor head trauma or are associated with coma.[20,21]

One study[22] showed that patients with sporadic hemiplegic migraine had symptoms indistinguishable from FHM but significantly different from migraine with aura. This gives extra weight to the notion that sporadic hemiplegic migraine should be classified with FHM.[12–14] Migraine in a parent may also present after onset in the child.

FAMILIAL HEMIPLEGIC MIGRAINE: A CHANNELOPATHY

Familial hemiplegic migraine is due to mutations of various channelopathy genes, including the *CACNA1A* gene, that encodes the *1A subunit of the voltage-dependent P/Q-type

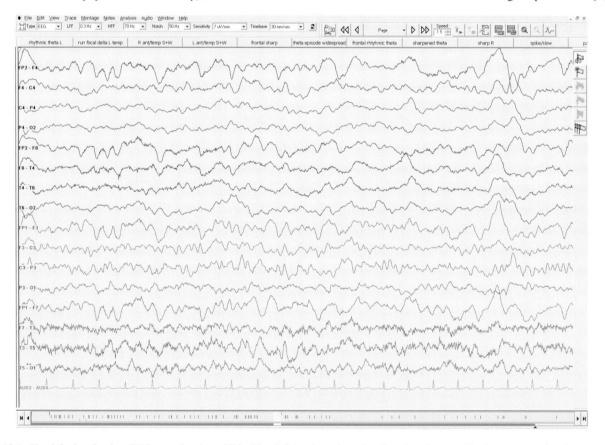

Fig. 12.1. Hemiplegic migraine: EEG recording in a child with a left hemiparesis and no imaging changes. Bipolar montage showing an asymmetry of activity with diffuse slowing and reduced fast activity over the contralateral, right hemisphere (upper half of the EEG). (Courtesy of Dr David Allen, Department of Neurophysiology, Southampton General Hospital, UK).

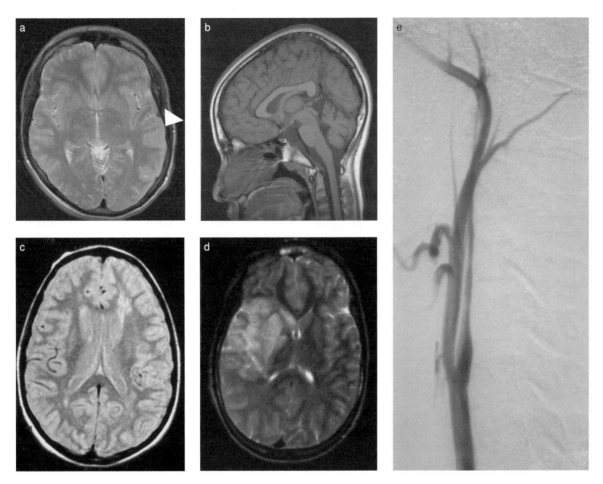

Fig. 12.2. MRI from children presenting with migraine and focal signs. (a) Parietal swelling (arrow) in a boy presenting with acute hemiparesis and headache. (b) Cerebellar atrophy in a girl with recurrent episodes of hemiplegic migraine and a *CACNA1A* mutation. (c) Subcortical infarction in a boy with migraine and CADASIL. (d) Large middle cerebral infarct in a child with a carotid dissection (e) who had fallen off his skateboard 5 days previously and was not scanned acutely because the previous year he had had an episode of facial weakness for 16 hours which had resolved completely.

calcium channel,[14,23] *ATP1A2* that encodes the *2 subunit of the Na^+/K pump,[14,24] and the *SCN1A* gene.[14] For *CACNA1A* (Fig. 12.4), a transition from G to A was identified resulting in an arginine to glutamine substitution (R192Q) within the fourth segment of the first membrane-spanning domain (IS4). The highly conserved S4 segment is thought to be part of the voltage sensor. The second mutation occurred within the pore-forming (P) hairpin loop of the second domain in *CACNA1A* replacing a threonine residue for methionine (T666M). The conserved P-segments, located between each S5 and S6, are involved in the ion-selectivity of ion channels and present binding sites for toxins.[24] Two other mutations were located in the sixth transmembrane spanning segments of repeats II and IV. The IIS6 mutation was a T-to-C transition at codon 714, resulting in a valine-to-alanine substitution (V714A). The IVS6 mutation was an A-to-C transversion at codon 1811 that resulted in a substitution of isoleucine for leucine (I1811L) and was found in two independent FHM families. The S6 mutations do not actually change the neutral-polar nature of the amino acids residues, but the original residues are conserved in all calcium channel α_1 subunit genes

described.[25] Residues in the S6 transmembrane segments may be of influence in the inactivation of the calcium channel.[26]

Subsequently, more *CACNA1A* missense mutations have been found associated with FHM (Fig. 12.4).[14] Some of these cause pure FHM and others have been associated with FHM plus cerebellar ataxia; these latter mutations may also be found in sporadic patients with hemiplegic migraine.[12–14]

Pathophysiology of hemiplegic migraine

Two important issues need to be considered: firstly, what is pathophysiology of aura, and secondly, what is the role of the cranial vessels in aura and more generally in migraine?

MIGRAINE AURA

Migraine aura is accompanied by a spreading oligaemia first reported by Olesen's pioneering studies,[27,28] and supported and extended by the elegant work of the Boston Group.[29] Some remarkable observations of an initial hyperaemic phase secure the validity of comparisons of migraine aura with cortical spreading depression.[30,31] There are many similarities between the blood flow changes measured during aura, and the animal experimental

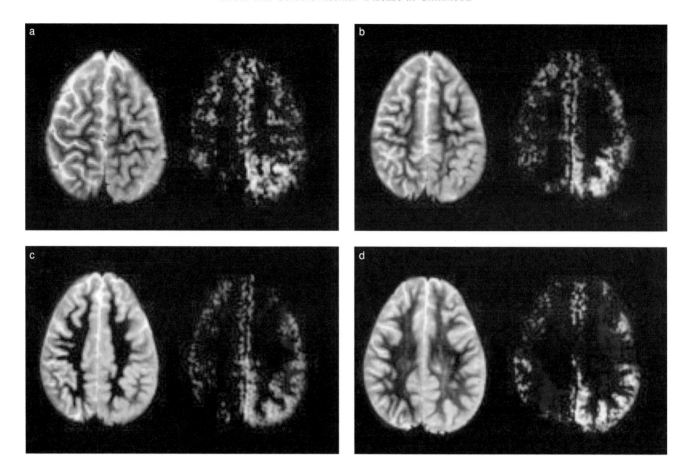

Fig. 12.3. This boy, whose mother subsequently developed migraine, initially presented at the age of 2 years with a left hemiparesis, from which he made a complete recovery, associated with only slight right hemisphere atrophy and no evidence of focal infarction on MRI. A year later he developed an acute right hemiparesis preceded by vomiting and irritability. An electroencephalogram showed an excess of slow activity in the hemisphere contralateral to the hemiparesis on both occasions. Axial T2-weighted images (left hand image in each pair) and diffusion-weighted images (right hand image in each pair) acquired 10 days after his initial presentation. (a–d) show images obtained from a descending series of slice positions starting near the top of the head. In each case, the T2-weighted images show areas of swollen cortex without hyperintensity in the left parieto-occipital region (the apparent focal high signal in the white matter in the left hemisphere in (d) is due to partial volume of the upper part of the lateral ventricle, as evidenced by the lower slices). The corresponding diffusion-weighted images show signal hyperintensity in the equivalent anatomical locations to the areas of tissue swelling. The child has been on flunarizine with no recurrent episodes. His neurological deficit resolved completely over the following few months on each occasion but he was hyperactive (from Connelly A, Chong WK, Johnson CL, Ganesan V, Gadian DG, Kirkham FJ. Diffusion weighted magnetic resonance imaging of compromised tissue in stroke. Arch Dis Child. 1997;77(1):38–41).

phenomenon of cortical spreading depression (CSD).[14,32] Notably these include the following:

- Comparable rate of spread: a few millimetres per minute.
- Absent cerebral hypercapnic vasodilator response after CSD.
- Restriction of each phenomenon to one hemisphere.

However, the electrophysiological changes Leao[33] first noted have never been directly recorded in humans. Indeed needlestick injury which easily triggers CSD[34] fails to do so in human cortex at neurosurgery.[35] It seems likely that migraine aura is what it is, and that rat or cat CSD is similar, and perhaps unsurprisingly, not identical. It is perfectly clear that the aura process represents vasoneuronal coupling, i.e. brain blood flow reduces or increases with underlying brain metabolic activity. Thus oligaemia in migraine aura is entirely a physiological response to neuronal inactivity. It becomes a problem when it is persistent, or complicated by other predisposing factors to stroke, which should always be vigorously sought.

What has emerged very clearly from both the Copenhagen group and the Boston group is that the headache phase begins while oligaemia is still present.[28] There is good clinical evidence[35], and some experimental evidence,[36] that CSD is not always nociceptive per se. Indeed, it is entirely plausible that migraine aura is part of a multifaceted migraine pathophysiology that occurs independent of the pain and other sensory disturbance.[37] Is there any specific role of the vessels in migraine?

MIGRAINE AND THE CRANIAL VESSELS

The essential question is to what extent changes in vessel calibre are unique to migraine, or any form of primary headache. The classical *Wolffian* view, more a conclusion of his acolytes than of Wolff since he wrote of migraine as a brain disease,[38] was that migraine pain was a result of painful cranial vasodilatation. However, human imaging data demonstrates this is completely incorrect. In a study of

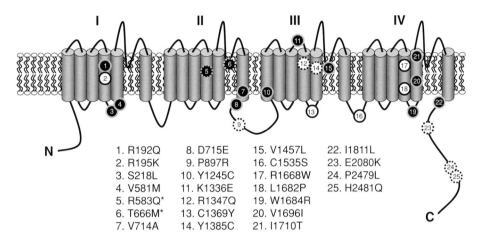

Fig. 12.4. Pure familial hemiplegic migraine (FHM) and FHM + cerebellar ataxia mutations in the *CACNA1A* α_{1A} calcium channel subunit gene. Symbols: circle with solid line, FHM; circle with dotted line, sporadic hemiplegic migraine (SHM); asterisk, mutation for which also SHM was reported; black circles, mutation was tested for functional consequences; white circle, mutation was not tested for functional consequences.

experimental head pain in which capsaicin was injected into the forehead of volunteers without headache[39] there was a bilateral activation pattern in midline structures over several planes, slightly lateralized to the left, anterior to the brainstem and posterior to the chiasmatic region. Superimposed on an MRI template, the location of the activation covers intracranial arteries, as well as the region of the cavernous sinus. Similarly, in studies of cluster headache[40] there is a strong activation again observed in the region of the cavernous sinus during pain.[41] This change might be interpreted as an increased venous inflow from the superior ophthalmic vein draining the ophthalmic artery[40] or a longer transit time for the tracer in this region possibly due to impeded venous drainage.

To further address this question magnetic resonance angiography (MRA) was performed using the same study design as in the cluster headache positron emission tomography study.[42] Using an image calculation tool, the angiographies were subtracted from each other and it was demonstrated that after nitroglycerine (NTG) inhalation, without headache, there was dilatation of the internal carotid arteries bilaterally compared to the resting state.[43] These vessels stayed dilated during the acute NTG-induced cluster headache that did not develop for a further 20–30 minutes. Moreover, dilatation has been observed in spontaneous (non-NTG associated) attacks.[43] Similarly, carotid dilatation occurs in migraine.[6] More importantly, it has been shown that injection of capsaicin into the forehead but not into the chin or leg, will produce ipsilateral carotid vasodilatation.[44] Such volunteers had neither migraine nor cluster headache, simply first (ophthalmic) division of trigeminal head pain. The somatotopically specific trigeminocerebrovascular dilator response is well described in animal studies.[45] Taken together it is clear that carotid diameter change in migraine is most likely to start as a reaction to probably perceived pain, and not as its cause.

Management of hemiplegic migraine

The essential areas to cover in the management of patient and families with hemiplegic migraine, are the following:

- Explaining the often familial nature of the problem, including appropriate investigation and warnings about triggers.
- Planning acute attack therapy.
- Discussion and instituting preventative therapy.

GENERAL ISSUES

The diagnosis of hemiplegic migraine opens the question of whether there is familial involvement. Spontaneous cases are well described in association with de novo mutations in ATP1A2 and CACNA1A[46] but we have often been faced with the index case. Genetic testing is not routine but some research centres, such as that in Leiden, will study appropriate families. Specific issues surround patients who have coma as part of the attack where relatively minor head trauma is implicated as a trigger.[47–50] The involvement of the P/Q voltage-gated calcium channel is now established,[51–56] and since death is a rare but recognized possibility, and environmental factors may play a role in determinity the clinical severity[56] it is important to have some clarification about risks. We advise these patients in the interim that activities at high risk for head trauma, such as contact sports, bicycle or horse riding, might be best avoided.

Whether to investigate otherwise typical cases of hemiplegic migraine is a vexed question. Not infrequently investigation is embarked upon when a first episode occurs and the prevailing sense of urgency and fear clouds the story. Many children are initially thought to have encephalitis, seizures or other conditions and neuroimaging and CSF examination are performed before the highly relevant family history is obtained. Although migraine by definition will yield little to investigation, unilateral slowing on EEG (Fig. 12.1) is a useful clue to the diagnosis[55] in a child with a typical presentation. However, attacks can be very disturbing to patients and those around them, and neuroimaging (Figs 12.2 and 12.3) is useful to exclude stroke or life-threatening oedema with brain shift. Cytotoxic oedema demonstrated on diffusion-weighted imaging[57] usually (but not always) reverses without infarction,[58,59] although there may be residual atrophy.[56–60] Patients who present with migraine with prolonged aura, who are at risk for sequelae, should be investigated for co-existent stroke risk factors (see Chapters 4, 5 and 6), including imaging of the carotid vessels and brain using magnetic resonance angiography.[61] Dissection of the extracranial vessels should be excluded using magnetic resonance techniques, particularly if there is a history of trauma even if previous episodes resolved completely.[62] Although conventional angiography may be abnormal,[63] because of the risk of triggering prolonged coma or seizures,[64] if there is a family or personal history of hemiplegic migraine or uni-lateral slowing on EEG, it should be avoided unless absolutely necessary, for example to exclude dissection. It is important to investigate commensurate with the concern of the family, who should understand the balance of risks. We have seen many patients repeatedly half-investigated, often with invasive tests, and feel the questions should be clearly resolved.

ACUTE ATTACK TREATMENTS

There is no established treatment of the aura phase of hemiplegic migraine.[65] Simple supportive measures including reassurance and, if necessary, intensive care for those with reduced level of consciousness, are vital. Triptans in migraine aura are probably safe[60–62] but in view of the difference in FHM pathophysiology and because in the larger sumatriptan studies treatment in aura compromised the headache response, their use should be avoided. Interestingly, in an open label study ketamine, a non-specific glutamate NMDA antagonist, improved half the patients with prolonged aura but did not at all affect the headache.[69] Verapamil appears to be beneficial in some patients.[70,71] It may be worth attempting improvement of clinical endpoints, such as depth of coma or associated seizures,[72] with anticonvulsants such as sodium valproate[65] or phenytoin[72] but there are currently few clinical series.

PREVENTIVE TREATMENTS

If hemiplegic migraine is frequent enough to interfere with life or is associated with prolonged aura, a migraine preventive, such as acetazolamide for those with familial hemiplegic migraine type 1 (FHM1)[73], or a beta-blocker (e.g. propranolol), tricyclic antidepressant (e.g. amitryptiline) or calcium channel blocker (e.g. flunarizine) for any FHM may be appropriate.[65] Our experience is that flunarizine is the treatment choice in hemiplegic migraine.[83] The use of any preventive needs to be balanced against the considerable disadvantage of taking medication every day for a period of several months, as benefit may not be obvious initially, and the view of the individual child is paramount.

Outcome

The majority of people who have an attack of hemiplegic migraine make a complete recovery and have no other neurological symptoms or signs outside attacks. However, detailed testing can reveal mild deficits in some children[57,74,75] and adults[76] and increased frequencies of epilepsy[77–81] and psychosis[82] have been reported in migraine with aura or familial hemiplegic migraine.

Acknowledgements

The work of PJG has been supported by the Sandler Family Trust.

REFERENCES

1. Olesen J, Tfelt-Hansen P, Welch KM. The Headaches, 2nd edn. Philadelphia: Lippincott, Williams and Wilkins, 2000.
2. Silberstein SD, Lipton RB, Goadsby PJ. Headache in Clinical Practice, 2nd edn. London: Martin Dunitz, 2002.
3. Weiller C, May A, Limmroth V, Juptner M, Kaube H, Schayck RV et al. Brain stem activation in spontaneous human migraine attacks. Nat Med 1995; 1(7):658–660.
4. Raskin NH, Hosobuchi Y, Lamb S. Headache may arise from perturbation of brain. Headache 1987; 27(8):416–420.
5. Goadsby PJ. Neurovascular headache and a midbrain vascular malformation: evidence for a role of the brainstem in chronic migraine. Cephalalgia 2002; 22(2):107–111.
6. Bahra A, Matharu MS, Buchel C, Frackowiak RS, Goadsby PJ. Brainstem activation specific to migraine headache. Lancet 2001; 357(9261):1016–1017.
7. Goadsby PJ, Lipton RB, Ferrari MD. Migraine: current understanding and management. N Engl J Med 2002; 346:257–270.
8. Goadsby PJ. Migraine pathophysiology. Headache 2005; 45(Suppl 1): S14–S24.
9. Classification and diagnostic criteria for headache disorders, cranial neuralgias and facial pain. Headache Classification Committee of the International Headache Society. Cephalalgia 1988; 8(Suppl 7): 1–96.
10. Olesen J. Revision of the International Headache Classification. An interim report. Cephalalgia 2001; 21:261.
11. Thomsen LL, Kirchmann M, Bjornsson A, Stefansson H, Jensen RM, Fasquel AC et al. The genetic spectrum of a population-based sample of familial hemiplegic migraine. Brain 2007; 130(Pt 2): 346–356.
12. de Vries B, Freilinger T, Vanmolkot KR, Koenderink JB, Stam AH, Terwindt GM et al. Systematic analysis of three FHM genes in 39 sporadic patients with hemiplegic migraine. Neurology 2007;69(23): 2170–2176.
13. Jen JC. Familial hemiplegic migraine, 2001 Jul 17. In: GeneReviews [Internet] (eds RA Pagon, TC Bird, CR Dolan, K Stephens). Seattle, WA: University of Washington, 1993–. Available from http://www.ncbi.nlm.nih.gov/bookshelf/br.fcgi?book=gene&part=fhm [updated 2009 Sep 8]
14. de Vries B, Frants RR, Ferrari MD, van den Maagdenberg AM. Molecular genetics of migraine. Hum Genet. 2009;126(1):115–132.
15. Gardner K, Barmada MM, Ptacek LJ, Hoffman EP. A new locus for hemiplegic migraine maps to chromosome 1q31. Neurology 1997; 49(5):1231–1238.
16. Ducros A, Joutel A, Vahedi K, Cecillon M, Ferreira A, Bernard E et al. Mapping of a second locus for familial hemiplegic migraine to 1q21-q23 and evidence of further heterogeneity. Ann Neurol 1997; 42(6):885–890.
17. Joutel A, Bousser MG, Biousse V, Labauge P, Chabriat H, Nibbio A et al. A gene for familial hemiplegic migraine maps to chromosome 19. Nat Genet 1993; 5(1):40–45.
18. Teh BT, Silburn P, Lindblad K, Betz R, Boyle R, Schalling M et al. Familial periodic cerebellar ataxia without myokymia maps to a 19-cM region on 19p13. Am J Hum Genet 1995; 56(6):1443–1449.
19. Ducros A, Denier C, Joutel A, Cecillon M, Lescoat C, Vahedi K et al. The clinical spectrum of familial hemiplegic migraine associated with mutations in a neuronal calcium channel. N Engl J Med 2001; 345(1):17–24.
20. Terwindt GM, Ophoff RA, Haan J, Frants RR, Ferrari MD. Familial hemiplegic migraine: a clinical comparison of families linked and unlinked to chromosome 19.DMG RG. Cephalalgia 1996; 16(3): 153–155.
21. Kors EE, Terwindt GM, Vermeulen FL, Fitzsimons RB, Jardine PE, Heywood P et al. Delayed cerebral edema and fatal coma after minor

head trauma: role of the CACNA1A calcium channel subunit gene and relationship with familial hemiplegic migraine. Ann Neurol 2001; 49(6):753–760.

22. Thomsen LL, Ostergaard E, Olesen J, Russell MB. Evidence for a separate type of migraine with aura: sporadic hemiplegic migraine. Neurology 2003; 60(4):595–601.

23. Ophoff RA, Terwindt GM, Vergouwe MN, van ER, Oefner PJ, Hoffman SM et al. Familial hemiplegic migraine and episodic ataxia type-2 are caused by mutations in the Ca^{2+} channel gene *CACNL1A4*. Cell 1996; 87(3):543–552.

24. Dunlap K, Luebke JI, Turner TJ. Exocytotic Ca^{2+} channels in mammalian central neurons. Trends Neurosci 1995; 18(2):89–98.

25. De FM, Marconi R, Silvestri L, Atorino L, Rampoldi L, Morgante L et al. Haploinsufficiency of ATP1A2 encoding the Na$^+$/K$^+$ pump alpha$_2$ subunit associated with familial hemiplegic migraine type 2. Nat Genet 2003; 33(2):192–196.

26. Stea A, Soong TW, Snutch TP. Voltage-gated calcium channels. In: Handbook of Receptors and Channels. Ligand and Voltage-Gated Ion Channels (ed RA North). Boca Raton, FL: CRC Press, 1995; 113–153.

27. Olesen J, Larsen B, Lauritzen M. Focal hyperemia followed by spreading oligemia and impaired activation of rCBF in classic migraine. Ann Neurol 1981; 9(4):344–352.

28. Olesen J, Friberg L, Olsen TS, Iversen HK, Lassen NA, Andersen AR et al. Timing and topography of cerebral blood flow, aura, and headache during migraine attacks. Ann Neurol 1990; 28(6):791–798.

29. Cutrer FM, Sorensen AG, Weisskoff RM, Ostergaard L, Sanchez Del RM, Lee EJ et al. Perfusion-weighted imaging defects during spontaneous migrainous aura. Ann Neurol 1998; 43(1):25–31.

30. Sanchez Del RM, Bakker D, Wu O, Agosti R, Mitsikostas DD, Ostergaard L et al. Perfusion weighted imaging during migraine: spontaneous visual aura and headache. Cephalalgia 1999; 19(8):701–707.

31. Jadjikhani N, Sanchez del Rio M, Bakker D, Wu O, Tootell RB, Fischl B. BOLD signal change in the occipital cortex during visual aura in migraine. Proc Soc Neurosci USA 1999; 25:1143.

32. Lauritzen M. Pathophysiology of the migraine aura. The spreading depression theory. Brain 1994; 117(Pt 1):199–210.

33. Leao AA. Spreading depression of activity in cerebral cortex. J Neurophys 1944; 7:359–390.

34. Goadsby PJ, Kaube H, Hoskin KL. Cerebral blood flow and metabolism are linked by nitric oxide during spreading depression. Aust N Z J Med 1993; 25:581.

35. McLachlan RS, Girvin JP. Spreading depression of Leao in rodent and human cortex. Brain Res 1994; 666(1):133–136.

36. Goadsby PJ, SNAP Database Study Group. The effect of migraine aura during an attack on the treatment outcome results from the sumatripan naratriptan aggregated patient (SNAP) database. Cephalalgia 2001; 21:416.

37. Ebersberger A, Schaible HG, Averbeck B, Richter F. Is there a correlation between spreading depression, neurogenic inflammation, and nociception that might cause migraine headache? Ann Neurol 2001; 49(1):7–13.

38. Goadsby PJ. The pathophysiology of headache. In: Wolff's Headache and Other Head Pain, 7th edn (eds SD Silberstein, RB Lipton, S Solomon). Oxford: Oxford University Press, 2001; 57–72.

39. Wolff HG. Headache and Other Head Pain, 1st edn. New York: Oxford University Press, 1948.

40. May A, Bahra A, Buchel C, Frackowiak RS, Goadsby PJ. Hypothalamic activation in cluster headache attacks. Lancet 1998; 352(9124):275–278.

41. Olsen J, Goadsby PJ. Cluster Headache and Related Conditions. Oxford: Oxford University Press; 1999.

42. Waldenlind E, Ekbom K, Torhall J. MR-angiography during spontaneous attacks of cluster headache: a case report. Headache 1993; 33(6):291–295.

43. May A, Buchel C, Bahra A, Goadsby PJ, Frackowiak RS. Intracranial vessels in trigeminal transmitted pain: a PET study. Neuroimage 1999; 9(5):453–460.

44. May A, Buchel C, Turner R, Goadsby PJ, Frackowiak RS. MR-angiography in facial and other pain: neurovascular mechanisms of trigeminal sensation. J Cereb Blood Flow Metab 1999; 21: 1171–1176.

45. Goadsby PJ, Knight YE, Hoskin KL, Butler P. Stimulation of an intracranial trigeminally-innervated structure selectively increases cerebral blood flow. Brain Res 1997; 751(2):247–252.

46. Riant F, Ducros A, Ploton C, Barbance C, Depienne C, Tournier-Lasserve E. De novo mutations in ATP1A2 and CACNA1A are frequent in early-onset sporadic hemiplegic migraine. Neurology. 2010;75(11):967–72.

47. Fitzsimons RB, Wolfenden WH. Migraine coma. Meningitic migraine with cerebral oedema associated with a new form of autosomal dominant cerebellar ataxia. Brain 1985; 108(Pt 3):555–577.

48. Snoek JW, Minderhoud JM, Wilmink JT. Delayed deterioration following mild head injury in children. Brain 1984; 107(Pt 1):15–36.

49. Tottene A, Pivotto F, Fellin T, Cesetti T, van den Maagdenberg AM, Pietrobon D. Specific kinetic alterations of human CaV2.1 calcium channels produced by mutation S218L causing familial hemiplegic migraine and delayed cerebral edema and coma after minor head trauma. J Biol Chem 2005; 280(18):17678–17686.

50. Munte TF, Muller-Vahl H. Familial migraine coma: a case study. J Neurol 1990; 237(1):59–61.

51. Vahedi K, Denier C, Ducros A, Bousson V, Levy C, Chabriat H et al. CACNA1A gene de novo mutation causing hemiplegic migraine, coma, and cerebellar atrophy. Neurology 2000; 55(7): 1040–1042.

52. Stam AH, Luijckx GJ, Poll-Thé BT, Ginjaar IB, Frants RR, Haan J et al. Early seizures and cerebral oedema after trivial head trauma associated with the CACNA1A S218L mutation. J Neurol Neurosurg Psychiatry 2009; 80(10):1125–1129.

53. Malpas TJ, Riant F, Tournier-Lasserve E, Vahedi K, Neville BG. Sporadic hemiplegic migraine and delayed cerebral oedema after minor head trauma: a novel de novo CACNA1A gene mutation. Dev Med Child Neurol 2010; 52(1):103–104.

54. Hart AR, Trinick R, Connolly DJ, Mordekar SR. Profound encephalopathy with complete recovery in three children with familial hemiplegic migraine. J Paediatr Child Health 2009; 45(3):154–157.

55. Chan YC, Burgunder JM, Wilder-Smith E, Chew SE, Lam-Mok-Sing KM, Sharma V et al. Electroencephalographic changes and seizures in familial hemiplegic migraine patients with the CACNA1A gene S218L mutation. J Clin Neurosci 2008; 15(8):891–894.

56. Romaniello R, Zucca C, Tonelli A, Bonato S, Baschirotto C, Zanotta N, Epifanio R, Righini A, Bresolin N, Bassi MT, Borgatti R. A wide spectrum of clinical, neurophysiological and neuroradiological abnormalities in a family with a novel CACNA1A mutation. J Neurol Neurosurg Psychiatry. 2010;81(8):840–3.

57. Connelly A, Chong WK, Johnson CL, Ganesan V, Gadian DG, Kirkham FJ. Diffusion weighted magnetic resonance imaging of compromised tissue in stroke. Arch Dis Child 1997; 77(1):38–41.

58. Ribeiro RT, Pinto MM, Villa TR, Gamba LT, Tengan CH, de Souza-Carvalho D. Migrainous infarction as a complication of sporadic hemiplegic migraine in childhood. Arq Neuropsiquiatr. 2009;67(3B): 906–8.

59. Toldo I, Cecchin D, Sartori S, Calderone M, Mardari R, Cattelan F, Laverda AM, Drigo P, Battistella PA. Multimodal neuroimaging in a child with sporadic hemiplegic migraine: A contribution to understanding pathogenesis. Cephalalgia. 2010. [Epub ahead of print] PubMed PMID: 21172953.

60. Butteriss DJ, Ramesh V, Birchall D. Serial MRI in a case of familial hemiplegic migraine. Neuroradiology 2003; 45(5):300–303.

61. Zajac A, Herman-Sucharska I, Kubik A, Skowronek-Ba**2**a B, Gergont A, Szafirska M. MRI and MRA data in children with migraine with aura. Przegl Lek 2007; 64(11):934–936.

62. Ganesan V, Kirkham FJ. Carotid dissection causing stroke in a child with migraine. BMJ 1997; 314(7076):291–292.

63. Zeiler K, Wessely P, Holzner F. The cerebral angiogram in patients with complicated migraine. Wien Klin Wochenschr 1985; 97(16): 667–672.

64. Holzner F, Wessely P, Zeiler K, Ehrmann L. Cerebral angiography in complicated migraine – reactions, incidents. Klin Wochenschr 1985; 63(3):116–122.

65. Gelfand AA, Fullerton HJ, Goadsby PJ. Child neurology: Migraine with aura in children. Neurology. 2010;75(5):e16–9.

66. Bates D, Ashford E, Dawson R, Ensink FB, Gilhus NE, Olesen J et al. Subcutaneous sumatriptan during the migraine aura. Sumatriptan Aura Study Group. Neurology 1994; 44(9):1587–1592.

67. Artto V, Nissila M, Wessman M, Palotie A, Farkkila M, Kallela M. Treatment of hemiplegic migraine with triptans. Eur J Neurol 2007; 14(9):1053–1056.

68. Dowson A. Can oral 311C90, a novel 5-HT1D agonist, prevent migraine headache when taken during an aura? Eur Neurol 1996; 36(Suppl 2):28–31.

69. Kaube H, Herzog J, Käufer T, Dichgans M, Diener HC. Aura in some patients with familial hemiplegic migraine can be stopped by intranasal ketamine. Neurology 2000; 55(1):139–141.

70. Yu W, Horowitz SH. Treatment of sporadic hemiplegic migraine with calcium-channel blocker verapamil. Neurology 2003; 60(1): 120–121.

71. Hsu DA, Stafstrom CE, Rowley HA, Kiff JE, Dulli DA. Hemiplegic migraine: hyperperfusion and abortive therapy with intravenous verapamil. Brain Dev 2008; 30(1):86–90.

72. Zangaladze A, Asadi-Pooya AA, Ashkenazi A, Sperling MR. Sporadic hemiplegic migraine and epilepsy associated with CACNA1A gene mutation. Epilepsy Behav 2010; 17(2):293–295.

73. Omata T, Takanashi JI, Wada T, Arai H, Tanabe Y. Genetic diagnosis and acetazolamide treatment of familial hemiplegic migraine. Brain Dev. 2010 Jun 11. [Epub ahead of print]

74. Enoki H, Takeda S, Hirose E, Matsubayashi R, Matsubayashi T. Unilateral spatial neglect in a child with hemiplegic migraine. Cephalalgia 2006; 26(9):1165–1167.

75. Guerin AA, Feigenbaum A, Donner EJ, Yoon G. Stepwise developmental regression associated with novel CACNA1A mutation. Pediatr Neurol 2008; 39(5):363–364.

76. Dodick DW, Roarke MC. Crossed cerebellar diaschisis during migraine with prolonged aura: a possible mechanism for cerebellar infarctions. Cephalalgia 2008; 28(1):83–86.

77. Ludvigsson P, Hesdorffer D, Olafsson E, Kjartansson O, Hauser WA. Migraine with aura is a risk factor for unprovoked seizures in children. Ann Neurol 2006; 59(1):210–213.

78. de Vries B, Stam AH, Kirkpatrick M, Vanmolkot KR, Koenderink JB, van den Heuvel JJ et al. Familial hemiplegic migraine is associated with febrile seizures in an FHM2 family with a novel de novo ATP1A2 mutation. Epilepsia 2009; 50(11):2503–2504.

79. Gallanti A, Tonelli A, Cardin V, Bussone G, Bresolin N, Bassi MT. A novel de novo nonsense mutation in ATP1A2 associated with sporadic hemiplegic migraine and epileptic seizures. J Neurol Sci 2008; 273(1–2):123–126.

80. Castro MJ, Stam AH, Lemos C, de Vries B, Vanmolkot KR, Barros J et al. First mutation in the voltage-gated Nav1.1 subunit gene SCN1A with co-occurring familial hemiplegic migraine and epilepsy. Cephalalgia 2009; 29(3):308–313.

81. Gargus JJ, Tournay A. Novel mutation confirms seizure locus SCN1A is also familial hemiplegic migraine locus FHM3. Pediatr Neurol 2007; 37(6):407–410.

82. Spranger M, Spranger S, Schwab S, Benninger C, Dichgans M. Familial hemiplegic migraine with cerebellar ataxia and paroxysmal psychosis. Eur Neurol 1999; 41(3):150–152.

83. Prabhakar P, Mohammed BP, Goadsby PJ. An audit in to the efficacy and tolerability of flunarizine in the treatment of childhood migraine. Journal of Headache and Pain 2010; 11(Suppl 1):74.

13
ALTERNATING HEMIPLEGIA OF CHILDHOOD

Jean Aicardi and Fenella J. Kirkham

Introduction

Alternating hemiplegia of childhood (AHC) is a puzzling disorder that combines episodic paroxysmal manifestations including dystonic crises with hemiplegic episodes, in addition to other neurological features, especially epileptic seizures. The hemiplegic attacks were the first recognized feature and the condition was named after them.[1] Progressively, other symptoms were reported, including abnormalities of ocular motor function,[2] dystonia and choreoathetosis, either paroxysmal or permanent,[2,3] quadriplegic episodes and autonomic dysfunction.[4] These features proved to be an integral part of the clinical picture of AHC and serve to separate the condition from other forms of episodic hemiplegia, especially hemiplegic migraine to which AHC was initially thought to be related. Indeed, probably only three of the original cases of Verret and Steele[1] actually belonged to AHC, while the other five cases were likely to represent hemiplegic migraine of early onset or a different type of alternating hemiplegia.[5]

AHC is a rare disorder; less than 150 cases had been reported[4,6–8] until recently when two articles from European study reported respectively on 103 and 157 cases, emphasizing the early onset (neonatal in 20 infants) and the non-progressive course of the disorder.[9,10] Mikati et al[11] collected 71 cases in the USA and were able to perform a detailed study of 44 of these patients. The disease is usually sporadic. Our personal series now includes 15 girls and 15 boys. Only five of these 30 patients had a family history of migraine and two of epileptic seizures. The frequency of a familial history of migraine is higher in several published series where it was found in 25%[10] to over 50%[8] of cases, although we systematically enquired about such a history. None of our patients had a family history of a similar disorder. However, Mikati et al[12] and Kanavakis et al[13] reported two families with several affected members in two or more generations, suggesting the likelihood of a genetic factor in at least some families. Two pairs of affected twins are also known but have not been reported so far to my knowledge. No cause for the disorder has been recognized.

Several infants had a history of neurological abnormalities. Nine were remarkably hypotonic at birth and four of these underwent a muscle biopsy on this account with normal results. A similar history is suggested in other reports[7,8,11,14] although muscle abnormalities were sometimes found. Five infants were reported to have had 'neonatal convulsions' although the possibility of early tonic seizures cannot be excluded.

The onset of AHC is always in childhood and, in most cases, the first manifestations appear within the first year of life, at times as early as the first few days[9]. The first definite attack of AHC appeared in the first 6 months of life in all but three of our patients and before 3 months in most. A later onset has been reported in a few of the patients reported by Mikati et al[11] (up to 6–7 years) and by Andermann et al,[15] although, in this latter case the disorder observed may have been distinct from the typical form. Despite these atypical cases, it is possible to describe a common clinical picture based on 30 personally observed patients.

Clinical findings

The clinical picture is generally stereotyped. The symptoms and signs can be schematically described under two types: *paroxysmal* and *non-paroxysmal*. The paroxysmal manifestations are usually observed in the first year of life while the non-paroxysmal features usually develop after months or years. Atypical cases are uncommon but have been reported in the past decade[15–17] and emphasized recently by Mikati et al,[11] suggesting that the condition might be heterogeneous.

Interestingly, the onset is usually not marked by hemiplegias.[9] In a majority of patients personally seen, these appeared after the age of 5–6 months and were preceded by other manifestations, making the diagnosis difficult. The most common initial feature was represented by paroxysmal eye movements[9] or tonic or dystonic attacks, suggesting the diagnosis of epilepsy, as was the case in 27 of our patients. Eventually, all patients have repeated attacks of hemiplegia or hemiparesis involving alternatively either side of the body. However, hemiplegias are never the sole clinical manifestation of the disorder and are always associated with, and often preceded by, other manifestations. Table 13.1 indicates the frequency of the different paroxysmal features in our patients. Dystonic attacks, episodes of diplegia or quadriplegia and abnormal eye movements were almost constant features, whereas epileptic seizures were present in 19–28% and dysautonomic features, especially dyspnoeic attacks, were seen in 7–48% of the children.

The frequency of non-paroxysmal features is shown in Table 13.1, illustrating that choreoathetosis and ataxia are extremely common, at least in patients followed for a sufficient length of time. These clinical findings, in addition to their unusual conjunction, also have individual peculiarities that make them quite distinctive and are described below.

PAROXYSMAL FEATURES

There are several types of attacks that recur frequently, at least once or twice a week in most cases. The exact frequency

TABLE 13.1
Clinical findings in 30 cases (15 boys, 15 girls) of alternating hemiplegia of childhood.
Age of onset of attacks: 3 days to 13 months (neonatal onset probable in four
infants diagnosed with neonatal convulsions)

Features	Number
Paroxysmal features	
Onset with dystonic attacks	15
Onset with bouts of hemiplegia	5
Hemiplegic episodes	30 (shifting bilateral involvement in 24)
Quadriplegic attacks	28
Tonic attacks	27 (unilateral in all cases; bilateral attacks in 9)
Paroxysmal nystagmus	24 (unilateral in 17)
Paroxysmal strabismus	11
Screaming, apparent pain	29
Vasomotor disturbances	23 (pallor, flushing, coldness, sometimes unilateral)
Disappearance with sleep	30
Paroxysmal respiratory disturbances	15
Non-paroxysmal features	
Learning disability/learning difficulties	26
Neurological signs:	
Choreoathetosis	29
Ataxia	27
Pyramidal tract signs	8

is sometimes difficult to assess, especially for hemiplegic episodes, because brief attacks sometimes occur in clusters and long episodes may be interrupted by brief periods of partial or total recovery. Paroxysmal phenomena are precipitated by a variety of stimuli in a large proportion or possibly in all cases. Most commonly reported are emotional triggers (e.g. birthday or Christmas parties) and fatigue. Medical examination frequently provokes an attack. Hot baths, cold and hot weather and bright lights are commonly reported precipitants.

Tonic or dystonic attacks are usually the earliest manifestation of AHC. They may occur as early as a few days of age and in most cases during the first year, especially its first half. In rare children, they can occur later but in virtually all cases before 3.5 years.[4,11] Unilateral attacks are most frequent, with rotation and tilting of the head to the affected side and stiffening of one side of the body which may be extreme, sometimes resulting in a vibratory tremor. Eye deviation to the same side is present. Bilateral tonic attacks feature arching of the back and upward deviation of gaze. The onset of attacks is sudden associated with fussiness and crying as if in pain. Dystonic attacks are brief, usually lasting only a few minutes but a few may recur in rapid succession for up to a few hours. They are often associated with dyspnoeic hemiplegic episodes.

Hemiplegic episodes
Hemiplegic episodes rarely occur as an isolated manifestation, especially in the early period, but often follow a dystonic attack so that they are often misdiagnosed as Todd paralysis. Their frequency and duration vary considerably. All our personal patients had monthly episodes or more, at least during a part of the evolution of the disorder, and most had weekly or more frequent episodes. Some children, however, had unexplained episodes of remission, lasting weeks, months, and even up to

2 years in one case. Brief episodes lasted a few minutes to a few hours, whereas long attacks could last several hours to several days, up to 2 weeks with an average length of 6–8 days. In some patients, paralysis occupied up to 50% of their time awake. In some children, there was a clear predominance on one side and this has also been reported by other investigators. Remarkably, the intensity of hemiplegia was fluctuating, occasionally disappearing briefly. In most cases, no pyramidal signs were present but they have been seen in several cases.[4,11,18] Dystonic posturing often alternated with flaccid weakness and usually resulted from attempts to move the hemiparetic arm. A disturbance of speech, apparently of motor origin, was experienced by some children whichever side was involved.

The effect of sleep is remarkable and mentioned in all reports.[2,11,18] Symmetrical movements are resumed within a few minutes of the child falling asleep. In long-lasting attacks, paralysis would reappear in the same location 10–30 minutes after awakening. This phenomenon is of crucial diagnostic importance and every effort should be made to elicit this information from the parents without suggesting the expected response. Many parents take advantage of the brief remission following sleep to feed the child, which may be difficult otherwise in severe and, especially, in bilateral attacks. Episodes of hemiplegia may disappear abruptly, especially when brief, but usually progressively over hours or days in more prolonged episodes.

Bilateral episodes are a very specific feature of AHC and occur in virtually all cases. As described below, they may appear in two different circumstances, either in the course of a hemiplegic episode at the time when hemiplegia, having started on one side, shifts to the opposite one (shifting attacks), or constituting the whole attack from onset.[18] In the case of shifting episodes, the duration of bilateral involvement is variable. At that point, feeding difficulties, such as choking on food,

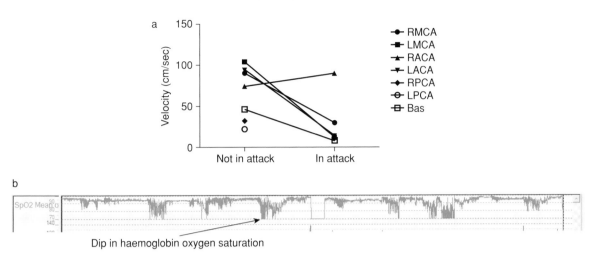

Fig. 13.1. (a) Velocities measured using transcranial Doppler in the right (R) and left (L) middle (MCA) and anterior (ACA) arteries in a 2-year-old child with alternating hemiplegia before and during an attack involving the right side. Velocities in the basilar, contralateral MCA and ACA and ipsilateral MCA are substantially reduced during the attack compared with baseline and are below the lower limit of normal (40cm/s for the MCA and ACA and 30cm/s for the basilar). The signal from the posterior cerebral arteries could not be obtained during the attack. This girl developed frequent bilateral episodes and also had severe obstructive sleep apnoea with dips in oxygen saturation (b); after adenotonsillectomy her bilateral episodes were very infrequent.

may occur. Respiratory problems may also appear (Fig. 13.1). Episodes of quadriplegia from onset may have special characteristics. These include marked facial involvement with amimia, profound, diffuse hypotonia and considerable feeding and respiratory problems.[17] Such episodes (see below) may be extremely severe and, when prolonged, may be followed by a considerable behavioral and cognitive deterioration, usually with slow recovery. Quadriplegic attacks can fluctuate in severity with waves of transient improvement, and paralysis temporarily disappears on awakening. However, it is not always possible, in our experience, to separate clearly attacks of bilateral involvement according to their mode of installation and shifting attacks may raise similar problems.

Dysponeic episodes: Laboured, noisy breathing is commonly observed, especially during bilateral episodes, as are irregularities in respiratory rhythm. In a minority of cases, severe dyspnoeic attacks can be life threatening. Such episodes probably include a spasmodic element and are associated with intercostal retraction and stridor. It seems likely that such episodes can be responsible for sudden death.[18] In one of our patients such dramatic attacks were considerably alleviated by tonsillectomy after documentation of obstructive sleep apnoea (Fig. 13.1).

Ocular motor phenomena can also be seen very early in life and are often the first recognized symptom. They were observed during the neonatal period in four of my patients. They are characterized by nystagmus, most often unilateral, or acute strabismus (see below). The nystagmus may be bilateral and of large amplitude and occasionally persist for long periods (days), although most episodes are of short duration (30 seconds to 3 minutes). Fusco and Vigevano[18] have demonstrated in some cases that the ocular involvement is in fact complex. They showed there was complete paralysis of one eye, while coarse nystagmus was evident in the opposite globe. Such features are reminiscent of what is seen in the so-called 'one-and-a half'

syndrome, which is thought to be due to involvement of the oculomotor pathways in the brainstem. Like other paroxysmal features of AHC, abnormal eye movement may appear as a part of a dystonic/hemiplegic episode or occur in isolation.

Other autonomic phenomena are frequent during or between attacks and variably include sweating, peripheral cyanosis, diarrhoea, abdominal distention, fever, mydriasis, pallor or flushing, the latter three being unilateral in some cases. Headache is present in a significant proportion of older children and vomiting in a few. Patients often yawn and appear sleepy but cannot get to sleep and appear extremely uncomfortable and fussy. The onset of attacks is sudden, associated with fussiness and crying as if in pain.

Epileptic seizures

It is not clear that epileptic seizures are a feature of AHC. The frequency of epileptic seizures in AHC patients varies with the reports from a low of 19%[10] to a high of 60%.[7] In a few cases,[9] ictal EEG recorded typical partial seizures with a characteristic sequence of fast rhythms and spikes in patients who had only some slowing of EEG rhythms during hemiplegic episodes. However, the actual incidence of epileptic seizures is difficult to assess because the dystonic episodes of AHC may be suggestive of epilepsy and because true epileptic seizures may appear only late in the course of the disorder. In three of my patients, clonic seizures, undoubtedly epileptic in nature, appeared at the peak of a hemiplegic attack, on the same side, whereas in five, they were apparently generalized and occurred independently. Status epilepticus occurred in two children.

Non-paroxysmal Features

Non-paroxysmal features of AHC are virtually constant but of quite variable severity and their date of appearance is unpredictable.

Delayed development or learning disability is present in most patients but is of very variable degree. Only four of our personal patients had a normal or borderline development and 90% of those of Mikati et al[11] were developmentally delayed. A majority of affected children have moderate to severe cognitive disability and approximately 15–20% do not develop communication skills. Patients with early onset of AHC are more affected than those with late paroxysmal manifestations. No detailed neuropsychological assessment has been reported, so the cognitive and psychological specificities are not known.

Delay in motor milestones is the rule. In my series, independent walking was acquired at an average age of 44 months and three patients had not achieved walking at 4 years of age. Fine motor control remains poor in all cases.

Fixed neurological abnormalities include gross hypotonia in most cases. Hypotonia was recognized very early in life, even at birth in several patients. Four of my patients had a muscle biopsy performed for severe hypotonia in their first year of life. No significant histological abnormality was recognized. *Choreo-athetotic movements* involving the face, trunk and limbs were almost invariably noted in our series, with variable intensity. This is at variance with the series of Mikati et al,[11] in which the symptom was recorded in only 50% of cases The reasons for this discrepancy are unclear, but duration of follow-up was variable and, in our series, all patients were personally examined. In addition, a dystonic component with the assumption of abnormal postures and slow torsional movements was present in many children. *Cerebellar ataxia* was also present in most cases. It was essentially static in type and may be difficult to assess because of the interference of abnormal movements with balance and normal voluntary movements. A minority of patients developed pyramidal tract signs and weakness on one side or bilaterally. In our experience, almost all children older than 5 years had developed fixed neurological signs.

Clinical course

The course of AHC is difficult to schematize as the severity of symptoms, frequency and duration of episodes and ultimate degree of neurodevelopmental disturbances are so variable. Longitudinal data are limited but although there is considerable variability, and the overall course of AHC seems to be progressive, at least in its initial period. Despite the recent report of Panagiotakaki et al (2010) that the course is non-progressive, there is no doubt that the clinical symptomatology is changing with time in the first years of course and that several attacks, at least, may be followed by obvious neurological and cognitive deterioration that may be regressive but whose outcome is not yet entirely clear. Longitudinal studies during the period including psychometric testing and repeat brain imaging are clearly needed. However, the onset may sometimes be in the neonatal period and in spite of the fact that 10–30% of infants may be hypotonic and delayed from a very early age,[4,11] the clinical findings may change with time. The course can be divided into two periods. An initial period with florid manifestations extends over the first 12–18 months of life, in which abnormal ocular motor abnormalities and dystonic attacks usually predominate, whereas hemiplegic episodes are not a major part of the symptomatology and may be absent altogether. Developmental delay is mild or even undetectable. A second phase features the complete clinical picture with repeated hemiplegias, often of long duration and often shifting from one side to the opposite, and quadriplegic attacks, sometimes with severe autonomic manifestations. Severe attacks, especially quadriplegias, are at times followed by definite loss of previously acquired milestones and an impression of cognitive deterioration.

Although mental function then slowly improves, no detailed follow-up study of cognitive and behavioural development is available to decide whether full recovery eventually results. In a third phase, although the hemiplegic attacks continue, the associated features tend to become less prominent. However, in a number of cases no clear difference between the second and third phases is apparent. There is, however, an overall decrease of IQ which may also result from absence of new acquisitions resulting from motor problems and from educational disadvantage. Later in the course, usually after 4–7 years of age, the frequency of hemiplegic and quadriplegic episodes may decrease but they have typically persisted up to adulthood in patients followed up to age 30 years. Neurological deficits become prominent. In most of our personal cases, choreoathetosis, dystonia or ataxia were present by 5 years of age although their appearance was often later than the florid period of paroxysmal attacks – usually between the ages of 2 and 5 years. All abnormalities then seem to remain static (e.g. in the father and paternal grandmother of the patient of Mikati et al after age 40 years), although complications such as pulmonary infections, choking and nutritional problems often supervene in severe cases and can result in early death;[20] however, one patient[21] first developed paroxysmal ataxia at 23 years of age.

The ultimate outcome of AHC is rather poor. Virtually all children have at least some degree of learning difficulties which are compounded by the high incidence of ataxia, choreoathetosis and dystonia to produce a severe educational disability. Only occasional children have normal or borderline cognitive function. Some may additionally exhibit severe behavioural disorders as was the case in three of my patients. A significant proportion have major disabilities including inability to walk, talk and swallow and have severe learning disability.

ATYPICAL FORMS

In some cases, a less stereotyped picture obtains. The most common atypical feature is a late onset of paroxysmal events after the first 18 months of life up to the age of 3–4 years.[11,12,15–17,21,22] Such a 'late' onset was observed by Mikati et al[12] in their familial cases and later in a few other patients.[11] In an occasional patient, the appearance of hemiplegic episodes is even later (up to 8 years) although dystonic attacks may have started during the first semester phase.[11] In late onset cases, the severity of the disease and of developmental delay tend to be milder.

A familial form of AHC has been reported in five members of the same pedigree in three generations.[12] In this family, the disorder may have been associated with a balanced translocation 46,XY,t(3;q)(p26;q34) that was found in four affected patients. Although the symptoms were typical in five patients, the onset tended to be late at 2 or 3 years of age and the severity was less than in usual, non-familial forms.

Another familial case has been reported by Kanavakis et al[13] in a Greek pedigree with six affected members in two generations (the mother and her brother in the first generation and four affected sons in the second). Another possible case (unpublished case quoted with the kind permission of Professor T. Deonna and Dr A. Ziegler, Lausanne, Switzerland) concerns a girl with a characteristic picture of AHC having started with dystonic and hemiparetic attacks at 3.5 years whose mother had had hemiplegic and dystonic episodes of short duration starting at age 12 years. The clinical picture in the mother was, however, not typical.

Other reported possible atypical variants of AHC include the cases of infantile hypotonia with paroxysmal dystonia,[16] those of benign familial nocturnal alternating hemiplegia[15] and of symptomatic alternating paroxysmal dystonia and hemiplegia.[17] For those cases, the diagnosis of AHC remains dubious as some of the most characteristic features of the condition, such as alleviation by sleep, were absent. However, a case with typical features other than late onset was diagnosed with Glut-1 deficiency[22] and this condition should be excluded.

Laboratory findings

The paucity of abnormal laboratory findings in AHC patients is in striking contrast with the florid clinical manifestations.

Routine biochemical studies have been negative in all patients studied except for low CSG glucose in the case with Glut-1 deficiency.[22] Serum and urinary amino and organic acids, plasma and CSF lactate and pyruvate levels, as well as CSF endorphin values, and histological and histochemical study of muscle and liver biopsies are usually normal. However, an increase of lipids or subsarcolemmal mitochondrial clusters have been found in some cases.[11] Karyotypes were normal (except in Mikati's family).

Electrophysiological studies have also been of little help. Interictal EEG is normal in most cases although in late stages interictal paroxysms may be present. Ictal tracings may show a mild to moderate slowing over the hemisphere involved that disappears rapidly on falling asleep. The most important finding is the absence of epileptic discharges. These may be present when typical epileptic seizures, mostly clonic in type, are recorded; recorded seizures have been focal, with repetitive spikes becoming slower as the discharge proceeds.[29] Evoked potentials have been normal in several cases.[24] Nerve conduction velocities, when measured, have been normal.

Neuroimaging, especially magnetic resonance imaging, does not show abnormalities although, in some cases studied late, a mild degree of atrophy may be found.[4,7] Progressive microcephaly has been reported clinically.[11] No change in

signal is recognized. Progressive atrophy of the cerebellar vermis has been reported.[24,25]

Pulsed Doppler study of the carotid artery contralateral to the hemiplegia showed an increased flow velocity (47cm/s) in one child and no difference in two other patients.[4] Single-photon emission computed tomography has given variable results with either hyper- or hypo-perfusion of the involved hemisphere.[25–27] The most likely explanation of these conflicting results is that there is decreased perfusion during the initial phase of the attack, followed by compensatory hyperperfusion during the recovery phase.[11,28] Only very few positron emission tomography studies are available and the data are difficult to interpret. Reduced glucose metabolism or cerebellar hypometabolism have been demonstrated in a few cases. Phosphorus magnetic resonance spectroscopy of muscles and proton magnetic resonance spectroscopy of the brain may show some evidence of mitochondrial dysfunction.[29,30] Thus, there may be a primary mitochondrial dysfunction in muscle although this may fluctuate and remains difficult to interpret. Indeed, the reality of mitochondrial abnormalities in AHC has been questionned.[31] The low *N*-acetylaspartate/creatine (NAA/Cr) ratio in the brain probably reflects some neuronal loss.

Differential diagnosis

Despite its highly distinctive features, the diagnosis of AHC is still commonly missed, especially during the early months of the disease. This is mostly because most physicians think of hemiplegic episodes as being the hallmark of the disorder, which often is not the case sometimes for long periods. Failure to appreciate that more specific symptoms than simply alternating or recurrent hemiplegia, which can be observed in many different conditions (Table 13.2), can be the predominant, and at times the only manifestation, is not yet widely appreciated.

Epilepsy is the most common misdiagnosis of AHC. Lateralized tonic attacks, followed by transient unilateral weakness, are often misinterpreted as seizures followed by Todd paralysis.

Additionally, vibratory tremor accompanying dystonic events can be mistaken for clonic activity and genuine epileptic seizures can also be an early feature of AHC. This misdiagnosis is often maintained for years despite the absence of true clonic jerking and of paroxysmal EEG abnormalities. Antiepileptic agents are ineffective and not indicated, unless the occurrence of real epileptic seizures can be demonstrated; video-EEG recording is very useful for this purpose.

Hemiplegic migraine has also been misdiagnosed as AHC, as probably happened in some of the first reported cases (see Chapter 12), and differentiation may be difficult in infants and young children who cannot express pain precisely. Hemiplegic migraine differs from AHC clinically by the absence of dystonic and ocular phenomena, and of quadriplegic episodes. In addition, it is not followed by neurologic sequelae or mental retardation. Some rare types, such as familial hemiplegic migraine due to a mutation of a calcium channel on chromosome 19q, may be associated with progressive cerebellar

TABLE 13.2
Differential diagnosis of alternating hemiplegia of childhood

Epilepsy
Postictal (Todd's) paralysis
Inhibitory seizures
Epileptic encephalopathies

Migraine and related conditions
Hemiplegic migraine (with or without recognized gene mutation)
Basilar migraine
Migraine – coma and atypical forms

Paroxysmal dyskinesias
Atypical kinesigenic or exercise-induced dyskinesias
Non-kinesigenic paroxysmal choreoathetosis
Paroxysmal torticollis of infancy
Paroxysmal episodic ataxias (especially type 2)

Metabolic diseases
Mitochondrial disorders, especially mitonchondrial encephalomyelopathy
    with lactic acidosis and stroke-like episodes (MELAS)
Leigh subacute encephalomyopathy
Pyruvate dehydrogenase deficiency
Ornithine transcarbamylase and other ammonia cycle enzyme deficiencies
Intermittent forms of organic acids and amino acids disorders Glut-1
    deficiency

Vascular diseases and blood coagulation abnormalities
Vascular (arteriovenous) malformations
Multiple emboli, e.g. atrial myxomas
Hereditary haemorrhagic telangiectasia (Osler–Weber–Rendu disease)
Cutis marmorata, livedo reticularis, Sneddon disease
Homocystinuria
Thrombocythaemia

Demyelinating diseases
Acute disseminated encephalomyelitis (chronic forms)
Multiple sclerosis
Schilder disease

ataxia, or other neurological features,[32,33] but not with bilateral paralysis and cognitive difficulties.

Paroxysmal dyskinesias of kinesigenic or choreoathetotic types have a number of similarities to AHC. The occurrence of episodes of dystonia or other abnormal movements, especially in the non-kinesigenic forms, may resemble episodes of AHC especially at onset when hemiplegia may not appear or be very brief. In some types of dyskinesia, interictal symptoms such as ataxia can follow the acute episodes. No other disorder, however, exhibits such features as quadriplegia and typical ocular manifestations that are probably pathognomonic.

All other conditions listed in Table 13.2 usually do not represent major diagnostic problems and their circumstances of occurrence and associated manifestations are quite different. However, rare cases of cutis marmorata congenita,[34] and perhaps of Osler–Weber–Rendu disease,[35] may raise some difficulties. Likewise, some of the features of AHC may suggest the possibility of mitochondrial disorders such as MELAS[11] but no actual infarct has ever been detected in AHC and the biochemical features of mitochondrial disorders are never found.

Treatment
No satistactory therapy for AHC is currently available but families require the support of a multidisciplinary team and

access to appropriate emergency services when necessary.[36] Antiepileptic agents are ineffective, except against true epileptic seizures when present. However, the benzodiazepines, especially clonazepam, may be effective in occasional cases, perhaps more so when combined with flunarizine.

Flunarizine, a calcium channel blocker, has proved to be of some value[4,8,11,37] in 50–85% of patients at doses of 3–15mg/day. The main effect seems to be a reduction of the duration and severity of the attacks rather than a decrease in their frequency. In some cases, a highly significant reduction of the time with paralysis is obtained. However, total disappearance of the attacks is very rare and recurrences have been observed in the few cases in which complete remission had been reached. Whether reduction in the frequency of attacks in cases of successful treatment with flunarizine protects the patients against neurodevelopmental sequelae is currently unknown. It has not prevented the late appearance of cerebellar ataxia and atrophy in the case of Nezu et al.[21] Undesirable side-effects, especially extrapyramidal symptoms and signs which have been reported in adults, have not been observed to my knowledge in the treatment of AHC in children. However, We recently saw a patient in whom the onset of treatment was associated with a marked increase in frequency and severity of dystonic attacks. These eventually were considerably improved with slow resumption of treatment.

Other agents such as haloperidol have been used and may also produce a reduction in the frequency of attacks.[38] However, no controlled study is available and side-effects may occur in the long term.

Encouraging results were reported in one boy treated with memantine, a derivative of amantadine hydrochloride,[39] with a dramatic response, and in two patients with the antiparkinsonian agent amantadine hydrochloride itself.[40] One of these patients experienced a marked decrease in the frequency of attacks that lasted almost 3 years. Both drugs are non-competitive inhibitors of NMDA receptors. These preliminary results, together with developing evidence that glutamate and NMDA receptors may influence the pathogenesis of AHC, suggest that glutamate toxicity plays a pathogenic role in AHC.[39,41] More experience with these and similar agents is needed.

A different approach to the treatment of AHC is represented by intermittent therapy of the incipient attacks. Administration of chloral hydrate rectally has been used by Siemes[42] and interrupted the hemiplegia without side-effects and not inducing sleep if a low dose was used (i.e. 300mg dissolved in sesame oil). A similar method using niaprazine by oral route has been proposed by Veneselli et al.[43] In one of our cases, oxygen was administered during attacks.

A recent report of successful treatment of a teenage girl with aripiprazole also reviews the pharmacology of successful and unsuccessful management strategies,[44] concluding that there is some evidence for benefit for those modulating dopamine or histamine pathways.

Comments

The clinical features of AHC are quite characteristic in a vast majority of cases. However, some reported cases exhibit significant differences to the usual forms. *Benign familial nocturnal alternating hemiplegia of childhood*[5,15] features hemiplegic episodes arising from sleep, usually of brief duration (2–20 minutes) and unassociated with dystonic features. Cognitive deterioration is not a feature. *Infantile hypotonia and paroxysmal dystonia*[16] was regarded as a possible variant of alternating hemiplegia but hemiplegic attacks occurred in only one of the reported cases. In one of the three affected children of this family, a few brief and mild bilateral attacks were observed. The patient described by Hart et al[17] had repeated hemiplegic episodes and dystonia but also permanent tremor and marked bilateral spasticity, so the nosological situation is difficult to determine. While all these children had features suggestive of AHC, there were also significant differences. They may represent only phenotypic variations of the same disease or belong to different entities. This cannot be decided in the absence of a reliable biological or genetic marker.

The causes and mechanism(s) of the disorder remain elusive. Although AHC was initially considered as a migraine variant, a number of its features are difficult to reconcile with migraine, especially the severity of the condition and the alterations of neurological examination, cognition and behaviour. The incidence of a family history of migraine, although variably appreciated, appears to be less than reported in migraine patients.

The possibility of a vascular mechanism involving especially the brainstem is suggested by the alternative side involvement and by the ocular motor symptoms that might be accounted for by a focal disturbance selectively involving vascularization of the median longitudinal fasciculus. It is supported by demonstration in some cases of hypoperfusion of the involved hemisphere followed by transition to iso- then hyperperfusion during hemiplegic attacks.[21,25,26,45] However, the findings have been conflicting, with some studies finding episodes of hypoperfusion during attacks (Fig. 13.1)[45] are non-specific and may well be secondary to a primary neural dysfunction.

The possibility of a mitochondrial disorder, suggested by similarities to the MELAS syndrome or other, less well classified cases of probable mitochondrial cause, has not been confirmed by direct demonstration, even though phosphorus MRS in muscle was occasionally shown to be consistent with mitochondrial dysfunction, and muscle pathology was suggestive in a few patients.[11,29,30] Such anomalies have not been fully characterized and they may well be secondary to an unknown undetermined aetiology.[31]

Evidence suggesting a possible toxicity of glutamate mediated through NMDA receptors[41] is mainly inferential.

The recent demonstration that some cases of autosomal dominant hemiplegic migraine are due to mutations affecting a subunit of a P/Q type voltage-gated calcium channel suggests the hypothesis that a 'channelopathy' might also be responsible for AHC. Channelopathies and AHC share several features: episodic occurrence, frequency of triggering factors, association of paralysis and positive motor phenomena. Such a hypothesis would account for many of the characteristics of AHC, especially its paroxysmal nature and the prominence of dystonic manifestations. Fixed deficits, including permanent nystagmus, ataxia and progressive cerebellar atrophy, can be observed in addition to the episodic features in some cases of familial hemiplegic migraine due to mutations of the CaCNLA4 gene on chromosome 19q.[33] This suggests that neurological sequelae can occur in ionic channels disorders. The recent recognition of familial forms of AHC, although rare, would be in line with such a hypothesis. Likewise, several epilepsy syndromes have been shown to be due to channelopathies and the frequent occurrence of epileptic seizures could be explained on this basis. It is now clear that the same mutations in ionic channel proteins can be variably associated with either epileptic seizures or with paroxysmal movement disorders.[46–49] It is possible that the response to flunarizine and to other strategies, including steroids[51] and airway management (Fig. 13.1), involve an effect on ion channels or any alteration in their function by hypoxic exposure. Moreover, acquired channel disorders do occur, the most common example being myasthenia gravis. Although attractive, this hypothesis is currently unproven and but further work along these lines is clearly indicated. Hopefully, this could lead to the discovery of more effective therapies.

REFERENCES

1. Verret S, Steele JC. Alternating hemiplegia in childhood: a report of eight patients with complicated migraine beginning in infancy. Pediatrics 1971; 47(4):675–680.
2. Dittrich J, Havlova M, Nevsimalova S. Paroxysmal hemipareses in childhood. Dev Med Child Neurol 1979; 21(6):800–807.
3. Krageloh I, Aicardi J. Alternating hemiplegia in infants: report of five cases. Dev Med Child Neurol 1980; 22(6):784–791.
4. Bourgeois M, Aicardi J, Goutieres F. Alternating hemiplegia of childhood. J Pediatr 1993; 122(5 Pt 1):673–679.
5. Chaves-Vischer V, Picard F, Andermann E, Dalla BB, Andermann F. Benign nocturnal alternating hemiplegia of childhood: six patients and long-term follow-up. Neurology 2001; 57(8):1491–1493.
6. Campistol PJ, San Fito A, Pineda A, Fernandez-Alvarez E. Hemiplegia alternant en la infancia: forma de presentacion, evolucion y tratamiento. Ann Esp Pediatr 1990; 32(4):336–368.
7. Sakuragawa N. Alternating hemiplegia in childhood: 23 cases in Japan. Brain Dev 1992; 14(5):283–288.
8. Silver K, Andermann F. Alternating hemiplegia of childhood: a study of 10 patients and results of flunarizine treatment. Neurology 1993; 43(1):36–41.
9. Sweney MT, Silver K, Gerard-Blanluet M, Pedespan JM, Renault F, Arzimanoglou A et al. Alternating hemiplegia of childhood: early characteristics and evolution of a neurodevelopmental syndrome. Pediatrics 2009; 123(3):e534e–541.
10. Panagiotakaki E, Gobbi G, Neville B, Ebinger F, Campistol J, Nevsímalová S, Laan L, Casaer P, Spiel G, Giannotta M, Fons C, Ninan M, Sange G, Schyns T, Vavassori R, Poncelin D; ENRAH Consortium, Arzimanoglou A. Evidence of a non-progressive course of alternating hemiplegia of childhood: study of a large cohort of children and adults. Brain. 2010;133(Pt 12):3598–610.
11. Mikati MA, Kramer U, Zupanc ML, Shanahan RJ. Alternating hemiplegia of childhood: clinical manifestations and long-term outcome. Pediatr Neurol 2000; 23(2):134–141.

12. Mikati MA, Maguire H, Barlow CF, Ozelius L, Breakefield XO, Klauck SM et al. A syndrome of autosomal dominant alternating hemiplegia: clinical presentation mimicking intractable epilepsy; chromosomal studies; and physiologic investigations. Neurology 1992; 42(12):2251–2257.

13. Kanavakis E, Xaidara A, Papathanasiou-Klontza D, Papadimitriou A, Velentza S, Youroukos S. Alternating hemiplegia of childhood: a syndrome inherited with an autosomal dominant trait. Dev Med Child Neurol 2003; 45(12):833–836.

14. De Stefano N, Silver K, Andermann F, Arnold DL. Mitochondrial dysfunction in patients with alternating hemiplegia of childhood. In: Alternating Hemiplegia of Childhood (eds F Andermann, J Aicardi, F Vigevano). New York: Raven Press, 1995; 115–121.

15. Andermann E, Andermann F, Silver K, Levin S, Arnold D. Benign familial nocturnal alternating hemiplegia of childhood. Neurology 1994; 44(10):1812–1814.

16. Andermann F, Ohtahara S, Andermann E, Camfield P, Kobayashi K. Infantile hypotonia and paroxysmal dystonia: a variant of alternating hemiplegia of childhood? Mov Disord 1994; 9(2):227–229.

17. Hart YM, Tampieri D, Andermann E, Andermann F, Connolly M, Farrell K. Alternating paroxysmal dystonia and hemiplegia in childhood as a symptom of basal ganglia disease. J Neurol Neurosurg Psychiatry. 1995;59(4):453–4.

18. Fusco L, Vigevano F. Alternating hemiplegia of childhood: clinical findings during attacks. In: Alternating Hemiplegia of Childhood (eds F Andermann, J Aicardi, F Vigevano). New York: Raven Press, 1995; 29–41.

19. Otakaki E, Gobbi G, Neville B, Ebinger F, Campistol J, Nevsímalová S, Laan L, Casaer P, Spiel G, Giannotta M, Fons C, Ninan M, Sange G, Schyns T, Vavassori R, Poncelin D; ENRAH Consortium, Arzimanoglou A. Evidence of a non-progressive course of alternating hemiplegia of childhood: study of a large cohort of children and adults. Brain. 2010;133(Pt 12):3598–3610.

20. Dalla BB, Fontana E, Colamaria V. Alternating hemiplegia of childhood: epilepsy and electroencephalographic investigations. In: Alternating Hemiplegia of Childhood (eds F Andermann, J Aicardi, F Vigevano). New York: Raven Press, 1995; 75–87.

21. Bourgeois M, Nevsimalova S, Aicardi J, Andermann F. Alternating hemiplegia of childhood: long-term outcome. In: Alternating Hemiplegia of Childhood (eds F Andermann, J Aicardi, F Vigevano). New York: Raven Press, 1995; 49–54.

22. Nezu A, Kimura S, Ohtsuki N, Tanaka M, Tada H. Alternating hemiplegia of childhood: report of a case having a long history. Brain Dev 1997; 19(3):217–221.

23. Rotstein M, Doran J, Yang H, Ullner PM, Engelstad K, De Vivo DC. Glut1 deficiency and alternating hemiplegia of childhood. Neurology. 2009; 73(23):2042–4.

24. Di Capua M, Bertini E. Evoked potentials and blink reflex in alternating hemiplegia of childhood. In: Alternating Hemiplegia of Childhood (eds F Andermann, J Aicardi, F Vigevano). New York: Raven Press, 1995; 95–98.

25. Saito Y, Sakuragawa N, Sasaki M, Sugai K, Hashimoto T. A case of alternating hemiplegia of childhood with cerebellar atrophy. Pediatr Neurol 1998; 19(1):65–68.

26. Zupanc ML, Dobkin JA, Perlman SB. ^{123}I-iodoamphetamine SPECT brain imaging in alternating hemiplegia. Pediatr Neurol 1991; 7(1):35–38.

27. Aminian A, Strashun A, Rose A. Alternating hemiplegia of childhood: studies of regional cerebral blood flow using ^{99m}Tc-hexamethyl-propylene amine oxime single-photon emission computed tomography. Ann Neurol 1993; 33(1):43–47.

28. Mikati M, Fishman AJ. Positron emission tomography in children with alternating hemiplegia of childhood. In: Alternating Hemiplegia of Childhood (eds F Andermann, J Aicardi, F Vigevano). New York: Raven Press, 1995; 109–114.

29. Zupanc ML, Perlman SB, Rust RS. Single photon emission computed tomography studies in alternating hemiplegia of childhood. In: Alternating Hemiplegia of Childhood (eds F Andermann, J Aicardi, F Vigevano). New York: Raven Press, 1995; 97–107.

30. Arnold DL, Silver K, Andermann F. Evidence for mitochondrial dysfunction in patients with alternating hemiplegia of childhood. Ann Neurol 1993; 33(6):604–607.

31. Kemp GJ, Taylor DJ, Barnes PR, Wilson J, Radda GK. Skeletal muscle mitochondrial dysfunction in alternating hemiplegia of childhood. Ann Neurol 1995; 38(4):681–684.

32. Kyriakides T, Drousiotou A. No structural or biochemical evidence for mitochondrial cytopathy in a case of alternating hemiplegia of childhood. Ann Neurol 1994; 36(5):805–806.

33. Vahedi K, Joutel A, Van BP, Ducros A, Maciazeck J, Bach JF et al. A gene for hereditary paroxysmal cerebellar ataxia maps to chromosome 19p. Ann Neurol 1995; 37(3):289–293.

34. Greenberg DA. Calcium channels in neurological disease. Ann Neurol 1997; 42(3):275–282.

35. Baxter P, Gardner-Medwin D, Green SH, Moss C. Congenital livedo reticularis and recurrent stroke-like episodes. Dev Med Child Neurol 1993; 35(10):917–921.

36. Myles ST, Needham CW, LeBlanc FE. Alternating hemiparesis associated with hereditary hemorrhagic telangiectasia. Can Med Assoc J 1970; 103(5):509–511.

37. Neville BG, Ninan M. The treatment and management of alternating hemiplegia of childhood. Dev Med Child Neurol 2007; 49(10):777–780.

38. Casaer P. Flunarizine in alternating hemiplegia in childhood. An international study in 12 children. Neuropediatrics 1987; 18(4):191–195.

39. Salmon MA, Wilson J. Drugs for alternating hemiplegia. Lancet 1984; 2:980.

40. Korinthenberg R. Is infantile alternating hemiplegia mediated by glutamate toxicity and can it be treated with memantine? Neuropediatrics 1996; 27(5):277–278.

41. Sone K, Oguni H, Katsumori H, Funatsuka M, Tanaka T, Osawa M. Successful trial of amantadine hydrochloride for two patients with alternating hemiplegia of childhood. Neuropediatrics 2000; 31(6):307–309.

42. Rho JM, Chugani HT. Alternating hemiplegia of childhood: insights into its pathophysiology. J Child Neurol 1998; 13(1):39–45.

43. Siemes H. Rectal chloral hydrate for alternating hemiplegia of childhood. Dev Med Child Neurol 1990; 32(10):931.

44. Veneselli E, Biancheri R. Alternating hemiplegia of childhood: treatment of attacks with chloral hydrate and niaprazine. Eur J Pediatr 1997; 156(2):157–158.

45. Haffejee S, Santosh PJ. Treatment of alternating hemiplegia of childhood with aripiprazole. Dev Med Child Neurol 2009; 51(1):74–77.

46. Bode H, Wick H. Abnormal cerebral hemodynamics during attacks of alternating hemiplegia. Childs Nerv Syst 1992; 8(4):231–233.

47. Szepetowski P, Rochette J, Berquin P, Piussan C, Lathrop GM, Monaco AP. Familial infantile convulsions and paroxysmal choreoathetosis: a new neurological syndrome linked to the pericentromeric region of human chromosome 16. Am J Hum Genet 1997; 61(4):889–898.

48. Lee WL, Tay A, Ong HT, Goh LM, Monaco AP, Szepetowski P. Association of infantile convulsions with paroxysmal dyskinesias (ICCA syndrome): confirmation of linkage to human chromosome 16p12–q12 in a Chinese family. Hum Genet 1998; 103(5):608–612.

49. Guerrini R, Bonanni P, Nardocci N, Parmeggiani L, Piccirilli M, De FM et al. Autosomal recessive rolandic epilepsy with paroxysmal exercise-induced dystonia and writer's cramp: delineation of the syndrome and gene mapping to chromosome 16p12–11.2. Ann Neurol 1999; 45(3):344–352.

50. Eunson LH, Rea R, Zuberi SM, Youroukos S, Panayiotopoulos CP, Liguori R et al. Clinical, genetic, and expression studies of mutations in the potassium channel gene KCNA1 reveal new phenotypic variability. Ann Neurol 2000; 48(4):647–656.

51. Wong V, Ho GC, Yeung HW, Ma KM. Alternating hemiplegia syndrome: electroencephalogram, brain mapping, and brain perfusion SPECT scan study in a Chinese girl. J Child Neurol. 1993; 8(3):221–226.

14
INBORN METABOLIC DISEASE AND ACUTE FOCAL NEUROLOGY

Robert Surtees and Fenella J. Kirkham

Introduction

Common metabolic problems can be associated with focal neurological disturbance in childhood.[1] In addition to the neonatal hypoglycaemia, which typically affects the white matter,[2] acute hemiparesis is well recognized in the context of hypoglycaemia secondary to idiopathic diabetes mellitus in children and adolescents, and is usually transient.[3,4] Seizures, coma behavioural disturbance, confusion and aphasia have all been described in addition to ataxia and hemiparesis.[3–5] One-third of the patients with insulin-dependent diabetes mellitus (IDDM) in one survey had experienced acute neurological symptoms of this type. Permanent sequelae have been documented, however, with hemispheric swelling acutely and subsequent unilateral atrophy (Fig. 14.1).[5] Recurrence may occur.[4]

Inborn errors of metabolism can cause acute focal neurological symptoms and signs (metabolic stroke).[6,7] The mechanisms which lead to metabolic stroke can be divided broadly into those associated with vascular disease and those that can cause brain tissue injury in areas that are selectively vulnerable. The latter may be associated with permanent damage (metabolic stroke) or the injury may be reversible (stroke-like episodes).

Suspicion of metabolic stroke is usually raised when the symptoms, signs or neuroimaging show an apparent infarct that is not confined to a single vascular territory. However, metabolic diseases can cause large cerebral vessel disease or the typical territories may be selectively vulnerable to a particular inborn error of metabolism, thus presenting as a typical stroke. There may be additional clues pointing to a metabolic disease, such as a family history of unexplained illness or sudden unexpected death in infancy. Often there are earlier unexplained symptoms in the child that may be gastrointestinal (anorexia, vomiting, failure to thrive) or neurological (developmental delay, seizures). The symptoms may be associated with a mild metabolic disturbance. The presence of these should heighten suspicion of a metabolic disease.

Many inborn errors of metabolism are treatable, some with very good outcomes if treated early. Because of this and because distinctive clinical features may not be apparent at the time of a metabolic stroke, it is recommended that individual inborn errors of metabolism known to cause metabolic stroke are screened for and further investigated as necessary. The individual disorders, screening tests and diagnostic investigations are given in Tables 14.1 and 14.2. The individual disorders will be considered further below.

Some inborn errors of metabolism can cause thrombocytopenia or a coagulopathy and this may result in cerebral haemorrhage.[8,9] These and their investigation are listed in Table 14.3, but are not hereafter considered further. Those metabolic conditions which appear to cause stroke through a coagulopathy, for example carbohydrate deficient glycoprotein syndromes, are dealt with under symptomatic stroke (see Chapter 15).

Inborn errors of metabolism causing stroke through vascular mechanisms

HOMOCYSTINURIA

Homocysteine is a highly chemically reactive thiol amino acid. Its sulphydryl group will readily form a disulphide bond with other free sulphydryl groups. Thus homocysteine can bind to itself to form the dimer homocystine, bind to free cysteine to form mixed disulphide and bind to proteins. Amino acid analysers normally measure concentrations of homocystine. If homocystine, mixed disulphide and protein-bound homocysteine are all chemically reduced and the resultant homocysteine concentrations are measured, this is termed total homocysteine.

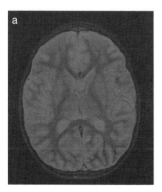 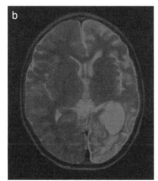

Fig. 14.1. MRI scans in a 4-year-old boy with recent onset of insulin dependent diabetes who presented in coma with hypoglycaemia. He had frequent seizures and raised intracranial pressure (opening 17, maximum 28 mmHg). (a) On admission showing diffuse swelling in the left cerebral cortex, with mild midline shift to the right. (b) Follow up 2 years later, when he had a right hemiplegia, right homonymous hemianopia, developmental delay, seizures and behavioural difficulties, showing left hemisphere atrophy.

TABLE 14.1
Inborn errors of metabolism that cause stroke through vascular mechanisms

Metabolic disorder	Screening tests	Diagnostic tests
Homocystinuria caused by β-cystathionine synthase deficiency	Plasma total homocysteine and methionine	Enzyme activity Mutation analysis of gene
Homocystinuria caused by remethylation defects	Plasma total homocysteine and methionine, plasma or red cell folates, serum vitamin B12, urine organic acids, blood spot acylcarnitine esters	Skin fibroblast enzyme activity or complementation Mutation analysis of gene (some)
Menkes disease	Plasma copper and serum caeruloplasmin	Skin fibroblast copper uptake Mutation analysis of gene
Fabry disease		White cell α-galactosidase A activity
Mitochondrial encephalopathies	Plasma and CSF lactate Plasma alanine	Enzyme activity Mutation analysis of gene

The pathways of homocysteine metabolism are shown in Fig. 14.2. Inborn errors affecting three enzymes (or the synthesis of their vitamin co-factors) are known to cause homocystinuria: 5,10-methylenetetrahydrofolate reductase (MTHFR); methionine synthase (MS); and cystathionine β-synthase (CBS). In addition, methionine adenosyltransferase deficiency, asymptomatic heterozygotes for CBS deficiency and protein variants (caused by genetic polymorphisms) of MTHFR and CBS can all cause raised plasma homocysteine (hyperhomocysteinaemia), but not homocystinuria. The clinical features of MTHFR and MS deficiencies are very similar and these are here grouped together, for the sake of brevity, as remethylation defects.

Homocystinuria caused by cystathionine
β-synthase deficiency

Classic homocystinuria has ocular, skeletal and central nervous system complications in addition to vascular disease. Undiagnosed patients with homocystinuria can present with stroke (Fig. 14.3),[10–14] typically with arterial occlusion and/or dissection,[11,13,15] although venous sinus thrombosis has also been described.[16] Typically, patients are tall with an increased arm span to height ratio, pes cavus, a high arched palate, and sometimes arachnodactyly and osteoporosis. Learning disability and psychiatric disturbances are common. High myopia and ectopia lentis frequently (probably universally) will develop. In addition to stroke, other thromboembolic events occur in around 70% of patients before the age of 20 years.[17] Treatment of classic homocystinuria (see below) greatly reduces the risk of thromboembolic disease.[18] Patients with classic homocystinuria can vary widely in their manifestation of these findings and in the rate of their acquisition.

The biochemical hallmark of classic homocystinuria is a greatly increased plasma total homocysteine (up to 100 times normal) and an increased plasma methionine;[19] homocystinuria is also usually present. A firm diagnosis can often be made on the basis of the clinical and biochemical findings. If necessary, or if there is some doubt, the diagnosis can be made by measuring CBS activity in skin fibroblasts or mutation analysis of the *CBS* gene.

Approximately half of patients with classic homocystinuria will be pyridoxine-responsive. This is investigated by examining the biochemical response to pyridoxine given in a dose of 100–200mg daily for one week. If the patient is pyridoxine-responsive, plasma methionine concentrations will normalize and plasma total homocysteine concentration will fall below 50μM. In pyridoxine-responsive classic homocystinuria, treatment with pyridoxine largely prevents the development of further complications. For complex reasons not elaborated here, pyridoxine treatment in pyridoxine-responsive classic homocystinuria can cause folate depletion and patients are usually given supplemental folic acid. If there is no response to pyridoxine, treatment is more difficult and consists of dietary restriction of methionine and the use of the methyl-donor betaine.[19] With such treatment, plasma methionine will normalize and plasma total homocysteine will decrease to between 50 and 100μM, but usually not to lower values.

It is also important to provide an "emergency regime" to try and prevent thrombosis at times of physical stress (such as surgery). Here it is important to maintain normal hydration with intravenous fluids and to treat with anti-platelet agents such as low dose aspirin.

Homocystinuria caused by remethylation defects

Remethylation defects are caused by inborn errors of cobalamin and tetrahydrofolate metabolism.[19] They are much rarer causes of homocystinuria than CBS deficiency, and only rarely present as stroke.[19]

The remethylation defects comprise biochemically three groups of disorders:

1. Inborn errors of intracellular cobalamin metabolism causing combined functional methylmalonylCoA mutase and methionine synthase deficiencies (termed cblC, cblD and cblF) which cause homocystinuria and methylmalonic aciduria.

TABLE 14.2
Inborn errors of metabolism that cause stroke through non-vascular mechanisms

Metabolic disorder	Screening tests	Diagnostic tests
Organic Acidaemias		
Glutaric aciduria	Urine organic acids Blood acylcarnitine species	Enzyme activity Mutation analysis of gene
Maple syrup urine disease	Urine organic acids Blood acylcarnitine species	Enzyme activity Mutation analysis of gene
Propionic acidaemia	Urine organic acids Blood acylcarnitine species	Enzyme activity Mutation analysis of gene
Methylmalonic acidaemia	Urine organic acids Blood acylcarnitine species	Enzyme activity Mutation analysis of gene
Isovaleric acidaemia	Urine organic acids Blood acylcarnitine species	Enzyme activity Mutation analysis of gene
Methylcrotonyl aciduria	Urine organic acids Blood acylcarnitine species	Enzyme activity Mutation analysis of gene
3-Hydroxy-3-methylglutaryl-coA lysase deficiency	Urine organic acids Blood acylcarnitine species	Enzyme activity Mutation analysis of gene
Hyperammonaemias		
Ornithine carbamoyltransferase deficiency	Blood ammonia Plasma amino acids Urine orotic acid	Mutation analysis of gene
Arginosuccinic aciduria	Blood ammonia Plasma amino acids Urine orotic acid	Enzyme activity Mutation analysis of gene
Arginase deficiency	Blood ammonia Plasma amino acids Urine orotic acid	Enzyme activity Mutation analysis of gene
Citrullinaemia	Blood ammonia Plasma amino acids Urine orotic acid	Enzyme activity Mutation analysis of gene
Mitochondrial		
Oxidative phosphorylation defects	Plasma and CSF lactate Plasma alanine	Enzyme activity Mutation analysis of gene
Fat oxidation defects	Urine organic acids Blood acylcarnitine species	Enzyme activity Mutation analysis of gene
Others		
Hartnup disease	Urine amino acids	
Porphyrias	Blood, urine and faecal porphyrins	Enzyme activity Mutation analysis of gene
Tyrosinaemia type 1	Plasma amino acids Urine succinylacetone	Enzyme activity Mutation analysis of gene
Sulphite oxidase and molybdenum cofactor deficiency		
Phosphoglycerate kinase deficiency		
Purine nucleoside phosphorylase deficiency		

2. Inborn errors of intracellular cobalamin metabolism causing functional methionine synthase deficiency (cblE and cblG) which cause homocystinuria alone.
3. An inborn error of the folate cycle enzyme 5,10-methylenetetrahydrofolate reductase which also causes homocystinuria alone.

Each has very similar clinical features that vary with the age of onset (and presumably therefore the severity of the defect). Isolated thromboembolic events have only been described in the later onset childhood and adult variants of these disorders.[20]

Remethylation defects are characterized by a raised plasma total homocysteine (ten times normal) and a reduced

TABLE 14.3
Inborn errors of metabolism that might predispose to cerebral haemorrhage

Metabolic disease	Screening tests	Diagnostic tests
Coagulopathy		
Congenital disorders of glycation	Serum transferrin glycoforms	Enzyme activity
	Clotting factor assay	Mutation analysis of gene
Galactosaemia	Urine reducing substances	Red cell enzyme activity
		Mutation analysis of gene
Tyrosinaemia type 1	Plasma tyrosine	Enzyme activity
	Urine succinylacetone	Mutation analysis of gene
α_1-Antitrypsin deficiency		Enzyme activity
Wilson disease	Plasma copper and serum	
	caeruloplasmin, haemolytic anaemia	Mutation analysis of gene
Fat oxidation defects	Urine organic acids	Fibroblast enzyme activity
	Blood acylcarnitine species	Mutation analysis of gene
Mitochondrial cytopathies	Plasma and CSF lactate	Muscle or fibroblast enzyme activity
	Plasma alanine	Mutation analysis of gene
Thrombocytopenia		
Organic acidurias	Urine organic acids	Enzyme activity
	Blood acylcarnitine species	Mutation analysis of gene
Remethylation defects	Urine organic acids	Skin fibroblast enzyme activity
	Blood acylcarnitine species	or complementation
	Plasma total homocysteine	Mutation analysis of gene
Gaucher disease	Blood film	White cell β-glucosidase
Pearson syndrome	Blood film	Large scale rearrangement or
	Pancreatic function	deletion mitochondrial DNA

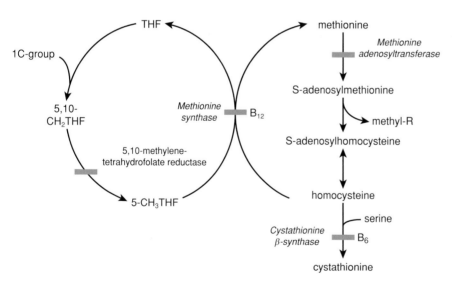

Fig. 14.2. Biochemical pathways of homo-cysteine metabolism. THF, tetrahydrofolate; 1C-group, a single carbon group (normally a methylene group derived from serine); CH_2, methylene; CH_3 methyl; B_{12}, methylcoba-lamin; methyl-R, a methylated acceptor; B6, pyridoxal phosphate. The B-group vitamin co-factors are shown in bold. The grey blocks show the sites at which an inborn error of metabolism can cause homocystinuria.

(or low normal) plasma methionine. Serum and red cell folate are decreased in 5,10-methylenetetrahydrofolate reductase deficiency, but serum cobalamins are normal or even increased in inborn errors of intracellular cobalamin metabolism. Definitive diagnosis depends upon studies of fibroblast single carbon metabolism.[21] Treatment is often difficult and is based upon pharmacological doses of cobalamin or folinic acid and the methyl-donor betaine.

CYSTINOSIS

Cystinosis is an autosomal recessive condition, with an incidence of around 1 per 100 000 live births, in which the transport of cystine out of lysosomes is impaired, typically because of a deletion in the cystinosin gene on chromosome 17; this can be treated with cysteamine. There is renal tubular acidosis and Fanconi syndrome, with eventually end-stage renal disease, usually by the teenage years. Dialysis and

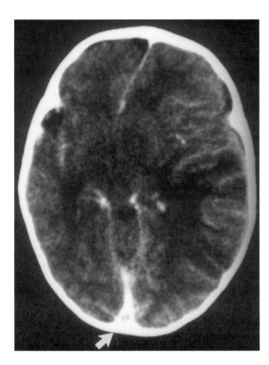

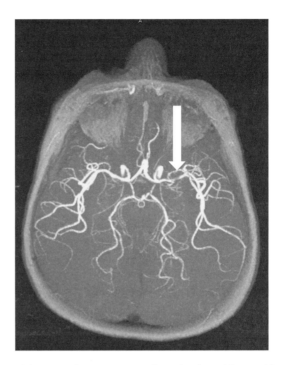

Fig. 14.3. Contrast cranial CT scan showing haemorrhagic infarct in the left hemisphere with massive oedema and shift of the midline in a previously well 6 month old boy. Contrast enhancement suggestive of thrombosis of the longitudinal sinus was also present (arrow). He died of massive cerebral oedema. Homocystinuria due to cystathionine β-synthase deficiency was diagnosed by metabolite analysis and confirmed by enzymatic activity measurement in a postmortem liver biopsy.

Fig. 14.4. Magnetic resonance angiography in a 14-year-old girl with cystinosis who presented with a left hemiparesis and had maximum transcranial Doppler velocities on the right of 194cm/s and on the left of 78cm/s. Although the MRI was normal (not shown), there is abnormal signal in the right middle cerebral artery (arrow) compatible with turbulence of blood flow or narrowing of this vessel. Over the subsequent few days, the velocities on the right decreased to 112cm/s and the hemiparesis disappeared.

transplantation prolongs life to at least the patient's early forties but cystine continues to accumulate systemically. In addition to cerebral atrophy[22] and idiopathic intracranial hypertension,[23] stroke and stroke-like episodes have been described and there may be cerebrovascular disease (Fig. 14.4).[24–26] An adolescent with a stroke in a vascular distribution had hyperhomocysteinamia and was also homozygous for the thermolabile variant of the MTHFR gene.[26]

FABRY DISEASE

Fabry disease is a lysosomal storage disorder that causes accumulation of the glycosphingolipid globotriaosylceramide in blood vessel endothelial cells, and, to some extent, in the vascular smooth muscle. It is an X-linked disorder and caused by deficiency of the lysosomal hydrolase α-galactosidase A.

First symptoms of Fabry disease usually start in late childhood, typically episodes of agonizing, burning pain in the palms or soles radiating up the affected limb.[27] These "crises" last from minutes to days. In addition, there may be more constant painful paraesthesiae affecting the same areas. It is not known whether the pain is caused by nerve ischaemia or autonomic dysfunction. Skin telangiectasia (angiokeratoma corporis diffusa) and characteristic lens and corneal opacities develop at around the same time. Renal and cardiac involvement occur next and may play a role in the development of

neurological complications.[28] Left ventricular hypertrophy is demonstrable on echocardiography in childhood.[29] Stroke and other cerebral ischaemic syndromes are said to occur relatively late in the disease[30,31] but in fact the diagnosis is often made after the first stroke.[32] Clinically silent lesions can be seen on MRI in the grey and white matter from the mid twenties onwards.[33] Stroke can be a presenting feature of Fabry disease in heterozygote females[34,35] as well as males.[34] The diagnosis should be considered in those presenting with stroke in young adulthood, particularly with posterior circulation disease,[36] although it is rarely the diagnosis[37] and the youngest patient reported so far was 19 at the time of stroke[35] so that in large databases of patients presenting in childhood, stroke has not been reported.[38] The diagnosis of Fabry disease is made by demonstrating deficiency of α-galactosidase A in white cells or by mutational analysis of the GLA gene, which was found in 2% of young adults with stroke in Portugal.[39,40]

Until recently, the treatment of Fabry disease was symptomatic. In some cases the episodes of neurogenic pain can be ameliorated by using phenytoin or carbamazepine (and gabapentin and amitriptyline anecdotally). Renal dialysis or transplantation is used to manage end-stage renal failure. More recently, enzyme replacement therapy has been undergoing clinical trials with encouraging success.[35,41]

MENKES DISEASE

Menkes disease is an X-linked disorder of copper transport and is caused by diverse mutations in a copper-transport gene, ATP7A, which causes copper deficiency. Menkes disease primarily affects the brain and the connective tissues, due to deficiency of important cuproenzymes (such as copper-zinc superoxide dismutases, cytochrome c oxidase, dopamine β-hydroxylase, tyrosinase, lysyl oxidase and peptidylglycine α-amidating monoxygenase and other copper transport enzymes). This results in a distinct clinical phenotype from around 3 months of age.[42] The male infants usually present with seizures, loss of developmental milestones or failure to thrive. They have pale skin and a cherubic face, scant eyebrows and sparse, white, fragile hair that resembles steel wool (Fig. 14.5). Light microscopy of the hair shaft reveals pili torti and fractures and is often the first screening investigation. Other connective tissue abnormalities may cause: Wormian bones, osteoporosis and metaphyseal dysplasia; diverticulae of the bladder and other organs; subdural haematomas; and tortuosity and occlusion of the intracranial vasculature.[43] However, the mechanisms of cerebral infarction in Menkes disease are far from clear and may not simply be based upon the cerebrovascular disease but also may have a metabolic component arising from the reduced cytochrome c oxidase activity (see below).[44] Cerebral and cerebellar degeneration continue and the neurological deficits become profound and cause death in early childhood.

Menkes disease is suspected from the distinctive clinical picture, light microscopy of hair and very low concentrations of serum caeruloplasmin and plasma copper. It can be difficult to diagnose in the first few months of life when plasma copper levels are naturally reduced. The diagnosis is made by demonstrating a defect in copper export in skin fibroblasts or mutation analysis of the gene.[45,46]

Treatment for Menkes disease relies on early diagnosis. Parenteral copper therapy can restore liver copper concentrations, but does not affect the impaired transport into the brain and has been considered to have little or no effect on the progressive neurodegenerative disease.[47] However, after screening boys at risk, 12 newborns were treated with copper within 22 days of birth[48] and survival at a median follow-up of 4.6 years was 92%, as compared with 13% at a median follow-up of 1.8 years for a historical control group of 15 late-diagnosis and late-treatment patients. Two of the 12 patients had normal neurodevelopment and brain myelination, both with mutations providing partial ATPase activity.[48]

Inborn errors of metabolism causing stroke through non-vascular mechanisms

Some organic acidaemias, urea cycle disorders and other inborn errors of metabolism can cause metabolic stroke (Table 14.2). Some mitochondrial disorders can also cause metabolic stroke (such as Leigh syndrome) whilst others can cause stroke-like episodes (such as MELAS). The mechanisms by which these occur are largely unknown. In the organic acidaemias and urea cycle disorders, metabolic stroke usually occurs within an episode of metabolic decompensation and it is likely that accumulation of a toxic metabolite causes infarction of a selectively vulnerable area of the brain. By contrast, mitochondrial disorders are liable to cause infarction because of deficient energy supply and by the generation of oxygen free radicals, again in brain areas selectively vulnerable. In some conditions, such as methylmalonic acidaemia, general vascular mechanisms may also have a role. In decompensated methylmalonic acidaemia, there is massive excretion of methylmalonate in the urine as its sodium and potassium salts, resulting in electrolyte loss. This can cause hypovolaemia which may cause ischaemia to already vulnerable areas of the brain.

ORGANIC ACIDAEMIAS

The organic acidaemias are a group of disorders characterized by increased excretion of individual organic acids (formed from vitamin, amino acid and fat metabolism) in the urine. The metabolic pathways involved in the three described in the text are shown in Fig. 14.6.

Methylmalonic acidaemia

This is caused by a defect in the conversion of methylmalonylCoA to succinylCoA (Fig. 14.6). This reaction is catalysed by methylmalonylCoA mutase, which requires 5′-deoxyadenosylcobalamin as a cofactor. Isolated methylmalonic acidaemia may have a defect in the apoenzyme causing reduced (mut⁻) or absent (mut⁰) activity, or a defect in the synthesis of adenosylcobalamin (cblA, cblB or cblH).[49] Inborn errors of cobalamin metabolism that cause deficiencies of both 5′-deoxyadenosyl- and methyl-cobalamin (cblC, cblD and cblF) have their clinical picture dominated by the remethylation defect and are briefly considered above.

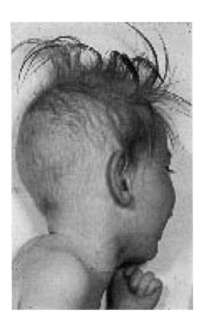

Fig. 14.5. Abnormal hair in Menkes' disease.

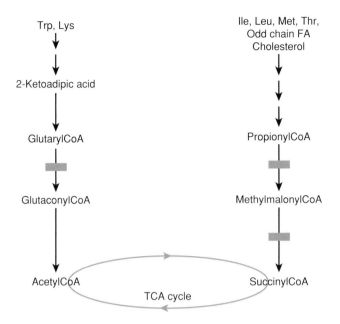

Fig. 14.6. The pathways of glutarylCoA and propionylCoA catabolism. FA, fatty acids; Ile, isoleucine; Leu, leucine; Lys, lysine; Met, methionine; TCA, tricarboxylic acid; Thr, threonine; Trp, tryptophan. The grey blocks show the site of the metabolic blocks.

Patients with isolated methylmalonic acidaemia commonly present in the first year of life with recurrent episodes of vomiting, failure to thrive, muscular hypotonia and encephalopathy. Acute, possibly focal, neurological syndromes can arise following acute metabolic decompensation (metabolic stroke).[50] This is normally associated with bilateral damage to the putamina and results in dystonia or complex movement disorders,[50–56] but can be asymptomatic.[57] However, cerebral hemisphere involvement can also cause diplegia or tetraplegia of pyramidal tract origin.[58]

Patients with methylmalonic acidaemia who have a defect in the synthesis of adenosylcobalamin often respond to high doses of cobalamin with a greater than 50% reduction in the urinary excretion of methylmalonate. These cobalamin-responsive patients (particularly if the disease onset is after the first month of life) have a much better neurological prognosis.[58,59]

The diagnosis is suspected by finding massive excretion of methylmalonic acid in the urine on organic acid analysis. Confirmation is by demonstrating reduced enzyme activity in skin fibroblasts. Gene mutation analysis is also becoming increasingly available.[50–59]

Propionic acidaemia
This is caused by an autosomal recessive defect in the conversion of propionylCoA to methylmalonylCoA (Fig. 14.6). The reaction is catalysed by propionylCoA carboxylase, which requires biotin as a cofactor. As a result of the enzyme deficiency, propionic acid, propionylglycine and propionylcarnitine accumulate in the blood and abnormal metabolites, including propionylglycine, propionylcarnitine, 3-hydroxypropionate and methylcitrate, are excreted in the urine.

Approximately half of the patients present in the neonatal period with lethargy, feeding difficulties, vomiting, tachypnoea and progressive encephalopathy.[60] The rest present later, usually with an acute encephalopathy. Occasionally, propionic acidaemia may present as a stroke.[60,61]

Metabolic stroke, affecting the basal ganglia symmetrically, appears to be a relatively common complication of propionic acidaemia. This normally occurs during metabolic decompensation in treated patients[62,63] but can occur without metabolic decompensation.[64] Usually the metabolic stroke manifests as a movement disorder (usually chorea, sometimes dystonia), but can be asymptomatic.[65]

The diagnosis is usually suspected by finding the characteristic metabolites on urinary organic acid analysis. Diagnosis is confirmed by enzyme activity analysis in cultured fibroblasts or by mutation analysis of the propionylCoA carboxylase subunit genes.

Glutaric aciduria type 1
Glutaric aciduria type 1 is an autosomal recessive inherited disorder of organic acid metabolism caused by deficiency of glutarylCoA dehydrogenase which catalyses the conversion of glutarylCoA to glutaconylCoA (Fig. 14.6). Glutaric aciduria type 1 characteristically presents as an acute encephalopathy between the ages of 3 and 18 months, with metabolic stroke involving the putamina and resulting in a subsequent movement disorder (usually a mixture of chorea and dystonia with the latter predominating).[66] Usually the metabolic stroke is symmetrical bilaterally, but it can be unilateral (Fig. 14.7). The encephalopathy (called an encephalitic crisis) is frequently precipitated by an intercurrent febrile illness. There is often a preceding history of developmental delay and macrocephaly

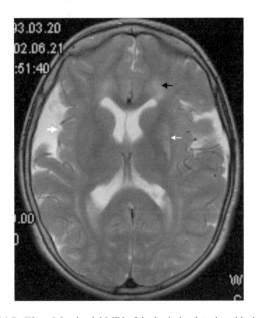

Fig. 14.7. T2-weighted axial MRI of the brain in glutaric aciduria type 1. There is signal abnormality in the left putamen (white arrow) and periventricular white matter (black arrow) and frontotemporal atrophy (broad white arrow).

may have become evident in the second half of the first year of life. However, there may be considerable phenotypic variability[67] Cranial imaging findings are almost pathognomic with "fronto-temporal atrophy" and signal abnormalities in the deep cerebral white matter as well as metabolic stroke always involving the putamina (Fig. 14.7). A recent study in an Amish population of 35 children with glutaric aciduria type 1[68] found wide middle cerebral (MCA), internal carotid and basilar arteries in all. In non-injured patients, MCA velocities were 18–26% below control values throughout late infancy and early childhood, whereas brain-injured children had an early velocity peak (18 months) and low values thereafter. Perfusion CT in six patients showed that tissue blood flow did not undergo a normal developmental surge. The three children (two non-injured) studied non-acutely had low cerebral blood flow (CBF), prolonged mean transit time (MTT), elevated cerebral blood volume (CBV) and high MTT/CBF and CBV/CBF ratios, compatible with low perfusion pressure and limited autoregulatory reserve with optimal substrate extraction at any given flow in steady state but risk of inadequate CBF for increased metabolic demand, for example during infections.

The diagnosis is important to make because there is some evidence that neonatal screening and treatment (dietary with supplemental carnitine) can prevent some of the neurological complications.[69] The characteristic metabolites found in urine (glutaric acid, 3-hydroxyglutaric acid and glutaconic acid) may not always be present and glutarylcarnitine concentration in blood should also be examined. The diagnosis is confirmed by enzyme studies in cultured fibroblasts or by mutation analysis.[70]

UREA CYCLE DEFECTS

The major function of the urea cycle is the detoxification of ammonia by incorporating it, bicarbonate and aspartate to form urea, which is excreted in the urine. The major biochemical marker of urea cycle defects is the accumulation of ammonia (and its transamination product glutamine). Acute neurological symptoms occurring in urea cycle defects are thought to be secondary to cerebral oedema caused by accumulation of glutamine, but ammonia is known to have many different effects on the brain that are not mutually exclusive, and more subtle effects may be responsible for some neurological symptoms.[71]

Ornithine carbamoyltransferase deficiency
Ornithine carbamoyltransferase (OCT) deficiency deficiency is the most common urea cycle defect. It is an X-linked disorder, but there is also a high incidence of manifesting heterozygotes in girls. Biochemically OCT deficiency impairs synthesis of citrulline, arginine and urea and causes accumulation of nitrogen as ammonia, alanine and glutamine and the diversion of carbamoyl phosphate into pyrimidine synthesis via orotic acid.

Affected hemizygous males usually present in the neonatal period with severe hyperammonaemic encephalopathy that is often fatal despite vigorous treatment. As a result of lyonization the clinical phenotype in heterozygote females is variable, even within one kindred. The most severely affected females present in the first year of life, some in the neonatal period, with persistent vomiting, developmental delay and failure to thrive. During acute exacerbations neurological symptoms such as headaches, irritability, ataxia and alterations in consciousness predominate. The illness has a characteristic fluctuating course with symptoms being aggravated by intercurrent infection or any other stress that precipitates protein catabolism. Some patients have few symptoms but may still develop severe encephalopathy unexpectedly.[72] Affected males who have residual enzyme activity usually present later in life in a similar way to the females.[73] OCT deficiency can also present as stroke (Fig. 14.8).[74–82]

The diagnosis is suspected by finding hyperammonaemia with raised glutamine and reduced arginine on plasma amino acid analysis, and the excretion of orotic acid in the urine. The glutamine may be detectable on proton magnetic resonance spectroscopy.[76] Demonstration of the enzyme deficiency requires either hepatic or gut biopsy and thus the diagnosis is usually made by mutation analysis.[83] Treatment is dietary.[84]

Arginase deficiency
Arginase deficiency is the least common urea cycle defect and prevents the catabolism of arginine to ornithine and urea. This leads to the accumulation of arginine and guanidino compounds derived from arginine, mild hyperammonaemia and increased urinary excretion of orotic acid, uracil and uridine.

Typically, children present with learning disability and a progressive diplegia with episodes of hyperammonaemic encephalopathy precipitated by incidental infections.[85] Seizures can also occur. There is often a preceding history of irritability, anorexia and delayed developmental milestones. Arginase deficiency can present as a stroke (personal observation).

The diagnosis is suspected from the biochemical findings and is confirmed by measuring red cell arginase 1 activity.

Citrullinaemia
Focal seizures and weakness with neuroimaging suggestive of focal ischaemia has been reported in citrullinaemia.[86] Plasma ammonia concentration is high and serum amino acid analyses reveals markedly elevated citrulline concentration.

MITOCHONDRIAL ENCEPHALOPATHIES

Mitochondrial encephalopathies are a diverse group of brain disorders caused by defective oxidative phosphorylation due to deficiencies of the respiratory chain. Oxidative phosphorylation is a ubiquitous pathway that supplies most organs and tissues with energy. The individual complexes of the respiratory chain are encoded for by both the nuclear and mitochondrial genomes. Thus, theoretically, defective oxidative phosphorylation can give rise to any symptom, at any age, in any organ with any mode of inheritance.[87] The mitochondrial encephalopathies are progressive, neurodegenerative disorders.

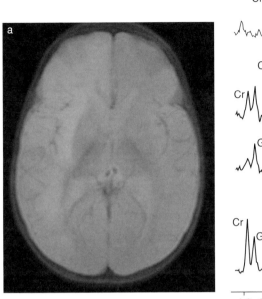

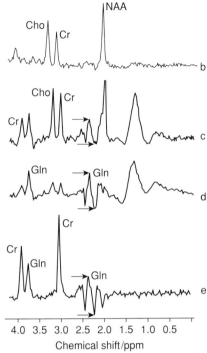

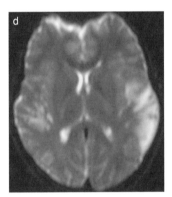

Fig. 14.8. (a) MRI scan showing right hemispheric swelling in a 9-month-old girl with a previous history of failure to thrive and nocturnal vomiting who developed a left hemiparesis. Her ammonia was 220 µmol/L and the diagnosis of ornithine carbamoyl transferase deficiency in a manifesting female heterozygote was made after her urinary orotic acid was found to be raised. (b–e) Magnetic spectroscopy from a normal infant of the same age (b), the girl with OCT deficiency on admission (c), the same girl 1 week later (d) and a phantom with glutamine (e). Glutamine peaks are seen in (c), (d) and (e) but not in (b). Cho, choline; Cr, creatine; Gln, glutamine; NAA, *N*-acetylaspartate.

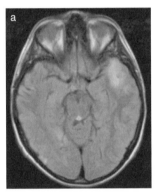
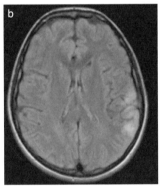
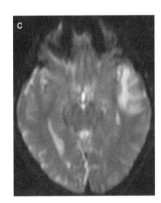

Fig. 14.9. MRI from a 6-year-old boy who presented with an episode of headache, vomiting and photophobia and was found to have a left hemianopia the previous year who on this occasion presented with dysphasia. There is abnormal signal on T2-weighted imaging (a,b) within the right temporal and occipital lobes compatible with previous infarction and a large area of abnormal signal involving both cortex and white matter of the left temporal lobe with mild mass effect and restricted diffusion (c,d). Plasma and CSF lactate were raised and genetic testing confirmed the 3242 mitochondrial mutation associated with mitochondrial encephalopathy with lactic acidosis and stroke-like episodes (MELAS).

Mitochondrial myopathy, encephalopathy with lactic acidosis and stroke-like episodes (MELAS)

MELAS is characterized by the stroke-like episodes, which normally start between 3 and 40 years of life. These present with hemianopia, blindness or hemiplegia, and are associated with infarcts visible on CT or MRI scans of the brain.[88–90] These infarcts commonly affect the occipital, posterior temporal and parietal lobes (Fig. 14.9). Usually the cerebral cortex is preferentially affected, the lesion often spreading across different vascular territories. Initially, the stroke-like episodes recover over a few hours or days with resolution of both symptoms and the neuroimaging lesions. However, the stroke-like episodes are recurrent and eventually result in permanent brain tissue damage causing seizures, dementia, hemiparesis, hemianopia,

hearing loss and early death. Imaging abnormalities also progress with cortical atrophy and basal ganglia calcification. The stroke-like episodes appear to be caused by both transient energy failure in the cortex and by a mitochondrial angiopathy. Patients can also have short stature, migraine-like headaches, psychosis, retinal degeneration, progressive external ophthalmoplegia, ataxia, endocrine involvement and cardiomyopathy. The skeletal myopathy is often not symptomatic or has minor symptoms such as exercise intolerance, but can present as rhabdomyolysis.[91]

Plasma, cerebrospinal fluid and brain lactate concentrations are usually raised in MELAS. A muscle biopsy often shows ragged red fibres, but these are not invariably identified. Approximately 80% of patients with MELAS have a heteroplasmic mitochondrial DNA A3243G mutation in the tRNA (Leu (UUR)) gene; this may not be evident in rapidly dividing tissues such as blood and may require analysis of muscle. Other mutations and mutations in other tRNA genes[92-94] and the POLG1 gene[95] can also be found.

L-arginine may improve endothelial function and lead to improvement in conscious level after stroke-like episodes in MELAS.[96,97] Long-term outcome is not independently related to neurological presentation and many of these patients have a good quality of life.[98]

Conclusions

Inborn errors of metabolism are an infrequent cause of stroke. However, they are important to diagnose because some are treatable, and all have genetic implications. Although most inborn errors of metabolism should have clinical features that will alert one to the possibility, this is not always the case. Children with stroke should be systematically biochemically screened for the possibility of metabolic disease.

REFERENCES

1. Pavlakis SG, Kingsley PB, Bialer MG. Stroke in children: genetic and metabolic issues. J Child Neurol 2000; 15(5):308–315.
2. Burns CM, Rutherford MA, Boardman JP, Cowan FM. Patterns of cerebral injury and neurodevelopmental outcomes after symptomatic neonatal hypoglycemia. Pediatrics 2008; 122(1):65–74.
3. Pocecco M, Ronfani L. Transient focal neurologic deficits associated with hypoglycaemia in children with insulin-dependent diabetes mellitus. Italian Collaborative Paediatric Diabetologic Group. Acta Paediatr 1998; 87(5):542–544.
4. Kossoff EH, Ichord RN, Bergin AM. Recurrent hypoglycemic hemiparesis and aphasia in an adolescent patient. Pediatr Neurol 2001; 24(5):385–386.
5. Christiaens FJ, Mewasingh LD, Christophe C, Goldman S, Dan B. Unilateral cortical necrosis following status epilepticus with hypoglycemia. Brain Dev 2003; 25(2):107–112.
6. Testai FD, Gorelick PB. Inherited metabolic disorders and stroke part 2: homocystinuria, organic acidurias, and urea cycle disorders. Arch Neurol 2010; 67(2):148–153.
7. Testai FD, Gorelick PB. Inherited metabolic disorders and stroke part 1: Fabry disease and mitochondrial myopathy, encephalopathy, lactic acidosis, and strokelike episodes. Arch Neurol 2010; 67(1):19–24.
8. Dave P, Curless RG, Steinman L. Cerebellar hemorrhage complicating methylmalonic and propionic acidemia. Arch Neurol 1984; 43(12):1293–1296.
9. Fischer AQ, Challa VR, Burton BK, McLean WT. Cerebellar hemorrhage complicating isovaleric acidemia: a case report. Neurology 1981; 31(6):746–748.
10. Taly AB, Nagaraja D, Subhash MN. Homocystinuria – a cause for stroke in the young. J Assoc Physicians India 1986; 34(8):598–599.
11. Lu CY, Hou JW, Wang PJ, Chiu HH, Wang TR. Homocystinuria presenting as fatal common carotid artery occlusion. Pediatr Neurol 1996; 15(2):159–162.
12. Cardo E, Campistol J, Vilaseca A, Caritg J, Ruiz S, Kirkham F et al. Stroke in infancy in a child with homocystinuria. Dev Med Child Neurol 1999; 41(2):132–135.
13. Kelly PJ, Furie KL, Kistler JP, Barron M, Picard EH, Mandell R et al. Stroke in young patients with hyperhomocysteinemia due to cystathionine beta-synthase deficiency. Neurology 2003; 60(2):275–279.
14. Linnebank M, Junker R, Nabavi DG, Linnebank A, Koch HG. Isolated thrombosis due to the cystathionine beta-synthase mutation c.833T>C (1278T). J Inherit Metab Dis 2003; 26(5):509–511.
15. Weiss N, Demeret S, Sonneville R, Guillevin R, Bolgert F, Pierrot-Deseilligny C. Bilateral internal carotid artery dissection in cystathionine beta-synthase deficiency. Eur Neurol 2006; 55(3):177–178.
16. Buoni S, Molinelli M, Mariottini A, Rango C, Medaglini S, Pieri S et al. Homocystinuria with transverse sinus thrombosis. J Child Neurol 2001; 16(9):688–690.
17. Mudd SH, Skovby F, Levy HL, Pettigrew KD, Wilcken B, Pyeritz RE et al. The natural history of homocystinuria due to cystathionine beta-synthase deficiency. Am J Hum Genet 1985; 37(1):1–31.
18. Yap S. Classical homocystinuria: vascular risk and its prevention. J Inherit Metab Dis 2003; 26(2–3):259–265.
19. Surtees R, Bowron A, Leonard J. Cerebrospinal fluid and plasma total homocysteine and related metabolites in children with cystathionine beta-synthase deficiency: the effect of treatment. Pediatr Res 1997; 42(5):577–582.
20. Surtees R. Cobalamin and folate responsive disorders. In: Vitamin Responsive Conditions in Paediatric Neurology (ed Bacter P). London: McKeith Press, 2001; 96–109.
21. Visy JM, Le CP, Chadefaux B, Fressinaud C, Woimant F, Marquet J et al. Homocystinuria due to 5,10-methylenetetrahydrofolate reductase deficiency revealed by stroke in adult siblings. Neurology 1991; 41(8):1313–1315.
22. Fink JK, Brouwers P, Barton N, Malekzadeh MH, Sato S, Hill S et al. Neurologic complications in long-standing nephropathic cystinosis. Arch Neurol 1989; 46(5):543–548.
23. Nesterova G, Gahl W. Nephropathic cystinosis: late complications of a multisystemic disease. Pediatr Nephrol 2007; 147(4):247–250.
24. van Lierde A, Colombo D, Rossi LN. Hemiparesis in a girl with cystinosis and renal transplant. Eur J Pediatr 1994; 153(9): 702–703.
25. Broyer M, Tete MJ, Guest G, Bertheleme JP, Labrousse F, Poisson M. Clinical polymorphism of cystinosis encephalopathy. Results of treatment with cysteamine. J Inherit Metab Dis 1996; 19(1):65–75.
26. Merouani A, Genest J, Jr., Rozen R, Lambert M, Mitchell GA, Dubois J et al. Cerebral vascular complication and hyperhomocysteinemia in a cystinotic uremic child. Pediatr Nephrol 1999; 13(1):73–76.
27. Ramaswamy V, Miller SP, Barkovich AJ, Partridge JC, Ferriero DM. Perinatal stroke in term infants with neonatal encephalopathy. Neurology 2004; 62(11):2088–2091.
28. Burlina AP, Manara R, Caillaud C, Laissy JP, Severino M, Klein I et al. The pulvinar sign: frequency and clinical correlations in Fabry disease. J Neurol 2008; 255(5):738–744.
29. Ries M, Gupta S, Moore DF, Sachdev V, Quirk JM, Murray GJ et al. Pediatric Fabry disease. Pediatrics 2005; 115(3):e344–e355.
30. Fowler B, Jakobs C. Post- and prenatal diagnostic methods for the homocystinurias. Eur J Pediatr 1998; 157(Suppl 2):S88–S93.
31. Schiffmann R. Natural history of Fabry disease in males: preliminary observations. J Inherit Metab Dis 2001; 24(Suppl 2):15–17.
32. Sims K, Politei J, Banikazemi M, Lee P. Stroke in Fabry disease frequently occurs before diagnosis and in the absence of other clinical events: natural history data from the Fabry Registry. Stroke 2009; 40(3):788–794.
33. Crutchfield KE, Patronas NJ, Dambrosia JM, Frei KP, Banerjee TK, Barton NW et al. Quantitative analysis of cerebral vasculopathy in patients with Fabry disease. Neurology 1998; 50(6):1746–1749.
34. Grewal RP. Stroke in Fabry's disease. J Neurol 1994; 241(3):153–156.
35. Giacomini PS, Shannon PT, Clarke JT, Jaigobin C. Fabry's disease presenting as stroke in a young female. Can J Neurol Sci 2004; 31(1):112–114.
36. Rolfs A, Bottcher T, Zschiesche M, Morris P, Winchester B, Bauer P et al. Prevalence of Fabry disease in patients with cryptogenic stroke: a prospective study. Lancet 2005; 366(9499):1794–1796.
37. Brouns R, Sheorajpanday R, Braxel E, Eyskens F, Baker R, Hughes D et al. Middelheim Fabry Study (MiFaS): a retrospective Belgian study on the prevalence of Fabry disease in young patients with cryptogenic stroke. Clin Neurol Neurosurg 2007; 109(6):479–484.
38. Ramaswami U, Whybra C, Parini R, Pintos-Morell G, Mehta A, Sunder-Plassmann G et al. Clinical manifestations of Fabry disease in children: data from the Fabry Outcome Survey. Acta Paediatr 2006; 95(1):86–92.

39. Baptista MV, Ferreira S, Pinho-E-Melo, Carvalho M, Cruz VT, Carmona C et al. Mutations of the GLA gene in young patients with stroke. The PORTYSTROKE Study – Screening Genetic Conditions in PORTuguese Young STROKE Patients. Stroke 2010; 41(3):431–436.

40. Brouns R, Thijs V, Eyskens F, Van den Broeck M, Belachew S, Van Broeckhoven C, et al; for the BeFaS Investigators. Belgian Fabry Study. Prevalence of Fabry Disease in a Cohort of 1000 Young Patients With Cerebrovascular Disease. Stroke. 2010; 41(5):863–868.

41. Ries M, Clarke JT, Whybra C, Timmons M, Robinson C, Schlaggar BL et al. Enzyme-replacement therapy with agalsidase alfa in children with Fabry disease. Pediatrics 2006; 118(3):924–932.

42. Desnick RJ. Enzyme replacement and enhancement therapies for lysosomal diseases. J Inherit Metab Dis 2004; 27(3):385–410.

43. Menkes JH. Menkes disease and Wilson disease: two sides of the same copper coin. Part I: Menkes disease. Eur J Paediatr Neurol 1999; 3(4):147–158.

44. Barkovich AJ, Good WV, Koch TK, Berg BO. Mitochondrial disorders: analysis of their clinical and imaging characteristics. AJNR Am J Neuroradiol 1993; 14(5):1119–1137.

45. Goldstein DS, Holmes CS, Kaler SG. Relative efficiencies of plasma catechol levels and ratios for neonatal diagnosis of Menkes disease. Neurochem Res 2009; 34(8):1464–1468.

46. Tonnesen T, Horn N. Prenatal and postnatal diagnosis of Menkes disease, an inherited disorder of copper metabolism. J Inherit Metab Dis 1989; 12(Suppl 1):207–214.

47. Tumer Z, Tonnesen T, Horn N. Detection of genetic defects in Menkes disease by direct mutation analysis and its implications in carrier diagnosis. J Inherit Metab Dis 1994; 17(3):267–270.

48. Kaler SG, Holmes CS, Goldstein DS, Tang J, Godwin SC, Donsante A et al. Neonatal diagnosis and treatment of Menkes disease. N Engl J Med 2008; 358(6):605–614.

49. Watkins D, Matiaszuk N, Rosenblatt DS. Complementation studies in the cblA class of inborn error of cobalamin metabolism: evidence for interallelic complementation and for a new complementation class (cblH). J Med Genet 2000; 37(7):510–513.

50. Nicolaides P, Leonard J, Surtees R. Neurological outcome of methylmalonic acidaemia. Arch Dis Child 1998; 78(6):508–512.

51. Thompson GN, Christodoulou J, Danks DM. Metabolic stroke in methylmalonic acidemia. J Pediatr 1989; 115(3):499–500.

52. Heidenreich R, Natowicz M, Hainline BE, Berman P, Kelley RI, Hillman RE et al. Acute extrapyramidal syndrome in methylmalonic acidemia: "metabolic stroke" involving the globus pallidus. J Pediatr 1988; 113(6):1022–1027.

53. de Sousa C, Piesowicz AT, Brett EM, Leonard JV. Focal changes in the globi pallidi associated with neurological dysfunction in methylmalonic acidaemia. Neuropediatrics 1989; 20(4):199–201.

54. Shevell MI, Matiaszuk N, Ledley FD, Rosenblatt DS. Varying neurological phenotypes among muto and mut- patients with methylmalonylCoA mutase deficiency. Am J Med Genet 1993; 45(5):619–624.

55. Roodhooft AM, Baumgartner ER, Martin JJ, Blom W, Van Acker KJ. Symmetrical necrosis of the basal ganglia in methylmalonic acidaemia. Eur J Pediatr 1990; 149(8):582–584.

56. Burlina AP, Manara R, Calderone M, Catuogno S, Burlina AB. Diffusion-weighted imaging in the assessment of neurological damage in patients with methylmalonic aciduria. J Inherit Metab Dis 2003; 26(5):417–422.

57. Peters HL, Nefedov M, Lee LW, Abdenur JE, Chamoles NA, Kahler SG et al. Molecular studies in mutase-deficient (MUT) methylmalonic aciduria: identification of five novel mutations. Hum Mutat 2002; 20(5):406.

58. Dobson CM, Wai T, Leclerc D, Kadir H, Narang M, Lerner-Ellis JP et al. Identification of the gene responsible for the cblB complementation group of vitamin B_{12}-dependent methylmalonic aciduria. Hum Mol Genet 2002; 11(26):3361–3369.

59. Zwickler T, Lindner M, Aydin HI, Baumgartner MR, Bodamer OA, Burlina AB et al. Diagnostic work-up and management of patients with isolated methylmalonic acidurias in European metabolic centres. J Inherit Metab Dis 2008; 31(3):361–367.

60. Surtees RA, Matthews EE, Leonard JV. Neurologic outcome of propionic acidemia. Pediatr Neurol 1992; 8(5):333–337.

61. Shigematsu Y, Mori I, Nakai A, Kikawa Y, Kuriyama M, Konishi Y et al. Acute infantile hemiplegia in a patient with propionic acidaemia. Eur J Pediatr 1990; 149(9):659–660.

62. Perez-Cerda C, Merinero B, Marti M, Cabrera JC, Pena L, Garcia MJ et al. An unusual late-onset case of propionic acidaemia: biochemical investigations, neuroradiological findings and mutation analysis. Eur J Pediatr 1998; 157(1):50–52.

63. Burlina AB, Ogier H, Korall H, Trefz FK. Long-term treatment with sodium phenylbutyrate in ornithine transcarbamylase-deficient patients. Mol Genet Metab 2001; 72(4):351–355.

64. Haas RH, Marsden DL, Capistrano-Estrada S, Hamilton R, Grafe MR, Wong W et al. Acute basal ganglia infarction in propionic acidemia. J Child Neurol 1995; 10(1):18–22.

65. Strauss KA, Puffenberger EG, Robinson DL, Morton DH. Type I glutaric aciduria, part 1: natural history of 77 patients. Am J Med Genet C Semin Med Genet 2003; 121C(1):38–52.

66. Zafeiriou DI, Zschocke J, Ugoustidou-Savvopoulou P, Mauromatis I, Sewell A, Kontopoulos E et al. Atypical and variable clinical presentation of glutaric aciduria type I. Neuropediatrics 2000; 31(6):303–306.

67. Hoffmann GF, Zschocke J. Glutaric aciduria type I: from clinical, biochemical and molecular diversity to successful therapy. J Inherit Metab Dis 1999; 22(4):381–391.

68. Strauss KA, Donnelly P, Wintermark M. Cerebral haemodynamics in patients with glutaryl-coenzyme A dehydrogenase deficiency. Brain 2010; 133(Pt 1):76–92.

69. Boneh A, Beauchamp M, Humphrey M, Watkins J, Peters H, Yaplito-Lee J. Newborn screening for glutaric aciduria type I in Victoria: treatment and outcome. Mol Genet Metab 2008; 94(3):287–291.

70. Zschocke J, Quak E, Guldberg P, Hoffmann GF. Mutation analysis in glutaric aciduria type I. J Med Genet 2000; 37(3):177–181.

71. Butterworth RF. Effects of hyperammonaemia on brain function. J Inherit Metab Dis 1998; 21(Suppl 1):6–20.

72. Gilchrist JM, Coleman RA. Ornithine transcarbamylase deficiency: adult onset of severe symptoms. Ann Intern Med 1987; 106(4):556–558.

73. Drogari E, Leonard JV. Late onset ornithine carbamoyl transferase deficiency in males. Arch Dis Child 1988; 63(11):1363–1367.

74. Kendall BE, Kingsley DP, Leonard JV, Lingam S, Oberholzer VG. Neurological features and computed tomography of the brain in children with ornithine carbamoyl transferase deficiency. J Neurol Neurosurg Psychiatry 1983; 46(1):28–34.

75. Lacey DJ, Duffner PK, Cohen ME, Mosovich L. Unusual biochemical and clinical features in a girl with ornithine transcarbamylase deficiency. Pediatr Neurol 1986; 2(1):51–53.

76. Connelly A, Cross JH, Gadian DG, Hunter JV, Kirkham FJ, Leonard JV. Magnetic resonance spectroscopy shows increased brain glutamine in ornithine carbamoyl transferase deficiency. Pediatr Res 1993; 33(1):77–81.

77. Bajaj SK, Kurlemann G, Schuierer G, Peters PE. CT and MRI in a girl with late-onset ornithine transcarbamylase deficiency: case report. Neuroradiology 1996; 38(8):796–799.

78. Christodoulou J, Qureshi IA, McInnes RR, Clarke JT. Ornithine transcarbamylase deficiency presenting with strokelike episodes. J Pediatr 1993; 122(3):423–425.

79. Mamourian AC, du PA. Urea cycle defect: a case with MR and CT findings resembling infarct. Pediatr Radiol 1991; 21(8):594–595.

80. De Grauw TJ, Smit LM, Brockstedt M, Meijer Y, vd Klei-von Moorsel J, Jakobs C. Acute hemiparesis as the presenting sign in a heterozygote for ornithine transcarbamylase deficiency. Neuropediatrics 1990; 21(3):133–135.

81. Keegan CE, Martin DM, Quint DJ, Gorski JL. Acute extrapyramidal syndrome in mild ornithine transcarbamylase deficiency: metabolic stroke involving the caudate and putamen without metabolic decompensation. Eur J Pediatr 2003; 162(4):259–263.

82. Nicolaides P, Liebsch D, Dale N, Leonard J, Surtees R. Neurological outcome of patients with ornithine carbamoyltransferase deficiency. Arch Dis Child 2002; 86(1):54–56.

83. Azevedo L, Vilarinho L, Teles EL, Amorim A. Ornithine transcarbamylase deficiency: a novel splice site mutation in a family with meiotic recombination and a new useful SNP for diagnosis. Mol Genet Metab 2002; 76(1):68–70.

84. Berry GT, Steiner RD. Long-term management of patients with urea cycle disorders. J Pediatr 2001; 138(1 Suppl):S56–S60.

85. Prasad AN, Breen JC, Ampola MG, Rosman NP. Argininemia: a treatable genetic cause of progressive spastic diplegia simulating cerebral palsy: case reports and literature review. J Child Neurol 1997; 12(5):301–309.

86. Choi JH, Kim H, Yoo HW. Two cases of citrullinaemia presenting with stroke. J Inherit Metab Dis 2006; 29(1):182–183.

87. Munnich A, Rustin P. Clinical spectrum and diagnosis of mitochondrial disorders. Am J Med Genet 2001; 106(1):4–17.

88. Iizuka T, Sakai F, Kan S, Suzuki N. Slowly progressive spread of the stroke-like lesions in MELAS. Neurology 2003; 61(9):1238–1244.

89. Kolb SJ, Costello F, Lee AG, White M, Wong S, Schwartz ED et al. Distinguishing ischemic stroke from the stroke-like lesions of MELAS using apparent diffusion coefficient mapping. J Neurol Sci 2003; 216(1):11–15.

90. Abe K, Yoshimura H, Tanaka H, Fujita N, Hikita T, Sakoda S. Comparison of conventional and diffusion-weighted MRI and proton MR spectroscopy in patients with mitochondrial encephalomyopathy, lactic acidosis, and stroke-like events. Neuroradiology 2004; 46(2):113–117.

91. Kwon JH, Kim JS. Rhabdomyolysis in a patient with MELAS syndrome. Eur Neurol 2003; 50(2):123–124.

92. Sakuta R, Honzawa S, Murakami N, Goto Y, Nagai T. Atypical MELAS associated with mitochondrial tRNA(Lys) gene A8296G mutation. Pediatr Neurol 2002; 27(5):397–400.

93. Tzen CY, Thajeb P, Wu TY, Chen SC. Melas with point mutations involving tRNALeu (A3243G) and tRNAGlu(A14693g). Muscle Nerve 2003; 28(5):575–581.

94. Melone MA, Tessa A, Petrini S, Lus G, Sampaolo S, di Fede G et al. Revelation of a new mitochondrial DNA mutation (G12147A) in a MELAS/MERFF phenotype. Arch Neurol 2004; 61(2):269–272.

95. Deschauer M, Tennant S, Rokicka A, He L, Kraya T, Turnbull DM et al. MELAS associated with mutations in the POLG1 gene. Neurology 2007; 68(20):1741–1742.

96. Koga Y, Akita Y, Junko N, Yatsuga S, Povalko N, Fukiyama R et al. Endothelial dysfunction in MELAS improved by l-arginine supplementation. Neurology 2006; 66(11):1766–1769.

97. Koga Y, Akita Y, Nishioka J, Yatsuga S, Povalko N, Katayama K et al. MELAS and L-arginine therapy. Mitochondrion 2007; 7(1–2):133–139.

98. Debray FG, Lambert M, Chevalier I, Robitaille Y, Decarie JC, Shoubridge EA et al. Long-term outcome and clinical spectrum of 73 pediatric patients with mitochondrial diseases. Pediatrics 2007; 119(4):722–733.

15
SYMPTOMATIC STROKE

15.1 Cardiac Disorders

Vijeya Ganesan

Epidemiology

With advances in the treatment of congenital and acquired heart disease, the proportion of affected children experiencing stroke has probably reduced over the last 150 years, although in many series they still comprise the largest subgroup. In the 1960s, the Joint Committee for Stroke Facilities reported up to half of childhood strokes were due to cardiac disorders.[1] More recent single and multicentre series have reported lower frequencies for ischaemic stroke[2–13] and population-based data suggest that 5–30% of children with ischaemic or haemorrhagic stroke have cardiac disease.[3,14–19] Symptomatic venous sinus thrombosis and haemorrhagic or ischaemic (Figs 15.1–15.10) stroke is six times as common in children with heart disease and affects those with acyanotic and cyanotic disorders equally, with the majority occurring in those who have had surgery, typically in the first two postoperative weeks.[20] The frequency in the postoperative period is 5.4 strokes per 1000 children undergoing procedures, with those undergoing repeat procedures at particularly increased risk[21] but pre- or postoperative silent or covert infarction is much commoner[22] and it is now becoming clear that brain development is compromised in utero in children with complex lesions.[23–25] Although usually stroke occurs in a child who is already known to have a cardiac lesion, occasionally it may be the presenting feature of congenital or acquired heart disease.

Stroke in children with congenital heart disease

Of children with congenital cardiac anomalies, the risk of stroke is greatest in major cyanotic congenital heart disease such as Fallot's tetralogy or transposition of the great arteries.[26,27] Overall, around 3% of children with untreated cyanotic congenital cardiac disease suffer stroke, usually before the age of 2 years.[28] Despite improvements in cardiac surgery, children with surgically corrected cardiac defects remain at risk of developing stroke.[29–31] Although children undergoing cardiac surgery are at risk of global cerebral ischaemia (see Chapter 17, Section 17.4), focal neurological deficits are well recognized in the immediate postoperative period and may result in long-term neurological sequelae.[32] For some anomalies, the risk is higher; for example, the incidence of combined early and late postoperative stroke in children undergoing the Fontan procedure is in the region of 2–8%.[31,33] Arterial[31] and venous[34,35] strokes have been documented, the latter usually in the immediate postoperative period, presumably in the context of venous congestion and hypertension. Risk factors for delayed embolic stroke include the presence of a pulmonary band[36] and/or a persistent right-to-left shunt at atrial level.[33,37] This is now a rare occurrence except peri-procedurally, probably because most patients receive long-term aspirin prophylaxis.[38]

PERIOPERATIVE STROKE IN CHILDREN WITH CONGENITAL HEART DISEASE

Children with cardiac disease may have strokes at catheterization or surgery or apparently spontaneously pre- or post-surgery. In addition to underlying aetiologies associated with both cardiac and cerebrovascular disease, risk factors associated with to stroke in children who have had cardiac surgery include the following:

1. Preoperative factors, e.g. iron deficiency[26,27] and the degree of oxygen desaturation,[26] as well as the need for catheterization with or without balloon septostomy[39] or dilatation.

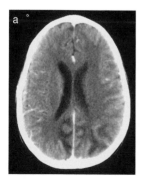 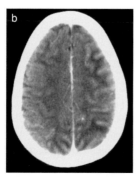 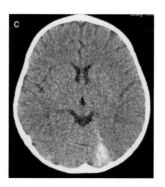

Fig. 15.1. (a,b) MRI showing subarachnoid haemorrhage with bilateral oedema in a post-operative patient with complex congenital heart disease. (courtesy of Dr Dawn Saunders) (c) MRI showing supratentorial haemorrhage in a post-operative patient with complex congenital heart disease. Sagittal sinus thrombosis should be excluded.

2. Intra-operative factors, e.g. cerebral oxygenation[22] and air embolus.[40]
3. Postoperative factors, such as hypotension, the presence of foreign material within the heart, stasis of blood in vascular stumps or alterations in intra-cardiac haemodynamics, shunts, cardiac arrhythmias and elevated systemic venous pressure resulting in systemic venous thrombosis.[22,31–33]

INADEQUATE PERFUSION/OXYGENATION BEFORE, DURING AND AFTER SURGERY

Infarction in children with congenital heart disease may not follow a typical arterial or venous distribution and it may be difficult to distinguish focal from global brain insults. Patients with ventricular dysfunction and poor cardiac output may develop borderzone infarction due to perfusion failure.[41] In addition, it has been clear for some time from pathological studies that injury predominantly involving the white matter, usually in a distribution compatible with periventricular leukomalacia (PVL), is common in infants dying of congenital heart disease or its treatment. These pathological studies suggest that in infants dying below the age of 3 months, white matter damage predominates[42,43] while in older children, damage to the hippocampus and global or focal cortical necrosis are more likely, in a pattern similar to that seen in adults.

A recent neuropathological study of 38 infants who died after cardiac surgery confirmed that cerebral white matter damage (PVL) was the most significant lesion in both severity and incidence.[44] Although no significant relationship was found between infant variables, such as age at time of surgery, or operative variables, such as duration of deep hypothermic circulatory arrest, and severity of brain damage, there was a tendency for neonates to be at greater risk for acute PVL, which the authors suggested reflected the greater vulnerability of the immature white matter to hypoxic-ischaemic damage, which can occur pre-, intra- or postoperatively.

It has recently been demonstrated using magnetic resonance imaging (MRI) that *surviving* term neonates with congenital cardiac disease are also at risk of injury to the white matter without involvement of the grey matter in a distribution similar to PVL as seen in preterm infants.[45–49] A study of neonates with transposition of the great arteries or single ventricle anatomy showed that nearly a third had abnormal white matter on magnetic resonance diffusion tensor imaging, in addition to magnetic resonance spectroscopy evidence of delayed maturation.[49] Another MRI study of neonates born at >36 weeks' gestation before and after surgical correction of complex congenital heart disease (of both cyanotic and acyanotic types) revealed that approximately one-quarter of infants' MRI scans prior to surgery demonstrated either damage to the white matter adjacent to the ventricles or evidence of infarcts.[45] Early postoperative MRI showed that two-thirds of infants had new lesions or worsening of existing PVL lesions, although on repeated scanning many of these had resolved. However, abnormal MRI was documented in 2/17 (13%) of those rescanned at 1 year.[45] Licht et al[50] studied 60 children with a variety of

congenital heart anomalies, of whom 13 had white matter damage pre-operatively; interestingly it was commoner in males. New or more extensive damage to the white matter is also reported postoperatively in the majority of series.[45–47] In the series from the Children's Hospital of Philadelphia, PVL was reported in 54% of 105 neonates with complex congenital heart disease scanned 6–14 days postoperatively, particularly in association with perioperative hypoxia and hypotension.[46] Twelve (11%) of these patients were born preterm but gestational age was not a significant predictor of PVL. There are few follow-up data but PVL may be associated with cognitive problems (see Fig. 17.10).

CARDIOEMBOLISM

Stroke in children with cardiac disease is commonly embolic. Material which may embolize from the heart includes thrombus, calcific material (aortic stenosis), tumour (atrial myxoma) or infected matter (bacterial endocarditis).[51] Emboli may also pass from the veins of the extremities or pelvis through a right to left shunt (see below).

Clinical features of cardioembolic stroke

Criteria for the diagnosis of cardioembolic stroke rely on circumstantial evidence rather than a definite criterion standard.[51,52] Pure cortical syndromes (e.g. transient aphasia or transient global amnesia) are rarely recognized in children and the frequency of these events in this age group is unknown.

Classically, embolic stroke results in a very abrupt neurological event,[53] associated with occlusion of a vessel and infarction of the distal territory (Figs 15.2–15.4) with a variable degree of subsequent improvement (due to dissolution of the embolus and the degree of subsequent recanalization; Fig. 5.9). However this clinical pattern is probably not a reliable means of distinguishing embolic from thrombotic strokes in adults and is even less so in children, in whom the exact clinical course is often unclear. Other suggestive clinical features include recurrent events within a short period and evidence of systemic embolic disease. The exact clinical syndrome will depend on the vessel which is occluded by the embolus. Emboli of varying sizes may occlude any size of vessel and therefore may be associated with a variety of clinical stroke syndromes including major territorial stroke, pure cortical syndromes or lacunar syndromes. Imaging evidence of cortical, large subcortical or cerebellar infarcts or infarcts in multiple vascular territories would be supportive of embolic stroke.[51] Haemorrhagic infarction may suggest an embolic aetiology, as dissolution of the embolic material and subsequent reperfusion may result in haemorrhage into the initial area of infarction.

It may be very difficult to prove or disprove an embolic mechanism in a child with prior heart disease and there is a good case for a comprehensive workup, including cerebrovascular imaging, in those in whom there is doubt. For example, in the Great Ormond Street series,[5,54] 31 children were known to have structural cardiac abnormalities (due to a variety of major congenital cardiac malformations) before an index arterial ischaemic stroke (AIS). Intracardiac thrombus was seen

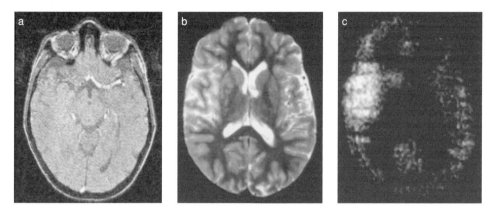

Fig. 15.2. MRI from a 9-year-old boy with double inlet univentricular heart and transposition who had undergone a Glenn and Blalock procedures 7 days before presenting with decreased vision in the right eye, right-sided jerking, vomiting and a left hemiparesis, 8 hours before the scan. The right terminal internal carotid bifurcation is occluded by embolus (a) and there is swelling in the middle cerebral artery territory on T2-weighted imaging (b). The extent of the ischaemia is well demonstrated on diffusion-weighted imaging (c), which is usually abnormal within minutes of an ischaemic insult.

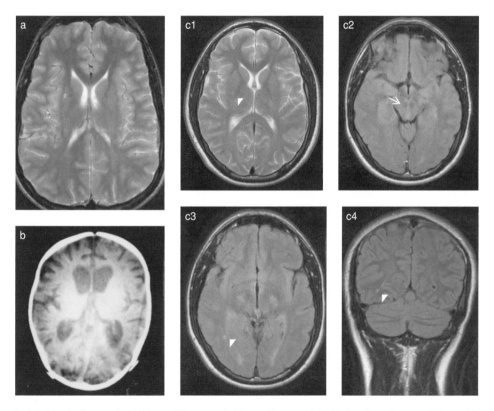

Fig. 15.3. Focal and global brain damage in children with congenital heart disease. (a) MRI showing a lacunar infarct with normal vessels in a teenager who developed Tourette syndrome postoperatively. (b) Bilateral cerebral atrophy in a child who had status epilepticus after emergency surgery for total anomalous pulmonary venous drainage with atrial and ventricular septal defects. She had a spastic quadriparesis and severe learning difficulties at follow-up. (c) Brain ischaemia in a child who presented with worsening heart failure at the age of 3 months and required emergency surgery for total anomalous pulmonary venous drainage. There are two areas of infarction secondary to emboli or to venous sinus thrombosis, in addition to signal change in the corticospinal tracts.

on transthoracic echocardiography (TTE) *before* the AIS in two but although TTE was conducted soon after the AIS in all 31, intracardiac thrombus was not identified in any others[5] while on cerebrovascular imaging, undertaken in 20, four had stenosis, two had dissection (Figs 15.5 and 15.6) and two had moyamoya (Figs 15.7 and 15.8).[54]

PRIMARY ARTERIAL DISEASE

It is important to consider the possibility of co-existent arterial disease such as arterial dissection,[55,56] aneurysm,[57] arteriovenous malformation[58] or moyamoya[59] in children with structural abnormalities of the heart, as these may have specific treatment implications. Primary cerebrovascular disease is

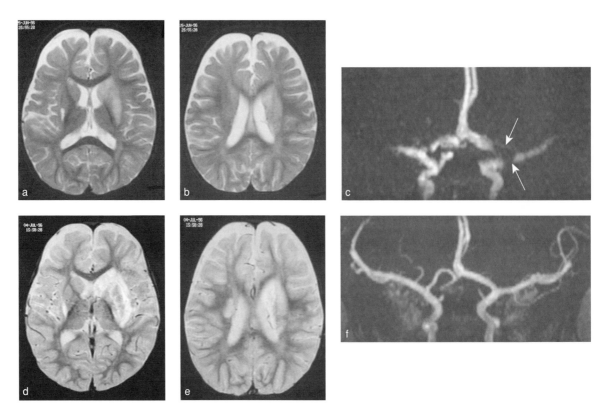

Fig. 15.4. MRI in a 2-year-old child with heart failure secondary to supraventricular tachycardia who presented with a right hemiparesis and had thrombus documented in the left atrial appendage on echocardiography. (a,b) T2-weighted MRI shows an acute infarct in right head of caudate and left striatum (caudate and lentiform nucluei). There is a small linear established infarct in the right posterior putamen and external capsule. (c) The magnetic resonance angiography reveals absence of flow of the left terminal internal carotid and proximal middle and anterior cerebral arteries. (d,e) Following treatment with heparin, the clot was no longer seen in the heart. Nine days later there is more mass effect and areas of decreased T2 signal indicating haemorrhagic transformation with the left sided infarct. There is an additional new infarct in the right corona radiata. (f) Flow within the circle of Willis has been restored following clot lysis (courtesy of Dr Dawn Saunders).

particularly associated with anomalies of the left ventricular outflow tract such as coarctation of the aorta[60,61] (Figs 15.7 and 15.8), bicuspid aortic valve[55] (Fig. 15.6) and patent ductus arteriosus.[62] Genetic syndromes which are associated with both structural cardiac and cerebrovascular abnormalities include Down[63] (Fig. 15.7), Williams[64] (Fig. 15.8), Noonan,[65] cardio-facio-cutaneous,[66] Alagille,[67] Aarskog–Scott[68] and PHACES[69] (Fig. 15.9) syndromes and these associated conditions are not uncommon in large series.[5]

CEREBRAL VENOUS THROMBOSIS
Polycythaemia, dehydration and anaemia may specifically result in cerebral venous thrombosis and secondary venous infarction[27,35,70–74] (Fig. 15.1; see Chapter 7). Recognizing patterns of infarction more suggestive of venous rather than arterial injury is the key to diagnosis but this can be challenging even with MRI.

OTHER MECHANISMS OF STROKE IN CARDIAC DISEASE
Both congenital and acquired cardiac arrhythmias may also predispose to stroke.[75,76] Acquired cardiac disease such as cardiomyopathies,[77] atrial myxomas[78] (see Chapter 5) and myocardial infarction[79] have also been described in association with ischaemic stroke. Left atrial myxoma is a rare but treatable

condition which may cause up to 1% of stroke in young adults[80–82] (see Chapter 5). Mitral valve prolapse affects 5–7% of all children but is rarely associated with stroke in this age group[83,84] and its relevance to pathogenesis of stroke remains unproven.[80]

Treatment

ACUTE MANAGEMENT (see Chapter 16)
Anticoagulation may be life-saving in venous sinus thrombosis (see Chapters and 16), which should be actively excluded and managed in acutely ill patients with coma and seizures as well as hemiparesis. The risk of spontaneous haemorrhagic transformation of cardioembolic strokes may be of concern if anticoagulation is considered in the acute period. This has been shown to occur in up to 40% of cases and usually occurs within the first 2–4 days after the stroke. Haemorrhagic transformation is more common in patients with large infarcts and is particularly hazardous in these patients as bleeding may result in significant mass effect. If this occurs and the patient is unconscious he or she should be referred for urgent consideration of surgical decompression (see Chapter 16). In patients who present acutely and who have large infarcts, it is prudent to delay initiation of anticoagulation for at least 48 hours.[52] Use

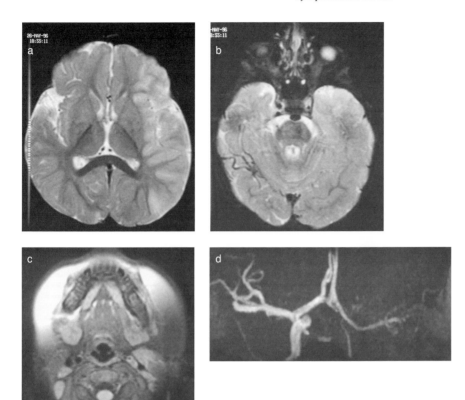

Fig. 15.5. MRI in a 1-year-old child with pulmonary atresia with intact septum who had a Blalock–Taussig shunt in the neonatal period and had signs of Horner's syndrome since then. The child presented acutely with a right hemiparesis and more obvious right Horner syndrome. (a,b) An acute, predominantly cortical, left middle cerebral artery territory infarct with no haemorrhage. (c) The crescent of haematoma surrounding a narrow left cervical internal carotid artery characteristic of a dissection. (d) Nearly absent flow within the distal left internal carotid artery and reduced flow within the proximal anterior and middle cerebral artery, presumably supplied mostly from the right internal carotid artery via the circle of Willis (courtesy of Dr Dawn Saunders).

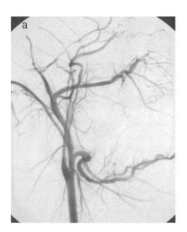
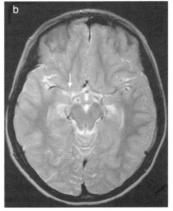
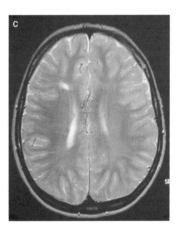

Fig. 15.6. Extracranial dissection in a child with aortic stenosis. (a) Right common carotid injection of a cerebral angiogram depicting the characteristic rat's tail appearance of a dissection of the internal carotid artery from the carotid bulb to its termination. (b) Axial T2-weighted imaging showing low flow in the right middle cerebral artery (arrow) and (c) a small infarct in the right deep watershed region.

of low molecular weight heparin should be considered as this is associated with a lower risk of bleeding complications than conventional intravenous heparin.

Since stroke in children with congenital heart disease commonly occurs after invasive procedures, affected children are often inpatients at the onset of neurological symptoms, This, along with rapid recognition of the significance of their symptoms, means that they may be candidates for hyperacute treatments. Although there have been case reports of the successful use of recombinant tissue plasminogen activator in such

a child,[85] this treatment cannot be recommended currently (see Chapter 16). The risk of bleeding associated with thrombolysis is likely to be significant and, in the absence of any clear indicators of the prognosis without treatment, the benefit remains undefined.

Prevention of recurrence (see Chapter 17, Section 17.1)
The risk of recurrent events should be considered on a case by case basis taking into account the underlying cardiac disease, for example dilated cardiomyopathy carries a stroke risk

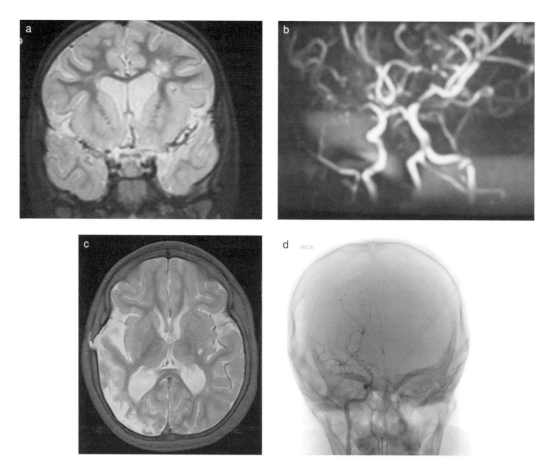

Fig. 15.7. A 4-year-old girl with Down syndrome who developed an acute right-sided hemiparesis in the context of an upper respiratory tract infection for which she required oxygen supplementation. In the past, she had had an aortic coarctation and atrio-ventricular septal repair in infancy, idiopathic thrombocytopenic purpura at the age of 18 months and recurrent upper respiratory tract infection with associated pallor. Transcranial Doppler showed right and left internal carotid/middle cerebral artery (ICA/MCA) velocities of 250 and 180cm/s respectively. Magnetic resonance imaging: bilateral watershed white matter infarction. (a) magnetic resonance angiography demonstrated bilateral occlusive vasculopathy with collateralization, worse on the right side. Arterial disease was confined to the terminal ICA and proximal A1 and M1 segments. (b) Her haemoglobin was 80g/L with elevated reticulocytes. Bone marrow examination showed active tri-lineage haematopoiesis consistent with recent maturation arrest but no leukaemic cells. She was started on aspirin. She represented with recurrent anaemia after a further upper respiratory tract infection with a haemoglobin of 47g/L and a marked reticulocytosis (495% of red blood cells, normal <100%) and a raised lactate dehydrogenase (878iu/L, normal <500iu/L). Warm IgG and C3d antibodies were detected and Coombs test was positive, confirming autoimmune haemolytic anaemia (Evans syndrome). Right and left MCA velocities increased to 300 and 290cm/s respectively. Overnight pulse oximetry: mean and minimum oxyhaemoglobin saturations of 93% and 73% respectively, normalizing with 1L/min nasal oxygen. Echocardiography showed slightly elevated right ventricular pressures (55mmHg) but no intracardiac clot. She had a further stroke (c) and formal arteriography prior to revascularization surgery (extracranial–intracranial bypass) showed MCA stenosis with collateralization (d) (courtesy of Dr Mary Gawne-Cain and Dr Andrea Whitney).

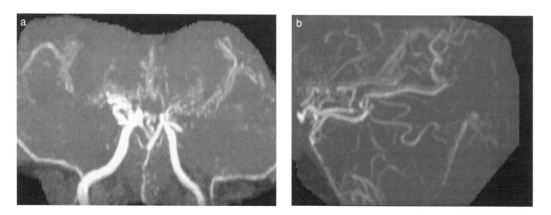

Fig. 15.8. Severe vasculopathy with moyamoya collaterals in a child with Williams syndrome and transient ischaemic attacks.

250

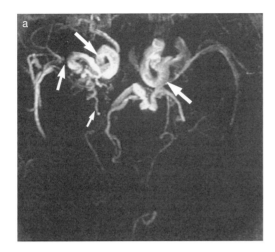
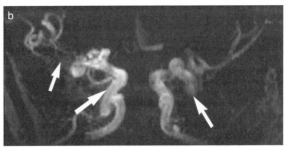
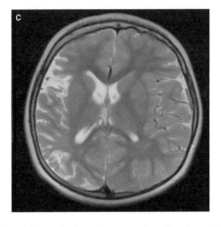

Fig. 15.9. Magnetic resonance angiogram shown in transverse axial (a) and frontal (b) projections demonstrating dilated, ectatic, terminal internal carotids arteries bilaterally in a child with PHACES who had had repair of coarctation at the age of 9 months and presented with a left hemiparesis 4 months later. Collateral vessels from the posterior circulation are shown on the right (small arrows), as well as a gap in perfusion in the right M2 region (medium arrow).[223] He had ischaemic injury in the borderzones between the middle and anterior and middle and posterior artery territories (c).

of 5% per year.[80] Similarly, it is difficult to categorically stipulate the nature or duration of anticoagulation. There is little evidence that anticoagulation has any advantage over aspirin for prevention of late stroke after the Fontan or Glenn procedure,[31,37,38] except perhaps in those with a family history suggestive of thrombophilia.[86]

Given that the relationship between patent foramen ovale and childhood stroke is unproven, and the lack of evidence for an advantage over aspirin prophylaxis in studies of adults[87] (see Chapter 5), there does not seem any justification for anticoagulating this group of children. The role of transcatheter closure is contentious and as yet undefined (see Chapter 5).

15.2 Genetically Determined Vasculopathies and Stroke Syndromes without Neurocutaneous Stigmata

Fenella J. Kirkham and Nomazulu Dlamini

Down syndrome

Down syndrome is a chromosomal disorder most commonly secondary to trisomy of chromosome 21, although translocations also occur. Genes coded on chromosome 21, including APP, CBS, SOD-1, BACE-2 and S100β, are upregulated in Down syndrome. These children have a number of complications including poor growth, leukaemia, hypothyroidism, atlanto-axial instability, epilepsy and learning difficulties. There is a wide range of cognitive ability in Down syndrome, ranging from children with no language to children with IQs in the low average range who function in mainstream school, at least in the primary years.

STROKE ASSOCIATED WITH DOWN SYNDROME
In a clinic population, the prevalence of new focal neurological deficits was 1.4%.[88] Patients with Down syndrome are at risk of embolus from their cardiac disease,[63,89,90] with the risk of 'top-of-the-basilar' syndrome from a posterior circulation embolus[91] as well as hemiparesis from a middle cerebral artery infarct.[92] Mycotic aneurysm[93,94] and abscess[88] may manifest if the emboli are infected. Patients with Down syndrome may also have venous sinus thrombosis[88,95–97] and this may be a particular risk at the time of cardiac surgery in infancy, although the diagnosis is often missed because these children are often too sick to undergo imaging. Posterior leukencephalopathy has been reported after immunosuppression with steroids[98,99] and cortical laminar necrosis in the context of hypoxaemia.[100] After trauma, patients with Down syndrome are at risk of epidural and subdural[88] haemorrhage as well as spinal cord injury.[88] However, the single most common cause in Down syndrome patients with focal neurological signs is arterial disease, particularly involving the intracranial

vessels[88,92] (Fig. 15.7). Most reports have been of moyamoya syndrome[63,101–124] and the typical presentation is with hemiparesis, but seizures,[120,125] visual loss,[126] chorea[127] and subarachnoid haemorrhage[128] have been reported and moyamoya can occasionally present perinatally.[129] Predominantly unilateral carotid and middle cerebral artery arterial stenosis without progressive collaterals has also been documented[130] but whether this is an early manifestation of disease which will progress to moyamoya syndrome is not clear. Involvement of the posterior circulation, including the posterior cerebral, basilar and vertebral arteries, may be more common than in primary moyamoya disease.[112,131] Pathologically, there is intimal thickening with collagen deposition, a histological feature characteristic of moyamoya disease,[131,132] but a major difference is that the cerebral vessels are of normal size.[131] Although presentation with haemorrhage in adolescence and adulthood[128] has been reported, the majority have had their first symptoms of focal ischaemia in infancy or early childhood.[92]

PATHOPHYSIOLOGY

There is evidence for systemic endothelial dysfunction, as measured by flow-mediated vasodilatation in the forearm, in patients with Down syndrome[133] but atherosclerosis is relatively uncommon and blood pressure is usually lower than in the general population. Arterial vasculopathy and moyamoya collaterals in Down syndrome may be related to proteins encoded on chromosome 21, immune dysregulation or prothrombotic disorders. As for childhood stroke in general, presentation in the context of infection is common, and sleep-disordered breathing may add to the risk.[134] The precise role of infection, both acute, for example upper respiratory tract infection, measles and chickenpox,[123,135,136] and chronic, remains to be elucidated. Dysregulation of the interferon system and upregulation of inflammatory cytokines may be important.[137] Autoimmunity has been implicated, as co-existent Graves disease has been reported.[118,138] Hyperlipidaemia[139] and prothrombotic abnormalities, such as antiphospholipid antibodies[140] and protein C deficiency,[122] have been reported but their role in pathogenesis is uncertain. Other associations with Down syndrome which might play a role in aetiology or in determining stroke subtype include poor nutrition,[141] lack of exercise,[142] atlanto-axial instability,[127] oxidative stress,[143,144] regulation of angiogenesis,[145] reduced tissue plasminogen activator inhibitor,[146] coeliac disease and tissue repair by tissue transglutaminase,[147,148] polycythaemia[149] and anaemia (iron deficiency and haemolytic).[150]

RELATIONSHIP WITH DEMENTIA

Although presenile dementia of the Alzheimer type is a common complication of Down syndrome, particularly in those with certain characteristics of the APP gene, apolipoprotein E4, oestrogen deficiency (including male sex), hyperhomocysteinaemia and evidence for inflammation, there appears to be an inverse relationship with the propensity to atherosclerosis.[151] There have been no prospective studies looking at the association between cognitive decline and cerebrovascular disease in children with Down syndrome.

Williams–Beuren syndrome

PATHOPHYSIOLOGY

Williams–Beuren syndrome[152,153] is usually caused by a sporadic autosomal dominant deletion involving 21 genes on chromosome 7q11.23, including the elastin gene, which may be confirmed by FISH studies.[154,155] Histopathologically, the vessels show localized dysplasia, which may be progressive. It appears that the lack of vessel wall elasticity is compensated for by proliferation of vascular smooth muscles cells which in turn leads to thickened intima-media with narrowing of the lumen. Carotid intima-media thickness is increased and distensibility decreased in children[156] and adults[157] with Williams syndrome.

CLINICAL FEATURES

Children characteristically have elfin facies with a turned up nose and thick lips. There is usually a stellate iris and dental enamel hypoplasia. Some children are hypercalcaemic in infancy, although the proportion is probably as low as 6%.[158] Some have cardiac disease, most often supervalvular aortic stenosis and peripheral pulmonary stenosis but also ventricular septal defects, patent ductus arteriosus and mitral valve prolapse. Renal anomalies, including nephrocalcinosis and stenoses, are well-recognized. Coeliac disease is more common than in the general population.[159] Hypertension is commonly a feature and adults may have raised cholesterol. Sudden death affects 1 in 1000 per year. Although sociability and verbal skills are usually preserved, learning difficulties are usually severe with IQs in the range 40–80 and there are specific problems with visual perception and memory, probably related to hippocampal abnormality. Seizures may occur.

STROKE

Ischaemic[64,160–162] and haemorrhagic[158,163,164] stroke have been reported in Williams syndrome, although it is relatively rare in large series.[158] Intracranial stenoses, often accompanied by moyamoya collaterals, have been well documented on magnetic resonance angiography[64,160–162,165] (Fig. 15.8), as well as at autopsy,[163] although digital subtraction arteriography is sometimes normal[162,164] and, in addition to the possibility of cardiogenic embolus, acute vasospasm may play a role.[162] Carotid occlusion, which was probably embolic in the context of intracardiac thrombus, has been reported in an adult.[166] Stroke is a cause of death in Williams syndrome.[158,163,164] Coronary vasospasm may also be important in sudden death from myocardial ischaemia, which often follows procedures involving anaesthesia and catheterization.[167] Now that non-invasive diagnostic procedures are available, cardiac catheterization and cerebral angiography should be avoided unless required for intervention, for example before revascularization for moyamoya.

Turner syndrome

Carotid occlusion and dissection and intracranial vasculopathy have been described in occasional children and young adults with stroke and Turner syndrome[168] but it is not clear that this occurs more commonly than in the general population.

Noonan syndrome

Ischaemic and haemorrhagic stroke have been reported in Noonan syndrome.[169–173] Aneurysms, arteriovenus malformations and moyamoya disease have all been reported and may affect both the anterior and the posterior circulation.

Alagille syndrome

PATHOPHYSIOLOGY

Alagille syndrome usually presents with liver disease secondary to paucity of the bile ducts, which is usually caused by mutations in the Jagged-1 gene (about half of which are inherited) in the Notch signaling pathway. Jagged 1 plays a role in signaling during embryonic development,[174] specifically in relation to vascular remodeling.[67]

CLINICAL FEATURES

Facies are characteristic. The majority of children present in the first year of life with liver disease. Biopsy shows paucity of the interlobular ducts associated with cholestasis. Cardiac murmur usually secondary to pulmonary artery anomalies, butterfly vertebrae and renal disease are common. Frequent otitis media,[175] mastoiditis and sinusitis[176] have been documented.

STROKE AND CEREBROVASCULAR DISEASE

Intracerebral, subdural and subarachnoid bleeding is common,[67,175,177,178] in some cases related to aneurysm and in others, with normal arterial imaging,[67] perhaps related to venous sinus thrombosis in the context of trauma or post liver transplant. In one series haemorrhagic or ischaemic stroke occurred in 14% of patients and accounted for 25% of the deaths,[178] while around 40% of patients (23% of asymptomatic) have cerebrovascular disease.[176] The vasculopathy is often progressive and normal angiography does not exclude the possibility of later stroke.[176] Unilateral or bilateral internal carotid stenosis, and with the development of collaterals, is the commonest form of cerebrovascular disease and frank moyamoya has been documented.[67,179–181] Internal carotid,[67,182] basilar and middle cerebral aneurysms[176] may be missed on screening magnetic resonance angiography (MRA) and probably develop over time rather than being congenital.[176] Other abnormalities on MRI include periventricular leukomalacia, Chiari I malformation and increased signal in the globus pallidus.[176] Benign intracranial hypertension, perhaps related to venous sinus thrombosis in the context of the frequent head and neck infections, has been reported.[176]

Marfan syndrome

Marfan syndrome is a dominantly inherited disorder of connective tissue caused by a deficiency of the glycoprotein fibrillin. Microscopic examination of the cerebral arteries shows widespread changes with intimal proliferation, medial degeneration and fragmentation of the internal elastic lamina. In the pre-genomic era, case reports suggested that people with Marfan syndrome have an increased risk of intracranial aneurysms[183] but the diagnosis was clinical and may have been in doubt, for example not excluding homocystinuria where the habitus is similar. In one autopsy series, of seven patients, each of two patients (one with aortic dissection and one with subarachnoid haemorrhage) had one or more intracranial aneurysms. It has also been suggested that carotid dissection and bicuspid aortic valve were likely mechanisms for ischaemic stroke. However, several large studies of patients with Marfan syndrome did not mention ruptured intracranial aneurysms and the current consensus is that, although there may be primary cerebrovascular disease in Marfan's, it is very rarely the cause of stroke. Two recent series have confirmed a lack of association. Of 135 patients in the Amsterdam Marfan clinic, no patient had a symptomatic intracranial aneurysm or was admitted with a ruptured intracranial aneurysm during a period in which 826 patients with symptomatic intracranial aneurysms were admitted. During follow-up of 129 of the 135 patients with Marfan syndrome (2850 retrospective patient observation years and 581 prospective patient observation years), none presented a symptomatic intracranial aneurysm.[184] In another retrospective series, 18 (3.5%) patients had a focal neurological event at a mean age of 40 years over an 8-year period. Fifteen patients had ischaemia, the majority of whom had aortic dissection as well as high-risk cardiac lesions, for example atrial fibrillation or prosthetic heart valves. Transient events, typically visual disturbance or parasthesias, occurred in 13 and there were two ischaemic infarcts. Anticoagulants were a risk factor in two of the three haemorrhagic strokes.[185] One child had a subdural haemorrhage of uncertain aetiology, presenting with a seizure and autonomic dysfunction.[185] There was no excess of bicuspid aortic valve in those with stroke.[185] Spinal cord infarction in two patients was related to aortic dissection, at least in part.[185]

Ehlers–Danlos syndrome (EDS) type IV

Ehlers–Danlos syndrome (EDS) type IV is an autosomal dominant disorder caused by mutations in the COL3A 1 gene encoding chains of type III procollagen. Individuals with this disorder tend to have fragile skin, easy bruising, increased joint mobility, easily dislocated knees and sometimes deformities of the foot and are predisposed to rupture of arteries and the bowel. Carotid intima-media thickness is reduced but there is an increase in wall stress across the vessel, which may increase the propensity to aneurysm and dissection.[186]

STROKE AND CEREBROVASCULAR DISEASE

EDS type IV has been reported in a sudden infant death accompanied by intracranial haemorrhage but no aneurysm.[187] In a 5-year-old child who underwent computed tomography for a febrile seizure, the diagnosis was made on skin biopsy after an asymptomatic basilar aneurysm was noted.[188] Angiography revealed multiple aneurysms and a middle cerebral artery stenosis with reduced flow distally. Presentation in childhood is exceptionally unusual and other conditions, such as Loeys–Dietz syndrome,[189] should be excluded. In a series of 202 individuals with EDS type IV from 121 families in which the diagnosis was confirmed by biochemical or molecular studies, 19 individuals had cerebrovascular complications, including intracranial aneurysms with secondary haemorrhage, spontaneous carotid-cavernous sinus fistula, and cervical artery dissection at a mean age of 28.3 (range 17–48) years. Conventional angiography may cause complications, so non-invasive procedures such as Doppler and MRA should be used where possible. On transcranial Doppler sonography, compared with 29 controls, the pulsatility index was decreased in a patient with EDS and an aneurysm and a possible link between aneurysm risk and reduced cerebrovascular resistance was suggested.[190] Anticoagulation therapy may result in increased bruising or bleeding and should be used with caution.

Congenital disorders of glycosylation or carbohydrate deficient glycoprotein syndromes

This family of autosomal recessive conditions involving defective glycosylation of *N*-glycosylated proteins are associated with developmental delay, seizures, hypertonia and stroke-like episodes.[191,192] The patients characteristically have a large jaw, almond-shaped eyes, a squint, inverted nipples and buttock fat pads. The coagulation proteins undergo post-translational glycosylation and a wide variety of abnormalities of the coagulation pathway have been described in carbohydrate deficient glycoprotein (CDG) syndromes and there is now some evidence for an association with the stroke-like episodes.[193] About half of the children with CDG type 1A have stroke-like episodes. They commonly present around the age of 3 and CT is usually negative but ischaemic stroke and oedema followed by focal necrosis were reported in separate episodes in one child.[192] Recovery is usually complete, although permanent hemiparesis has been recorded.[194]

Osteopetrosis

There are several forms of osteopetrosis which leads to severe thickening of the skull, anaemia and extramedullary haematopoeisis. Both the autosomal dominant and recessive forms are associated with internal carotid and vertebral stenosis and with dural venous sinus narrowing, and occasionally aneurysms perhaps related to bony overgrowth.[195] Stroke is rare but may affect the middle cerebral artery territory.[196] Bone marrow transplantation may be offered to some of these patients and stroke is a risk in this situation, perhaps in relation to immunosuppression and the infection risk.[5]

Schimke immunoosseous dysplasia

Schimke[197] described a form of spondyloepiphyseal dysplasia associated with progressive renal disease and immunodeficiencies, now known as immunoosseous dysplasia, characterized by flattened vertebral bodies and platyspondyly, a dysplastic pelvic skeleton involving iliac bones, hypoplastic acetabulae and femurs which present epiphyseal dysplasia, while similar findings may be found in upper limbs. It is secondary to mutations in the SMARCAL1 gene, which encodes a chromatin remodelling protein.[198,199]

The reported children with spondyloepiphyseal dysplasia had a history of short stature, growing below the 3rd percentile, with specific facies including a nose with a depressed bridge and bulbous tip, a long upper lip and fine hair. Cyclical lymphopenia may affect the CD4 T-cell lymphocyte subpopulation, with normal ratio CD4/CD8, and recurrent infections but low levels of immunogiobulin (Ig) and IgG subclasses, a feature of this syndrome or secondary to renal loss with the associated steroid-resistant nephrotic syndrome. Other complications are hypothyroidism, hypertension, hypercholesterolaemia and premature atherosclerosis. Stroke and transient ischaemic attacks have been documented in association with a widespread cerebral vasculopathy (Fig. 15.10)[200] and it is likely that brain development is affected in addition to formation of the cerebral vessels.[201]

COL4A1 mutations

Autosomal dominant mutations of COL4A1 on chromosome 13q34, encoding the alpha$_1$ chain of type IV collagen, have been associated with familial perinatal intracerebral haemorrhage with subsequent porencephaly in infants (Fig. 15.11)[202] and lacunar strokes and leukoaraiosis in adults;[203] other associated manifestations include nephropathy, cramps, intracranial aneurysm and intracranial haemorrhage (including microbleeds).[204] There is a wide spectrum of involvement[205] but COL4A1 should be excluded in children presenting with stroke if there is a family history suggesting autosomal dominant inheritance.[206]

CADASIL

CADASIL is a genetic condition associated with mutations in the NOTCH3 gene, a transmembrane protein expressed in vascular smooth muscle cells, which presents with migraine, neuropsychiatric impairments and subcortical infarction, usually in adults.[207] Children are usually diagnosed when there is a family history[208,209] but may present with hemiparesis and a history of headaches[210] and may not have abnormalities of MRI or MRA at presentation.[211] For the occasional child who presents with stroke,[210] the pattern of infarction is an unusual one and may be a clue to the diagnosis.[212]

Grange syndrome

This syndrome of brachydactyy and syndactyy with hypertension, renal stenosis, bone fragility, mild to moderate learning disability and occlusive disease of the carotid circulation, often with cardiac involvement, for example patent foramen ovale or aortic stenosis, is likely to be autosomal recessive.[213–215] Although the cerebral vasculopathy is not typical of moyamoya, the vessel wall may stain for basic fibrobastic growth factor.[214]

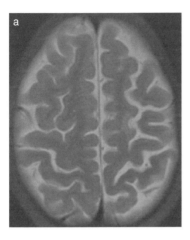
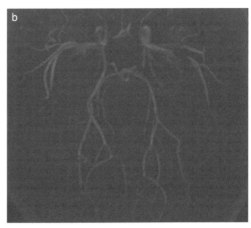

Fig. 15.10. MRI from a 5-year-old girl who had been followed up since the age of 3 years because of her growth failure and nephrotic syndrome. She had a characteristic face with a long upper lip and fine hair and small pigmented spots were found mostly in the neck, axillas and groin which increased in number with age. She had a waddling gait. At this stage she presented with nephrotic syndrome with mild hypertension resistant to steroids and immunosuppressive therapy with cycles of cyclophosphamide. Renal function deteriorated over the next months. Immunodeficiency was apparent with recurrent lymphopenia with low CD4 lymphocyte T cell levels. She also had decreased immunoglobulin levels, affecting mainly IgG and IgG subclasses. She had a pulmonary embolus requiring long-term warfarin therapy. A probable diagnoses of Schimke immunoosseous dysplasia was made. She had recurrent right- and left-sided transient ischaemic attacks characterized by headache, speech disturbance and weakness of the right upper limb associated with hypertension. (a) MRI shows atrophy and abnormal signal return of the white matter in the left frontal lobe, involving the premotor cortex consistent with ischaemic injury. (b) MRA demonstrates some evidence of flow disturbance at the level of the terminal carotid arteries bilaterally. Transcranial Doppler was normal. Conventional angiography showed a widespread vasculopathy with variation in calibre of vessels as well as focal stenoses in the proximal major branches with irregularity of the distal vertebral and basilar arteries (not shown). She also had recurrent transient ischaemic attacks and died after a cerebellar haemorrhage.

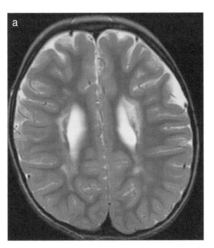
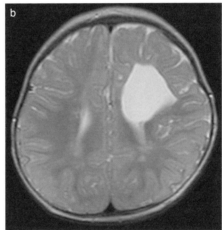

Fig. 15.11. COL4A mutation. (a) Periventricular leukomalacia in an 18-month-old boy who subsequently developed basal ganglia abnormalities. (b) Periventricular leukomalacia in his younger brother and a more focal porencephalic cyst in the left frontal region probably associated with haemorrhage in the perinatal period.

Mutations in smooth muscle alpha-actin (*ACTA2*)

Alpha-actin is a major component of the contractile apparatus of vascular smooth muscle cells located throughout the arterial system. The major role of vascular smooth muscle cells is to contract in response to the stretch caused by pulsatile blood flow. Heterozygous mutation carriers of ACTA2 are susceptible to diffuse and diverse vascular diseases including thoracic aortic aneurysms and dissections, premature coronary artery disease, ischaemic strokes, moyamoya and fusiform aneurysms[216] as a result of excessive proliferation of smooth muscle cells causing occlusive disease, or enlargement of the arteries. Ischaemic strokes may occur as young as 5 years of age, and moyamoya predisposes to both ischaemic and haemorrhagic stroke. The presence of livedo reticularis may be an additional clinical clue to this condition and is caused by occlusion of the dermal arteries.[217]

The role of anticoagulant or anti-thrombotic therapy is not established in this group. Re-vascularization surgery has been reported in two children with a clinically characterized syndrome of dolichoectasia, patent ductus arteriosus and pupillary abnormality.[62] This has recently been associated with a missense mutation in *ACTA2* (DM Mielewicz, personal communication). However, although they are an important cause of thoracic aortic aneurysms and dissections,[218] *ACTA2* mutation is a relatively rare cause of moyamoya.[219]

15.3 Genetically Determined Vasculopathies and Stroke Syndromes with Neurocutaneous Syndromes

Fenella J. Kirkham

PHACE(S)

This is a neurocutaneous disorder comprising a cervicofacial haemangioma with one or more of a posterior fossa malformation, arterial, cardiac and eye abnormalities or a sternal pit (PHACE(S)). Hypopituitarism and hypothyroidism are occasional associations.[220–222] Cardiac associations include aortic arch anomalies, particularly coarctation.[223,224] Patients with large facial cutaneous haemangiomas usually have cerebrovascular disease (Fig. 15.9) or structural malformations, including cortical dysplasia.[225] Its underlying basis is unknown and it is likely to comprise a heterogeneous group but is not unusual in series of stroke in infancy and childhood[5,226] and is occasionally fatal.[227] The cerebral arteriopathy of PHACES includes dysplasia or hypoplasia as well as steno-occlusive disease[69] and some may progress to aneurysm formation.[69,225] The initial cerebral vascular changes almost certainly occur by the fifth gestational week[69] and the pathophysiology may involve cellular proliferation and apoptosis.[228] The haemangioma should prompt consideration of this diagnosis and screening for the associated anomalies.

Neurofibromatosis type 1

CLINICAL FEATURES

Neurofibromatosis type 1 (NF1) is a neurocutaneous condition, with an incidence of around 1 in 3000, which is usually diagnosed in the first 2 years of life when the café-au-lait patches become obvious. Axillary freckling and Lisch nodules of the iris are diagnostic in young children in whom the café-au-lait patches are emerging. Neurological complications are common in neurofibromatosis and include hydrocephalus, epilepsy, headache, radiculopathy and polyneuropathy as well as tumours.[229] Children tend to manifest optic pathway tumours, cerebral gliomas and spinal compression due to intraspinal neurofibromas, while in adulthood the predominant neurological features are chronic pain and malignant peripheral nerve sheath tumours. Stroke is a well recognized complication of neurofibromatosis and occurs both spontaneously and after treatment for brain tumours (see Chapter 15), particularly radiotherapy for optic glioma[230] (see Fig. 6.9b), although stroke is uncommon overall, with prevalences of 0.7% of adults[229] and 0.3% in a recent series of children.[231] White matter disease has also been reported in around 1% of cases.[229] There are many case reports of cerebrovascular complications, but although populations have not been screened with vascular imaging, in the modern era this complication is relatively rare.[231] The

onset of seizures should prompt the exclusion of cerebrovascular disease as epilepsy affects <5% of patients.[229]

PATHOPHYSIOLOGY

The NF1 gene is on chromosome 17q11.2 and the protein product for that gene, neurofibromin, a tumour suppressor, has been identified in the endothelium of the cerebral vessels and in the smooth muscle of the aorta in animal models. The pathophysiology of the vasculopathy is not fully understood but neurofibromin may help to maintain the integrity of the endothelial layer and if it is reduced, as it is in neurofibromatosis, vascular smooth muscles may prolifiate.

CEREBROVASCULAR DISEASE AND STROKE

Occasionally stroke can be the presenting symptom of neurofibromatosis in infants;[232] pathologically there is marked intimal and medial hyperplasia.[233] The majority of case reports have been of children presenting with focal signs. In Rosser's series[231] of 353 children, 316 underwent MRI for routine screening for brain tumours. MRA was undertaken when there was clinical or radiological suspicion of cerebrovascular disease. At a mean age of 7.3 (range 1–13) years, eight children (2.5%) were found to have abnormal cerebral vessels including moyamoya (N=2), narrowing (N=1) or stenosis (N=1), occlusion (N=1), ectasia (N=1), hypoplasia (N=1) and aneurysm (N=1).[231] This is likely to be an underestimate of the prevalence of cerebrovascular disease because vascular imaging was not undertaken routinely. Two patents had had silent infarction in territories supplied by the abnormal vessels and one, who had moyamoya, had presented with acute hemiparesis. For the other five children the vasculopathy was an incidental finding. At follow up for a mean of 5.8 years (range 10 months to 9 years), only the child who presented with the stroke and moyamoya had three further strokes as well as developing epilepsy. None of the other children with vasculopathy as an incidental finding presented with a stroke. In another series of 419 children with NF1 in which two-thirds were investigated with MRI and MRA, there was a minimum prevalence of 6% (N=17) and in one-third of these cases, the vasculopathy was progressive.[234]

INTRACRANIAL ARTERIAL OCCLUSIVE DISEASE INCLUDING MOYAMOYA

Stenotic vasculopathy typically affects the anterior circulation[231,235] but posterior circulation involvement has been reported.[231,236] Young age and co-diagnosis with optic glioma are associated with cerebral vasculopathy.[234] Around one-third of children with NF1 undergoing radiotherapy for optic glioma will develop cerebrovascular disease, which is usually symptomatic within the first few years after treatment.[237] Sporadic cases are also well recognized[231,234,238,239] and it is possible that those who develop cerebrovascular disease after radiotherapy were predisposed.[240] In one series of children undergoing surgery for moyamoya, of 16 patients with NF1, 13 had had cranial irradiation.[241]

Aneurysms of the anterior[242] and posterior[243,244] circulation have been reported and may be difficult to manage because of the fragility of the vascular wall. However, there is controversy over whether there is an association between NF1 and intracranial aneurysms. Of 925 patents undergoing aneurysm surgery in one centre, none had NF1 and none of the 25 autopsied patents with NF1 had an intracranial aneurysm.[245] However, incidental aneurysms were found in two out of 31 (5%) of patients with NF1 referred for imaging to exclude tumours compared with 0/526 controls with tumours without NF1.[246] Although saccular aneurysms are seen, the cases seen may be atypical,[247,248] perhaps as the result of prior dissection,[246] or associated with moyamoya.[249,250]

OTHER CEREBROVASCULAR DISEASE

Presentation in adulthood in association with an arteriovenous malformation or arteriovenous fistula has also been documented.[244,251] Vertebral occlusion in the context of basilar impression has been reported in an adult.[252]

MODIFIABLE RISK FACTORS

Hypertension

Some of these patients are hypertensive[253,254] and the blood pressure may need to be reduced very slowly to avoid the possibility of rapid neurological deterioration.[253] In a recent series of patients with a mean age of 11 (SD) years, 16% were hypertensive and 19% had cardiac abnormalities. Early diagnosis and management of hypertension might be an important component in preventing the development of vasculopathy in patients with neurofibromatosis.[255] Although the hypertension may be related to the presence of neurofibromin in aortic smooth muscle, renal artery stenosis and phaeochromocyta should be excluded.[254]

RADIOTHERAPY

In patients with NF1 and optic glioma, radiotherapy is often delayed at least until the child reaches the age of 5, but in view of the mortality and morbidity for the tumour, treatment may be required. If this is the case, screening for cerebrovascular disease using MRA at the time of repeat MRI is warranted from the first year after treatment[237] and regularly thereafter as stroke can occur up to 10 years after treatment.[256]

Tuberous sclerosis

PATHOPHYSIOLOGY

Tuberous sclerosis is a dominantly inherited condition involving genes on chromosomes 9 and 16 and characterized by the presence of hamartomas in the skin, brain, heart and kidneys. White patches (hypomelanotic macules) which fluoresce under Wood's light are characteristic and children often also have facial angiofibroma and shagreen patches.

STROKE

Acute hemiparesis in a child with tuberous sclerosis is more likely to be a Todd paresis secondary to a prolonged focal seizure than to be a cerebral infarction. Although cardiac rhabdomyomas occur in two-thirds of the children with tuberous sclerosis complex, only a few of these children have developed a stroke[257] and the risk of embolism is so low that neither surgery nor anticoagulation is usually warranted.[258] However strokes have been reported.[259] White matter abnormalities are very common on MRI[260] and are usually related to supratentorial cortical tubers. Nevertheless in one series in 20% the white matter abnormalities were not related to the tubers and in one case had the appearances of infarction; this patient had presented with an acute episode compatible with a stroke.[260]

CEREBROVASCULAR DISEASE

Cerebrovascular disease has also been recognized occasionally, with moyamoya syndrome reported from Japan[261] and Germany[262] and increasing recognition of aneurysms involving the internal carotid and vertebrobasilar arteries.[263–266] The majority of aneurysms have been reported as incidental findings either on screening with CT or MRI (Fig. 15.12)[267,268] or at autopsy[269] but presentation with visual loss has been well documented.[270,271] Transient ischaemic attacks involving the arm and leg have been described in young children, so any change in neurological signs should prompt appropriate neuroimaging. One infant presenting with seizures and intraventicular haemorrhage in the context of a subependymal tuber had also a large fusiform aneurysm of the internal carotid artery and ectasia of the adjacent anterior and middle cerebral arteries.[272] Patients with giant intracranial aneurysms may not manifest some of the features of tuberous sclerosis such as facial angiofibroma, epilepsy and learning disability, although most

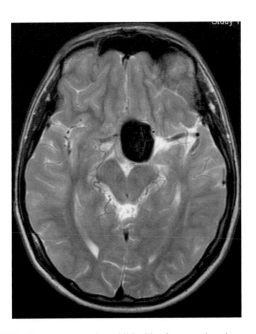

Fig. 15.12. Giant aneurysm in a child with tuberous sclerosis presenting with headaches.

of the cases have had skin manifestations such as shagreen patches and hypomelanotic macules. Case reports have recognized the link with renal cystic disease[273] and aneurysms have been reported alongside renal cysts in patients with TSC2 and PKD1 deletions.[274]

MANAGEMENT

There is little evidence that the majority of aneurysms haemorrhage but appropriate management may lead to relief of symptoms. One infant with a giant mid-basilar aneurysm underwent successful ablation using Guglielmi detachable coils.[266]

Incontinentia pigmenti

PATHOPHYSIOLOGY

Incontinentia pigmenti or Bloch–Sulzberger syndrome is an X-linked dominant disorder which is most commonly diagnosed in girls and their mothers, at least in part because the disease is so severe in boys that many die in utero or in early infancy. Mutations in the nuclear factor-KB essential modulator protein (NEMO) gene on *XQ28* cause the disease but the phenotype correlates poorly with mutation type or domain affected, probably at least in part because of skewed X-inactivation.[275] Many cases are sporadic and central nervous system manifestations affect up to 30% of this group, with motor findings in addition to developmental delay and microcephaly. It has been postulated that the neurological features are secondary to an inflammatory-apoptotic process which parallels the skin changes.[276]

CLINICAL FEATURES

Girls typically present in infancy with a blistering rash which lasts about 6 weeks and is characterized by inflammation and apoptosis. The rash initially consists of vesicles, then of hyperkeratosis with verrucous elements, and then becomes hyperpigmentated followed by atrophy along the lines of Blaschko. Dentition is abnormal in 90% and the skeletal system in 40%. Many patients have no neurological manifestations but seizures are relatively common and may be difficult to control.

NEONATAL STROKE

Presentation in the neonatal period with bilateral cerebral ischaemia, particularly affecting the white matter, has also been documented.[276–279] One patient had an MRI with signal characteristics suggestive of presence of blood products consistent with microvascular haemorrhage into the ventricular white matter. A magnetic resonance angiogram performed 6 days later showed considerably decreased branching of the intracerebral vessels and poor filling within the distal middle and proximal cerebral artery branches.[276] Despite widespread abnormality on MRI, patients presenting in the neonatal period may develop normally.[279] Similar processes in the retina may lead to blindness[280] and changes in the retinal vasculature may be a good marker for intracranial vascular pathology.[281]

Ischaemic stroke secondary to middle cerebral artery occlusion has been described in a 4-year-old girl.[282] Single photon emission computed tomography (SPECT) shows reduced cerebral blood flow consistent with infarction.[283] In a prospective series of seven patients (four related) undergoing prospective MRI, five had abnormal imaging consistent with small vessel occlusion, one of whom had reduced middle cerebral artery flow on MRA and increased lactate on magnetic resonance spectroscopy while the others had normal MRA.[281] Recurrence has been reported.[284] An adult patient had a right supraclinoid internal carotid aneurysm.

Sneddon syndrome

Sneddon[285] first described the association of cerebral manifestations in adults with generalized livedo racemosa (cutis marmorata-telangiectasia congenita), a dermatological condition with a 'fishnet' appearance which does not change with temperature. Livedo reticularis is a similar skin condition which is worse in cold conditions.[286] The incidence of Sneddon syndrome is 4/1 000 000 but the association may be under-diagnosed as livedo reticularis is a common cause of presentation to a dermatologist and appears to be associated with migraine.[287] Those with both appear to be at high risk of stroke[288] and livedo reticularis may be a marker for stroke risk in migraineurs.[289] Most cases are sporadic, although families with apparent autosomal dominant[290] or recessive[291] inheritance have been described.

Patients with Sneddon syndrome may present with transient ischaemic attacks or occasionally with stroke in childhood or young adulthood. The diagnosis is based on skin biopsy, which shows abnormality of the medium-sized vessels. The condition is likely to be secondary to an abnormal production of elastic-tissue-degrading enzymes or a constitutional abnormality of the elastic tissue, characterized by arteriolar changes with deterioration of the internal elastic lamina. The majority of young adults have normal extracranial and intracranial large vessels. Intermittent obstruction and recanalization of the medium-sized cerebral arteries is thought to be the pathogenic mechanism, although venous sinus thrombosis and microembolism may also play a role.

Baxter et al[292] reported three patients who presented with livideo reticularis in infancy that were followed into adolescence. All had frequent recurrent transient stroke-like hemipareses, affecting either side of the body, associated with ipsilateral pain, headache, visual symptoms, dysphasia, seizures, confusion and progressive intellectual failure. Extracerebral involvement included gastrointestinal bleeding, glaucoma, local tissue hypertrophy and renal involvement with hypertension. One developed progressive spasticity. Attacks were more frequent in winter and there was an abnormal peripheral vascular response to temperature change. Polycythaemia, circulating immune complexes and high anticardiolipin IgG were also features.[292] At least three other cases have been described in childhood, two with moyamoya (see Fig. 6.9a)[293,294] and one with white matter disease.[295]

Adults often present with stroke or transient ischaemic events and may have cerebral infarction on neuroimaging, typically in the white matter. Progressive leukoencephalopathy occurs and was commoner than recurrent infarction in a vascular distribution in a recent longitudinal series.[296] In parallel, headaches, vertigo and transient ischaemic attacks involving the posterior circulation as well as the middle cerebral artery territory are commoner than recurrent clinical stroke at follow-up.[296] Cerebral microemboli have been demonstrated on transcranial Doppler monitoring.[297] Atrial myxoma is an occasional association and some patients have mitral valve prolapse.[298] Moyamoya syndrome and arteriovenous malformation have been reported.[293,294] Haemorrhage has been described occasionally[299,300] but vascular imaging does not usually reveal a cause. Involvement of medium-sized arteries has been demonstrated on cerebral angiography[301] with retinal and ophthalmic artery occlusion,[291] but the majority of patients have normal large vessels on MRA.[296,302] In an autopsied case, there were multiple small, predominantly cortical, infarcts, with focal hyperplasia and fibrotic occlusion of arterial vessels in the superficial white matter, cortex and leptomeninges with a very occasional arterial thrombus.[303] Hypertension and seizures may be a prominent feature at presentation. Adults with Sneddon syndrome can develop psychiatric symptoms[304] including depression,[305] memory deficit[306] or dementia without antecedent clinical stroke, commonly in association with a hypercoagulable condition.[307] MRI usually shows fronto-temporal[304] or parieto-occipital infarction[308] or atrophy,[307] with reduced cerebral blood flow in a similar distribution. In one child, there was bilateral thalamic involvement[309] and in another, diffuse white matter abnormality.[295] Mechanisms accounting for these distributions include venous sinus thrombosis[310] or vascular 'watershed' ischaemia as well as involvement of the middle-sized arteries.[301] In one adult presenting with stroke, a leptomeningeal biopsy showed granulomatous infiltration suggesting that an inflammatory process plays a role in at least some cases.

Around 40–80% of patients have intermittently raised antiphospolipid antibodies,[298,311,312] and this may be part of the pathophysiology of the condition although this remains controversial. The antiphospholipid antibodies may simply be secondary to the abnormality of the endothelium and the exposure of endothelial phospholipids to circulating antibodies. In the French study, seizures, mitral regurgitation on echocardiogram and thrombocytopenia were more common in those who had raised antiphospolipid antibodies,[312] but there was no difference in the proportion of those with systemic venous thrombosis or in the distribution of lesions on MRI.[298] Other prothrombotic disorders, including the factor V Leiden mutation[313] and protein Z deficiency,[314] may play a role and anti-endothelial antibodies are raised in around one-third.[315]

INVESTIGATION

Patients presenting with cerebral symptoms associated with livedo reticularis should undergo MRI, MRA and magnetic resonance venography acutely to establish the vascular pathology. Patients should have an echocardiogram and full prothrombotic screening is justified.

MANAGEMENT

Anticoagulation may be of benefit if there is evidence of venous sinus thrombosis but most of these patients are managed with antiplatelet agents. Patients with moyamoya may require revascularization.[294]

Pigmented and depigmented naevi and hypomelanosis of Ito

Cerebrovascular disease, typically intracranial or spinal arteriovenous malformation or anomalous intracranial circulation, has occasionally been reported in linear sebaceous naevus[316,317] and in other forms of epidermal naevus.[318–324] They are occasionally familial[325] and haemorrhage may occur.[323]

Cerebrobovascular abnormalities described in hypomelanosis of Ito include arteriovenous malformation[326] and leptomeningeal angiomatosis.[327]

Vascular naevi

In Cobb syndrome, which typically presents with paraparesis in late childhood, there is vascular lesion of the spinal cord involving the same metamere as the epidermal naevus, although the skin lesion may not be obvious.[328–330] This may be part of the spectrum of conditions that includes PHACES and Sturge–Weber syndrome.[331]

Bonnet–Dechaume–Blanc or Wyburn–Mason syndrome

About 30–50% of those with Bonnet–Dechaume–Blanc or Wyburn–Mason syndrome,[332–334] the association of retinal vascular malformations with arteriovenous malformation of the midbrain and visual pathways, also have an ipsilateral facial haemangioma. Symptoms referable to the arteriovenous malformations often begin in childhood, typically visual loss,[333,334] although pituitary failure, epilepsy and haemorrhage[333–335] may also occur. The intracranial arteriovenous malformations may be inaccessible to surgery or stereotactic radiotherapy and as many never haemorrhage, a conservative approach is usually taken if they are found in a child undergoing neuroimaging because of visual failure, but for those with haemorrhage where there is likely to be a significant recurrence risk, endovascular techniques have been used to embolize[333] as for arteriovenous malformations in the general population, but with a high risk of neurological morbidity.

PTEN mutations

Cerebral arteriovenous malformations have been described in adults with Cowden syndrome[336] and children with Bannayan–Riley–Ruvalcaba syndrome,[337] who also have macrocephaly and autistic features. A study of PTEN mutation carriers in the UK showed that they are one condition with variable expression and age-related penetrance[338] which means that families of the children diagnosed need to be aware of the predisposition to cancer associated with the condition. Most males with the condition have penile freckling.[339] In one series from a referral centre, intracranial developmental venous anomalies were found in 8/9 of patients who had brain MRI with contrast.[339]

Hereditary haemorrhagic telangiectasia (Osler–Weber–Rendu disease)

PATHOPHYSIOLOGY

Hereditary haemorrhagic telangiectasia (HHT; Osler–Weber–Rendu disease) is an autosomal dominant condition with high penetrance. The incidence is between 1 in 2500 and 1 in 8000. Two chromosomes have been implicated and the mutations impair blood vessel growth and repair. The HHT1 mutation on chromosome 9 alters the coding sequence of endoglin, whereas for HHT2, the mutation on chromosome 12 alters the coding sequence of the activin receptor-like kinase 1.[340] Both encode receptor proteins in the transforming growth factor-β (TGF β) pathway, which has an important role in cellular proliferation, differentiation, migration and adhesion. There are artery-to-vein connections in the solid organs – small (telangietases) and large (arteriovenous malformations) – predisposing to shunting and haemorrhage. The arteriovenous malformations are considered to be congenital although they may enlarge at a later stage. Age at presentation is very variable although the reasons for this are presently unknown.

CLINICAL FEATURES

HHT often presents with nose bleeds with a mean age of onset of 12 years and a mean number of episodes per month of 18. Mucocutaneous telangiectasia becomes increasingly obvious in adulthood, usually in the context of a family history.

CEREBROVASCULAR DISEASE

Arteriovenous malformations are relatively common in the cerebral circulation (>10% of patients) and may present with seizures, headache or haemorrhage at any age, including infancy and childhood, i.e. before the skin manifestations or nosebleeds.[341]

STROKE

Overall, patients with HHT have an odds ratio of around 7.6 of suffering from stroke compared with family members without the condition.[342] Male and female patients with HHT have 20 and 6 times the risk of cerebral haemorrhage compared with the general population.[343] The incidence of haemorrhage is similar to that of patients with arteriovenous malformations (AVMs) without HHT.[343] In addition to the risk of haemorrhagic stroke from the AVMs, ischaemic stroke or abscess may arise after embolism from the pulmonary arteriovenous malformations (PAVMs), which occur in about a quarter of patients. Migraine is commoner in those with PAVMs. In fact,

the risk of intracranial haemorrhage is low among people with HHT and outcome is usually good but pulmonary arteriovenous fistulae are a much more frequent cause of neurological symptoms in this population. For example, in the Mayo Clinic series,[344] of 321 patients over a 20-year period, 12 patients (3.7%) had a history of cerebral vascular malformations. Ten patients had arteriovenous malformations, one had a dural arteriovenous fistula and one had a cavernous malformation. Seven patients (2.1%) presented with intracranial haemorrhage at a mean age of 25 years, two presented with seizures alone and three were discovered incidentally. All patients with a history of intracranial haemorrhage were classified as Rankin grade I or II at a mean follow-up interval of 6.0 years. A history of cerebral infarction or transient ischaemic attack was found in 30% of patients with HHT and a pulmonary arteriovenous fistula.[344] Cerebral AVMs are probably more common in families with members with pulmonary AVMs. Multiple, cortical, micro-AVMs or arteriovenous fistulae harboring single feeding arteries and single draining veins should raise clinical suspicion of HHT.[345] Although the mean age at stroke is around the age of 40,[343] both haemorrhagic and ischaemic stroke have been recognized during childhood, and clinical presentation is sometimes with CNS haemorrhage or ischaemic stroke.[341,346] A total of 75 central nervous system manifestations of HHT were found in the series of 50 symptomatic children referred to Bicêtre in Paris;[347] seven spinal cord arteriovenous fistulae that were all present in the paediatric age group (mean age: 2.2 years) and 34 cerebral arteriovenous fistulae with a mean age at presentation of 3 years. Of 127 patients referred to the HHT clinic in Toronto, three had neurological symptoms secondary to bleeding from spinal (N=2, both with HHT type 2) or cerebral AVMs.[346] Of 75 patients in a large UK series, 18 had presumed embolic strokes and 22 had cerebral abscesses, while the rest presented with haemorrhagic stroke.[343] In addition to AVMs of the brain and spine, these patients may occasionally have aneurysms.

SCREENING AT DIAGNOSIS AND IN CHILDREN

Identification of a mutation in an index family member allows pre-clinical screening; this may be performed on cord blood for an infant whose parent is known to be affected.[340] Screening for the cerebral AVMs with MRI with and without gadolinium contrast is justified as the haemorrhagic risk is significant and most of the vascular lesions are amenable to treatment.[340,342,343,348,349] Folz[350] screened six individuals with a family history and suspicion of HHT and found vascular lesions of the brain in two patients and of the lung in two. In the Toronto clinic, a cerebral AVM was found in 1 of 11 neurologically asymptomatic children.[346] Screening for pulmonary AVMs[342] with contrast echocardiography is recommended at least once at around the age of 10 years and more detailed imaging with chest CT to delineate the AVMs if a shunt is found. It is also possible to screen for pulmonary AVMs using pulse oximetry lying and sitting as oxygen saturation is higher on lying down due to gravity, because the AVMs are usually in the lower part of the lung.

MANAGEMENT

Cerebral AVMs occasionally regress spontaneously[351,352] but in view of the risk of haemorrhage, are usually treated with interventional neuroradiology, surgical extirpation and stereotactic radiotherapy and often a combination of two or three of these techniques. Pulmonary AVMs with feeder vessels larger than 3mm diameter should be treated, usually by transcatheter embolization.

Pseudoxanthoma elasticum

CLINICAL FEATURES

Pseudoxanthoma elasticum (PXE) has a prevalence of 1 in 70 000 to 1 in 100 000 live births and the phenotype is broad. The skin is thin and is rather like that of a plucked chicken, with characteristic yellow-orange papules in the flexures. Upper gastrointestinal haemorrhage is very common, and occurred in 17/94 patients followed up in one series (in one during aspirin use)[353] and may lead to acute and chronic anaemia. Angioid streaking of the retina is typical[354] and optic disc drusen are 50 times more common than in the general population.[355] Peripheral and cerebral vessels calcify.

AETIOLOGY AND PATHOPHYSIOLOGY

The hereditary forms are caused by mutations in the *ABCC6* gene on chromosome 16p13.1, and although dominant forms may occur are typically autosomal recessive. However, this is also considered to be at least in part an acquired condition, as the skin changes and retinal angioid streaking have also been documented in congenital anaemias, including thalassaemia[356] and sickle cell disease.[354,357] The vascular changes are characterized by proteoglycan accumulation and elastic fibres in the vessel wall are swollen, fragmented and calcified. Increased compressibility of the carotid wall has been demonstrated;[358] this tends to increase with age in patients under the age of 40 and reduces thereafter. Carotid intima-media thickness is increased[359] but the hypertrophy is external and there is no encroachment on the lumen. In adults, the pathology appears to behave like a slowly progressive premature atherosclerosis, perhaps related to accumulation of lipids in the arterial wall.[359]

ISCHAEMIC AND HAEMORRHAGIC STROKE

In a review, Schievink[57] considered that the typical vascular diseases in PXE were intracranial aneurysms, which have been described in the internal carotid artery,[360] and cerebral ischaemia caused by premature arterial occlusive disease. However, in a series of 100 patients from the Netherlands, no patient with PXE had a symptomatic intracranial aneurysm as the presenting symptom over 3168 retrospective patient observation years and 1602 prospective patient observation years.[353] Only one patient presented with an ischaemic stroke but during follow-up (*N*=94, mean follow-up 17.1 years, range 1–49 years), this patient suffered a recurrence and seven patients had a new ischaemic stroke. All were caused by small-vessel disease. The relative risk of ischaemia in PXE under 65 years compared with the general population was 3.6 (95% confidence interval 3.3–4.0). Adults may have vascular disease with large artery calcification and stenosis leading to transient ischaemic attacks and occasionally to ischaemic and haemorrhagic stroke.[361–368] However, lacunar infarction compatible with small vessel disease is characteristic and hypertension may be a risk factor. Seizures are more common than in the general population and may herald stroke.[363] Presentation may be rather protracted, with slow onset of cognitive loss and seizures[362] before more obvious transient ischaemic attacks and strokes, but the majority of people with PXE have no neuropsychological or psychiatric problems.[369] An abnormal network connecting the external and internal carotid circulations, similar to the rete mirabile typical of mammals such as cats, has been documented in adults[370,371] and adolescents[372] with PXE. Atherosclerosis leading to myocardial ischaemia and intermittent claudication have been described in children.[373,374] Stroke in association with carotid occlusion has been reported alongside severe cardiac involvement.[375] In one adolescent, recurrent stroke associated with right carotid hypoplasia was considered to be thromboembolic,[376] although dissection might have been another possibility. Moyamoya has been reported in a child with the typical skin manifestations of elastosis perforans serpiginosa who had two amino acid substitutions close to a critical region of the *ABCC6* gene, although a direct link remained unproven.[377] Visual loss in an 18-year-old girl was secondary to optic nerve head ischaemia in the context of acute anaemia after a gastrointestinal haemorrhage.[378]

DIAGNOSIS

The dermatological diagnosis is not easy and is sometimes made a long time after the initial vascular presentation.[379] A high index of suspicion is required. Although expensive, particularly as there are a large number of *ABCC6* mutations, genetic testing may be informative although there are few data on genotypic–phenotypic correlations.

MANAGEMENT

Antiplatelet and anticoagulant therapy should be avoided in patients with PXE in view of the risk of upper gastrointestinal haemorrhage. Acute bleeding should be managed with urgent volume replacement and transfusion to avoid the risk of global cerebral and ophthalmic ischaemia.

15.4 Congenital and Acquired Anaemias

Dimitrios Zafeiriou, Mara Prengler, Steven Pavlakis and Fenella J. Kirkham

Introduction

Stroke is a well-recognized complication of sickle cell disease and iron deficiency is a common association with arterial[5] and venous[74] stroke in childhood. A variety of neurological complications have been described in childhood in other congenital and acquired haemolytic and aplastic anaemias including β-thalassaemia, hereditary spherocytosis, haemoglobin Alesha,[380] haemoglobin Sabine,[381] Evans syndrome, Diamond–Blackfan syndrome and Fanconi anaemia. Early clinical descriptions allowed some insight into the natural history of these conditions, but vascular imaging was rarely performed, as conventional angiography was considered too invasive. Now that magnetic resonance imaging, including angiography and venography, can be performed in the acute phase, various stroke syndromes are being documented, although clinico-radiological associations remain uncertain in many cases. The effects of treatment and longer survival have proved difficult to tease out. There are very few contemporary population-based or cohort studies, so although it is clear that neurological events occur in the anaemias, figures for incidence or prevalence are scanty (Table 15.1). In fact anaemia may actually protect against arteriosclerotic events,[382] perhaps because cholesterol levels are lower.[383] Haemorrhage and other mechanisms for ischaemic events, including venous sinus thrombosis[74] and posterior leukoencephalopathy,[384] may play a more prominent role.

There are a number of mechanisms for the development of cerebrovascular disease and neurological symptoms, including transient ischaemic episodes and stroke, in these patients. Acute hypoxia may cause injury if cerebral blood flow is already close to the ischaemic threshold.[385,386] Recent evidence suggests that intravascular haemolysis renders the endothelium vulnerable by increasing free haemoglobin and red cell arginase that interferes with the bioavailability of endothelial nitric oxide.[387] In addition, chronic hypoxia tends to upregulate processes that lead to the adhesion of red cells, white cells and platelets to the endothelium, associated with inflammation.[388] Evidence is emerging that various degrees of exposure to, and compensation for, hypoxia leads eventually to irreversible stenosis and occlusion of arteries.[386,389–391] Right to left shunting through a patent foramen ovale (PFO) is a well-recognized cause of sustained and intermittent hypoxia,[392–394] and is a potentially treatable cause of stroke and migraine in young adults.[395] However, the possibility that PFO is a risk factor for overt or covert infarction in anaemias has received little attention until recently.[396–398] For both arteriopathy and venous sinus thrombosis in the context of anaemia, the clinical triggers for the neurological event[74,386] and the role of additional genetic pro-thrombotic disorders, such as the methylene tetrahydrofolate reductase C677T polymorphism, factor V Leiden and prothrombin 20210, require further investigation.

In addition, haemodynamic factors are likely, in part, important for the development of ischaemia and stroke. In sickle cell disease, the anaemia results in secondary hyperaemia, hypervolaemia and vasodilatation[399] and these haemodynamic insufficiencies are likely to play a role. In chronic anaemia, the brain blood flow is likely maximized, so any perturbation may result in flow insufficiency and stroke.

Aessopos[356] pointed out that some patients with beta-thalassaemia develop skin and ocular signs structurally indistinguishable from those of pseudoxanthoma elasticum,[400] although they do not appear to share the same ATP-binding cassette gene (ABCC6),[401] and long-term changes to elastic tissue is more likely to be related to oxidative damage.[402] The skin changes of pseudoxanthoma elasticum are more prominent clinically and pathologically in the various forms of β-thalassaemia[402] but ocular angioid streaks are seen in haemoglobin C,[403] sickle cell[404] and β-thalassaemia[405,406] trait as well as β-thalassaemia intermedia,[407,408] hereditary spherocytosis, congenital dyserythropoietic anaemia types I[409] and III[410] and the haemoglobin H form of α-thalassaemia.[411] They become more common with increasing age in homozygous sickle cell disease[412,413] as well as β-thalassaemia.[408] Subclinical changes in elastin anatomy (elastorrhexis) may be seen in extrasplenic and intrasplenic arteries of patients requiring surgery in the context of haemolytic anaemia.[414] Chronic connective tissue disorders may render patients vulnerable to the development of cerebral vascular disease as they age.

Congenital disorders of haemoglobin

β-Thalassaemia

β-Thalassaemia major (BTM) is a congenital haemolytic disorder caused by a partial or complete deficiency of beta-globin chain synthesis. Homozygous carriers of beta-globin gene defects suffer from severe anaemia and other serious complications from early childhood. The disease is treated with chronic blood transfusion. Despite the difficulties associated with treatment, standards of care for BTM patients have improved in recent years, resulting in a dramatic increase in the average life expectancy. As a consequence, previously undescribed complications have emerged. β-Thalassaemia intermedia (BTI) is characterized by a milder clinical course, a haemoglobin level of more than 7g/dl, an onset at ages over 2 years and growth problems, as well as a moderate blood transfusion requirement; there may be a need for chelation therapy but typically in older patients.

Thrombosis affects around 5% of patients with β-thalassaemia and a significant proportion are cerebral. As early as 1972, Logothetis[415] described a stroke syndrome in two patients and neurological deficits compatible with transient ischaemic attacks (TIAs) in about 20% of a total of 136 patients. An Italian multicentre study of 735 patients with BTM reported 16 individuals with a cerebral thromboembolic event.[416] In a Russian series of 42 patients, the peak age for cerebral complications was 6–12 years and the majority were TIAs rather than strokes,[417] often associated with haemolytic crises.[418] In TIAs, SPECT may reveal focal hypoperfusion when MRI is negative.[419] Clinically there appear to be at least three clinical stroke syndromes associated with β-thalassaemia.

Firstly, TIAs referable to the posterior circulation may be relatively common in thalassaemia major, probably in relation to the severity of the anaemia. In Logothetis's[415] series of patients

TABLE 15.1
Neurological complications of anaemia

Underlying cause	PXE	Thrombus	Embolus	Haemorrhage SAH	Haemorrhage ICH	Aneurysm	AVM	TIAs A	TIAs P	Stenosis EC	Stenosis IC	Moyamoya	VST	PT	PL	Cortical laminar necrosis	Covert
Haemoglobin SS	+	+	?	+	+	+		+	+	+	+	+	+	+	+	+	++
Haemoglobin SC													+	+	+	+	
Haemoglobin Sβ-thalassaemia																	++
Haemoglobin AS												+	+				
Thalassaemia major	+		+						+				+	+	+		++
Thalassaemia intermedia										+		+					
Thalassaemia minor (trait)			+														
Pyruvate kinase deficiency			+								+						
Hereditary spherocytosis			?								?	+	?				
Paroxysmal nocturnal haemoglobinuria												+	+				
Fanconi				+	+							+					
Blackfan–Diamond			+			Multiple						+					+
Acquired aplastic														+	?		
Acquired haemolytic											+		+				

A, anterior; AVM, arteriovenous malformation; EC, extracranial; IC, intracranial; ICH, intracranial haemorrhage; P, posterior; PL, periventricular leukomalacia or posterior leukoencephalopathy; PT, pseudotumour cerebri; PXE, pseudoxanthoma elasticum; SAH, subarachnoid haemorrhage; VST, venous sinus thrombosis; TIAs, transient ischaemic attacks.

in a moderately intensive transfusion regimen, dizziness, visual symptoms and fainting were documented in 20% of the patients, usually during the second half of the intertransfusional period. Recurrent TIAs and stroke have been reported in a 15-year-old boy with heterozygosity for β-thalassaemia and factor V Leiden, as well as slightly decreased plasma levels of proteins C and S.[419] It seems that additional prothrombotic risk factors may cause significant thrombophilia in patients with β-thalassaemia minor.

Secondly, acute neurological symptoms have been well documented at the time of a large transfusion with a substantial increase in haematocrit from a low baseline, either during or within the first few days after the transfusion and usually associated with an acute rise in blood pressure. Most of these patients have large spleens and many were undergoing preoperative transfusion before splenectomy for hypersplenism[420] or developed neurological symptoms and signs postoperatively.[415] In a prospective series, preoperative haematocrit was lower in the 16 who developed hypertension compared with the 84 who did not; three of these patients had convulsions despite prophylaxis and one had permanent sequelae.[421] These patients are also characterized by short stature and iron overload.[420] The patient develops headache and vomiting often accompanied by seizures and sometimes by hemiparesis or visual symptoms. Purpura, haematuria and pink tears were reported in one young case.[422] Acute intracerebral and subarachnoid haemorrhage have also been described in these patients.[420,421,423–428] The pathology resembles that seen after hypertensive encephalopathy, one of the causes of posterior leukoencephalopathy. Patients who have had EEG have had slowing and/or discharges in the parietal and occipital regions, compatible with posterior leukoencephalopathy, although acute neuroimaging was not performed in parallel.[429] At autopsy the brains is markedly oedematous and congested and there are visible and microscopic focal or perivascular cerebral haemorrhages. Microdissecting aneurysms characteristic of hypertensive cerebral haemorrhage may be seen but large vessel disease has not been detected.

There may be a role for a combination of furosemide and captopril in reducing the risk of perioperative hypertension.[430,431] Intracranial haemorrhage at an interval of a few days after the last transfusion has also been described in chronically transfused older patients.[428,432] An acute transfusion increases haematocrit and cerebral volume. Since the volume is already increased, a further increase in maximally dilated vessels might result in brain haemorrhages. Any transfusions should be done carefully or by a partial exchange technique in order to decrease the risk of intracranial haemorrhage.

Thirdly, both arterial ischaemic and haemorrhagic stroke has been documented in β-thalassaemia major as well as in β-thalassaemia intermedia.[433,434] The majority of patients appear to have cardioembolic stroke in the context of cardiomyopathy secondary to the iron overload.[356,416,435] Diabetes, chronic liver disease and hypothyroidism may also play a role.[416] Wong[436] reported two patients with extracranial carotid disease and arterial stroke and a case was reported[434] of middle cerebral artery occlusion (Fig. 15.13) in a 1 year old whose mother had been transfused in pregnancy for a refractory anaemia; both mother and child were heterozygous for the β-thalassaemia mutation IVS-I-1; the child was also homozygous for the MTHFR C677T mutation. Moyamoya has been reported in β-thalassaemia[437–439] and Sβ-thalassaemia,[440] albeit much less commonly than in sickle cell disease. It may, however, be very difficult to distinguish venous from arterial thrombosis in these patients, particularly as imaging may not be undertaken in the acute phase or include vascular imaging.[416,441,442] However, recurrence has been reported rarely,[435] perhaps because life expectancy for patients with multiple complications of thalassaemia is relatively short;[356] diagnosing stroke syndromes has not hitherto been a priority but may become so as survival improves with improved chelation.

Apart from these three clinically distinct syndromes in thalassaemic patients, of special merit is the ocurrence of silent infarcts in patients with thalassaemia intermedia, similar to those observed in the sickle cell syndromes. Manfre[443] found that

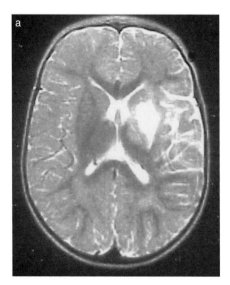
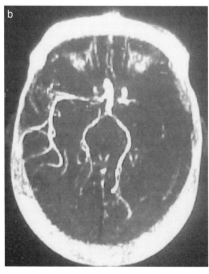

Fig. 15.13. (a) One-year-old child with β-thalassaemia trait who presented with a left hemiparesis. Axial T2-weighted MRI showing ischaemic infarction in the right internal capsule, putamen and thalamus. (b) MRA showing occlusion of the M1 segment of the right middle cerebral artery.[434]

37.5% of 16 patients with thalassaemia intermedia tested demonstrated abnormal findings consistent with silent infarcts in MRI; brain damage increased with age and inversely correlated with haemoglobin level. Other groups have found prevalences of 25–60%; risk factors include increasing age and lack of transfusion.[444,445] MRI is likely to be a useful tool in identifying patients with silent infarction at risk for clinical stroke.

Other mechanisms may play a role. Intradural extramedullary haematopoesis may be very striking[446] and mechanical factors secondary to bone marrow hyperplasia in the skull may be a risk factor for stroke. Isolated seizures occurred in 7% but recurrent seizures (1%) were probably no commoner than in the general population; however, terminal convulsions have been reported.[447] Venous sinus thrombosis has also been reported in β-thalassaemia[74] and some of the seizures and transient focal neurological deficits might be related to sinus thrombosis or cortical vein thrombosis with subsequent recanalization and full recovery.[429]

HYPERCOAGULABLE STATE IN BTM AND BTI

Among other complications, profound haemostatic changes have been observed in patients with BTM and BTI. The presence of a higher than normal incidence of thromboembolic events, mainly in BTI, and the existence of prothrombotic haemostatic abnormalities in a considerable number of BTM but also BTI patients,[448] even from a very early age,[449] have led to the recognition of a hypercoagulable state in these patients, irrespective of splenectomy.[450] Despite several publications reporting thromboembolic complications in BTM, very few comprehensive reviews or systematic studies exist to date.[451]

Patients with BTM have low levels of proteins S and C, and demonstrate enhanced platelet consumption and platelet, monocyte, granulocyte and endothelial activation. Increased levels of activation peptides TAT, F12, FPA and D-dimer are suggestive of continuous thrombin generation and enhanced fibrinolysis.[451] The markers of platelet and coagulation activation are persistently and consistently elevated in most thalassaemic patients, even in the absence of thromboembolic events. Several aetiological factors have been suggested. Changes in the lipid maintainance composition of the abnormal thalassaemic red bloood cells and haemosiderosis contribute to thrombin generation and activation of blood cells and the vascular endothelium. Thrombosis is largely a subclinical process in thalassaemia, manifest as platelet and fibrin thrombi in the microvasculature in the lungs and the brain at autopsy, but the exact pathophysiology is still unclear. Central venous line placement for chelation,[452] APC resistence[453] and protein C deficiency[454] are additional risk factors described in thalassaemic patients with thrombosis.

There may be intellectual problems, probably related to chronic hypoxia, which may be reflected in the EEG spectrum.[455] Evoked potential studies may reveal subclinical neuropathology involving the peripheral nervous system, the visual pathway and sensorineural hearing which are usually related to iron toxicity as measured by ferritin concentration and the presence of diabetes mellitus.[456–458]

Acquired aplastic anaemias

Many acquired aplastic anaemias in childhood are secondary to infections, such as parvovirus,[459] and it may be difficult to distinguish the neurological effects of the sudden drop in haemoglobin from those due to invasion of the organism. Infections may be an independent risk factor for stroke. For example, in the general population, in addition to meningoencephalitis, associated with ataxia and ventricular dilatation on imaging,[460] stroke in an arterial distribution has been reported in a child with a recent parvovirus infection; haematology has generally not been presented in these cases. Stroke after parvovirus B19 infection has also been reported in a 7-year-old male; however, there was no anaemia.[461] In a series of 10 patients with sickle cell disease with neurological complications in the context of aplastic crisis secondary to parvovirus, eight presented with seizures and two with cortical blindness, while five had a hemiparesis. Four had CSF pleiocytosis compatible with aseptic meningitis.[462] Only one of the four undergoing arteriography had arterial disease while three of the ten had abnormal parenchymal imaging involving the temporal, parietal and occipital regions and therefore compatible with venous sinus thrombosis or posterior leukoencephalopathy as well as arterial stroke, particularly as presentation was with seizures and/or cortical blindness and outcome was good. Pseudotumour cerebri has also been documented in acquired aplastic anaemia.[463] One patient in the Great Ormond Street series with aplastic anaemia and sickle cell trait had a small infarct in the basal ganglia from which he made a full recovery[5]. Stroke (arterial or thrombotic) has been repeatedly reported as a complication of various therapeutic regimens for acquired anaemia, a subject beyond the scope of this chapter.

Congenital aplastic anaemias

FANCONI ANAEMIA

Fanconi anaemia is an autosomal recessive condition caused by mutations in one of at least seven genes. Clinical manifestations include radial deformity, often with absent thumbs, short stature, aplastic anaemia, and a high risk of acute myeloid leukaemia and solid tumours.[464] Neurological involvement includes microcephaly, neural tube defects, agenesis of the corpus callosum, holoprosencephaly, acqueduct stenosis and hydrocephalus.[465] Intracerebral haemorrhage occurs as part of the natural history[466] and after bone marrow transplantation.[467–469] Moyamoya has been reported occasionally,[470,471] with a prevalence of 2/434 cases in one cohort.[471]

DIAMOND–BLACKFAN SYNDROME

Seizures have been reported occasionally in the Diamond–Blackfan syndrome, for example after a poorly matched transfusion and bolus steroids in one patient in whom CT was normal[472] and after cyclophosphamide in another in whom neuroimaging was not performed.[473] These settings are ones in which posterior leukoencephalopathy has been described but is commonly missed when MRI is not available.

In addition to one teenager with multiple cerebral aneurysms,[474] presumed perinatal infarction apparently secondary to a middle cerebral artery embolus has been documented in a boy with Blackfan–Diamond presenting with anaemia at 4 months and hemiparesis at 10 months.[475] He also had a patent foramen ovale with a left-to-right shunt at the time of echocardiography at the age of 5 months as well as heterozygosity for the methylenetetrahydrofolate reductase gene. One patient presenting in the neonatal period with acute collapse sufficient to cause renal damage had posterior infarction documented on MRI when she presented with seizures and fluctuating ataxia at the time of worsening anaemia in her teens (see Fig. 15.24a).

Acquired haemolytic anaemias

Haemolytic-Uraemic Syndrome

Coma occurring as a complication of haemolytic-uraemic syndrome (HUS) is of grave prognostic significance,[476] particularly if the patient's respiratory pattern is abnormal.[477] The following pathologies have been described: hypoxic-ischaemic damage and cerebral oedema,[478] multiple microvascular thrombi[479] and major cerebral vessel thrombosis[480] (Fig. 15.14). Intracranial pressure was raised in three children with the latter pathology and is probably worth monitoring in all deeply unconscious children with the condition, as the prognosis is not necessarily poor[481] even for those with focal infarction demonstrated on CT,[482–484] and some morbidity and mortality may be prevented by careful attention to fluid and electrolyte balance, guided by intracranial pressure measurement. Dialysis and supportive treatment with repeated infusions of fresh frozen plasma are the mainstay of treatment, and although plasma exchange is beneficial in those with thrombotic thrombocytopenic purpura, which was thought to be related, there is little evidence that additional therapy has any advantage in haemolytic-uraemic syndrome.[485] Neuroradiology may demonstrate diffuse cerebral oedema, large vessel infarctions, diffuse multiple small infarcts and focal or multiple haemorrhages.[486–488] Rarely, cerebral infarcts may occur with recurrence of HUS after renal transplantation[489] and moyamoya has been described.[490] However, for almost all children discharged from hospital without apparent neurological symptomatology after an episode of acute HUS, there is no increased risk of subsequent learning, behavioural or attention problems.[491]

Autoimmune Haemolytic Anaemias and Evans Syndrome

Warm IgG autoimmune haemolytic anaemia (AIHA) is a relatively common disorder in children, rarely revealing an underlying disorder and usually resolving with minimal treatment.[492] When associated with immune thrombocytopenic pupura, either serially or in parallel, it is known as Evans syndrome. Ischaemic stroke has been reported with warm IgM AIHA;[493,494] one patient who also had Down syndrome had moyamoya (Fig. 15.8)[123] Venous sinus thrombosis and pseudotumour cerebri have been diagnosed in patients with a warm autoimmune haemolytic anaemia who were eventually diagnosed as having systemic lupus erythematosus.[74,495] Venous sinus thrombosis occurs occasionally in Evans syndrome[496,497] and intracerebral haemorrhage has been reported in a patient treated with long-term steroids who developed aspergillosis.[498]

Paroxysmal Nocturnal Haemoglobinuria

Thrombosis, including involvement of the cerebral venous sinuses, is well documented in this acquired clonal stem cell disorder, leading to a deficient biosynthesis of surface proteins in haematopoetic cells, and moyamoya has been reported in an 11-year-old girl with recurrent cerebrovascular accidents.[499] Fatal cerebral ischaemic infarctions have been reported in young patients with paroxysmal nocturnal haemoglobonuria;[500,501] in one series four out of the nine patients died within a week after

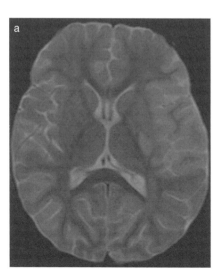 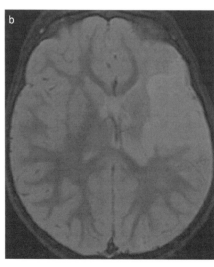

Fig. 15.14. (a,b) Middle cerebral artery territory infarct with occlusion of the proximal middle cerebral artery in a child with haemolytic-uraemic syndrome.

the initial thrombotic or arterial events with no difference in treatment between favourable and unfavourable outcome.[500]

Hereditary haemolytic anaemias

PYRUVATE KINASE DEFICIENCY

Red cell pyruvate kinase deficiency is the commonest glycolytic enzyme abnormality causing non-spherocytic haemolytic anaemia and is associated with a wide variation in the degree of haemolysis, although the anaemia is usually mild and transfusion and splenectomy are rarely required. Patients have high levels of 2,3 dihydrophosphoglycerate so the haemoglobin oxygen affinity curve is right-shifted. One young non-splenectomized adult has been reported to have had occlusion of a middle cerebral artery and infarction in the ipsilateral hemisphere soon after clinical presentation with symptoms of the anaemia.[502] There was evidence of intravascular haemolysis with low haptoglobin and high lactate dehydrogenase. Thromboembolism has also been reported after splenectomy.[503] Moyamoya has been reported in a 13-year-old Greek girl who presented with neonatal onset of anaemia, haemolytic and aplastic crises especially during infections, stroke and progressive psychomotor retardation, who in addition to the pyruvate kinase deficiency also had raised serum lipoprotein(a) concentration and homozygosity for the *C677T* mutation of the methylene-tetrahydrofolate reductase gene.[504]

HEREDITARY SPHEROCYTOSIS

Hereditary spherocytosis, a heterogeneous disorder caused by mutations in the genes encoding the proteins of the red cell membrane, is the commonest genetic cause of haemolysis in those of Northern European extraction, with an incidence of around 1 in 2000.[505] Moyamoya has been reported[506,507] and in one case transient ischaemic attacks appeared to coincide with haemolytic crises and stopped after splenectomy.[507] In addition to systemic thrombosis, cerebrovascular accident has also been reported after splenectomy.[508] Large vessel occlusion has been reported in adults[509] and a young woman presented with transient sensory symptoms and had normal parenchymal and vascular imaging but reduced flow in the parietal region, perhaps representing venous ischaemia.[510] However, for adults over 40 who have not had a splenectomy, the risk of vascular events is reduced fivefold compared with controls, probably because of the reduced cholesterol seen in association with anaemia.[382]

SICKLE CELL DISEASE

Introduction

Sickle cell disease (SCD) is a group of inherited haemoglobinopathies[511] common among peoples of Equatorial African ancestry but not confined to that population.[512] The condition is caused by a mutation in the gene for globin, an essential component of the haemoglobin molecule (Hb), which is located inside the red blood cells and carries oxygen to every cell in the body. The pattern of inheritance is autosomal

recessive and the homozygous state (HbSS) is known as sickle cell anaemia.[512]

Normal adult haemoglobin (Hb), HbA, consists of two α and two β polypeptides chains ($\alpha_2\beta_2$). HbA comprises about 97% of the Hb in adults. Two other haemoglobins, HbA$_2$ ($\alpha_2\delta_2$) and fetal haemoglobin (HbF) ($\alpha_2\gamma_2$), are found in smaller amounts (1.5–3% and <1%, respectively).[513] The mutation which produces HbS is the substitution of valine for glutamic acid at the sixth position of the β-globin chain (β6Glut→Val). Haemoglobin S behaves like normal haemoglobin when fully oxygenated but at low oxygen tension, the hydrophobic valine residue polymerizes resulting in gel formation. As a consequence, the red cell has an increased density and elongated sickle shape, becoming less pliable.[512,514,515] The rigid and deformed sickle cell is damaged by mechanical stress during the passage through the vasculature (especially in small blood vessels), resulting in a chronic haemolytic anaemia with red cell destruction (two to eight times higher than normal). The rate of red cell production and destruction in sickle cell anaemia is influenced by infection, drugs and other factors, and if the balance is disturbed, anaemic crisis may result.[514]

Other double heterozygote variants of the SCD syndromes include SCD (inheritance of one HbS with one gene for Hb C), the next in frequency after sickle cell anaemia. Co-inheritance of a β-thalassaemia gene with HbS causes HbSβ$^+$-thalassaemia with 3–25% HbA, or HbSβ^0-thalassaemia without HbA.[511,512,516] Clinically, sickle cell anaemia (HbSS) and HBSβ^0-thalassaemia tend to run a severe course, whereas haemoglobin SCD and HbSβ$^+$-thalassaemia have milder manifestations.[512]

Although the sickle gene mutation is most common in equatorial Africa, it is also found in the Mediterranean regions of Europe and Turkey.[517] The carrier state of the sickle cell gene (one β^5 globin gene and a normal β globin gene) is defined as sickle cell trait[512] and protects against malaria, as sickle cells are a hostile environment for the parasite,[514] although exact mechanisms are still debated. In SCD, carrier frequency is between 5% and 40% in the populations where the frequency of the gene is high.[511,512]

The phenotype may be influenced by the different β-haplotypes (the nucleotide 5′ and 3′ sickle cell gene sequence). There are three major African and African American haplotypes: Senegal, Benin and Bantu (or Central African Republic).[512] In addition, there is an independent haplotype in India and Saudi Arabia.[511] The sickle gene is distributed worldwide as a consequence of the slave trade and economic migration.[518]

Molecular sickling

The mechanism of molecular sickling in SCD, which is very important for the physiopathology of the complications, including cerebrovascular disease, is complex. HbSS behaves like normal haemoglobin (HbA) when fully oxygenated, but at low oxygen tensions, the hydrophobic valine residue polymerizes resulting in gel formation,[514,519] although this is less in the presence of HbA and HbF.[514,520] High concentration of

HbSS results in increased sickling with hypoxia, acidosis or infection[521,522] and the rigid cell may sludge in small blood vessels.[514] In addition, the endothelial surface may be damaged and become more adhesive to red and white cells and platelets,[388,514,523–525] which is a candidate mechanism for endothelial injury and vaso-occlusion in SCD,[522,524,526–529] perhaps resulting in the formation of a nidus of blood cells, and eventually leading to long-term arterial narrowing. There is probably an important additional effect of infection (Fig. 15.15) and it has been suggested that SCD should be seen as an inflammatory disease of the blood vessels.[528]

Nitric oxide, synthesized from L-arginine in endothelial cells, is a critical mediator of vascular integrity. Nitric oxide regulates mainly vasomotor tone and has powerful vasodilatory functions.[523] Disturbance of endothelial function in relation to the free haemoglobin and arginase released during haemolysis may reduce nitric oxide levels, allowing unopposed vasoconstriction instead of vasodilatation, which may contribute to the genesis of cerebrovascular disease in SCD.[523,530,531]

Non-neurological problems of sickle cell disease
There are a large number of complications of sickle cell disease. Patients with SCD present with symptoms secondary to two main mechanisms: haemolytic anaemia and vaso-occlusion.[512,514] The leading causes of death among very young children with SCD are firstly acute anaemia (caused by splenic sequestration and aplastic crisis due to viral infection) and, secondly, bacterial infection, particularly secondary to pneumoccocal meningitis or pneumonia (as the spleen becomes non-functional).[532] There is also substantial morbidity from early infancy due to vaso-occlusive events, which cause painful bone crisis, abdominal pain, acute chest syndrome and neurological events.[514] The median age at death for males with homozygous

sickle cell anaemia is 42–53 years and for females 48–58 years; survival is better for those with HbSC disease.[532,533] In older children and adults, death often occurs secondary to chronic organ damage, particularly pulmonary or renal failure,[532] although stroke is also an important cause.[534]

There is a high prevalence of snoring and sleep apnoea, apparently secondary to enlarged tonsils and adenoids, in children with sickle cell disease,[535,536] in addition to low daytime haemoglobin oxygen saturation.[537] Hypoxia triggers potentially adaptive changes leading to increased vascular tone and red and white cell and platelet adhesion,[388,525] as well as polymerization, gel formation and potassium efflux associated with increased cell density.[514,538]

Neurological complications of sickle cell disease
(Table 15.2, Figs 15.16–15.26)
In one North American study in which the overall incidence for childhood stroke was 1.29/100 000 per year (ischaemic 0.58/100 000/year and haemorrhagic 0.71/100 000/year), the commonest cause was SCD (39%),[539] with an incidence of 285–310/100 000/year,[539,540] which is similar to that found in general populations of elderly adults. However, in older adults with SCD, the rate may be three times as high.[540] In patients with sickle cell disease, the lifetime risk of stroke is between 25% and 30%.[534,541] Approximately 75% of the infarcts are ischaemic and the remainder are haemorrhagic,[542] although the latter group may be underestimated as intracranial bleeding may be a cause of sudden death.

Hemiparesis is the typical presentation of ischaemic stroke. Patients with prior infarction are at increased risk of haemorrhage as they age.[542] Infarction is common in mid-childhood, between 2 and 10 years of age. Stroke incidence decreases to a minimum between the ages of 20 and 29 years, but there is a further peak after the age of 35. Haemorrhage

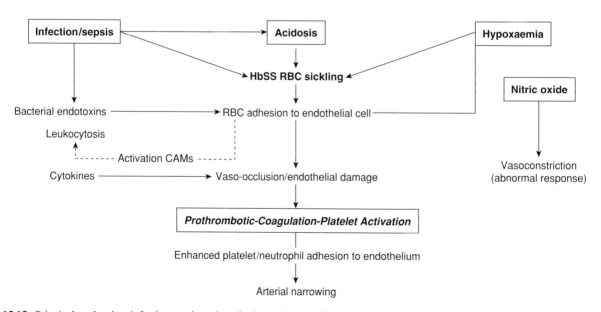

Fig. 15.15. Principal molecular, infectious and prothrombotic mechanisms involved in the genesis of cerebrovascular disease in sickle cell disease. CAMs, cell adhesion molecules; HbSS, sickle cell anaemia; RBC, red blood cell.[519]

TABLE 15.2

Neurological syndromes complicating sickle cell disease

Clinical syndrome	Context	Symptoms and signs	Parenchymal imaging	Pathophysiology
Acute anterior ischaemic stroke (if signs last for >24 hours)	'Out-of-the-blue' in a previously well child or adult	Acute weakness, usually one arm and leg	Focal ischaemia in MCA territory or anterior border zone	Arterial disease, typically stenosis or occlusion of distal ICA, proximal MCA and ACA. Exclude dissection
Acute anterior TIA (if signs last for <24 hours)	'Out-of-the-blue' in a previously well child or adult	Acute weakness, usually one arm and leg	May be normal or show 'covert' infarction	Exclude venous sinus thrombosis, dissection, stenosis, moyamoya
Acute posterior TIA (if signs last for <24 hours)	'Out-of-the-blue' in a previously well child or adult	Dizziness, ataxia, diplopia, VIth nerve palsy, visual disturbance	May be normal or show 'covert' infarction	Exclude venous sinus thrombosis, dissection, stenosis, moyamoya
Acute haemorrhagic stroke	Often following acute complications requiring transfusion or steroids	Altered mental status, headache, stiff neck, coma, seizures, hemiplegia	Subarachnoid or intracerebral haemorrhage	Exclude venous sinus thrombosis, moyamoya, aneurysm
Posterior reversible encephalopathy syndrome (PRES)	Acute chest syndrome, acute a anaemia (aplastic/sequestration), infection, after surgery, after immunosuppression	Altered mental status, headache, reduced level of consciousness, coma, confusion, seizures, visual symptoms (e.g. blindness), or focal signs	Acute: global or focal oedema, posterior leukencephalopathy, borderzone ischaemia, acute demyelination. Follow-up: normal or borderzone infarction	Arterial imaging may be normal; exclude poor cardiac function; exclude venous sinus thrombosis, including straight sinus, in the acute phase as this often recanalizes
Seizures	Fever, chest crisis, priapism, nephrotic syndrome, blood transfusion	Often none. Coma, confusion, visual loss, or focal signs	Often no abnormality; risk factor for covert infarction	Exclude venous sinus thrombosis, RPLS and arterial disease in distal ICA, proximal MCA and ACA[8]
Acute psychosis	'Out-of-the-blue' in previously well patient	Hallucinations, disinhibition	Normal or 'covert' infarction	Exclude pernicious anaemia, venous sinus thrombosis, hypoxia
Acute paraplegia	'Out-of-the-blue' in previously well patient, occasionally with pneumococcal meningitis	Weakness in legs and sometimes arms, acute retention	Spinal cord infarction	Exclude vasculopathy or embolus, extramedullary haemopoeisis
Acute visual disturbance	'Out-of-the-blue' in previously well patient, postoperative[123]	Blurred vision, blindness, bumping into objects	Often no abnormality; posterior leukencephalopathy, borderzone ischaemia	Parieto-occipital infarction: arterial or venous. Retinal artery occlusion secondary to embolus (?PFO). White matter/borderzone changes secondary to acute change BP. Idiopathic intracranial hypertension
Acute severe headache	'Out-of-the-blue' in a previously well adult or child	Reduced level of consciousness, coma, stiff neck, focal signs	Subarachnoid or intracerebral haemorrhage; ischaemia	Exclude aneurysm, venous sinus thrombosis, dissection, moyamoya, vasospasm
Chronic migrainous headache	Severe headache (patient lies down in dark room), often a family history	Occasional confusion, visual field loss or hemiparesis	Normal or 'covert' infarction	Exclude sleep-disordered breathing. Consider PFO
Chronic non-migrainous headache	Often early morning, mild	Usually none (exclude signs of raised ICP)	Exclude space occupying lesion	Exclude sleep-disordered breathing
'Soft neurological signs'	Insidious onset, often associated with poor progress at school	Motor abnormalities (e.g. on Zurich scale), diplegia, mild bilateral dystonia	'Covert' infarction white matter	Arterial imaging may be normal. Exclude sleep-disordered breathing
Poor school progress	Insidious onset	Cognitive difficulties, particularly affecting attention, executive function and arithmetic	Associated with 'covert' infarction but T2-weighted MRI may be normal	Exclude moyamoya but arterial imaging often normal. Exclude deafness, sleep-disordered breathing
'Covert' infarction	Routine screening	May be cognitive difficulties and/or motor abnormalities	Typically white matter of deep borderzone, may affect basal ganglia/grey matter in borderzone	Residua of previous venous or arterial pathology or 'reversible neurological syndrome'. Consider PFO
Deafness	Routine screening or poor attention, often not noticed by patient, may be sudden	Tympanometry, audiometry to differentiate conductive and sensorineural	Middle ear effusion, cholesteatoma, ossicle abnormalities associated with sensorineural deafness	Conductive: infection. Sensorineural: chronic hypoxia?

ACA, anterior cerebral artery; BP blood pressure; ICA, internal carotid artery; ICP, intracranial pressure; MCA, middle cerebral artery; PFO patent foramen ovale; RPLS, reversible posterior leukoencephalopathy; TIA, transient ischaemic attack.

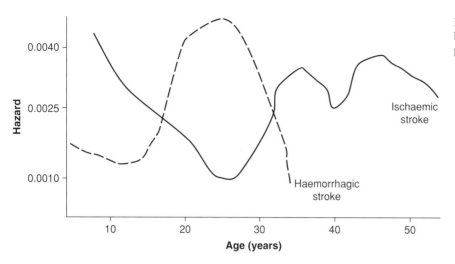

Fig. 15.16. Hazard rates of infarctive and haemorrhagic stroke in haemoglobin SS patients by age.[534]

has the highest incidence in young adults (20–30 years) but is not uncommon in children[534] (Fig. 15.16). Recurrence of stroke occurs in up 67% without blood transfusion therapy.[542]

Cerebral infarction may be symptomatic or asymptomatic (silent or covert infarct). Acute neurological symptoms and

signs are common in sickle cell disease and, as well as stroke (Figs 15.17 and 15.18), include transient ischaemic accident (TIA)[386] (Figs 15.19 and 15.20), headaches[543,544] (Figs 15.21 (See also colour plate 6) and 15.22), seizures[386,545] (Fig. 15.23) and coma[546] (Figs 15.17, 15.22 and 15.24). Altered mental

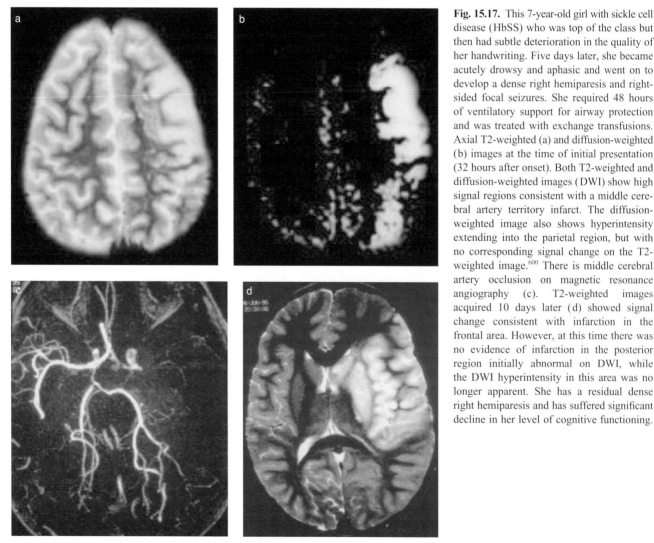

Fig. 15.17. This 7-year-old girl with sickle cell disease (HbSS) who was top of the class but then had subtle deterioration in the quality of her handwriting. Five days later, she became acutely drowsy and aphasic and went on to develop a dense right hemiparesis and right-sided focal seizures. She required 48 hours of ventilatory support for airway protection and was treated with exchange transfusions. Axial T2-weighted (a) and diffusion-weighted (b) images at the time of initial presentation (32 hours after onset). Both T2-weighted and diffusion-weighted images (DWI) show high signal regions consistent with a middle cerebral artery territory infarct. The diffusion-weighted image also shows hyperintensity extending into the parietal region, but with no corresponding signal change on the T2-weighted image.[600] There is middle cerebral artery occlusion on magnetic resonance angiography (c). T2-weighted images acquired 10 days later (d) showed signal change consistent with infarction in the frontal area. However, at this time there was no evidence of infarction in the posterior region initially abnormal on DWI, while the DWI hyperintensity in this area was no longer apparent. She has a residual dense right hemiparesis and has suffered significant decline in her level of cognitive functioning.

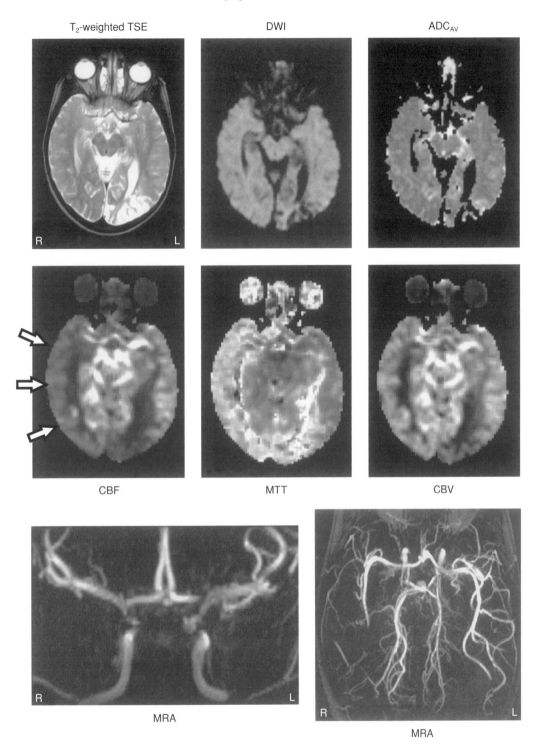

T2-weighted TSE   DWI   ADCAV

CBF   MTT   CBV

MRA   MRA

Fig. 15.18. This child presented with an acute flaccid right-sided hemiparesis 5 weeks prior to the scan. He had had a limp briefly 4 years previously and, in clinic prior to the stroke, had 'soft' neurological signs with increased tone in the left leg. On examination at the time of the scan, there was evidence of a bilateral movement disorder, with a diplegic gait and poor hand function bilaterally. Transcranial Doppler ultrasound showed velocities of 149/191cm/s in the right and left internal carotid artery/middle cerebral artery, respectively. Magnetic resonance angiography was abnormal, with severe turbulence in the terminal internal carotid artery bilaterally and moyamoya collaterals on the right (bottom row). The T2-weighted imaging shows a left occipital infarct with moderate lobar atrophy (top row, left). Diffusion-weighted imaging (top row, middle) showed abnormality within the same regions as the T2-weighted scans and with apparent diffusion coefficient (ADC) values (top row, right) suggesting that none of the areas of infarction was recent. Perfusion imaging showed reduced cerebral blood flow (CBF), increased mean transit time (MTT) and decreased cerebral blood volume (CBV) in the same region as the infarct in the left occipital region (middle row), and there was also reduced CBF and increased MTT beyond the areas of infarction in the left temporooccipital region (middle row) and throughout the right hemisphere (arrows). Despite regular blood transfusion, the child had a further transient ischaemic attack 7 months later.[543]

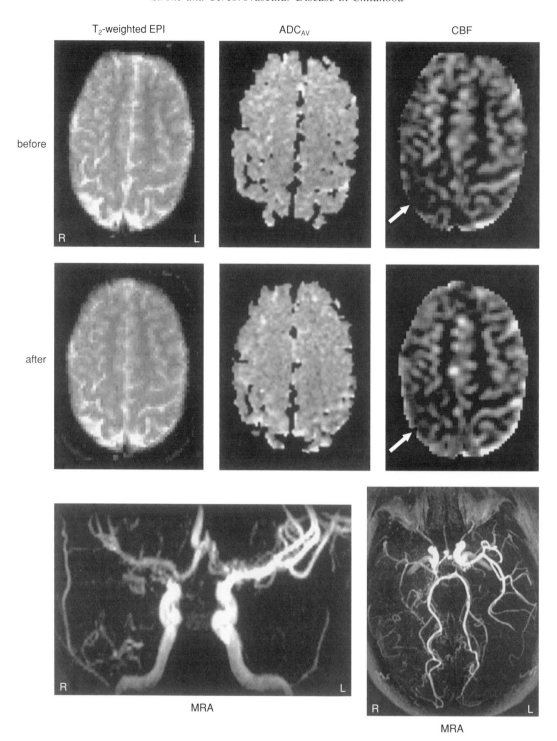

Fig. 15.19. This 15-year-old boy with HbSb0 thalassaemia was transfused regularly to maintain HbS <20%, as he had experienced three reversible ischaemic neurological deficits (left hemiparesis on one occasion and two episodes of right facial weakness) and most recently (14 months previously) a transient ischaemic attack (left-sided numbness and tingling). On transcranial Doppler, internal carotid artery (ICA) – middle cerebral artery (MCA) velocity was low on the right, and there was difficulty tracking the MCA bilaterally. On magnetic resonance angrography (bottom row), there was grade 2 turbulence in the right terminal ICA, A1, M1 and M2 and in the left M1. On T2-weighted imaging, there were multiple infarcts in the borderzones bilaterally. The image included here (top row, left) shows atrophy in the right parietooccipital region. Diffusion imaging showed abnormalities only in regions of chronic infarct (apparent diffusion coefficient maps shown in top and middle rows, centre). On perfusion imaging, there was decreased cerebral blood flow (arrow, top row, right; also decreased cerebral blood volume and increased mean transit time, not shown) outside the areas of infarction in the right parietal region immediately prior to transfusion, which appeared to have improved after transfusion (arrow, middle row, right).[543]

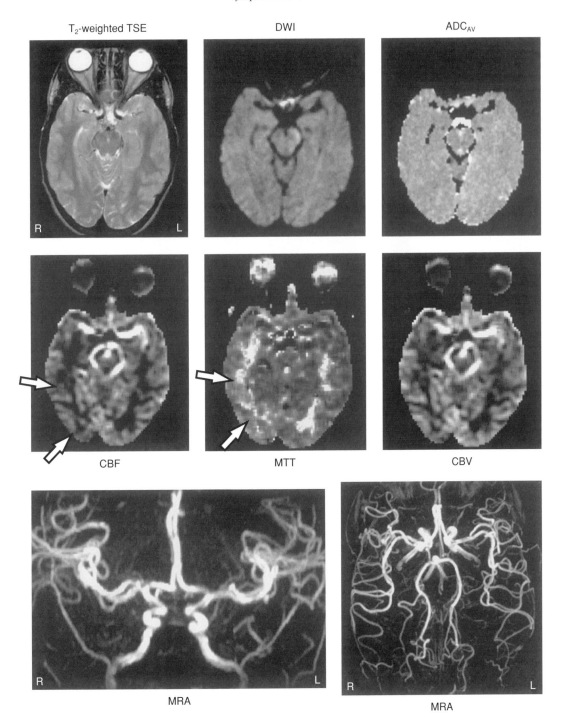

Fig. 15.20. This 13-year-old boy had had visual hallucinations (described as seeing monsters) since the age of 3 years and headaches since the age of 6 years. At the time of the scan, his headaches had become more frequent and tended to occur on waking. The T2-weighted and diffusion imaging were normal (top row), as was magnetic resonance angiography of the circle of Willis (bottom row). Perfusion imaging showed an area of reduced cerebral blood flow (middle row, left; arrows) and cerebral blood volume, and increased mean transit time (middle row, center; arrows) in the right temporo-occipital region.[543]

status – with or without reduced level of consciousness, headache, seizures, visual loss or focal signs – can occur in numerous contexts, including infection (Figs 15.23 and 15.24), shunted hydrocephalus (Fig. 15.23), acute chest syndrome (ACS)[384] (Fig. 15.23), acute anaemia,[547] after surgery,[548,549] transfusion[550] or immunosuppression,[551] (Fig. 15.23) and apparently spontaneously.[547] In one large series of patients with ACS, 3% of children had neurological symptoms at presentation, and these symptoms developed in a further 7–10% as a complication of ACS.[552] These patients are classified clinically as having had a cerebrovascular accident,[534] although there is a wide differential of focal and generalized vascular and non-vascular pathologies, often

273

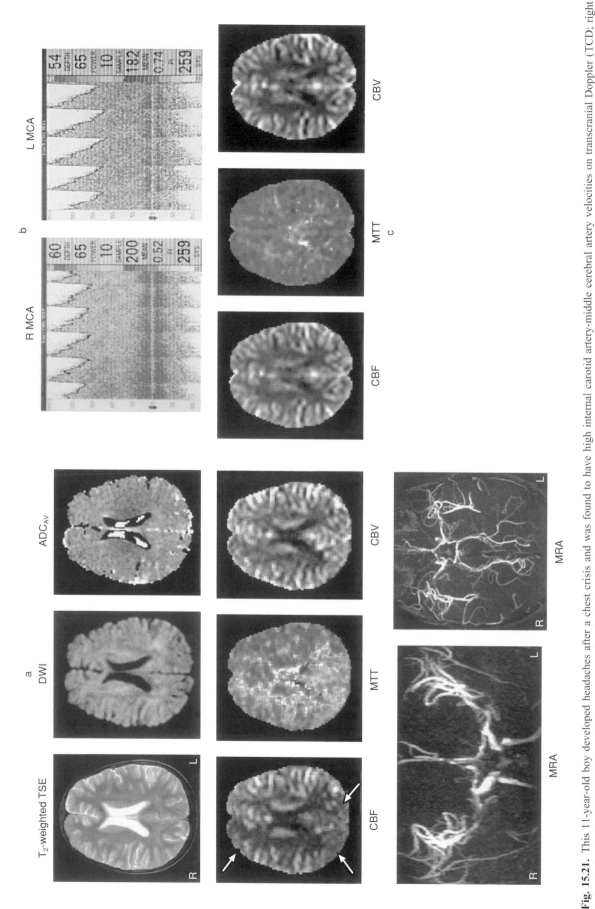

Fig. 15.21. This 11-year-old boy developed headaches after a chest crisis and was found to have high internal carotid artery–middle cerebral artery velocities on transcranial Doppler (TCD: right 200cm/s, left 182cm/s) (b). (a) Magnetic resonance results obtained at the time of initial presentation. Magnetic resonance angiography (MRA) showed turbulence in the M2 segments bilaterally (grade 2 on the right and 1 on the left) and in the P1 segment on the right (grade 2: a, top row). T2-weighted and diffusion-weighted imaging were normal (a, top row) but perfusion imaging showed reduced cerebral blood flow (CBF), high mean transit time (MTT) and decreased cerebral blood volume (CBV) throughout the right hemisphere and posteriorly on the left (arrows, a, middle row). The patient was transfused on the basis of the TCD and severely abnormal perfusion imaging findings; his headaches improved and he has not had a subsequent event. (b,c) Magnetic resonance perfusion data obtained after 1 year of monthly transfusions, when his MRA and TCD had returned to normal. There are no abnormalities of CBF, CBV or MTT; 6 months after discontinuation of the transfusion regimen, his TCD, MRA and perfusion imaging remained normal. (See colour plate 6)

274

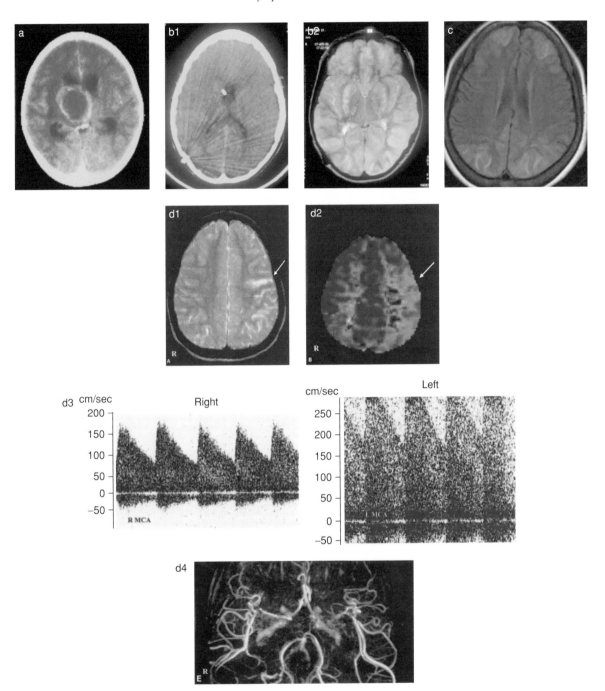

Fig. 15.22. MRI in patients with sickle cell disease presenting with acute seizures. (a) CT showing abscess in an 18-month-old boy with homozygous sickle cell anaemia. (B1) Child with haemoglobin sickle cell disease who had had an intraventricular haemorrhage despite a term birth, which may have been secondary to venous sinus thrombosis, requiring a shunt in infancy for post-haemorrhagic hydrocephalus. At the age of 9, he presented with headache, and CT performed 10 days after presentation in (a) shows definite cerebral oedema; the dense appearance of the straight sinus (arrow) raises the possibility of sinus venous thrombosis, but is not diagnostic. (b2) He then developed seizures and became unconscious; the MRI shows widespread cerebral oedema and there was no filling of the venous sinuses (not shown) due either to propagation of the venous clot or to the oedema. He fulfilled the criteria for brain death. (c) MRI showing bilateral borderzone ischaemia in a 25-year-old woman with homozygous sickle cell anaemia who collapsed soon after discharge for a chest crisis. She made a full neurological recovery. (d1) Seven-year-old girl with sickle cell anaemia (HbSS) and seizures (facial twitching and blank spells) who had also had a right hemiparesis; abnormal T2-weighted MRI (left precentral cortex infarct; d1, arrow) and perfusion MRI (dynamic susceptibility contrast-MRI with intravenous gadolinium (DSC-MRI)) with extensive cortical and subcortical perfusion abnormalities in the left frontal, parietal and temporal regions with an increase in the mean transit time (MTT) of the passage of the gadolinium bolus (MTT maps; d2, arrow) and a severe decrease in the cerebral blood flow (not shown). Transcranial Doppler ultrasound (TCD) shows normal right middle cerebral artery (MCA) velocities (137cm/s; d3) and abnormal mean left middle cerebral artery (MCA) velocities (250cm/s; d3). Abnormal MRA showed an abnormal left MCA (d4, arrow). The electroencephalogram showed epileptic activity mainly over the left central-temporal regions (not shown).

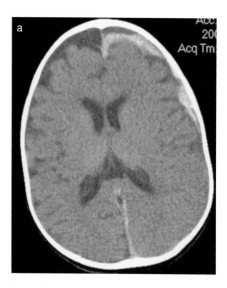
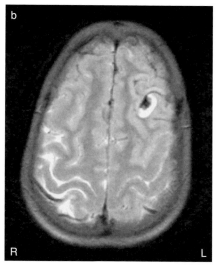

Fig. 15.23. Haemorrhagic stroke in sickle cell anaemia. (a) Subdural haemorrhage in a 6-month-old infant. (b) Intracerebral haemorrhage in a previously well child with sickle cell anaemia who presented with acute headache.

distinguished using acute magnetic resonance techniques (Figs 15.23 and 15.24),[553] with important management implications.

Coma in SCD may be due to intracranial haemorrhage[554,555] (Fig. 15.22), although extensive middle cerebral artery infarction with oedema can also have a similar presentation[556] (Fig. 15.17). In addition, children with SCD can present with central nervous system infections such as meningitis, bacterial abscess (Fig. 15.23) and cerebral tuberculoma. The incidence of central nervous system infections has decreased with penicillin prophylaxis and immunization.[514,554] Severe headache can also be a symptom of intracranial haemorrhage: subdural (Fig. 15.22a), intraparenchymal (Fig. 15.22b), subarachnoid or intraventricular.[554] Other symptoms of cerebral infarction include dysphasia, difficulty with gait[547] and 'soft neurological signs'.[554,557,558] Patients with SCD may also have single and recurrent seizures,[545,559,560] chronic headaches,[544,561–564] myelopathy and neuropathy.[514,519,554,565–568] Venous sinus thrombosis (Figs 15.23b and 15.24h; see Fig. 7.6c) and pseudotumor cerebri have also been reported.[74,514,554,561,562,569,570] Hyperventilation, for example during an EEG, occasionally provokes transient and permanent neurological deficits, usually involving the posterior circulation territory.[571]

Cerebrovascular disease in sickle cell disease
(Figs 15.25–15.27)

Pathology
Endothelial hyperplasia and thrombi in large and small vessels are associated with brain infarcts in autopsied patients with SCD.[572–574] These data are compatible with those obtained in living patients: between 60% and 95% of patients with SCD and stroke who underwent conventional angiography had large artery occlusive disease with intimal narrowing or complete occlusion of the intracranial portion of the internal carotid artery and proximal middle cerebral and anterior cerebral arteries.[575–579]

Not all patients who die after developing neurological symptoms have large vessel disease, however.[548] In addition to the typical small necrotic lesions in the border between the cortex and the subcortical white matter, acute demyelination[548] and venous sinus thrombosis[573,580,581] have also been documented.

Mechanism of small and large blood vessel disease
There are at least two mechanisms involved in the development of cerebral infarction in SCD (Fig. 15.27). The first mechanism is the large blood vessel disease with endothelial hyperplasia and risk of arterio-arterial thromboembolism. The abnormal red cells and increased blood flow at the level of the cerebral large vessel bifurcation in sickle patients may cause damage secondary to turbulence in the large vessel with thrombus formation and endothelial hyperplasia.[514] The arterial narrowing may cause a relative hypoperfusion in vulnerable regions of the brain[546] leading to middle cerebral artery territory (Fig. 15.17) or borderzone infarcts (anterior, posterior or deep watershed infarcts) (Fig. 15.24C) in the territory between branches of a central vessel (such as the internal carotid artery (ICA)).[386] The borderzone between two fields is vulnerable if blood pressure decreases. One of the most vulnerable regions of the human brain is the anterior borderzone of the frontal lobe between the territories of the middle and anterior cerebral arteries.[582,583] There is a parallel with non-SCD adult patients with large vessel disease (i.e. ICA stenosis), who suffer borderzone infarcts when suffering from acute haemodynamic insufficiency, such as severe heart disease, hypotension or syncope.[514,584] In addition, the risk of borderzone stroke in SCD patients may be increased by narrowing of the central large vessel or its branches, which is common in SCD.

The second mechanism is considered to be the sludging of the dense sickle cells in the small blood vessels of the brain, such as the small distal penetrating arteries of the cortex or lenticulostriates supplying the basal ganglia, although there is

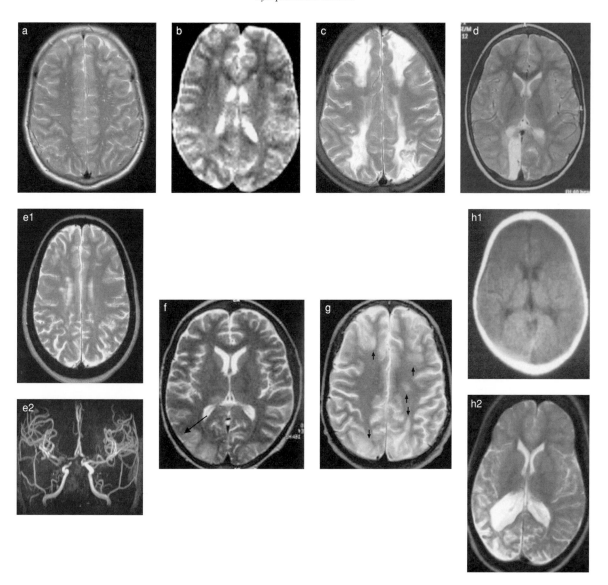

Fig. 15.24. Patterns and mechanisms of 'covert' or 'silent' infarction in anaemias. Axial T2-weighted magnetic resonance imaging. (a) Borderzone infarcts in a child with Blackfan–Diamond syndrome and seizures who had collapsed with a very low haemoglobin in infancy. (b) Infarcts in a child with sickle cell anaemia (SCA) and focal tonic seizures. (c) Infarction in both anterior and posterior arterial borderzones in an 8-year-old boy with previously uncomplicated SCA who developed seizures and coma after surgery to drain a painful swelling of his left cheek, associated with fever, after a fall. (d) Left occipital infarct in a boy with SCA who had a chest crisis the previous year and had had frequent seizures at that time. (e1) Silent infart in the deep white matter in a boy with HbSβ⁰-thalassaemia who also had ipsilateral middle cerebral artery signal dropout on magnetic resonance angiography (e2). (f) Signal change in the left posterior occipital (arrow) and bilateral high parietal regions ('reversible posterior leukoencephalopathy') with hippocampal involvement in a woman with previously uncomplicated SCA who presented aged 18 years old with acute chest syndrome. (g) Signal change in the grey and white matter ('reversible posterior leukoencephalopathy') (arrows) in a 9-year-old boy with SCA who had been treated with ciclosporin for nephrotic syndrome. (h1) Empty delta sign compatible with venous sinus thrombosis in an 18-month-old girl with SCA and pneumococcal meningitis. The child developed intractable epilepsy with multiple seizure types which eventually responded to topiramate. MRI 12 years later showed bilateral parieto-occipital infarction (h2).

little direct evidence. Cerebral blood flow rates and red blood cell oxygen content are lower in these vessels.[514,585] These conditions may lead to sickling and vaso-occlusion, which may explain the presence of infarcts in sickle cell patients without large vessel disease. In any given patient with SCD, either or both mechanisms may play a role in the development of cerebral infarction.

The role of other mechanisms, such as venous sinus thrombosis (Figs 15.23b and 15.24h; see Fig. 7.6c),[74,569,580,581,586]

posterior leukoencephalopathy (Figs 15.24f and 15.24g),[384,551,587] watershed ischaemia, acute cerebral oedema and demyelination,[588] in the development of central nervous system pathology has not been extensively explored.[589] These pathologies appear to be largely reversible and may be missed if patients do not receive emergency magnetic resonance imaging, as exchange transfusion in the local hospital is usually the priority.

As the patient with SCD ages, the progressive narrowing of the large vessels may be associated with aneurysmal dilatation

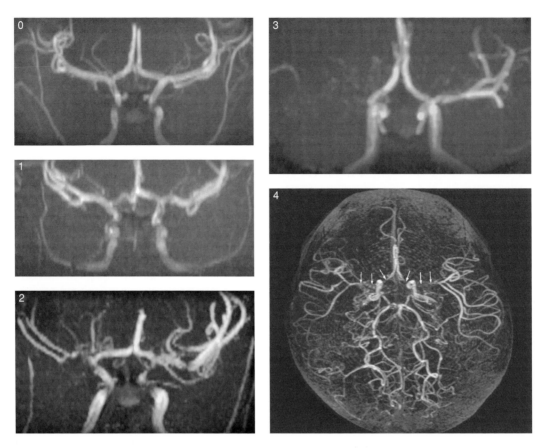

Fig. 15.25. Magnetic resonance angiography grading of turbulence or signal dropout in the intracranial vessels. (0) Normal or grade 0. (1) Grade 1 turbulence in an asymptomatic child with SCA and silent infarction. (2) Grade 1 turbulence in an asymptomatic child with SCA and a normal MRI. (3) Grade 2 turbulence in the right terminal internal cerebral artery, A1, M1 and M2 and in the left M1 in a boy with HbSβ⁰-thalassaemia. (4) Moyamoya in a child with SCA and recurrent transient ischaemic attacks.

(Fig. 15.26),[590–592] or the development of compensatory but fragile collaterals, defined as moyamoya syndrome[593–595] (Figs 15.25 and 15.26). Both entities may lead to intracranial haemorrhage in young adults, although in children with intracranial bleeding arterial imaging is usually normal.[555]

Parenchymal MRI in sickle cell disease: stroke and clinically silent disease

Ischaemia

There is a predilection for brain infarction in the borderzone areas of the brain demonstrated in several studies using T2-weighted MRI of the brain (Fig. 15.24C).[554,596–598] In a recent study using voxel-based morphometry, compared with controls there was evidence of damage in the white matter of the borderzones even in patients with sickle cell anaemia and normal T2-weighted MRI (Fig. 15.28. See also colour plate 5)).[599] For an acute focal neurological event, T2-weighted MRI is usually abnormal within a few hours while diffusion-weighted MRI (Fig. 15.17b) can show ischaemic regions within minutes – before irreversible infarction has occurred – and can distinguish between infarction and reversible phenomena including penumbral ischaemia (Fig. 15.17b) and posterior leukoencephalopathy[384,551,553,600] (Figs 15.23, 15.24, 15.30 and 15.35).

Silent infarction is found in up 40% of sickle cell patients without clinical symptoms,[514,601–606] including those with sickle β-thalassaemia (Fig. 15.24). The high prevalence of silent infarcts on MRI in children with SCD compared with children with non-sickle stroke[607] probably at least in part reflects the chronicity of the vascular compromise in this population. Silent infarction is associated with significant and progressive cerebrovascular disease, such as moyamoya syndrome or cerebral vasculitis, rarely in those with cryptogenic childhood stroke, whereas it is common in sickle cell disease.[608,609] Patients with SCD and overt or silent infarction are more likely to have abnormal psychometric testing[601,610,611] (Fig. 15.28. (See also colour plate 5), see Chapter 17, Section 17.5).

Quantitative T1 MRI (qT1 MRI) may add sensitivity to the conventional MRI study. Abnormal qT1 MRI is found in frontal and thalamic regions[612] in children with SCD who are 4 years of age and younger.[613,614] In contrast to other authors,[599,615] Steen's work demonstrated selective damage in the grey rather than in the white matter,[613] with evidence of loss of volume in the central as well as the cortical grey matter.[616] Those with abnormal grey matter and haematocrit lower than 27% (normal haematocrit is 34–40% for non-sickle children of similar age[617]) were more likely to have abnormal psychometric testing.[613,618] Another group has also

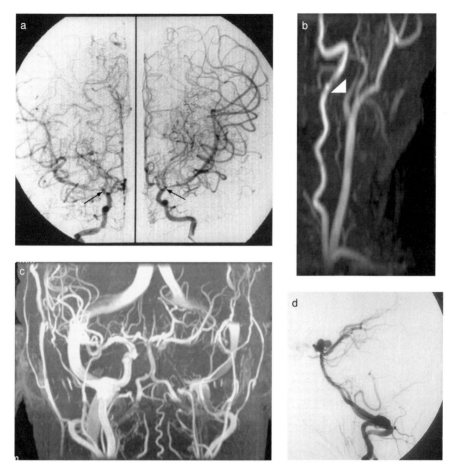

Fig. 15.26. Other cerebrovascular disease in sickle cell disease. (a) Conventional arteriogram showing moyamoya. (b) Tapering occlusion compatible with internal carotid dissection. (c) Occlusion of the internal carotid in the neck. (d) Posterior circulation aneurysm.

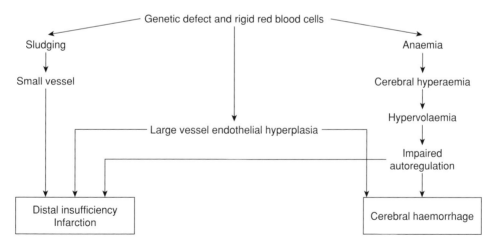

Fig. 15.27. Proposed pathophysiology of cerebrovascular disease in sickle cell disease.[514]

found a direct association between the volume of grey matter and IQ in SCD.[619] Chronic anaemic hypoxia in patients with SCD may compromise brain tissue and intellectual development in the absence of cerebrovascular disease,[620] although cerebrovascular disease is associated with the degree of brain injury visible on standard MRI.[621]

Haemorrhage

Intraparenchymal (Fig. 15.22), intraventricular, subarachnoid and occasionally subdural (Fig. 15.22) haemorrhages have all been described in patients with SCD.[555] Haemorrhage has the highest incidence in young adults with a peak between 20 and 30 years (Fig. 15.16).[534] Patients with prior infarction are at

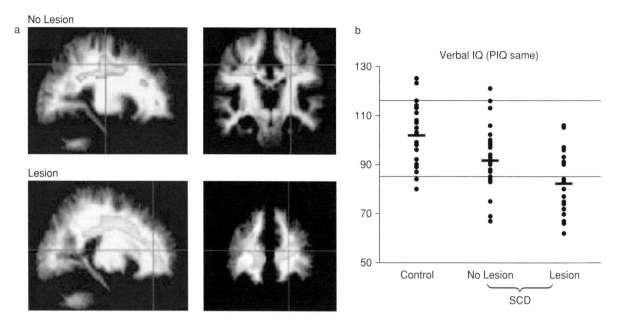

Fig. 15.28. (a,b) Voxel-based morphometry comparison of white matter density between controls and patients with sickle cell anaemia (SCA) with and without covert infarction. Regions of reduced white matter density in those with SCA and covert infarction are displayed on the mean white matter segment. The white matter abnormality distribution is similar to that in the patient with overt stroke shown in Fig. 15.18c and in the patient with apparently reversible ischaemia in Fig. 15.17c. The patients with covert lesions have lower verbal (and performance; not shown) IQ than those with no covert lesion, who have lower verbal (and performance; not shown) IQ than sibling controls; part of the explanation for which the voxel-based morphometry data provides evidence, is that there is tissue damage not visible on T2-weighted MRI. PIQ, performance IQ.[599] (See colour plate 5).

increased risk of haemorrhage as they age.[542] Subarachnoid and intracerebral haemorrhage occur in the context of acute hypertension and may be associated with corticosteroid use, recent transfusion or bone marrow transplantation.[555] Cerebral haemorrhage in older patients is commonly related to aneurysm formation.[592] The aneurysms which rupture are typically located at the bifurcations of major vessels, particularly in the vertebrobasilar circulation (Fig. 15.26). Intraparenchymal bleeding may be associated with large vessel vasculopathy, especially if moyamoya formation is present.[594] Venous sinus thrombosis[622] and reversible posterior leukencephalopathy[384] may also be associated with haemorrhage. There are reports of epidural haematomata in the absence of significant head trauma in SCD, probably related to hypervascular areas of bone.[623]

MRI and MR angiography studies may not be adequate to exclude an aneurysm and conventional contrast angiography may be required (see below). Vasospasm after subarachnoid haemorrhage may be diagnosed using transcranial Doppler ultrasound.

Vascular studies

Conventional cerebral angiography

Conventional cerebral angiography has been used in a relatively small proportion of patients with stroke and SCD, because of the risks of inducing crisis with the contrast medium, as well as of stroke, but large vessel disease is common.[575,577,624,625] This investigation should be undertaken after consultation

with a multidisciplinary team, including an experienced neuro-radiologist and a haematologist with an interest in haemoglobinopathies. Conventional angiography is the required diagnostic technique to visualize aneurysms,[590–592] where treatment may be required to reduce the risk of rebleeding, and for those in whom revascularization surgery for moyamoya may be an option.

Magnetic resonance angiography (Figs 15.25 and 15.26)
MRA abnormalities are associated with subclinical infarction when flow turbulence involves a long segment (6mm) and there is reduced distal flow.[626] In SCD, MRA can be up to 85% accurate when compared with conventional angiography.[627] Turbulence or signal dropout on MRA may be graded as mild, moderate and severe (Fig. 15.25), but there are few data looking at the relationship with the degree of arterial stenosis on conventional angiography.[543,628] In the STOP study, MRA was undertaken at baseline in 100 patients, 47 in the transfusion arm and 53 in the standard care arm, and was normal in 75 patients, or demonstrated stenosis in 25 that was mild in 4 and severe in 21.[629] In the standard care arm, 4 of 13 patients with abnormal MRA findings had strokes compared with 5 of 40 patients with normal MRA findings (p=0.03).[629]

MRA can detect cerebrovascular disease in very young children. In one study,[630] MRA abnormalities were found in 3 out of 29 patients from 7 to 48 months of age, although there were none with MRA abnormalities in the 23 studied at baseline for the BABY HUG trial.[631]

Ectasia of the basilar and intracranial circulations has also been documented and is associated with low haematocrit.[632,633] Bhattacharya et al[634] described four cases of extracranial occlusion in children with sickle cell anaemia. The radiological features were suggestive of dissection in one child who was scanned acutely (Fig. 15.26), and in the others were similar to the intracranial large vessel stenotic lesions typically seen in the intracranial distal ICA, and proximal MCA and ACA. Extracranial carotid artery occlusion or dissection should be considered in children with sickle cell anaemia presenting with symptoms of stroke, and imaging of the neck vessels should be part of the routine investigation of these patients.

Transcranial Doppler ultrasound (Fig. 15.18)

Transcranial Doppler ultrasound (TCD) may be used to measure the time averaged maximum velocities (TAMV) in the intracranial arteries (distal interior carotid (ICA) and middle (MCA), anterior and posterior (PCA) cerebral arteries) which are typically affected in SCD. Increased TCD velocities may be associated with a reduced artery diameter, or increased CBF in the presence of anaemia;[399] the possibility that these may be distinguished may be explored by comparing with velocities in the basilar artery,[635] which is rarely involved in SCD. A submandibular approach allows the detection of post-bulb extracranial carotid stenosis.[636–638]

In sickle cell anaemia, stenosis on digital subtraction arteriography may be detected when the distal ICA/MCA velocities are between 140 and 190cm/s; velocities more than 190cm/s are associated with marked artery stenosis on angiography.[579] ICA/MCA TAMV equal to or greater than 200cm/s are associated with a 40% risk of stroke over a 3-year period.[639] The STOP study has demonstrated that TCD is a useful tool for screening and detection of patients at risk of stroke in the sickle population. Children with TCD MCA or ICA TAMV ≥200cm/s are at high risk of first stroke over the subsequent few years (13% per year) if they do not receive indefinite regular blood transfusion therapy.[639–642] Those with 'conditional' TCD studies, i.e. with velocities between 170 and 200cm/s are also at higher risk of stroke than those with velocities <170cm/s.[643] Since the STOP trial ended prematurely because there was a very large advantage in favour of blood transfusion, screening and transfusion for those with velocities >200cm/s has been recommended as standard care in the USA and the UK.[644] Recent epidemiological evidence suggests there has been a parallel fall in the incidence of stroke in SCD[645,646] and that this strategy is cost effective.[647]

TCD may detect cerebrovascular disease at an earlier stage than MRA; the highest risk of stroke is in children in whom both are abnormal, whose cerebrovascular disease rarely improves without blood transfusion[629] and even then does not normalize completely.[648] ICA/MCA velocities are higher than control even in infancy[649] but those in the conditional range are rare and abnormal velocities have not so far been documented so there are no data as yet on the range predicting stroke risk in this age group. There are few data on regional cerebral blood flow in acutely symptomatic patients, but the available studies suggest that, as expected, those with vessel occlusion have an area of reduced CBF distally.[546] Studies have shown a good correlation between abnormally high TCD velocities and xenon CBF studies, conventional angiography[579] and MRA.[628,629,650,651]. However, there are very few data on the natural history in the 2–7% of patients with abnormally low velocities.[629,648,652]

Predictors of ICA/MCA velocity and/or abnormal TCD include haemoglobin,[653] haematocrit,[654] haemoglobin oxygen saturation,[635,655] markers of haemolysis including reticulocyte count,[656] aspartate transaminase[653] and lactate dehydrogenase.[657]

Cerebral blood flow studies in sickle cell disease (Fig. 15.29)

Global and focal perfusion

Xenon inhalation. Studies of *global* cerebral blood flow (CBF) have shown that neurologically asymptomatic patients with SCD usually have *global* cerebral hyperaemia secondary to anaemia and may fail to increase CBF with hypercapnia.[658] Studies with xenon[133] demonstrated that CBF in patients with SCD was 68% greater than in controls;[597,658] this increase was inversely related to haematocrit level[658] (Fig. 15.29A). The degree of hyperaemia is also related to the HbS percentage.[659] However, this hyperaemia may not be seen in tissue which is already compromised (e.g. abnormal white matter[660] or focal infarction), or in patients with acute neurological symptoms. For example, a study using xenon[133] demonstrated diffusely decreased perfusion in patients with stupor, coma and seizures.[546] There are few data on *regional* CBF in asymptomatic or acutely symptomatic patients, but the available studies suggest that, as expected, those with vessel occlusion have an area of *focally* reduced CBF distally,[546] which may extend outside the territory of any visible infarction.[661]

Positron emission tomography. Studies of *regional* CBF, for example using positron emission tomography (PET), have also shown *focal* changes in CBF in SCD patients, such as an increase in regional CBF;[662] or more extensive regional abnormalities than those demonstrated on MRI.[663] Another PET study showed abnormal regional cerebral metabolic rates for glucose in the frontal lobes of asymptomatic sickle cell patients with normal CT.[583]

Single photon emission computed tomography. Of 21 Kuwaiti patients undergoing single photon emission computed tomography (SPECT) using ^{99m}Tc-HMPAO as the tracer, seven (age 11–22 years) had brain perfusion deficits, mostly in the frontal lobe either alone or in combination with abnormalities in the temporal and/or parietal lobe.[664] Other studies have also shown abnormalities.[665] Two patients had silent infarction on MRI, one with SPECT abnormality and one without. In another study, focal perfusion deficits were seen in 12.5% of 48 children with symptomatic SCD on SPECT with acetazolamide testing, independent of reduced global cerebrovascular

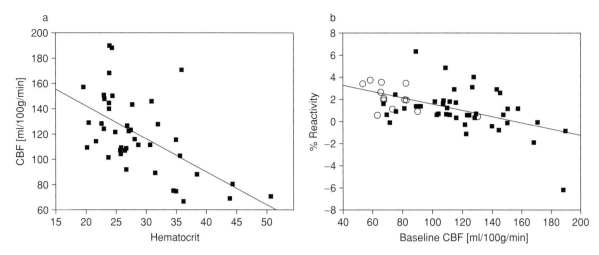

Fig. 15.29. Cerebral blood flow in patients with sickle cell disease (SCD).[399] (a) Baseline cerebral blood flow as a function of haematocrit. The continuous line depicts the linear regression. (b) Hypercapnic reactivity against its best predictor, normocapnic blood flow. SCD patients (filled squares) and controls (open circles) seem to fall on an identical regression line, which is linear up to about blood flow levels of 150ml per 100g/min but drops precipitously after that.

reserve, which was documented reproducibly in 69% on administration of acetazolamide.[666] Abnormal SPECT has been demonstrated in patients with SCD and psychiatric presentations.[667,668]

Perfusion MRI. Perfusion MRI (dynamic susceptibility contrast MRI), using a contrast agent (gadolinium-diethylenetriamine penta-acetic acid), demonstrated perfusion deficits associated with central nervous system events (such as stroke, TIA, severe headaches and coma) in symptomatic patients with SCD (Figs 15.18–15.21. See also colour plate 6).[543] These symptoms persisted in a significant proportion of patients despite transfusion therapy.[669] Patients with TIA had abnormal perfusion when other neuroimaging modalities were normal.[543] Perfusion abnormalities were associated with MRA turbulence, a marker of cerebrovascular disease.[543,670] Kirkham et al[543] demonstrated that all the patients with severe turbulence or occlusion on MRA had perfusion abnormalities, but also there were perfusion abnormalities in some patients with normal MRA and TCD. TCD velocities higher than 200cm/s are associated with perfusion abnormality[543] as well as risk of stroke,[639,640] but there is also an association between abnormal perfusion and moderately increased TCD velocities (>170 but <200cm/s)[543].

Another technique to measure cerebral blood flow is *continuous arterial spin-labelling (CASL) perfusion MR*, which allows quantification of regional CBF by using magnetically labelled water molecules in arterial blood, without the need of exogenous agents. In a study in children with SCD who had not had acute neurological events and had not received chronic transfusion, Oguz et al[671] demonstrated that mean CBF values were significantly higher in sickle patients than in controls (non-sickle) and, in four patients, the baseline CBF was significantly decreased in territories seen as unaffected on conventional MRI and MRA. Strouse et al[672] found grey matter CBF to be 112+/−36ml/100g/min in 24 children with

SCD and there was an inverse relationship between CBF and performance IQ. Van den Tweel et al[673] found that, although regional cerebal blood flow (rCBF) measured using CASL was of similar magnitude in SCD patients and controls in the frontal, middle and posterior territories, 58% of those with SCD demonstrated a left–right asymmetry of rCBF of >11.7ml/100g/min in one or more vascular territories whereas none of the controls did.

Cerebrovascular reserve and autoregulation
In addition, SCD patients have reduced vascular reserve capacity, which may be demonstrated using various CBF techniques and a vasodilatory stimulus, for example hypercapnia,[399,674] acetazolamide[666] or rapid eye movement sleep.[675] Whereas the normal response is to increase CBF in response to a vasodilatory stimulus such as hypercapnia,[676] SCD patients have a reduced or even negative response (Fig. 15.29B), related to the anaemia and the resultant adaptive vasodilatation and perhaps also to abnormal NO mechanisms.[399] Autoregulation may also be abnormal, with a reduced ability to buffer the effects of increased blood pressure.[677]

Effect of blood transfusion therapy on cerebrovascular disease and perfusion. The effect of blood transfusion therapy on cerebrovascular disease and perfusion has not been studied in depth, although Russell et al[577] demonstrated improvement in the vasculopathy in a few of their patients, as well as a reduction of the recurrence risk. However, in a series of 43 sickle patients on chronic transfusion therapy, 43% had moyamoya collaterals and 41% of the patients experienced recurrent cerebrovascular events despite transfusion.[594] In another series, in one patient with chronic cerebrovascular disease, perfusion abnormalities had improved on a study performed a few days after transfusion compared with the appearances immediately before (Fig. 15.19).[543] Another patient with evidence of bilateral cerebrovascular disease, with high velocities on TCD and turbulence on MRA in association with a widespread perfusion abnormality throughout both hemispheres, had completely normal MRI, MRA and perfusion MRI one year later (Fig. 15.21. See also colour plate 6).[543] However, in a larger study, the same authors found that perfusion did not improve in the short or long term in the majority of patients on a blood transfusion programme.[669] It is possible that chronic inflammation or infection is associated with progressive CVD and recurrence of CNS events despite a monthly transfusion regimen to keep the HbS less than 30%.[528,678] The effect of blood transfusion on the cerebral vasculature and cerebral perfusion is still uncertain.

Risk factors for stroke and cerebrovascular disease in sickle cell disease (Table 15.3)

Clinical risk factors

There are several risk factors that predispose individuals with sickle cell disease to develop cerebral infarction.[679,680] Patients with SC disease and sickle/β^+-thalassaemia are less likely to develop neurological symptoms, while those with homozygous sickle cell anaemia and sickle cell/β^0-thalassaemia have a more severe course with a higher risk of cerebrovascular events.[512,534,554] Age is an important risk factor as the highest incidence of first infarctive stroke is in the first years of life (2–5 years).[534]

Patients with clinical stroke have lower steady state haemoglobin concentrations, higher white cell count and higher reticulocyte counts.[534,681,682] Children with SCD have a reduction of protein S and C levels but there is little evidence that these prothrombotic abnormalities predict stroke.[683,684] Other clinical risk factors for stroke include relative hypertension,[685,686] painful crisis, infection, early dactylitis and other systemic illnesses.[554,682,687] Daytime and nocturnal oxygen desaturation in children with SCD appears to be associated with stroke, other central nervous system (CNS) events and cerebrovascular disease,[386,389,688–690] and asthma may also be a risk factor.[691] Dowling and his colleagues found a patent foramen ovale in a quarter of children with stroke in the context of SCD, typically those whose neurological symptoms had started during a painful crisis and had included headache, but the prevalence is probably similar to that in the general population (see Chapter 5).[398] Epilepsy is predicted by dactylitis and male gender.[692]

The largest multicentre study to date (the Cooperative Study of Sickle Cell Disease)[534] suggested that the predictors of ischaemic and haemorrhagic clinical stroke and silent infarction might be different. Independent risk factors for ischaemic stroke were previous TIA, lower steady-state-haemoglobin concentrations, recent acute chest syndrome and higher blood pressure, while those for haemorrhagic stroke included a low haemoglobin concentration and a high white cell count.[534] Risk factors for silent infarction were a low pain rate, history of seizures, leukocytosis and the Senegal β^s-globin haplo-

type,[602] but the severity of the anaemia was not independently associated. In the baseline studies from the silent infarct transfusion trial, low fetal haemoglobin and high blood pressure were risk factors for silent infarction.[606]

Infection and inflammation

Infection and chronic inflammation is a recurring theme in the pathophysiology of the neurological complications in sickle cell disease. Evidence of systemic inflammation is very common in sickle cell crisis with increased numbers of activated monocytes, platelets, endothelial cells and adhesion molecules and increased C-reactive protein[528,678,693] (Fig. 15.21. See also colour plate 6). As well as the evidence that leukocytosis is a risk factor for stroke, silent infarction and low IQ,[534,602,672,681,694] cerebrovascular episodes often appear to be precipitated by infections including pneumococcal meningitis,[695] *Parvovirus* aplastic anaemia[462] and *Mycoplasma pneumoniae*.[588] The role of chronic infection (e.g. secondary to *Chlamydia pneumoniae*[696] or tonsillitis[697]) remains controversial. This group of patients is also relatively immunodeficient, in part secondary to splenic autoinfarction or surgical removal of the spleen.

Genetic predisposition

There appears to be a familial predisposition to stroke[698] and to high blood flow velocities[699,700] in SCD, indicating that genetic factors probably play a role in stroke risk. Siblings might, however, also share adverse environmental conditions, including poverty, air pollution and poor nutrition. There is considerable interest currently in looking at epistatic polymorphisms as additional risk factors for stroke in SCD.[701] As well as the evidence for a possible effect of Senegal β^s-globin haplotype,[602] genetic modulators of the immune[702] and host inflammatory[703,704] responses might also be important in the development of cerebrovascular disease and stroke. There is evidence of human leukocyte antigen susceptibility for stroke in SCD.[541]

Sebastiani and her colleagues[705] have recently used Bayesian modelling to examine the association with sickle-related stroke of SNPs in candidate genes They found 31 SNPs in 11 genes, including bone morphogenetic protein 6 (*BMP6*), three genes involved in the transforming growth factor β (TGF-β) signalling pathway and SELP (selectin P (granule membrane protein 140kDa, antigen CD62)), which is known to be associated with stroke in the general population – all of these factors appeared to directly affect stroke risk. They also identified SNPs in a further nine genes, including endothelin-1, which is close to *BMP6* on chromosome 6 and is upregulated during acute hypoxia, that appeared to be acting indirectly. When validated in a separate population, this combination of genes, interacting with the percentage of haemoglobin F, was found to be 98.2% accurate at separating those with from those without stroke, with all seven of the strokes correctly classified.

Nutritional factors

Poor diet may also affect stroke risk, probably interacting with different genetic polymorphisms.[679] If nutritional factors do

TABLE 15.3
Risk factors for stroke in sickle cell disease

Risk factor	Ischaemic stroke	Haemorrhagic stroke	Silent infarct	Cognitive difficulties	Management	Randomized trial
Clinical						
Previous stroke	+	?	+	+	Monthly transfusion to HbS<30% / Aneurysm clipping for haemorrhage / Hydroxyurea?	SWITCH
Previous transient ischaemic event	+	–	?	?	TCD screening (see below)	None
Previous seizures	?	?	+	?	TCD screening (see below)	None
Previous meningitis	+	?	?	?	TCD screening (see below)	None
Hypertension	+	+	–	?	Antihypertensives?	None
Dactylitis in first year of life	+	?	?	?	Prophylactic hydroxyurea??	BABY HUG
Recent chest crisis (+/–thrombocytopenia)	+	?	?	?	Maintain steady state oxyhaemoglobin saturation	None
Asthma	+	?	?	?	Bronchodilators?	None
Obstructive sleep apnoea	+	?	?	?	Adenotonsillectomy?	None
Short stature	?	?	?	+	Nutrition	None
Recent blood transfusion	?	+	?	?	Avoid large increase Hb/BP	None
Recent corticosteroids	?	+	?	?	Avoid increase BP	None
Recent non-steroidal antinflammatory	?	+	?	?	Avoid decrease in platelets	None
Laboratory						
Low haemoglobin	+	+	+	+	Transfusion for aplastic crisis/splenic sequestration	None
High white cell count	+	+	+	+	Penicillin prophylaxis	None
High platelet count	–	–	–	?	?	Aspirin (START)
High pocked red cell count (splenic dysfunction)	+	?	+	?	Penicillin prophylaxis	None
High AST (haemolysis)	+	?	–	?	?	None
High LDH (haemolysis)	+	?	?	?	?	None
Absence of α-thalassaemia (lower haemoglobin)	+	?	–	?	?	None
Low haemoglobin F	+	?	+	?	Hydroxyurea	None
High homocysteine	+	?	?	?	Pyridoxine and folate	None
Low oxyhaemoglobin saturation	+	+	?	+	Overnight CPAP/O$_2$	Pilot (POMS)
Neuroimaging						
TCD velocity >170 but <200cm/s	+	–	?	?	Regular repeat TCD	None
TCD velocity >200cm/s	+	–	?	+	Indefinite transfusion	STOP and STOP2
Stenosis of intracranial arteries	+	?	?	?	?	None
Moyamoya	+	+	?	+	Revascularization	None
Aneurysm	–	+	–	–	Coils at arteriography	None
Previous silent infarction	+	?	+	+	Transfusion	Phase III in progress (SITT)
Perfusion abnormality	?	?	?	+	?	None

AST, aspartate aminotransferase; BABY HUG, Pediatric Hydroxyurea in Sickle Cell Anemia; CPAP/O$_2$, continuous positive airways pressure/oxygen; LDH, lactate dehydrogenase; POMS, Prevention of Morbidity in Sickle Cell Disease; START, Sickle Cell Two center Aspirin Response Trial; STOP, Stroke Prevention Trial in Sickle Cell Anemia; SWITCH, Stroke With Transfusions Changing to Hydroxyurea, SITT, Silent Infarct Transfusion Trial, TCD, transcranial Doppler ultrasound.

+, yes; –, no; ?, unknown.

indeed contribute to stroke risk in patients with SCD, this might explain certain geographical variations that have been observed. For example, although Greek patients with Sβ₀-thalassaemia have silent infarction (Fig. 15.13), high TCD velocities and cognitive problems appear to be rare[516] and this might be related to the Mediterranean diet.

Parenchymal and vascular imaging

Neuroimaging, cerebral angiography and TCD may help to predict stroke risk. Silent infarcts on MRI are associated with a higher risk of clinical stroke (14-fold)[604,706] and progressive infarction.[604] Cerebral angiography demonstrating severe arterial stenosis (≥75%) has been related to infarction, and moderate to severe arterial stenosis with deep white matter ischaemic lesions[578,707]. On MRA, signal dropout or turbulence in the cerebral vessels may also be related to infarction.[543,628] TCD studies demonstrated that patients with SCD who had MCA velocities of 200cm/s or higher had a 40% stroke risk over 3 years unless they received regular blood transfusion.[639–642]

Oxygen desaturation, hypoxia and anaemia

Hypoxia may be a risk factor for stroke by increasing haemoglobin gel formation and red cell adhesion, predisposing to molecular sickling and vaso-occlusion.[386,519] Acute worsening of anaemia and hypoxia is associated with a higher stroke risk.[524,534,708] In addition, acute chest syndrome is a risk factor for stroke,[534] and this respiratory complication is associated with hypoxia and may cause CNS events. Nocturnal oxygen desaturation is common in SCD in young children secondary to upper airway obstruction,[535,536,709,710] and appears to be associated with CNS events such as stroke, TIA and seizures.[389,688,689] A study demonstrated the association of nocturnal oxygen desaturation and increased numbers of platelet-erythrocyte complexes and monocytes, which enhance molecular sickling[525] and may predispose to vaso-occlusion. Endothelial attraction and adhesion of white cells, platelets, red cells and reticulocytes through upregulation of leukotriene B₄, L-selectin, P-selectin and vascular cellular adhesion molecule-1 (VCAM-1), as well as von Willebrand factor, may also be increased in chronic oxygen desaturation[388,711] and recent evidence suggest that low daytime saturations also predict transcranial Doppler velocities[635,655] and stroke.[690]

The mechanisms of sickling and increased red cell adhesion in association with hypoxia may be associated with red cell nidus formation and endothelial damage, leading to hyperplasia and arterial narrowing.[386,390] Interestingly, resting end-tidal pCO_2 was higher in three patients when they were on a transfusion regimen that reduced their HbS to <20% than when it was allowed to rise,[659] suggesting that hyperventilation may be a compensatory mechanism, perhaps for the hypoxia accompanying high HbS levels; this would in turn tend to reduce cerebral blood flow. The combination of hypocapnia and the development of CVD might be associated with perfusion abnormalities in those patients with SCD and chronic oxygen desaturation.

Stroke recurrence (see Chapter 17, Section 17.1)

In untreated patients, the risk of recurrence ranges from 60% to 92% in patients with sickle cell anaemia.[542,576,577,681,712–716] With regular blood transfusion, around 10% of patients experience a recurrence,[706] which is commoner in those whose stroke did not occur in the context of an acute illness[717] and if moyamoya collaterals are demonstrated angiographically.[594,595] Clinically covert reinfarction is typical of SCD with an incidence of 7.06/100 patient-years[605] and commonly progresses after symptomatic stroke despite regular transfusion.[718]

Therapy for stroke in sickle cell disease

Early management of stroke

Ischaemic stroke. Transfusion therapy is the mainstay of treatment for stroke in SCD. The aim is to reduce the percentage of sickle haemoglobin and increase levels of haemoglobin A, thus reducing the deleterious effects of sickling whilst improving tissue oxygenation. Studies of regional CBF using inhaled xenon[133] demonstrated that transfusion therapy reduced the cerebral hyperaemia in asymptomatic patients with SCD,[658] and that decreased CBF can be reversed by blood transfusion in patients with acute neurological problems.[546] For acutely sick patients (e.g. with severe acute chest or neurological symptoms), treatment is usually simple or partial exchange–blood transfusion, avoiding rapid fluid shifts.[719] The risk of recurrent stroke appears to be reduced in those who undergo exchange transfusion after the first stroke.[720]

A chronic intermittent transfusion programme, aiming to keep the HbS below 30% (see Chapter 16), decreases the risk of stroke recurrence.[514,519,706,719,721] After stroke, blood transfusion is recommended for life;[511,707] however, its side effects (such as antibody formation, blood-borne infections and iron overload) and the practical difficulties (time in hospital, nightly desferrioxamine injections) make it difficult for patients to tolerate this therapy in the long term. Prophylactic transfusion is recommended for patients with SCD and elevated TCD velocities (>200cm/s), as the Stroke Prevention Trial in Sickle Cell Anaemia (STOP and STOP2) clearly showed a reduction in strokes in this group.[641,642]

The aim of an intensive blood transfusion regimen is to keep the HbS level less than the range 20–30%. Moderate transfusion regimens, maintaining HbS between 45% and 50%, were associated with a higher CBF than seen with the traditional regimen, an effect apparently related in part to the haemoglobin and in part to the percentage of sickle haemoglobin.[659] Although there were no neurological complications, the effect of the associated hyperaemia over time is unknown.[659] A study with MRA showed that blood transfusion might help to reverse CVD by increasing the lumen of the blood vessel.[722]

Hydroxyurea may be an alternative treatment for those who have a low tolerance for blood transfusion. The drug increases the production of fetal haemoglobin and decreases sickling.[723–725] However, in one study, 19% of patients receiving hydroxyurea had stroke recurrence[725] and in a pilot study of young children there were also recurrent CNS events.[726] Nevertheless, recent data from a larger series with longer follow-up suggests that hydroxyurea is an effective alternative to blood transfusion, particularly if there is overlap; although there were more strokes in the SWITCH trial. Transcranial Doppler velocities may also be reduced into the low risk range on hydroxyurea.[728]

Adenotosillectomy may improve nocturnal oxygen desaturation in those with adenotonsillar hypertrophy and symptoms of upper airway obstruction,[536,678,689] although this may not necessarily reduce transcranial Doppler velocities[729] or the risk of neurological complications.[389] With respect to oxygen therapy, sickle cell adhesion may be transient[522,529] and may be reversed with hyperoxia.[524] One study showed that inhaled oxygen (50% O_2) in sickle cell patients produced a significant reduction in the number of irreversibly sickled cells compared to those who received air, but no effect on duration of painful crisis.[730] Further trials are necessary to evaluate the benefits of oxygen therapy or overnight repiratory support (e.g. with auto-adjusting positive airways pressure[389,731,732]) for cardiovascular[733] and cerebral[732] function.

In those patients with SCD and moyamoya syndrome, revascularization techniques (encephaloduroarteriosynangiosis or extracranial–intracranial bypass) may help to improve cerebral blood perfusion and stabilize the progression of cerebrovascular disease.[593,734] Recent series of patients with SCD and moyamoya who underwent indirect surgical revascularization adds further evidence that with careful pre-, peri- and postoperative management, this procedure is safe and probably reduces the risk of recurrent stroke. Despite regular blood transfusion, cognitive deterioration has also been reported in children with SCD and moyamoya.[735] Two groups from the USA recently reported encouraging results in terms of safety in 12 children with SCD and moyamoya who underwent indirect revascularization, although one postoperative stroke was reported in each series, at 24 hours and 3 weeks, respectively.[736,737] A further 10 patients undergoing direct and indirect surgical revascularization of 15 hemispheres (six direct) have been reported in an abstract from from the UK.[738] There were no strokes in the postoperative period but two of these patients had intraventricular haemorrhage in addition to one with an ischaemic stroke within the first postoperative year. Follow-up MRI after relatively short periods has not demonstrated recurrent covert infarction in any of these 34 revascularized patients but these patients will need to be compared with those on optimal regular blood transfusion regimens for stroke.[718] In part at least because indefinite blood transfusion and iron chelation are a heavy burden for children with SCD and many are non-compliant, revascularization is an attractive option. However, it should be compared with other treatment options, including hydroxyurea, antiplatelet agents, bone marrow transplantation, management of sleep-related breathing disorders and possibly statins for secondary prevention of stroke in SCD.

Bone marrow transplantation and allogenic umbilical cord blood stem cell transplantation may have the potential to prevent progression of cerebrovascular disease and stroke.[739–744] Other therapies such as short-chain fatty acids,[724] inhaled nitric oxide[745] and arginine supplementation[746] are currently under investigation. The blockade of endothelial α-V-β-3 integrin or other anti-adhesion therapies (directed to platelet integrin receptors or intravenous γ-globulin) may help to prevent vaso-occlusion.[747–749]

Haemorrhagic stroke. Patients with SCD and intracranial haemorrhage require immediate transfer to an intensive care unit with neurosurgery on site in case craniectomy is required. Urgent neurology and haematology consultations should also be obtained, in view of the wide differential diagnosis and high early mortality of up to 25%. Although published cases are rare, there is no contra-indication to management of haemorrhage as for non-sickle stroke, with general support including intensive care, and evacuation of space-occupying clot. In the acute phase, the main priorities are to prevent cerebral herniation if the blood collection is space-occupying, to reverse any coagulopathy, to exclude sinovenous thrombosis, and to treat any associated vasospasm; for example, in subarachnoid haemorrhage with volume expansion and possibly with a calcium channel blocker such as nimodipine.

As treatment appears to reduce mortality in the general adult population,[750] anticoagulation or thrombolysis may be considered for venous sinus thrombosis which fails to respond to general measures such as rehydration and treatment of infection. Interventional neuroradiology with coils has been successfully employed for the management of aneurysms in sickle cell disease[751] and may be an alternative to clipping at surgery.[752] Patients should be managed at centres where a multidisciplinary team includes a neurosurgeon with vascular expertise as well as an interventional neuroradiologist.

Primary stroke prevention

There is class A evidence for the role of blood transfusions in preventing first stroke in children with sickle cell anaemia and high blood flow velocities on TCD. The Stroke Prevention Trial in Sickle Cell Anaemia (STOP) showed a clear benefit for prophylactic transfusion in children with blood flow velocities of >200cm/s.[641] A large proportion of the treated patients apparently received unnecessary transfusion, however, as only 15% of the non-transfused children went on to have a stroke despite apparently very high velocities. This is an important issue, as transfusion is associated with risks of infection and alloimmunization, and many children and their families find regular blood transfusion and chelation therapy burdensome. A subsequent study, STOP II, has, however, shown that it is essential to continue to transfuse long term even if the TCD velocities return to the normal range, as the risk of stroke or reversion to high-risk TCD velocities is unacceptably high.[642] The fall in the incidence of stroke in SCD in California[645] and East London[646] is probably related to the introduction of TCD screening and prophylactic transfusion. However, TCD screening is currently not universally available and cannot therefore be mandated currently. In addition, there is evidence that adults with SCD do not have high TCD velocities and programmes of TCD screening and prophylactic transfusion are probably not appropriate for older age groups.

Prevention and management of cognitive problems
Cognitive problems are an important complication of sickle cell disease[753–755] (see Chapter 17, Section 17.5) and are often severe[756] and progressive in those with overt stroke with or without moyamoya.[735,757] There are very few data on their prevention or amelioration but blood transfusion[758] and hydroxyurea[759] may have a beneficial effect. The role of revascularization in preventing cognitive deterioration in moyamoya associated with sickle cell disease[735] has not been formally evaluated. Educational rehabilitation is also feasible[760,761] and treatment of sleep-related breathing disorders may improve attention and processing speed,[732] but for both of these interventions, larger randomized controlled trials will be required before they can be recommended.

15.5 Immunodeficiency and Bone Marrow Transplantation

Fenella J Kirkham

Stroke has been documented in children with primary immunodeficiency[5] in addition to being a complication of bone marrow transplantation[98,468,469,494,762] and immunoglobulin therapy.[763] Ciclosporin-related posterior leukoencephalopathy is an important mechanism[551] (Fig. 15.30) but cerebrovascular disease may also develop.[762]

15.6 Premature Ageing Syndromes (Progerias)

Fenella J. Kirkham

Hutchinson–Gilford progeria

Hutchinson–Gilford progeria (HGPS)[764,765] is a syndrome with an incidence of about 1 in 4 000 000.[766–768] Most affected patients are sporadic and the disease is caused by autosomal dominant de novo point mutations.[769,770] Rarely the condition is secondary to uniparental disomy[769] or deletions[771] of the LMNA gene on chromosome 1. Pathologically there is severe reduction in smooth muscle cells with reduction of the intima-media thickness,[768] and in some patients there may be premature arteriosclerosis.[768,772] Inheritance is typically from the germ line of the father, who is often older than average. A recessive form secondary to a missense mutation of the same gene has also been described.[773] Mutations result in activation of a cryptic splice site within exon 11 and to synthesis of a truncated lamin A protein which deletes 50 amino acids near the carboxy terminus[769] and progressively accumulates in the cell nucleus.[774] Transcription of a large number of genes is abnormal and there are mesodermal and mesenchymal abnormalities which appear to be involved with tissue proliferation.[775] Fibroblasts from individuals with HGPS have severe morphological abnormalities in nuclear envelope structure. In vitro, the accumulation has been reversed by corrective splicing at the genomic level[776] and by farnesyltransferase inhibition[237,777,778] and this might lead to prevention of the rapidly progressive ageing process in patients, as well as increasing understanding of the ageing process in general.[767]

Children are normal at birth but present in the first year with poor growth and premature ageing with characteristic scleroderma-like skin, midfacial cyanosis, alopecia, narrow and

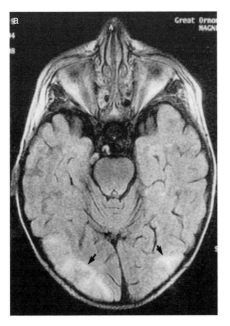
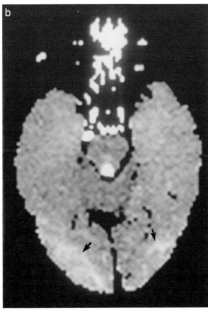

Fig. 15.30. Axial magnetic resonance images of a 4-year-old boy who presented with lethargy and focal seizures secondary to ciclosporin therapy on day 30 after bone marrow transplantation for severe combined immunodeficiency. The T2 signal abnormalities correspond to areas of increased diffusion, suggesting that these areas of cerebral oedema were caused by extravasation of fluid and not cerebral ischaemia. (a) A fluid-attenuated inversion-recovery image shows confluent cortical and juxtacortical signal alteration in both occipital lobes (arrows). (b) The apparent diffusion coefficient map at the same level reveals increased diffusion in the regions of prolonged T2 signal.

beaked nose, prominent scalp veins, hypertension and loss of subcutaneous fat.[766,779] Growth is poor and skeletal abnormalities include hypoplasia and dysplasia, persistent open fontanelle, severe osteolysis and pathological fractures. Intelligence is normal, at least in the early years. Total cholesterol, low density lipoprotein (LDL) and high density lipoprotein (HDL) cholesterol, triglyceride, and median C-reactive protein levels are not different from controls but HDL cholesterol and adiponectin fall with age,[780] while prothrombin times are prolonged and platelet counts and serum phosphorus levels elevated.[781] The development of atherosclerosis is probably related directly to the nuclear ageing process, rather than to the changes in lipid profile. Progressive cardiovascular and cerebrovascular diseases are usually the cause of death by age 13 years.[781,782]

The strokes reported occured at a median of age 9 (range 4–14) years. Some patients present acutely with seizures or hemiparesis while others appear to have recurrent transient ischaemic episodes, with headaches and vertigo as well as limb weakness.[768] The cerebrovascular disease characteristically involves the proximal internal carotid arteries and sometimes the vertebrobasilar arteries.[783,784] Carotid stenosis or occlusion is typical but aneurysms have been described.[785] Subclinical cerebrovascular disease may be diagnosed using MRA and subclinical infarction has been detected on MRI. If children present with clinical stroke and/or seizures, the infarction appears to be larger and in some cases the possibility of cardiac embolus has been raised. The differential diagnosis for hemiparesis in a child with progeria includes extradural[786] and subdural haematomas, probably related to fragile arteriosclerotic arteries and fragile veins.

Other premature ageing syndromes (progerias)

Other premature ageing syndromes such as Werner syndrome (adult progeria; mean age at presentation 39 years),[787] Wiedemann–Rautenstrauch syndrome (neonatal progeria)[788] and deBarsy syndrome[789] may be associated with cognitive difficulties. Childhood stroke is rarely diagnosed in these syndromes; for the Wiedemann–Rautenstrauch neonatal form, early death may preclude this manifestation. Multiple haemorrhages after trauma, possibly related to amyloid angiopathy, have been described in a 49 year old with Werner syndrome.[790] There is some clinical overlap, in age of onset, between syndromes related to the WRN gene, a DNA helicase, and those in which LMNA mutations are found.[787,791]

15.7 Stroke in Children with Cancer

Fenella J. Kirkham

One in a thousand young adults is a cancer survivor; about one-third had leukaemia and 10–15% had a brain tumour. Thus, quality of life and any resulting long-term disabilities in these individuals have become important public health issues. In terms of life-years lost by death from cancer, a suboptimal treatment in childhood has a high and much greater impact on society than in adults (average 68 years lost per case of childhood cancer, compared to 10 years for adult cancers). For example, the incidence of medulloblastoma is 0.7 per 100 000 children under 14 years per annum. This equates to some 1000 cases per annum in Europe. With a current estimated survival of 70% and 50–90% of survivors being affected by one or more disability, it can be predicted that 20 000 life-years per year will be lost and a burden of 30 000–50 000 life-years of disability will be gained by this group of children alone. The overall incidence of stroke is 5.9 per 1000 patient-years, 100-fold higher than in the general paediatric population.[792] Common vascular diagnoses include venous sinus thrombosis, particularly in leukaemia,[793,794] and arterial stenosis and occlusion, moyamoya, aneurysm, mineralizing microangiopathy, vascular malformations and stroke-like migraines, usually but not always associated with radiotherapy (Figs 15.31–15.33).[795] Any measures that together increase treatment efficacy and decrease long-term disability would carry huge advantages in human and economic terms.

Cerebrovascular disease and stroke

STROKE SYNDROMES

Perioperative stroke

Stroke may occur immediately after brain tumour surgery, either as a direct effect of surgical interference with the cerebral vessels or secondary to sinovenous thrombosis if the patient becomes relatively dehydrated.[796–800] Since thrombophilia and systemic venous thrombosis are both common in patients with brain tumour[801,802] this complication may be more common than has been documented to date as the symptoms and signs may be masked by those of the tumour. Reversible posterior leukencephalopathy in the context of fluctuations in blood pressure has also been reported after surgery for a posterior fossa tumour.[803]

Non-perioperative stroke

Non-perioperative stroke has been well described and has an incidence of 4.03 per 1000 years of follow up.[804] Cerebrovascular disease and arterial stroke are well-recognized associations with suprasellar tumours including optic and hypothalamic glioma, germinoma, pituitary adenoma and craniopharyngioma.[230,240,805–814] Occasionally cerebrovascular disease has been described in tumours in other locations, such as brainstem glioma[814] and medulloblastoma/primitive neuroectodermal tumour (MB/PNET).[815–817]

The basal cerebral vessels are usually stenosed or occluded and there is often a network of collateral vessels similar to those seen in primary moyamoya. The pathology appears to be endothelial proliferation and thickening of the tunica intima and tunica muscularis of the internal carotid and basal cerebral

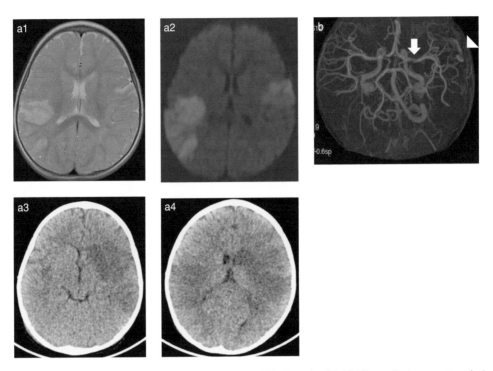

Fig. 15.31. (a) Progressive bilateral infarction in a child with acute myeloid leukaemia. (b) Middle cerebral artery stenosis (vertical arrow) in a child with transient ischaemic attacks after cranial irradiation for acute lymphoblastic leukaemia. The transient ischaemic attacks stopped after revascularization surgery (extracranial–intracranial bypass) (arrowhead).

arteries.[818] There may, however, be significant radiological and pathological differences from primary moyamoya.[819] The majority of patients present with TIA or infarctive stroke but haemorrhagic stroke secondary to aneurysm has been described.[820]

RISK FACTORS FOR CEREBROVASCULAR DISEASE AND STROKE

Risk factors include age at presentation,[792] the nature of the tumour, the extent of debulking surgery, whether the radiotherapy field covers the circle of Willis[792] and the radiotherapy dose.[256,792,804] Vasculopathy appears to be commoner with optic glioma than with other tumours[804] but some series have reported no cases. In a large series from one centre, radiotherapy was the strongest risk factor, with chemotherapy of borderline significance.[804] In midline tumours, such as craniopharyngioma, hypothalamic or optic glioma, stroke may occur even in children who have not received radiotherapy.[804] Encasement of the cerebral vessels by tumour, which may necessitate additional surgery and handling of the vessels, appears to increase the risk. It is possible that there are angiogenic growth factors related to the tumour.[821] Patients may have vascular risk factors[822,823] and the process may be one of accelerated atherosclerosis.[823] There is evidence for abnormal flow-mediated dilatation after radiotherapy, which suggests that the mechanism of vascular damage may involve nitric oxide bioavailability.[824] Genetic predisposition to vascular disease appears to be a risk factor, particularly neurofibromatosis type 1 (NF1),[230,240,825] which is associated with vasculopathy in the absence of tumour or radiation,[235] perhaps related to the gene for familial moyamoya

disease close to the NF1 gene on chromosome 17[826] or to the predisposition of patients with NF1 to hypertension.[254] Other predisposing factors may include those for thrombosis, such as hyperfibrinogenaemia and the factor V Leiden mutation[171,827–829] and for atherogenesis, such as hypertension,[5,830] diabetes,[823] hyperhomocysteinaemia[829,831] or hyperlipidaemia,[822,829] although there are very few data available at the present.[804] Cholesterol levels do appear to be higher in patients with brain tumours at the time of diagnosis than in the general population[832–834] and hypertriglyceridaemia has also been reported.[835] Although there may be no aetiological link in terms of oncogenesis,[834] dyslipidaemia may play a role in cerebrovascular disease. The secondary endocrine problems, such as hypopituiarism and Cushing syndrome, and their treatment (e.g. with growth hormone), may have as yet unidentified effects on endothelial function and the risk of small or large vessel disease.[836] It is also possible that relative immunodeficiency, exposure to infection and the host reaction to it play a role in triggering or exacerbating radiation-induced vascular disease, as they appear to do in other aetiologies for childhood stroke.[5] Anaemia or hypoxia may also be risk factors for cerebrovacular disease and stroke in children with brain tumours[837] and leukaemia.[74] The relative importance of various risk factors may vary with age, ethnicity and underlying diagnosis, as is the case in childhood stroke in general,[5] but there is a good case for investigating for vascular risk factors not related to the tumour or it treatment, as recurrence and outcome are related to the number of risk factors[4] and many are modifiable.[838]

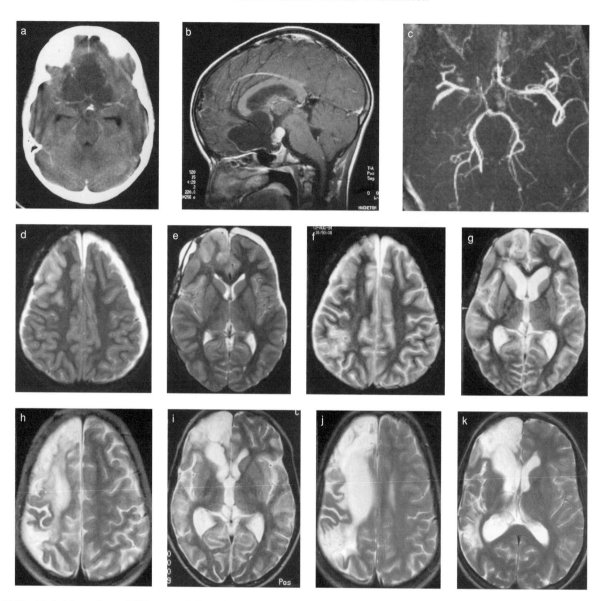

Fig. 15.32. (a) Axial unenhanced CT scan and (b) sagittal post-contrast T1-weighted MRI showing a large craniopharyngioma in a 10-year-old girl with a family history of hypercholesterolaemia. Calcification in the cyst wall is seen on the axial CT scan. The tumour exerts pressure on and displaces the chiasm posterosuperiorly and inferiorly involves the pituitary fossa. The anterior cerebral arteries are elevated and splayed and the middle cerebral arteries are attenuated by the cyst. The cyst was drained for immediate relief of pressure effects, and 3 weeks later she underwent a right frontal craniotomy for removal of the cystic and enhancing solid component (D,H). Ten days after surgery, she developed a left hemiparesis. (c) Magnetic resonance angiography showed complete loss of signal, indicating marked reduction in flow within the proximal right middle cerebral artery and reduced flow within the insular branches of the middle cerebral artery. (d,e) MRI obtained 3 days later showed bilateral shallow subdural collections over the frontal convexities, which are a common complication of craniotomy, and right frontal cortical oedema. (f,g) One month later, a repeat MRI showed a new right frontoparietal infarct in the middle cerebral artery territory. (h,i) Eighteen months later she had a further episode of left hemiparesis and there was further extension of the infarction along the middle and posterior cerebral artery border zone. (j,k) She continued to experience frequent headaches and seizures. The final scan, 5 years after the original presentation, shows maturation of the anterior and middle cerebral artery territory infarction. Right carotid angiography performed 18 months after the first stroke was normal (not shown). (Courtesy of Dr Dawn Saunders).

Diffuse brain damage

EFFECTS OF RADIOTHERAPY

It is increasingly clear that there is a significant cost in terms of neurological, behavioural and cognitive sequelae for children who survive brain tumours. This appears to be due to a widespread effect of radiotherapy on neuronal, glial and endothelial cells.

Pathology

The available evidence suggests that the oligodendrocytes and endothelial cells are involved in radiation damage.[839] Injury to the endothelium of the small vessels may result in a cascade of events leading to increased vascular permeability and fibrinoid necrosis of the vessel wall.[840] In rabbits with hypercholesterolaemia, 5Gy of radiation caused small- and medium-sized vessel disease, with deposition of lipophages and

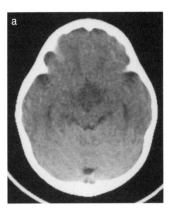

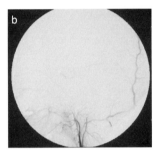
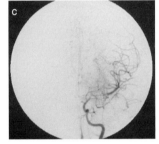

Fig. 15.33. (a) CT scan showing a hypothalamic glioma in a boy aged 22 months. He was treated with radiotherapy and presented 3 years later with left- and right-sided transient hemipareses and seizures. MRI showed multiple areas of altered signal in the left frontal and temporal white matter. Formal angiography showed poor filling of the main vessels (b) with collateral formation (c). (Courtesy of Dr Dawn Saunders).

changes to the elastic structure.[841] Similar changes may occur in humans.[842,843] Large vessels may also be infiltrated by fat-laden macrophages.[844] Some, but not all, of the changes secondary to radiotherapy may be visualized on conventional MRI.[845] Full scale IQ, factual knowledge, verbal and performance thinking (but not sustained attention or verbal memory) in patients with posterior fossa tumours is related to the volume of normal appearing white matter (NAWM).[846] Compared with controls with low grade cerebellar tumours, the volume of NAWM is lower in those treated with chemotherapy as well as radiotherapy.[847] The rate of loss of NAWM volume was 23% lower in those receiving 24Gy than in those receiving 36Gy.[848] Quantitative T1 mapping shows an effect on white matter at doses >20Gy and on grey matter at doses >60Gy.[722]

Imaging also provides some evidence for a small vessel vasculopathy. Lacunar infarcts were seen in 25/421 children who had radiotherapy or chemotherapy for brain tumour but in none of those treated with surgery alone,[849] but IQ was not lower in those with lacunes than in age- and diagnosis-matched controls. Fourteen patients had craniospinal irradiation and 11 had local radiotherapy only. The strongest predictor of lacunar infarction was age <5 years at the time of radiotherapy. Cerebral calcification shows high rather than low intensity on T1, suggesting a mineralizing microangiopathy.[850] Magnetic resonance spectroscopy has also been performed in children who have undergone brain irradiation. In one study of children with leukaemia, the *N*-acetyl aspartate/creatine ratio was not

related to age at diagnosis but progressively decreased with time since diagnosis.[851] However, in another study, proton spectroscopy markers were not different from control in 14 children irradiated for ALL or tumour and only choline: water related to full scale IQ.[852]

There is also evidence for reduced cerebral blood flow and metabolic rate in association with neurological and cognitive sequelae. For patients with leukaemia treated with radiotherapy and chemotherapy, there is evidence for reduced glucose metabolism in the white matter and thalami.[853] In adults, SPECT may show focal perfusion deficits which correlate with neuropsychological deficit in patients who have undergone radiotherapy.[854] PET may help to distinguish between post-surgical or radiation damage and recrudescence of the tumour[855,856] and a case report suggests that diffusion-weighted MRI may also be useful in this context.[857]

Other risk factors for diffuse brain damage
Neurological and cognitive function may also be affected by the associated hormonal deficiency. Calcification of the basal ganglia was seen in 5% of brain tumours in a Dutch centre and was associated with larger IQ loss and a higher incidence of hypothyroidism and growth hormone deficiency, which might possibly have an aetiological role.[858] As discussed above, hypopituitarism may be associated with dyslipidaemias.[835] In adults, there is some evidence for an additional effect of anticonvulsants, especially carbamazepine,[859] and this possibility should be examined in children; it is certainly sensible to avoid polypharmacy for epilepsy.

TREATMENT OF RADIATION NECROSIS

Steroids
Steroids may improve the symptoms of radiation necrosis, probably by reducing local cerebral oedema.[860] It has also been suggested that the radiation-associated vasculopathy is in part an autoimmune phenomenon, which may be exacerbated by co-existing infection and may be treatable with steroids.[861] The presently available steroids would, however, produce unacceptable side effects if used long term.

Hyperbaric oxygenation
There have been isolated reports of improvement in radiation necrosis with hyperbaric oxygenation performed soon after diagnosis,[862,863] but an animal study showed no benefit[864,864] and this therapy has not been further pursued.

PREVENTION OF STROKE AND DIFFUSE BRAIN DAMAGE
There have been studies looking at the possibility of reducing the radiation dosage without increasing the mortality for the tumour. Substitution with chemotherapy has been investigated in the most vulnerable (<3 years age) patients and where 5-year survival rates are already very high (e.g. leukaemias). Increasing the poorer 5-year survival rates (60%) in children with brain tumours, without increasing intellectual morbidity,

291

is being attempted by substituting more aggressive chemotherapy, and/or the reduction, hyperfractionation or more focal (stereotactic) application of the cranial irradiation dose. However, these strategies carry their own risks of potentially compromising cure rates and causing later additive toxicity after salvage therapy. An alternative strategy is to attempt neuroprotection in those at highest risk, but at present these patients are difficult to identify and there is no evidence-based therapy which reduces the brain injury associated with the treatment of brain tumours.

Early diagnosis and optimal surgical technique

There are still unacceptable delays in the diagnosis of brain tumours in some children[865] and strategies to enable earlier diagnosis must be instituted as part of clinical governance. The surgical management of children with brain tumours is usually conducted by experienced neurosurgeons in centres with a large number of patients, but audit and research into the optimal strategy for each tumour type and presentation must continue.

Reduction of the radiation dose

The toxicity of radiotherapy may be reduced by reducing the dose or altering the fractionation.[866] As part of a controlled trial for low grade medulloblastoma, Mulhern[847] provided evidence that a dose of 36Gy was associated with greater neuropsychological decline than 23.4Gy and that this effect was greater in younger children. For children with posterior fossa tumours, Grill[867] found that the mean IQ was most strongly related to the dose of craniospinal irradiation, with full scale IQs of 84.5, 76.9 and 63.7 for doses of 0, 25Gy and 35Gy respectively and significant loss of verbal comprehension for those with the higher dosage. Kieffer-Renaux,[868] from the same group, found in a controlled trial of 25 vs 36Gy of whole brain irradiation that the higher dose of radiation was associated with more verbal and performance deficits in children with medulloblastoma. Fuss[869] pooled data from 1938 children and found that, for whole brain irradiation, IQ<85 was related to dose and age so that for those <3, the critical dose was 24Gy and for those >6, it was 36Gy. Partial brain irradiation had a measurable effect only at doses >50Gy. Reduced dose radiotherapy for medulloblastoma was associated with a decline in IQ in the whole group of approximately 4 points/year, i.e. still substantial but better than previous studies using a higher dose.[870] Certain subgroups may be more vulnerable, so that, for example, verbal IQ declined more in females, non-verbal IQ declined more in those treated at a younger age, and full scale IQ declined most in those with a higher IQ at baseline. Another recent study using lower doses of radiation for medulloblastoma also shows a loss of 2.55 IQ points/year of follow-up;[871] the raw scores suggested that the ongoing problem is a failure to learn new information.

The main concern currently is that any preservation of cognitive performance may be bought at the expense of a lower cure rate. For standard risk medulloblastoma, 5-year survival was lower with 24Gy of CST than with 36Gy,[872] but survival with adjuvant chemotherapy may be better.[873] However, tumour progression may be commoner in those in whom radiotherapy is delayed.[874] The management of medulloblastoma in very young children and in those with disseminated disease is difficult, as the majority of children progress despite chemotherapy and then require radiotherapy; there is a progressive reduction in IQ of −3.9 points/year whether or not radiotherapy is required.[873]

Prevention of the vasculopathy: reduction of risk factors for cerebrovascular disease

There is evidence from animal studies and early pathological data in humans that small and large vessel disease occurs after irradiation for brain tumours, but the relative importance of this vasculopathy compared with direct damage to neurones and glial cells has received little attention. This is unfortunate, since at the present there is considerable interest in reducing the impact of genetic and environmental risk factors for cerebrovascular disease in the context of stroke and of vascular dementia. Some of these strategies are low risk for the patient, for example folate supplementation for hyperhomocysteinaemia.[831] There is considerable evidence from adult studies that control of hypertension reduces the risk of stroke recurrence and it is possible that raised blood pressure is important in the cognitive decline seen after radiotherapy for brain tumours in children[875] (see Chapter 5).

Since patients with brain tumours have higher cholesterol levels than the general population[832–834] and there is evidence from animal studies that the pathophysiology of radiation vasculopathy includes accumulation of lipids;[841] variation in lipid profiles might account for part of the risk of cerebrovascular disease and dementia. In elderly adults, there is a little evidence that prophylaxis with HMG-CoA reductase inhibitors (statins) reduces the risk of vascular dementia[876] and there is a possibility that statin prophylaxis might reduce the cognitive consequences associated with radiotherapy. There are concerns over the risk of oncogenesis, cerebral haemorrhage and the effect of widespread apoptosis with the use of statins.[875] There would then be an important question to be answered as to whether statins might have adverse effects by promoting tumour growth through angiogenesis,[877] or might have a beneficial effect by reducing tumour bulk because the rate-limiting step in the mevalonate pathway (hepatic hydroxymethyl glutaryl coenzyme A reductase) is inhibited, reducing the synthesis of cell wall lipids and inducing apoptosis,[878] although not arrest of the cellular proliferation.[479] Phase I/II trials have shown that statins may be tolerated in adults with very malignant brain tumours[879] and in children with hypercholesterolaemia,[880,881] but a considerable amount of preclinical work would be needed before their use could be considered for children with malignant brain tumours.

Rehabilitation, cognitive therapy and education

In children who have had a brain tumour, with or without an overt stroke, academic and social failure may reinforce cognitive and behavioural difficulties,[882] but encouragingly remediation may allow improvement, for example in literacy.[883] Adults receiving surgery and radiotherapy may experience a reduction in full-scale IQ which may recover in those who return to work early. Late improvement may also be seen in children, perhaps secondary to targeted education for specific learning difficulties. Appropriate rehabilitation with physiotherapy, occupational therapy and reintegration into school is therefore essential.

15.8 Inflammatory Vasculopathies

Fenella J. Kirkham

Takayasu arteritis

Takayasu arteritis is a systemic granulomatous inflammation of the aorta and its branches, including the common carotid arteries (Fig. 15.34), which has an incidence of 1 per million per year. It is commoner in women, typically of Mexican or South Asian extraction,[884] but may present in childhood[885] with headache, seizures, ptosis secondary to intraorbital mass, visual disturbance, dizziness, TIA or stroke,[886,887] and has been described in patients as young as 6 months of age.[888] Signs include absent carotid or radial pulses, cervical bruits, asymmetrical blood pressure measurements and fever. Diagnosis can be supported by MRA, but the most accurate assessment requires aortography. In a recent series of 24 children, four had had a hemiparesis.[885] There are HLA haplotypes, especially HLAB5201, which predispose[889] and the current concept of aetiology is that Takayasu arteritis is an unusual autoimmune reaction, possibly involving tumour necrosis factor-α, to infections such as chronic tonsillitis, tuberculosis, chronic

hepatitis B or C or inflammatory diseases such as thyroiditis, Crohn disease and ulcerative colitis.[890–892] In the acute phase of disease, there are systemic symptoms such as fever, weight loss, malaise, elevated C-reactive protein levels and a high ESR.[893,894] The tuberculin test result may be positive. Vascular bruit is typical and most patients have stenoses, occlusions or aneurysmal changes of the aorta and its main branches. Around a fifth of patients present with symptoms referable to cerebrovascular disease, although most have transient symptoms rather than disabling stroke.[895] The diagnosis is often delayed in younger patients[884,896] but hypertension or a high ESR should raise suspicion.[894] Extra- and intra-cranial cerebrovascular disease and microemboli can be detected non-invasively using ultrasound techniques[895,897,898] as well as MR, CT and conventional angiography.[886,891] The angiographic manifestations can be classified as type I, cervicobrachial; type II, thoracoabdominal; type III, peripheral; and type IV, generalized. Saccular and fusiform aneurysms have been documented in children[891] and there may be intracranial vessel involvement.[899] Hypertension is common at presentation[894] and congestive heart failure, left ventricular hypertrophy, and coronary, pulmonary and renal artery involvement may develop. Complications include myocardial infarction, ischaemic and haemorrhagic stroke,[893,900] aortic valve disease requiring replacement, and death, typically due to renovascular hypertension or secondary atherosclerotic complications. Medical therapy prevents progression in most patients, who usually respond to steroids with or without immunosuppression (cyclophosphamide initially and longer term azathioprine or methotrexate).[896] Drugs reducing the effect of tumour necrosis factor-α, such as infliximab, may play a role.[901] Vascular surgery may be indicated and is often effective in controlling hypertension,[896,902,903] although restenosis is common.

Polyarteritis nodosa

This condition tends to affect middle aged patients and has an annual prevalence of 6.3 per 100 000. Stroke occurs in around 15% of patients, occasionally in children,[904–906] ischaemic stroke particularly. Lacunar stroke and leukariosis secondary to small vessel disease is particularly common in adults.[907] Patients may also have intracranial haemorrhage secondary to aneurysm formation or small vessel vasculitis; there may be aneurysms elsewhere, for example in the renal circulation (Fig. 15.35).[908] The use of corticosteroids may be a risk factor for stroke in polyarteritis nodosa and anti-platelet agents are recommended as prophylaxis.[907] The mechanisms of stroke in polyarteritis nodosa include direct involvement of the arterial wall in the vascular process and atherosclerotic disease, perhaps precipitated in part by associated hypertension.

Systemic lupus erythematosus

Neurological complications are common at presentation with systemic lupus erythematosus in childhood.[909] Typical symptoms include headache, behavioural disorders including confusion, depression, anxiety and psychosis, lethargy, diplopia,

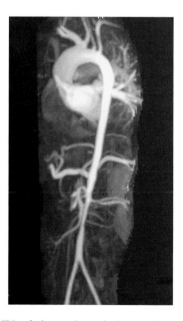

Fig. 15.34. MRI of the aortic arch in an adolescent girl with Takayasu arteritis.

blurred vision, memory alteration, dizziness and altered consciousness. The most frequently observed neurological signs are cranial nerve palsy, ataxia, papilloedema, nystagmus, meningism, chorea, tremor, rigidity, myelopathy, neuropathy and cortical blindness. Presentation with seizures, status epilepticus or coma is not uncommon. More subtle presentations include progressive cognitive dysfunction and idiopathic intracranial hypertension. Ischaemic or haemorrhagic stroke is obvious in 15–30% of those with neurological complications and may be associated with arterial abnormality including occlusion (Fig. 15.36), moyamoya[910] and vasculitis, but in most of the presentations the possibility of venous sinus thrombosis (see Fig. 7.6A,B),[74,911] or stenosis[912] should be excluded. Embolism from a left-sided valve abnormality (Libman–Sacks endocarditis) or through a shunt from systemic deep venous thrombosis is a likely mechanism for arterial occlusion. Valvular vegetations are generally located on the atrial side of the mitral valve or on the arterial side of the aortic valve. The presence of the lupus anticoagulant on laboratory testing is associated with cerebrovascular disease at the time of diagnosis and chorea thereafter.[913] Anticoagulation is usually appropriate for those with venous sinus thrombosis.[74] The use of prednisolone and cyclophosphamide for the management of the cerebrovascular disease is controversial[914].

Nephrotic syndrome

The majority of the cases published recently have had a diagnosis of cerebral venous sinus thrombosis[99,915–921] but arterial stroke has occasionally been reported.[922–924] Iron deficiency may be a risk factor but if there are prothrombotic risk factors, anticoagulation during relapses is recommended because of the risk of recurrence.[925]

Inflammatory bowel disease

Neurological complications of inflammatory bowel disease in childhood have been recognized increasingly as having a vascular basis over the past decade[926,927] and there is an excess of ischaemic strokes in young patients with Crohn disease compared with the general population.[928] In childhood, the majority of the cases reported have had cerebral venous sinus thrombosis[927,929–932] and this may precede diagnosis,[933] be the presenting syndrome[931] or diagnosed many years lafter surgery.[934] Posterior leukoencephalopathy has been documented in children in relation to immunosuppression in inflammatory bowel disease[935] (Fig. 15.37) and arterial disease is not uncommon in adults.[936–938] In a recent series of 154 patients newly diagnosed with inflammatory bowel disease, one-third with ulcerative colitis,[4] (2.6%) had cerebral thromboembolism over a 5-year period, all patients with additional risk factors.[926]

Henoch–Schönlein purpura

Coma, convulsions and focal neurological signs may complicate Henoch–Schönlein purpura secondary to intracerebral haemorrhage,[939–946] arteriopathy, venous sinus thrombosis and posterior leukoencephalopathy.[946] In children with stroke in an arterial distribution, both middle and posterior cerebral arteries are typically involved.[946] Children are usually treated with immunomodulatory therapy: steroids, immunoglobulin, plasma exchange and cyclophosphamide.[946] Intracerebral haemorrhage is typically in the parieto-occipital region and may be secondary to venous sinus thrombosis; most cases can be managed conservatively but occasionally surgical drainage is required.[939]

Antiphosphatidylethanolamine antibody was found in the CSF of one patient with Henoch–Schönlein purpura with a stroke but not in two controls or two patients with Henoch–Schönlein

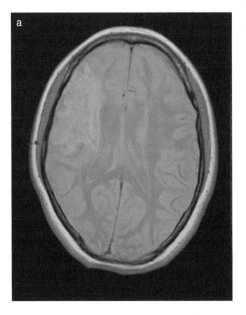
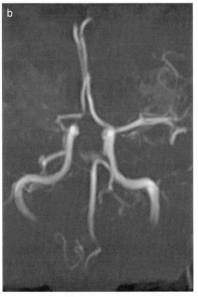

Fig. 15.35. MRI showing large middle cerebral artery territory infarct (a) and middle cerebral artery occlusion (b) in a 12-year-old who had had idiopathic intracranial hypertension 2 years before and chorea 1 year before. She was diagnosed with systemic lupus erythematosus and was anticoagulated and immunosuppressed.

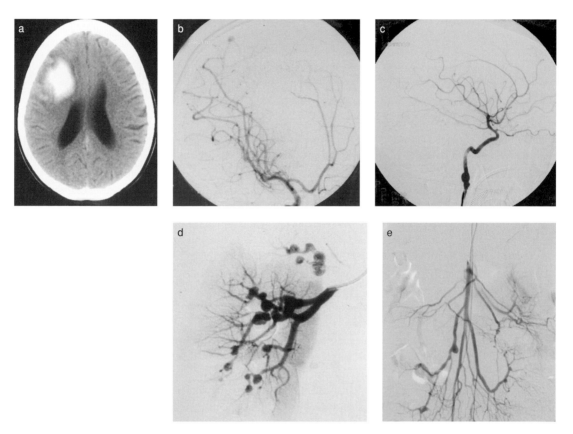

Fig. 15.36. (a) Digital subtraction arteriography from a child who presented with an intracranial haemorrhage. The intracranial vessels are normal except for a small area (b) but there is an aneurysm in the internal carotid (c) and multiple aneurysms in the kidney (d) and systemic vessels (e). She fulfilled the criteria for polyarteritis nodosa and was immunosuppressed.

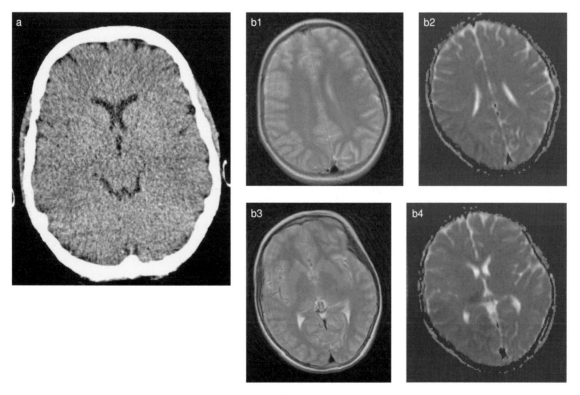

Fig. 15.37. Transient focal ischaemia in inflammatory bowel disease. (a) CT scan showing mild effacement of the sulci in an immunosuppressed child with Crohn disease who became hypertensive and had four generalized tonic-clonic seizures after a blood transfusion for a post-ileostomy drop in haemoglobin. (b) MRI in another girl with Crohn disease who presented with diarrhoea and vomiting and a week later developed a left hemiparesis which recovered after 48 hours. MRI shows cortical oedema in the right parietal region. Diffusion-weighted imaging shows asymmetry with signal change in the right parietal region and posterior thalamus. In both cases the imaging is compatible with posterior reversible encephalopathy syndrome (PRES).

purpura without stroke, suggesting that there may be a specific autoimmune mechanism.[947]

Idiopathic thrombocytopenic purpura

Cerebral haemorrhage is a much feared complication of idiopathic thrombocytopenic purpura (ITP) and, although rare, continues to be a problem in the acute phase and occasionally over the longer term,[948–954] particularly at platelet counts of below 10 000.[951] Younger patients are more likely to have intracerebral, while older ones tend to have subdural haemorrhage.[955] The mortality rate of intracerebral haemorrhage associated with ITP has historically been similar to that occurring spontaneously, i.e. up to half are fatal (see Chapter 8), although the survival rate has been better in younger patients and recent series[950] and subdural haemorrhage has a good prognosis. Occasional patients also harbour arteriovenous malformations[948,956] and intracranial haemorrhage may also predict the eventual development of systemic lupus erythematosus.[950] Treatment with steroids, immunoglobulin[957] and, if necessary, splenectomy does not always prevent this complication.[950] If intracranial haemorrhage occurs, emergency management with steroids, splenectomy, immunoglobulin and neurosurgical intervention may be required. Although the platelet count may increase more rapidly with immunoglobulin therapy,[957] therefore potentially reducing the risk of intracranial haemorrhage, venous sinus thrombosis has been reported.[958] Cerebral infarction has also been recognized in patients who have had ITP and both ischaemic and haemorrhagic stroke may be associated with anticardiolipin antibodies and the eventual emergence of systemic lupus erythematosus. Patients who have had ITP may also develop Coombs positive autoimmune haemolytic anaemia and Evans syndrome which is a cause of childhood stroke (Fig. 15.7).[123]

Kawasaki disease

Kawasaki disease may be associated with cerebral infarction, both clinical[904,959–961] and subclinical,[962] as well as subdural effusion,[963] and posterior circulation involvement with facial palsy and meningism.[964] In addition to the risk of embolic stroke in the context of coronary aneurysms, which probably extends at least a year after initial presentation,[961] late formation of cerebral aneurysms has also been reported.[965] Subclinical hypoperfusion may be quite common, occurring in six out of 21 patients in one series.[966] Early recognition of the characteristic blistering of the hands and feet and appropriate management with immunoglobulin probably prevents most of the complications, although stroke has been described despite early intervention and may even be related to high dose immunoglobulin therapy.[967]

Behçet disease

Behçet disease is a rare condition which is commoner in people of Mediterranean origin, affects both sexes equally and is related to the HLAB5101 haplotype. The characteristic presentation is with oral and genital ulcers but thrombosis including cerebral venous thrombosis[968] occurs in up to 25% of adults, perhaps more commonly in those who also have genetic prothrombotic risk factors such as factor V Leiden. Other neurological complications in adults include seizures, ischaemic stroke secondary to occlusion and haemorrhagic stroke in the context of aneurysm.[969] Neurological complications, including cerebral venous thrombosis, idiopathic intracranial hypertension and spinal cord involvement,[970,971] are less common in children but are occasionally the presenting features,[972–980] which means that the diagnosis should always be considered during follow-up as well as at presentation, as it may be difficult to exclude. Immunosuppression, colchicine and thalidomide are used to treat Behçet disease.[975]

Susac syndrome

The combination of microangiopathy of the brain, retina and inner ear described by Susac and his collegues,[981–984] which typically presents in young women but is diagnosed in men (ratio 1:3), has been reported in adolescents[985,986] and in children as young as 9.[984] MRI typically shows multifocal supratentorial white matter lesions including the corpus callosum, often with a 'hub-and-spoke' appearance. The deep grey nuclei (basal ganglia and thalamus) are involved in the majority and there is usually also parenchymal enhancement and sometimes leptomeningeal enhancement.[983] It is considered to be an autoimmune condition affecting the small vessels and anti-endothelial antibodies have been found in serum but not CSF, which reduced after steroid therapy.[987] Serial fluorescein angiograms are important to monitor subclinical disease activity, which appears as multifocal hyperfluorescence intermittently, and any response to treatment, which is usually immunomodulation with steroids, immunoglobulin, cyclophosphamide, tacrolimus, microphenolate or rituximab.[984,986,988]

15.9 Summary

Fenella J. Kirkham

This chapter has covered the commoner symptomatic causes of stroke and cerebrovascular disease that have been documented in childhood and are not discussed elsewhere in this book but it is not comprehensive; the reader is referred to other sources for more detail.[989–991] Neuroimaging undertaken in the acute stage of neurological presentations including coma, headache and seizures, as well as focal signs, has led to the realization that the pathophysiology of the cerebral complications of childhood diseases is commonly vascular. Recently, there has been increased awareness of the high proportion of patients with a family history, especially for the aneurysms[992] and arteriovenous malformations[993] underlying the majority of haemorrhagic strokes (see Chapter 8), and rapid progress in understanding the genetic basis of ischaemic stroke in addition.[994] Many children and families may have a specific diagnosis in the years to come rather than an eponymous syndrome. However, management strategies are not necessarily evidence based and collaborative efforts will be needed to achieve progress.

REFERENCES

1. Gold AP, Challenor YB, Gilles FH, Kilal SP, Leviton A, Rollins EI. Report of Joint Committee for Stroke Facilities: IX. Strokes in Children (Part 1). Stroke 1973; 4:835–894.
2. Higgins JJ, Kammerman LA, Fitz CR. Predictors of survival and characteristics of childhood stroke. Neuropediatrics 1991; 22(4):190–193.
3. Mancini J, Girard N, Chabrol B, Lamoureux S, Livet MO, Thuret I et al. Ischemic cerebrovascular disease in children: retrospective study of 35 patients. J Child Neurol 1997; 12(3):193–199.
4. Lanthier S, Carmant L, David M, Larbrisseau A, de Veber G. Stroke in children: the coexistence of multiple risk factors predicts poor outcome. Neurology 2000; 54(2):371–378.
5. Ganesan V, Prengler M, McShane MA, Wade AM, Kirkham FJ. Investigation of risk factors in children with arterial ischemic stroke. Ann Neurol 2003; 53(2):167–173.
6. Brankovic-Sreckovic V, Milic-Rasic V, Jovic N, Milic N, Todorovic S. The recurrence risk of ischemic stroke in childhood. Med Princ Pract 2004; 13(3):153–158.
7. Bowen MD, Burak CR, Barron TF. Childhood ischemic stroke in a nonurban population. J Child Neurol 2005; 20(3):194–197.
8. Aydinli N, Tatli B, Caliskan M, Ozmen M, Citak A, Unuvar A et al. Stroke in childhood: experience in Istanbul, Turkey. J Trop Pediatr 2006; 52(3):158–162.
9. Auvichayapat N, Tassniyom S, Hantragool S, Auvichayapat P. The etiology and outcome of cerebrovascular diseases in Northeastern Thai children. J Med Assoc Thai 2007; 90(10):2058–2062.
10. Lee YY, Lin KL, Wang HS, Chou ML, Hung PC, Hsieh MY et al. Risk factors and outcomes of childhood ischemic stroke in Taiwan. Brain Dev 2008; 30(1):14–19.
11. Wang JJ, Shi KL, Li JW, Jiang LQ, Caspi O, Fang F et al. Risk factors for arterial ischemic and hemorrhagic stroke in childhood. Pediatr Neurol 2009; 40(4):277–281.
12. Del BF, Spalice A, Ruggieri M, Greco F, Properzi E, Iannetti P. Stroke in children: inherited and acquired factors and age-related variations in the presentation of 48 paediatric patients. Acta Paediatr 2009; 98:1130–1136.
13. Rasul CH, Mahboob AA, Hossain SM, Ahmed KU. Predisposing factors and outcome of stroke in childhood. Indian Pediatr 2009; 46(5):419–421.
14. Giroud M, Lemesle M, Gouyon JB, Nivelon JL, Milan C, Dumas R. Cerebrovascular disease in children under 16 years of age in the city of Dijon, France: a study of incidence and clinical features from 1985 to 1993. J Clin Epidemiol 1995; 48(11):1343–1348.
15. Strater R, Vielhaber H, Kassenbohmer R, von Kreis R, Gobel U, Nowak-Gottl U. Genetic risk factors of thrombophilia in ischaemic childhood stroke of cardiac origin. A prospective ESPED survey. Eur J Pediatr 1999; 158 Suppl 3:S122–S125.
16. Williams AN, Davies P, Eunson PD, Kirkham FJ, Green SH. Stroke and cerebrovascular disease: Brimingham Children's Hospital 1993–1998. Dev Med Child Neurol 2002; 45:10.
17. Williams AN, Kirkham FJ. Childhood stroke, stroke-like illness and cerebrovascular disease. Stroke 2004; 35:311.
18. Chung B, Wong V. Pediatric stroke among Hong Kong Chinese subjects. Pediatrics 2004; 114(2):e206–e212.
19. Salih MA, Abdel-Gader AG, Al-Jarallah AA, Kentab AY, Alorainy IA, Hassan HH et al. Stroke in Saudi children. Epidemiology, clinical features and risk factors. Saudi Med J 2006; 27(Suppl 1):S12–S20.
20. Fox C, Johnston SC, Sidney S, Fullerton H. Congenital heart disease increases childhood stroke risk six-fold: results of a population-based case-control study. Stroke (International Stroke Conference 2010 Oral Presentations) 2010; 41(4):e17–e18.
21. Domi T, deVeber G, Shroff M, Kouzmitcheva E, MacGregor DL, Kirton A. Corticospinal tract pre-wallerian degeneration: a novel outcome predictor for pediatric stroke on acute MRI. Stroke 2009; 40(3):780–787.
22. McQuillen PS, Barkovich AJ, Hamrick SE, Perez M, Ward P, Glidden DV et al. Temporal and anatomic risk profile of brain injury with neonatal repair of congenital heart defects. Stroke 2007; 38(2 Suppl):736–741.
23. Miller SP, McQuillen PS, Hamrick S, Xu D, Glidden DV, Charlton N et al. Abnormal brain development in newborns with congenital heart disease. N Engl J Med 2007; 357(19):1928–1938.
24. Berman JI, Hamrick SE, McQuillen PS, Studholme C, Xu D, Henry RG et al. Diffusion-weighted imaging in fetuses with severe congenital heart defects. AJNR Am J Neuroradiol 2010; Feb 11 (epub ahead of print).
25. McQuillen PS, Miller SP. Congenital heart disease and brain development. Ann N Y Acad Sci 2010; 1184:68–86.
26. Phornphutkul C, Rosenthal A, Nadas AS, Berenberg W. Cerebrovascular accidents in infants and children with cyanotic congenital heart disease. Am J Cardiol 1973; 32(3):329–334.
27. Cottrill CM, Kaplan S. Cerebral vascular accidents in cyanotic congenital heart disease. Am J Dis Child 1973; 125(4):484–487.
28. Tyler HR, Clark DB. Cerebrovascular accidents in patients with congenital heart disease. Trans Am Neurol Assoc 1956;(81st Meeting):26–30.
29. McConnell JR, Fleming WH, Chu WK, Hahn FJ, Sarafian LB, Hofschire PJ et al. Magnetic resonance imaging of the brain in infants and children before and after cardiac surgery. A prospective study. Am J Dis Child 1990; 144(3):374–378.
30. Fallon P, Aparicio JM, Elliott MJ, Kirkham FJ. Incidence of neurological complications of surgery for congenital heart disease. Arch Dis Child 1995; 72(5):418–422.
31. du Plessis AJ, Chang AC, Wessel DL, Lock JE, Wernovsky G, Newburger JW et al. Cerebrovascular accidents following the Fontan operation. Pediatr Neurol 1995; 12(3):230–236.
32. Ferry PC. Neurologic sequelae of cardiac surgery in children. Am J Dis Child 1987; 141(3):309–312.
33. Day RW, Boyer RS, Tait VF, Ruttenberg HD. Factors associated with stroke following the Fontan procedure. Pediatr Cardiol 1995; 16(6):270–275.
34. Graser F. Non-inflammatory venous thrombosis, especially of the cerebral sinuses, as a complication of congenital heart disease. Z Kinderheilkd 1951; 70(2):142–147.
35. Wilson WR, Greer GE, Tobias JD. Cerebral venous thrombosis after the Fontan procedure. J Thorac Cardiovasc Surg 1998; 116(4):661–663.
36. Chun DS, Schamberger MS, Flaspohler T, Turrentine MW, Brown JW, Farrell AG et al. Incidence, outcome, and risk factors for stroke after the Fontan procedure. Am J Cardiol 2004; 93(1):117–119.
37. Mahnke CB, Boyle GJ, Janosky JE, Siewers RD, Pigula FA. Anticoagulation and incidence of late cerebrovascular accidents following the Fontan procedure. Pediatr Cardiol 2005; 26(1):56–61.
38. Barker PC, Nowak C, King K, Mosca RS, Bove EL, Goldberg CS. Risk factors for cerebrovascular events following fontan palliation in patients with a functional single ventricle. Am J Cardiol 2005; 96(4):587–591.
39. McQuillen PS, Hamrick SE, Perez MJ, Barkovich AJ, Glidden DV, Karl TR et al. Balloon atrial septostomy is associated with pre-operative stroke in neonates with transposition of the great arteries. Circulation 2006; 113(2):280–285.
40. Buompadre MC, Arroyo HA. Accidental cerebral venous gas embolism in a young patient with congenital heart disease. J Child Neurol 2008; 23(1):121–123.
41. Liu AY, Zimmerman RA, Haselgrove JC, Bilaniuk LT, Hunter JV. Diffusion-weighted imaging in the evaluation of watershed hypoxic-ischemic brain injury in pediatric patients. Neuroradiology 2001; 43(11):918–926.
42. Bozoky B, Bara D, Kertesz E. Autopsy study of cerebral complications of congenital heart disease and cardiac surgery. J Neurol 1984; 231(3):153–161.

43. Terplan KL. Brain changes in newborns, infants and children with congenital heart disease in association with cardiac surgery. Additional observations. J Neurol 1976; 212(3):225–236.

44. Kinney HC, Panigrahy A, Newburger JW, Jonas RA, Sleeper LA. Hypoxic-ischemic brain injury in infants with congenital heart disease dying after cardiac surgery. Acta Neuropathol 2005; 110(6):563–578.

45. Mahle WT, Tavani F, Zimmerman RA, Nicolson SC, Galli KK, Gaynor JW et al. An MRI study of neurological injury before and after congenital heart surgery. Circulation 2002; 106(12 Suppl 1):I109–I114.

46. Galli KK, Zimmerman RA, Jarvik GP, Wernovsky G, Kuypers MK, Clancy RR et al. Periventricular leukomalacia is common after neonatal cardiac surgery. J Thorac Cardiovasc Surg 2004; 127(3):692–704.

47. Partridge SC, Vigneron DB, Charlton NN, Berman JI, Henry RG, Mukherjee P et al. Pyramidal tract maturation after brain injury in newborns with heart disease. Ann Neurol 2006; 59(4):640–651.

48. Licht DJ, Wang J, Silvestre DW, Nicolson SC, Montenegro LM, Wernovsky G et al. Preoperative cerebral blood flow is diminished in neonates with severe congenital heart defects. J Thorac Cardiovasc Surg 2004; 128(6):841–849.

49. Miller SP, McQuillen PS, Hamrick S, Xu D, Glidden DV, Charlton N et al. Abnormal brain development in newborns with congenital heart disease. N Engl J Med 2007; 357(19):1928–1938.

50. Licht DJ, Agner S, Montenegro LM, Nicolson SC, Silvestre DW, Tabbutt S et al. Pre-operative MRI abnormalities are common in full term infants with severe CHD and resemble legions in pre-term infants. Neuropediatrics 2006; 26(1):129.

51. Cardiogenic brain embolism. The second report of the Cerebral Embolism Task Force. Arch Neurol 1989; 46(7):727–743.

52. Hart RG. Cardiogenic embolism to the brain. Lancet 1992; 339(8793):589–594.

53. Braun KP, Rafay MF, Uiterwaal CS, Pontigon AM, deVeber G. Mode of onset predicts etiological diagnosis of arterial ischemic stroke in children. Stroke 2007; 38(2):298–302.

54. Murugan V, Kirkham F. Characteristics of children with underlying cardiac defects who developed arterial ischaemic stroke. Cerebrovasc Dis 2008; 25(Suppl 2):98.

55. Schievink WI, Mokri B. Familial aorto-cervicocephalic arterial dissections and congenitally bicuspid aortic valve. Stroke 1995; 26:1935–1940.

56. Ganesan V, Kirkham FJ. Carotid dissection causing stroke in a child with migraine. BMJ 1997; 314(7076):291–292.

57. Schievink WI, Mokri B, Piepgras DG, Gittenberger-de Groot AC. Intracranial aneurisms and cervicophalic arterial dissections associated with congenital heart disease. Neurosurgery 1996; 39:685–690.

58. Tomlinson FH, Piepgras DG, Nichols DA, Rufenacht DA, Kaste SC. Remote congenital cerebral arteriovenous fistulae associated with aortic coarctation. Case report. J Neurosurg 1992; 76(1):137–142.

59. Lutterman J, Scott M, Nass R, Geva T. Moyamoya syndrome associated with congenital heart disease. Pediatrics 1998; 101(1 Pt 1):57–60.

60. Tyler HR, Clark DB. Neurologic complications in patients with coarctation of aorta. Neurology 1958; 8(9):712–718.

61. Hudaoglu O, Kurul S, Cakmakci H, Men S, Yis U, Dirik E. Aorta coarctation presenting with intracranial aneurism rupture. J Paediatr Child Health 2006; 42(7–8):477–479.

62. Khan N, Schinzel A, Shuknecht B, Baumann F, Ostergaard JR, Yonekawa Y. Moyamoya angiopathy with dolichoectatic internal carotid arteries, patent ductus arteriosus and pupillary dysfunction: a new genetic syndrome? Eur J Neurol 2004; 51(2):72–77.

63. Pearson E, Lenn NJ, Cail WS. Moyamoya and other causes of stroke in patients with Down syndrome. Pediatr Neurol 1985; 1(3):174–179.

64. Ardinger RH, Jr, Goertz KK, Mattioli LF. Cerebrovascular stenoses with cerebral infarction in a child with Williams syndrome. Am J Med Genet 1994; 51(3):200–202.

65. Schuster JM, Roberts TS. Symptomatic moyamoya disease and aortic coarctation in a patient with Noonan's syndrome: strategies for management. Pediatr Neurosurg 1999; 30(4):206–210.

66. Ishiguro Y, Kubota T, Takenaka J, Maruyama K, Okumura A, Negoro T et al. Cardio-facio-cutaneous syndrome and moyamoya syndrome. Brain Dev 2002; 24(4):245–249.

67. Kamath BM, Spinner NB, Emerick KM, Chudley AE, Booth C, Piccoli DA et al. Vascular anomalies in Alagille syndrome: a significant cause of morbidity and mortality. Circulation 2004; 109(11):1354–1358.

68. Diluna ML, Amankulor NM, Johnson MH, Gunel M. Cerebrovascular disease associated with Aarskog–Scott syndrome. Neuroradiology 2007; 49(5):457–461.

69. Heyer GL, Dowling MM, Licht DJ, Tay SK, Morel K, Garzon MC et al. The cerebral vasculopathy of PHACES syndrome. Stroke 2008; 39(2):308–316.

70. Terplan KL. Patterns of brain damage in infants and children with congental heart disease. Association with catheterization and surgical procedures. Am J Dis Child 1973; 125(2):176–185.

71. Wu YW, Miller SP, Chin K, Collins AE, Lomeli SC, Chuang NA et al. Multiple risk factors in neonatal sinovenous thrombosis. Neurology 2002; 59(3):438–440.

72. Gurgey A, Ozyurek E, Gumruk F, Celiker A, Ozkutlu S, Ozer S et al. Thrombosis in children with cardiac pathology: frequency of factor V Leiden and prothrombin G20210A mutations. Pediatr Cardiol 2003; 24(3):244–248.

73. Smilari P, Romeo MG, Sciacca P, Scalzo G, Gallo C, Mattia C et al. Cerebral venous sinuses thrombosis in an infant with supramitral obstructive membrane associated with partial anomalous pulmonary venous return. Minerva Pediatr 2005; 57(2):111–116.

74. Sebire G, Tabarki B, Saunders DE, Leroy I, Liesner R, Saint-Martin C et al. Cerebral venous sinus thrombosis in children: risk factors, presentation, diagnosis and outcome. Brain 2005; 128(Pt 3):477–489.

75. Zapson DS, Riviello JJ, Jr, Bagwell S. Supraventricular tachycardia leading to stroke in childhood. J Child Neurol 1995; 10(3):239–241.

76. Casta A, Talabi A, Coulter DL, Sapire DW. Capsular stroke in congenital complete heart block. Eur J Pediatr 1982; 139(1):71–72.

77. Biller J, Love BB. Cardiac disorders and stroke in children and young adults. In: Stroke in Children and Young Adults (eds J Biller). Newton: Butterworth-Heinemann, 1994; 83–102.

78. Landers C, Baumann R, Cottrill CM. Embolic strokes in an 8-year-old girl. Neurology 2000; 55(1):146.

79. Nakashima M, Takashima S, Hashimoto K, Shiraishi M. Association of stroke and myocardial infarction in children. Neuropediatrics 1982; 13(1):47–49.

80. Chambers JB, de Belder MA, Moore D. Echocardiography in stroke and transient ischaemic attack. Heart 1997; 78(Suppl 1):2–6.

81. Al-Mateen M, Hood M, Trippel D, Insalaco SJ, Otto RK, Vitikainen KJ. Cerebral embolism from atrial myxoma in pediatric patients. Pediatrics 2003; 112(2):e162–e167.

82. Mariano A, Pita A, Leon R, Rossi R, Gouveia R, Teixeira A et al. Primary cardiac tumors in children: a 16-year experience. Rev Port Cardiol 2009; 28(3):279–288.

83. Grotta J. Cerebrovascular disease in young patients. Thromb Haemost 1997; 78(1):13–23.

84. Rice GP, Ebers GC, Bondar RL, Boughner DR. Mitral valve prolapse: a cause of stroke in children? Dev Med Child Neurol 1981; 23(3):352–356.

85. Gruber A, Nasel C, Lang W, Kitzmuller E, Bavinzski G, Czech T. Intra-arterial thrombolysis for the treatment of perioperative childhood cardioembolic stroke. Neurology 2000; 54(8):1684–1686.

86. Germanakis I, Sfyridaki C, Papadopoulou E, Raissaki M, Rammos S, Sarris G et al. Stroke following Glenn anastomosis in a child with inherited thrombophilia. Int J Cardiol 2006; 111(3):464–467.

87. Homma S, Sacco RL, Di Tullio MR, Sciacca RR, Mohr JP. Effect of medical treatment in stroke patients with patent foramen ovale: patent foramen ovale in Cryptogenic Stroke Study. Circulation 2002; 105(22):2625–2631.

88. Worley G, Shbarou R, Heffner AN, Belsito KM, Capone GT, Kishnani PS. New onset focal weakness in children with Down syndrome. Am J Med Genet A 2004; 128A(1):15–18.

89. Ishida S, Date M, Doi Y, Sato T, Sugino M, Kimura F et al. Recurrent cerebral embolism in a young adult with Down's syndrome. A case report. J Neurol 2004; 251(10):1275–1277.

90. Caner I, Olgun H, Buyukavci M, Tastekin A, Ors R. A giant thrombus in the right ventricle of a newborn with Down syndrome: successful treatment with rt-PA. J Pediatr Hematol Oncol 2006; 28(3):120–122.

91. Baram TZ, Fishman MA. 'Top of the basilar' artery stroke in an adolescent with Down's syndrome. Arch Neurol 1985; 42(3):296.

92. Junqueira PA, Moura-Ribeiro MV. Moyamoya and Down syndrome: study conducted by meta-analysis. Arq Neuropsiquiatr 2002; 60(2-A):274–280.

93. Diab KA, Richani R, Al KA, Mikati M, Dbaibo GS, Bitar FF. Cerebral mycotic aneurysm in a child with Down's syndrome: a unique association. J Child Neurol 2001; 16(11):868–870.

94. Ozawa H, Toba M, Nakamoto N, Noma S, Ichiyama T, Takahashi H. Increased cytokine levels in a cerebral mycotic aneurysm in a child with Down's syndrome. Brain Dev 2005; 27(6):434–436.

95. Tarlaci S, Sagduyu A. Cerebral venous thrombosis in Down's syndrome. Clin Neurol Neurosurg 2001; 103(4):242–244.

96. del-Rio CG, Orozco AL, Perez-Higueras A, Camino LM, Al-Assir I, Ruiz-Moreno M. Moyamoya disease and sagittal sinus thrombosis in a child with Down's syndrome. Pediatr Radiol 2001; 31(2):125–128.

97. Williams M, Nand S. Superior sagittal sinus thrombosis in a child with Down syndrome. J Paediatr Child Health 2003; 39(3):226–228.

98. Antunes NL, Small TN, George D, Boulad F, Lis E. Posterior leukoencephalopathy syndrome may not be reversible. Pediatr Neurol 1999; 20(3):241–243.

99. Kim BS, Lee SH, Lee JE, Chung SW, Kim YO, Choi KB et al. Posterior leukoencephalopathy syndrome during steroid therapy in a Down syndrome patient with nephrotic syndrome. Nephron 2001; 87(3):289–290.

100. Takeda K, Takahashi S, Higano S, Kurihara N, Haginoya K, Shirane R et al. Cortical laminar necrosis in a patient with moyamoya disease associated with Down syndrome: MR imaging findings. Radiat Med 1997; 15(1):59–63.

101. Schultze G, Piefke S, Molzahn M. Blood pressure in terminal renal failure. Fluid spaces and the renin-angiotensin-system. Nephron 1980; 25(1):15–24.

102. Nishimura M, Takakura H, Ieshima A, Eda I, Ohno K, Takashima S. A case of Down syndrome with moyamoya disease. No To Hattatsu 1985; 17(1):71–75.

103. Fukushima Y, Kondo Y, Kuroki Y, Miyake S, Iwamoto H, Sekido K et al. Are Down syndrome patients predisposed to Moyamoya disease? Eur J Pediatr 1986; 144(5):516–517.

104. Storm W, Uhlenbrock D. Magnetic resonance imaging of moyamoya disease in a child with Down's syndrome. J Ment Defic Res 1989; 33(Pt 6):507–510.

105. Outwater EK, Platenberg RC, Wolpert SM. Moyamoya disease in Down syndrome. AJNR Am J Neuroradiol 1989; 10(5 Suppl):S23–S24.

106. Goldstein EM, Singer HS. Moyamoya-like disease in Down's syndrome. Pediatr Neurosurg 1990; 16(1):14–16.

107. Berg JM, Armstrong D. On the association of moyamoya disease with Down's syndrome. J Ment Defic Res 1991; 35(Pt 4):398–403.

108. Vicari S, Albertini G. Moyamoya disease in Down's syndrome: a report of two cases. J Ment Defic Res 1991; 35(Pt 4):392–397.

109. Fukuyama Y, Osawa M, Kanai N. Moyamoya disease (syndrome) and the Down syndrome. Brain Dev 1992; 14(4):254–256.

110. Arevalo CE, Marchezzotti A, Haessler A, Lanosa R. Moyamoya disease and Down syndrome. Medicina (B Aires) 1993; 53(5):473.

111. Gadoth N. On the problem of essential and secondary moyamoya and vascular dysplasia in Down syndrome. Brain Dev 1993; 15(4):317–318.

112. Cramer SC, Robertson RL, Dooling EC, Scott RM. Moyamoya and Down syndrome. Clinical and radiological features. Stroke 1996; 27(11):2131–2135.

113. Park M, Raila FA, Russell WF. Moyamoya disease in an adult with Down syndrome: comparison of magnetic resonance angiography and conventional angiography. South Med J 1996; 89(1):89–92.

114. Soto-Ares G, Hamon-Kerautret M, Leclerc X, Vallee L, Pruvo JP. Moyamoya associated with Down syndrome. J Radiol 1996; 77(6):441–444.

115. Dai AI, Shaikh ZA, Cohen ME. Early-onset Moyamoya syndrome in a patient with Down syndrome: case report and review of the literature. J Child Neurol 2000; 15(10):696–699.

116. De Borchgrave V, Saussu F, Depre A, de Barsy T. Moyamoya disease and Down syndrome: case report and review of the literature. Acta Neurol Belg 2002; 102(2):63–66.

117. Fung CW, Kwong KL, Tsui EY, Wong SN. Moyamoya syndrome in a child with Down syndrome. Hong Kong Med J 2003; 9(1):63–66.

118. Vila-Herrero E, Padilla-Parrado F, Vega-Perez J, Garcia-Casares N, Heras-Perez JA, Romero-Acebal M. Moya-moya syndrome and arterial dysplasia associated to Down syndrome. Rev Neurol 2004; 39(10):943–945.

119. Jea A, Smith ER, Robertson R, Scott RM. Moyamoya syndrome associated with Down syndrome: outcome after surgical revascularization. Pediatrics 2005; 116(5):e694–e701.

120. Erguven M, Deveci M, Turgut T. Moyamoya disease and Down syndrome. Indian J Pediatr 2005; 72(8):697–699.

121. Bhalala US, Parekh PR. Moyamoya syndrome in a child with Down syndrome. Indian J Pediatr 2005; 72(7):635–637.

122. Gururaj A, Hardy D, Al-Gazali LI, Sztriha L, Roos A, Nork M. Are the strokes in moyamoya syndrome associated with Down syndrome due to protein C deficiency? Brain Dev 2002; 24(7):719–722.

123. Whitney A, Morgan M, Gawne-Cain M, Kirkham FJ. Stroke in a child with Down syndome and haemolytic anaemia; a pathophysiological explanation? Dev Med Child Neurol 2006; 48(Suppl 107):33.

124. Boggs S, Hariharan SL. An uncommon presentation of stroke in a child with trisomy 21. Pediatr Emerg Care 2008; 24(4):230–232.

125. Cornelio-Nieto JO, vila-Gutierrez G, Ferreyro-Irigoyen R, Alcala H. Acute hemiplegia in childhood and alternating hemiconvulsions secondary to Moya-Moya disease. Report of a case associated with Down's syndrome. Bol Med Hosp Infant Mex 1990; 47(1):39–42.

126. Schrager GO, Cohen SJ, Vigman MP. Acute hemiplegia and cortical blindness due to moya moya disease: report of a case in a child with Down's syndrome. Pediatrics 1977; 60(1):33–37.

127. Takanashi J, Sugita K, Honda A, Niimi H. Moyamoya syndrome in a patient with Down syndrome presenting with chorea. Pediatr Neurol 1993; 9(5):396–398.

128. Aylett SE, Britton JA, De Sousa CM. Down syndrome and moyamoya disease: presentation with subarachnoid hemorrhage. Pediatr Neurol 1996; 14(3):259–261.

129. Pysden K, Fallon P, Moorthy B, Ganesan V. Presumed perinatal stroke in a child with Down syndrome and moyamoya disease. Dev Med Child Neurol 2010; 52(2):212–214.

130. Gaggero R, Donati PT, Curia R, De NM. Occlusion of unilateral carotid artery in Down syndrome. Brain Dev 1996; 18(1):81–83.

131. Nagasaka T, Shiozawa Z, Kobayashi M, Shindo K, Tsunoda S, Amino A. Autopsy findings in Down's syndrome with cerebrovascular disorder. Clin Neuropathol 1996; 15(3):145–149.

132. Mito T, Becker LE. Vascular dysplasia in Down syndrome: a possible relationship to moyamoya disease. Brain Dev 1992; 14(4):248–251.

133. Cappelli-Bigazzi M, Santoro G, Battaglia C, Palladino MT, Carrozza M, Russo MG et al. Endothelial cell function in patients with Down's syndrome. Am J Cardiol 2004; 94(3):392–395.

134. Loughlin GM, Wynne JW, Victorica BE. Sleep apnea as a possible cause of pulmonary hypertension in Down syndrome. J Pediatr 1981; 98(3):435–437.

135. Takasugi H, Maemoto T, Kitazawa K, Honda A. A case of Down syndrome with moyamoya syndrome presenting extensive multiple cerebral infarction during measles infection. No To Hattatsu 2000; 32(1):39–43.

136. Morino M, Yamano H, Sasaki N. Role of varicella virus and anti-cardiolipin antibodies in the development of stroke in a patient with Down syndrome associated with Moyamoya syndrome. Pediatr Int 2009; 51(2):300–302.

137. Franciotta D, Verri A, Zardini E, Andreoni L, De Amici M, Moratti R et al. Interferon-gamma- and interleukin-4-producing T cells in Down's syndrome. Neurosci Lett 2006; 395(1):67–70.

138. Leno C, Mateo I, Cid C, Berciano J, Sedano C. Autoimmunity in Down's syndrome: another possible mechanism of Moyamoya disease. Stroke 1998; 29(4):868–869.

139. Nishida Y, Akaoka I, Nishizawa T, Maruki M, Maruki K. Hyper-lipidaemia in patients with Down's syndrome. Atherosclerosis 1977; 26(3):369–372.

140. Gatenby P, Tucko R, Andrews C, O'Neil R. Antiphospholipid antibodies and stroke in Down syndrome. Lupus 2003; 12(1):58–62.

141. Thiel R, Fowkes SW. Can cognitive deterioration associated with Down syndrome be reduced? Med Hypotheses 2005; 64(3):524–532.

142. Dodd KJ, Shields N. A systematic review of the outcomes of cardiovascular exercise programs for people with Down syndrome. Arch Phys Med Rehabil 2005; 86(10):2051–2058.

143. Pastore A, Tozzi G, Gaeta LM, Giannotti A, Bertini E, Federici G et al. Glutathione metabolism and antioxidant enzymes in children with Down syndrome. J Pediatr 2003; 142(5):583–585.

144. Garcez ME, Peres W, Salvador M. Oxidative stress and hematologic and biochemical parameters in individuals with Down syndrome. Mayo Clin Proc 2005; 80(12):1607–1611.

145. Yao YG, Duh EJ. VEGF selectively induces Down syndrome critical region 1 gene expression in endothelial cells: a mechanism for feedback regulation of angiogenesis? Biochem Biophys Res Commun 2004; 321(3):648–656.

146. Hopkins WE, Fukagawa NK, Sobel BE, Schneider DJ. Plasminogen activator inhibitor type 1 in adults with Down syndrome and protection against macrovascular disease. Am J Cardiol 2000; 85(6):784–786.

147. Carlsson A, Axelsson I, Borulf S, Bredberg A, Forslund M, Lindberg B et al. Prevalence of IgA-antigliadin antibodies and IgA-antiendomysium antibodies related to celiac disease in children with Down syndrome. Pediatrics 1998; 101(2):272–275.

148. Agardh D, Nilsson A, Carlsson A, Kockum I, Lernmark A, Ivarsson SA. Tissue transglutaminase autoantibodies and human leucocyte antigen in Down's syndrome patients with coeliac disease. Acta Paediatr 2002; 91(1):34–38.

149. Lappalainen J, Kouvalainen K. High hematocrits in newborns with Down's syndrome: a hitherto undescribed finding. Clin Pediatr (Phila) 1972; 11(8):472–474.

150. Melnyk AR, Adams BW, Suarez CR. Down syndrome complicated by hemoglobin S/beta+ thalassemia. Atypical expression of coexistent disease. Clin Pediatr (Phila) 1990; 29(6):331–335.

151. Lott IT, Head E. Alzheimer disease and Down syndrome: factors in pathogenesis. Neurobiol Aging 2005; 26(3):383–389.

152. Williams JC, Barratt-Boyes BG, Lowe JB. Supravalvular aortic stenosis. Circulation 1961; 24:1311–1318.

153. Beuren AJ, Apitz J, Harmjanz D. Supravalvular aortic stenosis in association with mental retardation and a certain facial appearance. Circulation 1962; 26:1235–1240.

154. Lowery MC, Morris CA, Ewart A, Brothman LJ, Zhu XL, Leonard CO et al. Strong correlation of elastin deletions, detected by FISH, with Williams syndrome: evaluation of 235 patients. Am J Hum Genet 1995; 57(1):49–53.

155. Nickerson E, Greenberg F, Keating MT, McCaskill C, Shaffer LG. Deletions of the elastin gene at 7q11.23 occur in approximately 90% of patients with Williams syndrome. Am J Hum Genet 1995; 56(5):1156–1161.

156. Aggoun Y, Sidi D, Levy BI, Lyonnet S, Kachaner J, Bonnet D. Mechanical properties of the common carotid artery in Williams syndrome. Heart 2000; 84(3):290–293.

157. Lacolly P, Boutoyrie P, Glukhova M, Daniel Lamaziere JM, Plouin PF, Bruneval P et al. Disruption of the elastin gene in adult Williams syndrome is accompanied by a paradoxical reduction in arterial stiffness. Clin Sci (Lond) 2002; 103(1):21–29.

158. Amenta F, Barili P, Bronzetti E, Felici L, Mignini F, Ricci A. Localization of dopamine receptor subtypes in systemic arteries. Clin Exp Hypertens 2000; 22(3):277–288.

159. Giannotti A, Tiberio G, Castro M, Virgilii F, Colistro F, Ferretti F et al. Coeliac disease in Williams syndrome. J Med Genet 2001; 38(11):767–768.

160. Kaplan P, Levinson M, Kaplan BS. Cerebral artery stenoses in Williams syndrome cause strokes in childhood. J Pediatr 1995; 126(6):943–945.

161. Putman CM, Chaloupka JC, Eklund JE, Fulbright RK. Multifocal intracranial occlusive vasculopathy resulting in stroke: an unusual manifestation of Williams syndrome. AJNR Am J Neuroradiol 1995; 16(7):1536–1538.

162. Wollack JB, Kaifer M, LaMonte MP, Rothman M. Stroke in Williams syndrome. Stroke 1996; 27(1):143–146.

163. Kawai M, Nishikawa T, Tanaka M, Ando A, Kasajima T, Higa T et al. An autopsied case of Williams syndrome complicated by moyamoya disease. Acta Paediatr Jpn 1993; 35(1):63–67.

164. Kalbhenn T, Neumann LM, Lanksch WR, Haberl H. Spontaneous intracerebral hemorrhage and multiple infarction in Williams–Beuren syndrome. Pediatr Neurosurg 2003; 39(6):335–338.

165. Soper R, Chaloupka JC, Fayad PB, Greally JM, Shaywitz BA, Awad IA et al. Ischemic stroke and intracranial multifocal cerebral arteriopathy in Williams syndrome. J Pediatr 1995; 126(6):945–948.

166. Blanc F, Wolff V, Talmant V, Attali P, Germain P, Flori E et al. Late onset stroke and myocardial infarction in Williams syndrome. Eur J Neurol 2006; 13(12):e3–e4.

167. Bird LM, Billman GF, Lacro RV, Spicer RL, Jariwala LK, Hoyme HE et al. Sudden death in Williams syndrome: report of ten cases. J Pediatr 1996; 129(6):926–931.

168. Fuentes K, Silveira DC, Papamitsakis NI. Spontaneous carotid artery dissection in a patient with Turner syndrome. Cerebrovasc Dis 2007; 24(6):543–544.

169. Hara T, Sasaki T, Miyauchi H, Takakura K. Noonan phenotype associated with intracerebral hemorrhage and cerebral vascular anomalies: case report. Surg Neurol 1993; 39(1):31–36.

170. Hinnant CA. Thromboembolic infarcts occurring after mild traumatic brain injury in a paediatric patient with Noonan's syndrome. Brain Inj 1994; 8(8):719–727.

171. Ganesan V, Kirkham FJ. Noonan syndrome and moyamoya. Pediatr Neurol. 1997;16(3):256–8.

172. Robertson S, Tsang B, Aftimos S. Cerebral infarction in Noonan syndrome. Am J Med Genet 1997; 71(1):111–114.

173. Wilms H, Neubauer B, Deuschl G, Zunker P. Cerebral occlusive artery disease in Noonan syndrome. Cerebrovasc Dis 2002; 14(2):133–135.

174. Piccoli DA, Spinner NB. Alagille syndrome and the Jagged1 gene. Semin Liver Dis 2001; 21(4):525–534.

175. Quiros-Tejeira RE, Ament ME, Heyman MB, Martin MG, Rosenthal P, Hall TR et al. Variable morbidity in Alagille syndrome: a review of 43 cases. J Pediatr Gastroenterol Nutr 1999; 29(4):431–437.

176. Emerick KM, Krantz ID, Kamath BM, Darling C, Burrowes DM, Spinner NB et al. Intracranial vascular abnormalities in patients with Alagille syndrome. J Pediatr Gastroenterol Nutr 2005; 41(1):99–107.

177. Berard E, Triolo V. Intracranial hemorrhages in Alagille syndrome. J Pediatr 2000; 136(5):708–710.

178. Emerick KM, Rand EB, Goldmuntz E, Krantz ID, Spinner NB, Piccoli DA. Features of Alagille syndrome in 92 patients: frequency and relation to prognosis. Hepatology 1999; 29(3):822–829.

179. Rachmel A, Zeharia A, Neuman-Levin M, Weitz R, Shamir R, Dinari G. Alagille syndrome associated with moyamoya disease. Am J Med Genet 1989; 33(1):89–91.

180. Woolfenden AR, Albers GW, Steinberg GK, Hahn JS, Johnston DC, Farrell K. Moyamoya syndrome in children with Alagille syndrome: additional evidence of a vasculopathy. Pediatrics 1999; 103(2):505–508.

181. Connor SE, Hewes D, Ball C, Jarosz JM. Alagille syndrome associated with angiographic moyamoya. Childs Nerv Syst 2002; 18(3–4):186–190.

182. Moreau S, Bourdon N, Jokic M, de Rugy MG, Babin E, Valdazo A et al. Alagille syndrome with cavernous carotid artery aneurysm. Int J Pediatr Otorhinolaryngol 1999; 50(2):139–143.

183. Schievink WI, Mokri B. Aortic dissection decades following internal carotid artery dissection – report of two cases. Angiology 1997; 48:985–988.

184. van den Berg JS, Limburg M, Hennekam RC. Is Marfan syndrome associated with symptomatic intracranial aneurysms? Stroke 1996; 27(1):10–12.

185. Wityk RJ, Zanferrari C, Oppenheimer S. Neurovascular complications of Marfan syndrome: a retrospective, hospital-based study. Stroke 2002; 33(3):680–684.

186. Boutouyrie P, Germain DP, Fiessinger JN, Laloux B, Perdu J, Laurent S. Increased carotid wall stress in vascular Ehlers–Danlos syndrome. Circulation 2004; 109(12):1530–1535.

187. Byard RW, Cutz E. Sudden and unexpected death in infancy and childhood due to pulmonary thromboembolism. An autopsy study. Arch Pathol Lab Med 1990; 114(2):142–144.

188. Kato N, Hirano T, Kawaguchi T, Ishida M, Shimono T, Yada I et al. Aneurysmal degeneration of the aorta after stent-graft repair of acute aortic dissection. J Vasc Surg 2001; 34(3):513–518.

189. Loeys BL, Schwarze U, Holm T, Callewaert BL, Thomas GH, Pannu H et al. Aneurysm syndromes caused by mutations in the TGF-beta receptor. N Engl J Med 2006; 355(8):788–798.

190. Holzschuh M, Woertgen C, Brawanski A. Transcranial Doppler sonography in a patient with Ehlers–Danlos syndrome: case report. Neurosurgery 1996; 39(1):170–172.

191. Miossec-Chauvet E, Mikaeloff Y, Heron D, Merzoug V, Cormier-Daire V, de LP et al. Neurological presentation in pediatric patients with congenital disorders of glycosylation type Ia. Neuropediatrics 2003; 34(1):1–6.

192. Ishikawa N, Tajima G, Ono H, Kobayashi M. Different neuro-radiological findings during two stroke-like episodes in a patient with a congenital disorder of glycosylation type Ia. Brain Dev 2009; 31(3):240–243.

193. Arnoux JB, Boddaert N, Valayannopoulos V, Romano S, Bahi-Buisson N, Desguerre I et al. Risk assessment of acute vascular events in congenital disorder of glycosylation type Ia. Mol Genet Metab 2008; 93(4):444–449.

194. Kjaergaard S, Schwartz M, Skovby F. Congenital disorder of glycosylation type Ia (CDG-Ia): phenotypic spectrum of the R141H/F119L genotype. Arch Dis Child 2001; 85(3):236–239.

195. Makin GJ, Coates RK, Pelz D, Drake CG, Barnett HJ. Major cerebral arterial and venous disease in osteopetrosis. Stroke 1986; 17(1):106–110.

196. Tasdemir HA, Dagdemir A, Celenk C, Albayrak D. Middle cerebral arterial occlusion in a child with osteopetrosis major. Eur Radiol 2001; 11(1):145–147.

197. Schimke RN, Horton WA, King CR, Martin NL. Chondroitin-6-sulfate mucopolysaccharidosis in conjunction with lymphopenia, defective cellular immunity and the nephrotic syndrome. Birth Defects Orig Artic Ser 1974; 10(12):258–266.

198. Boerkoel CF, Takashima H, John J, Yan J, Stankiewicz P, Rosenbarker L et al. Mutant chromatin remodeling protein SMAR-CAL1 causes Schimke immuno-osseous dysplasia. Nat Genet 2002; 30(2):215–220.

199. Elizondo LI, Cho KS, Zhang W, Yan J, Huang C, Huang Y et al. Schimke immuno-osseous dysplasia: SMARCAL1 loss-of-function and phenotypic correlation. J Med Genet 2009; 46(1):49–59.

200. Boerkoel CF, O'Neill S, Andre JL, Benke PJ, Bogdanovic R, Bulla M et al. Manifestations and treatment of Schimke immuno-osseous dysplasia: 14 new cases and a review of the literature. Eur J Pediatr 2000; 159(1–2):1–7.

201. Deguchi K, Clewing JM, Elizondo LI, Hirano R, Huang C, Choi K et al. Neurologic phenotype of Schimke immuno-osseous dysplasia and neurodevelopmental expression of SMARCAL1. J Neuropathol Exp Neurol 2008; 67(6):565–577.

202. Breedveld G, de Coo, I, Lequin MH, Arts WF, Heutink P, Gould DB et al. Novel mutations in three families confirm a major role of COL4A1 in hereditary porencephaly. J Med Genet 2006; 43(6):490–495.

203. Gould DB, Phalan FC, van Mil SE, Sundberg JP, Vahedi K, Massin P et al. Role of COL4A1 in small-vessel disease and hemorrhagic stroke. N Engl J Med 2006; 354(14):1489–1496.

204. Volonghi I, Pezzini A, Del ZE, Giossi A, Costa P, Ferrari D et al. Role of COL4A1 in basement-membrane integrity and cerebral small-vessel disease. The COL4A1 Stroke Syndrome. Curr Med Chem 2010; 17(13):1317–1324.

205. Alamowitch S, Plaisier E, Favrole P, Prost C, Chen Z, Van AT et al. Cerebrovascular disease related to COL4A1 mutations in HANAC syndrome. Neurology 2009; 73(22):1873–1882.

206. Shah S, Kumar Y, McLean B, Churchill A, Stoodley N, Rankin J et al. A dominantly inherited mutation in collagen IV A1 (COL4A1) causing childhood onset stroke without porencephaly. Eur J Paediatr Neurol 2010; 14(2):182–187.

207. Desmond DW, Moroney JT, Lynch T, Chan S, Chin SS, Mohr JP. The natural history of CADASIL: a pooled analysis of previously published cases. Stroke 1999; 30(6):1230–1233.

208. Hartley J, Westmacott R, Decker J, Shroff M, Yoon G. Childhood-onset CADASIL: clinical, imaging, and neurocognitive features. J Child Neurol 2010; 25(5):623–627.

209. Gong M, Rueschendorf F, Marx P, Schulz H, Kraft HG, Huebner N et al. Clinical and genetic features in a family with CADASIL and high lipoprotein(a) values. J Neurol 2010; 257:1240–1245.

210. Granild-Jensen J, Jensen UB, Schwartz M, Hansen US. Cerebral auto-somal dominant arteriopathy with subcortical infarcts and leukoen-cephalopathy resulting in stroke in an 11-year-old male. Dev Med Child Neurol 2009; 51(9):754–757.

211. Golomb MR, Sokol DK, Walsh LE, Christensen CK, Garg BP. Recurrent hemiplegia, normal MRI, and NOTCH3 mutation in a 14-year-old: is this early CADASIL? Neurology 2004; 62(12):2331–2332.

212. Fattapposta F, Restuccia R, Pirro C, Malandrini A, Locuratolo N, Amabile G et al. Early diagnosis in cerebral autosomal dominant arteriopathy with subcortical infarcts and leukoencephalopathy (CADASIL): the role of MRI. Funct Neurol 2004; 19(4):239–242.

213. Grange DK, Balfour IC, Chen SC, Wood EG. Familial syndrome of progressive arterial occlusive disease consistent with fibromuscular dysplasia, hypertension, congenital cardiac defects, bone fragility, brachysyndactyly, and learning disabilities. Am J Med Genet 1998; 75(5):469–480.

214. Weymann S, Yonekawa Y, Khan N, Martin E, Heppner FL, Schinzel A et al. Severe arterial occlusive disorder and brachysyn-dactyly in a boy: a further case of Grange syndrome? Am J Med Genet 2001; 99(3):190–195.

215. Wallerstein R, Augustyn AM, Wallerstein D, Elton L, Tejeiro B, Johnson V et al. A new case of Grange syndrome without cardiac findings. Am J Med Genet A 2006; 140(12):1316–1320.

216. Guo DC, Papke CL, Tran-Fadulu V, Regalado ES, Avidan N, Johnson RJ et al. Mutations in smooth muscle alpha-actin (ACTA2) cause coronary artery disease, stroke, and Moyamoya disease, along with thoracic aortic disease. Am J Hum Genet 2009; 84(5):617–627.

217. Guo DC, Pannu H, Tran-Fadulu V, Papke CL, Yu RK, Avidan N et al. Mutations in smooth muscle alpha-actin (ACTA2) lead to thoracic aortic aneurysms and dissections. Nat Genet 2007; 39(12):1488–1493.

218. Morisaki H, Akutsu K, Ogino H, Kondo N, Yamanaka I, Tsutsumi Y et al. Mutation of ACTA2 gene as an important cause of familial and nonfamilial nonsyndromatic thoracic aortic aneurysm and/or dis-section (TAAD). Hum Mutat 2009; 30(10):1406–1411.

219. Shimojima K, Yamamoto T. ACTA2 is not a major disease-causing gene for moyamoya disease. J Hum Genet 2009; 54(11):687–688.

220. Goddard DS, Liang MG, Chamlin SL, Svoren BM, Spack NP, Mulliken JB. Hypopituitarism in PHACES association. Pediatr Dermatol 2006; 23(5):476–480.

221. Ghosh A, Tibrewal SR, Thapa R. PHACES syndrome with congenital hypothyroidism. Indian Pediatr 2007; 44(2):144–147.

222. Mussa A, Corrias A, Baldassarre G, Biamino E, Silengo M. Congenital hypothyroidism, cerebellar atrophy, and the incomplete phenotypic expression of PHACES syndrome. Endocr J 2008; 55(1):231.

223. Hsia TY, Kirkham F, Waldman A, Tsang V. The implications of extensive cerebral vascular dysplasia in surgical repair of coarcta-tion of the aorta and ventricular septal defect. J Thorac Cardiovasc Surg 2001; 121(5):998–1001.

224. Bronzetti G, Giardini A, Patrizi A, Prandstraller D, Donti A, Formigari R et al. Ipsilateral hemangioma and aortic arch anoma-lies in posterior fossa malformations, hemangiomas, arterial anoma-lies, coarctation of the aorta, and cardiac defects and eye abnormalities (PHACE) anomaly: report and review. Pediatrics 2004; 113(2):412–415.

225. Oza VS, Wang E, Berenstein A, Waner M, Lefton D, Wells J et al. PHACES association: a neuroradiologic review of 17 patients. AJNR Am J Neuroradiol 2008; 29(4):807–813.

226. Drolet BA, Dohil M, Golomb MR, Wells R, Murowski L, Tamburro J et al. Early stroke and cerebral vasculopathy in children with facial hemangiomas and PHACE association. Pediatrics 2006; 117(3):959–964.

227. Prieto ES, Santos-Juanes J, Medina VA, Concha TA, Rey GC, Sanchez Del RJ. Death from cerebrovascular infarction in a patient with PHACES syndrome. J Am Acad Dermatol 2004; 51(1):142–143.

228. Bhattacharya JJ, Luo CB, Alvarez H, Rodesch G, Pongpech S, Lasjaunias P. PHACES syndrome: a review of eight previously unreported cases with late arterial occlusions. Neuroradiology 2004; 46(3):227–233.

229. Creange A, Zeller J, Rostaing-Rigattieri S, Brugieres P, Degos JD, Revuz J et al. Neurological complications of neurofibromatosis type 1 in adulthood. Brain 1999; 122(Pt 3):473–481.

230. Okuno T, Prensky AL, Gado M. The moyamoya syndrome associated with irradiation of an optic glioma in children: report of two cases and review of the literature. Pediatr Neurol 1985; 1(5):311–316.

231. Rosser TL, Vezina G, Packer RJ. Cerebrovascular abnormalities in a population of children with neurofibromatosis type 1. Neurology 2005; 64(3):553–555.

232. Hornstein L, Borchers D. Stroke in an infant prior to the development of manifestations of neurofibromatosis. Neurofibromatosis 1989; 2(2):116–120.

233. Woody RC, Perrot LJ, Beck SA. Neurofibromatosis cerebral vasculopathy in an infant: clinical, neuroradiographic, and neuropathologic studies. Pediatr Pathol 1992; 12(4):613–619.

234. Rea D, Brandsema JF, Armstrong D, Parkin PC, deVeber G, MacGregor D et al. Cerebral arteriopathy in children with neurofibromatosis type 1. Pediatrics 2009; 124:e476–e483.

235. Tomsick TA, Lukin RR, Chambers AA, Benton C. Neurofibromatosis and intracranial arterial occlusive disease. Neuroradiology 1976; 11(5):229–234.

236. Gebarski SS, Gabrielsen TO, Knake JE, Latack JT. Posterior circulation intracranial arterial occlusive disease in neurofibromatosis. AJNR Am J Neuroradiol 1983; 4(6):1245–1246.

237. Capell BC, Erdos MR, Madigan JP, Fiordalisi JJ, Varga R, Conneely KN et al. Inhibiting farnesylation of progerin prevents the characteristic nuclear blebbing of Hutchinson–Gilford progeria syndrome. Proc Natl Acad Sci USA 2005; 102(36):12879–12884.

238. Horikawa M, Utunomiya H, Hirotaka S, Yamada S, Ohtaki E, Matsuishi T. Case of von Recklinghausen disease associated with cerebral infarction. J Child Neurol 1997; 12(2):144–146.

239. Kwong KL, Wong YC. Moyamoya disease in a child with neurofibromatosis type-1. J Paediatr Child Health 1999; 35(1):108–109.

240. Kestle JR, Hoffman HJ, Mock AR. Moyamoya phenomenon after radiation for optic glioma. J Neurosurg 1993; 79(1):32–35.

241. Scott RM, Smith JL, Robertson RL, Madsen JR, Soriano SG, Rockoff MA. Long-term outcome in children with moyamoya syndrome after cranial revascularization by pial synangiosis. J Neurosurg 2004; 100(2 Suppl Pediatrics):142–149.

242. Zhao JZ, Han XD. Cerebral aneurysm associated with von Recklinghausen's neurofibromatosis: a case report. Surg Neurol 1998; 50(6):592–596.

243. Miyazaki T, Ohta F, Daisu M, Hoshii Y. Extracranial vertebral artery aneurysm ruptured into the thoracic cavity with neurofibromatosis type 1: case report. Neurosurgery 2004; 54(6):1517–1520.

244. Schievink WI, Piepgras DG. Cervical vertebral artery aneurysms and arteriovenous fistulae in neurofibromatosis type 1: case reports. Neurosurgery 1991; 29(5):760–765.

245. Conway JE, Hutchins GM, Tamargo RJ. Lack of evidence for an association between neurofibromatosis type I and intracranial aneurysms: autopsy study and review of the literature. Stroke 2001; 32(11):2481–2485.

246. Schievink WI, Riedinger M, Maya MM. Frequency of incidental intracranial aneurysms in neurofibromatosis type 1. Am J Med Genet A 2005; 134A(1):45–48.

247. Siqueira Neto JI, Silva GS, De Castro JD, Santos AC. Neurofibromatosis associated with moyamoya arteriopathy and fusiform aneurysm: case report. Arq Neuropsiquiatr 1998; 56(4):819–823.

248. Muhonen MG, Godersky JC, VanGilder JC. Cerebral aneurysms associated with neurofibromatosis. Surg Neurol 1991; 36(6):470–475.

249. Sasaki J, Miura S, Ohishi H, Kikuchi K. Neurofibromatosis associated with multiple intracranial vascular lesions: stenosis of the internal carotid artery and peripheral aneurysm of the Heubner's artery; report of a case. No Shinkei Geka 1995; 23(9):813–817.

250. Sobata E, Ohkuma H, Suzuki S. Cerebrovascular disorders associated with von Recklinghausen's neurofibromatosis: a case report. Neurosurgery 1988; 22(3):544–549.

251. Hattori S, Kiguchi H, Ishii T, Nakajima T, Yatsuzuka H. Moyamoya disease with concurrent von Recklinghausen's disease and cerebral arteriovenous malformation. Pathol Res Pract 1998; 194(5):363–369.

252. Piovesan EJ, Scola RH, Werneck LC, Zetola VH, Novak EM, Iwamoto FM et al. Neurofibromatosis, stroke and basilar impression. Case report. Arq Neuropsiquiatr 1999; 57(2B):484–488.

253. Pellock JM, Kleinman PK, McDonald BM, Wixson D. Childhood hypertensive stroke with neurofibromatosis. Neurology 1980; 30(6):656–659.

254. Virdis R, Balestrazzi P, Zampolli M, Donadio A, Street M, Lorenzetti E. Hypertension in children with neurofibromatosis. J Hum Hypertens 1994; 8(5):395–397.

255. Lama G, Graziano L, Calabrese E, Grassia C, Rambaldi PF, Cioce F et al. Blood pressure and cardiovascular involvement in children with neurofibromatosis type1. Pediatr Nephrol 2004; 19(4):413–418.

256. Bitzer M, Topka H. Progressive cerebral occlusive disease after radiation therapy. Stroke 1995; 26(1):131–136.

257. Gomez MR. Strokes in tuberous sclerosis: are rhabdomyomas a cause? Brain Dev 1989; 11(1):14–19.

258. Butany J, Nair V, Naseemuddin A, Nair GM, Catton C, Yau T. Cardiac tumours: diagnosis and management. Lancet Oncol 2005; 6(4):219–228.

259. Larrode PP, Pascual Millan LF, Morales AF, Ayuso BT, Bello DS. Cerebral infarction and convulsive crises in a forme fruste of tuberous sclerosis. Rev Clin Esp 1986; 179(9):477–478.

260. Griffiths PD, Bolton P, Verity C. White matter abnormalities in tuberous sclerosis complex. Acta Radiol 1998; 39(5):482–486.

261. Imaizumi M, Nukada T, Yoneda S, Takano T, Hasegawa K, Abe H. Tuberous sclerosis with moyamoya disease. Case report. Med J Osaka Univ 1978; 28(3–4):345–353.

262. Kramer HH, Karch D, Seibert H. Moyamoya like vascular disease in tuberous sclerosis (author's transl). Monatsschr Kinderheilkd 1981; 129(10):595–597.

263. Blumenkopf B, Huggins MJ. Tuberous sclerosis and multiple intracranial aneurysms: case report. Neurosurgery 1985; 17(5):797–800.

264. Copley DJ. Case of the season. Diagnosis: intracranial aneurysms in a patient with tuberous sclerosis. Semin Roentgenol 1985; 20(2):107–109.

265. Beltramello A, Puppini G, Bricolo A, Andreis IA, El-Dalati G, Longa L et al. Does the tuberous sclerosis complex include intracranial aneurysms? A case report with a review of the literature. Pediatr Radiol 1999; 29(3):206–211.

266. Jones BV, Tomsick TA, Franz DN. Guglielmi detachable coil embolization of a giant midbasilar aneurysm in a 19-month-old patient. AJNR Am J Neuroradiol 2002; 23(7):1145–1148.

267. Brill CB, Peyster RG, Hoover ED, Keller MS. Giant intracranial aneurysm in a child with tuberous sclerosis: CT demonstration. J Comput Assist Tomogr 1985; 9(2):377–380.

268. Martin N, de BT, Cambier J, Marsault C, Nahum H. MRI evaluation of tuberous sclerosis. Neuroradiology 1987; 29(5):437–443.

269. Ho KL. Intraventricular aneurysm associated with tuberous sclerosis. Arch Neurol 1980; 37(6):385–386.

270. Davidson S. Tuberous sclerosis with fusiform aneurysms of both internal carotid arteries manifested by unilateral visual loss and papilledema. Bull Los Angeles Neurol Soc 1974; 39(3):128–132.

271. Guttman M, Tanen SM, Lambert CD. Visual loss secondary to a giant aneurysm in a patient with tuberous sclerosis. Can J Neurol Sci 1984; 11(4):472–474.

272. Spangler WJ, Cosgrove GR, Moumdjian RA, Montes JL. Cerebral arterial ectasia and tuberous sclerosis: case report. Neurosurgery 1997; 40(1):191–193.

273. Snowdon JA. Cerebral aneurysm, renal cysts and hamartomas in a case of tuberous sclerosis. Br J Urol 1974; 46(5):583.

274. Longa L, Scolari F, Brusco A, Carbonara C, Polidoro S, Valzorio B et al. A large TSC2 and PKD1 gene deletion is associated with renal and extrarenal signs of autosomal dominant polycystic kidney disease. Nephrol Dial Transplant 1997; 12(9):1900–1907.

275. Fusco F, Bardaro T, Fimiani G, Mercadante V, Miano MG, Falco G et al. Molecular analysis of the genetic defect in a large cohort of IP patients and identification of novel NEMO mutations interfering with NF-kappaB activation. Hum Mol Genet 2004; 13(16):1763–1773.

276. Hennel SJ, Ekert PG, Volpe JJ, Inder TE. Insights into the pathogenesis of cerebral lesions in incontinentia pigmenti. Pediatr Neurol 2003; 29(2):148–150.

277. Shuper A, Bryan RN, Singer HS. Destructive encephalopathy in incontinentia pigmenti: a primary disorder? Pediatr Neurol 1990; 6(2):137–140.

278. Fiorillo L, Sinclair DB, O'Byrne ML, Krol AL. Bilateral cerebrovascular accidents in incontinentia pigmenti. Pediatr Neurol 2003; 29(1):66–68.

279. Porksen G, Pfeiffer C, Hahn G, Poppe M, Friebel D, Kreuz F et al. Neonatal seizures in two sisters with incontinentia pigmenti. Neuropediatrics 2004; 35(2):139–142.

280. Goldberg MF. The blinding mechanisms of incontinentia pigmenti. Trans Am Ophthalmol Soc 1994; 92:167–176.

281. Lee YS, Jung KH, Roh JK. Diagnosis of moyamoya disease with transcranial Doppler sonography: correlation study with magnetic resonance angiography. J Neuroimaging 2004; 14(4):319–323.

282. Pellegrino RJ, Shah AJ. Vascular occlusion associated with incontinentia pigmenti. Pediatr Neurol 1994; 10(1):73–74.

283. Kasai T, Kato Z, Matsui E, Sakai A, Nishida T, Kondo N et al. Cerebral infarction in incontinentia pigmenti: the first report of a case evaluated by single photon emission computed tomography. Acta Paediatr 1997; 86(6):665–667.

284. Cartwright MS, White DL, Miller LM, III, Roach ES. Recurrent stroke in a child with incontinentia pigmenti. J Child Neurol 2009; 24(5):603–605.

285. Sneddon IB. Cerebro-vascular lesions and livedo reticularis. Br J Dermatol 1965; 77:180–185.

286. Wohlrab J, Frances C, Sullivan KE. Strange symptoms in Sneddon's syndrome. Clin Immunol 2006; 119(1):13–15.

287. Tietjen GE, Al-Qasmi MM, Gunda P, Herial NA. Sneddon's syndrome: another migraine-stroke association? Cephalalgia 2006; 26(3):225–232.

288. Tietjen GE, Al-Qasmi MM, Shukairy MS. Livedo reticularis and migraine: a marker for stroke risk? Headache 2002; 42(5):352–355.

289. Tietjen GE, Gottwald L, Al-Qasmi MM, Gunda P, Khuder SA. Migraine is associated with livedo reticularis: a prospective study. Headache 2002; 42(4):263–267.

290. Bolayir E, Kececi H, Akyol M, Tas A, Polat M. Sneddon's syndrome and antithrombin III. J Dermatol 1999; 26(8):532–534.

291. Rehany U, Kassif Y, Rumelt S. Sneddon's syndrome: neuroophthalmologic manifestations in a possible autosomal recessive pattern. Neurology 1998; 51(4):1185–1187.

292. Baxter P, Gardner-Medwin D, Green SH, Moss C. Congenital livedo reticularis and recurrent stroke-like episodes. Dev Med Child Neurol 1993; 35(10):917–921.

293. Gruppo RA, DeGrauw TJ, Palasis S, Kalinyak KA, Bofinger MK. Strokes, cutis marmorata telangiectatica congenita, and factor V Leiden. Pediatr Neurol 1998; 18(4):342–345.

294. Richards KA, Paller AS. Livedo reticularis in a child with moyamoya disease. Pediatr Dermatol 2003; 20(2):124–127.

295. Parmeggiani A, Posar A, De Giorgi LB, Sangiorgi S, Mochi M, Monari L et al. Sneddon syndrome, arylsulfatase A pseudodeficiency and impairment of cerebral white matter. Brain Dev 2000; 22(6):390–393.

296. Boesch SM, Plorer AL, Auer AJ, Poewe W, Aichner FT, Felber SR et al. The natural course of Sneddon syndrome: clinical and magnetic resonance imaging findings in a prospective six year observation study. J Neurol Neurosurg Psychiatry 2003; 74(4):542–544.

297. Sitzer M, Sohngen D, Siebler M, Specker C, Rademacher J, Janda I et al. Cerebral microembolism in patients with Sneddon's syndrome. Arch Neurol 1995; 52(3):271–275.

298. Tourbah A, Piette JC, Iba-Zizen MT, Lyon-Caen O, Godeau P, Frances C. The natural course of cerebral lesions in Sneddon syndrome. Arch Neurol 1997; 54(1):53–60.

299. De Fusco M, Marconi R, Silvestri L, Atorino L, Rampoldi L, Morgante L et al. Haploinsufficiency of ATP1A2 encoding the Na+/K+ pump alpha2 subunit associated with familial hemiplegic migraine type 2. Nat Genet 2003; 33(2):192–196.

300. Serrano-Pozo A, Gomez-Aranda F, Franco-Macias E, Serrano-Cabrera A. Cerebral haemorrhage in Sneddon's syndrome: case report and literature review. Rev Neurol 2004; 39(8):731–733.

301. Rebollo M, Val JF, Garijo F, Quintana F, Berciano J. Livedo reticularis and cerebrovascular lesions (Sneddon's syndrome). Clinical, radiological and pathological features in eight cases. Brain 1983; 106 (Pt 4):965–979.

302. Stockhammer G, Felber SR, Zelger B, Sepp N, Birbamer GG, Fritsch PO et al. Sneddon's syndrome: diagnosis by skin biopsy and MRI in 17 patients. Stroke 1993; 24(5):685–690.

303. Hilton DA, Footitt D. Neuropathological findings in Sneddon's syndrome. Neurology 2003; 60(7):1181–1182.

304. Kume M, Imai H, Motegi M, Miura AB, Namura I. Sneddon's syndrome (livedo racemosa and cerebral infarction) presenting psychiatric disturbance and shortening of fingers and toes. Intern Med 1996; 35(8):668–673.

305. Bolayir E, Yilmaz A, Kugu N, Erdogan H, Akyol M, Akyuz A. Sneddon's syndrome: clinical and laboratory analysis of 10 cases. Acta Med Okayama 2004; 58(2):59–65.

306. Mesa D, Franco M, Suarez de LJ, Munoz J, Rus C, Delgado M et al. Prevalence of patent foramen ovale in young patients with cerebral ischemic accident of unknown origin. Rev Esp Cardiol 2003; 56(7):662–668.

307. Adair JC, Digre KB, Swanda RM, Hartshorne MF, Lee RR, Constantino TM et al. Sneddon's syndrome: a cause of cognitive decline in young adults. Neuropsychiatry Neuropsychol Behav Neurol 2001; 14(3):197–204.

308. Karagulle AT, Karadag D, Erden A, Erden I. Sneddon's syndrome: MR imaging findings. Eur Radiol 2002; 12(1):144–146.

309. Charles PD, Fenichel GM. Sneddon and antiphospholipid antibody syndromes causing bilateral thalamic infarction. Pediatr Neurol 1994; 10(3):262–263.

310. Viswanathan KN, Anandan S, Sreenivas S, Kumar KS, Raman S. A 30-year-old man with stroke and skin lesions. Postgrad Med J 2000; 76(891):49–51.

311. Kalashnikova LA, Nasonov EL, Aleksandrova EN, Kosheleva NM, Reshetniak TM, Salozhin KV. Antibodies to phospholipids and ischemic disorders of cerebral circulation in young age. Zh Nevrol Psikhiatr Im S S Korsakova 1997; 97(6):59–65.

312. Frances C, Papo T, Wechsler B, Laporte JL, Biousse V, Piette JC. Sneddon syndrome with or without antiphospholipid antibodies. A comparative study in 46 patients. Medicine (Baltimore) 1999; 78(4):209–219.

313. Besnier R, Frances C, Ankri A, Aiach M, Piette JC. Factor V Leiden mutation in Sneddon syndrome. Lupus 2003; 12(5):406–408.

314. Ayoub N, Esposito G, Barete S, Soria C, Piette JC, Frances C. Protein Z deficiency in antiphospholipid-negative Sneddon's syndrome. Stroke 2004; 35(6):1329–1332.

315. Frances C, Le TM, Salohzin KV, Kalashnikova LA, Piette JC, Godeau P et al. Prevalence of anti-endothelial cell antibodies in patients with Sneddon's syndrome. J Am Acad Dermatol 1995; 33(1):64–68.

316. Zhu I, Weston WL. Nevus sebaceous and stroke. Arch Dermatol 2005; 141(5):648–649.

317. Okuda K, Matsui T, Kitaguchi M, Kihara M, Takahashi M. A case of linear sebaceous nevus syndrome associated with a cerebrovascular anomaly. Rinsho Shinkeigaku 1998; 38(5):471–473.

318. Baker RS, Ross PA, Baumann RJ. Neurologic complications of the epidermal nevus syndrome. Arch Neurol 1987; 44(2):227–232.

319. Kang WH, Koh YJ, Chun SI. Nevus sebaceus syndrome associated with intracranial arteriovenous malformation. Int J Dermatol 1987; 26(6):382–384.

320. Leno C, Sedano MJ, Combarros O, Berciano J. Congenital giant pigmented nevus and intracranial arteriovenous malformation. Surg Neurol 1989; 31(5):407–408.

321. Nuno K, Mihara M, Shimao S. Linear sebaceous nevus syndrome. Dermatologica 1990; 181(3):221–223.

322. Dobyns WB, Garg BP. Vascular abnormalities in epidermal nevus syndrome. Neurology 1991; 41(2 (Pt 1)):276–278.

323. Kotulska K, Jurkiewcz E, Jozwiak S, Kuczynski D. Epidermal nevus syndrome and intraspinal hemorrhage. Brain Dev 2006; 28(8):541–543.

324. Kara B, Inan N, Bayramgurler D, Altintas O, Akbulut A. Epidermal nevus syndrome with azygos anterior cerebral artery. Pediatr Neurol 2008; 39(4):283–285.

325. Meschia JF, Junkins E, Hofman KJ. Familial systematized epidermal nevus syndrome. Am J Med Genet 1992; 44(5):664–667.

326. Urgelles E, Pascual-Castroviejo I, Roche C, Moneo JL, Martinez MA, Vega A. Arteriovenous malformation in hypomelanosis of Ito. Brain Dev 1996; 18(1):78–80.

327. Garcia Muret MP, Puig L, Allard C, Alomar A. Hypomelanosis of Ito with Sturge–Weber syndrome-like leptomeningeal angiomatosis. Pediatr Dermatol 2002; 19(6):536–540.

328. Pascual-Castroviejo I, Frutos R, Viano J, Pascual-Pascual SI, Gonzalez P. Cobb syndrome: case report. J Child Neurol 2002; 17(11):847–849.

329. Matullo KS, Samdani A, Betz R. Low-back pain and unrecognized Cobb syndrome in a child resulting in paraplegia. Orthopedics 2007; 30(3):237–238.

330. Clark MT, Brooks EL, Chong W, Pappas C, Fahey M. Cobb syndrome: a case report and systematic review of the literature. Pediatr Neurol 2008; 39(6):423–425.

331. Krings T, Geibprasert S, Luo CB, Bhattacharya JJ, Alvarez H, Lasjaunias P. Segmental neurovascular syndromes in children. Neuroimaging Clin N Am 2007; 17(2):245–258.

332. Schmidt D, Pache M, Schumacher M. The congenital unilateral retinocephalic vascular malformation syndrome (Bonnet–Dechaume–Blanc syndrome or Wyburn–Mason syndrome): review of the literature. Surv Ophthalmol 2008; 53(3):227–249.

333. Luo CB, Lasjaunias P, Bhattacharya J. Craniofacial vascular malformations in Wyburn–Mason syndrome. J Chin Med Assoc 2006; 69(12):575–580.

334. Dayani PN, Sadun AA. A case report of Wyburn–Mason syndrome and review of the literature. Neuroradiology 2007; 49(5):445–456.

335. Chan WM, Yip NK, Lam DS. Wyburn–Mason syndrome. Neurology 2004; 62(1):99.

336. Turnbull MM, Humeniuk V, Stein B, Suthers GK. Arteriovenous malformations in Cowden syndrome. J Med Genet 2005; 42(8):e50.

337. Srinivasa RN, Burrows PE. Dural arteriovenous malformation in a child with Bannayan–Riley–Ruvalcaba syndrome. AJNR Am J Neuroradiol 2006; 27(9):1927–1929.

338. Lachlan KL, Lucassen AM, Bunyan D, Temple IK. Cowden syndrome and Bannayan–Riley–Ruvalcaba syndrome represent one condition with variable expression and age-related penetrance: results of a clinical study of PTEN mutation carriers. J Med Genet 2007; 44(9):579–585.

339. Tan WH, Baris HN, Burrows PE, Robson CD, Alomari AI, Mulliken JB et al. The spectrum of vascular anomalies in patients with PTEN mutations: implications for diagnosis and management. J Med Genet 2007; 44(9):594–602.

340. Bayrak-Toydemir P, Mao R, Lewin S, McDonald J. Hereditary hemorrhagic telangiectasia: an overview of diagnosis and management in the molecular era for clinicians. Genet Med 2004; 6(4):175–191.

341. Morgan T, McDonald J, Anderson C, Ismail M, Miller F, Mao R et al. Intracranial hemorrhage in infants and children with hereditary hemorrhagic telangiectasia (Osler–Weber-Rendu syndrome). Pediatrics 2002; 109(1):E12.

342. Kjeldsen AD, Oxhoj H, Andersen PE, Green A, Vase P. Prevalence of pulmonary arteriovenous malformations (PAVMs) and occurrence of neurological symptoms in patients with hereditary haemorrhagic telangiectasia (HHT). J Intern Med 2000; 248(3):255–262.

343. Easey AJ, Wallace GM, Hughes JM, Jackson JE, Taylor WJ, Shovlin CL. Should asymptomatic patients with hereditary haemorrhagic telangiectasia (HHT) be screened for cerebral vascular malformations? Data from 22 061 years of HHT patient life. J Neurol Neurosurg Psychiatry 2003; 74(6):743–748.

344. Maher CO, Piepgras DG, Brown RD, Jr, Friedman JA, Pollock BE. Cerebrovascular manifestations in 321 cases of hereditary hemorrhagic telangiectasia. Stroke 2001; 32(4):877–882.

345. Matsubara S, Mandzia JL, Ter BK, Willinsky RA, Faughnan ME. Angiographic and clinical characteristics of patients with cerebral arteriovenous malformations associated with hereditary hemorrhagic telangiectasia. AJNR Am J Neuroradiol 2000; 21(6):1016–1020.

346. Mei-Zahav M, Letarte M, Faughnan ME, Abdalla SA, Cymerman U, Maclusky IB. Symptomatic children with hereditary hemorrhagic telangiectasia: a pediatric center experience. Arch Pediatr Adolesc Med 2006; 160(6):596–601.

347. Krings T, Ozanne A, Chng SM, Alvarez H, Rodesch G, Lasjaunias PL. Neurovascular phenotypes in hereditary haemorrhagic telangiectasia patients according to age. Review of 50 consecutive patients aged 1 day–60 years. Neuroradiology 2005; 47(10):711–720.

348. Khurshid I, Downie GH. Pulmonary arteriovenous malformation. Postgrad Med J 2002; 78(918):191–197.

349. McDonald JE, Miller FJ, Hallam SE, Nelson L, Marchuk DA, Ward KJ. Clinical manifestations in a large hereditary hemorrhagic telangiectasia (HHT) type 2 kindred. Am J Med Genet 2000; 93(4):320–327.

350. Folz BJ, Zoll B, Alfke H, Toussaint A, Maier RF, Werner JA. Manifestations of hereditary hemorrhagic telangiectasia in children and adolescents. Eur Arch Otorhinolaryngol 2006; 263(1):53–61.

351. Cloft HJ. Spontaneous regression of cerebral arteriovenous malformation in hereditary hemorrhagic telangiectasia. AJNR Am J Neuroradiol 2002; 23(6):1049–1050.

352. Leung KM, Agid R, Terbrugge K. Spontaneous regression of a cerebral arteriovenous malformation in a child with hereditary hemorrhagic telangiectasia. Case report. J Neurosurg 2006; 105(5 Suppl):428–431.

353. van den Berg JS, Hennekam RC, Cruysberg JR, Steijlen PM, Swart J, Tijmes N et al. Prevalence of symptomatic intracranial aneurysm and ischaemic stroke in pseudoxanthoma elasticum. Cerebrovasc Dis 2000; 10(4):315–319.

354. Donaldson EJ. Angioid streaks. Aust J Ophthalmol 1983; 11(1):55–58.

355. Coleman K, Ross MH, Mc Cabe M, Coleman R, Mooney D. Disk drusen and angioid streaks in pseudoxanthoma elasticum. Am J Ophthalmol 1991; 112(2):166–170.

356. Aessopos A, Farmakis D, Karagiorga M, Rombos I, Loucopoulos D. Pseudoxanthoma elasticum lesions and cardiac complications as contributing factors for strokes in beta-thalassemia patients. Stroke 1997; 28(12):2421–2424.

357. Van MK, Hintz S, Rhine W, Benitz W. The use of inhaled nitric oxide in the premature infant with respiratory distress syndrome. Minerva Pediatr 2006; 58(5):403–422.

358. Boutouyrie P, Germain DP, Tropeano AI, Laloux B, Carenzi F, Zidi M et al. Compressibility of the carotid artery in patients with pseudoxanthoma elasticum. Hypertension 2001; 38(5):1181–1184.

359. Germain DP, Boutouyrie P, Laloux B, Laurent S. Arterial remodeling and stiffness in patients with pseudoxanthoma elasticum. Arterioscler Thromb Vasc Biol 2003; 23(5):836–841.

360. Munyer TP, Margulis AR. Pseudoxanthoma elasticum with internal carotid artery aneurysm. AJR Am J Roentgenol 1981; 136(5):1023–1024.

361. Messis CP, Budzilovich GN. Pseudoxanthoma elasticum. Report of an autopsied case with cerebral involvement. Neurology 1970; 20(7):703–709.

362. Goto K. Involvement of central nervous system in pseudoxanthoma elasticum. Folia Psychiatr Neurol Jpn 1975; 29(3):263–277.

363. Iqbal A, Alter M, Lee SH. Pseudoxanthoma elasticum: a review of neurological complications. Ann Neurol 1978; 4(1):18–20.

364. Galle G, Galle K, Huk W, Taghavy A. Stenoses of the cerebral arteries in pseudoxanthoma elasticum (author's transl). Arch Psychiatr Nervenkr 1981; 231(1):61–70.

365. Liedholm LJ, Duchek M, Monestam E. Pseudoxanthoma elasticum – unusual cause of stroke and eye complications. Lakartidningen 1992; 89(30–31):2521–2523.

366. Hirano T, Hashimoto Y, Kimura K, Uchino M. Lacunar brain infarction in patients with pseudoxanthoma elasticum. Rinsho Shinkeigaku 1996; 36(5):633–639.

367. Manfredi M, Beltramello A, Mazzilli S, Magni E, Gandolfini M, Donati E. Stroke and pseudoxanthoma elasticum. Acta Neurol Belg 2000; 100(1):48–50.

368. Aralikatti AK, Lee MW, Lipton ME, Kamath GG. Visual loss due to cerebral infarcts in pseudoxanthoma elasticum. Eye 2002; 16(6):785–786.

369. Heaton RK, Vogt AT, Neldner KH, Reeve EB. Neuropsychological findings with pseudoxanthoma elasticum. Acta Med Scand 1978; 203(3):215–221.

370. Rios-Montenegro EN, Behrens MM, Hoyt WF. Pseudoxanthoma elasticum. Association with bilateral carotid rete mirabile and unilateral carotid-cavernous sinus fistula. Arch Neurol 1972; 26(2):151–155.

371. Araki Y, Imai S, Saitoh A, Ito T, Shimizu K, Yamada H. A case of carotid rete mirabile associated with pseudoxanthoma elasticum: a case report. No To Shinkei 1986; 38(5):495–500.

372. Yasuhara T, Sugiu K, Kakishita M, Date I. Pseudoxanthoma elasticum with carotid rete mirabile. Clin Neurol Neurosurg 2004; 106(2):114–117.

373. Schachner L, Young D. Pseudoxanthoma elasticum with severe cardiovascular disease in a child. Am J Dis Child 1974; 127(4):571–575.

374. Hacker SM, Ramos-Caro FA, Beers BB, Flowers FP. Juvenile pseudoxanthoma elasticum: recognition and management. Pediatr Dermatol 1993; 10(1):19–25.

375. Barrie L, Mazereeuw-Hautier J, Garat H, Bonafe JL. Early pseudoxanthoma elasticum with severe cardiovascular involvement. Ann Dermatol Venereol 2004; 131(3):275–278.

376. Pieczuro A, Lozza M. Cerebrovascular disease and pseudoxanthoma elasticum: apropos of a case. Riv Neurol 1981; 51(5):261–273.

377. Meyer S, Zanardo L, Kaminski WE, Horn P, Schmitz G, Hohenleutner U et al. Elastosis perforans serpiginosa-like pseudoxanthoma elasticum in a child with severe Moya Moya disease. Br J Dermatol 2005; 153(2):431–434.

378. Yap EY, Gleaton MS, Buettner H. Visual loss associated with pseudoxanthoma elasticum. Retina 1992; 12(4):315–319.

379. Araki Y, Yokoyama T, Sagawa N, Okuno S, Hoshino Y, Sando Y et al. Pseudoxanthoma elasticum diagnosed 25 years after the onset of cardiovascular disease. Intern Med 2001; 40(11):1117–1120.

380. Brockmann K, Stolpe S, Fels C, Khan N, Kulozik AE, Pekrun A. Moyamoya syndrome associated with hemolytic anemia due to Hb Alesha. J Pediatr Hematol Oncol 2005; 27(8):436–440.

381. Pavlovic S, Kuzmanovic M, Urosevic J, Poznanic J, Zoranovic T, Djordjevic V et al. Severe central nervous system thrombotic events in hemoglobin Sabine patient. Eur J Haematol 2004; 72(1):67–70.

382. Schilling RF, Gangnon RE, Traver M. Arteriosclerotic events are less frequent in persons with chronic anemia: evidence from families with hereditary spherocytosis. Am J Hematol 2006; 81(5):315–317.

383. Rahimi Z, Merat A, Haghshenass M, Madani H, Rezaei M, Nagel RL. Plasma lipids in Iranians with sickle cell disease: hypo-cholesterolemia in sickle cell anemia and increase of HDL-cholesterol in sickle cell trait. Clin Chim Acta 2006; 365(1–2):217–220.

384. Henderson JN, Noetzel MJ, McKinstry RC, White DA, Armstrong M, DeBaun MR. Reversible posterior leukoencephalopathy syndrome and silent cerebral infarcts are associated with severe acute chest syndrome in children with sickle cell disease. Blood 2003; 101(2):415–419.

385. Miyamoto O, Auer RN. Hypoxia, hyperoxia, ischemia, and brain necrosis. Neurology 2000; 54(2):362–371.

386. Kirkham FJ, Datta AK. Adaptation to hypoxia during development and pattern of neurological presentation and cognitive disability. Dev Sci 2006; 9:411–427.

387. Gladwin MT, Kato GJ. Cardiopulmonary complications of sickle cell disease: role of nitric oxide and hemolytic anemia. Hematology Am Soc Hematol Educ Program 2005; 51–57.

388. Setty BN, Stuart MJ, Dampier C, Brodecki D, Allen JL. Hypoxaemia in sickle cell disease: biomarker modulation and relevance to pathophysiology. Lancet 2003; 362(9394):1450–1455.

389. Kirkham FJ, Hewes DK, Prengler M, Wade A, Lane R, Evans JP. Nocturnal hypoxaemia and central-nervous-system events in sickle-cell disease. Lancet 2001; 357(9269):1656–1659.

390. Kirkham FJ, Bynevelt M, Hewes DK, Cox TC, Evans JP, Connelly A. Nocturnal hypoxaemia and intracranial vessel turbulence on magnetic resonance angiography in children with sickle cell disease. Stroke 2002; 33:345.

391. Baguet JP, Hammer L, Levy P, Pierre H, Launois S, Mallion JM, Pépin JL. The severity of oxygen desaturation is predictive of carotid wall thickening and plaque occurrence. Chest. 2005;128(5):3407–12.

392. Shnaider H, Shiran A, Lorber A. Right ventricular diastolic dysfunction and patent foramen ovale causing profound cyanosis. Heart 2004; 90(6):e31.

393. Shanoudy H, Soliman A, Raggi P, Liu JW, Russell DC, Jarmukli NF. Prevalence of patent foramen ovale and its contribution to hypoxemia in patients with obstructive sleep apnea. Chest 1998; 113(1):91–96.

394. Soliman A, Shanoudy H, Liu J, Russell DC, Jarmukli NF. Increased prevalence of patent foramen ovale in patients with severe chronic obstructive pulmonary disease. J Am Soc Echocardiogr 1999; 12(2):99–105.

395. Finsterer J, Sommer O, Stiskal M, Stollberger C, Baumgartner H. Closure of a patent foramen ovale: effective therapy of migraine and occipital stroke. Int J Neurosci 2005; 115(1):119–127.

396. Kirkham FJ, Salmon AP, Khambadkone S. A hole in the heart: a hole in the head? Arch Dis Child 2011; in press doi: 10.1136/adc.2010.208470

397. Dowling MM, Quinn CT, Rogers ZR, Journeycake JM. Stroke in sickle cell anemia: alternative etiologies. Pediatr Neurol 2009; 41(2):124–126.

398. Dowling MM, Lee N, Quinn CT, Rogers ZR, Boger D, Ahmad N et al. Prevalence of intracardiac shunting in children with sickle cell disease and stroke. J Pediatr 2009; 156(4):645–650.

399. Prohovnik I, Hurlet-Jensen A, Adams R, De VD, Pavlakis SG. Hemodynamic etiology of elevated flow velocity and stroke in sickle-cell disease. J Cereb Blood Flow Metab 2009; 29(4):803–810.

400. Baccarani-Contri M, Bacchelli B, Boraldi F, Quaglino D, Taparelli F, Carnevali E et al. Characterization of pseudoxanthoma elasticum-like lesions in the skin of patients with beta-thalassemia. J Am Acad Dermatol 2001; 44(1):33–39.

401. Hamlin N, Beck K, Bacchelli B, Cianciulli P, Pasquali-Ronchetti I, Le SO. Acquired pseudoxanthoma elasticum-like syndrome in beta-thalassaemia patients. Br J Haematol 2003; 122(5):852–854.

402. Aessopos A, Farmakis D, Loukopoulos D. Elastic tissue abnormalities resembling pseudoxanthoma elasticum in beta thalassemia and the sickling syndromes. Blood 2002; 99(1):30–35.

403. McBrayer GM, Semes L, Stephens GG. Angioid streaks and AC hemoglobinopathy – a newly discovered association. J Am Optom Assoc 1993; 64(4):250–253.

404. Gerde LS. Angioid streaks in sickle cell trait hemoglobinopathy. Am J Ophthalmol 1974; 77(4):462–464.

405. Kinsella FP, Mooney DJ. Angioid streaks in beta thalassaemia minor. Br J Ophthalmol 1988; 72(4):303–304.

406. O'Donnell BF, Powell FC, O'Loughlin S, Acheson RW. Angioid streaks in beta thalassaemia minor. Br J Ophthalmol 1991; 75(10):639.

407. Gartaganis S, Ismiridis K, Papageorgiou O, Beratis NG, Papanastasiou D. Ocular abnormalities in patients with beta thalassemia. Am J Ophthalmol 1989; 108(6):699–703.

408. Aessopos A, Stamatelos G, Savvides P, Kavouklis E, Gabriel L, Rombos I et al. Angioid streaks in homozygous beta thalassemia. Am J Ophthalmol 1989; 108(4):356–359.

409. Roberts E, Madhusudhana KC, Newsom R, Cullis JO. Blindness due to angioid streaks in congenital dyserythropoietic anaemia type I. Br J Haematol 2006; 133(5):456.

410. Sandstrom H, Wahlin A, Eriksson M, Holmgren G, Lind L, Sandgren O. Angioid streaks are part of a familial syndrome of dyserythropoietic anaemia (CDA III). Br J Haematol 1997; 98(4):845–849.

411. Daneshmend TK. Ocular findings in a case of haemoglobin H disease. Br J Ophthalmol 1979; 63(12):842–844.

412. Condon PI, Serjeant GR. Ocular findings of elderly cases of homozygous sickle-cell disease in Jamaica. Br J Ophthalmol 1976; 60(5):361–364.

413. Hamilton AM, Pope FM, Condon PI, Slavin G, Sowter C, Ford S et al. Angioid streaks in Jamaican patients with homozygous sickle cell disease. Br J Ophthalmol 1981; 65(5):341–347.

414. Tsomi K, Karagiorga-Lagana M, Karabatsos F, Fragodimitri C, van Vliet-Konstantinidou C, Premetis E et al. Arterial elastorrhexis in beta-thalassaemia intermedia, sickle cell thalassaemia and hereditary spherocytosis. Eur J Haematol 2001; 67(3):135–141.

415. Logothetis J, Constantoulakis M, Economidou J, Stefanis C, Hakas P, Augoustaki O et al. Thalassemia major (homozygous beta-thalassemia). A survey of 138 cases with emphasis on neurologic and muscular aspects. Neurology 1972; 22(3):294–304.

416. Borgna PC, Carnelli V, Caruso V, Dore F, De Mattia D, Di Palma A et al. Thromboembolic events in beta thalassemia major: an Italian multicenter study. Acta Haematol 1998; 99(2):76–79.

417. Mutalimova AB. Features of cerebrovascular disorders in children with beta-thalassemia major. Zh Nevrol Psikhiatr Im S S Korsakova 1975; 75:1484–1489.

418. Mutalimova AB. Pathomorphology of the nevous system in beta thalassemia major. Arkh Patol 1976; 38:33–37.

419. Engelborghs S, Pickut BA, De Deyn PP. Recurrent transient ischemic attacks in a 15-year-old boy with beta-thalassemia minor and thrombophilia. Contribution of perfusion SPECT to clinical diagnosis. Acta Neurol Belg 2003; 103(2):99–102.

420. Wasi P, Na-Nakorn S, Pootrakul P, Sonakul D, Piankijagum A, Pacharee P. A syndrome of hypertension, convulsion, and cerebral haemorrhage in thalassaemic patients after multiple blood-transfusions. Lancet 1978; 2(8090):602–604.

421. Suwanchinda V, Tengapiruk Y, Udomphunthurak S. Hypertension perioperative splenectomy in thalassemic children. J Med Assoc Thai 1994; 77(2):66–70.

422. Yetgin S, Hicsonmez G. Hypertension, convulsions, and purpuric skin lesions after blood-transfusion. Lancet 1979; 1(8116):610.

423. Constantopoulos A, Matsaniotis N. Hypertension, convulsion, and cerebral haemorrhage in thalassaemic patients after multiple blood transfusions. Helv Paediatr Acta 1980; 35(3):269–271.

424. Chuansumrit A, Isarangkura P, Hathirat P, Thirawarapan S. A syndrome of post-transfusion hypertension, convulsion and cerebral hemorrhage in beta-thalassemia Hb E disease: a case report with high plasma renin activity. J Med Assoc Thai 1986; 69(Suppl 2):1–5.

425. Thirawarapan SS, Snongchart N, Fucharoen S, Tanphaichitr VS, Dhorranintra B. Study of mechanisms of post-transfusion hypertension in thalassaemic patients. Southeast Asian J Trop Med Public Health 1989; 20(3):471–478.

426. Michaeli J, Mittelman M, Grisaru D, Rachmilewitz EA. Thromboembolic complications in beta thalassemia major. Acta Haematol 1992; 87(1–2):71–74.

427. Gurgey A, Kalayci O, Gumruk F, Cetin M, Altay C. Convulsion after blood transfusion in four beta-thalassemia intermedia patients. Pediatr Hematol Oncol 1994; 11(5):549–552.

428. Incorpora G, Di Gregorio F, Romeo MA, Pavone P, Trifiletti RR, Parano E. Focal neurological deficits in children with beta-thalassemia major. Neuropediatrics 1999; 30(1):45–48.

429. Sinniah D, Vignaendra V, Ahmad K. Neurological complications of beta-thalassaemia major. Arch Dis Child 1977; 52(12):977–979.

430. Suwanchinda V, Pirayavaraporn S, Yokubol B, Tengapiruk Y, Laohapensang M, Udomphunthurak S. Does furosemide prevent hypertension during perioperative splenectomy in thalassemic children? J Med Assoc Thai 1995; 78(10):542–546.

431. Suwanchinda V, Tanphaichitr V, Pirayavaraporn S, Somprakit P, Laohapensang M. Hemodynamic responses to captopril during splenectomy in thalassemic children. J Med Assoc Thai 1999; 82(7):666–671.

432. Lee KF. Fatal intra-cranial haemorrhage in 2 cases of beta-thalassaemia major. Med J Malaysia 1995; 50(1):110–113.

433. Karimi M, Yavarian M, Afrasiabi A, Dehbozorgian J, Rachmilewitz E. Prevalence of beta-thalassemia trait and glucose-6-phosphate dehydrogenase deficiency in Iranian Jews. Arch Med Res 2008; 39(2):212–214.

434. Brankovic-Sreckovic V, Milic RV, Djordjevic V, Kuzmanovic M, Pavlovic S. Arterial ischemic stroke in a child with beta-thalassemia trait and methylentetrahydrofolate reductase mutation. J Child Neurol 2007; 22(2):208–210.

435. Singh R, Venketasubramanian N. Recurrent cerebral infarction in beta thalassaemia major. Cerebrovasc Dis 2004; 17(4):344–345.

436. Wong V, Yu YL, Liang RH, Tso WK, Li AM, Chan TK. Cerebral thrombosis in beta-thalassemia/hemoglobin E disease. Stroke 1990; 21(5):812–816.

437. Mukherjee A. Moyamoya disease and beta-thalassemia. J Assoc Physicians India 1995; 43(10):710–711.

438. Peerless SJ. Risk factors of moyamoya disease in Canada and the USA. Clin Neurol Neurosurg 1997; 99(Suppl 2):S45–S48.

439. Sanefuji M, Ohga S, Kira R, Yoshiura T, Torisu H, Hara T. Moyamoya syndrome in a splenectomized patient with beta-thalassemia intermedia. J Child Neurol 2006; 21(1):75–77.

440. Salih MA, Murshid WR, Al-Salman MM, Abdel-Gader AG, Al-Jarallah AA, Alorainy IA et al. Moyamoya syndrome as a risk factor for stroke in Saudi children. Novel and usual associations. Saudi Med J 2006; 27(Suppl 1):S69–S80.

441. Senanayake MP, Lamabadusuriya SP. Cerebral thrombosis in beta-thalassaemia major. Indian J Pediatr 2001; 68(11):1081–1082.

442. Caksen H, Odabas D, Akbayram S, Faik OA, Arslan S, Cesur Y et al. Silent stroke in a case of beta-thalassemia major associated with chronic renal failure and diabetes mellitus. J Child Neurol 2003; 18(11):798–800.

443. Manfre L, Giarratano E, Maggio A, Banco A, Vaccaro G, Lagalla R. MR imaging of the brain: findings in asymptomatic patients with thalassemia intermedia and sickle cell-thalassemia disease. AJR Am J Roentgenol 1999; 173(6):1477–1480.

444. Metarugcheep P, Chanyawattiwongs S, Srisubat K, Pootrakul P. Clinical silent cerebral infarct (SCI) in patients with thalassemia diseases assessed by magnetic resonance imaging (MRI). J Med Assoc Thai 2008; 91(6):889–894.

445. Taher AT, Musallam KM, Nasreddine W, Hourani R, Inati A, Beydoun A. Asymptomatic brain magnetic resonance imaging abnormalities in splenectomized adults with thalassemia intermedia. J Thromb Haemost 2010; 8(1):54–59.

446. Parano E, Pavone V, Di GF, Pavone P, Trifiletti RR. Extraordinary intrathecal bone reaction in beta-thalassaemia intermedia. Lancet 1999; 354(9182):922.

447. Dhechakaisaya S, Shuangshoti S, Susakares A. Extramedullary hematopoiesis of cranial dura mater and choroid plexus and terminal convulsions in a patient with thalassemia-hemoglobin E disease. J Med Assoc Thai 1979; 62(9):503–511.

448. Moratelli S, De Sanctis V, Gemmati D, Serino ML, Mari R, Gamberini MR et al. Thrombotic risk in thalassemic patients. J Pediatr Endocrinol Metab 1998; 11(Suppl 3):915–921.

449. Eldor A, Durst R, Hy-Am E, Goldfarb A, Gillis S, Rachmilewitz EA et al. A chronic hypercoagulable state in patients with beta-thalassaemia major is already present in childhood. Br J Haematol 1999; 107(4):739–746.

450. Cappellini MD, Robbiolo L, Bottasso BM, Coppola R, Fiorelli G, Mannucci AP. Venous thromboembolism and hypercoagulability in splenectomized patients with thalassaemia intermedia. Br J Haematol 2000; 111(2):467–473.

451. Eldor A, Rachmilewitz EA. The hypercoagulable state in thalassemia. Blood 2002; 99(1):36–43.

452. Finkelstein Y, Yaniv I, Berant M, Zilber R, Garty BZ, Epstein O et al. Central venous line thrombosis in children and young adults with thalassemia major. Pediatr Hematol Oncol 2004; 21(5):375–381.

453. Giordano P, Sabato V, Schettini F, De Mattia D, Iolascon A. Resistance to activated protein C as a risk factor of stroke in a thalassemic patient. Haematologica 1997; 82(6):698–700.

454. Levin C, Zalman L, Shalev S, Mader R, Koren A. Legg-Calve–Perthes disease, protein C deficiency, and beta-thalassemia major: report of two cases. J Pediatr Orthop 2000; 20(1):129–131.

455. Micheloyannis S, Papadaki F, Jannopoulos A. The effect of blood transfusion on alpha EEG activity in thalassemic patients. Eur Neurol 1991; 31(3):131–135.

456. Wong V, Li A, Lee AC. Neurophysiologic study of beta-thalassemia patients. J Child Neurol 1993; 8(4):330–335.

457. Zafeiriou DI, Kousi AA, Tsantali CT, Kontopoulos EE, Ugoustidou-Savvopoulou PA, Tsoubaris PD et al. Neurophysiologic evaluation of long-term desferrioxamine therapy in beta-thalassemia patients. Pediatr Neurol 1998; 18(5):420–424.

458. Economou M, Zafeiriou DI, Kontopoulos E, Gompakis N, Koussi A, Perifanis V, Athanassiou-Metaxa M. Neurophysiologic and intellectual evaluation of beta-thalassemia patients. Brain Dev. 2006;28(1):14–18.

459. Qian XH, Zhang GC, Jiao XY, Zheng YJ, Cao YH, Xu DL et al. Aplastic anaemia associated with parvovirus B19 infection. Arch Dis Child 2002; 87(5):436–437.

460. Barah F, Vallely PJ, Chiswick ML, Cleator GM, Kerr JR. Association of human parvovirus B19 infection with acute meningoencephalitis. Lancet 2001; 358(9283):729–730.

461. Guidi B, Bergonzini P, Crisi G, Frigieri G, Portolani M. Case of stroke in a 7-year-old male after parvovirus B19 infection. Pediatr Neurol 2003; 28(1):69–71.

462. Wierenga KJ, Serjeant BE, Serjeant GR. Cerebrovascular complications and parvovirus infection in homozygous sickle cell disease. J Pediatr 2001; 139(3):438–442.

463. Jeng MR, Feusner J, Skibola C, Vichinsky E. Central venous catheter complications in sickle cell disease. Am J Hematol 2002; 69(2):103–108.

464. Tischkowitz MD, Hodgson SV. Fanconi anaemia. J Med Genet 2003; 40(1):1–10.

465. Pavlakis SG, Frissora CL, Giampietro PF, Davis JG, Gould RJ, Adler-Brecher B et al. Fanconi anemia: a model for genetic causes of abnormal brain development. Dev Med Child Neurol 1992; 34(12):1081–1084.

466. Rogers PC, Desai F, Karabus CD, Hartley PS, Fisher RM. Presentation and outcome of 25 cases of Fanconi's anemia. Am J Pediatr Hematol Oncol 1989; 11(2):141–145.

467. Tezcan I, Tuncer M, Uckan D, Cetin M, Alikasifoglu M, Ersoy F et al. Allogeneic bone marrow transplantation in Fanconi anemia from Turkey: a report of four cases. Pediatr Transplant 1998; 2(3):236–239.

468. Bleggi-Torres LF, de Medeiros BC, Werner B, Neto JZ, Loddo G, Pasquini R et al. Neuropathological findings after bone marrow transplantation: an autopsy study of 180 cases. Bone Marrow Transplant 2000; 25(3):301–307.

469. Uckan D, Cetin M, Yigitkanli I, Tezcan I, Tuncer M, Karasimav D et al. Life-threatening neurological complications after bone marrow transplantation in children. Bone Marrow Transplant 2005; 35(1):71–76.

470. Cohen N, Berant M, Simon J. Moyamoya and Fanconi's anemia. Pediatrics 1980; 65(4):804–805.

471. Pavlakis SG, Verlander PC, Gould RJ, Strimling BC, Auerbach AD. Fanconi anemia and moyamoya: evidence for an association. Neurology 1995; 45(5):998–1000.

472. Jabr FI, Aoun E, Azar C, Taher A. Diamond–Blackfan anemia responding to valproic acid. Blood 2004; 104(10):3415.

473. Nagarajan R, Peters C, Orchard P, Rydholm N. Report of severe neurotoxicity with cyclophosphamide. J Pediatr Hematol Oncol 2000; 22(6):544–546.

474. Trivedi RA, Kirkpatrick PJ. Arteriovenous malformations of the cerebral circulation that rupture in pregnancy. J Obstet Gynaecol 2003; 23(5):484–489.

475. Daniels SR, Loggie JM, Schwartz DC, Strife JL, Kaplan S. Systemic hypertension secondary to peripheral vascular anomalies in patients with Williams syndrome. J Pediatr 1985; 106(2):249–251.

476. Bale JF, Jr, Brasher C, Siegler RL. CNS manifestations of the hemolytic-uremic syndrome. Relationship to metabolic alterations and prognosis. Am J Dis Child 1980; 134(9):869–872.

477. Bos AP, Donckerwolcke RA, van Vught AJ. The hemolytic-uremic syndrome: prognostic significance of neurological abnormalities. Helv Paediatr Acta 1985; 40(5):381–389.

478. Rooney JC, Anderson RM, Hopkins IJ. Clinical and pathologic aspects of central nervous system involvement in the haemolytic uraemic syndrome. Proc Aust Assoc Neurol 1971; 8:67–75.

479. Schmidt S, Gudinchet F, Meagher-Villemure K, Maeder P. Brain involvement in haemolytic-uraemic syndrome: MRI features of coagulative necrosis. Neuroradiology. 2001;43(7):581–585.

480. Trevathan E, Dooling EC. Large thrombotic strokes in hemolytiuremic syndrome. J Pediatr 1987; 111(6 Pt 1):863–866.

481. Steele K. Bilateral axillary vein thrombosis. Ulster Med J 1983; 52(1):71–72.

482. Crisp DE, Siegler RL, Bale JF, Thompson JA. Hemorrhagic cerebral infarction in the hemolytic-uremic syndrome. J Pediatr 1981; 99(2):273–276.

483. Steinberg A, Ish-Horowitcz M, El-Peleg O, Mor J, Branski D. Stroke in a patient with hemolytic-uremic syndrome with a good outcome. Brain Dev 1986; 8(1):70–72.

484. Nakahata T, Tanaka H, Tateyama T, Ueda T, Suzuki K, Osari S et al. Thrombotic stroke in a child with diarrhea-associated hemolytic-uremic syndrome with a good recovery. Tohoku J Exp Med 2001; 193(1):73–77.

485. Michael M, Elliott EJ, Ridley GF, Hodson EM, Craig JC. Interventions for haemolytic uraemic syndrome and thrombotic thrombocytopenic purpura. Cochrane Database Syst Rev 2009; (1):CD003595.

486. Jeong YK, Kim IO, Kim WS, Hwang YS, Choi Y, Yeon KM. Hemolytic uremic syndrome: MR findings of CNS complications. Pediatr Radiol. 1994;24(8):585–586.

487. Hahn JS, Havens PL, Higgins JJ, O'Rourke PP, Estroff JA, Strand R. Neurological complications of hemolytic-uremic syndrome. J Child Neurol 1989; 4(2):108–113.

488. Theobald I, Kuwertz-Broking E, Schiborr M, Heindel W. Central nervous system involvement in hemolytic uremic syndrome (HUS) – a retrospective analysis of cerebral CT and MRI studies. Clin Nephrol 2001; 56(6):S3–S8.

489. Mochon M, Kaiser BA, deChadarevian JP, Polinsky MS, Baluarte HJ. Cerebral infarct with recurrence of hemolytic-uremic syndrome in a child following renal transplantation. Pediatr Nephrol 1992; 6(6):550–552.

490. Singla M, John E, Hidalgo G, Grewal D, Macmillan C. Moyamoya vasculopathy in a child after hemolytic uremic syndrome: a possible etiopathogenesis. Neuropediatrics 2008; 39(2):128–130.

491. Schlieper A, Orrbine E, Wells GA, Clulow M, McLaine PN, Rowe PC. Neuropsychological sequelae of haemolytic uraemic syndrome. Investigators of the HUS Cognitive Study. Arch Dis child 1999; 80(3):214–220.

492. Norton A, Roberts I. Management of Evans syndrome. Br J Haematol 2006; 132(2):125–137.

493. Friedmann AM, King KE, Shirey RS, Resar LM, Casella JF. Fatal autoimmune hemolytic anemia in a child due to warm-reactive immunoglobulin M antibody. J Pediatr Hematol Oncol 1998; 20(5):502–505.

494. Nowak-Wegrzyn A, King KE, Shirey RS, Chen AR, McDonough C, Lederman HM. Fatal warm autoimmune hemolytic anemia resulting from IgM autoagglutinins in an infant with severe combined immunodeficiency. J Pediatr Hematol Oncol 2001; 23(4):250–252.

495. Vargiami E, Zafeiriou DI, Gombakis NP, Kirkham FJ, Athanasiou-Metaxa M. Hemolytic anemia presenting with idiopathic intracranial hypertension. Pediatr Neurol. 2008;38(1):53–54.

496. Shiozawa Z, Ueda R, Mano T, Tsugane R, Kageyama N. Superior sagittal sinus thrombosis associated with Evans' syndrome of haemolytic anaemia. J Neurol 1985; 232(5):280–282.

497. Yilmaz S, Oren H, Irken G, Turker M, Yilmaz E, Ada E. Cerebral venous thrombosis in a patient with Evans syndrome: a rare association. Ann Hematol 2005; 84(2):124–126.

498. Cleri DJ, Moser RL, Villota FJ, Wang Y, Husain SA, Nadeem S et al. Pulmonary aspergillosis and central nervous system hemorrhage as complications of autoimmune hemolytic anemia treated with corticosteroids. South Med J 2003; 96(6):592–595.

499. Lin HC, Chen RL, Wang PJ. Paroxysmal nocturnal hemoglobinuria presenting as moyamoya syndrome. Brain Dev 1996; 18(2):157–159.

500. Audebert HJ, Planck J, Eisenburg M, Schrezenmeier H, Haberl RL. Cerebral ischemic infarction in paroxysmal nocturnal hemoglobinuria report of 2 cases and updated review of 7 previously published patients. J Neurol 2005; 252(11):1379–1386.

501. Naithani R, Mahapatra M, Dutta P, Kumar R, Pati HP, Choudhry VP. Paroxysmal nocturnal hemoglobinuria in childhood and adolescence – a retrospective analysis of 18 cases. Indian J Pediatr 2008; 75(6):575–578.

502. Pincus M, Stark RA, O'Neill JH. Ischaemic stroke complicating pyruvate kinase deficiency. Intern Med J 2003; 33(9–10):473–474.

503. Chou R, DeLoughery TG. Recurrent thromboembolic disease following splenectomy for pyruvate kinase deficiency. Am J Hematol 2001; 67(3):197–199.

504. Skardoutsou A, Voudris KA, Mastroyianni S, Vagiakou E, Magoufis G, Koukoutsakis P. Moya moya syndrome in a child with pyruvate kinase deficiency and combined prothrombotic factors. J Child Neurol 2007; 22(4):474–478.

505. Bolton-Maggs PH. Hereditary spherocytosis; new guidelines. Arch Dis Child 2004; 89(9):809–812.

506. Holz A, Woldenberg R, Miller D, Kalina P, Black K, Lane E. Moyamoya disease in a patient with hereditary spherocytosis. Pediatr Radiol 1998; 28(2):95–97.

507. Tokunaga Y, Ohga S, Suita S, Matsushima T, Hara T. Moyamoya syndrome with spherocytosis: effect of splenectomy on strokes. Pediatr Neurol 2001; 25(1):75–77.

508. Bruguier A, Clement MC, Texier P, Ponsot G. Cerebral ischemic accident and hereditary spherocytosis. Arch Fr Pediatr 1983; 40(8):653–654.

509. van Hilten JJ, Haan J, Wintzen AR, van de Nes JC, Heuvelmans JH, Aarts PA et al. Cerebral infarction in hereditary spherocytosis. Stroke 1989; 20(12):1755–1756.

510. Monge-Argiles JA, Lopez-Garcia MD, Ortega-Ortega MD, Kahn-Mesia EI, Perez-Vicente JA, Morales-Ortiz A et al. Ischemic cerebral infarction due to factor V Leiden, hereditary spherocytosis and smoking. Rev Neurol 2005; 40(2):125–126.

511. Ballas SK. Sickle cell disease: clinical management. Baillières Clin Haematol 1998; 11(1):185–214.

512. Serjeant GR. Sickle-cell disease. Lancet 1997; 350(9079):725–730.

513. Murphy MF. Diseases of the blood. In: Clinical Medicine (eds P Kumar, M Clark). London: WB Saunders, 1994; 1151–1153.

514. Pavlakis SG, Prohovnik I, Piomelli S, DeVivo DC. Neurologic complications of sickle cell disease. Adv Pediatr 1989; 36:247–276.

515. Alavi JB. Sickle cell anemia. Pathophysiology and treatment. Med Clin North Am 1984; 68(3):545–556.

516. Zafeiriou DI, Prengler M, Gombakis N, Kouskouras K, Economou M, Kardoulas A et al. Central nervous system abnormalities in asymptomatic young patients with Sbeta-thalassemia. Ann Neurol 2004; 55(6):835–839.

517. Ranney HM. Historical milestones. In: Sickle Cell Disease: Basic principles and clinical practice (eds SH Embury, RP Hebbel, N Mohondas, MH Steinberg). New York: Raven Press, 1994; 1–5.

518. Nagel RL. Origins and dispersion of the sickle gene. In: Sickle Cell Disease: Basic principles and clinical practice (eds SH Embury, RP Hebbel, N Mohondas, MH Steinberg). New York: Raven Press, 1994; 353–380.

519. Prengler M, Pavlakis SG, Prohovnik I, Adams RJ. Sickle cell disease: the Neurological Complications. Ann Neurol 2002; 51:543–552.

520. Franco RS, Yasin Z, Lohmann JM, Palascak MB, Nemeth TA, Weiner M et al. The survival characteristics of dense sickle cells. Blood 2000; 96(10):3610–3617.

521. Keidan AJ, Noguchi CT, Player M, Chalder SM, Stuart J. Erythrocyte heterogeneity in sickle cell disease: effect of deoxygenation on intracellular polymer formation and rheology of sub-populations. Br J Haematol 1989; 72(2):254–259.

522. Sultana C, Shen Y, Rattan V, Johnson C, Kalra VK. Interaction of sickle erythrocytes with endothelial cells in the presence of endothelial cell conditioned medium induces oxidant stress leading to transendothelial migration of monocytes. Blood 1998; 92(10):3924–3935.

523. French JA, Kenny D, Scott JP, Hoffmann RG, Wood JD, Hudetz AG et al. Mechanisms of stroke in sickle cell disease: sickle erythrocytes decrease cerebral blood flow in rats after nitric oxide synthase inhibition. Blood 1997; 89(12):4591–4599.

524. Nath KA, Shah V, Haggard JJ, Croatt AJ, Smith LA, Hebbel RP et al. Mechanisms of vascular instability in a transgenic mouse model of sickle cell disease. Am J Physiol Regul Integr Comp Physiol 2000; 279(6):R1949–R1955.

525. Inwald DP, Kirkham FJ, Peters MJ, Lane R, Wade A, Evans JP et al. Platelet and leucocyte activation in childhood sickle cell disease: association with nocturnal hypoxaemia. Br J Haematol 2000; 111(2):474–481.

526. Westerman MP, Green D, Gilman-Sachs A, Beaman K, Freels S, Boggio L et al. Antiphospholipid antibodies, proteins C and S, and coagulation changes in sickle cell disease. J Lab Clin Med 1999; 134(4):352–362.

527. Green D. Thrombosis in sickle cell disease. J Lab Clin Med 1999; 134(4):329–330.

528. Belcher JD, Marker PH, Weber JP, Hebbel RP, Vercellotti GM. Activated monocytes in sickle cell disease: potential role in the activation of vascular endothelium and vaso-occlusion. Blood 2000; 96(7):2451–2459.

529. Wajer SD, Taomoto M, McLeod DS, McCally RL, Nishiwaki H, Fabry ME et al. Velocity measurements of normal and sickle red blood cells in the rat retinal and choroidal vasculatures. Microvasc Res 2000; 60(3):281–293.

530. Kato GJ, Hsieh M, Machado R, Taylor J, Little J, Butman JA et al. Cerebrovascular disease associated with sickle cell pulmonary hypertension. Am J Hematol 2006; 81(7):503–510.

531. Kato GJ, Taylor JG. Pleiotropic effects of intravascular haemolysis on vascular homeostasis. Br J Haematol 2009; 148(5):690–701.

532. Platt OS, Brambilla DJ, Rosse WF, Milner PF, Castro O, Steinberg MH et al. Mortality in sickle cell disease. Life expectancy and risk factors for early death. N Engl J Med 1994; 330(23):1639–1644.

533. Wierenga KJ, Hambleton IR, Lewis NA. Survival estimates for patients with homozygous sickle-cell disease in Jamaica: a clinic-based population study. Lancet 2001; 357(9257):680–683.

534. Ohene-Frempong K, Weiner SJ, Sleeper LA, Miller ST, Embury S, Moohr JW et al. Cerebrovascular accidents in sickle cell disease: rates and risk factors. Blood 1998; 91(1):288–294.

535. Sidman JD, Fry TL. Exacerbation of sickle cell disease by obstructive sleep apnea. Arch Otolaryngol Head Neck Surg 1988; 114(8):916–917.

536. Samuels MP, Stebbens VA, Davies SC, Picton-Jones E, Southall DP. Sleep related upper airway obstruction and hypoxaemia in sickle cell disease. Arch Dis Child 1992; 67(7):925–929.

537. Homi J, Levee L, Higgs D, Thomas P, Serjeant G. Pulse oximetry in a cohort study of sickle cell disease. Clin Lab Haematol 1997; 19(1):17–22.

538. Steinberg MH. Management of sickle cell disease. N Engl J Med 1999; 340(13):1021–1030.

539. Earley CJ, Kittner SJ, Feeser BR, Gardner J, Epstein A, Wozniak MA et al. Stroke in children and sickle-cell disease: Baltimore-Washington Cooperative Young Stroke Study. Neurology 1998; 51(1):169–176.

540. Strouse JJ, Jordan LC, Lanzkron S, Casella JF. The excess burden of stroke in hospitalized adults with sickle cell disease. Am J Hematol 2009; 84(9):548–552.

541. Styles LA, Hoppe C, Klitz W, Vichinsky E, Lubin B, Trachtenberg E. Evidence for HLA-related susceptibility for stroke in children with sickle cell disease. Blood 2000; 95(11):3562–3567.

542. Powars D, Wilson B, Imbus C, Pegelow C, Allen J. The natural history of stroke in sickle cell disease. Am J Med 1978; 65(3):461–471.

543. Kirkham FJ, Calamante F, Bynevelt M, Gadian DG, Evans JP, Cox TC et al. Perfusion magnetic resonance abnormalities in patients with sickle cell disease. Ann Neurol 2001; 49(4):477–485.

544. Niebanck AE, Pollock AN, Smith-Whitley K, Raffini LJ, Zimmerman RA, Ohene-Frempong K et al. Headache in children with sickle cell disease: prevalence and associated factors. J Pediatr 2007; 151(1):67–72.

545. Prengler M, Pavlakis SG, Boyd S, Connelly A, Calamante F, Chong WK et al. Sickle cell disease: ischemia and seizures. Ann Neurol 2005; 58(2):290–302.

546. Huttenlocher PR, Moohr JW, Johns L, Brown FD. Cerebral blood flow in sickle cell cerebrovascular disease. Pediatrics 1984; 73(5):615–621.

547. Dowling MM, Quinn CT, Rogers ZR, Buchanan GR. Acute silent cerebral infarction in children with sickle cell anemia. Pediatr Blood Cancer 2010; 54(3):461–464.

548. Kimmelstiel P. Vascular occlusion and ischemic infarction in sickle cell disease. Am J Med Sci 1948; 216:11–19.

549. Makani J. Stroke in sickle cell disease in Africa: case report. East Afr Med J 2004; 81(12):657–659.

550. Hamdan JM, Mallouh AA, Ahmad MS. Hypertension and convulsions complicating sickle cell anaemia: possible role of transfusion. Ann Trop Paediatr 1984; 4(1):41–43.

551. Coley SC, Porter DA, Calamante F, Chong WK, Connelly A. Quantitative MR diffusion mapping and ciclosporine-induced neurotoxicity. AJNR Am J Neuroradiol 1999; 20(8):1507–1510.

552. Vichinsky EP, Neumayr LD, Earles AN, Williams R, Lennette ET, Dean D et al. Causes and outcomes of the acute chest syndrome in sickle cell disease. National Acute Chest Syndrome Study Group. N Engl J Med 2000; 342(25):1855–1865.

553. Gadian DG, Calamante F, Kirkham FJ, Bynevelt M, Johnson CL, Porter DA et al. Diffusion and perfusion magnetic resonance imaging in childhood stroke. J Child Neurol 2000; 15(5):279–283.

554. Adams RJ. Neurological complications. In: Sickle Cell Disease: Basic principles and clinical practice (eds SH Embury, RP Hebbel, N Mohondas, MH Steinberg). New York: Raven Press, 1994; 599–621.

555. Strouse JJ, Hulbert ML, DeBaun MR, Jordan LC, Casella JF. Primary hemorrhagic stroke in children with sickle cell disease is associated with recent transfusion and use of corticosteroids. Pediatrics 2006; 118(5):1916–1924.

556. Koshy M, Thomas C, Goodwin J. Vascular lesions in the central nervous system in sickle cell disease (neuropathology). J Assoc Acad Minor Phys. 1990;1(3):71–78.

557. Mercuri E, Faundez JC, Roberts I, Flora S, Bouza H, Cowan F et al. Neurological 'soft' signs may identify children with sickle cell disease who are at risk for stroke. Eur J Pediatr 1995; 154(2):150–156.

558. Melek I, Akgul F, Duman T, Yalcin F, Gali E. Neurological soft signs as the stroke risk in sickle cell disease. Tohoku J Exp Med 2006; 209(2):135–140.

559. Kehinde MO, Temiye EO, Danesi MA. Neurological complications of sickle cell anemia in Nigerian Africans – a case-control study. J Natl Med Assoc 2008; 100(4):394–399.

560. Kirkham FJ, Murugan V. Epidemiology and semiology of seizures in sickle cell anemia and association with cerebrovascular disease and stroke. Epilepsia 2008; 49(7):186.

561. Henry M, Driscoll MC, Miller M, Chang T, Minniti CP. Pseudotumor cerebri in children with sickle cell disease: a case series. Pediatrics 2004; 113(3 Pt 1):e265–e269.

562. Segal L, Discepola M. Idiopathic intracranial hypertension and sickle cell disease: two case reports. Can J Ophthalmol 2005; 40(6):764–767.

563. Palermo TM, Platt-Houston C, Kiska RE, Berman B. Headache symptoms in pediatric sickle cell patients. J Pediatr Hematol Oncol 2005; 27(8):420–424.

564. Silva GS, Vicari P, Figureiredo MS, Junior HC, Idagawa MH, Massaro AR. Migraine-mimicking headache and sickle cell disease: a transcranial Doppler study. Cephalalgia 2006; 26(6):678–683.

565. Shields RW, Jr, Harris JW, Clark M. Mononeuropathy in sickle cell anemia: anatomical and pathophysiological basis for its rarity. Muscle Nerve 1991; 14(4):370–374.

566. Danesi MA. Acquired aetiological factors in Nigerian Epileptics (an investigation of 378 patients). Trop Geogr Med 1983; 35(3):293–297.

567. Liu JE, Gzesh DJ, Ballas SK. The spectrum of epilepsy in sickle cell anemia. J Neurol Sci 1994; 123(1–2):6–10.

568. Gregory G, Olujohungbe A. Mandibular nerve neuropathy in sickle cell disease. Local factors. Oral Surg Oral Med Oral Pathol 1994; 77(1):66–69.

569. van Mierlo TD, van den Berg HM, Nievelstein RA, Braun KP. An unconscious girl with sickle-cell disease. Lancet 2003; 361(9352):136.

570. Sidani CA, Ballourah W, El Dassouki M, Muwakkit S, Dabbous I, Dahoui H et al. Venous sinus thrombosis leading to stroke in a patient with sickle cell disease on hydroxyurea and high hemoglobin levels: treatment with thrombolysis. Am J Hematol 2008; 83:818–820.

571. Prengler M, Pavlakis SG, Boyd S, Connelly A, Calamante F, Chong WK et al. Sickle cell disease and electroencephalogram hyperventilation. Ann Neurol 2006; 59:214–215.

572. Bridgers WH. Cerebrovascular disease accompanying sickle cell anemia. Am J Pathol 1939; 15:353–361.

573. Rothman SM, Fulling KH, Nelson JS. Sickle cell anemia and central nervous system infarction: a neuropathological study. Ann Neurol 1986; 20(6):684–690.

574. Koshy M, Thomas C, Goodwin J. Vascular lesions in the central nervous system in sickle cell disease (neuropathology). J Assoc Acad Minor Phys. 1990;1(3):71–78.

575. Stockman JA, Nigro MA, Mishkin MM, Oski FA. Occlusion of large cerebral vessels in sickle-cell anemia. N Engl J Med 1972; 287(17):846–849.

576. Wilimas J, Goff JR, Anderson HR, Jr, Langston JW, Thompson E. Efficacy of transfusion therapy for one to two years in patients with sickle cell disease and cerebrovascular accidents. J Pediatr 1980; 96(2):205–208.

577. Russell MO, Goldberg HI, Hodson A, Kim HC, Halus J, Reivich M et al. Effect of transfusion therapy on arteriographic abnormalities and on recurrence of stroke in sickle cell disease. Blood 1984; 63(1):162–169.

578. Zimmerman RA, Gill F, Goldberg HI, Bilaniuk LT, Hackney DB, Johnson M et al. MRI of sickle cell cerebral infarction. Neuroradiology 1987; 29(3):232–237.

579. Adams RJ, Nichols FT, Figurueroa R, McKie V, Lott T. Transcranial Doppler correlation with cerebral angiography in sickle cell disease. Stroke 1992; 23(8):1073–1077.

580. Garcia JH. Thrombosis of cranial veins and sinuses: brain parenchymal effects. In: Cerebral Sinus Thrombosis: experimental and clinical aspects (eds KM Einhaupl, O Kempski, A Baethmann). Plenum Press; 1990.

581. Di Rolo C, Jourdan C, Terrier A, Artru F. Sickle cell anemia and internal cerebral vein thrombosis. Ann Fr Anesth Reanim 1997; 16(8):967–969.

582. Torvik A. The pathogenesis of watershed infarcts in the brain. Stroke 1984; 15(2):221–223.

583. Rodgers GP, Clark CM, Larson SM, Rapoport SI, Nienhuis AW, Schechter AN. Brain glucose metabolism in neurologically normal patients with sickle cell disease. Regional alterations. Arch Neurol 1988; 45(1):78–82.

584. Bogousslavsky J, Regli F. Borderzone infarctions distal to internal carotid artery occlusion: prognostic implications. Ann Neurol 1986; 20(3):346–350.

585. Kaul DK, Fabry ME, Nagel RL. Vaso-occlusion by sickle cells: evidence for selective trapping of dense red cells. Blood 1986; 68(5):1162–1166.

586. Oguz M, Aksungur EH, Soyupak SK, Yildirim AU. Vein of Galen and sinus thrombosis with bilateral thalamic infarcts in sickle cell anaemia: CT follow-up and angiographic demonstration. Neuroradiology 1994; 36(2):155–156.

587. Khademian Z, Speller-Brown B, Nouraie SM, Minniti CP. Reversible posterior leuko-encephalopathy in children with sickle cell disease. Pediatr Blood Cancer 2009; 52(3):373–375.

588. Lee KH, McKie VC, Sekul EA, Adams RJ, Nichols FT. Unusual encephalopathy after acute chest syndrome in sickle cell disease: acute necrotizing encephalitis. J Pediatr Hematol Oncol 2002; 24(7):585–588.

589. Upadhyaya VS, Bynevelt M, Cox TC, Chong K, Ganesan V, Prengler M et al. Generalized radiological abnormality associated with acute neurological presentations in sickle cell disease. Dev Med Child Neurol 2004; 47(Suppl 101): 17.

590. Rinkel GJ, van GJ, Wijdicks EF. Subarachnoid hemorrhage without detectable aneurysm. A review of the causes. Stroke 1993; 24(9):1403–1409.

591. Diggs LW, Brookoff D. Multiple cerebral aneurysms in patients with sickle cell disease. South Med J 1993; 86(4):377–379.

592. Preul MC, Cendes F, Just N, Mohr G. Intracranial aneurysms and sickle cell anemia: multiplicity and propensity for the vertebrobasilar territory. Neurosurgery 1998; 42(5):971–977.

593. Vernet O, Montes JL, O'Gorman AM, Baruchel S, Farmer JP. Encephaloduroarterio-synangiosis in a child with sickle cell anemia and moyamoya disease. Pediatr Neurol 1996; 14(3):226–230.

594. Dobson SR, Holden KR, Nietert PJ, Cure JK, Laver JH, Disco D et al. Moyamoya syndrome in childhood sickle cell disease: a predictive factor for recurrent cerebrovascular events. Blood 2002; 99(9):3144–3150.

595. Inusa B, Prengler M, Pohl KR, Saunders D, Bynevelt M, Cox T et al. Risk factors for stroke recurrence in sickle cell disease. Br J Haematol 2007; 137(1): 73–74.

596. Pavlakis SG, Bello J, Prohovnik I, Sutton M, Ince C, Mohr JP et al. Brain infarction in sickle cell anemia: magnetic resonance imaging correlates. Ann Neurol 1988; 23(2):125–130.

597. Kugler S, Anderson B, Cross D, Sharif Z, Sano M, Haggerty R et al. Abnormal cranial magnetic resonance imaging scans in sickle-cell disease. Neurological correlates and clinical implications. Arch Neurol 1993; 50(6):629–635.

598. Moser FG, Miller ST, Bello JA, Pegelow CH, Zimmerman RA, Wang WC et al. The spectrum of brain MR abnormalities in sickle-cell disease: a report from the Cooperative Study of Sickle Cell Disease. AJNR Am J Neuroradiol 1996; 17(5):965–972.

599. Baldeweg T, Hogan AM, Saunders DE, Telfer P, Gadian DG, Vargha-Khadem F et al. Detecting white matter injury in sickle cell disease using voxel-based morphometry. Ann Neurol 2006; 59(4):662–672.

600. Connelly A, Chong WK, Johnson CL, Ganesan V, Gadian DG, Kirkham FJ. Diffusion weighted magnetic resonance imaging of compromised tissue in stroke. Arch Dis Child 1997; 77(1):38–41.

601. Armstrong FD, Thompson RJ, Jr, Wang W, Zimmerman R, Pegelow CH, Miller S et al. Cognitive functioning and brain magnetic resonance imaging in children with sickle cell disease. Neuropsychology Committee of the Cooperative Study of Sickle Cell Disease. Pediatrics 1996; 97(6 Pt 1):864–870.

602. Kinney TR, Sleeper LA, Wang WC, Zimmerman RA, Pegelow CH, Ohene-Frempong K et al. Silent cerebral infarcts in sickle cell anemia: a risk factor analysis. The Cooperative Study of Sickle Cell Disease. Pediatrics 1999; 103(3):640–645.

603. Bernaudin F, Verlhac S, Freard F, Roudot-Thoraval F, Benkerrou M, Thuret I et al. Multicenter prospective study of children with sickle cell disease: radiographic and psychometric correlation. J Child Neurol 2000; 15(5):333–343.

604. Miller ST, Macklin EA, Pegelow CH, Kinney TR, Sleeper LA, Bello JA et al. Silent infarction as a risk factor for overt stroke in children with sickle cell anemia: a report from the Cooperative Study of Sickle Cell Disease. J Pediatr 2001; 139(3):385–390.

605. Pegelow CH, Macklin EA, Moser FG, Wang WC, Bello JA, Miller ST et al. Longitudinal changes in brain magnetic resonance imaging findings in children with sickle cell disease. Blood 2002; 99(8):3014–3018.

606. Sarnaik S, Casella JF, Barton B, Afif M, Airewele G, Berman B et al. Elevated systolic blood pressure and low fetal hemoglobin are risk factors for silent cerebral infarcts in children with sickle cell anemia. Blood 2010; 114(Suppl);262.

607. Ganesan V, Prengler M, Wade A, Kirkham FJ. Clinical and radiological recurrence after childhood arterial ischemic stroke. Circulation 2006; 114(20):2170–2177.

608. Dlamini N, Saunders DE, Bynevelt M, Hewes DK, Cox TC, Chong K et al. Covert cerebral infarction on MRI in a UK-based population of children with sickle cell disease. Neurology 2009; 72(11):A135.

609. Thangarajh M, Fuchs D, McKinstry RC, Noetzel MJ, Casella JF, Vendt BA et al. Silent cerebral infarcts are not associated with magnetic resonance imaging-defined intracranial vasculopathy or with elevated transcranial Doppler measurements in children with sickle cell anemia. Neurology 2009; 72(11):A268–A269.

610. DeBaun MR, Schatz J, Siegel MJ, Koby M, Craft S, Resar L et al. Cognitive screening examinations for silent cerebral infarcts in sickle cell disease. Neurology 1998; 50(6):1678–1682.

611. Watkins KE, Hewes DK, Connelly A, Kendall BE, Kingsley DP, Evans JE et al. Cognitive deficits associated with frontal-lobe infarction in children with sickle cell disease. Dev Med Child Neurol 1998; 40(8):536–543.

612. Steen RG, Langston JW, Reddick WE, Ogg R, Chen G, Wang WC. Quantitative MR imaging of children with sickle cell disease: striking T1 elevation in the thalamus. J Magn Reson Imaging 1996; 6(1):226–234.

613. Steen RG, Langston JW, Ogg RJ, Xiong X, Ye Z, Wang WC. Diffuse T1 reduction in grey matter of sickle cell disease patients: evidence of selective vulnerability to damage? Magn Reson Imaging 1999; 17(4):503–515.

614. Steen RG, Hunte M, Traipe E, Hurh P, Wu S, Bilaniuk L et al. Brain T1 in young children with sickle cell disease: evidence of early abnormalities in brain development. Magn Reson Imaging 2004; 22(3):299–306.

615. Schatz J, Buzan R. Decreased corpus callosum size in sickle cell disease: relationship with cerebral infarcts and cognitive functioning. J Int Neuropsychol Soc 2006; 12(1):24–33.

616. Steen RG, Emudianughe T, Hunte M, Glass J, Wu S, Xiong X et al. Brain volume in pediatric patients with sickle cell disease: evidence of volumetric growth delay? AJNR Am J Neuroradiol 2005; 26(3):455–462.

617. Camitta B. The anemias. In: Nelson Textbook of Pediatrics (eds WE Nelson, RE Behrman, RM Kliegman, AM Arvin). Philadelphia: WB Saunders Company, 1996; 1379.

618. Steen RG, Xiong X, Mulhern RK, Langston JW, Wang WC. Subtle brain abnormalities in children with sickle cell disease: relationship to blood hematocrit. Ann Neurol 1999; 45(3):279–286.

619. Chen R, Pawlak MA, Flynn TB, Krejza J, Herskovits EH, Melhem ER. Brain morphometry and intelligence quotient measurements in children with sickle cell disease. J Dev Behav Pediatr 2009; 30(6):509–517.

620. Steen RG, Miles MA, Helton KJ, Strawn S, Wang W, Xiong X et al. Cognitive impairment in children with hemoglobin SS sickle cell disease: relationship to MR imaging findings and hematocrit. AJNR Am J Neuroradiol 2003; 24(3):382–389.

621. Steen RG, Xiong X, Langston JW, Helton KJ. Brain injury in children with sickle cell disease: prevalence and etiology. Ann Neurol 2003; 54(5):564–572.

622. Sébire G, Tabarki B, Saunders DE, Leroy I, Liesner R, Saint-Martin C et al. Venous sinus thrombosis in children. Brain 2005; 128(3):477–489.

623. Naran AD, Fontana L. Sickle cell disease with orbital infarction and epidural hematoma. Pediatr Radiol 2001; 31(4):257–259.

624. Adeloye A, Odeku E. Nervous system in sickle cell disease. Afr J Med Sci 1970; 1:33.

625. Borosh TC, Weiner WJ. Large vessel disease in sickle cell anemia. J Neurol Neurosurg Psychiatr 1986; 39:1236.

626. Gilliams A, McMahon L, Weinberg G, Carter A. MRA of the intracranial circulation in asymptomatic patients with sickle cell disease. Pediatr Radiol 1998; 28:283.

627. Kandeel AY, Zimmerman RA, Ohene-Frempong K. Comparison of magnetic resonance angiography and conventional angiography in sickle cell disease: clinical significance and reliability. Neuroradiology 1996; 38(5):409–416.

628. Seibert JJ, Glasier CM, Kirby RS, Allison JW, James CA, Becton DL et al. Transcranial Doppler, MRA, and MRI as a screening examination for cerebrovascular disease in patients with sickle cell anemia: an 8-year study. Pediatr Radiol 1998; 28(3):138–142.

629. Abboud MR, Cure J, Granger S, Gallagher D, Hsu L, Wang W et al. Magnetic resonance angiography in children with sickle cell disease and abnormal transcranial Doppler ultrasonography findings enrolled in the STOP study. Blood 2004; 103(7):2822–2826.

630. Wang WC, Langston JW, Steen RG, Wynn LW, Mulhern RK, Wilimas JA et al. Abnormalities of the central nervous system in very young children with sickle cell anemia. J Pediatr 1998; 132(6):994–998.

631. Wang WC, Pavlakis SG, Helton KJ, McKinstry RC, Casella JF, Adams RJ et al. MRI abnormalities of the brain in one-year-old children with sickle cell anemia. Pediatr Blood Cancer 2008; 51(5):643–646.

632. Steen RG, Langston JW, Ogg RJ, Manci E, Mulhern RK, Wang W. Ectasia of the basilar artery in children with sickle cell disease: relationship to hematocrit and psychometric measures. J Stroke Cerebrovasc Dis 1998; 7(1):32–43.

633. Steen RG, Reddick WE, Glass JO, Wang WC. Evidence of cranial artery ectasia in sickle cell disease patients with ectasia of the basilar artery. J Stroke Cerebrovasc Dis 1998; 7(5):330–338.

634. Bhattacharya A, Newell H, Evanson J, Kirkham F, Telfer P. Extracranial carotid artery occlusion in children with sickle cell disease. Br J Haematol 2007; 137(1):217.

635. Quinn CT, Variste J, Dowling MM. Haemoglobin oxygen saturation is a determinant of cerebral artery blood flow velocity in children with sickle cell anaemia. Br J Haematol 2009; 145(4):500–505.

636. Gorman MJ, Nystrom K, Carbonella J, Pearson H. Submandibular TCD approach detects post-bulb ICA stenosis in children with sickle cell anemia. Neurology 2009; 73(5):362–365.

637. Jordan LC, Strouse JJ. Will submandibular TCD prevent stroke in children with sickle cell anemia? Neurology 2009; 73(5):340–341.

638. Deane CR, Goss D, Bartram J, Pohl KR, Height SE, Sibtain N et al. Extracranial internal carotid arterial disease in children with sickle cell anemia. Haematologica 2010; Mar 10 95(8):1287–1292.

639. Adams RJ, McKie VC, Carl EM, Nichols FT, Perry R, Brock K et al. Long-term stroke risk in children with sickle cell disease screened with transcranial Doppler. Ann Neurol 1997; 42(5):699–704.

640. Adams R, McKie V, Nichols F, Carl E, Zhang DL, McKie K et al. The use of transcranial ultrasonography to predict stroke in sickle cell disease. N Engl J Med 1992; 326(9):605–610.

641. Adams RJ, McKie VC, Hsu L, Files B, Vichinsky E, Pegelow C et al. Prevention of a first stroke by transfusions in children with sickle cell anemia and abnormal results on transcranial Doppler ultrasonography. N Engl J Med 1998; 339(1):5–11.

642. Adams RJ, Brambilla D. Discontinuing prophylactic transfusions used to prevent stroke in sickle cell disease. N Engl J Med 2005; 353(26):2769–2778.

643. Adams RJ, Brambilla DJ, Granger S, Gallagher D, Vichinsky E, Abboud MR et al. Stroke and conversion to high risk in children screened with transcranial Doppler ultrasound during the STOP study. Blood 2004; 103(10):3689–3694.

644. deVeber G, Kirkham F. Guidelines for the treatment and prevention of stroke in children. Lancet Neurol 2008; 7(11):983–985.

645. Fullerton HJ, Adams RJ, Zhao S, Johnston SC. Declining stroke rates in Californian children with sickle cell disease. Blood 2004; 104(2):336–339.

646. Telfer P, Coen P, Chakravorty S, Wilkey O, Evans J, Newell H et al. Clinical outcomes in children with sickle cell disease living in England: a neonatal cohort in East London. Haematologica 2007; 92(7):905–912.

647. Mazumdar M, Heeney MM, Sox CM, Lieu TA. Preventing stroke among children with sickle cell anemia: an analysis of strategies that involve transcranial Doppler testing and chronic transfusion. Pediatrics 2007; 120(4):e1107–e1116.

648. Minniti CP, Gidvani VK, Bulas D, Brown WA, Vezina G, Driscoll MC. Transcranial Doppler changes in children with sickle cell disease on transfusion therapy. J Pediatr Hematol Oncol 2004; 26(10):626–630.

649. Hogan AM, Kirkham FJ, Prengler M, Telfer P, Lane R, Vargha-Khadem F et al. An exploratory study of physiological correlates of neurodevelopmental delay in infants with sickle cell anaemia. Br J Haematol 2006; 132(1):99–107.

650. Siegel MJ, Luker GD, Glauser TA, DeBaun MR. Cerebral infarction in sickle cell disease: transcranial Doppler US versus neurologic examination. Radiology 1995; 197(1):191–194.

651. Verlhac S, Bernaudin F, Tortrat D, Brugieres P, Mage K, Gaston A et al. Detection of cerebrovascular disease in patients with sickle cell disease using transcranial Doppler sonography: correlation with MRI, MRA and conventional angiography. Pediatr Radiol 1995; 25(Suppl 1):S14–S19.

652. Kotecha K, Prengler M, Saunders DE, Hewes DK, Kirkham FJ, Telfer P. Change over time of transcranial Doppler cerebral blood flow velocity and the relationship with turbulence on magnetic resonance angiography in patients with sickle cell disease. Blood 2005; 106:3799.

653. Rees DC, Dick MC, Height SE, O'Driscoll S, Pohl KR, Goss DE et al. A simple index using age, hemoglobin, and aspartate transaminase predicts increased intracerebral blood velocity as measured by transcranial Doppler scanning in children with sickle cell anemia. Pediatrics 2008; 121(6):e1628–e1632.

654. Brass LM, Pavlakis SG, DeVivo D, Piomelli S, Mohr JP. Transcranial Doppler measurements of the middle cerebral artery. Effect of hematocrit. Stroke 1988; 19(12):1466–1469.

655. Makani J, Kirkham FJ, Komba A, Jala-Agbo T, Otieno G, Fegan G et al. Risk factors for high cerebral blood flow velocity and death in Kenyan children with sickle cell anaemia: role of haemoglobin oxygen saturation and febrile illness. Br J Haematol 2009; 145(4):529–532.

656. Silva CM, Giovani P, Viana MB. High reticulocyte count is an independent risk factor for cerebrovascular disease in children with sickle cell anemia. Pediatr Blood Cancer. 2011;56(1):116–121.

657. O'Driscoll S, Height SE, Dick MC, Rees DC. Serum lactate dehydrogenase activity as a biomarker in children with sickle cell disease. Br J Haematol 2008; 140(2):206–209.

658. Prohovnik I, Pavlakis SG, Piomelli S, Bello J, Mohr JP, Hilal S et al. Cerebral hyperemia, stroke, and transfusion in sickle cell disease. Neurology 1989; 39(3):344–348.

659. Hurlet-Jensen AM, Prohovnik I, Pavlakis SG, Piomelli S. Effects of total hemoglobin and hemoglobin S concentration on cerebral blood flow during transfusion therapy to prevent stroke in sickle cell disease. Stroke 1994; 25(8):1688–1692.

660. Helton KJ, Paydar A, Glass J, Weirich EM, Hankins J, Li CS et al. Arterial spin-labeled perfusion combined with segmentation techniques to evaluate cerebral blood flow in white and grey matter of children with sickle cell anemia. Pediatr Blood Cancer 2009; 52(1):85–91.

661. Numaguchi Y, Haller JS, Humbert JR, Robinson AE, Lindstrom WW, Gruenauer LM et al. Cerebral blood flow mapping using stable xenon-enhanced CT in sickle cell cerebrovascular disease. Neuroradiology 1990; 32(4):289–295.

662. Herold S, Frackowiak RS, Neil-Dwyer G. Studies on cerebral blood flow and oxygen metabolism in patients with established cerebral infarcts undergoing omental transposition. Stroke 1987; 18(1):46–51.

663. Powars DR, Conti PS, Wong WY, Groncy P, Hyman C, Smith E et al. Cerebral vasculopathy in sickle cell anemia: diagnostic contribution of positron emission tomography. Blood 1999; 93(1):71–79.

664. Al-Kandari FA, Owunwanne A, Syed GM, Ar MR, Elgazzar AH, Shiekh M et al. Regional cerebral blood flow in patients with sickle cell disease: study with single photon emission computed tomography. Ann Nucl Med 2007; 21(8):439–445.

665. Yalcin H, Melek I, Okuyucu E, Reyhan M, Akgül F, Serarslan G, Duman T, Yalçin F. Sickle cell disease with regional silent cerebral infarction detected by SPECT. Clin Nucl Med. 2007;32(11):842–843.

666. Kedar A, Drane WE, Shaeffer D, Nicole M, Adams C. Measurement of cerebrovascular flow reserve in pediatric patients with sickle cell disease. Pediatr Blood Cancer 2006; 46(2):234–238.

667. Parsa MA, Mehregany D, Schulz SC. Psychiatric manifestation of sickle cell disease and findings on single photon emission computed tomography. Psychosomatics 1992; 33(2):239–241.

668. Gomes de AP, Zanetti MV, Elkis H. Refractory psychotic symptoms in a patient with homozygous sickle cell disease: a 24-month follow-up. Prog Neuropsychopharmacol Biol Psychiatry 2008; 32(1):301–303.

669. Prengler M, Calamante F, Connelly A, Saunders D, Chong WK, Davies SC et al. Blood transfusion in sickle cell disease does not necessarily improve cerebral perfusion in the short or long term. Dev Med Child Neurol 2003; 46:10.

670. Tzika AA, Massoth RJ, Ball WS, Jr, Majumdar S, Dunn RS, Kirks DR. Cerebral perfusion in children: detection with dynamic contrast-enhanced T2*-weighted MR images. Radiology 1993; 187(2):449–458.

671. Oguz KK, Golay X, Pizzini FB, Freer CA, Winrow N, Ichord R et al. Sickle-cell disease: continuous arterial spin-labelling perfsion MR imaging in children. Radiology 2003; 227(2):567–574.

672. Strouse JJ, Cox CS, Melhem ER, Lu H, Kraut MA, Razumovsky A et al. Inverse correlation between cerebral blood flow measured by continuous arterial spin-labeling (CASL) MRI and neurocognitive function in children with sickle cell anemia (SCA). Blood 2006; 108(1):379–381.

673. van den Tweel XW, Nederveen AJ, Majoie CB, van der Lee JH, Wagener-Schimmel L, van Walderveen MA, Poll The BT, Nederkoorn PJ, Heijboer H, Fijnvandraat K. Cerebral blood flow measurement in children with sickle cell disease using continuous arterial spin labeling at 3.0-Tesla MRI. Stroke. 2009;40(3):795–800.

674. Nur E, Kim YS, Truijen J, van Beers EJ, Davis SC, Brandjes DP et al. Cerebrovascular reserve capacity is impaired in patients with sickle cell disease. Blood 2009; 114(16):3473–3478.

675. Kehn-Alafun T, Callaghan B, Dingle-Gavlak J, Laverty A, Lane R, Kirkham FJ. Changes in cerebral blood flow velocity during sleep in children with sickle cell anaemia. Dev Med Child Neurol 2005; 48(Suppl 104):15.

676. Kirkham FJ, Padayachee TS, Parsons S, Seargeant LS, House FR, Gosling RG. Transcranial measurement of blood velocities in the basal cerebral arteries using pulsed Doppler ultrasound: velocity as an index of flow. Ultrasound Med Biol 1986; 12(1):15–21.

677. Kim YS, Nur E, van Beers EJ, Truijen J, Davis SC, Biemond BJ et al. Dynamic cerebral autoregulation in homozygous sickle cell disease. Stroke 2009; 40(3):808–814.

678. Prengler M, Ganesan V, Dick MC. Risk factors for recurrent transient ischaemic event and stroke in sickle cell disease. Dev Med Child Neurol 2001; 43:27.

679. Kirkham FJ. Therapy insight: stroke risk and its management in patients with sickle cell disease. Nat Clin Pract Neurol 2007; 3(5):264–278.

680. Wang WC. Central nervous system complications of sickle cell disease in children: an overview. Child Neuropsychol 2007; 13(2):103–119.

681. Balkaran B, Char G, Morris JS, Thomas PW, Serjeant BE, Serjeant GR. Stroke in a cohort of patients with homozygous sickle cell disease. J Pediatr 1992; 120(3):360–366.

682. Miller ST, Sleeper LA, Pegelow CH, Enos LE, Wang WC, Weiner SJ et al. Prediction of adverse outcomes in children with sickle cell disease. N Engl J Med 2000; 342(2):83–89.

683. Tam DA. Protein C and protein S activity in sickle cell disease and stroke. J Child Neurol 1997; 12(1):19–21.

684. Liesner R, Mackie I, Cookson J, McDonald S, Chitolie A, Donohoe S et al. Prothrombotic changes in children with sickle cell disease: relationships to cerebrovascular disease and transfusion. Br J Haematol 1998; 103(4):1037–1044.

685. Rodgers GP, Walker EC, Podgor MJ. Is 'relative' hypertension a risk factor for vaso-occlusive complications in sickle cell disease? Am J Med Sci 1993; 305(3):150–156.

686. Pegelow CH, Colangelo L, Steinberg M, Wright EC, Smith J, Phillips G et al. Natural history of blood pressure in sickle cell disease: risks for stroke and death associated with relative hypertension in sickle cell anemia. Am J Med 1997; 102(2):171–177.

687. Osuntokun BO. Undernutrition and infectious disorders as risk factors in stroke (with special reference to Africans). Adv Neurol 1979; 25:161–174.

688. Robertson PL, Aldrich MS, Hanash SM, Goldstein GW. Stroke associated with obstructive sleep apnea in a child with sickle cell anemia. Ann Neurol 1988; 23(6):614–616.

689. Davies SC, Stebbens VA, Samuels MP, Southall DP. Upper airways obstruction and cerebrovascular accident in children with sickle cell anaemia. Lancet 1989; 2(8657):283–284.

690. Quinn CT, Sargent JW. Daytime steady-state haemoglobin desaturation is a risk factor for overt stroke in children with sickle cell anaemia. Br J Haematol 2008; 140(3):336–339.

691. Nordness ME, Lynn J, Zacharisen MC, Scott PJ, Kelly KJ. Asthma is a risk factor for acute chest syndrome and cerebral vascular accidents in children with sickle cell disease. Clin Mol Allergy 2005; 3(1):2.

692. Ali SB, Reid M, Fraser R, MooSang M, Ali A. Seizures in the Jamaica cohort study of sickle cell disease. Br J Haematol. 2010;151(3):265–272.

693. Swerlick RA, Eckman JR, Kumar A, Jeitler M, Wick TM. Alpha 4 beta 1-integrin expression on sickle reticulocytes: vascular cell adhesion molecule-1-dependent binding to endothelium. Blood 1993; 82(6):1891–1899.

694. Hogan AM, Telfer P, Kirkham FJ. The impact of infection in early childhood on intellectual function in adolescence: evidence from children with sickle cell disease. Br J Haematol 2007; 137(1):29.

695. de Montalembert M, Beauvais P, Bachir D, Galacteros F, Girot R. Cerebrovascular accidents in sickle cell disease. Risk factors and blood transfusion influence. French Study Group on Sickle Cell Disease. Eur J Pediatr 1993; 152(3):201–204.

696. Goyal M, Miller ST, Hammerschlag MR, Gelling M, Gaydos CA, Hardick J et al. Is *Chlamydia pneumoniae* infection associated with stroke in children with sickle cell disease? Pediatrics 2004; 113(4):e318–e321.

697. Ajulo SO. The significance of recurrent tonsillitis in sickle cell disease. Clin Otolaryngol Allied Sci 1994; 19(3):230–233.

698. Driscoll MC, Hurlet A, Styles L, McKie V, Files B, Olivieri N et al. Stroke risk in siblings with sickle cell anemia. Blood 2003; 101(6):2401–2404.

699. Kwiatkowski JL, Hunter JV, Smith-Whitley K, Katz ML, Shults J, Ohene-Frempong K. Transcranial Doppler ultrasonography in siblings with sickle cell disease. Br J Haematol. 2003;121(6):932–937.

700. Hsu LL, Miller ST, Wright E, Kutlar A, McKie V, Wang W et al. Alpha thalassemia is associated with decreased risk of abnormal transcranial Doppler ultrasonography in children with sickle cell anemia. J Pediatr Hematol Oncol 2003; 25(8):622–628.

701. Kirkham FJ. Is there a genetic basis for pediatric stroke? Curr Opin Pediatr 2003; 15(6):547–558.

702. Taylor JG, Tang D, Foster CB, Serjeant GR, Rodgers GP, Chanock SJ. Patterns of low-affinity immunoglobulin receptor polymorphisms in stroke and homozygous sickle cell disease. Am J Hematol 2002; 69(2):109–114.

703. Hoppe C, Klitz W, Noble J, Vigil L, Vichinsky E, Styles L. Distinct HLA associations by stroke subtype in children with sickle cell anemia. Blood 2003; 101(7):2865–2869.

704. Hoppe C, Cheng S, Grow M, Silbergleit A, Klitz W, Trachtenberg E et al. A novel multilocus genotyping assay to identify genetic predictors of stroke in sickle cell anaemia. Br J Haematol 2001; 114(3):718–720.

705. Sebastiani P, Ramoni MF, Nolan V, Baldwin CT, Steinberg MH. Genetic dissection and prognostic modeling of overt stroke in sickle cell anemia. Nat Genet 2005; 37(4):435–440.

706. Pegelow CH, Adams RJ, McKie V, Abboud M, Berman B, Miller ST et al. Risk of recurrent stroke in patients with sickle cell disease treated with erythrocyte transfusions. J Pediatr 1995; 126(6):896–899.

707. Powars DR. Management of cerebral vasculopathy in children with sickle cell anaemia. Br J Haematol 2000; 108(4):666–678.

708. Banka RS, Goldberg HI, Russel MO, Slater R, Reivich M. Regional cerebral blood flow in children with stroke secondary to sickle cell vascular disease. Acta Neurol Scand Suppl 1977; 64:482–483.

709. Walsh JW, Stevens DB, Young AB. Traumatic paraplegia in children without contiguous spinal fracture or dislocation. Neurosurgery 1983; 12(4):439–445.

710. Scharf MB, Lobel JS, Caldwell E, Cameron BF, Kramer M, De MJ et al. Nocturnal oxygen desaturation in patients with sickle cell anemia. JAMA 1983; 249(13):1753–1755.

711. Krishnan S, Siegel J, Pullen G, Jr, Hevelow M, Dampier C, Stuart M. Increased von Willebrand factor antigen and high molecular weight multimers in sickle cell disease associated with nocturnal hypoxemia. Thromb Res 2008; 122(4):455–458.

712. Portnoy BA, Herion JC. Neurological manifestations in sickle-cell disease, with a review of the literature and emphasis on the prevalence of hemiplegia. Ann Intern Med 1972; 76(4):643–652.

713. Wood DH. Cerebrovascular complications of sickle cell anemia. Stroke 1978; 9(1):73–75.

714. Moohr JW, Wilson H, Pang EJ. Strokes and their management in sickle cell disease. In: Comparative Clinical Aspects of Sickle Cell Disease (eds W Fried). Amsterdam: Elsevier, 1982; 101–111.

715. Njamnshi AK, Mbong EN, Wonkam A, Ongolo-Zogo P, Djientcheu VD, Sunjoh FL et al. The epidemiology of stroke in sickle cell patients in Yaounde, Cameroon. J Neurol Sci 2006; 250(1–2):79–84.

716. Fatunde OJ, Lagunju IA, Adeniyi OF, Orimadegun AE. Non-traumatic paraplegia in Nigerian children presenting at the University College Hospital, Ibadan. Afr J Med Med Sci 2006; 35(1):37–41.

717. Scothorn DJ, Price C, Schwartz D, Terrill C, Buchanan GR, Shurney W et al. Risk of recurrent stroke in children with sickle cell disease receiving blood transfusion therapy for at least five years after initial stroke. J Pediatr 2002; 140(3):348–354.

718. Hulbert ML, McKinstry RC, Lacey JL, Moran CJ, Panepinto JA, Thompson AA et al. Silent cerebral infarcts occur despite regular blood transfusion therapy after first stroke in children with sickle cell disease. Blood 2010; 117(3):772–779.

719. Kirkham FJ, DeBaun MR. Stroke in children with sickle cell disease. Curr Treat Options Neurol 2004; 6(5):357–375.

720. Hulbert ML, Scothorn DJ, Panepinto JA, Scott JP, Buchanan GR, Sarnaik S et al. Exchange blood transfusion compared with simple

transfusion for first overt stroke is associated with a lower risk of subsequent stroke: a retrospective cohort study of 137 children with sickle cell anemia. J Pediatr 2006; 149(5):710–712.

721. Uchida K, Rackoff WR, Ohene-Frempong K, Kim HC, Reilly MP, Asakura T. Effect of erythrocytapheresis on arterial oxygen saturation and hemoglobin oxygen affinity in patients with sickle cell disease. Am J Hematol 1998; 59(1):5–8.

722. Steen RG, Koury BSM, Granja CI, Xiong X, Wu S, Glass JO et al. Effect of ionizing radiation on the human brain: white matter and grey matter T1 in pediatric brain tumor patients treated with conformal radiation therapy. Int J Radiat Oncol Biol Phys 2001; 49(1):79–91.

723. Goldberg MA, Brugnara C, Dover GJ, Schapira L, Charache S, Bunn HF. Treatment of sickle cell anemia with hydroxyurea and erythropoietin. N Engl J Med 1990; 323(6):366–372.

724. Kaul DK, Fabry ME, Costantini F, Rubin EM, Nagel RL. In vivo demonstration of red cell-endothelial interaction, sickling and altered microvascular response to oxygen in the sickle transgenic mouse. J Clin Invest 1995; 96(6):2845–2853.

725. Ware RE, Zimmerman SA, Schultz WH. Hydroxyurea as an alternative to blood transfusions for the prevention of recurrent stroke in children with sickle cell disease. Blood 1999; 94(9):3022–3026.

726. Wang WC, Wynn LW, Rogers ZR, Scott JP, Lane PA, Ware RE. A two-year pilot trial of hydroxyurea in very young children with sickle-cell anemia. J Pediatr 2001; 139(6):790–796.

727. Ware RE, Zimmerman SA, Sylvestre PB, Mortier NA, Davis JS, Treem WR et al. Prevention of secondary stroke and resolution of transfusional iron overload in children with sickle cell anemia using hydroxyurea and phlebotomy. J Pediatr 2004; 145(3):346–352.

728. Zimmerman SA, Schultz WH, Burgett S, Mortier NA, Ware RE. Hydroxyurea therapy lowers transcranial Doppler flow velocities in children with sickle cell anemia. Blood 2007; 110(3):1043–1047.

729. Hogan AM, Hill CM, Bucks R, Telfer P, Kirkham FJ. Adenotonsillectomy is not associated with reduction of middle cerebral artery velocity in sickle cell disease. Pediatrics 2007; 120:236–237.

730. Zipursky A, Robieux IC, Brown EJ, Shaw D, O'Brodovich H, Kellner JD et al. Oxygen therapy in sickle cell disease. Am J Pediatr Hematol Oncol 1992; 14(3):222–228.

731. Kirkham FJ, Lerner NB, Noetzel M, DeBaun MR, Datta AK, Rees DC et al. Trials in sickle cell disease. Pediatr Neurol 2006; 34(6):450–458.

732. Marshall MJ, Bucks RS, Hogan AM, Hambleton IR, Height SE, Dick MC et al. Auto-adjusting positive airway pressure in children with sickle cell anemia: results of a phase I randomized controlled trial. Haematologica 2009; 94(7):1006–1010.

733. Johnson MC, Kirkham FJ, Redline S, Rosen CL, Yan Y, Roberts I et al. Left ventricular hypertrophy and diastolic dysfunction in children with sickle cell disease are related to asleep and waking oxygen desaturation. Blood 2010; 116(1):16–21.

734. Ganesan V. Moyamoya: to cut or not to cut is not the only question. A paediatric neurologist's perspective. Dev Med Child Neurol. 2010;52(1):10–13.

735. Hogan AM, Kirkham FJ, Isaacs EB, Wade AM, Vargha-Khadem F. Intellectual decline in children with moyamoya and sickle cell anaemia. Dev Med Child Neurol 2005; 47(12):824–829.

736. Hankinson TC, Bohman LE, Heyer G, Licursi M, Ghatan S, Feldstein NA et al. Surgical treatment of moyamoya syndrome in patients with sickle cell anemia: outcome following encephaloduroarteriosynangiosis. J Neurosurg Pediatr 2008; 1(3):211–216.

737. Smith ER, McClain CD, Heeney M, Scott RM. Pial synangiosis in patients with moyamoya syndrome and sickle cell anemia: perioperative management and surgical outcome. Neurosurg Focus 2009; 26(4):E10.

738. Ganesan V. Surgical revascularization for moyamoya in sickle cell disease. Dev Med Child Neurol 2007; 49(S1):3.

739. Walters MC, Storb R, Patience M, Leisenring W, Taylor T, Sanders JE et al. Impact of bone marrow transplantation for symptomatic sickle cell disease: an interim report. Multicenter investigation of bone marrow transplantation for sickle cell disease. Blood 2000; 95(6):1918–1924.

740. Walters MC, Patience M, Leisenring W, Eckman JR, Scott JP, Mentzer WC et al. Bone marrow transplantation for sickle cell disease. N Engl J Med 1996; 335(6):369–376.

741. Nietert PJ, Abboud MR, Silverstein MD, Jackson SM. Bone marrow transplantation versus periodic prophylactic blood transfusion in sickle cell patients at high risk of ischemic stroke: a decision analysis. Blood 2000; 95(10):3057–3064.

742. Gore L, Lane PA, Quinones RR, Giller RH. Successful cord blood transplantation for sickle cell anemia from a sibling who is human leukocyte antigen-identical: implications for comprehensive care. J Pediatr Hematol Oncol 2000; 22(5):437–440.

743. Steen RG, Helton KJ, Horwitz EM, Benaim E, Thompson S, Bowman LC et al. Improved cerebrovascular patency following therapy in patients with sickle cell disease: initial results in 4 patients who received HLA-identical hematopoietic stem cell allografts. Ann Neurol 2001; 49(2):222–229.

744. Hsieh MM, Kang EM, Fitzhugh CD, Link MB, Bolan CD, Kurlander R et al. Allogeneic hematopoietic stem-cell transplantation for sickle cell disease. N Engl J Med 2009; 361(24):2309–2317.

745. Gladwin MT, Schechter AN, Shelhamer JH, Pannell LK, Conway DA, Hrinczenko BW et al. Inhaled nitric oxide augments nitric oxide transport on sickle cell hemoglobin without affecting oxygen affinity. J Clin Invest 1999; 104(7):937–945.

746. Romero JR, Suzuka SM, Nagel RL, Fabry ME. Arginine supplementation of sickle transgenic mice reduces red cell density and Gardos channel activity. Blood 2002; 99(4):1103–1108.

747. Kaul DK, Hebbel RP. Hypoxia/reoxygenation causes inflammatory response in transgenic sickle mice but not in normal mice. J Clin Invest 2000; 106(3):411–420.

748. Harlan JM. Introduction: anti-adhesion therapy in sickle cell disease. Blood 2000; 95(2):365–367.

749. Hertel CE, Kuypers F, Larkin S, Styles L. IVIG: a potential anti-adhesion therapy for sickle cell disease. The National Sickle Cell Disease Program 2001; 96.

750. Stam J, de Bruijn S, deVeber G. Anticoagulation for cerebral sinus thrombosis. Stroke 2003; 34(4):1054–1055.

751. McQuaker IG, Jaspan T, McConachie NS, Dolan G. Coil embolization of cerebral aneurysms in patients with sickling disorders. Br J Haematol 1999; 106(2):388–390.

752. Cheatham ML, Brackett CE. Problems in management of subarachnoid hemorrhage in sickle cell anemia. J Neurosurg 1965; 23(5):488–493.

753. Schatz J, Finke RL, Kellett JM, Kramer JH. Cognitive functioning in children with sickle cell disease: a meta-analysis. J Pediatr Psychol 2002; 27(8):739–748.

754. Hogan AM, Pit-ten CI, Vargha-Khadem F, Prengler M, Kirkham FJ. Physiological correlates of intellectual function in children with sickle cell disease: hypoxaemia, hyperaemia and brain infarction. Dev Sci 2006; 9(4):379–387.

755. Berkelhammer LD, Williamson AL, Sanford SD, Dirksen CL, Sharp WG, Margulies AS et al. Neurocognitive sequelae of pediatric sickle cell disease: a review of the literature. Child Neuropsychol 2007; 13(2):120–131.

756. Cohen MJ, Branch WB, McKie VC, Adams RJ. Neuropsychological impairment in children with sickle cell anemia and cerebrovascular accidents. Clin Pediatr (Phila) 1994; 33(9):517–524.

757. Hogan A, Telfer P, Prengler M, Saunders D, Wade AM, Vargha-Khadem F et al. Intellectual function in children with sickle cell anemia: longitudinal data from the East London Cohort. Br J Haematol 2008; 141(1):111.

758. Kral MC, Brown RT. Transcranial Doppler ultrasonography and executive dysfunction in children with sickle cell disease. J Pediatr Psychol 2004; 29(3):185–195.

759. Puffer E, Schatz J, Roberts CW. The association of oral hydroxyurea therapy with improved cognitive functioning in sickle cell disease. Child Neuropsychol 2007; 13(2):142–154.

760. Hijmans CT, Fijnvandraat K, Grootenhuis MA, van Geloven N, Heijboer H, Peters M, Oosterlaan J. Neurocognitive deficits in children with sickle cell disease: a comprehensive profile. Pediatr Blood Cancer. 2010 Dec 15. [Epub ahead of print]

761. King AA, White DA, McKinstry RC, Noetzel M, DeBaun MR. A pilot randomized education rehabilitation trial is feasible in sickle cell and strokes. Neurology 2007; 68(23):2008–2011.

762. Abboud MR, Jackson SM, Barredo J, Holden KR, Cure J, Laver J. Neurologic complications following bone marrow transplantation for sickle cell disease. Bone Marrow Transplant 1996; 17(3):405–407.

763. Dalakas MC, Clark WM. Strokes, thromboembolic events, and IVIg: rare incidents blemish an excellent safety record. *Neurology* 2003; 60(11):1736–1737.

764. Hutchinson J. Case of continuous absence of hair, with atrophic condition of the skin and it's appendages, in a boy who's mother had been almost continually bald from alopecia areata from the age of six. Lancet 1886; 1:923.

765. Gilford H. Ateleiosis and progeria: continuous youth and premature old age. BMJ 1904; 2:914–918.

766. DeBusk FL. The Hutchinson–Gilford progeria syndrome. Report of 4 cases and review of the literature. J Pediatr 1972; 80(4):697–724.

767. Pollex RL, Hegele RA. Hutchinson–Gilford progeria syndrome. Clin Genet 2004; 66(5):375–381.

768. Hennekam RC. Hutchinson–Gilford progeria syndrome: review of the phenotype. Am J Med Genet A 2006; 140(23):2603–2624.

769. Eriksson M, Brown WT, Gordon LB, Glynn MW, Singer J, Scott L et al. Recurrent de novo point mutations in lamin A cause Hutchinson–Gilford progeria syndrome. Nature 2003; 423(6937):293–298.

770. Cao H, Hegele RA. LMNA is mutated in Hutchinson–Gilford progeria (MIM 176670) but not in Wiedemann–Rautenstrauch progeroid syndrome (MIM 264090). J Hum Genet 2003; 48(5):271–274.

771. Delgado LW, Rojas MA, Ortiz LR, Martinez BC, Rojas-Atencio A, Quintero M et al. Del(1)(q23) in a patient with Hutchinson–Gilford progeria. Am J Med Genet 2002; 113(3):298–301.

772. Al-Shali KZ, Hegele RA. Laminopathies and atherosclerosis. Arterioscler Thromb Vasc Biol 2004; 24(9):1591–1595.

773. Plasilova M, Chattopadhyay C, Pal P, Schaub NA, Buechner SA, Mueller H et al. Homozygous missense mutation in the lamin A/C gene causes autosomal recessive Hutchinson–Gilford progeria syndrome. J Med Genet 2004; 41(8):609–614.

774. Goldman RD, Shumaker DK, Erdos MR, Eriksson M, Goldman AE, Gordon LB et al. Accumulation of mutant lamin A causes progressive changes in nuclear architecture in Hutchinson–Gilford progeria syndrome. Proc Natl Acad Sci USA 2004; 101(24):8963–8968.

775. Csoka I, Csanyi E, Zapantis G, Nagy E, Feher-Kiss A, Horvath G et al. In vitro and in vivo percutaneous absorption of topical dosage forms: case studies. Int J Pharm 2005; 291(1–2):11–19.

776. Scaffidi P, Misteli T. Reversal of the cellular phenotype in the premature aging disease Hutchinson–Gilford progeria syndrome. Nat Med 2005; 11(4):440–445.

777. Glynn MW, Glover TW. Incomplete processing of mutant lamin A in Hutchinson–Gilford progeria leads to nuclear abnormalities, which are reversed by farnesyltransferase inhibition. Hum Mol Genet 2005; 14(20):2959–2969.

778. Toth JI, Yang SH, Qiao X, Beigneux AP, Gelb MH, Moulson CL et al. Blocking protein farnesyltransferase improves nuclear shape in fibroblasts from humans with progeroid syndromes. Proc Natl Acad Sci USA 2005; 102(36):12873–12878.

779. Sevenants L, Wouters C, De Sandre-Giovannoli A, Devlieger H, Devriendt K, van den Oord JJ et al. Tight skin and limited joint movements as early presentation of Hutchinson–Gilford progeria in a 7-week-old infant. Eur J Pediatr 2005; 164(5):283–286.

780. Gordon LB, Harten IA, Patti ME, Lichtenstein AH. Reduced adiponectin and HDL cholesterol without elevated C-reactive protein: clues to the biology of premature atherosclerosis in Hutchinson–Gilford Progeria Syndrome. J Pediatr 2005; 146(3):336–341.

781. Merideth MA, Gordon LB, Clauss S, Sachdev V, Smith AC, Perry MB et al. Phenotype and course of Hutchinson–Gilford progeria syndrome. N Engl J Med 2008; 358(6):592–604.

782. Rosman NP, Anselm I, Bhadelia RA. Progressive intracranial vascular disease with strokes and seizures in a boy with progeria. J Child Neurol 2001; 16(3):212–215.

783. Dyck JD, David TE, Burke B, Webb GD, Henderson MA, Fowler RS. Management of coronary artery disease in Hutchinson–Gilford syndrome. J Pediatr 1987; 111(3):407–410.

784. Smith AS, Wiznitzer M, Karaman BA, Horwitz SJ, Lanzieri CF. MRA detection of vascular occlusion in a child with progeria. AJNR Am J Neuroradiol 1993; 14(2):441–443.

785. Green LN. Progeria with carotid artery aneurysms: report of a case. Arch Neurol 1981; 38(10):659–661.

786. Mandera M, Larysz D, Pajak J, Klimczak A. Epidural hematomas in a child with Hutchinson–Gilford progeria syndrome. Childs Nerv Syst 2003; 19(1):63–65.

787. Hegele RA. Drawing the line in progeria syndromes. Lancet 2003; 362(9382):416–417.

788. Almeida P, Hernandez J, Marti M, Hernandez B. What syndrome is this? Wiedemann–Rautenstrauch syndrome. Pediatr Dermatol 2005; 22(1):75–78.

789. Guerra D, Fornieri C, Bacchelli B, Lugli L, Torelli P, Balli F et al. The De Barsy syndrome. J Cutan Pathol 2004; 31(9):616–624.

790. Yanagawa Y, Nakau H, Kita H, Shimizu A, Chigasaki H. Werner's syndrome associated with meningioma and a cerebrovascular disorder. No To Shinkei 1994; 46(11):1069–1074.

791. Chen L, Lee L, Kudlow BA, Dos Santos HG, Sletvold O, Shafeghati Y et al. LMNA mutations in atypical Werner's syndrome. Lancet 2003; 362(9382):440–445.

792. Campen CJ, Kranick SM, Kessler SK, Kasner SE, Ichord RN, Beslow LA et al. Late neurovascular events in pediatric brain tumour patients. Stroke (International Stroke Conference 2010 Oral Presentations) 2010; 41(4):e18.

793. Kieslich M, Porto L, Lanfermann H, Jacobi G, Schwabe D, Bohles H. Cerebrovascular complications of L-asparaginase in the therapy of acute lymphoblastic leukemia. J Pediatr Hematol Oncol 2003; 25(6):484–487.

794. Nowak-Gottl U, Ahlke E, Fleischhack G, Schwabe D, Schobess R, Schumann C et al. Thromboembolic events in children with acute lymphoblastic leukemia (BFM protocols): prednisone versus dexamethasone administration. Blood 2003; 101(7):2529–2533.

795. Morris B, Partap S, Yeom K, Gibbs IC, Fisher PG, King AA. Cerebrovascular disease in childhood cancer survivors: a Children's Oncology Group Report. Neurology 2009; 73(22):1906–1913.

796. Zimmerman RA, Bilaniuk LT, Hackney DB, Goldberg HI, Grossman RI. Magnetic resonance imaging of dural venous sinus invasion, occlusion and thrombosis. Acta Radiol Suppl 1986; 369:110–112.

797. Nadel L, Braun IF, Muizelaar JP, Laine FJ. Tumoral thrombosis of cerebral venous sinuses: preoperative diagnosis using magnetic resonance phase imaging. Surg Neurol 1991; 35(3):189–195.

798. Carvalho KS, Bodensteiner JB, Connolly PJ, Garg BP. Cerebral venous thrombosis in children. J Child Neurol 2001; 16(8):574–580.

799. deVeber G, Andrew M, Adams C, Bjornson B, Booth F, Buckley DJ et al. Cerebral sinovenous thrombosis in children. N Engl J Med 2001; 345(6):417–423.

800. Kiya K, Satoh H, Mizoue T, Kinoshita Y. Postoperative cortical venous infarction in tumours firmly adherent to the cortex. J Clin Neurosci 2001; 8(Suppl 1):109–113.

801. Ruud E, Holmstrom H, Natvig S, Wesenberg F. Prevalence of thrombophilia and central venous catheter-associated neck vein thrombosis in 41 children with cancer – a prospective study. Med Pediatr Oncol 2002; 38(6):405–410.

802. Goh KY, Tsoi WC, Feng CS, Wickham N, Poon WS. Haemostatic changes during surgery for primary brain tumours. J Neurol Neurosurg Psychiatry 1997; 63(3):334–338.

803. Moriarity JL, Jr, Lim M, Storm PB, Beauchamp NJ, Jr, Olivi A. Reversible posterior leukoencephalopathy occurring during resection of a posterior fossa tumor: case report and review of the literature. Neurosurgery 2001; 49(5):1237–1239.

804. Bowers DC, Mulne AF, Reisch JS, Elterman RD, Munoz L, Booth T et al. Nonperioperative strokes in children with central nervous system tumors. Cancer 2002; 94(4):1094–1101.

805. Painter MJ, Chutorian AM, Hilal SK. Cerebrovasculopathy following irradiation in childhood. Neurology 1975; 25(2):189–194.

806. Wright TL, Bresnan MJ. Radiation-induced cerebrovascular disease in children. Neurology 1976; 26(6 Pt 1):540–543.

807. Servo A, Puranen M. Moyamoya syndrome as a complication of radiation therapy. Case report. J Neurosurg 1978; 48(6):1026–1029.

808. Mori K, Takeuchi J, Ishikawa M, Handa H, Toyama M, Yamaki T. Occlusive arteriopathy and brain tumor. J Neurosurg 1978; 49(1):22–35.

809. Rajakulasingam K, Cerullo LJ, Raimondi AJ. Childhood moya-moya syndrome. Postradiation pathogenesis. Childs Brain 1979; 5(5):467–475.

810. Benoit P, Destee A, Verier A, Giraldon JM, Warot P. Post-radio-therapy stenosis of the supraclinoid internal carotid artery. Moyamoya network. Rev Neurol (Paris) 1985; 141(10):666–668.

811. Montanera W, Chui M, Hudson A. Meningioma and occlusive vasculopathy: coexisting complications of past extracranial radiation. Surg Neurol 1985; 24(1):35–39.

812. Lau YL, Milligan DW. Atypical presentation of craniopharyngioma associated with Moyamoya disease. J R Soc Med 1986; 79(4):236–237.

813. Beyer RA, Paden P, Sobel DF, Flynn FG. Moyamoya pattern of vascular occlusion after radiotherapy for glioma of the optic chiasm. Neurology 1986; 36(9):1173–1178.

814. Kitano S, Sakamoto H, Fujitani K, Kobayashi Y. Moyamoya disease associated with a brain stem glioma. Childs Nerv Syst 2000; 16(4):251–255.

815. Aihara N, Nagai H, Mase M, Kanai H, Wakabayashi S, Mabe H. Atypical Moyamoya disease associated with brain tumor. Surg Neurol 1992; 37(1):46–50.

816. Grenier Y, Tomita T, Marymont MH, Byrd S, Burrowes DM. Late postirradiation occlusive vasculopathy in childhood medulloblastoma. Report of two cases. J Neurosurg 1998; 89(3):460–464.

817. Maher CO, Raffel C. Early vasculopathy following radiation in a child with medulloblastoma. Pediatr Neurosurg 2000; 32(5):255–258.

818. Brant-Zawadzki M, Anderson M, DeArmond SJ, Conley FK, Jahnke RW. Radiation-induced large intracranial vessel occlusive vasculopathy. AJR Am J Roentgenol 1980; 134(1):51–55.

819. Aoki S, Hayashi N, Abe O, Shirouzu I, Ishigame K, Okubo T et al. Radiation-induced arteritis: thickened wall with prominent enhancement on cranial MR images report of five cases and comparison with 18 cases of Moyamoya disease. Radiology 2002; 223(3):683–688.

820. Maruyama K, Mishima K, Saito N, Fujimaki T, Sasaki T, Kirino T. Radiation-induced aneurysm and moyamoya vessels presenting with subarachnoid haemorrhage. Acta Neurochir (Wien) 2000; 142(2):139–143.

821. Harris OA, Chang SD, Harris BT, Adler JR. Acquired cerebral arteriovenous malformation induced by an anaplastic astrocytoma: an interesting case. Neurol Res 2000; 22(5):473–477.

822. Katoh M, Kamiyama H, Abe H, Aida T, Takikawa S, Kuroda S. Complete occlusion of right middle cerebral artery by radiation therapy after removal of pituitary adenoma: case report. No Shinkei Geka 1990; 18(9):855–859.

823. Sinsawaiwong S, Phanthumchinda K. Progressive cerebral occlusive disease after hypothalamic astrocytoma radiation therapy. J Med Assoc Thai 1997; 80(5):338–342.

824. Beckman JA, Thakore A, Kalinowski BH, Harris JR, Creager MA. Radiation therapy impairs endothelium-dependent vasodilation in humans. J Am Coll Cardiol 2001; 37(3):761–765.

825. Grill J, Couanet D, Cappelli C, Habrand JL, Rodriguez D, Sainte-Rose C et al. Radiation-induced cerebral vasculopathy in children with neurofibromatosis and optic pathway glioma. Ann Neurol 1999; 45(3):393–396.

826. Yamauchi T, Tada M, Houkin K, Tanaka T, Nakamura Y, Kuroda S et al. Linkage of familial moyamoya disease (spontaneous occlusion of the circle of Willis) to chromosome 17q25. Stroke 2000; 31(4):930–935.

827. Kenet G, Sadetzki S, Murad H, Martinowitz U, Rosenberg N, Gitel S et al. Factor V Leiden and antiphospholipid antibodies are significant risk factors for ischemic stroke in children. Stroke 2000; 31(6):1283–1288.

828. Bonduel M, Hepner M, Sciuccati G, Torres AF, Tenembaum S. Prothrombotic disorders in children with moyamoya syndrome. Stroke 2001; 32(8):1786–1792.

829. Nowak-Gottl U, Strater R, Heinecke A, Junker R, Koch HG, Schuierer G et al. Lipoprotein(a) and genetic polymorphisms of clotting factor V, prothrombin, and methylenetetrahydrofolate reductase are risk factors of spontaneous ischemic stroke in childhood. Blood 1999; 94(11):3678–3682.

830. Heikens J, Ubbink MC, van der Pal HP, Bakker PJ, Fliers E, Smilde TJ et al. Long term survivors of childhood brain cancer have an increased risk for cardiovascular disease. Cancer 2000; 88(9):2116–2121.

831. Prengler M, Sturt N, Krywawych S, Surtees R, Liesner R, Kirkham F. Homozygous thermolabile variant of the methylenetetrahydrofolate reductase gene: a potential risk factor for hyperhomocysteinaemia, CVD, and stroke in childhood. Dev Med Child Neurol 2001; 43(4):220–225.

832. Abramson ZH, Kark JD. Serum cholesterol and primary brain tumours: a case-control study. Br J Cancer 1985; 52(1):93–98.

833. Smith GD, Neaton JD, Ben-Shlomo Y, Shipley M, Wentworth D. Serum cholesterol concentration and primary malignant brain tumors: a prospective study. Am J Epidemiol 1992; 135(3):259–265.

834. Herrington LJ, Friedman DG. Serum chlesterol concentration and risk of brain cancer. BMJ 1995; 310:367–368.

835. Crook M, Robinson R, Swaminathan R. Hypertriglyceridaemia in a child with hypernatraemia due to a hypothalamic tumour. Ann Clin Biochem 1995; 32 (Pt 2):226–228.

836. Landin-Wilhelmsen K, Tengborn L, Wilhelmsen L, Bengtsson BA. Elevated fibrinogen levels decrease following treatment of acromegaly. Clin Endocrinol (Oxf) 1997; 46(1):69–74.

837. Kamuri K, Borbone J, Mackie S, Murugan V, Puttha R, Kennedy CR et al. Modifiable risk factors associated with cerebrovascular accidents in children with cerebral tumour. Eur J Paed Neurol 2009; 13(Suppl 1), S15.

838. Kirkham FJ, Prengler M, Hewes DK, Ganesan V. Risk factors for arterial ischemic stroke in children. J Child Neurol 2000; 15(5):299–307.

839. Schultheiss TE, Kun LE, Ang KK, Stephens LC. Radiation response of the central nervous system. Int J Radiat Oncol Biol Phys 1995; 31(5):1093–1112.

840. Glantz MJ, Burger PC, Friedman AH, Radtke RA, Massey EW, Schold SC, Jr. Treatment of radiation-induced nervous system injury with heparin and warfarin. Neurology 1994; 44(11):2020–2027.

841. Lamberts HB, de BW. Contributions to the study of immediate and early X-ray reactions with regard to chemo-protection. VII. X-ray-induced atheromatous lesions in the arterial wall of hypercholesterolaemic rabbits. Int J Radiat Biol 1963; 6:343–350.

842. Levinson SA, Close MB, Ehrenfeld WK, Stoney RJ. Carotid artery occlusive disease following external cervical irradiation. Arch Surg 1973; 107(3):395–397.

843. Murros KE, Toole JF. The effect of radiation on carotid arteries. A review article. Arch Neurol 1989; 46(4):449–455.

844. Glick B. Bilateral carotid occlusive disease. Following irradiation for carcinoma of the vocal cords. Arch Pathol 1972; 93(4):352–355.

845. Constine LS, Konski A, Ekholm S, McDonald S, Rubin P. Adverse effects of brain irradiation correlated with MR and CT imaging. Int J Radiat Oncol Biol Phys 1988; 15(2):319–330.

846. Mulhern RK, Palmer SL, Reddick WE, Glass JO, Kun LE, Taylor J et al. Risks of young age for selected neurocognitive deficits in medulloblastoma are associated with white matter loss. J Clin Oncol 2001; 19(2):472–479.

847. Mulhern RK, Reddick WE, Palmer SL, Glass JO, Elkin TD, Kun LE et al. Neurocognitive deficits in medulloblastoma survivors and white matter loss. Ann Neurol 1999; 46(6):834–841.

848. Reddick WE, Russell JM, Glass JO, Xiong X, Mulhern RK, Langston JW et al. Subtle white matter volume differences in children treated for medulloblastoma with conventional or reduced dose craniospinal irradiation. Magn Reson Imaging 2000; 18(7):787–793.

849. Fouladi M, Langston J, Mulhern R, Jones D, Xiong X, Yang J et al. Silent lacunar lesions detected by magnetic resonance imaging of children with brain tumors: a late sequela of therapy. J Clin Oncol 2000; 18(4):824–831.

850. Suzuki S, Nishio S, Takata K, Morioka T, Fukui M. Radiation-induced brain calcification: paradoxical high signal intensity in T1-weighted MR images. Acta Neurochir (Wien) 2000; 142(7):801–804.

851. Chan YL, Roebuck DJ, Yuen MP, Yeung KW, Lau KY, Li CK et al. Long-term cerebral metabolite changes on proton magnetic resonance spectroscopy in patients cured of acute lymphoblastic leukemia with previous intrathecal methotrexate and cranial irradiation prophylaxis. Int J Radiat Oncol Biol Phys 2001; 50(3):759–763.

852. Davidson A, Tait DM, Payne GS, Hopewell JW, Leach MO, Watson M et al. Magnetic resonance spectroscopy in the evaluation of neurotoxicity following cranial irradiation for childhood cancer. Br J Radiol 2000; 73(868):421–424.

853. Phillips PC, Moeller JR, Sidtis JJ, Dhawan V, Steinherz PG, Strother SC et al. Abnormal cerebral glucose metabolism in long-term survivors of childhood acute lymphocytic leukemia. Ann Neurol 1991; 29(3):263–271.

854. Dadparvar S, Hussain R, Koffler SP, Gillan MM, Bartolic EI, Miyamoto C. The role of Tc-99m HMPAO functional brain imaging in detection of cerebral radionecrosis. Cancer J 2000; 6(6):381–387.

855. Plowman PN, Saunders CA, Maisey M. On the usefulness of brain PET scanning to the paediatric neuro-oncologist. Br J Neurosurg 1997; 11(6):525–532.

856. Langleben DD, Segall GM. PET in differentiation of recurrent brain tumor from radiation injury. J Nucl Med 2000; 41(11):1861–1867.

857. Biousse V, Newman NJ, Hunter SB, Hudgins PA. Diffusion weighted imaging in radiation necrosis. J Neurol Neurosurg Psychiatry 2003; 74(3):382–384.

858. Lippens RJ, van Ooijen AG. Calcifications of the basal ganglia in children with brain tumours. Eur J Paediatr Neurol 1997; 1(2–3):85–89.

859. Nieder C, Leicht A, Motaref B, Nestle U, Niewald M, Schnabel K. Late radiation toxicity after whole brain radiotherapy: the influence of antiepileptic drugs. Am J Clin Oncol 1999; 22(6):573–579.

860. Martins AN, Johnston JS, Henry JM, Stoffel TJ, Di CG. Delayed radiation necrosis of the brain. J Neurosurg 1977; 47(3):336–345.

861. Groothuis DR, Mikhael MA. Focal cerebral vasculitis associated with circulating immune complexes and brain irradiation. Ann Neurol 1986; 19(6):590–592.

862. Hart GB, Mainous EG. The treatment of radiation necrosis with hyperbaric oxygen (OHP). Cancer 1976; 37(6):2580–2585.

863. Guy J, Schatz NJ. Hyperbaric oxygen in the treatment of radiation-induced optic neuropathy. Ophthalmology 1986; 93(8):1083–1088.

864. Poulton TJ, Witcofski RL. Hyperbaric oxygen therapy for radiation myelitis. Undersea Biomed Res 1985; 12(4):453–458.

865. Edgeworth J, Bullock P, Bailey A, Gallagher A, Crouchman M. Why are brain tumours still being missed? Arch Dis Child 1996; 74(2):148–151.

866. Habrand JL, de CR. Radiation therapy in the management of childhood brain tumors. Childs Nerv Syst 2001; 17(3):121–133.

867. Grill J, Renaux VK, Bulteau C, Viguier D, Levy-Piebois C, Sainte-Rose C et al. Long-term intellectual outcome in children with posterior fossa tumors according to radiation doses and volumes. Int J Radiat Oncol Biol Phys 1999; 45(1):137–145.

868. Kieffer-Renaux V, Bulteau C, Grill J, Kalifa C, Viguier D, Jambaque I. Patterns of neuropsychological deficits in children with medulloblastoma according to craniospatial irradiation doses. Dev Med Child Neurol 2000; 42(11):741–745.

869. Fuss M, Poljanc K, Hug EB. Full Scale IQ (FSIQ) changes in children treated with whole brain and partial brain irradiation. A review and analysis. Strahlenther Onkol 2000; 176(12):573–581.

870. Ris MD, Packer R, Goldwein J, Jones-Wallace D, Boyett JM. Intellectual outcome after reduced-dose radiation therapy plus adjuvant chemotherapy for medulloblastoma: a Children's Cancer Group study. J Clin Oncol 2001; 19(15):3470–3476.

871. Palmer SL, Goloubeva O, Reddick WE, Glass JO, Gajjar A, Kun L et al. Patterns of intellectual development among survivors of pediatric medulloblastoma: a longitudinal analysis. J Clin Oncol 2001; 19(8):2302–2308.

872. Thomas PR, Deutsch M, Kepner JL, Boyett JM, Krischer J, Aronin P et al. Low-stage medulloblastoma: final analysis of trial comparing standard-dose with reduced-dose neuraxis irradiation. J Clin Oncol 2000; 18(16):3004–3011.

873. Packer RJ, Goldwein J, Nicholson HS, Vezina LG, Allen JC, Ris MD et al. Treatment of children with medulloblastomas with reduced-dose craniospinal radiation therapy and adjuvant chemotherapy: A Children's Cancer Group Study. J Clin Oncol 1999; 17(7):2127–2136.

874. Tornesello A, Mastrangelo S, Piciacchia D, Bembo V, Colosimo C, Di Rocco C et al. Progressive disease in children with medulloblastoma/PNET during preradiation chemotherapy. J Neurooncol 1999; 45(2):135–140.

875. Cucchiara B, Kasner SE. Use of statins in CNS disorders. J Neurol Sci 2001; 187(1–2):81–89.

876. Jick H, Zornberg GL, Jick SS, Seshadri S, Drachman DA. Statins and the risk of dementia. Lancet 2000; 356(9242):1627–1631.

877. Ungvari Z, Pacher P, Csiszar A. Can simvastatin promote tumor growth by inducing angiogenesis similar to VEGF? Med Hypotheses 2002; 58(1):85–86.

878. Macaulay RJ, Wang W, Dimitroulakos J, Becker LE, Yeger H. Lovastatin-induced apoptosis of human medulloblastoma cell lines in vitro. J Neurooncol 1999; 42(1):1–11.

879. Larner J, Jane J, Laws E, Packer R, Myers C, Shaffrey M. A phase I–II trial of lovastatin for anaplastic astrocytoma and glioblastoma multiforme. Am J Clin Oncol 1998; 21(6):579–583.

880. de JS, Ose L, Szamosi T, Gagne C, Lambert M, Scott R et al. Efficacy and safety of statin therapy in children with familial hypercholesterolemia: a randomized, double-blind, placebo-controlled trial with simvastatin. Circulation 2002; 106(17):2231–2237.

881. Black DM. Statins in children: what do we know and what do we need to do? Curr Atheroscler Rep 2001; 3(1):29–34.

882. Riva D, Giorgi C. The neurodevelopmental price of survival in children with malignant brain tumours. Childs Nerv Syst 2000; 16(10–11):751–754.

883. Zucchinelli V, Bouffet E. Academic future of children treated for brain tumors. Single-center study of 27 children. Arch Pediatr 2000; 7(9):933–941.

884. Kerr G. Takayasu's arteritis. Curr Opin Rheumatol 1994; 6(1):32–38.

885. Jain S, Sharma N, Singh S, Bali HK, Kumar L, Sharma BK. Takayasu arteritis in children and young indians. Int J Cardiol 2000; 75(Suppl 1):S153–S157.

886. Kim HJ, Suh DC, Kim JK, Kim SJ, Lee JH, Choi CG et al. Correlation of neurological manifestations of Takayasu's arteritis with cerebral angiographic findings. Clin Imaging 2005; 29(2):79–85.

887. Brenner DA, Alberts MJ, Amarenco P. Clinical genetic issues in stroke. Handb Clin Neurol 2008; 92(ch 18):355–372.

888. Kohrman MH, Huttenlocher PR. Takayasu arteritis: a treatable cause of stroke in infancy. Pediatr Neurol 1986; 2(3):154–158.

889. Kimura A, Ota M, Katsuyama Y, Ohbuchi N, Takahashi M, Kobayashi Y et al. Mapping of the HLA-linked genes controlling the susceptibility to Takayasu's arteritis. Int J Cardiol 2000; 75(Suppl 1):S105–S110.

890. Ohta Y, Ohya Y, Fujii K, Tsuchihashi T, Sato K, Abe I et al. Inflammatory diseases associated with Takayasu's arteritis. Angiology 2003; 54(3):339–344.

891. McCulloch M, Andronikou S, Goddard E, Sinclair P, Lawrenson J, Mandelstam S et al. Angiographic features of 26 children with Takayasu's arteritis. Pediatr Radiol 2003; 33(4):230–235.

892. Etgen T, Winbeck K, Conrad B, Sander D. Hemiballism with insular infarction as first manifestation of Takayasu's arteritis in association with chronic hepatitis B. J Neurol 2003; 250(2):226–229.

893. Sheikhzadeh A, Tettenborn I, Noohi F, Eftekharzadeh M, Schnabel A. Occlusive thromboaortopathy (Takayasu disease): clinical and angiographic features and a brief review of literature. Angiology 2002; 53(1):29–40.

894. Fieldston E, Albert D, Finkel T. Hypertension and elevated ESR as diagnostic features of Takayasu arteritis in children. J Clin Rheumatol 2003; 9(3):156–163.

895. Hoffmann M, Corr P, Robbs J. Cerebrovascular findings in Takayasu disease. J Neuroimaging 2000; 10(2):84–90.

896. Vanoli M, Daina E, Salvarani C, Sabbadini MG, Rossi C, Bacchiani G et al. Takayasu's arteritis: A study of 104 Italian patients. Arthritis Rheum 2005; 53(1):100–107.

897. Cantu C, Pineda C, Barinagarrementeria F, Salgado P, Gurza A, Paola DP et al. Noninvasive cerebrovascular assessment of Takayasu arteritis. Stroke 2000; 31(9):2197–2202.

898. Kumral E, Evyapan D, Aksu K, Keser G, Kabasakal Y, Balkir K. Microembolus detection in patients with Takayasu's arteritis. Stroke 2002; 33(3):712–716.

899. Klos K, Flemming KD, Petty GW, Luthra HS. Takayasu's arteritis with arteriographic evidence of intracranial vessel involvement. Neurology 2003; 60(9):1550–1551.

900. Kim DS, Kim JK, Yoo DS, Huh PW, Cho KS, Kang JK. Takayasu's arteritis presented with subarachnoid hemorrhage: report of two cases. J Korean Med Sci 2002; 17(5):695–698.

901. Filocamo G, Buoncompagni A, Viola S, Loy A, Malattia C, Ravelli A et al. Treatment of Takayasu's arteritis with tumor necrosis factor antagonists. J Pediatr 2008; 153(3):432–434.

902. Kalangos A, Christenson JT, Cikirikcioglu M, Vala D, Buerge A, Simonet F et al. Long-term outcome after surgical intervention and interventional procedures for the management of Takayasu's arteritis in children. J Thorac Cardiovasc Surg 2006; 132(3):656–664.

903. Reddy E, Robbs JV. Surgical management of Takayasu's arteritis in children and adolescents. Cardiovasc J Afr 2007; 18(6):393–396.

904. Laxer RM, Dunn HG, Flodmark O. Acute hemiplegia in Kawasaki disease and infantile polyarteritis nodosa. Dev Med Child Neurol 1984; 26(6):814–818.

905. Engel DG, Gospe SM, Jr, Tracy KA, Ellis WG, Lie JT. Fatal infantile polyarteritis nodosa with predominant central nervous system involvement. Stroke 1995; 26(4):699–701.

906. Morfin-Maciel B, Medina A, Espinosa RF, Berron R, Huerta LJ. Central nervous system involvement in a child with polyarteritis nodosa and severe atopic dermatitis. Rev Alerg Mex 2002; 49(6):189–195.

907. Reichert-Penetrat S, Barbaud A, Antunes A, Borsa-Dorion A, Vidailhet M, Schmutz JL. An unusual form of Stevens–Johnson syndrome with subcorneal pustules associated with *Mycoplasma pneumoniae* infection. Pediatr Dermatol 2000; 17(3):202–204.

908. Goodwin F, Javaid K, Cooper C, Kennedy CR. Recurrent intracranial haemorrhage due to aneurysmal formation in a teenage girl: Lupus or PAN? Dev Med Child Neurol 2001; 43(12 Suppl):20.

909. Yu HH, Lee JH, Wang LC, Yang YH, Chiang BL. Neuropsychiatric manifestations in pediatric systemic lupus erythematosus: a 20-year study. Lupus 2006; 15(10):651–657.

910. El Ramahi KM, Al Rayes HM. Systemic lupus erythematosus associated with moyamoya syndrome. Lupus 2000; 9(8):632–636.

911. Lee MK, Kim JH, Kang HR, Rho HJ, Nam EJ, Kim SW et al. Systemic lupus erythematosus complicated with cerebral venous sinus thrombosis: a report of two cases. J Korean Med Sci 2001; 16(3):351–354.

912. Conen KL, Jeanneret C, Hecker B, Cathomas G, Biedermann BC. Acute occlusive large vessel disease leading to fatal stroke in a patient with systemic lupus erythematosus: arteritis or atherosclerosis? Arthritis Rheum 2006; 54(3):908–913.

913. Avcin T, Benseler SM, Tyrrell PN, Cucnik S, Silverman ED. A follow-up study of antiphospholipid antibodies and associated neuropsychiatric manifestations in 137 children with systemic lupus erythematosus. Arthritis Rheum 2008; 59(2):206–213.

914. Olfat MO, Al-Mayouf SM, Muzaffer MA. Pattern of neuropsychiatric manifestations and outcome in juvenile systemic lupus erythematosus. Clin Rheumatol 2004; 23(5):395–399.

915. Meena AK, Naidu KS, Murthy JM. Cortical sinovenous thrombosis in a child with nephrotic syndrome and iron deficiency anaemia. Neurol India 2000; 48(3):292–294.

916. Lin CC, Lui CC, Tain YL. Thalamic stroke secondary to straight sinus thrombosis in a nephrotic child. Pediatr Nephrol 2002; 17(3):184–186.

917. Rodrigues MM, Zardini LR, de Andrade MC, Mangia CM, Carvalhaes JT, Vilanova LC. Cerebral sinovenous thrombosis in a nephrotic child. Arq Neuropsiquiatr 2003; 61(4):1026–1029.

918. Gangakhedkar A, Wong W, Pitcher LA. Cerebral thrombosis in childhood nephrosis. J Paediatr Child Health 2005; 41(4):221–224.

919. Papachristou FT, Petridou SH, Printza NG, Zafeiriou DI, Gompakis NP. Superior sagittal sinus thrombosis in steroid-resistant nephrotic syndrome. Pediatr Neurol 2005; 32(4):282–284.

920. Fluss J, Geary D, deVeber G. Cerebral sinovenous thrombosis and idiopathic nephrotic syndrome in childhood: report of four new cases and review of the literature. Eur J Pediatr 2006; 165(10):709–716.

921. Balci YI, Tavil B, Fidan G, Ozaltin F. Cerebral sinovenous thrombosis in a child with steroid sensitive nephrotic syndrome. Eur J Pediatr 2007; 166(7):757–758.

922. Raghu V, Malik AK, Datta BN, Narang A, Mehta S. Focal glomerulosclerosis with cerebral infarction in a young nephrotic patient. Indian Pediatr 1981; 18(10):754–756.

923. Igarashi M, Roy S, III, Stapleton FB. Cerebrovascular complications in children with nephrotic syndrome. Pediatr Neurol 1988; 4(6):362–365.

924. Huemer M, Emminger W, Trattnig S, Freilinger M, Wandl-Vergesslich K. Kinking and stenosis of the carotid artery associated with homolateral ischaemic brain infarction in a patient treated with ciclosporin A. Eur J Pediatr 1998; 157(7):599–601.

925. Kenet G, Kirkham F, Niederstadt T, Heinecke A, Saunders D, Stoll M et al. Risk factors for recurrent venous thromboembolism in the European collaborative paediatric database on cerebral venous thrombosis: a multicentre cohort study. Lancet Neurol 2007; 6(7):595–603.

926. Barclay AR, Keightley JM, Horrocks I, Garrick V, McGrogan P, Russell RK. Cerebral thromboembolic events in pediatric patients with inflammatory bowel disease. Inflamm Bowel Dis 2009; 16(4):677–683.

927. Standridge S, de los Reyes E. Inflammatory bowel disease and cerebrovascular arterial and venous thromboembolic events in 4 pediatric patients: a case series and review of the literature. J Child Neurol 2008; 23(1):59–66.

928. Andersohn F, Waring M, Garbe E. Risk of ischemic stroke in patients with Crohn's disease: a population-based nested casecontrol study. Inflamm Bowel Dis 2009; (epub ahead of print).

929. Kao A, Dlugos D, Hunter JV, Mamula P, Thorarensen O. Anticoagulation therapy in cerebral sinovenous thrombosis and ulcerative colitis in children. J Child Neurol 2002; 17(7):479–482.

930. McQueen A. "I think she's just crazy". Lancet 2005; 365(9469):1513.

931. Ennaifer R, Moussa A, Mouelhi L, Salem M, Bouzaidi S, Debbeche R et al. Cerebral venous sinus thrombosis as presenting feature of ulcerative colitis. Acta Gastroenterol Belg 2009; 72(3):350–353.

932. Robison NJ, Dawlabani N, Lastra CR, Dhall G. Cerebral sinus thrombosis in a child with active ulcerative colitis and factor V Leiden. Pediatr Blood Cancer 2009; 52(7):867–869.

933. Jorens PG, Delvigne CR, Hermans CR, Haber I, Holvoet J, De Deyn PP. Cerebral arterial thrombosis preceding ulcerative colitis. Stroke 1991; 22(9):1212.

934. Yerby MS, Bailey GM. Superior sagittal sinus thrombosis 10 years after surgery for ulcerative colitis. Stroke 1980; 11(3):294–296.

935. Sood A, Midha V, Sood N. Reversible posterior leukoencephalopathy due to oral ciclosporine in severe ulcerative colitis. Indian J Gastroenterol 2003; 22(6):233–234.

936. Schluter A, Krasnianski M, Krivokuca M, Spielmann RP, Neudecker S, Hirsch W. Magnetic resonance angiography in a patient with Crohn's disease associated cerebral vasculitis. Clin Neurol Neurosurg 2004; 106(2):110–113.

937. Gobron C, Kaci R, Sokol H, Vahedi K, Lejoyeux P, Guillaud C et al. Unilateral carotid granulomatous arteritis and Crohn's disease. Rev Neurol (Paris) 2010; 166(5):542–546.

938. Harris D. Left middle cerebral artery infarct in a young man with Crohn's disease. J R Soc Med 2009; 102(10):443–444.

939. Altinors N, Cepoglu C. Surgically treated intracerebral hematoma in a child with Henoch–Schönlein purpura. J Neurosurg Sci 1991; 35(1):47–49.

940. Ng CC, Huang SC, Huang LT. Henoch–Schönlein purpura with intracerebral hemorrhage: case report. Pediatr Radiol 1996; 26(4):276–277.

941. Chiaretti A, Caresta E, Piastra M, Pulitano S, Di RC. Cerebral hemorrhage in Henoch–Schönlein syndrome. Childs Nerv Syst 2002; 18(8):365–367.

942. Imai T, Okada H, Nanba M, Kawada K, Kusaka T, Itoh S. Henoch–Schönlein purpura with intracerebral hemorrhage. Brain Dev 2002; 24(2):115–117.

943. Paolini S, Ciappetta P, Piattella MC, Domenicucci M. Henoch–Schönlein syndrome and cerebellar hemorrhage: report of an adolescent case and literature review. Surg Neurol 2003; 60(4):339–342.

944. Misra AK, Biswas A, Das SK, Gharai PK, Roy T. Henoch–Schönlein purpura with intracerebral haemorrhage. J Assoc Physicians India 2004; 52:833–834.

945. Wen YK, Yang Y, Chang CC. Cerebral vasculitis and intracerebral hemorrhage in Henoch–Schönlein purpura treated with plasmapheresis. Pediatr Nephrol 2005; 20(2):223–225.

946. Garzoni L, Vanoni F, Rizzi M, Simonetti GD, Simonetti BG, Ramelli GP et al. Nervous system dysfunction in Henoch–Schönlein syndrome: systematic review of the literature. Rheumatology (Oxford) 2009; 48(12):1524–1529.

947. Sokol DK, McIntyre JA, Short RA, Gutt J, Wagenknecht DR, Biller J et al. Henoch–Schönlein purpura and stroke: antiphosphatidylethanolamine antibody in CSF and serum. Neurology 2000; 55(9):1379–1381.

948. Lilleyman JS. Intracranial haemorrhage in idiopathic thrombocytopenic purpura. Paediatric Haematology Forum of the British Society for Haematology. Arch Dis Child 1994; 71(3):251–253.

949. Giroud M, Lemesle M, Madinier G, Manceau E, Osseby GV, Dumas R. Stroke in children under 16 years of age. Clinical and etiological difference with adults. Acta Neurol Scand 1997; 96(6):401–406.

950. Iyori H, Bessho F, Ookawa H, Konishi S, Shirahata A, Miyazaki S et al. Intracranial hemorrhage in children with immune thrombocytopenic purpura. Japanese Study Group on childhood ITP. Ann Hematol 2000; 79(12):691–695.

951. Butros LJ, Bussel JB. Intracranial hemorrhage in immune thrombocytopenic purpura: a retrospective analysis. J Pediatr Hematol Oncol 2003; 25(8):660–664.

952. Kühne T, Buchanan GR, Zimmerman S, Michaels LA, Kohan R, Berchtold W, Imbach P; Intercontinental Childhood ITP Study Group; Intercontinental Childhood ITP Study Group. A prospective comparative study of 2540 infants and children with newly diagnosed idiopathic thrombocytopenic purpura (ITP) from the Intercontinental Childhood ITP Study Group. J Pediatr. 2003;143(5):605–608.

953. Koçak U, Aral YZ, Kaya Z, Oztürk G, Gürsel T. Evaluation of clinical characteristics, diagnosis and management in childhood immune thrombocytopenic purpura: a single center's experience. Turk J Pediatr. 2007;49(3):250–255.

954. Paling A, Stefan DC. Idiopathic thrombocytopenic purpura in childhood: a 10-year audit. Hematology 2008; 13(3):175–180.

955. Lee MS, Kim WC. Intracranial hemorrhage associated with idiopathic thrombocytopenic purpura: report of seven patients and a meta-analysis. Neurology. 1998;50(4):1160–1163.

956. Downs LA, Thomas NJ, Comito MA, Meier AH, Dias MS. Idiopathic thrombocytopenic purpura complicated by an intracranial hemorrhage secondary to an arteriovenous malformation. Pediatr Emerg Care 2005; 21(5):309–311.

957. Beck CE, Nathan PC, Parkin PC, Blanchette VS, Macarthur C. Corticosteroids versus intravenous immune globulin for the treatment of acute immune thrombocytopenic purpura in children: a systematic review and meta-analysis of randomized controlled trials. J Pediatr 2005; 147(4):521–527.

958. Kayyali HR, Abdelmoity AT, Morriss MC, Graf WD. Cerebral venous thrombosis after immune thrombocytopenic purpura and anti-D immune globulin therapy. J Child Neurol 2008; 23(3):325–330.

959. Lapointe JS, Nugent RA, Graeb DA, Robertson WD. Cerebral infarction and regression of widespread aneurysms in Kawasaki's disease: case report. Pediatr Radiol 1984; 14(1):1–5.

960. Templeton PA, Dunne MG. Kawasaki syndrome: cerebral and cardiovascular complications. J Clin Ultrasound 1987; 15(7):483–485.

961. Levy DM, Silverman ED, Massicotte MP, McCrindle BW, Yeung RS. Longterm outcomes in patients with giant aneurysms secondary to Kawasaki disease. J Rheumatol 2005; 32(5):928–934.

962. Fujiwara S, Yamano T, Hattori M, Fujiseki Y, Shimada M. Asymptomatic cerebral infarction in Kawasaki disease. Pediatr Neurol 1992; 8(3):235–236.

963. Bailie NM, Hensey OJ, Ryan S, Allcut D, King MD. Bilateral subdural collections – an unusual feature of possible Kawasaki disease. Eur J Paediatr Neurol 2001; 5(2):79–81.

964. Sangermani R, Morello CA, Lucchini F, Posani L, Vergnaghi D. Recurrent infantile multifocal periostosis. Description of a case. Minerva Pediatr 1987; 39(11–12):545–547.

965. Tanaka S, Sagiuchi T, Kobayashi I. Ruptured pediatric posterior cerebral artery aneurysm 9 years after the onset of Kawasaki disease: a case report. Childs Nerv Syst 2007; 23(6):701–706.

966. Ichiyama T, Nishikawa M, Hayashi T, Koga M, Tashiro N, Furukawa S. Cerebral hypoperfusion during acute Kawasaki disease. Stroke 1998; 29(7):1320–1321.

967. Wada Y, Kamei A, Fujii Y, Ishikawa K, Chida S. Cerebral infarction after high-dose intravenous immunoglobulin therapy for Kawasaki disease. J Pediatr 2006; 148(3):399–400.

968. Wechsler B, Dell'lsola B, Vidailhet M, Dormont D, Piette JC, Bletry O et al. MRI in 31 patients with Behçet's disease and neurological involvement: prospective study with clinical correlation. J Neurol Neurosurg Psychiatry 1993; 56(7):793–798.

969. Le Thi HD, Wechsler B, Papo T, Piette JC, Bletry O, Vitoux JM et al. Arterial lesions in Behçet's disease. A study in 25 patients. J Rheumatol 1995; 22(11):2103–2113.

970. Yoshioka H, Matsubara T, Miyanomae Y, Kawase S, Akioka S, Sawada T. Spinal cord MRI in neuro-Behçet's disease. Neuroradiology 1996; 38(7):661–662.

971. Yesilot N, Mutlu M, Gungor O, Baykal B, Serdaroglu P, Akman-Demir G. Clinical characteristics and course of spinal cord involvement in Behçet's disease. Eur J Neurol 2007; 14(7):729–737.

972. Fujikawa S, Suemitsu T. Behçet disease in children: a nationwide retrospective survey in Japan. Acta Paediatr Jpn 1997; 39(2):285–289.

973. Kone-Paut I, Chabrol B, Riss JM, Mancini J, Raybaud C, Garnier JM. Neurologic onset of Behçet's disease: a diagnostic enigma in childhood. J Child Neurol 1997; 12(4):237–241.

974. Eldem B, Onur C, Ozen S. Clinical features of pediatric Behçet's disease. J Pediatr Ophthalmol Strabismus 1998; 35(3):159–161.

975. Kari JA, Bamashmous H, Lingawi S, Al-Sabban E, Akhtar M. Infantile nephrotic syndrome and congenital glaucoma. Pediatr Nephrol 2001; 16(11):894–897.

976. Alper G, Yilmaz Y, Ekinci G, Kose O. Cerebral vein thrombosis in Behçet's disease. Pediatr Neurol 2001; 25(4):332–335.

977. Budin C, Ranchin B, Glastre C, Fouilhoux A, Canterino I, David L. Neurologic signs revealing a Behçet's disease: two pediatric case reports. Arch Pediatr 2002; 9(11):1160–1162.

978. Besbas N, Ozyurek E, Balkanci F, Ozen S, Saatci I, Ozaltin F et al. Behçet's disease with severe arterial involvement in a child. Clin Rheumatol 2002; 21(2):176–179.

979. Chaloupka K, Baglivo E, Hofer M, Chizzolini C, Delavelle J, Rossillion B et al. Cerebral sinus thrombosis in Behçet disease: case report and review of the literature. Klin Monbl Augenheilkd 2003; 220(3):186–188.

980. Panicker JN, Vinayan KP, hsan Moosa NV, Elango EM, Kumar AA. Juvenile Behçet's disease: highlighting neuropsychiatric manifestations and putative genetic mechanisms. Clin Neurol Neurosurg 2007; 109(5):436–438.

981. Susac JO, Hardman JM, Selhorst JB. Microangiopathy of the brain and retina. Neurology 1979; 29(3):313–316.

982. Susac JO. Susac's syndrome: the triad of microangiopathy of the brain and retina with hearing loss in young women. Neurology 1994; 44(4):591–593.

983. Susac JO, Murtagh FR, Egan RA, Berger JR, Bakshi R, Lincoff N et al. MRI findings in Susac's syndrome. Neurology 2003; 61(12):1783–1787.

984. Susac JO, Egan RA, Rennebohm RM, Lubow M. Susac's syndrome: 1975–2005 microangiopathy/autoimmune endotheliopathy. J Neurol Sci 2007; 257(1–2):270–272.

985. Hahn JS, Lannin WC, Sarwal MM. Microangiopathy of brain, retina, and inner ear (Susac's syndrome) in an adolescent female presenting as acute disseminated encephalomyelitis. Pediatrics 2004; 114(1):276–281.

986. Rennebohm RM, Lubow M, Rusin J, Martin L, Grzybowski DM, Susac JO. Aggressive immunosuppressive treatment of Susac's syndrome in an adolescent: using treatment of dermatomyositis as a model. Pediatr Rheumatol Online J 2008; 6:3.

987. Jarius S, Neumayer B, Wandinger KP, Hartmann M, Wildemann B. Anti-endothelial serum antibodies in a patient with Susac's syndrome. J Neurol Sci 2009; 285(1–2):259–261.

988. Rennebohm RM, Egan RA, Susac JO. Treatment of Susac's syndrome. Curr Treat Options Neurol 2008; 10(1):67–74.

989. Caplan LR, Bogousslavsky J. Uncommon Causes of Stroke. Cambridge, UK: Cambridge University Press; 2008.

990. Lasjaunias P, in collaboration with Karel ter Brugge. Vascular Diseases in Neonates, Infants, and Children: interventional neuroradiology Management. Berlin: Springer; 1997.

991. Lasjaunias P, Berenstein A, Ter Brugge KG. Surgical Neuroangiography. Berlin: Springer; 2001.

992. Kim DH, Van GG, Milewicz DM. Incidence of familial intracranial aneurysms in 200 patients: comparison among Caucasian, African-American, and Hispanic populations. Neurosurgery 2003; 53(2):302–308.

993. Hanjani SA. The genetics of cerebrovascular malformations. J Stroke Cerebrovasc Dis 2002; 11(5):279–287.

994. Matarin M, Singleton A, Hardy J, Meschia J. The genetics of ischaemic stroke. J Intern Med 2010; 267(2):139–155.

16
ACUTE MANAGEMENT

Rebecca Ichord, Anne Yardumian, Fenella J. Kirkham and Gabrielle deVeber

Introduction

Stroke and cerebrovascular disease cause considerable anxiety to the paediatrician, at least in part because treatment protocols have not previously been well worked out, although there is evidence that adherence improves outcome in adults.[1] As there was historically no evidence that emergency management improved outcome for adults or children, there was no impetus towards the development of protocols for investigation or management. Although the evidence base is still very small, the situation has recently improved with the publication of the UK,[2] Chest[3] and American Stroke Association[4] guidelines, which have recently been compared (Tables 16.1 and 16.2).[5] Currently, the majority of patients have irreversible focal brain damage by the time of presentation to hospital, and therapeutic effort is usually concentrated on rehabilitation and the prevention of recurrence. There are no studies specifically examining the efficacy of acute treatments for stroke in children. In adults, as a result of controlled trials of thrombolysis,[6–8] there is now an increased awareness of the need for rapid assessment and appropriate management of people, including children, with acute arterial ischaemic stroke. This is the main focus of this chapter, and more detail on the management of other stroke syndromes, such as venous sinus thrombosis and haemorrhage, are available elsewhere in this volume.

Organization

There is little doubt that stroke units save adult lives and improve outcome in survivors[9,10] and the benefits continue for at least 10 years after admission.[11,12] By contrast, services for children with stroke are relatively poorly organized, and as the

TABLE 16.1

Comparison of AHA and other childhood stroke guidelines: acute treatment of childhood stroke by subtype. (Adapted from deVeber G, Kirkham F. Guidelines for the treatment and prevention of stroke in children. Lancet Neurol 2008; 7(11):983–985)

Subtype	UK guidelines 2004 recommendation	G	S	Chest guidelines 2008 recommendation	G	S	American Heart Association (AHA) 2008 Recommendation	G	S
Acute supportive measures	Maintain normal temperature and oxygen saturation	D	4	Not addressed			Control fever, maintain normal oxygenation, control systemic hypertension and normalize serum glucose	1-C	1
General	ASA 5mg/kg	WPC	1	UFH or LMWH or ASA 1–5mg/kg/day until cardioembolic and dissection excluded	1B	1	UFH or LMWH (1mg/kg/12h) up to 1 week until cause determined	2b-C	3
Sickle-cell disease	Exchange transfusion to HbS <30%	WPC	1	IV hydration and exchange transfusion to HbS<30%	1B	1	Exchange transfusion to HbS <30%	2a-B	2
Cardiac	Anticoagulation should be discussed by senior paediatric neurologist and paediatric cardiologist	WPC	1	LMWH 6+ weeks	2C	3	For cardiac embolism unrelated to PFO, and judged to have high recurrence risk: UFH or LMWH as a bridge to oral anticoagulation	2a-B	
							Alternative: UFH or LMWH as a bridge to maintenance LMWH	2a-C	2
Dissection	Anticoagulation for extracranial with no haemorrhage	WPC	1	LMWH 6+ weeks	2C	3	UFH or LMWH as a bridge to oral Anticoagulation	2a-C	2
tPA	Not recommended		1	Not recommended	1B	1	Not recommended	3-C	1
tPA in teens	Not addressed			Not addressed			No consensus on use		

Childhood defined as 28 days to 18 years (Chest), 1 month to 16 years (UK). G, Grade of Evidence/Recommendation; S, Strength of Evidence/Recommendation.
AIS, arterial ischaemic stroke; ASA, aspirin; ICH, intracranial haemorrhage; INR, international normalized ratio; LMWH, low molecular weight heparin;
UFH, unfractionated heparin; WPC, working-party consensus.

TABLE 16.2
Comparison of AHA and other childhood stroke guidelines: chronic treatment. (Adapted from deVeber G,
Kirkham F. Guidelines for the treatment and prevention of stroke in children. Lancet Neurol 2008; 7(11):983–985)

Subtype	UK guidelines 2004 recommendation	G	S	Chest guidelines 2008 recommendation	G	S	American Heart Association (AHA) 2008 recommendation	G	S
General	ASA 1–5mg/kg/day	WPC	1	Once dissection and cardioembolism are excluded, ASA 1–5mg/kg/day, 2+ years	1B	1	ASA 3–5mg/kg/day	2a-C	3
Dissection	Consider anticoagulation until evidence of vessel healing or up to 6 months	WPC	1	LMWH ongoing depending on radiographic results	2C	3	Intracranial or associated SAH: anticoagulation not recommended	3-C	1
							Extracranial: LMWH or warfarin 3–6 months ASA may be substituted	2a-C	
							ASA beyond 6 months	2a-C	
Cardiogenic embolism	Consider anticoagulation after discussion with the cardiologist managing the patient	WPC	1	LMWH ongoing depending on radiographic results	2C	3	LMWH or warfarin ≥ 1 year	2a-B	2
Prothrombotic states	Refer patient to a haematologist	WPC	1	Not addressed			Warfarin long term for selected hypercoagulable states	2a-C	2
Vasculopathy	Vasculopathy ASA 1–3mg/kg/day	WPC	1	Not addressed			Not addressed		
Moyamoya	Revascularization surgery	D	3	Revascularization surgery	1B	1	Revascularization surgery	1-B	1
Sickle-cell disease	Blood transfusion every 3–6 weeks to HbS 30%	C	3	Long-term transfusion programme	1B	1	Regular transfusion program	1-B	1
	After 3 years aim for HbS<50%	C	3	Not addressed			Not addressed		
	If no transfusion, hydroxyurea	C	3	Not addressed			If no transfusion, hydroxyurea	2b-B	2
	Consider bone-marrow transplant	B	2	Not addressed			Consider bone-marrow transplant	2b-C	3
Recurrent stroke on ASA	Consider anticoagulation	WPC	1	Change to clopidogrel or anticoagulation	2C	3	Not addressed		
Rehabilitation	Rehabilitation developmentally relevant and appropriate to home, community and school environment	D	4	Not addressed			Age-appropriate rehabilitation and psychological assessment of cognitive and language deficits	1-C	
Preventing atherosclerosis	Advise re preventable risk factors smoking, exercise and diet	D	4	Not addressed			Advise re diet, exercise, tobacco	2a-C	

SAH, subarachnoid haemorrhage. For definition of other abbreviations, see Table 16.1.

condition is much less common than in adults, paediatric stroke units are unlikely to be a health service priority in the immediate future. In part because of the relative rarity of childhood stroke, the wide range of pathologies and the lack of infrastructure, it has not yet proved possible to conduct large randomized trials of acute treatment in groups of children with similar pathologies. As 15–20% of children presenting with a focal neurological deficit have a non-vascular cause,[13,14] it is very difficult to design protocols which will cover all possibilities. Several units around the world have acquired expertise, however, and this chapter is an attempt to summarize the current position, with a conservative minimum care pathway

suggested for the individual child. Interventions considered are those for which there is either safety data or low risk for harm and evidence of benefit in adults, although none have been assessed by randomized controlled clinical trials in children and data from cohorts does not provide class A evidence of efficacy. Areas of controversy are highlighted, as these are priorities in terms of well-designed randomized controlled trials, particularly if there are significant risks inherent in the therapy. The evidence to date has come largely from studies in adults or from case series in children and must be evaluated in that light when attempting to design a management strategy for an individual child which can be justified to the parents.

There is, however, no longer an excuse for therapeutic nihilism, as although mortality may be lower than for adults, cerebrovascular disease is an important cause of chronic and sometimes progressive childhood disability (see Chapter 17). In all three sets of guidelines,[2–4] most recommendations receive only consensus support as the evidence base contains so few trials[5] (Tables 16.1 and 16.2). As part of the strategy leading up to the development of randomized trials, an international registry, the International Paediatric Stroke Study, has been set up,[15] and patients should be reported, particularly if they have undergone therapies with associated risks. In addition, emergency expert advice for acute management of childhood stroke may be available in individual countries.

General care measures (Tables 16.1 and 16.3)

Emergency management must proceed under appropriate protocols such as Advanced Paediatric Life Support so that the priority is to maintain the airway and cardiovascular function.[16] There are no studies which have specifically examined the effect of disruptions in homeostasis on stroke outcome in children but, based on principles which would be applied to the care of any acutely ill child, as well as from the evidence base in adults, temperature, glucose and oxygen saturation should be maintained within normal limits.[17] At the same time that blood is drawn for emergency chemistry and full blood count, an intravenous line should be sited for administration of isotonic intravenous fluids. The child's hydration status should be assessed and dehydration should be corrected; the rate and nature of fluid replacement depends on electrolyte status. Oxygen saturation, temperature, blood pressure and pulse must be measured regularly; at least hourly for the first 24 hours. Hypotension should be prevented and actively treated. There is evidence for worse outcome in adults with hypertension in the context of acute stroke[18] but there are inadequate data from studies in which patients have been randomized to blood pressure lowering agents or on the prevalence of hypertension in acute stroke in childhood. Hypertensive encephalopathy

and posterior reversible encephalopathy syndrome (PRES) are in the differential diagnosis in children and there is a danger of causing optic nerve and posterior circulation stroke by reducing blood pressure too quickly.[19,20] If significantly raised, blood pressure should therefore be reduced steadily over 24–48 hours. The Glasgow Coma Score should be recorded at hourly intervals until established at 15; a reduced coma score should lead to admission to paediatric intensive care and emergency management of raised intracranial pressure (see below). Patients with a deteriorating level of consciousness should be intubated and ventilated and transferred to the nearest neurosurgical unit in case they require drainage of a haematoma (see Chapter 8), ventriculostomy for hydrocephalus secondary to a large cerebellar infarct[21] or craniectomy for malignant middle cerebral artery territory infarction.[22] Seizures in the acute phase should be managed according to appropriate local, national or international guidelines for the management of acute seizures and status epilepticus.[23–25] Prophylactic compression stockings should be used to prevent deep vein thrombosis in patients with weak or paralysed legs. Infarct volume and outcome appear to be related to body temperature during the first few days of the stroke;[26,27] at present the evidence is inconclusive in children[28] and a direct causative effect remains unproven, but maintaining body temperature just below 37°C is unlikely to do harm. Apart from preventing fever, there is no neuroprotective strategy available at the present time which could be recommended for use in children.

Emergency neuroimaging (Figs 16.1–16.3; see Figs 4.1 and 4.2)

Apart from the lack of randomized controlled trials, the major barrier to evidence-based practice for childhood stroke is the wide range of pathologies, for each of which the current optimal strategy may be different. If emergency magnetic resonance imaging (MRI) is available, despite the need for general anaesthesia in most cases, it has advantages over computed tomography (CT) as, in addition to the essential exclusion

---

TABLE 16.3
Acute supportive care, convalescence and rehabilitation

Review with primary team measures for appropriate monitoring, nursing and general medical care, with attention to specific problems as follows:

- Airway, oxygenation: monitor haemoglobin oxygen saturation, make nil by mouth, provide support as needed for decreased airway protective reflexes from depressed consciousness or brainstem deficits. Careful attention to pulmonary care to prevent aspiration pneumonia.
- Fluids, nutrition: isotonic IV fluids, aim for normoglycaemia, normovolaemia; optimize nutrition early with nutrition consult and supplement as needed with parenteral or tube feedings. Consult speech therapy for feeding/swallow evaluation *prior to restarting oral feeds* for all patients with aphasia, facial weakness, large MCA strokes or significant brainstem deficits.
- Temperature regulation: aggressively prevent and treat hyperthermia (>37.0°C).
- Prevent secondary DVT from immobilization – low dose subcutaneous heparin and compression devices for profound or sustained immobility.
- Acquired infection: balance need for invasive monitoring against risk of acquired infection. Remove indwelling vascular and bladder catheters as soon as possible.
- Musculoskeletal and skin care: involve occupational therapists and physiotherapists early to assist nursing with care plans, positioning, splints, etc., to maintain range of movements and skin integrity.
- Family/social support: provide supportive services to family, and ask case manager to begin evaluating long-term care and placement options/procedures.
- Consult multidisciplinary rehabilitation team within the first 48–72 hours.

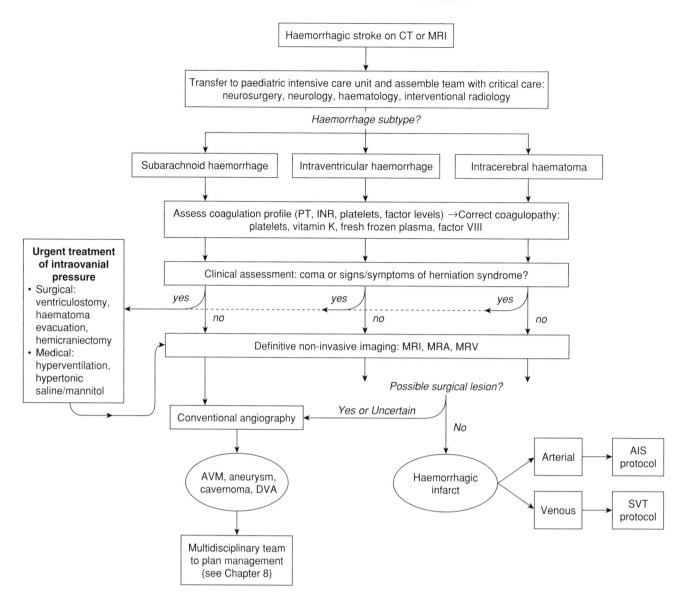

Fig. 16.1. Flow chart for the management of haemorrhagic stroke. AIS, arterial ischaemic stroke; AVM, arteriovenous malformation; DVA, developmental venous anomaly; INR, internal normalized ratio; MRA, magnetic resonance angiography; MRV, magnetic resonance venography; PT, prothrombin time; SUT, sinous venous thrombosis.

of haemorrhage, ischaemia may be documented within minutes (using diffusion-weighted imaging)[29,30] or hours (with T2-weighted imaging),[31] rather than days. In adults, ischaemic but uninfarcted tissue with 'misery perfusion' on perfusion MRI is a target for emergency reperfusion with thrombolysis, usually within a 3- to 6-hour time window, although for basilar artery thrombolysis with balloon angioplasty, there is evidence of benefit at least up to 12 hours.[32] The addition of fat-saturated T1-MRI of the neck,[33] magnetic resonance angiography (MRA) of the circle of Willis[34] and of the neck vessels and magnetic resonance venography (MRV)[35] allows definition of the vascular pathology which may guide management (Table 16.1; see Figs 4.1 and 4.2). Importantly, most of the conditions which mimic ischaemic stroke, such as acute disseminated encephalomyelitis (ADEM), metabolic disease (MELAS) and PRES,[36] may be recognized on MRI (see Figs 4.1 and 4.2), which may mean that a child is not exposed

to the unnecessary risks of antithrombotic therapy, but receives the appropriate evidence-based management strategy for the condition.

Up to 80% of children with an infarct in an arterial territory have large vessel disease demonstrable on MRA or MRI, for example stenosis, occlusion or dissection. Thrombosis in the large venous sinuses (sagittal, lateral, straight) may be diagnosed on MRV or CT venography (Fig. 16.3; see Figs 4.1 and 4.2), which is essential in patients with thalamic or cortical infarcts (particularly parietal and occipital). Although there is a 1% risk of stroke, patients with normal MRA and MRV and no evidence of dissection on fat-saturated MRI of the neck should undergo conventional angiography,[33,34,37] which is usually required for the diagnosis of small vessel vasculitis, cortical venous thrombosis and sometimes for the diagnosis of dissection, particularly in the posterior circulation.

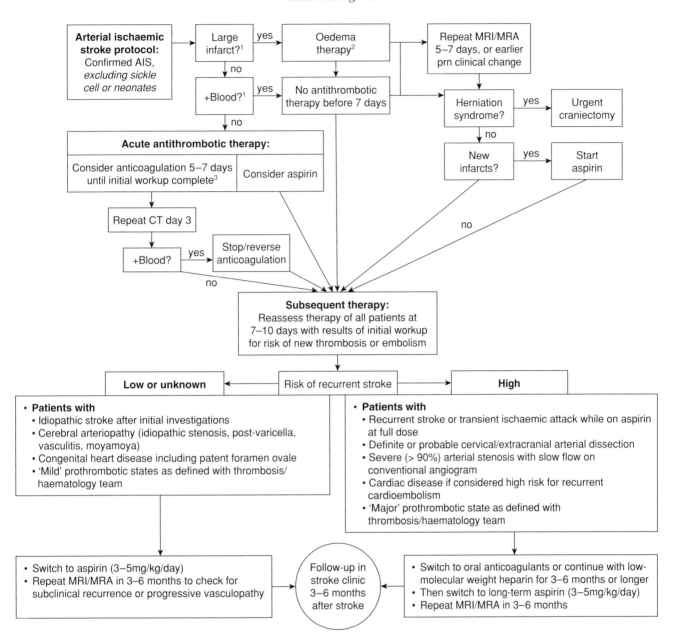

Fig. 16.2. Flow chart for the management of arterial ischaemic stroke (AIS).

[1] **+Blood** = anything more than scant or petechial blood; large infarct = R–L shift, or extensive sulcal effacement, or >1/3 of middle cerebral artery territory.

[2] **Therapy for oedema**: $Paco_2$ 35–45 mmHg, Na 15 0s/Osm 310; if evolving herniation consider craniectomy, hypothermia.

[3] **Anticoagulation therapy**: Always consult haematology team (thrombosis group) in concert with primary treating team. For sinovenous (venous sinus) thrombosis, start as soon as possible. For AIS, may start as early as 12–24 h. If 'large' infarct or blood present, start no sooner than 7 days. Contraindications for heparin or low-molecular-weight heparin include: platelets <50 000; recent intracranial haemorrhage (subdural, subarachnoid, intraventricular, etc); active systemic haemorrhage; major surgery within previous 24 h (negotiable if intracardiac clot), uncontrolled severe hypertension. Asprin is an alternative.

[4] **Thrombotic and embolic risk workup**: cardiac history and examination and electrocardiography in all cases; history of recent vascular instrumentation or immobilization, neck trauma or repeated Valsalva/vomiting; echocardiogram (transoesophageal if high suspicion, consider bubble study if patent foramen ovale present); peripheral vascular examination for signs of embolism or vasculopathy (e.g. hypertension, rash, coarctation); history of varicella; family history of thrombosis.

Laboratory investigations: chemistry, full blood count, coagulation screen; thrombophilia subdural, subarachnoid, intraventricular, regardless of presence of other stroke aetiology (except perhaps haemoglobinopathy). Consult haematology if results abnormal, or if positive family history of thrombophilia. See Figure 16.3 for thrombophilia workup. If stroke is not in typical vascular distribution, add workup for 'metabolic' stroke, including cerebrospinal fluid lactate, plasma lactate/pyruvate, plasma amino acids, urine organic acids. If acute febrile illness consider lumbar puncture, serology for mycoplasma, lyme disease. At later stages, obtain risk factor profiles to guide secondary prevention strategies: fasting cholesterol and lipid profiles; serum folate and iron levels.

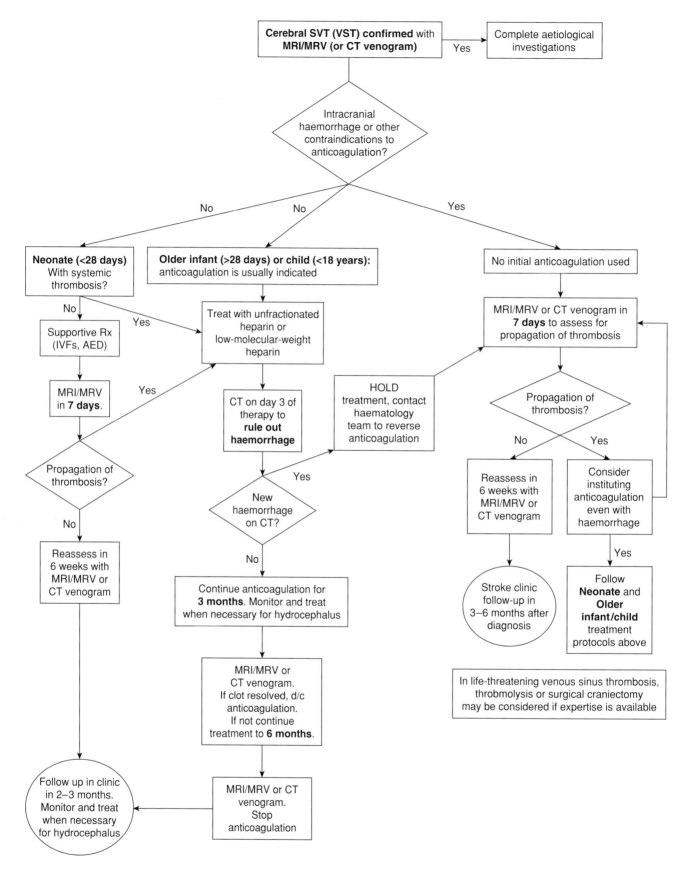

Fig. 16.3. Flow chart for the management of venous sinus (sinovenous) thrombosis (VST, SVT). AED, antiepileptic drugs. IVFs, intravenous fluids; MRV, magnetic resonance venography; Rx treat.

Specific measures

HAEMORRHAGIC STROKE (see Chapter 8; Fig. 16.1)
These patients require immediate transfer to a paediatric intensive care unit with neurosurgery on site in case craniotomy is required (Fig. 16.1) but paediatric neurology and haematology consultations should also be obtained, in view of the wide differential diagnosis and high early mortality of up to 25%. Structural arterial disorders, specifically arteriovenous malformations, aneurysms and cavernomas[38,39] (see Chapter 8), or sinovenous thrombosis[40] (see Chapter 7), or developmental venous anomalies, or coagulopathies[38,39] such as haemophilia, are the most common pathologies. In the acute phase, the main priorities are to prevent cerebral herniation if the blood collection is space-occupying, to reverse any thrombocytopenia or coagulopathy, to exclude sinovenous thrombosis, and to treat any associated vasospasm, for example in subarachnoid haemorrhage, with volume expansion. A randomized controlled trial in adults showed no benefit of early surgery compared with conservative management[41] but children with life-threatening herniation syndromes may benefit from craniectomy and haematoma drainage. Increase in haematoma size is associated with higher mortality and current efforts in adult studies are directed at methods of reducing this using blood pressure reduction,[42] but there is no evidence base in children.

Underlying coagulopathy is particularly common under the age of a year. Haemorrhagic disease of the newborn should be treated with vitamin K and disseminated intravascular coagulation with fresh frozen plasma. Protamine may be used if excess heparin has been given. Fresh platelet transfusion is required if the haemorrhage has occurred in the context of thrombocytopenia and factor VIII is the treatment for haemophilia. Factor VII cannot be recommended for intracranial haemorrhage as the encouraging results of a phase II trial[43] were not confirmed in a larger phase III study,[44] at least in part because of the risk of ischaemic complications, although it has been used in a few children with life-threatening bleeding with mixed results.[45–47]

Emergency vascular imaging should include an MR venogram as well as an MR angiogram, as 10% of haemorrhages in young adults are secondary to sinovenous thrombosis (SVT) and the underlying conditions for which there is a high mortality include those in which SVT has been described.[39] The management of SVT with haemorrhage in childhood is controversial (see below), but in two anticoagulant trials in adults,[48,49] new haemorrhage was not documented. Heparin should certainly be considered if there is deterioration in clinical status, for example intractable seizures, coma or CT or MRV evidence of propagation of thrombus (Fig. 16.3). Intravascular thromobolysis may occasionally be indicated[50,51] (see Chapter 7).

If there is an underlying arteriovenous malformation, the risk of rebleeding is 2–3% per year for life if untreated and a carefully considered decision over management needs to be made once the patient has recovered from the acute phase. Although less common, aneurysms are associated with a more significant rebleeding risk, particularly in the acute phase. Ideally, a vascular team with considerable experience should evaluate these children so that an individual management strategy, targeted at early spasm and preventing recurrent re-bleeding from the lesion, can be implemented (see Chapter 8).

ISCHAEMIC STROKE (Fig. 16.2)
Approximately half the children presenting with arterial ischaemic stroke,[13] and a similar proportion of those with sinovenous thrombosis,[35,39] have a known predisposing condition, particularly sickle cell disease, cardiac disease and bacterial meningitis. Some of these children are candidates for emergency management of the stroke, for example exchange transfusion for patients with sickle cell disease (see Chapter 15) or anticoagulation for venous sinus thrombosis (see Chapter 7) (Fig. 16.2 and Table 16.1). Ideally, neuroimaging to identify the pathology of the infarct and of the vascular disease should be performed either before or as therapy commences (see Figs 4.1 and 4.2).

Transfusion for emergency management of stroke in sickle cell disease (Table 16.4)
Transfusion therapy has evolved through haematological clinical experience[52–57] rather than being subject to rigorous evaluation by randomized controlled trial.[58] Transfusion improves tissue oxygenation,[59] allowing a reduction in the compensatory cerebral hyperaemia[60] and may occasionally be associated with improvement in the vasculopathy.[61,62] Haemoglobin should be measured at presentation with any neurological complication; if there has been any recent transfusion, the percentage of the haemoglobin (Hb) which is HbS/non-S (laboratories variably report either HbS% or non-S%, so both are given here) should also be quantified. Compatible red cells units (20ml/kg) should be made available as quickly as possible. In the UK red cell units are provided by the National Blood Service, and are screened for transmissible pathogens (hepatitis B by surface antigen; HIV 1 and 2, HTLV, and syphilis by antibody; hepatitis C by antibody and RNA). All donations are leucodepleted and some donations are tested for cytomegalovirus which may be required in selected patients – for example cytomegalovirus-negative patients who might be considered for later transplant. Units should be HbS negative.

Where no atypical antibodies are detected red cell units should be selected that are ABO, fully Rhesus (including C/c and E/e as well as D) and Kell compatible; that is, they should be negative for any ABO, Rhesus and Kell antigens that the patient lacks. A full red cell phenotype should be among the first blood tests an infant with sickle cell disease has, in order to allow provision of suitable units should the need arise. Where pre-transfusion testing detects atypical antibodies, the units must additionally be antigen negative for the antibodies detected. Selected units should be HbS negative. Any other testing and issuing of the products should be guided in accordance with the blood transfusion laboratory local policies and procedures.

TABLE 16.4
Exchange transfusion for stroke in sickle cell disease

Aims: HbS <30%; Hb 10–11g/dl; steady blood volume
Check: Hb, HbS, HbA
Cross match: 20ml/kg packed cells
1–2 intravenous lines, 100ml/h, 5–10ml/kg/aliquot
Monitor blood pressure, haemoglobin oxygen saturation, pulse, temperature every five minutes.

Initial Hb	<6g/dl	6–7g/dl	7–9g/dl	>9g/dl
	Out: nil	In: 5ml/kg saline	In: 10ml/kg saline	In: 15ml/kg saline
	In: 5ml/kg blood	Out: 5ml/kg blood	Out: 10ml/kg blood	Out: 15ml/kg blood
	Out: 5ml/kg blood	In: 5ml/kg blood	In: 5 ml/kg blood	In: 5ml/kg blood
	In: 5ml/kg blood	Out: 10ml/kg blood	Out: 10ml/kg blood	Out: 15ml/kg blood
		In: 5ml/kg blood	In: 5ml/kg blood	In: 5ml/kg blood
Blood so far	Out: 5ml/kg	Out: 15ml/kg	Out: 20ml/kg	Out: 30ml/kg
	In: 10ml/kg	In: 10ml/kg	In: 10ml/kg	In: 10ml/kg
Check Hb	<7g/dl	7–8g/dl	8–9g/dl	>9g/dl
	In: 10ml/kg saline	In: 15ml/kg saline	In: 15ml/kg saline	In: 20ml/kg saline
	Out: 5ml/kg blood	Out: 10ml/kg blood	Out: 15ml/kg blood	Out: 15ml/kg blood
	In: 5ml/kg blood	In: 5ml/kg blood	In: 5ml/kg blood	In: 5ml/kg blood
	Out: 10ml/kg blood	Out: 10ml/kg blood	Out: 10ml/kg blood	Out: 15ml/kg blood
Additional blood	Out: 15ml/kg	Out: 20ml/kg	Out: 25ml/kg	Out: 30ml/kg
	In: 5ml/kg	In: 5ml/kg	In: 5ml/kg	In: 5ml/kg

Check haemoglobin (Hb), calculate (11 − present Hb) × weight in kg × 3.5 to top up to Hb 10–11g/dl.
Saline exchange if Hb>14g/dl, further exchange if HbA% <80%.

If available, exchange rather than top-up transfusion is recommended by most haematologists, although there are no randomized data. The goal should be to begin the exchange transfusion within 2–4 hours of presentation with an acute neurological event, particularly if the deficit is persisting or progressing. Emergency exchange transfusion at the time of presentation with first stroke appears to reduce the risk of recurrence[63] by an unknown mechanism.

The aim of the exchange transfusion is to reduce the haemoglobin S percentage to <30% that is, non-S Hb >70% and raise the haemoglobin to 10–11g/dl with a haematocrit of >30% and this can be accomplished using a manual regime as outlined in Table 16.4 or using an automated cell separator for erythrocytapheresis. If manual exchange is performed, two or three procedures are usually required; automation usually allows the exchange to be completed in a single session but requires good venous access. Ideally two intravenous lines should be placed so that saline may be infused whilst blood is withdrawn in the other line, although it is possible to exchange through one large vein using a 20ml syringe and a three-way tap and a diaphragm bung into which the venesection bag needle is inserted. A central line is needed if peripheral access is impossible. The volumes for the exchange are calculated once the haemoglobin is known and are recalculated at the halfway stage depending on the repeat haemoglobin (Table 16.4). Exchange transfusion must be conducted slowly, in aliquots of 5–10ml/kg, and with caution in view of the occasional association with neurological deterioration, perhaps related to increasing viscosity[64] and/or blood pressure.[65–67] Aliquots should be recalculated to be no more than 5ml/kg if

the patient is acutely unwell or hypoxic. Once the exchange is complete, a top-up transfusion may be required to increase the haemoglobin to 10–11g/dl using the formula:

$$(11 - \text{present Hb}) \times \text{weight in kg} \times 3.5\text{ml}$$

The levels achieved by exchanging a certain volume of blood are to an extent predictable, but as in any biological system there is some individual variation. If at the end of the first exchange, the percentage of non-S haemoglobin is less than 70%, but the total Hb is too high to achieve that level by a simple top-up, then a further small exchange may be required. Thus, supposing that a post-exchange check gives an Hb level of 10g/dl, but non-S only 50%, it is necessary to venesect down to 8g/dl (thus 20% of blood volume, calculated at 70ml/kg, preceded by the same volume of saline infused) in order that a final top-up to 10g/dl will increase the non-S level by the required 20% up to 70%.

If the patient has had a neurological event in the context of severe anaemia (e.g. splenic sequestration or aplastic crisis), or if exchange transfusion is going to be delayed for more than 4 hours, urgent top-up blood transfusion by 2–3g/dl should be considered in the interim.

Historically, patients with stroke in the context of sickle cell disease have often been managed in local hospitals without access to neuroimaging or with access to CT only, although it has become clear that the pathology includes haemorrhage,[67] sinovenous thrombosis,[35,68–70] posterior reversible encephalopathy syndrome,[71,72] acute necrotizing encephalitis[73] and arterial dissection[74] as well as watershed infarction secondary to distal internal carotid, middle and anterior cerebral artery stenosis, and emergency MRI, MRA and MRV may guide management. Although published cases are rare, there is no known contraindication to management of haemorrhage, sinovenous thrombosis or dissection as outlined in the protocols for non-sickle stroke. Haemorrhage is commonly secondary to aneurysm,[75] sinovenous thrombosis[35] or moyamoya. Interventional neuroradiology with coils has been successfully employed for the management of aneurysms in sickle cell disease[76] and represents a reasonable alternative to clipping at surgery.[77]

Thrombolysis with tissue plasminogen activator

In adults with ischaemic stroke, the main focus of recent studies has been in looking at the possibility of minimizing the effect of the initial stroke by promoting hyper-acute recanalization of the occluded artery using thrombolysis. One controlled study of intravenous tissue plasminogen activator (tPA), conducted in adults who could be randomized and treated within 3 hours, showed significant benefit in terms of outcome at 3 months[6] with subsequent confirmation from observational studies.[78] Intra-arterial thrombolysis with urokinase within 6 hours of onset of stroke caused by middle cerebral artery occlusion onset improves outcome[79,80] and is considered to be an option for patients within 6 hours of stroke onset who are not candidates for intravenous tPA.[81] In a study of basilar occlusion in 619 adults, there was little evidence of advantage for intra-arterial thrombolysis over intravenous thrombolysis or antithrombotic treatment (antiplatelet agents or anticoagulation)[82] but all 27 patients given no treatment did badly and trials are needed. Mechanical thrombectomy with intra-arterial thrombolysis can be considered as a method to achieve patency if intravenous thrombolysis fails.[83] However, thrombolysis in adults carries at least a 2% risk of symptomatic haemorrhage,[78] associated with considerable mortality, and although some patients benefit when treated beyond 3 hours, the results

beyond a 6-hour time window have been very disappointing. The prognosis is poor for those with internal carotid occlusion.[84,85] Even with the reorganization of services for adults with acute stroke to enable emergency transport and triage, only about 5–20% of adult stroke patients fulfil the criteria for thrombolysis.

There have been no randomized controlled trials which address the use of tPA in the acute treatment of stroke in children. In fact, it appears that 2–4% of children presenting with stroke currently receive thrombolysis.[86,87] A few cases with good outcome have been published using intravenous or intra-arterial tPA for anterior circulation stroke.[84,88–97] For basilar occlusion, urokinase[32,84,98–102] or tPA[103,104] (Fig. 16.4) has often been combined with balloon angioplasty or other mechanical methods for thrombolysis. There is often considerable pressure to consider thrombolysis outside the time window in children, particularly if the child is unconscious or has a severe neurological deficit, if the stroke is iatrogenic or if there is basilar occlusion where the time window compatible with good recovery is longer.[32] Haemorrhage is a significant risk[87] and is probably higher with longer time to treatment. There appears to be a publication bias, with an excess of published cases to date treated according to the adult guidelines and with good outcome,[87] while overall mortality and morbidity are worse in the very high risk patients receiving tPA.[86]

Although children with a stroke often present to a doctor within 3 hours, because of the rarity of stroke, the low sensitivity of CT for acute infarction and the wide differential in this age group, the diagnosis of arterial occlusion is rarely made with any degree of certainty at this stage. In addition, mortality is lower and most children presenting with stroke can probably expect to lead independent lives as adults. It is therefore difficult to see a major role for thrombolysis in this age group at the present time, although a protocol has been developed for those over the age of 18 (Table 16.5). Very occasionally, if occlusive arterial thrombus is visualized, thrombolysis

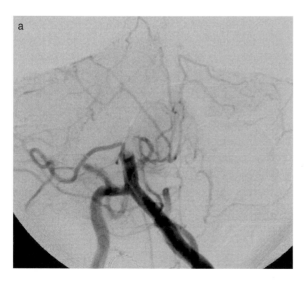
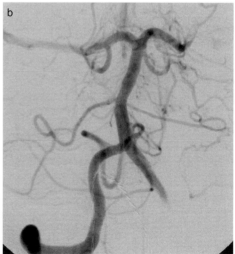

Fig. 16.4. (a) Basilar occlusion in a deeply unconscious 11-year-old boy with artery vertebral dissection after being hit with a schoolbag. (b) Basilar patency was restored after mechanical thrombolysis with intra-arterial tissue plasminogen activator 11 hours after presentation; outcome was good with mild ataxia only. (Images courtesy of Dr John Millar, consultant neuroradiologist, Southampton University Hospitals NHS Trust.)

TABLE 16.5
Tissue plasminogen activator (tPA) protocol for treatment of acute AIS in patients >18 years of age

Inclusion criteria

- Clinical diagnosis of ischaemic stroke, with onset* of symptoms within 4.5 hours of initiation of treatment for IV tPA; or within 6 hours of initiation of treatment for intra-arterial tPA or within 12 hours of initiation of treatment for basilar thrombosis. If unable to start IV tPA at less than 4.5 hours from symptom onset, or basilar thrombosis, arrange arteriogram for possible mechanical thrombolysis and/or intra-arterial tPA.
- CT (non-contrast) without evidence of haemorrhage.
- Clinical deficit is potentially life-threatening or significantly disabling.

Exclusion criteria

- Rapidly improving stroke symptoms, or *mild non-disabling deficit.*
- Seizure at onset of stroke (*relative contraindication, as post-ictal state may exacerbate apparent neurological deficit*).
- Symptoms suggestive of subarachnoid haemorrhage, even if CT is normal.
- *Severe neurological deficit, NIHSS > 22 (relative contraindication, expanded discussion with family about risk vs. benefit).*
- CT with evidence of haemorrhage.
- CT with evidence of hypodensity and/or effacement of cerebral sulci in >33% of middle cerebral artery territory (*relative contraindication, expanded discussion with family about risk vs. benefit*).
- Stroke or head trauma within prior 3 months.
- Any prior history of intracranial haemorrhage which may increase risk for recurrent haemorrhage.
- Major surgery within 14 days. (*No IV tPA. intra-arterial tPA negotiable with surgeon.*)
- Gastrointestinal or genitourinary bleeding within previous 21 days.
- Arterial puncture at a non-compressible site, or lumbar puncture within 7 days.
- Clinical presentation consistent with acute myocardial infarction or post-myocardial infarction pericarditis requires evaluation by cardiologist prior to treatment.
- Persistent systolic blood pressure (BP)>185 or diastolic BP>110mmHg (or disproportionately high for age), or requiring aggressive therapy to control BP.
- Platelets <100 000μl.
- Glucose < 50 or > 400mg/dl.
- Concurrent treatment with warfarin, *and* PT>15s, or INR>1.7.
- If known coagulopathy present, and PT>15s.
- On heparin therapy within 48 hours and with elevated PTT or INR>1.7.
- Pregnant or lactating female (*if uncertain, check HCG or expand discussion about risk*).

Administration and management

1. Mobilize stroke service: call paediatric neurology consultant, and adult stroke consultant as appropriate; and interventional neuroradiologist, intensivist and anaesthesiologists as appropriate.
2. Supportive care and preparation for therapy: cardiorespiratory monitoring, head of bed flat, IV isotonic fluids, place second IV line for possible tPA; send for laboratory investigations (full blood count, platelets, coagulation screen, chemistry, glucose, type and cross match).
3. Arrange urgent CT (within 1 hour).
4. For patients meeting inclusion criteria within 4.5 hours of symptoms onset, start IV tPA with paediatric neurologist attending and resident in attendance. Admit to paediatric intensive care unit (or cardiac intensive care unit if cardiac patient) when bed available.
5. For patients with anterior circulation stroke between >4.5h and <6h of symptom onset, discuss option of intra-arterial t-PA with adult stroke service. Supportive care, monitoring and preparation same as for IV t-PA.
6. For patients with posterior circulation stroke between >4.5h and <12h of symptom onset, discuss option of mechanical thrombolysis and intra-arterial t-PA with adult stroke service and interventional neuroradiologist. Supportive care, monitoring and preparation same as for IV t-PA.
7. Administration of IV t-PA: MUST BEGIN WITHIN 4.5H OF SYMPTOM ONSET*
   - Total dose: 0.9mg/kg (maximum dose is 90mg).
   - Administration: 10% of the dose as an IV bolus over 1 minute, remainder infused over 1 hour, via dedicated IV line for t-PA.
   - Hold other anticoagulation treatment for at least 24 hours (heparin, warfarin, aspirin, ticlopidine).
   - Monitor in intensive care unit for at least 48 hours for close neurological and cardiac monitoring.
   - Avoid invasive procedures (blood tests, lines, nasogastric tube) for at least 24 hours.

Major adverse effect: intracranial haemorrhage.
In event of suspected intracranial haemorrhage, immediately arrange for CT and laboratory investigations (PT, PTT, platelets, fibrinogen, type and cross), and prepare to give 6–8 units of cryoprecipitate (fibrinogen and factor VIII) and 6–8 units of platelets.

---

* Symptom onset = time when patient was last seen well. HCG, human chorionic gonadotrophin; INR, internal normalized ratio; NIHSS, National Institutes of Health Stroke Score; PT, prothrombin time; PTT, partial thromboplastin time.

with intravenous tPA given within 3 hours or intra-arterial tPA within 6 hours may be considered for middle cerebral artery occlusion or intra-arterial tPA within 12 hours for basilar artery occlusion, after detailed counselling and consultation with the family. Circumstances in which this may be justifiable include children known to be at risk (e.g. because of congenital heart disease) who suffer stroke in hospital and those who arrive at a centre with experience in the use of tPA within the relevant time window. However the use of thrombolysis in patients who have stroke in hospital and who have undergone a recent surgical procedure is very controversial. Transcranial Doppler thrombolysis[105] is an attractive option in children but more research into this and the role of mechanical thrombectomy is required.[106]

In sinovenous thrombosis, experience with thrombolysis is confined to case reports and small series.[51,107–110] There are no randomized data even in adults,[111,112] but it has been used in small series of seriously ill patients, including children, usually in coma and with extensive thrombosis of superficial and deep venous structures.[107–112] A non-randomized study comparing urokinase thrombolysis with heparin in adults suggested better functional outcome for the thrombolysed patients but higher risk of haemorrhage.[50]

Ideally, all children with stroke given tPA should be documented carefully in the International Paediatric Stroke Registry, so that complications and outcome can be documented and indications worked out.

Prevention of propagation of thrombus and early recurrence (Table 16.2)

The acute management of children without sickle cell disease who have stroke remains controversial and some physicians give no specific treatment. As outlined above, unless emergency MRI is available, there may be difficulty in distinguishing sinovenous thrombosis from arterial stroke, although there may be clinical clues. Although there are no epidemiologically based data, children with non-sickle arterial ischaemic stroke referred to teaching centres have an early recurrence risk for stroke of at least 10% (see Chapter 17) and an even higher risk of further transient ischemic attacks. For cerebral venous sinus thrombosis (CVST), although there may be spontaneous recanalization of thrombosed venous sinuses with general measures such as rehydration and correction of hypoxaemia,[35] propagation of sinovenous thrombosis may be associated with clinical deterioration and poor outcome, including death, in childhood[35] and recurrence occurs, albeit less often than in AIS.[113]

ANTICOAGULATION

The question of anticoagulation treatment for childhood stroke remains a difficult one. In adults with ischaemic stroke, probably mainly arterial, one trial suggested benefit.[114] In the very large International Stroke Trial[115] patients allocated to heparin had significantly fewer recurrent ischaemic strokes within 14 days (2.9% vs 3.8%), but this was offset by a similar-sized increase in haemorrhagic strokes (1.2% vs 0.4%), so the difference in death or non-fatal recurrent stroke (11.7% vs 12.0%) was not significant. As children are less at risk of haemorrhage, have an increased prevalence of prothrombotic disorders, and have a more frequent underlying arterial dissection or cardiac embolism, there may be a case for initial anticoagulation in non-haemorrhagic arterial ischaemic stroke[116] and it is widely used, particularly in dissection and in children with cardiac disease.[117] Two prospective cohort studies have assessed initial high dose (1.5mg/kg 12-hourly) low molecular weight heparin (LMWH) treatment in a total of 80 children with unselected arterial stroke, and reported no major haemorrhages; however in two patients there was subclinical haemorrhagic conversion of initially bland infarcts.[118,119] In another cohort series, in which physicians chose either low dose (1–1.5mg/kg/day) LMWH at prophylactic doses or aspirin for their patients, the long-term recurrence rates were similar.[120] Since this was not a randomized controlled trial, efficacy could not be assessed,[121] but there was no obvious bias in the physician's choice.[120]

For sinovenous thrombosis (Fig. 16.3), in adults a small controlled trial of intravenous unfractionated heparin showed reduction in mortality[48] and a larger controlled trial of subcutaneous LMWH showed a trend for benefit in terms of death and dependency.[49] It is the practice of many adult stroke centres to anticoagulate regardless of the presence of haemorrhage because of the very high risk in the absence of anticoagulation for clot propagation, expansion of infarction and ultimately herniation and death. Some paediatric neurologists have adopted this approach and always anticoagulate non-neonates (and sometimes neonates as well) even if there is already haemorrhagic infarction present. The exception is in children who have skull fractures as the cause of their thrombosis. The decision to treat is controversial when there is haemorrhage present, and an expanded discussion of risk versus benefit is in order. Some patients may be treated if the risk of witholding anticoagulation is considered to outweigh the risk of treatment. Non-recanalization is common[120] and is associated with recurrence[113] but it is not yet clear whether anticoagulation makes a difference to late patency rates. Several studies have also reported feasibility and safety of unfractionated intravenous or subcutaneous LMWH in neonatal or childhood SVT[35,40,113,122–125] and there is a little evidence for better cognitive outcome[35] as well as reduced recurrence.[113]

For dissection of the extracranial arteries, data available from studies in adults suggest that there is a relatively small risk of early recurrent events on antithrombotic treatment[126–131] and a controlled trial would be needed with around 2000 patients to determine whether anticoagulation had any benefit over antiplatelet agents in reducing this risk. In addition to recurrent events secondary to embolism, which may be more common in the posterior than in the anterior circulation,[130,131] recurrent dissection has been described in children.[130] Although antithrombotic treatment appears to reduce the risk of recurrence in the cases reported,[130] recurrent events may occur occasionally despite anticoagulation[37,130–132] or antiplatelet agents,[130] perhaps in relation to bony instability in the neck.[131] Stent placement carries considerable risk[129] although it has occasionally been undertaken in children.[133]

Providing there is no haemorrhage on brain imaging, anticoagulation should be considered in children with confirmed extracranial arterial dissection[134] or ischaemic stroke or cerebral venous sinus thrombosis (Fig. 16.3).[123] The use of anticoagulation in patients with cardiac embolism is controversial, and may be influenced by the cardiac pathology and by neurological and imaging findings. Individual patient management should involve senior clinicians in cardiology and neurology. There may also be a case for anticoagulating patients with known prothrombotic abnormalities.

Choice of antiplatelet or anticoagulant treatment in childhood ischaemic stroke: available data on safety and efficacy in terms of prevention of recurrence

In two very large controlled trials in adults,[115,135] aspirin appeared to be associated with a modest improvement in outcome, probably because of a reduction in early recurrence and the risk of haemorrhage appeared to be lower than with anticoagulants. Although there have been no controlled trials, antiplatelet or anticoagulant therapy is now commonly prescribed in acute stroke in children without sickle cell disease.[56,136–142] Aspirin at low to moderate dose appears to be safe in children with arterial ischaemic stroke (AIS).[120,137,138,143] In the German cohort,[138] physicians chose aspirin (5mg/kg/day) or LMWH as secondary prophylaxis for their patients; the risk of recurrent stroke (clinical event accompanied by infarction on imaging) was 10% in both arms. In the Hershey, Pennsylvania, cohort, nine were treated with LMWH (Enoxaparin) 1mg/kg or 60mg if >60kg and eight received other anticoagulation; no recurrences were reported.[139,140] There was one haemorrhagic transformation. In Barnes' series,[141] 28/95 patients were treated (16 antiplatelet, nine anticoagulation, two antiplatelet + anticoagulation, one thromolysis + anticoagulation). Three children were known to have recurred. There was no effect of treatment on outcome; data on recurrence were not examined as numbers were too small. In Soman's report[142] from the Toronto cohort, 17 children (13 recurrent stroke or transient ischaemic attack (TIA) on aspirin, four intolerant of aspirin) received clopidogril (nine alone, eight concurrent with aspirin). Two had subdural haemorrhages (both also on aspirin, both had marked cerebral atrophy: one moyamoya, one progeria vasculopathy). During follow-up for a mean of 1.69 years (range 1 month to 3 years), there were no further recurrent events. In Bonduel's series,[143] six died acutely, two (2%) of thrombosis and four from the underlying disease. All those with cardiac disease were warfarinized and there were no recurrences in this group. There were four (5%) second events in the 84 children without cardiac disease who were treated with aspirin; none of these patients had further events after warfarinization. There were no major haemorrhagic complications. Sixty-three (68%) had neurological sequelae. In Ganesan's[144] series, of 171 children with a first stroke who did not have sickle cell disease physicians chose to treat 64 with aspirin and 33 with anticoagulation, while 74 were not treated. Thirteen (6%) died, one after haemorrhagic transformation, three acutely of other causes, four at the time of clinical recurrence, five later after censoring at the time of recurrence. After adjusting for the presence of vasculopathy, there was a trend for reduction in risk of recurrence for aspirin (hazard ratio (HR), HR, 0.55, 95% confidence intervals (CI) 0.26–1.16, p=0.11) but not for anticoagulation (HR 1.06, 95% CI 0.45–2.59; p=0.89). In Fullerton's series,[145] overall there was no effect of antithrombotic treatment on the risk of recurrence (log rank, p=0.42) although only 9% of those treated with aspirin recurred, compared with 18% of those on no treatment (and 27% of those anticoagulated, perhaps because they were considered to be at higher risk of recurrence). In a recent French

series,[146] aspirin prophylaxis was prescribed for the majority of the children and recurrence was rare in the anterior circulation. Although there have been no studies assessing benefit in children, a moderate dose (3–5mg/kg/day) is reasonable, once there is radiological confirmation of arterial ischaemic stroke, except in patients with evidence of intracranial haemorrhage on imaging.

MANAGEMENT OF INTRACTABLE INTRACRANIAL HYPERTENSION

Early referral to a paediatric intensive care unit with access to neurosurgery is essential for children with stroke who have depressed or deteriorating conscious level or other signs of raised intracranial pressure. Intracranial pressure monitoring is of help in guiding medical management of intracranial hypertension with control of ventilation, fluid balance and temperature (Figs 16.1 and 16.2). If intracranial pressure continues to rise or there is evidence of transtentorial herniation, there is a good case for craniectomy in children presenting in coma with large ischaemic middle cerebral infarcts (Fig. 16.5), as this is almost always fatal if managed conservatively and there is evidence of benefit for those with stroke in the dominant as well as the non-dominant hemisphere in cohort studies[147] and three randomized trials involving adults younger than 60 years[148]. Case reports and small series have also reported benefit in childhood,[22,149–152] although there may be publication bias. Young age is one of the best predictors of survival and good outcome after this procedure.[153,154] In adults, a Glasgow Coma Score (GCS) of ≤7 was a predictor of poor outcome,[155] although independent outcome has been reported in children with a GCS as low as 7.[22] Technique, including size of the craniotomy and durotomy, removal of overlying temporal muscle and the creation of a vascular tunnel[156] may make a difference to the likelihood of good outcome. Neuroimaging criteria suggestive of poor outcome include attenuated corticomedullary contrast as well as evidence of midline shift and extent of infarction, particularly if the entire middle cerebral artery (MCA) territory is involved and/or there is extension of the infarction into the anterior or posterior cerebral artery territory.[153] A volume larger than 145cm^3 on diffusion-weighted imaging is also a good predictor and either CT or magnetic resonance perfusion may be used to define the extent of tissue at risk. Other early predictors include midline shift detected using transcranial Doppler duplex ultrasound,[157] high serum S100[158] or cellular fibronection, and reduced non-transmitter amino acids in the non-infarcted ipsilateral hemisphere on microdialysis. There is a little evidence from animal studies and human cohorts that early craniectomy, before signs of uncal herniation develop, is associated with better outcome but the difficulty is that these patients might have done well without surgery. Patients with hydrocephalus secondary to large cerebellar infarcts may need ventriculostomy instead of or as well as decompression.

Children with cerebral venous sinus thrombosis have a high risk of secondary complications, including status epilepticus, hydrocephalus[50,125] and raised intracranial pressure,[159,160] and

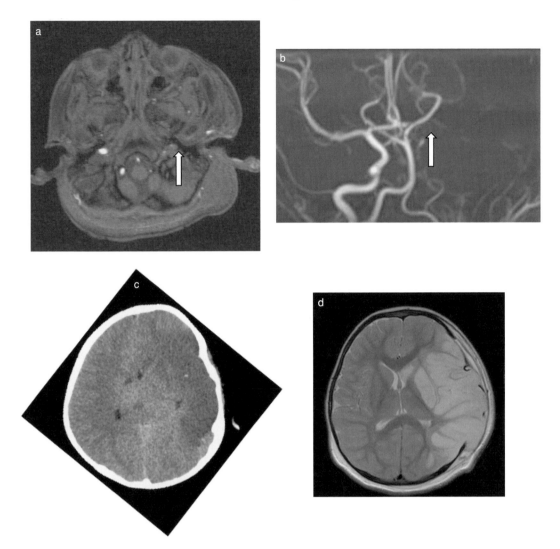

Fig. 16.5. Occlusion of the carotid artery in the neck on T1-weighted MRI of the neck (a) and magnetic resonance angiography of the neck (b) in an unconscious 2-year-old boy with a dense hemiparesis who had been running with a pencil in his mouth. There is a large middle cerebral artery territory infarct before (c) and after (d) surgical decompression. He woke up, and one year later was walking and talking although he had significant developmental and behavioural problems, at least in part related to his premorbid hyperactivity and a previous fall with a significant head injury.

may benefit from intensive care and monitoring of electroencephalography (EEG) and intracranial pressure as well as neuroimaging. There are no randomized data of surgical decompression in cerebral venous sinus thrombosis even in adults, but it has been used with apparent success in isolated cases or small series of seriously ill patients in coma and with extensive thrombosis of superficial and deep venous structures.[161,162]

MANAGEMENT OF NON-VASCULAR STROKE SYNDROMES
(see Figs 4.1 and 4.2)

Posterior reversible encephalopathy syndrome
This apparently reversible condition has been described in children with hypertension, including sickle cell disease, although it is clear that the clinical and radiological features may occur in patients with normal blood pressure. Other associated conditions include hypoglycaemia, human immunodeficiency virus and ciclosporin toxicity. The clinical hallmarks are visual dis-

turbance, seizures, headache and altered mental status. The majority of patients make a full clinical and radiological recovery after conservative measures, including very slow reduction of blood pressure and maintenance of normal oxygenation and glucose levels.

Acute disseminated encephalomyelitis
MRI may reveal acute demyelination in children presenting with acute focal neurological signs mimicking stroke. There is evidence that intravenous methyl prednisolone reduces the duration of the illness and perhaps reduces relapse rate and improves long-term outcome[163] and some children with progressive disease appear to benefit from immunoglobulin or plasmapheresis.[164]

Metabolic disease
Treatment is generally supportive in the acute stage and the priority is to make a diagnosis in case long-term therapy (e.g.

enzyme replacement for Fabry disease) is an option (see Chapter 14). Arginine appears to reduce the duration of the stroke-like episodes in MELAS[165,166] and may also improve endothelial function.[167]

Conclusion

For adults, the funded large randomized controlled trials have shown benefit for acute treatment with aspirin, thrombolysis and surgical decompression in arterial stroke and acute anti-coagulation with heparin in venous sinus thrombosis. The Cochrane collaboration has allowed the rapid dissemination of the available evidence base on acute management of stroke in adults. The concept of a 'brain attack' has received widespread publicity and many adults are now triaged very quickly. By contrast, even when a child has a predisposing condition such as a congenital heart malformation or sickle cell disease, lack of awareness that stroke occurs and that 'time is brain' means that currently the mean time to presentation is more than one day.[168] However, although the level of evidence is much less, the publication of guidelines for childhood stroke[2-4] is likely to lead to more consistent management for childhood stroke and international collaboration should eventually lead to adequately powered randomized controlled trials of new treatments which reduce mortality and morbidity and reduce recurrence.

REFERENCES

1. California Acute Stroke Pilot Registry Investigators. The impact of standardized stroke orders on adherence to best practices. Neurology 2005; 65(3):360–365.
2. Royal College of Physicians. Stroke in Childhood: Clinical Guidelines for Diagnosis, Management and Rehabilitation. 2004. http://www.rcplondon.ac.uk/pubs/. . ./childstroke/childstroke_guidelines.pdf
3. Monagle P, Chalmers E, Chan A, deVeber G, Kirkham F, Massicotte P et al. Antithrombotic therapy in neonates and children: American College of Chest Physicians Evidence-Based Clinical Practice Guidelines (8th Edition). Chest 2008; 133(6 Suppl):887S–968S.
4. Roach ES, Golomb MR, Adams R, Biller J, Daniels S, deVeber G et al. Management of stroke in infants and children: a scientific statement from a Special Writing Group of the American Heart Association Stroke Council and the Council on Cardiovascular Disease in the Young. Stroke 2008; 39(9):2644–2691.
5. deVeber G, Kirkham F. Guidelines for the treatment and prevention of stroke in children. Lancet Neurol 2008; 7(11):983–985.
6. The National Institute of Neurological Disorders and Stroke. rt-PA stroke study group. Tissue plasminogen activator for acute ischemic stroke. New Engl J Med 1995; 333:1581–1587.
7. Hacke W, Donnan G, Fieschi C, Kaste M, von KR, Broderick JP et al. Association of outcome with early stroke treatment: pooled analysis of ATLANTIS, ECASS, and NINDS rt-PA stroke trials. Lancet 2004; 363(9411):768–774.
8. Wardlaw JM, Murray V, Berge E, Del Zoppo GJ. Thrombolysis for acute ischaemic stroke. Cochrane Database Syst Rev 2009; Oct 7; (4):CD000213.
9. Indredavik B, Bakke F, Slordahl SA, Rokseth R, Haheim LL. Stroke unit treatment improves long-term quality of life: a randomized controlled trial. Stroke 1998; 29(5):895–899.
10. Stroke Unit Trialists' Collaboration. Organised inpatient (stroke unit) care for stroke. Cochrane Database Syst Rev 2007 Oct 17; (4):CD000197.
11. Indredavik B, Bakke F, Slordahl SA, Rokseth R, Haheim LL. Stroke unit treatment. 10-year follow-up. Stroke 1999; 30(8):1524–1527.
12. Drummond AE, Pearson B, Lincoln NB, Berman P. Ten year follow-up of a randomized controlled trial of care in a stroke rehabilitation unit. BMJ 2005; 331(7515):491–492.
13. Ganesan V, Prengler M, McShane MA, Wade AM, Kirkham FJ. Investigation of risk factors in children with arterial ischemic stroke. Ann Neurol 2003; 53(2):167–173.
14. Shellhaas RA, Smith SE, O'Tool E, Licht DJ, Ichord RN. Mimics of childhood stroke: characteristics of a prospective cohort. Pediatrics 2006; 118(2):704–709.
15. Golomb MR, Fullerton HJ, Nowak-Gottl U, deVeber G. Male predominance in childhood ischemic stroke: findings from the international pediatric stroke study. Stroke 2009; 40(1):52–57.
16. Pappachan J, Kirkham FJ. Cerebrovascular disease and stroke. Arch Dis Child 2008; 93(10):890–898.
17. ez-Tejedor E, Fuentes B. Homeostasis as basis of acute stroke treatment: stroke units are the key. Cerebrovasc Dis 2005; 20(Suppl 2):129–134.
18. Willmot M, Leonardi-Bee J, Bath PM. High blood pressure in acute stroke and subsequent outcome: a systematic review. Hypertension 2004; 43(1):18–24.
19. Taylor D, Ramsay J, Day S, Dillon M. Infarction of the optic nerve head in children with accelerated hypertension. Br J Ophthalmol 1981; 65(3):153–160.
20. Mak W, Chan KH, Cheung RT, Ho SL. Hypertensive encephalopathy: BP lowering complicated by posterior circulation ischemic stroke. Neurology 2004; 63(6):1131–1132.
21. Koh MG, Phan TG, Atkinson JL, Wijdicks EF. Neuroimaging in deteriorating patients with cerebellar infarcts and mass effect. Stroke 2000; 31(9):2062–2067.
22. Smith SE, Kirkham FJ, deVeber G, Millman G, Dirks PB, Wirrell E et al. Outcome following decompressive craniectomy for malignant middle cerebral artery infarction in children. Dev Med Child Neurol 2011;53(1):29–33.
23. Appleton R, Choonara I, Martland T, Phillips B, Scott R, Whitehouse W. The treatment of convulsive status epilepticus in children. The Status Epilepticus Working Party, Members of the Status Epilepticus Working Party. Arch Dis Child 2000; 83(5):415–419.
24. Prasad AN, Seshia SS. Status epilepticus in pediatric practice: neonate to adolescent. Adv Neurol 2006; 97:229–243.
25. Scott RC, Kirkham FJ. Clinical update: childhood convulsive status epilepticus. Lancet 2007; 370(9589):724–726.
26. Reith J, Jorgensen HS, Pedersen PM, Nakayama H, Raaschou HO, Jeppesen LL et al. Body temperature in acute stroke: relation to stroke severity, infarct size, mortality, and outcome. Lancet 1996; 347(8999):422–425.
27. Ginsberg MD, Busto R. Combating hyperthermia in acute stroke: a significant clinical concern. Stroke 1998; 29(2):529–534.
28. Prengler M, Ganesan V, Ghezzo A, Ng V, Wade A, Connelly A et al. Predictors of infarct volume and outcome in paediatric stroke. Dev Med. Child Neurol 1999; 41(Suppl 82):16.
29. Connelly A, Chong WK, Johnson CL, Ganesan V, Gadian DG, Kirkham FJ. Diffusion weighted magnetic resonance imaging of compromised tissue in stroke. Arch Dis Child 1997; 77(1):38–41.
30. Gadian DG, Calamante F, Kirkham FJ, Bynevelt M, Johnson CL, Porter DA et al. Diffusion and perfusion magnetic resonance imaging in childhood stroke. J Child Neurol 2000; 15(5):279–283.
31. Bryan RN, Levy LM, Whitlow WD, Killian JM, Preziosi TJ, Rosario JA. Diagnosis of acute cerebral infarction: comparison of CT and MR imaging. AJNR Am J Neuroradiol 1991; 12(4):611–620.
32. Grigoriadis S, Gomori JM, Grigoriadis N, Cohen JE. Clinically successful late recanalization of basilar artery occlusion in childhood: what are the odds? Case report and review of the literature. J Neurol Sci 2007; 260(1–2):256–260.
33. Ganesan V, Savvy L, Chong WK, Kirkham FJ. Conventional cerebral angiography in children with ischemic stroke. Pediatr Neurol 1999; 20(1):38–42.
34. Husson B, Rodesch G, Lasjaunias P, Tardieu M, Sebire G. Magnetic resonance angiography in childhood arterial brain infarcts: a comparative study with contrast angiography. Stroke 2002; 33(5):1280–1285.

35. Sebire G, Tabarki B, Saunders DE, Leroy I, Liesner R, Saint-Martin C et al. Cerebral venous sinus thrombosis in children: risk factors, presentation, diagnosis and outcome. Brain 2005; 128(Pt 3):477–489.

36. Pavlakis SG, Frank Y, Chusid R. Hypertensive encephalopathy, reversible occipitoparietal encephalopathy, or reversible posterior leukoencephalopathy: three names for an old syndrome. J Child Neurol 1999; 14(5):277–281.

37. Chabrier S, Husson B, Lasjaunias P, Landrieu P, Tardieu M. Stroke in childhood: outcome and recurrence risk by mechanism in 59 patients. J Child Neurol 2000; 15(5):290–294.

38. Al-Jarallah A, Al-Rifai MT, Riela AR, Roach ES. Nontraumatic brain hemorrhage in children: etiology and presentation. J Child Neurol 2000; 15(5):284–289.

39. Blom I, De Schryver EL, Kappelle LJ, Rinkel GJ, Jennekens-Schinkel A, Peters AC. Prognosis of haemorrhagic stroke in childhood: a long-term follow-up study. Dev Med Child Neurol 2003; 45(4):233–239.

40. deVeber G, Andrew M, Adams C, Bjornson B, Booth F, Buckley DJ et al. Cerebral sinovenous thrombosis in children. N Engl J Med 2001; 345(6):417–423.

41. Mendelow AD, Gregson BA, Fernandes HM, Murray GD, Teasdale GM, Hope DT et al. Early surgery versus initial conservative treatment in patients with spontaneous supratentorial intracerebral haematomas in the International Surgical Trial in Intracerebral Haemorrhage (STICH): a randomized trial. Lancet 2005; 365(9457):387–397.

42. Anderson CS, Huang Y, Wang JG, Arima H, Neal B, Peng B et al. Intensive blood pressure reduction in acute cerebral haemorrhage trial (INTERACT): a randomized pilot trial. Lancet Neurol 2008; 7(5):391–399.

43. Mayer SA, Brun NC, Begtrup K, Broderick J, Davis S, Diringer MN et al. Recombinant activated factor VII for acute intracerebral hemorrhage. N Engl J Med 2005; 352(8):777–785.

44. Mayer SA, Brun NC, Begtrup K, Broderick J, Davis S, Diringer MN et al. Efficacy and safety of recombinant activated factor VII for acute intracerebral hemorrhage. N Engl J Med 2008; 358(20):2127–2137.

45. Hubbard D, Tobias JD. Intracerebral hemorrhage due to hemorrhagic disease of the newborn and failure to administer vitamin K at birth. South Med J 2006; 99(11):1216–1220.

46. Hartmann M, Sucker C, Messing M. Recombinant activated factor VII in the treatment of near-fatal bleeding during pediatric brain tumor surgery. Report of two cases and review of the literature. J Neurosurg 2006; 104(1 Suppl):55–58.

47. Altuncu E, Berrak S, Bilgen H, Yurdakul Z, Canpolat C, Ozek E. Use of recombinant factor VIIa in a preterm infant with coagulopathy and subdural hematoma. J Matern Fetal Neonatal Med 2007; 20(8):627–629.

48. Einhaupl KM, Villringer A, Meister W, Mehraein S, Garner C, Pellkofer M et al. Heparin treatment in sinus venous thrombosis. Lancet 1991; 338(8767):597–600.

49. de Bruijn SF, Stam J. Randomized, placebo-controlled trial of anticoagulant treatment with low-molecular-weight heparin for cerebral sinus thrombosis. Stroke 1999; 30(3):484–488.

50. Wasay M, Bakshi R, Kojan S, Bobustuc G, Dubey N, Unwin DH. Nonrandomized comparison of local urokinase thrombolysis versus systemic heparin anticoagulation for superior sagittal sinus thrombosis. Stroke 2001; 32(10):2310–2317.

51. Wasay M, Bakshi R, Dai A, Roach S. Local thrombolytic treatment of cerebral venous thrombosis in three paediatric patients. J Pak Med Assoc 2006; 56(11):555–556.

52. Danielson CF. The role of red blood cell exchange transfusion in the treatment and prevention of complications of sickle cell disease. Ther Apher 2002; 6(1):24–31.

53. Kirkham FJ, DeBaun MR. Stroke in children with sickle cell disease. Curr Treat Options Neurol 2004; 6(5):357–375.

54. Platt OS. Prevention and management of stroke in sickle cell anemia. Hematology Am Soc Hematol Educ Program 2006;54–57.

55. Wang WC. The pathophysiology, prevention, and treatment of stroke in sickle cell disease. Curr Opin Hematol 2007; 14(3):191–197.

56. Carpenter J, Tsuchida T, Lynch JK. Treatment of arterial ischemic stroke in children. Expert Rev Neurother 2007; 7(4):383–392.

57. Kirkham FJ. Therapy insight: stroke risk and its management in patients with sickle cell disease. Nat Clin Pract Neurol 2007; 3(5):264–278.

58. Kirkham FJ, Lerner NB, Noetzel M, DeBaun MR, Datta AK, Rees DC et al. Trials in sickle cell disease. Pediatr Neurol 2006; 34(6):450–458.

59. Nahavandi M, Tavakkoli F, Wyche MQ, Trouth AJ, Tavakoli N, Perlin E. Effect of transfusion on cerebral oxygenation, flow velocity in a patient with sickle cell anemia and Moyamoya disease: a case report. Hematology 2006; 11(5):381–383.

60. Hurlet-Jensen AM, Prohovnik I, Pavlakis SG, Piomelli S. Effects of total hemoglobin and hemoglobin S concentration on cerebral blood flow during transfusion therapy to prevent stroke in sickle cell disease. Stroke 1994; 25(8):1688–1692.

61. Russell MO, Goldberg HI, Hodson A, Kim HC, Halus J, Reivich M et al. Effect of transfusion therapy on arteriographic abnormalities and on recurrence of stroke in sickle cell disease. Blood 1984; 63(1):162–169.

62. Kirkham FJ, Calamante F, Bynevelt M, Gadian DG, Evans JP, Cox TC et al. Perfusion magnetic resonance abnormalities in patients with sickle cell disease. Ann Neurol 2001; 49(4):477–485.

63. Hulbert ML, Scothorn DJ, Panepinto JA, Scott JP, Buchanan GR, Sarnaik S et al. Exchange blood transfusion compared with simple transfusion for first overt stroke is associated with a lower risk of subsequent stroke: a retrospective cohort study of 137 children with sickle cell anemia. J Pediatr 2006; 149(5):710–712.

64. Jan K, Usami S, Smith JA. Effects of transfusion on rheological properties of blood in sickle cell anemia. Transfusion 1982; 22(1):17–20.

65. Hamdan JM, Mallouh AA, Ahmad MS. Hypertension and convulsions complicating sickle cell anaemia: possible role of transfusion. Ann Trop Paediatr 1984; 4(1):41–43.

66. Siegel JF, Rich MA, Brock WA. Association of sickle cell disease, priapism, exchange transfusion and neurological events: ASPEN syndrome. J Urol 1993; 150(5 Pt 1):1480–1482.

67. Strouse JJ, Hulbert ML, DeBaun MR, Jordan LC, Casella JF. Primary hemorrhagic stroke in children with sickle cell disease is associated with recent transfusion and use of corticosteroids. Pediatrics 2006; 118(5):1916–1924.

68. Garcia JH. Thrombosis of cranial veins and sinuses: brain parenchymal effects. In: Cerebral Sinus Thrombosis: experimental and clinical aspects (eds KM Einhaupl, O Kempski, A Baethmann). New York: Plenum Press, 1990.

69. van Mierlo TD, van den Berg HM, Nievelstein RA, Braun KP. An unconscious girl with sickle-cell disease. Lancet 2003; 361(9352):136.

70. Ciurea SO, Thulborn KR, Gowhari M. Dural venous sinus thrombosis in a patient with sickle cell disease: case report and literature review. Am J Hematol 2006; 81(4):290–293.

71. Coley SC, Porter DA, Calamante F, Chong WK, Connelly A. Quantitative MR diffusion mapping and cyclosporine-induced neurotoxicity. AJNR Am J Neuroradiol 1999; 20(8):1507–1510.

72. Henderson JN, Noetzel MJ, McKinstry RC, White DA, Armstrong M, DeBaun MR. Reversible posterior leukoencephalopathy syndrome and silent cerebral infarcts are associated with severe acute chest syndrome in children with sickle cell disease. Blood 2003; 101(2):415–419.

73. Lee KH, McKie VC, Sekul EA, Adams RJ, Nichols FT. Unusual encephalopathy after acute chest syndrome in sickle cell disease: acute necrotizing encephalitis. J Pediatr Hematol Oncol 2002; 24(7):585–588.

74. Kirkham FJ, Hewes DK, Prengler M, Wade A, Lane R, Evans JP. Nocturnal hypoxaemia and central-nervous-system events in sickle-cell disease. Lancet 2001; 357(9269):1656–1659.

75. Preul MC, Cendes F, Just N, Mohr G. Intracranial aneurysms and sickle cell anemia: multiplicity and propensity for the vertebrobasilar territory. Neurosurgery 1998; 42(5):971–977.

76. McQuaker IG, Jaspan T, McConachie NS, Dolan G. Coil embolization of cerebral aneurysms in patients with sickling disorders. Br J Haematol 1999; 106(2):388–390.

77. Cheatham ML, Brackett CE. Problems in management of subarachnoid hemorrhage in sickle cell anemia. J Neurosurg 1965; 23(5):488–493.

78. Wahlgren N, Ahmed N, Davalos A, Ford GA, Grond M, Hacke W et al. Thrombolysis with alteplase for acute ischaemic stroke in the Safe Implementation of Thrombolysis in Stroke-Monitoring Study (SITS-MOST): an observational study. Lancet 2007; 369(9558): 275–282.

79. Furlan A, Higashida R, Wechsler L, Gent M, Rowley H, Kase C et al. Intra-arterial prourokinase for acute ischemic stroke. The PROACT II study: a randomized controlled trial. Prolyse in Acute Cerebral Thromboembolism. JAMA 1999; 282(21):2003–2011.

80. Ogawa A, Mori E, Minematsu K, Taki W, Takahashi A, Nemoto S et al. Randomized trial of intraarterial infusion of urokinase within 6 hours of middle cerebral artery stroke: the middle cerebral artery embolism local fibrinolytic intervention trial (MELT), Japan. Stroke 2007; 38(10):2633–2639.

81. Adams HP, Jr, del ZG, Alberts MJ, Bhatt DL, Brass L, Furlan A et al. Guidelines for the early management of adults with ischemic stroke: a guideline from the American Heart Association/American Stroke Association Stroke Council, Clinical Cardiology Council, Cardiovascular Radiology and Intervention Council, and the Atherosclerotic Peripheral Vascular Disease and Quality of Care Outcomes in Research Interdisciplinary Working Groups: The American Academy of Neurology affirms the value of this guideline as an educational tool for neurologists. Circulation 2007; 115(20):e478–e534.

82. Schonewille WJ, Wijman CA, Michel P, Rueckert CM, Weimar C, Mattle HP et al. Treatment and outcomes of acute basilar artery occlusion in the Basilar Artery International Cooperation Study (BASICS): a prospective registry study. Lancet Neurol 2009; 8(8):724–730.

83. Smith WS, Sung G, Saver J, Budzik R, Duckwiler G, Liebeskind DS et al. Mechanical thrombectomy for acute ischemic stroke: final results of the Multi MERCI trial. Stroke 2008; 39(4):1205–1212.

84. Arnold M, Steinlin M, Baumann A, Nedeltchev K, Remonda L, Moser SJ et al. Thrombolysis in childhood stroke: report of 2 cases and review of the literature. Stroke 2009; 40(3):801–807.

85. Fischer U, Anca D, Arnold M, Nedeltchev K, Kappeler L, Ballinari P et al. Quality of life in stroke survivors after local intra-arterial thrombolysis. Cerebrovasc Dis 2008; 25(5):438–444.

86. Janjua N, Nasar A, Lynch JK, Qureshi AI. Thrombolysis for ischemic stroke in children: data from the nationwide inpatient sample. Stroke 2007; 38(6):1850–1854.

87. Amlie-Lefond C, Chan AK, Kirton A, deVeber G, Hovinga CA, Ichord R et al. Thrombolysis in acute childhood stroke: design and challenges of the thrombolysis in pediatric stroke clinical trial. Neuroepidemiology 2009; 32(4):279–286.

88. Gruber A, Nasel C, Lang W, Kitzmuller E, Bavinzski G, Czech T. Intra-arterial thrombolysis for the treatment of perioperative childhood cardioembolic stroke. Neurology 2000; 54(8):1684–1686.

89. Thirumalai SS, Shubin RA. Successful treatment for stroke in a child using recombinant tissue plasminogen activator. J Child Neurol 2000; 15(8):558.

90. Carlson MD, Leber S, Deveikis J, Silverstein FS. Successful use of rt-PA in pediatric stroke. Neurology 2001; 57(1):157–158.

91. Noser EA, Felberg RA, Alexandrov AV. Thrombolytic therapy in an adolescent ischemic stroke. J Child Neurol 2001; 16(4):286–288.

92. Cannon BC, Kertesz NJ, Friedman RA, Fenrich AL. Use of tissue plasminogen activator in a stroke after radiofrequency ablation of a left-sided accessory pathway. J Cardiovasc Electrophysiol 2001; 12(6):723–725.

93. Kirton A, Wong JH, Mah J, Ross BC, Kennedy J, Bell K et al. Successful endovascular therapy for acute basilar thrombosis in an adolescent. Pediatrics 2003; 112:248–251.

94. Golomb MR, Rafay M, Armstrong D, Massicotte P, Curtis R, Hune S et al. Intra-arterial tissue plasminogen activator for thrombosis complicating cerebral angiography in a 17-year-old girl. J Child Neurol 2003; 18(6):420–423.

95. Ortiz GA, Koch S, Wallace DM, Lopez-Alberola R. Successful intravenous thrombolysis for acute stroke in a child. J Child Neurol 2007; 22(6):749–752.

96. Benedict SL, Ni OK, Schloesser P, White KS, Bale JF, Jr. Intra-arterial thrombolysis in a 2-year-old with cardioembolic stroke. J Child Neurol 2007; 22(2):225–227.

97. Tan M, Armstrong D, Birken C, Bitnun A, Caldarone CA, Cox P et al. Bacterial endocarditis in a child presenting with acute arterial ischemic stroke: should thrombolytic therapy be absolutely contraindicated? Dev Med Child Neurol 2009;51(2):151–154.

98. Cognard C, Weill A, Lindgren S, Piotin M, Castaings L, Moret J. Basilar artery occlusion in a child: 'clot angioplasty' followed by thrombolysis. Childs Nerv Syst 2000; 16(8):496–500.

99. Sungarian A, Duncan JA, III. Vertebrobasilar thrombosis in children: report of two cases and three recommendations for treatment. Pediatr Neurosurg 2003; 38(1):16–20.

100. Rosman NP, Adhami S, Mannheim GB, Katz NP, Klucznik RP, Muriello MA. Basilar artery occlusion in children: misleading presentations, "locked-in" state, and diagnostic importance of accompanying vertebral artery occlusion. J Child Neurol 2003; 18(7):450–462.

101. Yoshikawa H. Basilar artery infarction. Arch Dis Child 2005; 90(4):410.

102. Zaidat OO, Tolbert M, Smith TP, Alexander MJ. Primary endovascular therapy with clot retrieval and balloon angioplasty for acute basilar artery occlusion. Pediatr Neurosurg 2005; 41(6):323–327.

103. Bhatt A, Naravetla B, Farooq MU, Majid A, Kassab M, Gupta R. Treatment of a basilar artery occlusion with intra-arterial thrombolysis in a 3-year-old girl. Neurocrit Care 2008; 9(3):357–360.

104. Janmaat M, Gravendeel JP, Uyttenboogaart M, Vroomen PC, Brouwer OF, Luijckx GJ. Local intra-arterial thrombolysis in a 4-year-old male with vertebrobasilar artery thrombosis. Dev Med Child Neurol. 2009;51(2):155–158.

105. Tsivgoulis G, Eggers J, Ribo M, Perren F, Saqqur M, Rubiera M et al. Safety and efficacy of ultrasound-enhanced thrombolysis: a comprehensive review and meta-analysis of randomized and non-randomized studies. Stroke 2010;41(2):280–287.

106. Grunwald IQ, Walter S, Shamdeen MG, Dautermann A, Roth C, Haass A et al. New mechanical recanalization devices – the future in pediatric stroke treatment? J Invasive Cardiol 2010;22(2):63–66.

107. Griesemer DA, Theodorou AA, Berg RA, Spera TD. Local fibrinolysis in cerebral venous thrombosis. Pediatr Neurol 1994; 10(1):78–80.

108. Soleau SW, Schmidt R, Stevens S, Osborn A, MacDonald JD. Extensive experience with dural sinus thrombosis. Neurosurgery 2003; 52(3):534–544.

109. Liebetrau M, Mayer TE, Bruning R, Opherk C, Hamann GF. Intra-arterial thrombolysis of complete deep cerebral venous thrombosis. Neurology 2004; 63(12):2444–2445.

110. Mallick AA, Sharples PM, Calvert SE, Jones RW, Leary M, Lux AL et al. Cerebral venous sinus thrombosis: a case series including thrombolysis. Arch Dis Child. 2009;94(10):790–794.

111. Ciccone A, Canhao P, Falcao F, Ferro JM, Sterzi R. Thrombolysis for cerebral vein and dural sinus thrombosis. Cochrane Database Syst Rev 2004; (1):CD003693.

112. Einhäupl K, Stam J, Bousser MG, de Bruijn SF, Ferro JM, Martinelli I et al. EFNS guideline on the treatment of cerebral venous and sinus thrombosis in adult patients. Eur J Neurol 2010; 17(10):1229–1235.

113. Kenet G, Kirkham F, Niederstadt T, Heinecke A, Saunders D, Stoll M et al. Risk factors for recurrent venous thromboembolism in the European collaborative paediatric database on cerebral venous thrombosis: a multicentre cohort study. Lancet Neurol 2007; 6(7):595–603.

114. Kay R, Wong KS, Yu YL, Chan YW, Tsoi TH, Ahuja AT et al. Low-molecular-weight heparin for the treatment of acute ischemic stroke. N Engl J Med 1995; 333(24):1588–1593.

115. The International Stroke Trial (IST): a randomized trial of aspirin, subcutaneous heparin, both, or neither among 19435 patients with acute ischaemic stroke. International Stroke Trial Collaborative Group. Lancet 1997; 349(9065):1569–1581.

116. Bernard TJ, Goldenberg NA, Tripputi M, Manco-Johnson MJ, Niederstadt T, Nowak-Gottl U. Anticoagulation in childhood-onset arterial ischemic stroke with nonmoyamoya arteriopathy. Findings from the Colorado and German (COAG) Collaboration. Stroke 2009; 40(8):2869–2871.

117. Goldenberg NA, Bernard TJ, Fullerton HJ, Gordon A, deVeber GA, for the International Pediatric Stroke Study group. Antithrombotic

treatments, outcomes, and prognostic factors in acute childhood-onset arterial ischaemic stroke: a multicentre, observational, cohort study. Lancet Neurol 2009; 8(12):1120–1127.

118. Dix D, Andrew M, Marzinotto V, Charpentier K, Bridge S, Monagle P et al. The use of low molecular weight heparin in pediatric patients: a prospective cohort study. J Pediatr 2000; 136(4):439–445.

119. Ng W, Chan AK, Curtis RM, MacGregor D, Massicotte MP, Sofronas M et al. Safety of low molecular weight heparin at treatment doses in children with arterial ischemic stroke: a consecutive cohort study. Ann Neurol 2002; 52(3):132.

120. Strater R, Kurnik K, Heller C, Schobess R, Luigs P, Nowak-Gottl U. Aspirin versus low-dose low-molecular-weight heparin: antithrombotic therapy in pediatric ischemic stroke patients: a prospective follow-up study. Stroke 2001; 32(11):2554–2558.

121. deVeber G, Chan A. Aspirin versus low-molecular-weight heparin for ischemic stroke in children: an unanswered question. Stroke 2002; 33(8):1947–1948.

122. Moharir MD, Shroff M, Stephens D, Pontigon AM, Chan A, MacGregor D et al. Anticoagulants in pediatric cerebral sinovenous thrombosis: a safety and outcome study. Ann Neurol 2010; 67(5):590–599.

123. deVeber G, Chan A, Monagle P, Marzinotto V, Armstrong D, Massicotte P et al. Anticoagulation therapy in pediatric patients with sinovenous thrombosis: a cohort study. Arch Neurol 1998; 55(12):1533–1537.

124. deVeber G, Shroff M, Atre M, Chan AK, Adams M. Recanalization of neonatal cerebral sinovenous thrombosis: a follow-up study. Pediatr Res 2003; 53:A537.

125. Wasay M, Dai AI, Ansari M, Shaikh Z, Roach ES. Cerebral venous sinus thrombosis in children: a multicenter cohort from the United States. J Child Neurol 2008; 23(1):26–31.

126. Lyrer P, Engelter S. Antithrombotic drugs for carotid artery dissection. Cochrane Database Syst Rev 2003; (3):CD000255.

127. Beletsky V, Nadareishvili Z, Lynch J, Shuaib A, Woolfenden A, Norris JW. Cervical arterial dissection: time for a therapeutic trial? Stroke 2003; 34(12):2856–2860.

128. Arauz A, Hoyos L, Espinoza C, Cantu C, Barinagarrementeria F, Roman G. Dissection of cervical arteries: long-term follow-up study of 130 consecutive cases. Cerebrovasc Dis 2006; 22(2–3):150–154.

129. Chandra A, Suliman A, Angle N. Spontaneous dissection of the carotid and vertebral arteries: the 10-year UCSD experience. Ann Vasc Surg 2007; 21(2):178–185.

130. Fullerton HJ, Johnston SC, Smith WS. Arterial dissection and stroke in children. Neurology 2001; 57(7):1155–1160.

131. Ganesan V, Chong WK, Cox TC, Chawda SJ, Prengler M, Kirkham FJ. Posterior circulation stroke in childhood: risk factors and recurrence. Neurology 2002; 59(10):1552–1556.

132. Rafay MF, Armstrong D, deVeber G, Domi T, Chan A, MacGregor DL. Craniocervical arterial dissection in children: clinical and radiographic presentation and outcome. J Child Neurol 2006; 21(1):8–16.

133. Wolfe SQ, Mueller-Kronast N, ziz-Sultan MA, Zauner A, Bhatia S. Extracranial carotid artery pseudoaneurysm presenting with embolic stroke in a pediatric patient. Case report. J Neurosurg Pediatr 2008; 1(3):240–243.

134. Schievink WI. Spontaneous dissection of the carotid and vertebral arteries. N Engl J Med 2001; 344:898–906.

135. CAST: randomized placebo-controlled trial of early aspirin use in 20 000 patients with acute ischaemic stroke. CAST (Chinese Acute Stroke Trial. Collaborative Group). Lancet 1997; 349(9066):1641–1649.

136. Kuhle S, Mitchell L, Andrew M, Chan AK, Massicotte P, Adams M et al. Urgent clinical challenges in children with ischemic stroke: analysis of 1065 patients from the 1–800-NOCLOTS pediatric stroke telephone consultation service. Stroke 2006; 37(1):116–122.

137. Hung R, Chan AK, deVeber GA. Aspirin therapy for prevention of recurrent cerebral thrombo-embolic events in children: a prospective cohort study. Ann Neurol 2002; 52:S123.

138. Sträter R, Kurnik K, Heller C, Schobess R, Luigs P, Nowak-Göttl U. Aspirin versus low-dose low-molecular-weight heparin:

antithrombotic therapy in pediatric ischemic stroke patients: a prospective follow-up study. Stroke. 2001; 32(11):2554–2558.

139. Burak CR, Bowen MD, Barron TF. The use of enoxaparin in children with acute, nonhemorrhagic ischemic stroke. Pediatr Neurol 2003; 29(4):295–298.

140. Bowen MD, Burak CR, Barron TF. Childhood ischemic stroke in a nonurban population. J Child Neurol 2005; 20(3):194–197.

141. Barnes C, Newall F, Furmedge J, Mackay M, Monagle P. Arterial ischaemic stroke in children. J Paediatr Child Health 2004; 40(7):384–387.

142. Soman T, Rafay MF, Hune S, Allen A, MacGregor D, deVeber G. The risks and safety of clopidogrel in pediatric arterial ischemic stroke. Stroke 2006; 37(4):1120–1122.

143. Bonduel M, Sciuccati G, Hepner M, Pieroni G, Torres AF, Frontroth JP et al. Arterial ischemic stroke and cerebral venous thrombosis in children: a 12-year Argentinean registry. Acta Haematol 2006; 115(3–4):180–185.

144. Ganesan V, Prengler M, Wade A, Kirkham FJ. Clinical and radiological recurrence after childhood arterial ischemic stroke. Circulation 2006; 114(20):2170–2177.

145. Fullerton HJ, Wu YW, Sidney S, Johnston SC. Risk of recurrent childhood arterial ischemic stroke in a population-based cohort: the importance of cerebrovascular imaging. Pediatrics 2007; 119(3):495–501.

146. Toure A, Chabrier S, Plagne M-D, Presles E, des Portes V, Rousselle C. Neurological outcome and risk of recurrence depending on the anterior vs posterior arterial distribution in children with stroke. Neuropediatrics 2010; 40(3):126–128.

147. Gupta R, Connolly ES, Mayer S, Elkind MS. Hemicraniectomy for massive middle cerebral artery territory infarction: a systematic review. Stroke 2004; 35(2):539–543.

148. Vahedi K, Hofmeijer J, Juettler E, Vicaut E, George B, Algra A et al. Early decompressive surgery in malignant infarction of the middle cerebral artery: a pooled analysis of three randomized controlled trials. Lancet Neurol 2007; 6(3):215–222.

149. Carter BS, Ogilvy CS, Candia GJ, Rosas HD, Buonanno F. One-year outcome after decompressive surgery for massive non-dominant hemispheric infarction. Neurosurgery 1997; 40(6):1168–1175.

150. Simma B, Tscharre A, Hejazi N, Krasznai L, Fae P. Neurologic outcome after decompressive craniectomy in children. Intensive Care Med 2002; 28(7):1000.

151. Lee MC, Frank JI, Kahana M, Tonsgard JH, Frim DM. Decompressive hemicraniectomy in a 6-year-old male after unilateral hemispheric stroke. Case report and review. Pediatr Neurosurg 2003; 38(4):181–185.

152. Tan MA, Salonga AM, Jamora RD. Decompressive hemicraniectomy in a 2-year-old girl with a left middle cerebral artery infarct. Childs Nerv Syst 2006; 22(5):523–525.

153. Uhl E, Kreth FW, Elias B, Goldammer A, Hempelmann RG, Liefner M et al. Outcome and prognostic factors of hemicraniectomy for space occupying cerebral infarction. J Neurol Neurosurg Psychiatry 2004; 75(2):270–274.

154. Curry WT, Jr, Sethi MK, Ogilvy CS, Carter BS. Factors associated with outcome after hemicraniectomy for large middle cerebral artery territory infarction. Neurosurgery 2005; 56(4):681–692.

155. Kilincer C, Asil T, Utku U, Hamamcioglu MK, Turgut N, Hicdonmez T et al. Factors affecting the outcome of decompressive craniectomy for large hemispheric infarctions: a prospective cohort study. Acta Neurochir (Wien) 2005; 147(6):587–594.

156. Csokay A, Egyud L, Nagy L, Pataki G. Vascular tunnel creation to improve the efficacy of decompressive craniotomy in post-traumatic cerebral edema and ischemic stroke. Surg Neurol 2002; 57(2):126–129.

157. Gerriets T, Stolz E, Konig S, Babacan S, Fiss I, Jauss M et al. Sonographic monitoring of midline shift in space-occupying stroke: an early outcome predictor. Stroke 2001; 32(2):442–447.

158. Foerch C, Otto B, Singer OC, Neumann-Haefelin T, Yan B, Berkefeld J et al. Serum S100B predicts a malignant course of infarction in patients with acute middle cerebral artery occlusion. Stroke 2004; 35(9):2160–2164.

159. Canhao P, Ferro JM, Lindgren AG, Bousser MG, Stam J, Barinagarrementeria F. Causes and predictors of death in cerebral venous thrombosis. Stroke 2005; 36(8):1720–1725.

160. Petzold A, Smith M. High intracranial pressure, brain herniation and death in cerebral venous thrombosis. Stroke 2006; 37(2):331–332.

161. Stefini R, Latronico N, Cornali C, Rasulo F, Bollati A. Emergent decompressive craniectomy in patients with fixed dilated pupils due to cerebral venous and dural sinus thrombosis: report of three cases. Neurosurgery 1999; 45(3):626–629.

162. Keller E, Pangalu A, Fandino J, Konu D, Yonekawa Y. Decompressive craniectomy in severe cerebral venous and dural sinus thrombosis. Acta Neurochir Suppl 2005; 94:177–183.

163. Anlar B, Basaran C, Kose G, Guven A, Haspolat S, Yakut A et al. Acute disseminated encephalomyelitis in children: outcome and prognosis. Neuropediatrics 2003; 34(4):194–199.

164. Khurana DS, Melvin JJ, Kothare SV, Valencia I, Hardison HH, Yum S et al. Acute disseminated encephalomyelitis in children: discordant neurologic and neuroimaging abnormalities and response to plasmapheresis. Pediatrics 2005; 116(2):431–436.

165. Koga Y, Ishibashi M, Ueki I, Yatsuga S, Fukiyama R, Akita Y et al. Effects of L-arginine on the acute phase of strokes in three patients with MELAS. Neurology 2002; 58(5):827–828.

166. Kubota M, Sakakihara Y, Mori M, Yamagata T, Momoi-Yoshida M. Beneficial effect of L-arginine for stroke-like episode in MELAS. Brain Dev 2004; 26(7):481–483.

167. Koga Y, Akita Y, Junko N, Yatsuga S, Povalko N, Fukiyama R et al. Endothelial dysfunction in MELAS improved by L-arginine supplementation. Neurology 2006; 66(11):1766–1769.

168. Gabis LV, Yangala R, Lenn NJ. Time lag to diagnosis of stroke in children. Pediatrics 2002; 110(5):924–928.

17
RECURRENCE, OUTCOME AND REHABILITATION

17.1 Recurrence and Secondary Prevention

Vijeya Ganesan and Fenella J. Kirkham

Defining the risk of recurrent acute ischaemic stroke (AIS) in individual patients is challenging given the diverse range of risk factors which may be present in different combinations in each case. Recent studies have, however, identified several factors associated with high recurrence risk which will be discussed in detail below, followed by a discussion of potential preventative strategies.

Risk of recurrence

RECURRENCE AFTER FIRST AIS IN UNTREATED PATIENTS
In untreated children who suffer a first AIS outside the neonatal period, the risk of recurrence is 10–25% overall[1–15] but may be as low as 6% in those with no or one risk factors[6] or as high as 92% in patients with sickle cell disease (SCD) who receive no treatment.[16–24] In the context of SCD the risk of recurrence appears to be highest in children with a 'moyamoya' pattern of lenticulostriate collaterals[25] and in those in whom the original stroke does not occur in the context of an acute illness.[26] There are few long-term follow-up data for patients who develop AIS in the context of cardiac disease but both symptomatic and clinically silent recurrence have been described.[12] In symptomatic and cryptogenic cases of childhood AIS, recurrence is commoner if there are ≥2 risk factors,[6] in those with vasculopathy[15,27,28] (Fig. 17.1a) particularly if it is progressive[29]

or if moyamoya collaterals are demonstrated angiographically[2,5,11,14,25,30] and in those of low birth weight[14]. Children with vascular stenosis or moyamoya have a risk of recurrence as high as 66%.[14,15,29] However, the severity of recurrent symptoms associated with moyamoya varies considerably between patients; some have frequent but brief transient ischaemic attacks (TIAs) whereas others have fewer but more devastating recurrent strokes. Even if clinical recurrence is limited to a TIA there is a significant risk of deterioration in cognitive function.[31]

Chabrier et al[7] found that the risk of recurrence was related to stroke mechanism. In particular it was noted that patients with cardiac disease, moyamoya or systemic disease could have recurrence many years after the original stroke, whereas those with transient cerebral arteriopathy or dissection were more likely to have early recurrence. A more recent publication from the French group suggests that those with posterior circulation territory stroke are at particular risk.[32] Thus, comprehensive evaluation of children with AIS for potential risk factors may enable partial stratification of patients into high and low risk groups or according to likely timing of recurrence.

In the Great Ormond Street series, genetic thrombophilia was significantly commoner in children with cryptogenic stroke who recurred.[14] Data pooled from the Münster, Hospital for Sick Children, Toronto and Great Ormond Street cohorts found that patients with multiple prothrombotic disorders had

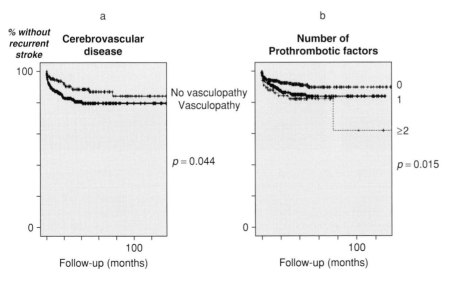

Fig. 17.1. Kaplan–Meier curves showing time to recurrent stroke for children (a) with and without vasculopathy and (b) with no, 1 or ≥2 prothrombotic disorders identified in data pooled from stroke databases from Münster, Toronto and London.[28] p values are for comparisons using the Log rank test.

337

a higher risk of recurrent infarction (Fig. 17.1b), independent of vasculopathy and underlying disorder.[28] Isolated antiphospholipid antibodies are not associated with recurrence[33] but the lupus anticoagulant may be and systematic lupus erythematosus (SLE), for which the recurrence risk is higher, should be considered in the clinical differential diagnosis as anticoagulation reduces the high recurrence risk.

RADIOLOGICAL RECURRENCE OF CEREBRAL INFARCTION

Clinically covert, or 'silent' reinfarction is typical of sickle cell disease with an incidence of 7.06/100 patient-years,[34] but also occurs in cryptogenic AIS.[14] Sixty of 179 patients who had repeat neuroimaging in the Great Ormond Street series[14] had re-infarction (Fig. 17.2), for which the risk factors were bilateral infarction at first stroke, underlying immunodeficiency, previous TIA and leukocytosis; the latter two were also risk factors for clinically covert re-infarction.

CEREBRAL VENOUS THROMBOSIS

Between 6% and 20% of children who have a cerebral venous sinus thrombosis will experience a recurrent symptomatic venous event, at least half of which are systemic rather than cerebral.[35] Predictors of recurrence in childhood include age >12 months (Fig. 17.3a), not anticoagulating in high risk situations[35] (Fig. 17.3b), failure to recanalize the thrombosed sinus or vein (Fig. 17.3c) and the prothrombin 20210 mutation, but there have been no trials of preventative strategies in children or adults.

Prevention of AIS recurrence

SURGICAL REVASCULARIZATION IN MOYAMOYA

Surgical cerebral revascularization is widely used as a treatment to prevent recurrent stroke in patients with moyamoya. The indications for and efficacy of revascularization remain controversial[36,37] because there is variation in the natural history and several series have reported good outcomes in untreated patients.[38,39] Individual surgical series have reported positive outcomes in terms of symptom reduction, prevention of further infarction and stabilization of cognitive function, and good outcomes after surgery were supported by the findings of a pooled analysis of the published data.[40] Thus it would seem prudent to refer children with a moyamoya pattern of arteriopathy to a specialist centre for consideration of revascularization.

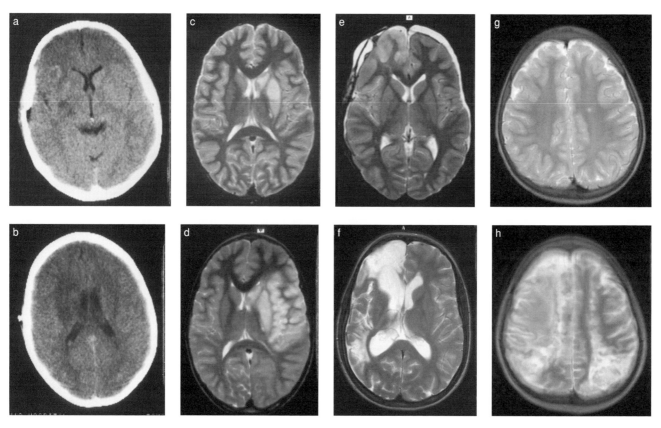

Fig. 17.2. Examples of recurrent strokes. (a,b) CT scans showing enlargement of a stroke in the midde cerebral artery territory in an 11-year-old boy whose transcranial Doppler and conventional arteriogram showed a tight stenosis of the middle cerebral artery.[507] (c,d) MRI scans showing enlargement of a stroke in the midde cerebral artery territory in an 8-year-old boy with middle cerebral artery stenosis on MR and digital subtraction arteriography who was heterozygous for factor V Leiden and prothrombin 20210 and homozygous for thermolabile methylene tetrahydrofolate reductase mutations. (e,f) MRI scans showing recurrent silent infarction within the borderzone in an 11-year-old child with familial hypercholesterolaemia who had her first stroke the day after she had had a craniopharyngioma removed. (g) Small silent infarct in the deep white matter of a 7-year-old boy with sickle cell anaemia. (h) Extensive bilateral stroke in the same boy with sickle cell anaemia 1 year later after a chest crisis.

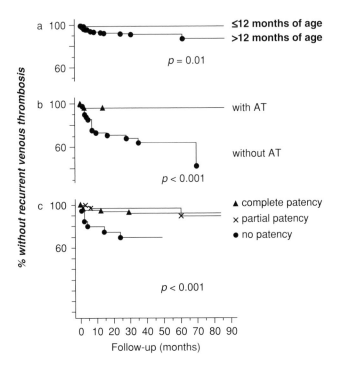

Fig. 17.3. Kaplan–Meier curves showing cumulative thrombosis-free survival with respect to age at first cerebral venous sinus thrombosis onset for children in the European collaborative study:[35] (a) aged ≤12 months and >12 months (●); (b) children with (▲) and without (●) anti-thrombotic therapy (AT) prior to recurrent venous thrombosis; (c) children with complete (▲), partial (×) and no (●) 3–6 months cerebral venous sinus patency. *p* values are for comparisons using the log rank test.

SICKLE CELL DISEASE

Blood transfusion has been shown to significantly reduce the risk of recurrent AIS in children with SCD[41] but up to 40% of patients may have recurrence despite transfusion.[25] In general the aim of regular blood transfusion is to maintain HbS% below 25% and to maintain haemoglobin between 10 and 14.5g/dl. A less intensive regime may be considered after 3 years, relaxing the target HbS% to <50% (see Chapters 15 and 16). Regular blood transfusion is associated with significant adverse effects and many patients find it an unacceptably onerous treatment. It is therefore encouraging that other treatments acting on a wide range of pathogenic mechanisms (e.g. hydroxyurea) are under active consideration.[42] There are case series of surgical revascularization in SCD patients with moyamoya syndrome[43–45] but the criteria for considering surgery have not yet been defined. Bone marrow transplantation stabilizes imaging abnormalities in patients with SCD;[46] in the UK AIS is an indication for considering bone marrow transplantation (BMT) in children with SCD but lack of related donors is a limiting factor. The effects of unrelated-donor stem cell transplantation or cord blood stem cell transplantation are under evaluation.[42]

ANTIPLATELET AND ANTICOAGULANT TREATMENT
IN CHILDHOOD STROKE: SAFETY AND PREVENTION
OF RECURRENCE

Whilst there is no direct evidence that either antiplatelet agents or anticoagulants reduce recurrence risk in children who have

had a first AIS, both are commonly prescribed and advocated in published clinical guidelines.[47] In the German cohort,[27,48] physicians chose aspirin (5mg/kg/day) or low-molecular-weight heparin as secondary prophylaxis for their patients; the risk of recurrent AIS (clinical event accompanied by infarction on imaging) was 10% in both arms. In the Hershey, Pennsylvania, cohort, nine were treated with LMWH (enoxaparin) 1mg/kg or 60mg if >60kg and eight received other anticoagulation; no recurrences were reported.[49,50] There was one haemorrhagic transformation. In Barnes'[10] series, 28/95 patients were treated (16 antiplatelet, nine anticoagulation, two antiplatelet + anticoagulation, one thrombolysis + anticoagulation). Three children were known to have recurred. There was no effect of treatment on outcome; data on recurrence were not examined as numbers were too small. Two Turkish studies in which at least half of the patients received prophylaxis reported low recurrence rates,[51,52] although as vascular imaging was rarely perfomed, it is possible that some of these patients had had venous sinus thrombosis, for which the recurrence risk is lower (see below). In Soman's[53] report from the Toronto cohort, 17 children (13 recurrent stroke or transient ischaemic attack (TIA) on aspirin, four intolerant of aspirin) received clopidogrel (nine alone, eight concurrent with aspirin). Two had subdural haemorrhages (both also on aspirin, both had marked cerebral atrophy: one moyamoya, one progeria vasculopathy). During follow-up for a mean of 1.69 years (range 1 month to 3 years), there were no further recurrent ischaemic events. In Bonduel's series,[54] six died acutely, two (2%) of thrombosis and four from the underlying disease. All those with cardiac disease were warfarinized and there were no recurrences in this group. There were four (5%) second events in the 84 children without cardiac disease who were treated with aspirin; none of these patients had further events after warfarinization. There were no major haemorrhagic complications. Sixty-three (68%) had neurological sequelae. In Ganesan's[14] series, of 171 children with a first stroke who did not have SCD, physicians chose to treat 64 with aspirin and 33 with anticoagulation, while 74 were not treated. Thirteen (6%) died, one after haemorrhagic transformation, three acutely of other causes, four at the time of clinical recurrence, and five later after censoring at the time of recurrence. After adjusting for the presence of vasculopathy, there was a trend for reduction in risk of recurrence for aspirin (hazard ratio, HR, 0.55, 95% confidence intervals (CI) 0.26–1.16, *p*=0.11) but not for anticoagulation (HR 1.06, 95% CI 0.45, 2.59; *p*=0.89). In Fullerton's series,[15] overall there was no effect of antithrombotic treatment on the risk of recurrence (log rank, *p*=0.42), although only 9% of those treated with aspirin recurred, compared with 18% of those on no treatment (and 27% of those anticoagulated, perhaps because they were considered to be at higher risk of recurrence). In the recent French series, the relatively low incidence of recurrence in those with anterior circulation stroke may have been related to aspirin prophylaxis.[55]

Current clinical guidelines recommend anti-platelet doses of aspirin in the majority of children presenting with first AIS,[56] reserving anticoagulation (usually with warfarin) for certain patient groups; these vary to some extent between the three sets of guidelines but include patients with cardioembolic stroke, extracranial dissection and cerebral venous thrombosis. There may also be a role for anticoagulation in children who develop recurrent AIS despite adequate antiplatelet therapy, although alternative stroke mechanisms (such as hypoperfusion due to occlusive arterial disease) should be considered.

SECONDARY PREVENTION FOR VENOUS SINUS THROMBOSIS AND EXTRACRANIAL DISSECTION

In the recent series of patients pooled from several European centres, non-administration of antithrombotic treatment in clinical risk situations and in children with idiopathic cerebral venous thrombosis (*N*=3) was significantly associated with higher recurrence (*p*<0.001). The mode of antithrombotic therapy administered, for example the use of UFH and warfarin, or of LMWH, did not influence thrombosis free survival (*p*=0.54).[35] Consideration should be given to anticoagulation during relapses in those with conditions which may lead to pro-thrombotic states with relapse, for example nephrotic syndrome and inflammatory bowel disease. Patients with the prothrombin 20210 mutation are at high risk of relapse and consideration should be given to longer-term anticoagulation in them.[35] There is a little evidence that stopping the use of oral contraceptives reduces the risk of recurrent cerebral venous thrombosis and there are several low risk strategies, such as improving the quality of the diet, which can be recommended.

In patients with extracranial arterial dissection, data from studies in adults suggest that there is a relatively small risk of early recurrent events on antithrombotic treatment[57,58] but a very large controlled trial would be needed to determine whether anticoagulation had any benefit over antiplatelet agents in reducing this risk. In addition to recurrent events, which may be more common in the posterior than in the anterior circulation,[59,60] recurrent dissection has been described in children.[59] Although antithrombotic treatment appears to reduce the risk in the cases reported,[59] recurrent events may occur occasionally despite anticoagulation[7,59–61] or antiplatelet agents,[59] perhaps in relation to bony instability in the neck.[60]

PATENT FORAMEN OVALE (see Chapter 5)

The role of closure of patent foramen ovale to prevent stroke recurrence in young stroke patients remains controversial.[62] The association with stroke or stroke recurrence is unproven in children but appears to be significant in young adults,[63] and is related to the degree of right to left shunting. Given the lack of evidence of an association in children, the risks and benefits of closure should be considered on an individual basis with detailed characterization of the defect as described in Chapter 5.

POSTERIOR CIRCULATION STROKE

As previously described mechanical factors related to the cervical spine may be associated with recurrence in patients with posterior circulation stroke. Patients should be evaluated with plain radiographs of the neck in flexion and extension, and neck

immobilization in a soft collar should be considered if there is evidence of subluxation.[60] Cushing et al[64] reported a high incidence of calcification of the arcuate ligament in children with vertebral dissection and advocated deroofing as a strategy to prevent recurrence.

DIET AND GENERAL ADVICE

Hyperhomocysteinaemia or genetic mutations predisposing to this are commonly found in children with AIS[65] and may be associated with a higher incidence of recurrence.[66] As folate supplementation is cheap and appears to be safe, our practice is to recommend this to children with hyperhomocysteinaemia or those who are homozygous for the thermolabile methylene tetrahydrofolate reductase gene mutation.

Advice on the importance of measures to reduce the long-term risk of vascular disease should not be neglected. Blood pressure should be measured and treated if elevated. Dietary advice is increasingly important in an era of increasing childhood obesity, as well as advice regarding regular exercise and avoidance of smoking.

17.2 Outcome after Stroke in Childhood

Anne Gordon, Lucinda Carr, Vijeya Ganesan, Fenella J. Kirkham and Gabrielle deVeber

Health outcomes

Stroke may affect many domains of health and well-being for the children themselves, and their families. A number of studies have reported the outcomes of childhood stroke. These studies are presented in this chapter for the two major types of stroke, ischaemic and haemorrhagic, separating neonatal from childhood stroke. More detail can be found throughout the book and specifically in the chapters on venous sinus thrombosis (see Chapter 7), neonatal stroke (see Chapter 9), haemorrhagic stroke (see Chapter 8), and outcomes for congenital heart disease (see Chapter 15, Sections 15.2 and 15.3) and sickle cell disease (see Chapter 15, Section 15.42).

OUTCOME

Optimizing the outcome of paediatric stroke is of prime concern to affected children and their parents, and to clinicians. Outcome can be considered at the level of the person, the activities they need to perform, and their interaction with their environment. In this chapter both the neurological and functional outcome of paediatric stroke will be reviewed. We have also drawn from our own clinical experience with children seen in tertiary level paediatric stroke services in Toronto, Canada, London, UK and Melbourne, Australia.

Definitions of health outcome

In measuring outcome following stroke, it is important to have a clear concept of health. Rudd[67] defined health outcomes as 'changes in health, health related status or risk factors affecting health, or lack of change when change is expected'. This may be as a result of the condition itself or from the interventions designed to prevent or treat it.

The World Health Organization's 'International Classification of Functioning, Disability and Health' (ICF)[68] provides a framework and common language for the description of health and health-related states. The old definitions of impairment, disability and handicap are now superceded by the umbrella terms of functioning and disability. The health and health-related domains in the ICF are described from the perspectives of the body, the individual and society at two levels, namely

- Body functions and structures
- Activities and participation.

The term 'functioning' in this classification describes positive or neutral aspects whilst 'disability' describes the problems that may entail. ICF also lists environmental factors, which may influence health. This framework enables the clinician to classify the nature of disability or functioning they are assessing. The paediatric stroke outcome literature, in line with the ICF, is now defining outcome in terms of impairments of body structures and functions, limitations in activities and restrictions in participation.

Optimally health outcome assessment should address the following:

- Epidemiology
- Symptoms, risk factors, causes and complications
- Impact on an individual's daily living
- Health-related quality of life (the individual's perceptions of health and well-being)
- The experiences of the individuals and their carers
- The impact of relevant interventions
- The costs and use of resources.[67,69]

These aspects should be considered within the context of the environment specific to the individual.

Measuring outcome in paediatric stroke

Much research on the sequelae of acquired neurological disorders in childhood has focused on the findings of health status measures of impairment (e.g. the presence of abnormal neurological signs). The trend is now to move away from a disease model to one that encompasses health and well-being. This is reflected in the development of health status measures that incorporate physical functioning, psychological well-being and social support items.[69] As yet there are still few validated measures suitable for children with acquired neurological conditions. Measurement tools for this population pose a number of challenges; these include the ability to address what may be a wide range of types and severities of functional disabilities across a broad range of development. To date this area of outcome research has not been satisfactorily addressed.[70]

Function may be assessed using a number of methodologies: direct physical testing, direct observation of behaviour, or interviewing the individual or a proxy/third party. Individuals will react differently to similar levels of impairment (at the level of body structures and functions), depending on their expectations, priorities and goals. In the assessment of children, proxy rating of a child's health by their carer may further complicate this. An additional difficulty lies in longitudinally tracking a child's health following stroke. As there are no single functional health measures validate for this population that can be used from infancy through to adulthood, and the child may 'grow into' new or increasing deficits over time with maturation, the methods and nature of data collected will change through the developmental process. The transition from parent-/carer-reported information in infancy and childhood and the individual's own rating of health in adolescence may also affect the conclusions drawn longitudinally about health functioning.

There is a paucity of literature on functional outcome measurements following paediatric stroke.[71] The best source of relevant information comes from literature on adult stroke and more general outcomes research in paediatric neurology, for example in patients with cerebral palsy. A review of outcome measures in acute adult stroke trials concluded that impairment measures were probably the best indicators of prognosis[72] and made a number of recommendations when selecting stroke outcome measures that may be applicable to children affected by stroke. These included the measurement of any interventions (medical, surgical, pharmacological), baseline environmental characteristics (family functioning, supports, socioeconomic status), and the ability to assess transitions in disability, non-parametrically if necessary, rather than by simply dichotomizing recovery. Further, given that activity and participation are the main concerns of individuals, these abilities should be the markers of recovery, not impairments.

One way of addressing this is by using qualitative research, which is likely to provide valuable longitudinal information on the subjective experiences of children with stroke.

ASSESSMENT OF DISABILITY

Thorough assessment is required before specific needs can be clarified, therapeutic goals established and the effectiveness of any interventions determined. To select the most appropriate tool, issues that should be considered are these:

- What are the domains measured by the tool (i.e. within the ICF framework)?
- Does the tool encompass one or more health components and within each component, single or multiple aspects?
- Are there comparative norms from the general population and the disabled population?
- What is the subject and administrative burden involved?
- Is the tool valid and reliable?[73]
- Are cultural or language adaptations available?[74]

DESCRIPTION OF MEASURES

Assessment tools may be generic or condition specific and often measure performance components (i.e. strength, range of motion) rather than functional ability. This may be due to ease of evaluation, credibility of evaluation and the application of these evaluations within the predominant biomedical model of current practice.[75] Assessment tools currently used in paediatric practice may be useful in evaluating children affected by stroke (for examples of neurological and motor assessment tools see Table 17.1). It should, however, be noted that few have been validated in detail for this population. In selecting assessment tools, it is worthwhile considering the purpose for which the tool was developed, for example descriptive measure of nature of disability, screening measure to determine if disability present, measure predictive of outcome. Those most commonly used in recent publications on the outcome for childhood stroke include the modified Rankin scale[8,30] and the Paediatric Stroke Outcome Measure.[76–78]

ISSUES SPECIFIC TO MEASURING OUTCOME AFTER CHILDHOOD STROKE

It is commonly perceived that following ischaemic stroke, outcome in children is generally favourable compared to that in adults. However, there is little objective evidence for this. Indeed when evaluating outcome in children there are a number of confounding factors:

1. Paediatric stroke is relatively rare and the underlying pathology is diverse. This makes it difficult to compare subjects with similar size of lesion, age of onset and location. The outcome will be influenced by the underlying diagnosis, by the nature of the stroke itself (haemorrhagic vs ischaemic vs metabolic) and by its severity. Many diagnoses carry co-existing neurological morbidity. For example, even in the absence of stroke, cognitive abilities are generally lower in children with sickle cell disease[79,80] and in those with neurofibromatosis type 1.[81] Children with sickle cell disease are at risk of 'silent' or covert cerebral infarction on MRI (see Chapter 15, Section 15.4), which affects up to 25% of those who have not had a stroke by mid-childhood. Although formal neurological examination is usually normal, there is a high sensitivity and specificity in abnormal MRI for predicting neurological 'soft' signs (Zurich Neuromotor Test)[82] and minor abnormalities of motor function (Movement ABC)[83] and these may be used as clinical screening tools. Thus it is not always possible to separate pre- and post-stroke functioning or to assume that pre-morbid functioning was normal. Fluctuations in function and acute decompensation may occur in some metabolic disorders, for example mitochondrial encephalopathy with lactic acidosis (MELAS). It is important that the natural history is recognized to ensure accurate assessment and realistic management plans.

2. In contrast to adults, children show an ongoing developmental trajectory. Subtle deficits may not be immediately apparent after a stroke but remain hidden until there is failure to meet standard 'milestones', social expectations or educational demands. Since comprehensive assessment is rarely possible in younger children, long-term monitoring of health and educational attainment is important to detect the need for intervention or support. Furthermore, with reduced learning capabilities and consequent failure to build on established milestones, long-term deficits may be cumulative.

3. The consequence of stroke in adults is the loss of premorbidly acquired skills and related independence. In children, the stroke may also impact the ability to learn new, more developmentally mature skills through the lifespan.

4. Expectations for children differ from adults. A child's ultimate level of function within their lifespan is not yet established and they are still perceived as dependents. Their families generally provide secure and nurturing environments to which they will return after a stroke even if there is considerable disability. In contrast to adults, very few children are in long-term residential care. Hurvitz's[84] study showed that of 50 paediatric stroke survivors, all were discharged home, although 36% were still requiring assistance in Activities of Daily Living (ADL). The amount and nature of assistance required in ADL over the course of recovery, and related carer burden, remain unknown in the paediatric stroke population. Further, the independent living (and working) potential for adults who have had a stroke in childhood is not known.

Many studies have attempted to predict eventual outcome on the basis of the underlying pathology, clinical features and scan changes. A number of descriptive studies have examined the outcome of paediatric stroke and evaluated the factors that are significant for prognosis; these are reviewed below (Tables 17.2–17.4). Such studies show that following cerebral infarction, 50–75% of children will have residual difficulties. Determinants of outcome include cognitive level,[85] ongoing epilepsy[86] and age at time of lesion.[87] With the given heterogeneity within the population of paediatric strokes and the relatively small scale of most published series, it is perhaps not surprising that robust predictors have not been identified. Although large anterior circulation ischaemic strokes are typically associated with poor outcome[87] (Fig. 17.4), the outcome in patients with small strokes, particularly subcortical infarcts, is much more variable.[88–90] However, in neonatal stroke imaging findings are more directly related to neuromotor outcome (see Chapter 9).[90,91]

Specific aspects of functional outcome following stroke

MORTALITY

The reported mortality after stroke in childhood varies widely between different series from around 3% to 23% (Tables 17.2, 17.3 and 17.4).[2,92–94] Mortality is higher in children with haemorrhagic rather than ischaemic stroke.[95] It appears to be higher in children with sickle cell disease,[17] although has probably been reduced by emergency transfusion nowadays, and in those who present with a depressed conscious level.[89,95,96]

TABLE 17.1

Examples of impairment and activity limitation measures with potential application for the paediatric stroke population

Tool	Domain assessed	Target population	Pros	Cons
Impairment measures				
Barry–Albright Dystonia Scale[153]	Impairment – dystonia	All ages and diagnostic groups	Adequate reliability	Need for further reliability and validity studies, especially for mild dystonia
Hand-Held Dynamometry	Impairment – strength	All ages; however, depends on manufacturer whether age norms available	For some muscle groups, more objective measure than manual muscle testing	Need for further reliability and validity studies in children
The Melbourne Assessment of Unilateral Upper Limb Function[154]	Impairment – upper limb	Children with cerebral palsy	Adequate reliability and validity	Reliability and validity testing limited to children with cerebral palsy.
Modified Ashworth Scale[155]	Impairment – spasticity	All ages and diagnostic groups	Scores have been found to correlate with measures of motor function in adults	Intra- and inter-observer reliability at elbow only
National Institutes of Health Stroke Scale – Pediatrics (NIHSS)[156]	Impairment – neurological	Paediatric stroke	Brief to administer	Undergoing validation in children (based on adult stroke NIHSS)
Pediatric Stroke Oucome Measure[104,157]	Impairment – neurological	Paediatric stroke. Birth to 18 years	Good interrater reliability. Correlation with standard measures of IQ and activity limitation. Canadian Occupational Performance Measure (COPM) Performance & Satisfaction scores, the Vineland Adaptive Behavior Composite and Full Scale IQ	Lengthy procedure. Need for further reliability and validity studies in children
Quality of Upper Extremity Skills Test (QUEST)[158]	Impairment – upper limb	Children with cerebral palsy	Assesses movement quality	Reliability and validity testing limited to children with cerebral palsy
Rankin scale,[159] Modified Rankin[160]	Global level of disability Impairment – activity Limitation – participation	Adult stroke	Simple, reliable. Good for overall assessment of disability. Moderate inter-observer. Used in children	Walking only explicit assessment criterion. Mixes objective and subjective items, which span impairment, activity, participation. Low sensitivity
Activity limitation measures				
Assisting Hand Assessment[161]	Activity limitation	Children 2.5–18 years	Good validity and reliability	Requires assessor training, and video for scoring
Bruininks-Oseretsky Test of Motor Proficiency[162]	Activity limitation	Evaluation of children with developmental delay and/or clumsiness	Reliability and validity for able-bodied children	Needs further assessment of usefulness for children with more significant motor problems. Lengthy administration
Jebsen Hand Function Test[163]	Activity limitation	Children over 5 years and adults	Used widely in variety of settings	Content validity has been questioned
Paediatric Evaluation of Disability Inventory (PEDI)[164]	Activity limitation	Functional capabilities of children 6 months to 7 years	Overall good reliability and content validity	Reliability increased when administered to both the parent/carer and primary health care professional
WeeFIM (Functional Independence Measure for Children)[165]	Activity limitation	Children 6 months to 7 years. Functional abilities and level of assistance required	Adequate overall reliability, good content validity	Specific training required for test users
Zurich Neuromotor Assessment[82]	Activity limitation	Children 5–18 years	Separate centiles for timed performance and associated movements. Intraobserver, interobserver, test–retest reliability for timed measurements moderate to high	Long-lasting developmental change, large interindividual variation. Associated movements: non-linear developmental course, sex difference

Good reliability = more than two well-designed reliability studies completed with adequate to excellent reliability values (>0.80). Adequate reliability = one or two well-designed studies complete with adequate to excellent reliability values (0.60–0.79). Good validity = more than two well-designed validity studies supporting the measures validity. Adequate validity = one or two well-designed validity studies supporting the measures validity.[75] NIHSS, National Institutes of Health Stroke Scale.

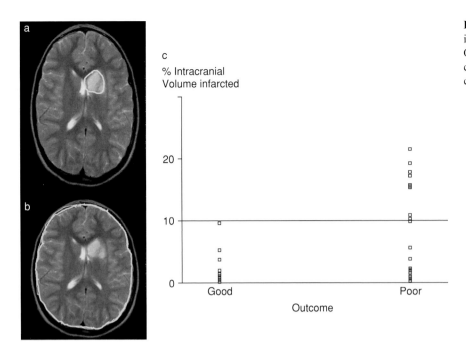

Fig. 17.4. Measurement of (a) volume of infarct and (b) intracranial volume.[88] (c) Outcome for childhood related to mean per cent intracranial volume (%ICV) infarcted calculated as (a/b)*100.

Ischaemic stroke

The mortality from ischaemic stroke is approximately 15–20%;[6,10,11,65,97] Table 17.2), with about half being stroke-related. Mortality was higher in those of black ethnicity in a US-wide study of deaths from 1979 to 1998[98] which reported no difference in sex ratio, but not in a Californian database of cases from 1991 to 2000 which found an excess of deaths in males.[97] Death can be due to the stroke itself, or to the childhood illnesses underlying the stroke, as in overwhelming sepsis or congenital heart disease.

Haemorrhagic stroke

The mortality from haemorrhagic stroke, including intracerebral haemorrhage and subarachnoid haemorrhage, is 5–40%[11,99–103] (Table 17.3), and in most studies is greater than that for ischaemic stroke. Again, there was an excess of deaths in those of black ethnicity and male sex in the US-wide study of deaths[98] but not in the Californian study.[97] In studies of combined ischaemic and haemorrhagic stroke types in children, haemorrhagic stroke type predicts death[95,96] (Table 17.4).

OUTCOME IN SURVIVORS

Ischaemic stroke

Although there were few large series before 1990, the frequencies of moderate or severe long-term neurological deficits may have decreased in the past 20 years to approximately 50–60% (Table 17.2).[7–9,30,87,104] Methodological variation between studies in terms of assessment and timing complicate the ability to draw conclusions; however the decrease in impairments seen may reflect the inclusion of a milder spectrum of disease now identifiable with newer generation CT and MRI. Improving outcomes may also reflect

the increasing tendency to treat children with antithrombotic agents. Guidelines for antithrombotic therapies for acute therapy or secondary prevention of arterial ischaemic stroke or sinovenous thrombosis have now been published,[15,32,105–109] and in the Canadian Registry from 40% to 60% of children received antithrombotic agents, depending on the stroke subtypes and age group.[76,104,105,108,109] Long-term, seizures occur in 15–20%.

Predictors of outcome include the presence of multiple aetiological risk factors, seizures at onset, extent of brain damage, arterial stroke type compared with sinovenous thrombosis, and for sinus thrombosis, the presence of venous infarcts.[6,76,104,108] Not surprisingly, need for rehabilitation also predicts poor outcome on a quality of life measure (Simple Questions) as well as a standardized neurological examination (the Paediatric Stroke Outcome Measure, PSOM).[77,104] The estimated recurrence rates for childhood arterial ischaemic stroke are less than 5% for neonates while for older infants and children, recurrent stroke occurs in around 10% with a further 10–25% experiencing further TIAs[14,15,48,93,103,104] (see Section 17.1). For cerebral sinovenous thrombosis recurrence rates are lower, 3–17% in older infants and children[35,108,110,111] (see Chapter 7).

Haemorrhagic stroke

In survivors of haemorrhagic stroke, neurological deficits (33–50%) and seizures (5–10%) appear to be less frequent than for survivors of ischaemic stroke.[99,100] Recurrent stroke also occurs in 10–20% of children with haemorrhagic stroke, and is often fatal.[99] In a population-based study, recurrence was documented in 13% of those with medical aetiologies, usually within the first week, and there was a 5-year cumulative recurrence rate of 13% for those with unoperated vascular malformations or tumours.[103]

TABLE 17.2
Summary of studies reporting outcome after ischaemic stroke in childhood, 1965–2009

Authors	Population	N follow-up/total	Median follow-up (years)[a]	Age at stroke	Normal	Mild deficit	Moderate deficit	Severe deficit	Motor deficit	Cognitive impairment	Epilepsy	Behavioural problems	Death	Recurrent stroke and TIA	Other outcomes	Predictors of poor outcome
Greer 1965[166]	Acute neurological disorders of infancy and childhood	12/23	>2	1mo-13y	1/12 (8%)	5 (42%)	6/12 (50%)		10/12 (83%)	4/12 (33%)	4/12 (33%)					
Aicardi 1969[167]	Acute hemiplegia without seizures at onset	23/33	c.3	6mo-13y		14/17 slight or normal		3/17		8/17 (47%)	2/33 (6%)		0			
Solomon 1970[116]	Acute hemiplegia	41							30 (73%)	17 (41%)	20 (49%)		3 (7%)		14/41 hyperkinetic behaviour	
Tibbles 1975[168]	Acute hemiplegia	10			4/10 (40%)				6/10 (60%)	0	0					
Schoenberg 1978[169]	Ischaemic stroke	38	c.5	1mo-13y	2 (6%)				31 (82%)	8 (21%)	5 (13%)		4 (12%)			
Blennow 1978[170]	Ischaemic stroke	13/14	5.8	2.5-19y	4	4	4				3		1	0		
Eeg-Olofsson 1983[171]	Ischaemic stroke	11		2-15y	3 (25%)			0	5	2	0		2 (18%)	0	1 hemianopia	
Isler 1984[93]	Acquired cerebral arterial occlusion	87			8 (9%)				69 (80%)	42 (49%)	39 (44%)		10 (11%)	15 (20%)		
Mazza 1985[172]	Ischaemic stroke	10	2	3mo-14y	1				9				1	1		
Dusser 1986[2]	Ischaemic stroke	41/44	Mean 3.33	6w-15y	8 (20%)				31/41 (76%)	11/41 (27%)	12/41 (29%)		0	4	2 hemianopia, 14 dystonia	Symptomatic, moyamoya
Wanifuchi 1988[94]	Ischaemic stroke not moyamoya	23		3mo-13y	5 (22%)	4 (17%)	9 (39%)	3 (13%)					2 (9%)			Trend for cardiac
Lanska 1991[118]	Ischaemic stroke	42	3	Neo-19y	10 (24%)				32 (76%)		8 (19%)		0			
Satoh 1991[173]	Ischaemic stroke	54	0.5	Neo-16y	30 (56%)				48 (89%)							
Inagaki 1992[174]	Ischaemic basal ganglia stroke	16			9 (56%)				5 (31%)		1				1 blind	
Broderick 1993[175]	Ischaemic stroke	7	0.08	2mo-14y	1 (14%)	2 (28%)	3 (43%)	1 (14%)	6 (86%)	1 (14%)	0	3	1 (14%)			
Powell 1994[176]	Subcortical infarction	29/104	>0.42	2mo-17y	12/29	11	6									
Giroud 1995[117]	Ischaemic stroke	17	4.1	2w-9y	5 (29%)				11 (65%)		2 (12%)		1 (6%)	0	8 dystonia	

345

TABLE 17.2 *(cont'd)*

Authors	Population	N follow-up/total	Median follow-up (years)[a]	Age at stroke	Normal	Mild deficit	Moderate deficit	Severe deficit	Motor deficit	Cognitive impairment	Epilepsy	Behavioural problems	Death	Recurrent stroke and TIA	Other outcomes	Predictors of poor outcome
Abram 1996[5]	Cryptogenic ischaemic stroke	42	7.4	9mo-18y	15 (37%)	12 (29%)	6 (14%)	8 (19%)	20 (48%)	16 (38%)	7 (17%)	5 (12%)	1 (2%)	7 (17%)	18 'poor', 24 'good'	Hemiparesis at 1 month, cortical infarct, moyamoya
Visudhiphan 1996[177]	Ischaemic stroke	38			10 (26%)								3 (7%)			
Brower 1996[b 178]	Basal ganglia and thalamic infarction	36	1.33	1d-13y (3 neonates)	14 (39%)	16 (44%)	1 (3%)	5 (14%)	15 (42%)		1 (3%)		0			
Giroud 1997[187]	Ischemic stroke	31									4		1	0	14 dystonia	
Andrew 1997[179]	Ischaemic stroke: Arterial Venous	155/165 41/49			35/155 25/41		94/155 10/41				16/155 3/41		10/155 3/41			
Mancini 1997[4]	Ischaemic stroke	35		2mo-17y	17 (49%)				10 (29%)	3 (9%)	4 (11%)		1 (3%)	4 (11%)	2/35 visually impaired	
Ganesan 1999[88]	MCA arterial ischaemic stroke	38		6mo-15y									2 (5)		24 'poor' 12 'good'	Infarct volume
Ganesan 2000[87]	Ischaemic stroke	90	3	3mo-16y	13 (14%)				66 (74%)	2/4 young 5/18 older	13 (15%)	33 (37)			53 'poor' 37 'good'	Lower age
Chabrier 2000[7]	Arterial ischaemic stroke	59	2.5	3mo-17y	16 (27%)		17 (29%)	26 (44%)					0	13 (22%)		Embolus, moyamoya, systemic disease
De Schryver 2000[8]	Ischaemic stroke	35/37 F/U 27/37 CNS	7	3mo-14y	11/27 (41%) MRS 0	5/27 (19%) MRS 1	11/27 (41%) MRS 2	0/27 MRS 3,4 or 5	16/27 (59%)	6 (24%) Raven's 3 (12%) vocab	9/35 (26%)		4/35	2 (6%) stroke + 8 (23%) TIAs	1 hemianopia, 1 sensory, 2 dysarthria	Cognitive: seizures Vocabulary: LMCA Raven's: MRS>0
DeVeber 2000[76]	Toronto PSOM Arterial: Neonate Older Venous: Neonate Older	161 33 90 19 19	mean 2.07 (SD, 1.49; range, 0.01 to 17.59)	0-17y	(39%)	(20%)	(25%)	(16%)		12 (13%)	12 (13%) 6 (23%)			11 (11%) 3 (3%) 2 (15%)	Headache 32 (33%) 9 (35%)	Independent: Arterial, associated neurological disorders, need for rehabilitation

346

Study	Stroke type	n	Age, mean/median (y)	Age range									Predictors of outcome
DeVeber 2000[76]	Toronto Euroquol	102			(45%)					(10%)	(19%)		Need for rehabilitation
deVeber 2000[104]	Arterial	660			(34%)				60	(10%)	(10%)		Seizures, infarcts
deVeber 2001[180]	Venous	160			(65%)				15	(20%)	(9%)		
Lanthier 2000[6]	Arterial ischaemic stroke	51 (46 AIS, 5 SVT)	1.9	1mo–18y	18 (35%)				23 (45%)	6 (12%)	8 (16%)	8 (16%)	Recurrence: multiple risk factors, death: recurrence
Delsing 2001[89]	Arterial ischaemic stroke	31		2mo–16y	9 (29%)	9 (29%)		9 (29%)		—	4 (16%)	7 (22%)	Coma, seizures, or both, cortical completed MCA stroke, trend for cardiac
Williams 2002[b][181]	Ischaemic stroke	56	1.25	0–18y (4 neonates)	11 (19%)					0			
Gordon 2002[77]	Arterial ischaemic stroke	17	2 (0.8–8.5)	4y (1–13y)	6 (35%)	7 (41%)	3 (18%)	1 (6%)	10 (59%)		10 (59%)		Extent brain damaged predicted motor
Rodrigues 2004[182]	Ischaemic stroke 2000–2002	15	Mean 4.9	1y 1mo–10y 8mo	2				13	6 severe, 4 mild		3 visual	Hypoperfusion on SPECT
Barnes 2004[b][10]	Arterial ischaemic stroke	83/95	1.6	1d–19y	15/83 (18%)		14/83 (17%)		54/83 (65%)	5/83 (6%)	14/95 (15%)		
Steinlin 2004[30]	Arterial ischaemic stroke MRS	20	7	6mo–16y	2/16 (10%) MRS 0	7/16 (44%) MRS 1	3/16 (19%) MRS 2	4/16 (25%) MRS 3	4/16 (25%)	2/20 (10%)	3/18 (15%)		
Steinlin 2005[9]	Arterial ischaemic stroke	38/40	>0.5	1mo–16y	10/38 (26%)	7/38 (18%)	16/38 (42%)	1 (3%)	24/38 (63%)	4/38 (11%)	1 (0.5%)		Size infarct, young age
Bowen 2005[50]	Ischaemic stroke	27	Mean 17	1y 4mo–17y	6 (22%)	9 (33%)	12 (44%)		21 (77%)	2 (7%)	2 (7%)	0	
Simma 2007[135]	Ischaemic stroke	15	3.7	11mo–14y	7 (47%)						0	1	
Gokben 2007[52]	Arterial ischaemic stroke	31	0.08–12	3mo–14y	6 (19%)						0	4	
Jordan 2007[183]	Arterial ischaemic stroke	55		0–18y							9 (16%)	7 (13%)	Death: critical illness
Lee 2008[184]	Ischaemic stroke	94		1mo–18y	41 (55%)						7 (9%)	12 (16%)	
Buompadre 2009[185]	Basal ganglia stroke	28			19 (68%)					0			

ᵃ Excluding acute deaths in first month. ᵇ Study included neonates. CHQ, Child Health Questionnaire; MCA, middle cerebral artery; MRS, modified Rankin scale; PSOM, Paediatric Stroke Outcome Measure; SPECT, single proton emmission tomography.

347

TABLE 17.3

Summary of studies reporting outcome after haemorrhagic stroke in childhood, 1965–2009

Authors	Population	N follow-up/total	Median follow-up (years)[a]	Age at stroke	Normal	Mild deficit	Moderate deficit	Severe deficit	Motor deficit	Cognitive impairment	Epilepsy	Behavioural problems	Death	Recurrent stroke and TIA	Other outcomes	Predictors of poor outcome
Schoenberg 1978[92]	Haemorrhagic stroke	31	c.5	1mo-18y	11 (35%)				4 (13%)	5 (16%)	2 (6%)		8 (26%)			
Eeg-Olofsson 1983[171]	Haemorrhagic stroke	14	1.5	6mo-15y	2 (14%)				5 (36%)	2 (14%)	1 (7%)		5 (36%)	0	1 hemianopia	Death: lumbar puncture
Mazza 1985[172]	Haemorrhagic stroke	15	1.5	1mo-16y	10				2		1		2		1 visual problems	
Broderick 1993[175]	Haemorrhagic stroke	9		3w-14y	1	2	2	2	4	4			2	0	1 poor vision	
Giroud 1995[117]	Haemorrhagic stroke	11	4.1	1w-16y	0				4	3	3		2	2	2 dystonia	
Visudhiphan 1996[177]	Haemorrhagic stroke	30			16 (52%)								2 (7%)			
Merino Arribas 1997[186]	Haemorrhagic stroke	21											4 (19%)			
Giroud 1997[187]	Haemorrhagic stroke	23									9		2	3	4 dystonia	
Al Jarrallah 2000*[100]	Haemorrhagic stroke	68			34 (50%)				17 (25%)	9; 5 aphasic	7 (10%)		6 (9%)		3 hydrocephalus	
Lanthier 2000*[6]	Haemorrhagic stroke	21	1.9	1mo-18y	8 (38%)				6 (29%)		2 (10%)		6 (29%)	2 (10%)		Death: recurrence
Williams 2002[182]	Haemorrhagic stroke	39	1.25	Neo-18y	20 (51%)								13 (34%)			
Blom 2003[99]	Haemorrhagic stroke MRS	51/56	10	1mo-16y	14/51 MRS 0	8/51 MRS 1	7/51 MRS 2	2/51 MRS 3	20/56	No skew IQ 15/51 difficulty	6/56		13 acute + 7 F/U (3 rec)			
Meyer-Heim 2003[101]	Haemorrhagic stroke	32/34	Mean 3	10w-17y		10/32 (31%) mild/normal	7/32 (22%)	7/32 (22%), 1 vegetative		9/13: 5 mild, 4 severe			8/32 (25%)	3 (9%)		Death: age <3 years, infratentorial, haematological, aneurysm
Simma 2007[135]	Haemorrhagic stroke	5	3.7	11m-14y	4 (80%)								0	0		
Fullerton 2007[103]	Haemorrhagic stroke	153	3.3	Neo-20y									8 acute + 3 F/U	11/116 (10%)		
Jordan 2009[188]	Haemorrhagic stroke	30	0.08	Neo-16y	21 (70%)									0		Volume of ICH > 4%

[a] Excluding acute deaths in first month. ICH, intracerebral haemorrhage; MRS, modified Rankin scale.

TABLE 17.4
Summary of studies reporting outcome after combined ischaemic and haemorrhagic stroke in childhood, 1965–2009

Authors	Population	N follow-up/total	Median follow-up (years)[a]	Age at stroke	Normal	Mild deficit	Moderate deficit	Severe deficit	Motor deficit	Cognitive impairment	Epilepsy	Behavioural problems	Death	Recurrent stroke and TIA	Other outcomes	Predictors of poor outcome
Higgins 1991[95]	Stroke	88/95	0.19	8-22y	20 (23%)				48 (54%)				20 (23%)			Death: coma, haemorrhage, Caucasian
Keidan 1994[96]	Cerebrovascular disease	45	4.2	8-18y	11 (30%)				23 (51%)	13 (29%)	13 (29%)		8 (18%)	5 (11%)		Death: coma haemorrhage
Obama 1994[189]	Stroke	35	0.5	5mo-15y	0				34 (97%)				1 (3%)			
De Moura-Ribiero 1999,[190] Guimaraes 2007[134]	Cerebrovascular disease; 27 ischaemic (5 haemorrhagic conversion); 15 haemorrhage (2 SAH)	42	4.33	Neo-13y	8 (19%)				24 (57%)	4/14 ischaemic	4 (10%)		2 (5%)		13 (31%): Other – visual, involuntary movements, cognitive	
Hurvitz 1999[84]	Stroke	50/73	6	7mo-18y						20 speech and language impaired			6		42 (84%) mobile independently; 38 (76%) ADL independent	ADL: young age, female, cardiac, hemiparesis, ischaemic
Hurvitz 2004[153]	Stroke	32/73	11.9	8mo-18y											32 mobile independently, mean VABS moderate-low	Anticonvulsants, ischaemic
Chung 2004[11]	Stroke	50 (36 AIS, 14 haemorrhages)	8.7	8-16y	22 (44%)	7 (14%)	3 (6%)	7 (15%)	10 (20%)	11 (22%)	7 (14%)		9 (18%)	5		Death: coma Morbidity: acute seizures
Salih 2006[13]	Stroke	95/104	3.33	8-12y	6/95 (6%)				73 (81%)	45 (50%)	52 (58%)		5 (5%)			
Auvichayapat 2007[191]	Cerebrovascular disease	109		6mo-16y									24 (22%)			
Lo 2008[78]	Stroke, PSOM	39		Neo-18y									0			
Rasul 2009[192]	Stroke	42/42		Neo-16y	22 (52%)								3 (7%)			
Emam[193]	Stroke	25			28%								28%			
Tham[194]	Stroke	20/26	3.3 (0.1-10)	3mo-18y	11 (42%)	6	2			2 mild, 2 severe			0	1		Coma, seizures, systemic, cortical and subcortical

[a] Excluding acute deaths in first month. ADL, Activities of Daily Living; AIS, arterial ischaemic stroke; MRS, modified Rankin scale; PSOM, Paediatric Stroke Outcome Measure; SAH, subarachnoid haemorrhage; VABS, Vineland Adaptive Behavior Scale.

EPILEPSY

The reported incidence of epilepsy after ischaemic stroke varies between 25% and 50%, most of which is limited to the acute stroke period (<14 days), and appears to be higher than in adults.[2,112] Cortical lesions and persistence of seizures beyond 2 weeks of the acute insult have previously been identified as risk factors for secondary epilepsy.[113,114] The incidence of secondary epilepsy in ischaemic stroke appears lower than that quoted in earlier reports of 'acute infantile hemiplegia'. This is probably due to exclusion of patients with hemiplegic syndromes such as HHE (hemiplegia, hemiconvulsions, epilepsy) in the former group and the short duration of follow-up in some studies. Epilepsy appears to be an important determinant of cognitive outcome[8,86] (see Section 17.3) and treatment itself may also affect behaviour and recovery.[115]

MOTOR FUNCTION

Some degree of long-term motor impairment affects up to 90% of children following a stroke.[2,8–10,87,92,116,117] Hemiparesis is typical since cerebral infarction most commonly affects the territory of the middle cerebral artery but the spectrum of motor impairment can vary widely. Children will usually regain ambulation after ischaemic stroke, unless they experience bilateral or secondary insults.[87,118] Hariman et al[119] found that although overall gross motor function was normal or only mildly impaired after stroke in 14 patients with sickle cell disease, nearly half had moderately severe dysfunction in the hand, especially in relation to complex tasks.

Pyramidal signs may initially predominate in children with striatocapsular infarcts, but subsequently the motor picture is often dominated by dystonia.[2,7,87] This is more likely in children having a stroke beyond the neonatal period.[90] Secondary dystonia following basal ganglia injury appears to be a phenomenon which is confined to childhood.[77,117,120] Our clinical experience suggests that hemidystonia is as common as spastic hemiparesis in children following a stroke, and that this may be a slowly emerging picture over several weeks to a year. Involuntary movements and posturing of the affected limb or limbs may interfere with cosmetic appearance as well as motor function, and both these factors are of concern to children and their families. The upper limb may be particularly functionally impaired, with dystonic spasms associated with muscular cramps and pain. In considering medical, orthotic or therapy intervention for hemidystonia, the expectations of the child and family with regard to impact on cosmesis and function, and ability to adhere to a treatment regime should be considered.[121] This will enable targeting of the most appropriate intervention, and measurement of any benefits with regard to the individual's daily life.

SENSORY FUNCTION

Impaired tactile, kinaesthetic and proprioceptive sensation in the affected limbs may further compromise manual dexterity and should be formally assessed in the hemiplegic child. When compared with congenital hemiplegia, sensory loss is generally more marked with hemiplegias acquired during childhood.[122] There is, however, little consensus on the optimal measurement tool for measuring hand sensibility.[123] In school-aged children with hemiplegic cerebral palsy, two-point discrimination, functional pick-up ability, and stereognosis of familiar objects were found to be useful assessments of tactile abilities.[124] Visual field defects may be present in over 25% of hemiplegic children[122] but have not been well described in children affected by stroke. The visual functional of all children presenting with stroke should be assessed in detail.[32,125]

SPEECH AND LANGUAGE

The effect of brain injury on language function is complex. Whilst initial clinical observation suggests that language function is usually spared after early (<5 years of age) brain injury, recent studies have challenged this assumption. Furthermore, it appears that relative preservation of verbal skills, when it does occur, may do so at the expense of visuospatial skills or reduction in overall IQ.[85,126]

Pure expressive aphasia is unusual in childhood and formal testing usually reveals an associated receptive component. The typical course of recovery is for an initial period of relatively rapid improvement which then tails off. The extent of the initial recovery is predictive of eventual outcome. Lees & Neville[127] found that children with acquired aphasia who did not attain at scores within −2 standard deviations from mean scores in an assessment of language comprehension at 6 months following stroke were likely to have significant long-term language difficulties. They noted that even children apparently functioning within the 'normal range' for speech and language may show qualitative impairments in speech and language function. Parents are often much more aware of these qualitative differences than of decreases in the developmental level of the child's language ability.[87] This area therefore merits formal evaluation, as significant difficulties may largely go unnoticed and could potentially benefit from educational or rehabilitative strategies.

Subtle abnormalities may be detectable on formal testing even in those with apparently pure subcortical stroke.[128,129] Gout et al[128] studied nine patients with left internal capsule, lenticular or thalamic infarction or a combination of these. Early aphasic manifestations following the deep cerebral infarcts affected language expression. These included mutism, non-fluent speech, word finding difficulties, and phonemic and semantic paraphasia. Speech comprehension was better preserved. Although there was improvement, only two patients fully recovered, both of whom had their strokes over the age of 6 years. Those who had their strokes aged <6 years had persistent dysfluency, word finding difficulties and written language learning impairment. Rowan et al[129] found that, compared with controls, children with basal ganglia stroke had lower scores on the Clinical Evaluation of Language Fundamentals (CELF-III); scores for the reduced expressive language scale scores approached statistical significance. Interestingly, no

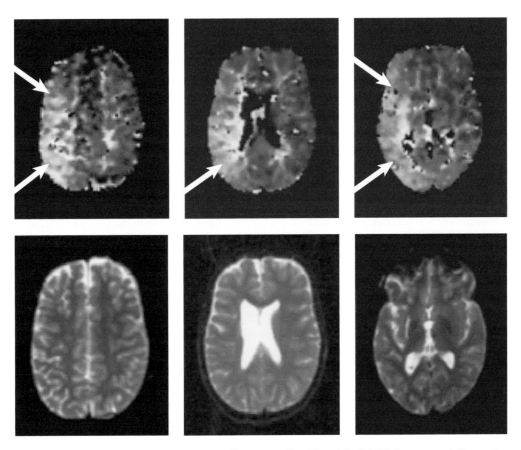

Fig. 17.5. Time to peak cerebral perfusion maps (top row) and corresponding T2-weighted MRI (bottom row) from a 5-year-old girl who sustained a right hemiparesis and global aphasia due to a traumatic internal carotid dissection, demonstrating haemodynamic abnormalities (seen as increased signal intensity in the images on the top row) affecting cortical language areas which are not infarcted in the images on the bottom row.[129]

evidence was found for differences related to side of injury for either the receptive, expressive or total language scales. However, the patients with left-hemisphere lesions showed large variations in performance in association with loss of grey and white matter in the cortex demonstrable using voxel-based morphometry. Three of these patients obtained CELF-III language scores that were greater than two standard deviations below the normal mean, suggesting that language performance in these patients was clinically abnormal; these patients also had perfusion abnormalities in cortical language areas with gadolinium-enhanced perfusion MRI (Fig. 17.5).[129]

COGNITIVE OUTCOME

There is considerable evidence for an effect of childhood stroke and cerebrovascular disease on cognitive function;[130] see Section 17.3). Most of the available neuropsychological studies are limited by their sample size and cross-sectional design, and sometimes by assumptions about the capacity of the immature brain to re-organize function. Despite these limitations, the available evidence largely reveals a mean level of intellectual and cognitive functioning in the low to low-average range.[8,130–136] Although the effect of stroke on IQ is generally minor,[8,130–134] mean scores may mask variability in intellectual and cognitive outcome associated with multiple

variables, such as the aetiology of stroke, for example trauma versus genetic predisposition.

Performance IQ is almost always more affected than verbal IQ[130,136] and visual-perceptual problems are more common than language difficulties whatever the side of the lesion.[136] In one study of children with congenital hemiplegia, performance IQ was an average of 13 points lower than verbal IQ, apparently reflecting specific visuospatial difficulties rather than an effect of the motor disability itself.[85] The severity of neurological impairment has been found predictive of IQ but side of lesion was not associated with full scale IQ or verbal-performance discrepancy in this study.[85] Similar findings have been demonstrated after childhood stroke.[131,136,137] Children with cortical and subcortical involvement have more cognitive problems than those with either cortical or subcortical involvement alone.[138] Some children have clear evidence of specific learning difficulties,[138] including problems with arithmetic and reduced processing speed and memory (digit span and working memory).[136,138] Although verbal IQ is usually within the normal range, there may be problems with verbal learning and memory[137] and other subtle language deficits which only emerge during discourse.[139] Children functioning at this level are at risk of learning difficulties, with co-existing everyday behavioural problems. There is evidence for late emergence of cognitive deficits after perinatal stroke, with IQ measured in the preschool period higher than that measured later.[140]

In direct contradiction to the idea that the young brain is more plastic and therefore has more capacity for recovery after injury, in all of these studies of childhood stroke, the younger the age at stroke, the worse the cognitive and behavioural outcomes,[138] with one study finding the best outcomes for those experiencing stroke in mid-childhood.[136] Although there is no doubt that in general outcome is better in children than in elderly adults, in a study matching site and size of lesion in children (mean age at stroke 3 years) and adults (mean age at stroke 53 years), the overall level of impairment judging by pair-by-pair qualitative profile analysis was not impressively different.[141] However, the pattern was somewhat different in terms of which domains of cognitive abilities were affected for children versus adults.

A particular concern is the lack of longitudinal data with follow-up into adulthood. This is necessary to distinguish between transient cognitive deficits, and late-developing effects that may only appear as level of educational demand increases and the transition into employment. In addition, systemic factors, such as hypotension, hypertension, heart failure, anaemia and hypoxia may play an important role in determining IQ before and after stroke in children with underlying conditions such as cardiac disease and anaemia (see Chapters 5 and 15).

BEHAVIOUR

In hemiplegic children, there is evidence of a significant excess of psychiatric morbidity including attention-deficit-hyperactivity disorder (ADHD), anxiety, mood disorder and personality change.[142,143] IQ is a significant predictor of behavioural and emotional problems in children with hemiplegia.[142,143] In a large study of 428 children with both congenital and acquired hemiplegia,[142] 61% were affected by psychiatric disorders when judged by individual assessment; the proportions when assessed by parental (54%) or teacher (42%) ratings were slightly lower. A subgroup of these children were studied more intensively (*N*=149), revealing that emotional (37%) and conduct (35%) disorders were most common, although pervasive (15%) and situational hyperactivity (20%) was also evident in large numbers. This cohort was followed up approximately 4 years later (*N*=328), and psychiatric problems were found to persist in a large number of children who had been identified as having emotional and behavioural problems at baseline (70%).[144] In a study comparing 29 children with stroke with children with orthopaedic diagnoses such as scoliosis or talipes equinovarus, Max et al[143] confirmed the relationship between full scale IQ and psychiatric disorder and found a trend for an effect of stroke severity. In a logistic regression looking at the risk factors for psychiatric morbidity in stroke patients, he found that neurological severity and family history of psychiatric disorder were independent predictors. It is likely that IQ is a marker for genetic or environmental effects on the brain which are also associated with psychiatric disorder; some may also be risk factors for cerebrovascular disease and stroke.

There is some evidence for an effect of the site of the lesion on whether or not there is psychiatric morbidity after stroke. ADHD symptoms were associated with lesions in the dopamine-rich posterior ventral putamen in 25 children in Max's series who had MRI imaging.[144] The same group[131,145] also reported that inattention and apathy are core features associated with ADHD after childhood stroke. Lesions within Posner's executive inattention network and its orbital frontal connections may be linked to important mechanisms in the expression of ADHD symptomatology after childhood stroke.[146]

These emotional and behavioural difficulties are likely to cause problems as the child returns to school[115] and may affect quality of life in the long term. Around half of children with hemiplegia have some degree of emotional or behavioural difficulties. These include conduct disorder, irritability, anxiety, hyperactivity and inattention. Considering children with ischaemic stroke specifically, around a third of parents of children who have had ischaemic stroke reported concerns about their child's behaviour.[5,87]

For children with congenital hemiplegia and childhood stroke, it is most important to consider both behavioural and cognitive factors when looking at school placement, since secondary behavioural problems may arise as a result of inappropriate educational placement. Peer issues are very common in schoolchildren and may cause considerable distress.[147,148] Although De Schryver[8] reported that 27/29 children who had had an ischaemic stroke rated themselves as being as happy as their peers, their parents reported that around a third experienced behaviour difficulties and difficult peer relationships. Hariman[119] found that social and personal adjustment was severely affected in 14 children who had had stroke as a result of sickle cell disease. The difficulties with peer relationships appear largely due to impaired social understanding on the part of the child who had had the stroke rather than peer responses to disability. The social difficulties very commonly experienced by adults with right hemisphere stroke are not universal after right hemisphere stroke in childhood, but there is a high degree of similarity between chronic neuropsychological and social function outcomes in adults and children with similarly located brain lesions due to unilateral stroke.[141]

The behavioural and psychiatric consequences of congenital and acquired childhood hemiplegia are described in detail by Goodman and Yude.[115] These are likely to result both from organic brain injury as well as from its secondary physical and social consequences. The possibility that there are modifiable risk factors has received little attention[149] but might be as important as it appears to be in reducing the risk of cognitive decline in adults with cerebrovascular disease, at least in part because of the reduction in recurrent stroke.

SOCIAL AND EDUCATIONAL EFFECTS

Goodman and Yude[115] found that behaviour problems in children with hemiplegia were associated with increased parental anxiety and depression. One of the main anxieties for parents is the concern about possible recurrence of stroke.[77] We have found that the psychological and social aspects of parental health could be adversely affected following stroke in their child, regardless of the presence of neurological impairment in the child. In addition the children themselves may have significant physical limitations in performing school-related activities and activities with friends.[77] Coordination of assessment and intervention between health and education professionals can help smooth the transition back to school for children following a stroke. The involvement of therapists, a psychologist, special educational needs teacher and specialist advisory teachers may be indicated. Areas of assessment may include physical accessibility of the school environment, the structure of educational materials, positioning in class with regard to a visual field deficit, and strategies for the child in talking with their peers about the stroke.

Of 90 children with childhood-onset ischaemic stroke whose parents were surveyed, 43 had had a statement of educational needs, 30 required additional help but were in mainstream school and 17 were in special education.[87] This corresponds with data from Delsing,[89] who reported that a third of surviving children from their group of patients with arterial ischaemic stroke had special educational needs.

Quality of Life
De Schryver[8] looked at quality of life in four domains (physical, functional, social and psychological) for 31 survivors a median of 7 years after childhood stroke. Seventeen had no difficulty with physical activities such as running, cycling and gymnastics. Half had remedial teaching at least initially, one-third had to repeat a school year and one-third had special educational needs. Behaviour was a problem in one-third. Three-quarters of the children thought they were as healthy as other children and almost all thought they were as happy.

Friefeld et al[150] used the parent and child forms for the PedsQL in 84 children with arterial ischemic stroke and 16 with cerebral sinovenous thrombosis at a mean age of 8.4 years, a mean of 4.4 years after their stroke. Both the parent-proxy and child self-report Health Related Quality of Life (HRQOL) scores were significantly reduced compared with normal children. The effect of stroke on school was of greatest concern for both parents and children, closely followed by the impact on emotional and social function, whereas scores in physical domain were better. The children with poor neurological recovery had the lowest mean PedsQL scores and their quality of life was significantly poorer compared with normative data of children with chronic health conditions.

In Simma's[135] follow-up study of 20 children seen at a median of 3.7 (range 0.4–18) years after ischaemic or haemorrhagic stroke, although nine children were assessed as having severe or moderate neurological deficits, only four children had a reduced quality of life on the parent form of the Child Health Questionnaire, summarized as the Physical Summary and Psychological Summary Score. Again, outcome was worse for those with young age at onset and for ischaemic stroke. Everts et al[136] studied 21 children from Bern or Berlin who had had an ischaemic stroke at a mean age of 7 years and were followed up after a median of 5 years (range 14 days to 14 years). Using the Kidscreen,[151] a quality of life measure validated in a number of European centres, certain aspects of quality of life were significantly reduced from the child's point-of-view (autonomy $p=0.003$; parents' relation $p=0.003$; social acceptance $p=0.037$), although most components were at the lower end of the normal range. From the parents' point of view the perception of social support and mood stability were reduced.

Activity Limitation
Activity limitations are evidently common after stroke in children, particularly later acquired stroke. Ganesan et al[87] found in 90 children with childhood-onset stroke that most had residual difficulties in home and educational activities, and that younger children at age of stroke had more functional limitations that older children.

A number of studies have assessed both quality of life and daily life activities of children following a stroke. In a study of 17 children and adolescents with middle cerebral artery territory cerebral infarction, the relationship between activity limitation scores on an author devised scale, standardized health-related quality of life assessment (Child Health Questionnaire), extent of brain damage, and results of a comprehensive neurological examination (Paediatric Stroke Outcome Measure) were investigated.[77] Activity limitation was evident in the domains of education, self-care and motor skills. There was very good interobserver agreement using the new activity limitation scale between the occupational therapist and paediatric neurologist (Cohen's kappa = 0.88). In comparison with population norms, the subjects scored below average in both physical and psychological health. There was a clear relationship between radiologically apparent extent of brain injury, degree of impairment and functional outcome.

Hurvitz et al[84] followed up 50 of a total of 76 patients with ischaemic or haemorrhagic stroke at a mean of 70 months after stroke and found that 84% were independently mobile and 76% were independent for all activities of daily living. Thirty-two of the same patients were located 5–6 years later, at a median age of 18 (range 9–37) years;[152] three had died and 29 were assessed on the Vineland Adaptive Behavior Scales, a structured interview undertaken with a relative or close friend, and the Satisfaction With Life Scale, usually completed at interview with the participant. The majority had good educational and mobility outcomes, with many completing college and gaining employment, although few were financially independent and communication, activities of daily living and socialization fell into the low–moderate range. Outcome was worse for those with a younger age of stroke onset and for those still requiring anticonvulsant medication.

Parent/Carer Health
Little attention has so far been paid to the impact of a stroke on family members. Anecdotally, it is apparent that the frequent

stress around the diagnosis of stroke, hospital admission and ongoing care needs impact the parents, siblings, friends and grandparents. Gordon et al[77] assessed parent health in a study of school-aged children who had childhood-onset stroke and found that parent health rated lower in the psychological/social subscales of the Short-Form 36 measure. The children of these parents were all at least one year post-stroke suggesting that the impact of the event and subsequent care may have long-reaching effects.

Conclusion

Data on outcome for stroke in childhood are now available but interpretation of published series and any comparison between them is difficult because of to non-standardized use of outcome measures. For those with a medical or health professional background interested in predicting and improving outcome, scales which describe impairment or activity limitation remain useful and dichotomizing into good and poor outcome allows logistic regression to be performed. The majority of paediatric stroke outcome research undertaken up until now has been limited by a focus on neurological impairments, and hampered by a lack of tools which measure beyond this domain, can be used across age ranges or compared with outcome in adults. However, for children with stroke and for their families, scales measuring and describing activity, participation and quality of life are more relevant. It has proved difficult to comprehensively evaluate activity and participation over such a wide age range. In addition to motor and sensory deficits, any cognitive and behavioural outcomes may also significantly affect educational and social opportunities, long-term participation and quality of life.

17.3 Ontogenetic Specialization of Hemispheric Function

Faraneh Vargha-Khadem, Elizabeth Isaacs, Kate Watkins and Mortimer Mishkin

Introduction

The division of labour between the two cerebral hemispheres has been recognized for over a century. In adults, the most impressive demonstration of this hemispheric specialization is the dramatic impairment in speech and language resulting from left hemisphere lesions that encroach on the perisylvian areas.[193,194] Although some degree of improvement in function may occur after the onset of pathology in these cases, the impairment is typically chronic and despite intensive efforts at rehabilitation, often remains severe enough to be referred to as an 'aphasia', rather than a 'dysphasia'. The complementary pattern of impairment, namely, a deficit in certain forms of visuospatial function, is produced in the adult by extensive right hemisphere lesions. Although in long-term follow-up these

problems are less obvious than the linguistic disorder and tend to interfere less with everyday activities, they nonetheless seriously limit the capacity for cognitive and behavioural function generally and for non-verbal intelligence specifically. These complementary impairments resulting from extensive lesions of the left and right hemisphere of the mature brain have long provided what is perhaps our major source of information regarding hemispheric specialization of function.

In contrast to the vast literature on the cognitive and behavioural consequences of unilateral lesions in adults, there are relatively few studies addressing this issue in children. The dearth of such studies in children is at least partly due to the fact that cerebral lesions sustained during fetal development, infancy or childhood are fortunately relatively rare. The low incidence rates, however, have commonly resulted in the collection of only small and heterogeneous study groups, allowing investigation of the effects of just one variable, usually hemispheric side of damage, even though cognitive outcome after injury is clearly the result of side of injury interacting with numerous other variables, including aetiology of the lesion, site and size of damage, age at injury, time since injury, age and developmental status at assessment, presence or absence of epilepsy and, if present, type of epilepsy, etc. Furthermore, except for two recent investigations,[195,196] the studies have been retrospective rather than longitudinal, and so have not taken into account the important changes in development and learning that are likely to occur after the onset of early lesions. Finally, few studies have examined the locus and extent of early injury in the detail made possible by modern non-invasive MRI techniques.

Despite these drawbacks in the existing literature, it is informative to review the studies on the consequences of early unilateral brain damage in order to trace the evolution of ideas concerning the ontogeny of hemispheric specialization. With that as the focus, we have excluded from this review other types of early damage that affect the development of specialized behavioural and cognitive abilities, in particular speech and language and other verbal functions, such as bilateral pathology (as in bilateral frontal opercular syndrome,[197] inherited forms of verbal dyspraxia)[198] and developmental disorders that are associated with widespread and multifocal pathology (as in specific language impairment,[199] dyslexia,[200] Williams syndrome[201] and autism).[202]

The equipotentiality view

Among the earliest studies on groups of children with unilateral hemispheric lesions are a series of reports in the 1960s by McFie,[203,204] Basser,[205] Alajouanine and Lhermitte[206] and Lenneberg.[207] Although McFie[204] concluded that the pattern of intellectual outcome in children with unilateral damage sustained after 1 year of age approximated the pattern observed in adults, namely, deficits in verbal intelligence after left hemisphere damage and in non-verbal intelligence after right hemisphere damage, in fact he failed to obtain any significant differences between the two groups on either type of measure.

Moreover, in long-term follow-up of a group of hemispherectomized children, McFie[203] found that, whereas verbal abilities were impaired more than non-verbal, this differential effect was independent of the side of the removal. Similarly, Basser[205] failed to demonstrate hemisphere-dependent effects in speech and language function after hemispherectomy. Alajouanine and Lhermitte[206] did report selective impairments in speech and written language following early acquired lesions of the left hemisphere, but they concluded that in long-term follow-up, the deficits had disappeared.

The results from these and other early group studies on the effects of early unilateral damage are concordant on two points: (1) compared with adults, children show an impressive degree of plasticity, such that by one or more years after injury, despite the chronicity of sensory and motor deficits, the majority of cases show normal or near normal levels of linguistic and intellectual ability; and (2) even in the presence of chronic behavioural and cognitive deficits, there is little evidence for differential hemispheric mediation of verbal and non-verbal functions.

Partly in an attempt to integrate the findings on preservation or recovery of function after early, focal, unilateral lesions, Lenneberg[207] proposed the *equipotentiality* model, which states that the two cerebral hemispheres are equipotential at the start but gradually acquire specialization with increasing age and learning experience, particularly for speech and language. According to this view, increasing functional specialization with increasing age is accompanied by a gradual decline in neural plasticity, such that, by about the age of puberty, hemispheric specialization becomes 'crystalized', at which point it resembles the adult pattern. If unilateral brain injury occurs at any time during the prepubertal period, then an intact right hemisphere, say, can mediate the speech and language functions of the left hemisphere. The earlier the lesion, however, the more effective the compensatory takeover, and consequently, the better the outcome.

This implication of the *equipotentiality* view, that specialized abilities like language should show different degrees of preservation depending on age at injury, has been difficult to test (for a detailed discussion of this issue, see Bates et al[195]). Although it is well documented that speech and language are rescued even after very extensive early lesions of the left hemisphere, the shape of the decline in this compensatory process as a function of increasing age at injury has been difficult to measure, mainly because groups of children with left and right hemispheric lesions sustained during each age level up to puberty have not been available for study. As a result, investigators have had to rely on case comparisons (e.g. Vargha-Khadem et al[208]) with all their attendant drawbacks (this issue is discussed further later in the chapter.)

The early specialization view

Lenneberg's model prevailed only until the mid 1970s, when a series of studies carried out on children with unilateral lesions,[209–212] including hemispherectomy,[213–216] obtained evidence of material-specific impairments corresponding to the hemispheric side of insult. This wave of studies helped launch the *early specialization* view of the two cerebral hemispheres, a view that proved to be highly influential, remaining in force at least throughout the 1980s.

To appreciate why the *early specialization* view held sway for so long, it is necessary to examine developments that were taking place during this same period in disciplines allied to paediatric neuropsychology. For example, in the field of linguistics, Chomsky[217,218] proposed the notion that language and grammar were *innate* properties and autonomous from other cognitive systems. This view of language was in line with Fodor's[219] model of the modular organization of cognition and is consistent with the data on adult patients with focal brain injury and selective impairments in specific cognitive processes. In this model, a modular deficit is a selective impairment in one area of cognitive function that cannot be explained in terms of a more general loss of cognitive ability. The mapping of the innate module for language to an anatomical region in the brain was provided by the studies of Geschwind & Levitsky,[220] Wada et al[221] and Witelson and Pallie,[222] whose postmortem examinations of the brains of both adults and newborns revealed an asymmetry favouring the left side in the length of the planum temporale within the Sylvian fissure. The availability of techniques and paradigms to measure a wide range of psychophysiological processes, such as long-latency evoked potentials,[223] heart rate deceleration[224] and non-nutritive sucking,[225,226] enabled researchers to investigate whether the anatomical asymmetries in normal infants led to differential responses to lateralized inputs of various types of stimuli. Most, though not all,[227–230] of these types of studies concluded that hemispheric specialization of function could indeed be demonstrated even in the neonate, thus supporting the notion that the left and right cerebral hemispheres were innately organized to preferentially process verbal and non-verbal information, respectively.

It was against this background that the wave of neuropsychological studies referred to earlier appeared. The main claim of these studies was that children with early left hemisphere disease or damage, despite the apparent recovery of their speech, continue to show subtle but selective impairments in both verbal intelligence and certain aspects of language. Thus, unlike early right hemidecortication, early left hemidecortication was found to cause deficits in comprehension of complex syntax, specifically of the word order in passive negative sentences.[213,214] Further, early acquired lesions on the left but not on the right were found to produce impairments not only in complex receptive grammar,[231] but also in expressive grammar,[232] lexical retrieval,[233] sentence repetition[231] and verbal fluency.[234] Frank dysphasic symptoms were observed by Hecaen[211] in long-term follow-up of a group of children with acquired left hemisphere lesions, although in this study comparative data were not provided for children with right hemisphere lesions. Even in cases with congenital injury, impairments after left as compared with right hemisphere damage were observed in speech and language as well as in writing and spelling.[210,235] Finally, our own initial study on hemiplegic children with congenital or acquired hemispheric lesions[236] revealed more impairments in receptive language and in lexical retrieval after left as compared with right hemisphere damage, although these differential findings were no longer evident when patients with seizures were excluded from the analysis.[86]

During the period in which the *early specialization* view prevailed, the majority of studies reported in the literature concentrated on language functions, although there were a few reports in which visuospatial functions had been examined either of small groups or of single cases in whom early neuropathology had led to hemispherectomy.[216,237–239] The most pronounced evidence of hemisphere-dependent impairment was obtained by Kohn and Dennis,[216] who found that right hemispherectomized patients (*N*=4) performed more poorly than left hemispherectomized patients (*N*=4), but only on those aspects of visuospatial function, such as map-reading, that are late-maturing in the normal child. It is worth noting, however, that a similar pattern of results, i.e. no impairment on simple visuospatial tasks but pronounced impairment on more demanding ones, was later reported by Ogden[238] in two patients with infantile hemiplegia and seizures who underwent *left* hemispherectomy during adolescence.

Although these neuropsychological studies supporting the *early specialization* view suffered from many methodological shortcomings (for critical reviews, see Bishop[240,241]), their message reinforced the idea that had been forming simultaneously in the other disciplines that the hemispheric division of labour for processing verbal and non-verbal material begins as early as birth or shortly after.

The ontogenetic specialization view

There is now a sizeable accumulation of reports on cognitive outcome in children with unilateral brain damage. For example, from 1977 to 2008, at least 10 different studies have appeared wherein groups of children with left or right hemisphere lesions were directly compared on the well-standardized verbal and performance measures of the Wechsler Intelligence Scales (Table 17.5). Unfortunately, again largely because of small and heterogeneous groups in many of the studies, the findings continue to be divergent, and so a clear consensus has still not emerged. It should be pointed out, however, that there is clear agreement between the findings in the two studies with the largest populations (Vargha-Khadem et al,[86] *N*=82; Goodman and Yude,[85] *N*=124), both of which report no significant differences between verbal and performance IQ as a function of hemispheric side of damage and more recent studies provide further evidence for this position.[242]

The studies on speech and language after early unilateral damage are even more difficult to assess, because, in addition to containing small and heterogeneous samples, they have used different and often non-standardized tests. In their review of numerous published and ongoing investigations spanning the period from 1961 to 1999, Bates et al[196] concluded that a clear

consensus had likewise not been reached regarding linguistic outcome. They acknowledged that delays in language production, particularly in expressive grammar, are more likely to occur in children with damage to the left hemisphere,[243–246] but these effects are neither robust nor stable. Furthermore, the most frequent reports regarding side-dependent effects were negative ones.[247] Finally, an ongoing Italian study[248] on groups of children with left or right hemisphere lesions and normal controls matched for age, sex and social class, concluded that there is little evidence for a difference between left-handed and right-handed children on most language measures.

Outcome studies of visuospatial ability after early unilateral cerebral damage are also difficult to evaluate. A leading group in this area[249,250] has obtained some evidence suggesting that the pattern of deficits in visuospatial processing in children with focal lesions resembles one that has been seen in adult patients with unilateral posterior lesions, namely, greater impairment in local processing after left-sided damage and in global processing after damage on the right. Like the linguistic impairments, however, the visuospatial deficits are neither robust nor consistently present on different measures. Furthermore, longitudinal follow-up revealed substantial recovery of function, such that by adolescence many of the patients had attained levels of performance that did not differ from those of normal controls.[251,252]

In discussing the ontogeny of hemispheric specialization, and cognizant of the importance of developmental plasticity and its compatibility with the equipotentiality hypothesis, but also of the undeniable fact that in the absence of brain damage the majority of individuals go on to demonstrate hemispheric specialization in adulthood, Satz et al[253] argued in favour of a middle ground between the extremes of equipotentiality and early specialization. This compromise position, which has been referred to as 'constrained plasticity',[195] we shall call *ontogenetic specialization*. Unlike the *equipotentiality* position, the mediating view assumes that hemispheric specialization has an anatomical basis that is genetically determined and further that, under normal circumstances, functional expression of this genetic disposition can begin to appear even very early in life. However, unlike the *early specialization* view, it also assumes that such functional expression is determined during development by the interaction between environmentally evoked neural activity and the special form of neural plasticity that appears to end during puberty.[207] Accordingly, early brain damage may counteract the genetic disposition by affecting and modifying the activity/plasticity interaction.

The *ontogenetic specialization* view fits well with research on the normal development of linguistic functions. Studies of event-related potentials (ERPs) have shown that whilst even very young infants, just like adults, are electrophysiologically sensitive to a range of acoustical features that characterize speech as opposed to non-speech sounds, such as temporal lag, voicing cue, etc., their ERP responses are not as clearly lateralized as they are in adults, suggesting that the two hemispheres may be more nearly equal in infancy than they

TABLE 17.5
Summary of results for verbal and performance IQ in children with left versus right hemisphere damage. (Adapted from Vargha-Khadem F, Isaacs E, Muter V. A review of cognitive outcome after unilateral lesions sustained during childhood. J Child Neurol 1994; 9(Suppl 2):67–73; Bates E, Vicari S, Trauner D. Neural mediation of language development: perspectives from lesion studies of infants and children. In: Neurodevelopmental Disorders (ed H Tager-Flusberg). Cambridge, MA: MIT Press, 1999; 533–581)

Study	N	Age at lesion onset	Time after lesion (years:months)	Seizure history (% incidence)	Verbal (VIQ)	Performance (PIQ)
Woods 1980[212]	L=27 R=23	Early = <1 year Late = >1 year	LE=17:02 RE=14:01 LLa=8:06 RLa=10:03	LE=27% RE=50% LL=19% RL=15%	LE < normal RE < normal LLa < normal RLa = normal	LE < normal RE < normal LLa < normal RLa < normal
Riva & Cazzaniga 1986[231]	L=22 R=26	Early = <1 year Late = <1 year	Early = 8:05 Late = 4:02	None	LE < normal RE = normal LLa = normal RLa = normal	LE < normal RE < normal LLa = normal RLa < normal
Riva et al 1987[279]	L=8 R=8	Not divided by age of lesion onset	L=6:08 R=4:06	L=37.5% R=37.5%	L < normal R = normal	L < normal R < normal
Nass et al 1989[280]	L=15 R=13	Pre/perinatal	L=6:07 R=8:05	Not indicated	L = normal R = normal	L < normal R < normal
Vargha-Khadem et al 1992[86]	L=42 R=40	Congenital/perinatal	L=12:03 R=11:05	2 seizure groups 2 non-seizure groups	L + S < normal L − S = normal R + S < normal R − S = normal	L + S < normal L − S < normal R + S < normal R − S < normal
Scarvie et al 1996[282]	L=8 R=9	Congenital/perinatal	L=9:0 R=11:2	L=62.5% R=55.5%	L < normal R < normal L VIQ = PIQ R VIQ > PIQ	L < normal R < normal L VIQ = PIQ R VIQ > PIQ
Goodman and Graham 1996[142]	L=51 R=73	Congenital/perinatal	(range 6–10 years)	~40%	L + R < normal L + R VIQ > PIQ	L + R < normal L + R PIQ < VIQ
Muter et al 1997[196]	L=23 R=15	Congenital/perinatal	L=4:09 R=4:09	L=35% R=27%	L + S < normal L − S = normal R + S < normal R − S = normal	L + S < normal L − S = normal R + S < normal R − S < normal
Bates et al 1998[195]	L=28 R=15	All congenital/ perinatal	L=5:04 R=5:05	L=40.7% R=46.7%	L < normal R < normal L = R	L < normal R < normal L = R
Max et al 2004[242]	L=13 R=16	Prenatal to 13 years	L=9:10 R=8:7	Not indicated	L < normal R = normal L = R	L < normal R < normal L = R

L, left-hemisphere damage; R, right-hemisphere damage; E, early lesion onset; La, late lesion onset; +S, with seizure history; S, without seizure history.

are later in their ability to process these types of distinctions.[254,255] Similarly, Dehaene-Lambertz and Baillet,[256] studying phonological processing with ERPs, found that infants, like adults, process phonemes categorically; but unlike adults, who show activation predominantly in the left temporal lobe,[257] infants show more bilaterally symmetrical processing, even though the voltages are higher on the left. A second study[256] pursued this question of phoneme processing in infants by contrasting the effects of a phonemic change with a voice change or, separately, a change in timbre. Results again indicated higher voltages over the left hemisphere for the phonetic change, but, unlike in adults, there was no greater asymmetry for the phonetic than for the non-phonetic discrimination. When and how this asymmetry in response to both phonetic and non-phonetic stimuli eventually turns into left hemisphere specialization for linguistic processing selectively remains an open question. A possible answer suggested by connectionist theorists,[258] and one that is consistent with the position favoured here, is that language experience itself propels the emerging specialization of the left hemisphere for this function.[258]

The *ontogenetic specialization* view also fits well with the increasing recognition that, in the aftermath of early brain injury, the ontogenetic trend toward hemispheric specialization is probably influenced by many variables that can counter this trend. Thus, one level of a variable, say a very small unilateral lesion, could well lead to a finding that accords with *early specialization*, while a level of the variable at the opposite extreme, in this case an extensive unilateral lesion, could result in a finding suggesting *equipotentiality*. The same could be true for widely divergent levels of many other variables.

In attempting to resolve the discrepancies in the literature, numerous authors have touched on this issue, raising questions about the role of such factors as age at lesion onset,[85,263] lesion site as well as size,[195,243,259–263] unsuspected contralateral pathology,[264] presence of seizures,[86,196] stage of development of the cognitive function under study,[243,265] age at testing,[262,265,266] elapsed time since onset of the pathology[195,259,262,267] and so on. However, none of these studies obtained definitive evidence regarding the role of such variables in tilting the results in favour of one or the other extreme theoretical position.

Effects of hemiplegia-causing lesions on intelligence

The above review of previous research suggests that the *ontogenetic specialization* hypothesis probably provides the best fit to the available data. At the same time, this plausible notion, namely, that functional specialization of the hemispheres emerges and becomes consolidated only gradually during the course of normal development, and so can be overridden in cases of early unilateral injury, still lacks direct empirical support from brain-lesion studies. As already pointed out, all previous brain-injury studies, our own included, were plagued by the presence of many uncontrolled and therefore potentially confounding variables. Because the total sample sizes were always relatively small, more homogeneous patient groups could not readily be formed, and so systematic investigation of these variables could not be undertaken. Among these variables, perhaps the most critical one for the issue under discussion is age at onset of injury. According to the *ontogenetic specialization* view, cognitive outcome after unilateral brain injury should vary depending on the age at which the damage occurred. Thus, congenital or very early acquired unilateral lesions should yield the same cognitive effects irrespective of lesion side, whereas comparable unilateral lesions sustained later in childhood, but before maturity, should begin to result in side-dependent deficits resembling those seen in brain-injured adults.

To test this prediction, we examined the IQ data obtained from the largest sample gathered to date of children who had suffered a single, non-progressive, unilateral hemispheric insult resulting in a hemiplegia.[268] The large sample size of 196 hemiplegic patients (left hemisphere, $N=106$; right, $N=90$) allowed us to compare the effects of hemispheric side of damage on standardized measures of verbal and non-verbal intelligence as a function of age at injury, while controlling for the important variable of seizure history.[86] The patient groups with unilateral left or right hemisphere insult were each divided further into three age-at-injury groups, namely, a group with congenital injury ($N=96$), one with early acquired injury (i.e. 1 month to <5 years; $N=46$) and a third with late acquired injury (i.e. 5–16 yrs; $N=54$). MR scans of patients representative of the congenital and acquired groups are shown in Fig. 17.6. Table 17.6 shows the main aetiological categories for both the early acquired and late acquired groups.

The six left and right hemisphere groups with congenital, early acquired or late acquired injury were each further divided into two groups on the basis of the presence (total $N=52$)

TABLE 17.6
Aetiology in 196 children with hemiplegia[268]

Aetiology	No. of patients <5 years	5–16 years	Total
CVA	27	32	59
HI	5	5	10
AVM	2	5	7
Tumour	2	4	6
Trauma	2	3	5
Other	1	3	4
RE	0	3	3
Cyst	1	0	1
Total	40	55	95

AVM, arteriovenous malformation; CVA, cerebrovascular accident; HI, hypoxia ischaemia; RE, Rasmussen encephalitis.

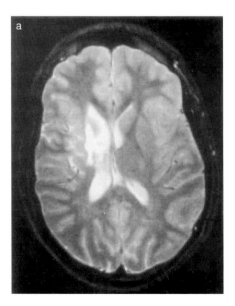 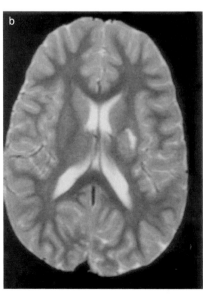

Fig. 17.6. Horizontal sections from MRI scans of two representative patients with strokes in the territory of the middle cerebral artery, each with lesion-severity ratings of 2 on a scale of 1–5. (a) Congenital lesion. (b) Acquired lesion.

or absence (total *N*=144) of a history of clinical seizures of cerebral origin, excluding febrile convulsions or uncontrolled seizures. The 12 patient groups formed on the basis of the foregoing classification, and the numbers for each, are listed in Table 17.6. All patients were given the age-appropriate Wechsler Intelligence Scales (WISC, WISC-R, WISC-III, Wechsler–Bellevue, WAIS, WAIS-R) to provide measures of verbal, performance and full scale intelligence (VIQ, PIQ, FSIQ).[269–272] The latter two scores were used as the dependent variables in an analysis of variance with repeated measures to determine the effects on verbal and non-verbal intelligence of the independent variables of hemispheric side of insult, age at insult and presence or absence of seizures. Whenever appropriate, post hoc comparisons between groups were carried out using Student's two-tailed *t*-tests.

EFFECTS OF SEIZURES ON IQ

In this study,[268] nearly all groups without seizures obtained mean VIQ and PIQ scores in the average range (90–109). By contrast, the groups with a history of seizures generally had lower scores on both measures, with means often falling in the low average range (80–89) or even below. Across the entire group of 196 patients, this difference yielded the only significant main effect, indicating that patients with a history of seizures scored reliably lower than patients without seizures on both IQ measures (mean difference = −8.2 points, *p*=0.002; Fig. 17.7). This strong impact of seizure history on IQ was totally independent of the effects of the other variables – side of injury and age at injury – in that there were no significant interactions with these other factors. Furthermore, it is interesting to note that these other variables did not independently exert any influence across the two types of IQ.

When the scores of the seizure and non-seizure groups were analysed separately, the main effect of IQ type was found to be significant, but in the non-seizure group only. As shown in Fig. 17.7, regardless of hemispheric side of insult, the mean VIQ score of those without a history of seizures was slightly but significantly higher than their mean PIQ score (mean diff. = 2.8 points, *p*=0.015) suggesting that, in the absence of seizures, priority is assigned to the preservation of verbal abilities. In the children with a history of seizures, however, this priority disappears.

EFFECTS OF HEMISPHERIC SIDE OF INSULT ON IQ

Across the entire group of patients (i.e. both those with and those without a history of seizures), there was a significant interaction between hemispheric side of injury and IQ type (*p*=0.025). Post hoc comparisons indicated that there were no significant differences between the left and right groups on either VIQ (mean difference = −3.1 points) or PIQ (mean difference = 0.7 points). Rather, the interaction resulted from the fact that, in the group with right hemisphere damage, VIQ was relatively better preserved than PIQ (mean difference = 4.2 points; *p*=0.008; Fig. 17.8A). The same analysis performed on the scores of the seizure and non-seizure groups separately showed similar patterns, but ones which fell just short of significance (*p*=0.071 and 0.055, respectively; Fig. 17.8B,C). None of the analyses indicated a comparable sparing of PIQ after left hemisphere insult (mean difference = 0.4 points). As indicated below, the relative sparing of VIQ after right hemisphere damage was due mainly to the results obtained in the group with injuries that were acquired late in childhood.

EFFECTS OF AGE AT INSULT ON IQ

Across the entire group of patients, there was a significant three-way interaction between age at insult, hemispheric side of insult and IQ type (*p*=0.025; Fig. 17.9). Post hoc analyses indicated that this interaction was due mainly to the results obtained in the group with late-acquired injuries, as follows. Firstly, the two-way interactions between side of injury and IQ type were analysed for each of the three age-at-injury groups separately; only the interaction in the late-acquired group was significant (*p*=0.008). Secondly, post hoc comparisons between VIQ and PIQ were run for each of the six side-of-injury by age-at-injury groups; again, the only difference that approached significance was the one for the right late-acquired group (mean difference = 5.9 points, *p*=0.056). The comparison for the left late-acquired group also fell short of significance (mean difference. = −5.2 points, *p*=0.101).

The three-way interactions between age at injury, side of injury and IQ type analysed separately for the seizure and non-seizure groups again revealed patterns of results similar to the one obtained for the group as a whole, but these interactions were not significant.

In both our studies of hemiplegic children,[85,268] seizures, even though their clinical manifestation is relatively well controlled by anticonvulsant medication, have a deleterious effect on intelligence. In the present study the seizure factor reduced both VIQ and PIQ by about 8 points in relation to patients without a history of seizures, and by about 12 points in relation to the hypothetical normal population means of 100. This deleterious effect was about the same regardless of which hemisphere was injured or when it was injured. Neither handedness, age at onset of chronic epilepsy, nor site of EEG abnormality are good predictors of language lateralization,[273] highlighting the

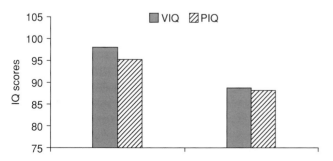

Fig. 17.7. Effects of seizures. Mean difference between the two groups, 8.2 IQ points, *p*=0.002. Mean VIQ–PIQ difference in non-seizure group, 2.8 IQ points; *p*=0.015. PIQ, performance intelligence; VIQ, verbal intelligence.

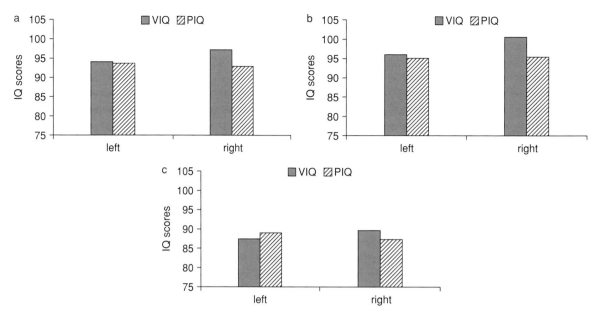

Fig. 17.8. Interaction between hemispheric side of injury and IQ type. (a) All patients (*N*=196, *p*=0.025). (b) Non-seizure patients (*N*=144, *p*=0.055). (c) Seizure patients (*N*=52, *p*=0.073). PIQ, Performance IQ; VIQ, Verbal IQ.

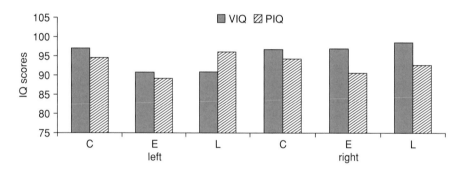

Fig. 17.9. Three-way interaction between age at injury, hemispheric side of injury and IQ type. All patients (*N*=196, *p*=0.025). C, congenital lesion; E, early acquired lesion; L, late acquired lesion.

need for links between cognitive neuroscience paradigms and techniques such as functional neuroimaging and traditional behavioural testing. By contrast, hemiplegia-causing lesions that did not result in seizures reduced VIQ and PIQ by only about 3 points in relation to the normal population means.

In the absence of the added burden of a history of seizures, there is a small but significant tendency for the preferential rescue of VIQ as compared with PIQ (mean scores of 98 and 95, respectively), with this effect also being independent of which hemisphere was injured and when it was injured. Thus, the net effect of an early hemiplegia-causing lesion that does not result in seizures is a slight selective lowering of PIQ (see also Satz et al[253]). The cost paid by non-verbal functions for the sparing of verbal functions was labelled 'crowding' by Hans-Lukas Teuber and his colleagues,[209,274,275] but this phenomenon was assumed to be hemisphere dependent, reflecting successful rescue of speech and language functions by a non-dominant hemisphere (usually the right) after sufficiently early lesions of the dominant hemisphere. The results

described above are consistent with previous reports from our group and others.[85,86,131,196,276] They are also consistent with the notion that PIQ is 'crowded out' by the higher-priority VIQ. However, the effect in our hemiplegic cases without a history of seizures is only a small one and is clearly independent of whether the hemispheric damage is on the left or the right. Moreover, inasmuch as only a small minority of our patients with left hemisphere damage give any evidence of a shift of speech and language functions to the right,[260] our results imply, in addition, that the 'crowding' effect occurs regardless of whether or not there is post-injury reorganization of speech and language functions. Finally, in the patients with a history of seizures, the electrographic abnormality, the anticonvulsant medication, or both, apparently interfere sufficiently with the functions of undamaged tissue, whether in the intact portions of the damaged hemisphere or in the undamaged hemisphere, such that the priority which would otherwise be given to VIQ gives way to the more serious challenge of rescuing intellectual functions overall.

EFFECTS OF HEMISPHERIC SIDE OF INJURY ON IQ

Unlike the results of large-scale investigations carried out on adults with unilateral cerebral lesions,[277,278] but like earlier findings on children with such lesions, as reported both in our own studies[86,126,130,196,268] and in many of the studies of others,[85,133,136,195,231,242,279–281] there was no significant effect of side of lesions on either VIQ or PIQ. In the adult studies, left hemisphere lesions were found to result in a discrepancy of 7–9 points in favour of PIQ, and right hemisphere lesions in an even larger discrepancy of 12 points in favour of VIQ.[277,278] In our study,[268] on the other hand, there was no discrepancy in IQ type after left-sided injuries, and only a 4-point discrepancy in favor of VIQ after right-sided injuries. The latter difference yielded the significant interaction between side of injury and IQ type. Although both Milner and Warrington and her colleagues emphasized that the discrepancy scores they observed in their large adult samples (955 cases in Milner's study[277] and 656 in the Warrington et al study[278]) were quite variable, they nevertheless suggested that these discrepancies could be used as a first approximation in characterizing the specialized functions of the two cerebral hemispheres. This conclusion, however, is only applicable to the effects of unilateral lesions in adults, in whom hemispheric specialization has already been established before the injury. Clearly, the same conclusion cannot be applied to the effects of hemispheric lesions in children, presumably because hemispheric specialization of cognitive function emerges only gradually during development. One practical byproduct of this difference in outcome after childhood versus adult brain injury is that, whereas a large discrepancy between VIQ and PIQ scores can provide an important clue to the lateralization of a focal lesion in an adult, it cannot do so either in a child with a congenital brain injury or in one with a brain injury sustained before the age of about five. The reason for suggesting this age as the tentative cutoff in the differential consequences of early versus late hemispheric damage derives from the final results to be discussed.

EFFECTS OF AGE AT INJURY ON IQ

In addition to the interaction of side of injury with IQ type, there was also a three-way interaction involving age at injury. The analyses based on this interaction revealed that, whereas there was no influence of lesion side on IQ type in either the congenital or early acquired groups, the group with lesions acquired at the age of five or later in childhood had a pattern of IQ scores that was at least qualitatively similar to the one that has been reported in adults (Fig. 17.9). In this age group only, there was a significant interaction between hemispheric side of injury and IQ type. Thus, in the patients with right hemisphere lesions, there was a VIQ–PIQ difference of 6 points, while in the patients with left hemisphere lesions, there was a PIQ–VIQ difference of 5 points. Although each of these discrepancy scores alone fell short of significance (i.e. only the interaction was reliable), and although each is roughly only half as large as that found after injuries acquired in adulthood (see above), the overall similarity in the pattern of results suggests

that hemispheric specialization starts to become consolidated at about age five, and then presumably becomes more firmly fixed gradually, i.e. less vulnerable to the effects of unilateral damage, throughout later childhood.

Conclusions

Overall, the results suggest that hemispheric specialization of cognitive function, at least as indicated by a dissociation between verbal and performance IQ in children with unilateral, hemiplegia-causing brain injuries, begins to appear only at about age five or later. Some cautions must of course be placed around this conclusion. First, the VIQ–PIQ discrepancies in the group with late-onset lesions were just at the borderline of detectability. It remains for future large-scale studies of children with unilateral lesions to determine whether more clearcut or even earlier hemispheric dissociations might appear on particular linguistic and visuospatial tests that may tap more selective, and so perhaps earlier maturing, aspects of hemispheric function. Second, the exact age at which specialization in IQ appears is still uncertain. All that can be said at present is that, at some point between ages 5 and 16, functional development is sufficiently advanced and/or developmental neural plasticity is sufficiently attenuated that some degree of specialized hemispheric processing can be observed after unilateral injury sustained during this developmental period. Both of the above circumstances, i.e. advanced functional development and attenuated plasticity, are probably present when the injury occurs close to puberty. However, at least two very different scenarios can be imagined when the injury occurs in the early part of the period, closer to age 5, and further cognitive development over many childhood years must still take place in the presence of unilateral damage. Under these circumstances, one possibility is that the consolidation of hemispheric specialization has already been set in motion and the two hemispheres will continue undeflected on that course during further development, constrained only by the functional limitation of the damaged hemisphere. The other possibility is that environmental pressure combines with a still high degree of developmental plasticity to partially override the genetic disposition toward hemispheric specialization, just as it apparently does more fully when the injury occurs before age 5. Deciding between these and other alternatives will require a more fine-grained analysis of age at lesion onset than the one carried out here. With these caveats, however, we can conclude that the results support at least the general notion of *ontogenetic specialization*, i.e. the gradual emergence and consolidation during development of hemispheric specialization for cognitive abilities.

When unilateral brain damage is incurred congenitally or even in early childhood before age 5, the anatomical disposition toward hemispheric specialization will be overridden by a fairly extensive, hemiplegia-causing lesion. In losing whatever cognitive advantage accrues to a clear division of labour between two normal hemispheres, the damaged brain may preserve the most effective performance possible of the cognitive functions that are under the greatest environmental demand.

Perhaps the prime example of environmental demand on children is social communication through speech and language. If an early unilateral lesion of either hemisphere encroaches on this function's normal neural substrates, which are centred on the perisylvian region, the young child will need to recruit additional neuronal resources from one or both hemispheres depending on the site and extent of the damage. This recruitment, enabled by developmental neural plasticity, may ensure enough neuronal tissue to satisfy the demands of speech and language development. However, this type of reorganization can occur only at the cost of other cognitive systems, which may be 'crowded out' and become diffusely represented because the neuronal resources needed for their development have been siphoned off by the higher priority function. The net effect of an early and extensive lesion of either hemisphere would thus be a non-specialized pattern of hemispheric organization for intellectual functions, differing from the pattern in the normal adult not only in being non-lateralized but also possibly lacking many of its *intra*hemispheric functional specializations.

Acknowledgements
Our work was supported in part by the Medical Research Council and The Wellcome Trust.

17.4 Neurodevelopmental Outcome in Children with Congenital Heart Defects

Amy Savage, Catherine Hill, Fenella J. Kirkham and Alexandra Hogan

Congenital heart disease is one of the commonest causes of stroke, yet there are relatively few publications on long-term cognitive outcome. In part, this is due to the wide range of underlying conditions and the other confounding factors, such as surgery, hypoxaemia and heart failure, which impact on motor function, cognition and behaviour in this group. This chapter therefore reviews the previous literature on cognitive outcome for congenital heart disease as background for future studies of outcome for stroke in this group of conditions.

Types of congenital heart disease and cognitive outcome
The term congenital heart defect (CHD) refers to a group of defects which are present at birth, and involve structural alterations to the heart itself or to the major blood vessels surrounding the heart. It is estimated that CHD affects approximately 1% of live births (and a higher percentage of those aborted spontaneously or stillborn), making CHD the most common birth defect.[283] Although the aetiology of CHD is often unknown and is presumed to be due to a combination of genetic and environmental factors, specific types of CHD are found to show an increased prevalence in the presence of chromosomal

abnormalities, such as Down syndrome.[284] Given the significant confound between chromosomal abnormalities and intellectual development, the vast majority of research in this field has excluded children with known chromosomal abnormalities or diagnosed genetic syndromes. From the point of view of childhood stroke, this is an omission, as recurrence and poor outcome are more likely in those with multiple risk factors.[6] However, very large studies would be required to explore the confounding effect of additional underlying pathology and in this review, the reader may assume that all studies discussed have excluded children with known chromosomal abnormalities or diagnosed genetic syndromes unless otherwise stated.

CHDs are primarily divided into two classes, depending upon their effect on the circulation of oxygenated blood: (1) cyanotic lesions refer to those defects where the lesion involves deoxygenated blood bypassing the lungs (a right to left shunt), and circulating haemoglobin is not fully saturated with oxygen; (2) acyanotic lesions in which the defect does not result in blood bypassing the pulmonary circulation, therefore hypoxaemia is not a problem unless there is a problem with the adequacy of gaseous exchange. The majority of patients with CHD have only mild lesions which do not require surgery and some of the most minor defects may correct themselves with time, as with small ventricular septal defects (VSD). However, a significant minority of patients will require surgical and/or medical treatment in order to correct the lesion or to treat the effects of the lesion on the circulation, and with advances in medicine, correction is now often undertaken during the neonatal period. A brief description of the most common types of CHD, their clinical implications, and their associated treatments is provided in Table 17.7.

In the past few decades, significant medical advances have resulted in dramatic improvements in survival rates for infants with CHD.[285] However, a growing body of evidence exists indicating that children born with CHD are at increased risk of developmental and intellectual deficits.[286] A recent review concluded that children with cyanotic lesions have more pronounced intellectual and cognitive impairment than those with acyanotic lesions, resulting in a full scale IQ score of between 8.3 and 9.3 points lower.[287] Children with acyanotic lesions typically perform better, but nevertheless show some impairments compared to healthy controls,[288] possibly due to reduced cerebral perfusion.[289] Children presenting in infancy with CHD of both cyanotic and acyanotic subtypes are often in heart failure and may become relatively hypotensive and acidotic, particularly as the ductus arteriosus closes. They are therefore vulnerable to global ischaemia ante-, peri- and postnatally. Those with cyanotic defects have chronic systemic and cerebral hypoxia unless they are able to undergo corrective surgery.

Effect of chronic hypoxaemia and heart failure on cognitive function
Research has consistently found a significantly lower level of global intellectual functioning in children with cyanotic CHD

TABLE 17.7
Common types of congenital heart defect

Name	Clinical description and treatment
Acyanotic subtypes	
Pulmonary stenosis or aortic stenosis	The pulmonary valve (which allows blood to flow from the right ventricle to the lungs) is defective, causing the heart to pump harder than normal to overcome the obstruction. In severe cases some cyanosis can occur. Surgery serves to open the valve satisfactorily, and can be a relatively routine procedure (balloon valvuloplasty) or require open heart surgery
Aortic stenosis	The aortic valve (which allows blood to flow from the left ventricle and the aorta) is defective, causing the heart difficulty in pumping blood around the body. Surgery serves to open the valve satisfactorily, and can be a relatively routine procedure (balloon valvuloplasty) or require open heart surgery
Coarctation of the aorta	The aorta is constricted, which obstructs blood flow to the body, and causes high blood pressure or poor circulation to the limbs. In severe cases congestive heart failure may occur. Surgery can usually be delayed until later in childhood, unless the symptoms are particularly severe. The surgical procedure is called balloon angioplasty
Atrial septal defects (ASD)	An opening exists between the two atria that allows some blood that has already been to the lungs back into the right atrium, instead of flowing out of the aorta and to the body. Many children with ASD have few symptoms and the hole often closes spontaneously, although open heart surgery is required in some cases
Ventricular septal defects (VSD)	An opening exists between the two ventricles, causing blood from the lungs to leak back into the right ventricle instead of being pumped around the body. This means that the heart has to work harder, and may enlarge. Surgery is required when the hole is too large, causing high blood pressure in the lungs or failure to thrive
Atroventricular canal (also called atrioventricular septal defect)	A large hole exists where the four chambers of the heart join, and often there are malformations of the tricuspid and mitral valves, causing blood to leak back into the right side of the heart. The heart must pump more blood than normal, and may enlarge. Infants with this condition may become undernourished and have damaged blood vessels in the lungs due to high blood pressure. Surgery must usually be carried out in infancy; the hole is closed and the valve is reconstructed. A band may also be placed around the pulmonary artery to reduce the blood flow to the lungs
Cyanotic subtypes	
Tetralogy of Fallot (TOF)	The major defect in TOF is a VSD, and a narrowing near the pulmonary valve. In addition, the right ventricle is more muscular than usual, and the aorta lies directly over the VSD. These defects allow blood to pass from the right to the left ventricle without going through the lungs, causing severe cyanosis or even unconsciousness. Surgery begins with positioning a shunt between the aorta and the pulmonary artery to increase blood flow to the lungs. Later open heart surgery involves closing the VSD and removing obstructing muscle
Transposition of the great arteries (TGA)	The positions of the aorta and pulmonary artery are reversed, causing blood returning to the heart from the body to be pumped back out to the body without being reoxygenated in the lungs. Infants born with TGA only survive if they have another defect allowing oxygenated blood to reach the body, such as an ASD or VSD. Surgery is always necessary and involves balloon atrial septostomy to improve the body's oxygen supply. An arterial switch or venous switch is used to create a tunnel inside the atria
Tricuspid atresia	The infant is born without a tricuspid valve, meaning that no blood can flow from the right atrium to the right ventricle. Infants only survive if they have another defect such as a VSD or ASD. Often a surgical shunting procedure is used to increase blood flow to the lungs; others need a pulmonary artery banding to reduce the blood flow to the lungs
Pulmonary atresia	The infant is born without a pulmonary valve, meaning that blood does not flow into the lungs. Survival is based on the presence of a defect in the heart walls, allowing some oxygenated blood to be pumped around the body. Early treatment often involves medication to keep this defect open, and is followed by surgery to increase blood flow to the lungs. Open heart surgery is most successful when the pulmonary artery and right ventricle are of normal size. Otherwise, a compensatory surgical procedure (Fontan procedure) is used to connect the right atrium directly to the pulmonary artery
Total anomalous pulmonary venous connection	The pulmonary veins are abnormally connected to the right atrium, causing oxygenated blood to be mixed with deoxygenated blood from the body. An ASD allows this mixture to pass through into the left side of the heart, from where it is pumped around the body. Because of the high degree of cyanosis, surgical repair must be carried out in early infancy
Hypoplastic left heart syndrome	The left side of the heart is dramatically underdeveloped. The condition becomes evident when the ductus arteriosus (a normal hole in the heart in the fetus) closes a few hours after birth, because this closure prevents blood from reaching the aorta. The defect is not correctable; some infants undergo a series of operations and others require a heart transplant

compared to healthy children[290,291] and a higher incidence of learning disability.[292] The central nervous system appears more vulnerable to injury in primary school aged children with uncorrected transposition of the great arteries or Fallot's tetralogy than in children whose cardiac anomalies spontaneously correct, and once central nervous system impairment was controlled for there was no difference between groups.[290] Others have suggested that chronic hypoxaemia may be the most significant factor responsible for the lower scores obtained by children with cyanotic CHD, given that significant differences in IQ scores between children with cyanotic CHD and children with acyanotic CHD have been demonstrated when the effects of age, social class, degree of sickness of the child at the time of testing and the type of test used have been taken into account.[293]

In a study of intellectual functioning and personality in children with CHD, Kramer et al[294] divided children into two groups according to the severity of their symptoms, irrespective of diagnostic group. The 'symptomatic' group, described as demonstrating limited physical capacity, consisted of 28 children who had undergone corrective surgery and 49 children who either had received palliation or did not require surgery. The asymptomatic group, whose physical capacity was described as 'normal', contained 25 children who had already undergone corrective surgery and 26 who had not. A healthy control group was selected from children presenting at clinics with innocent heart murmurs, a common condition without clinically significant symptoms.[295] Significant group differences were found on German adaptations of the Wechsler intelligence tests, such that children who were described as symptomatic obtained results that were significantly lower than both the asymptomatic children and the healthy control children. This result may be explained by physical limitations of the symptomatic children having a negative impact on cognitive development, or that physical ability is simply a proxy measure of brain vulnerability. Either way, it appears that the functional implications of having a heart defect may be a more important factor in children's cognitive outcome than the type of CHD per se.

As can be seen from the literature already described, cyanotic CHD appears to be a risk factor for neurodevelopmental impairment. The evidence regarding outcome for children with acyanotic CHD is less clear, and suggests that the risk of reduced intelligence may not be as high as that established for children with cyanotic CHD. However, a substantial proportion of the research regarding neurodevelopmental outcome in children with acyanotic CHD took place during the era in which death in infancy was a common outcome for children with serious forms. In attempting to understand the reasons that CHD can result in adverse cognitive outcome, it is necessary to consider the many potentially negative influences on brain development that occur when a child has CHD.

Brain growth and development is compromised in untreated cyanotic CHD. In an older series, where the mean age of operation was 8.3 months, occipitofrontal circumference (OFC) was 1.9 standard deviations below the mean for a normal population of the same age and sex, and 44% had an abnormally small OFC.[296] In another study, 14% of children operated on at a mean age of 13.3 months were microcephalic and 75% of children had an OFC below the 50% centile.[297] In both studies mean OFC increased significantly after operation. A more recent study has confirmed these findings, with 25% of children operated on between 1 month and 2 years (mean 6.7 months) having a head circumference below the 3rd centile; 71% of these patients had evidence of poor postnatal growth, with weight also below the 3rd percentile.[298]

These findings provided the justification for early surgical intervention for children with cyanotic CHD, which is now the rule. Indeed, children who underwent surgical correction for transposition of the great arteries before the age of 14 months obtained higher IQ scores at age 9 years than those children whose surgery was conducted later,[299] suggesting that the duration of hypoxia may be critical in determining later neurodevelopmental outcome. Increased duration of cyanosis appeared to cause a progressive impairment of cognitive functioning with an inverse correlation between age at repair and WPPSI IQ scores in children with transposition of the great arteries.[300] However, in Newburger's sample,[300] there was a significant relative deficit in perceptual-motor functioning, present even among those children who underwent surgical correction during the first year of life, demonstrating the vulnerability of infant neurological development to the effects of hypoxia. Since surgery for cyanotic CHD became feasible in the neonatal period and it was shown that age at operation had a significant effect on IQ,[300] surgery has been offered as early as possible. Interestingly, more recent research has failed to find a correlation between age at repair and IQ scores in children with cyanotic CHD.[291,301]

Research using the Bayley Scales of Infant Development with infants with CHD aged between 2 and 13 months who had not yet undergone any surgical intervention, found a strong independent relationship between the presence of congestive heart failure and developmental delay.[302] In addition, the presence of hypoxaemia (systemic arterial oxygen saturation <90%) was significantly related to motor functioning scores, suggesting that development may be compromised in infants with CHD because of their significant physical limitations, which cause restrictions on the infants' interactions with their environment. Similar conclusions were made by Linde et al[288] in their preoperative study of children with CHD. These authors found that children with cyanotic defects had marked impairments in gross motor functioning, and that in younger children the degree of physical incapacity was significantly associated with the level of developmental delay observed, indicating that being able to physically interact with one's environment may be crucial for normal development to occur. An alternative explanation for this result given by Linde and colleagues[288] suggested that the reliance on sensory-motor items in early-years tests may have caused this association. Moreover, Aisenberg and colleagues' study[302] did not include any long-term follow-up, and therefore it is not clear whether the developmental delays evident at the age of 2 months in these infants were transient, or an early signal that their later cognitive functioning would be compromised.

In a study designed to evaluate the effects of chronic hypoxia in children with CHD, Silbert et al[303] evaluated three groups of children aged between 4 and 8 years, on tests of intellectual, perceptual and motor functioning. A sample of children with cyanotic CHD were compared with children with acyanotic CHD who had experienced congestive heart failure, and a further group of children with acyanotic CHD who had not experienced any episodes of heart failure and had not received any cardiac medications. Stanford Binet IQ scores were significantly lower in children with cyanotic CHD than in children with acyanotic CHD. More specifically, children with cyanotic CHD performed more poorly in tests of perceptual skills and intellectual functioning than children with acyanotic

CHD who had experienced heart failure, and children with acyanotic CHD without a history of heart failure obtained the highest scores. Significant differences in gross (but not fine) motor functioning were also found between groups, with children with cyanotic CHD demonstrating specific difficulties on items requiring the use of lower limbs. In attempting to explain these findings, Silbert and colleagues[303] analysed data concerning the activity levels of children in each of the three groups, and found that children in the cyanotic group were most likely to restrict their own activity, and were most likely to have their activities restricted by their parents, than children in other groups. When these data were divided based on the children's level of physical activity, significant differences still existed in intellectual and perceptual functioning between children with cyanotic CHD and children with acyanotic CHD, suggesting that cyanosis has a significant effect on cognitive development irrespective of its effects on physical activity.

Clearly, biological factors directly related to CHD, such as acute hypoxic episodes related to cyanosis, or hypoxic-ischaemic insults due to reduced cerebral perfusion, may be responsible for changes to children's neurodevelopmental trajectory, but it is also important to consider whether more general effects associated with the presence of a chronic illness may be responsible for the documented cognitive deficit. Wray and Sensky[304] conducted a controlled prospective study of cognitive development in young children with CHD, and compared their performance on a range of developmental assessments with children requiring bone marrow transplants, in order to control for the effect of chronic illness on development. Prior to surgical interventions, children in the cyanotic CHD, acyanotic CHD and bone marrow transplant groups all scored within the normal range on intellectual assessments, but scored significantly lower than a healthy control group, suggesting that factors related to the presence of a chronic illness may have indeed influenced intellectual development. Following surgery and transplants, children with CHD still scored significantly lower than healthy controls, whereas results obtained from children who had had bone marrow transplants were not significantly different from healthy children, suggesting that there may be specific effects related to the presence of CHD which have a detrimental influence on cognitive development.

Preoperative studies

Relatively few studies of developmental functioning in infants with congenital heart defects have investigated neurodevelopmental status prior to corrective surgery. Techniques used during open-heart surgery in infants can often involve alterations to the blood supply (e.g. cardiopulmonary bypass), which have the potential to adversely influence neurological functioning.[305] The absence of information on baseline neurodevelopmental functioning prior to surgical intervention against which to compare postoperative assessment results makes it difficult to attribute observed abnormalities in this population directly to changes relating to CHD, as perioperative factors,

prolonged hypoxia, restricted physical capacity or a combination of all of these factors are often present in children with CHD.[306]

Dittrich et al[307] conducted prospective research on infants with CHD, and found that despite all infants having normal cranial ultrasound prior to surgery, 25 out of 68 infants were judged to have neurological abnormalities before surgery. The rate of neurological abnormalities was higher in those infants awaiting palliative surgery (6/10) compared with those awaiting corrective surgery (19/58), although interpretation of this finding is made difficult by the significant difference in group sizes. MRI has also been used to investigate the morphological features of the brain in infants and children before and after cardiac surgery. McConnell et al[308] found that one-third (5/15) demonstrated abnormal MRI findings before surgery, and only 2/15 children had normal MRI post-surgery. A recent MRI study of infants before and after surgical correction of complex CHD (of both cyanotic and acyanotic types) revealed that approximately one-quarter of infants' MRI scans prior to surgery either demonstrated damage to the white matter adjacent to the ventricles or evidence of infarcts.[309] Early postoperative MRI scans showed that two-thirds of infants had new lesions or worsening of existing lesions, although on repeated scanning at 3–6 months of age many of these had resolved. Presently the literature suggests that a relationship exists between white matter lesions and subsequent cognitive deficits in children who were born preterm,[310] but no such literature exists in infants with CHD, making it difficult to state conclusively what the clinical implications of these white matter abnormalities might be for later neuropsychological functioning.

A neuropathological study of 38 infants who died after cardiac surgery revealed that cerebral white matter damage (periventricular leukomalacia – PVL) was the most significant lesion in both severity and incidence.[311] Although no significant relationship was found between infant variables such as age at time of surgery and severity of brain damage or operative variables such as duration of deep hypothermic circulatory arrest and severity of brain damage, there was a tendency for neonates to be at greater risk for acute PVL, which the authors suggested reflected the greater vulnerability of the immature white matter to hypoxic-ischaemic damage, which can occur pre-, intra- or postoperatively. Further research is required to establish whether the abnormalities uncovered on pre- and postoperative MRI (Fig. 17.10) are indicative of significant neurodevelopmental problems for infants and children with CHD, or whether they might reflect transient intracranial venous hypertension.[312]

Research studying the oxygen saturation of neonates without pre-existing brain damage before, during and after cardiac surgery concluded that the preoperative neurological status of neonates had a significant impact on the postoperative neurological outcome.[313] On the basis of the finding that infants with lower preoperative regional cerebral oxygen saturation values tended to have lower developmental quotient scores

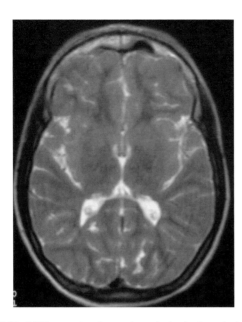

Fig. 17.10. MRI scan showing periventricular leukomalacia, worse on the left than the right, in a child born at term with pulmonary atresia with intact septum who has a mild right hemiparesis, a verbal IQ of 63 and a performance IQ of 46 with behavioural problems and executive dysfunction.

at 30–36 months, Toet and colleagues proposed that lack of preoperative brain damage may be a necessary requirement for normal neurodevelopmental outcome after cardiac surgery in infancy.

In one of the few studies to evaluate neurological functioning in infants with CHD before open-heart surgery, Limperopoulos et al[289] completed a neurobehavioural assessment and a neurological examination in 56 infants awaiting surgical repair. Infants with hypoplastic left heart syndrome, extracardiac abnormalities involving the central nervous system or known central nervous system insults were excluded. Twenty per cent of the infants had an abnormal neurobehavioural assessment result, and 56% demonstrated one or more abnormal findings, such as hypotonia or motor asymmetries, when examined by a neurologist. Interestingly, infants with acyanotic CHD were found to be at greater risk of having an abnormal neurological examination; Limperopoulos and colleagues suggested that this result may have occurred due to specific acyanotic defects causing reduced cardiac output, resulting in decreased cerebral perfusion and increasing the potential for hypoxic-ischaemic brain damage. The authors concluded that neurobehavioural abnormalities as measured using a standardized assessment were common in children with CHD pre-surgery, and argued that further investigation should be undertaken to focus on the causes of these neurological deficits as a priority.

Effect of surgery

Comparison of scores obtained on the Bayley Scales of Infant Development (BSID) recorded pre- and postoperatively in infants undergoing cardiac surgery with cardiopulmonary bypass have shown significant changes in neurodevelopmental

functioning after surgery.[305] The BSID is a standardized assessment tool designed to evaluate neurodevelopmental status in infancy and childhood, and yields two index scores, a Mental Development Index (MDI) and a Psychomotor Development Index (PDI); both index scores have a mean of 100 and a standard deviation of 15. Recent research by Robertson, Justo and colleagues with infants born with CHD found that 5.7% of the sample had PDI scores below the normal range prior to surgery, whereas only 57% of infants had both MDI and PDI scores that were within the normal range at 1 year follow-up.[305] This finding suggests that infants with CHD are at a significant risk of abnormal neurodevelopmental outcome due to the vulnerability of the infant brain to hypoxic-ischaemic insults. Infants with CHD are often exposed to multiple potential causes of hypoxia during the neonatal period, such as preoperative hypoxic periods due to cyanosis or reduced cerebral perfusion due to poor cardiac output or restricted blood flow, intra-operative insults due to cardiopulmonary bypass CPB and other life-support methods, and hypoxic incidents during postoperative recovery.

Robertson et al[305] assessed neurodevelopmental functioning at 18 months in 67 survivors of neonatal heart surgery. Children with the lowest Bayley MDI and PDI scores tended to have chromosomal or other congenital anomalies, such as chromosome 22q11 deletion syndrome or Down syndrome. Outcomes for the 85 children studied were recorded at 18 months as in-hospital death, post-discharge death, motor or sensory disability, motor or cognitive delay and intact survivors. One-quarter of the children studied were found to have motor or cognitive delay. A multivariate analysis model predicted 55% of variance in outcome: 23% was determined by preoperative, 18% from interoperative and 14% from postoperative factors. Robertson and colleagues found that the duration of pre-operative ventilation contributed most to the likelihood of an adverse outcome, and concluded that infants requiring respiratory support represented the most vulnerable proportion of the sample.[305] In contrast with previous research findings[314] neither socio-economic status nor parental education profiles predicted outcome in this study. The authors suggested that this lack of association may have occurred because environmental factors had perhaps not yet had a chance to exert a significant influence on neuropsychological functioning, or because the influence of having a major illness on neuropsychological functioning was much stronger at this young age.

The research findings presented thus far indicate that the neuropsychological development of infants with CHD may be adversely affected, with particularly compelling evidence for an association between cyanotic CHD and poorer neurodevelopmental outcome. However, few studies have systematically demonstrated that children with acyanotic CHD have an entirely normal neurodevelopmental trajectory. Prospective studies using neuroimaging have provided indications that neurological structures may be damaged by hypoxia-ischaemia even before infants undergo surgery, and that the risk of these insults is present in infants with both cyanotic and acyanotic

CHD. Results obtained on neurodevelopmental assessments pre- and post-surgery have highlighted that infants with CHD are exposed to a variety of risk factors that may be responsible for neurodevelopmental impairments; the most significant risk factor would appear to be hypoxia-ischaemia, which may be caused by cyanosis, reduced cerebral perfusion due to poor cardiac output or restricted blood flow, or hypoxic insults occurring during surgical procedures. It is also important to give consideration to factors related to the presence of any significant medical condition that may adversely affect development. These may include the effect of prolonged hospitalization on the level of environmental and social stimulation an infant receives, and the ongoing restrictions placed on an infant's interactions with objects in its environment when physical capacity is limited by illness.

At present there has been limited research which has studied preoperative baseline neuropsychological functioning in infants with CHD, and clearly neurological and neuropsychological morbidity may be significantly influenced when infants undergo open heart surgery. Most research has focused on evaluating the associations between surgery related variables and cognitive outcomes for children with CHD, in order to improve morbidity, and some of the findings related to intra-operative risk factors will now be discussed.

For most cardiac procedures, it is a major advantage to have low flow and pressure in the systemic circulation. This results in an easier operating environment, is associated with reduction in blood trauma from the pump oxygenator system and also reduces coronary collateral flow which will add to myocardial hypothermia and protection. The introduction of circulatory arrest to deep hypothermia allowed a field free of catheters and blood and therefore the development of anatomical correction for a number of CHD, including ventricular septal defect (VSD) and transposition of the great arteries (TGA). Circulatory arrest was first used for periods of only a few minutes, for example for the closure of an atrial septal defect (ASD), but was soon extended in attempts to repair previously untreatable CHD. Initially, there was very considerable concern at the high mortality, with brain damage in a significant proportion of survivors mainly due to damage to the basal ganglia. Surgical techniques improved and the duration of circulatory arrest could therefore be shortened, with corresponding reductions in mortality and morbidity. The initial research was almost always confined to adult populations because of ethical considerations and it has only recently been recognized that the best bypass technique for supporting a child during complex surgery for CHD may be very far from optimal in adults undergoing coronary artery bypass; it is now clear that excluding children from this type of data collection is unethical as animal and adult data may be misleading.

Haneda et al[315] conducted pre- and postoperative assessments on 161 infants and children, in order to assess the impact of cardiac surgery on intellectual functioning. Using the Gesell Developmental Schedule for Infants and the Binet Intelligence Test for Children in a repeated measures design, between 1 and 2 weeks before surgery, and 2 to 4 weeks afterwards, their results found that in general, postoperative scores showed a tendency to increase. Statistically significant increases were found in postoperative IQ scores for children who had undergone surgical correction of atrial or ventricular septal defects, TGA, tetralogy of Fallot or complete atrioventricular canal. Infants who experienced an extended period of circulatory arrest during surgery (>50 minutes) demonstrated a significant decrease in developmental quotient scores. Haneda and colleagues concluded that cardiac surgery did not normally significantly impair intellectual function, but that the application of circulatory arrest for periods of more than 50 minutes increased the risk of cerebral dysfunction post-surgery. Comparable results were obtained by Forbess et al[314] who found a trend towards lower full scale IQ scores in 5 year olds who had experienced periods of hypothermic circulatory arrest of longer than 39 minutes duration when undergoing cardiac surgery as infants, although the result was not statistically significant.

A comparison of 8-year neurodevelopmental outcomes for infants who received two different methods of vital organ support during cardiac surgery revealed that both groups showed IQ scores that were within the normal range and levels of academic achievement that were comparable.[316] However, despite demonstrating overall intellectual functioning that was within the normal range on standardized testing, more than a third of children in both samples had been identified as requiring additional educational support, and many showed relative deficits in specific areas of neuropsychological functioning, such as working memory, sustained attention and vigilance, and higher-order language skills. The comparison revealed that infants who underwent total circulatory arrest showed greater morbidity in the domain of motor functioning compared to those infants supported with low-flow cardiopulmonary bypass.

Sharma et al[317] evaluated a sample of 100 infants who underwent surgical correction of CHD using deep hypothermic bypass with and without circulatory arrest. Follow-up evaluations (carried out at approximately 4 years of age) found that operated infants had a mean mental performance quotient that was significantly below the mean of a demographically matched control group, but that there was no significant difference in outcomes between infants who had total circulatory arrest and those who did not. Similar findings were reported by Bellinger et al,[316] who found significantly greater morbidity in motor functioning in infants who had undergone total circulatory arrest during surgery, compared to those infants supported by low-flow cardiopulmonary bypass. These results suggest that, despite the majority of research findings documenting non-significant differences in global measures of cognitive functioning post-surgery between children with CHD and healthy controls, there are clearly long-term effects of life support techniques on specific aspects of neuropsychological functioning.

Wells et al[318] published data on a cohort of children who had undergone circulatory arrest, comparing IQ with their siblings and with a group of children with similar cardiac lesions who had undergone corrective surgery with moderate hypothermia and continuous cardiopulmonary bypass. The circulatory arrest group had significantly lower IQs than their siblings and than the moderate hypothermia group, with a reduction in IQ of 0.53 points per minute of circulatory arrest time. The only significant difference between a more recent group of children undergoing moderate hypothermic cardiopulmonary bypass for ASD repair and a group undergoing deep hypothermic circulatory arrest (DHCA) for repair of VSD, tetralogy of Fallot or transpostion was in motor reaction time, but IQ decreased 0.36 points per minute of arrest time in the DHCA group.[319] Wells et al[318] found verbal, quantitative and cognitive problems on the McCarthy scales and there is more recent evidence for language and behavioural difficulties,[320] but the most consistent finding has been moderate motor dysfunction.[320-323] There is increasing evidence that deep hypothermic circulatory arrest is associated with an increased risk of motor delay[324] and long-term neuropsychological sequelae,[316,323] and most surgeons have been avoiding this method unless the operation is technically impossible without it.

The safe ischaemic period for DHCA in young children is theoretically between 11 and 19 minutes at 28°C and 39 and 65 minutes at 18°C.[325] With a larger surface area:volume ratio and therefore more efficient brain cooling, infants can probably tolerate longer ischaemic periods than older children and adults.[325] Greeley's data[325] are concordant with animal experiments suggesting severe brain damage with periods of DHCA over 70 minutes[326] and the clinical data, which suggest that severe neurological sequelae are seen mainly in those children who have undergone circulatory arrest for over 60 minutes.[301,318] Although DHCA was still in use in some of the best centres in the world in 1991 (e.g. Aachen and Boston, where the randomized study was done), because of the Wells[318] data, by 1991, most surgeons operating using this technique were striving to limit the duration to a maximum of 1 hour. In the Boston study, in those infants with transposition with a VSD randomized to DHCA, the mean duration was 55 minutes (interquartile range 51–59 minutes). In Aachen, the mean time for DHCA for transposition was 51–67 minutes (mean 60±SD3.1).

The controlled trial conducted between April 1988 and February 1992 in Boston randomizing infants to circulatory arrest or low flow bypass showed an advantage for the latter particularly in terms of the reduction of seizures and EEG discharges post bypass and in terms of motor development at 1 year follow-up.[323] In fact, both groups received a period of DHCA, although this was shorter in those randomized to low flow CPB.[324]

Increasing concern over the risk of significant neurodevelopmental problems after circulatory arrest led to the development of alternative strategies. Many surgeons were using low-flow continuous cardiopulmonary bypass at deep hypothermia to repair all but the most complex congenital heart disease; if circulatory arrest is then required, the period of time is usually substantially reduced. It is technically feasible to perform the arterial switch operation at full pump flow with only 2 minutes of circulatory arrest for ASD closure.[327] There are, however, disadvantages in prolonging cardiopulmonary bypass time, especially in relation to the risk of embolism. In a contemporaneous audit of early neurological outcome conducted for 523 patients operated on in 1991 at Great Ormond Street Hospital, the risk of seizures, coma, neuro-ophthalmic sequelae and motor disorders in the immediate postoperative period was related to the duration of cardiopulmonary bypass. The Aachen series of neonatal switches for transposition performed between 1986 and 1992 had mean DHCA periods of 60±SD3 minutes (i.e. +2 SD 66 minutes) and cardiopulmonary bypass periods of 63.4±SD13.7 minutes (i.e. +2 SD 90.8 minutes). When followed up 8–13 years later, duration of cardiopulmonary bypass (CPB) predicted neurological and speech problems (relative risk 1.9 for every 10 minutes of CPB time)[328] and reduced quality of life.[328] In the Aachen series, in addition to the effect of preoperative hypoxia and acidosis, peri- and postoperative cardiovascular insufficiency independently predicted motor disability. These patients underwent cross-clamping for 53–96 minutes (65.7±SD8.1).

There have been several studies suggesting that neuro-developmental sequelae were commoner in children who had been cooled rapidly,[322,329] but this remains controversial.[330] Kern et al,[331] who compared two strategies for cooling within 20 minutes using α-stat, found that there was less jugular venous desaturation with rapid than with gradual core cooling, suggesting that there are advantages for the earlier institution of surface cooling, and lower blanket and water bath temperatures if cooling is to be achieved within this time frame. Eke et al[332] found no effect of rate of cooling on neurodevelopmental outcome in a group of infants undergoing heart transplantation for hypoplastic left heart with core cooling, but the average psychomotor index was 91 and mental index 88 in this population and the data may not be transferable to other conditions where the cognitive outcome is usually better than this. Hovels-Gurich[330] also found that rate of cooling was not a predictor of long-term neurological outcome, but all their patients were managed using a pH-stat strategy, which may allow more thorough cooling within a short time. There is also evidence for improved recovery of metabolic function after DHCA if the head is packed in ice.[333]

The speed and method of rewarming may also be critical.[334] During reperfusion after relative ischaemia, cerebral blood flow may be too low to meet an increase in the metabolic demand with increased temperature. In addition, mild hypothermia is protective after an ischaemic insult, whereas slight hyperthermia may enhance cerebral damage.[334] There may be a case for cold reperfusion before rewarming, particularly after DHCA.

There is evidence from adult studies that significant hypocapnia may have an adverse effect on neurological outcome and there may also be adverse effects in children. Reactivity of the cerebral circulation to carbon dioxide is preserved during moderate and deep hypothermia in most cases, and CBF may therefore fall to very low levels with hypocapnia, which might be critical if cerebral perfusion is already reduced at low pump flow. Jonas et al[335] found, in a retrospective survey of children undergoing the Senning procedure, that developmental score was directly related to arterial pCO_2 at the time of circulatory arrest. In practice, it is difficult to separate the direct effects of carbon dioxide tension from those of the predetermined pH strategy.

The weight of evidence indicates that neurodevelopmental outcomes for children born with CHD are different than those for healthy children, but this is not to suggest that there is consensus of opinion, or that the evidence is definitive. Forbess et al[314] found that children who had undergone surgical repair or palliation of CHD scored within one standard deviation of the normative population mean on tests of intellectual functioning. However, the authors concluded that despite apparently normal test results, children with CHD still demonstrated impairments in neurodevelopmental functioning, based on the finding that a significant proportion of the sample had received assistance from speech and language therapists or occupational therapists. Similar results have been reported by Wright & Nolan,[336] whose study compared a sample of children with corrected cyanotic CHD (TGA or tetrology of Fallot) and a control sample of children with innocent heart murmurs. Wright & Nolan found a higher incidence of referral for additional educational support among children with corrected CHD,[336] which is in concordance with the report by Bellinger et al[316] who found that one-third of children who had undergone cardiac surgery as infants had been identified as needing additional educational support, despite scoring within the normal range on standardized intellectual assessments. These findings all suggest that children with CHD may be at a disadvantage in their learning compared to their healthy peers, despite apparently normal test results.

In the study reported by Kramer and colleagues,[294] symptomatic children with CHD scored below asymptomatic children with CHD (symptomatic mean IQ 102.6, asymptomatic mean IQ 107.4), who scored less than healthy control children (mean IQ 114.2) on tests of intellectual functioning. Despite the significant difference in scores between symptomatic and healthy children, the mean score of the symptomatic group still fell within the normal range according to published test data. Kramer and colleagues concluded that the comparison with healthy control children reflected a true difference in intellectual functioning, and that the comparison with published test norms was no longer valid. Similar results have been reported by Wray & Sensky[304] and by Aram and colleagues,[293] who found significantly higher IQ scores in children with acyanotic CHD compared to children with cyanotic CHD, although both cardiac groups scored within the normal range according to test standardization samples. The lack of a control group in this study makes it difficult to establish the practical significance of this finding, but when put into the context of similar findings (e.g. the study by Kramer et al[294]) it appears reasonable to conclude that children with CHD as a group have a reduced level of intellectual functioning compared to healthy control children.

As yet, causal pathways explaining the association between CHD and neurodevelopmental problems remain under investigation. Long-term outcome studies are difficult and by the time they are undertaken, they may be rendered less relevant by changes in patient population and in surgical procedure. Bypass techniques evolved as various practical aspects of supporting patients during operations for heart disease were solved, and have varied widely from institution to institution in the absence of firm scientific evidence of the over-riding benefit of any one approach, at least in part because a change of protocol may increase the risk of human error. An adequate technical repair of the defect is often achievable, but every surgical variable may have an influence on the brain and is potentially a confound in any clinical study. Research has also been hampered by the fact that there are a wide variety of cardiac abnormalities which require surgical correction and the incidence of neurological complications varies with the underlying diagnosis, presumably partly because of the cardiac anatomy and partly because of the variance in surgical techniques appropriate to repair the lesion.

Relatively few studies have managed to observe infants preoperatively, but studies using prospective neuroimaging have indicated that significant damage may have already occurred prior to surgery taking place. Studies examining the relationship between age at corrective surgery (assumed to be a marker of the duration of chronic hypoxia) and neurodevelopmental outcome have not shown a clear benefit of earlier surgery, although there are many potential confounds to be considered. As cardiac surgical techniques have advanced, often the age at which such repairs are undertaken has reduced. In addition, greater understanding of the effects of specific life-support techniques on neurodevelopmental functioning has led to the selection of techniques which have been proven to reduce morbidity in this group, thereby resulting in a significant confound between age and cohort. Findings relating the duration of CPB to outcome have suggested a trend towards longer bypass resulting in increased morbidity; however, statistics demonstrate that the largest proportion of variance in outcome for infants with CHD can be attributed to preoperative factors. Taken together, these findings suggest that the severity of the defect may be confounded with the length of time on bypass, as more severe defects may require a greater period of time in order for the surgeon to complete the palliation or repair.

A further significant difficulty has arisen in assessing intellectual functioning in children with CHD, as selecting an appropriate control group against which to compare the children's results is fraught with complications. As noted by Forbess et al,[314] many of the heart defects are not conducive to the survival of the child without prompt surgical intervention, and with surgery now taking place in the neonatal period, this makes pre- and postoperative testing (to allow children to act as their own controls) extremely difficult. In addition, children with CHD may have a significantly different early infancy to healthy children; spending long periods of time in hospital potentially limits the level of stimulation they receive and restricts their social interactions, which may adversely affect their social and language development. There is also some evidence to suggest that parents of children with CHD may demonstrate higher anxiety levels than parents of healthy children,[288] and may restrict the activity level of their child[294] potentially placing further limitations on their child's development.

Outcomes for children with CHD are often reported using broad indicators of overall functioning, such as IQ scores. The research presented here suggests that these children perform significantly differently from healthy children; the IQ scores obtained by children with CHD may fall within the normal range, but are, on average, significantly lower than those obtained by healthy children. Some have suggested that this result has occurred due to the general increase in average test scores over time, and that comparisons with test norms are no longer valid.[337] There is also evidence to suggest that school-aged children with CHD are more likely to have been identified as experiencing problems with their learning than healthy children, further highlighting the significant differences in intellectual functioning.

As yet, few research studies have delineated which specific aspects of intellectual functioning are problematic for children with CHD as they grow up, nor have they been able to identify at an early age which children may later need additional educational support. Those few studies which have presented detailed neuropsychological profiles of older children with CHD have suggested that executive functioning, including working memory, sustained attention and higher order language skills, may be an area of relative deficit for children with CHD,[316] and is in concordance with findings from studies of the effects of hypoxia on intellectual functioning in adults (e.g. as a result of chronic obstructive pulmonary disease[338]).

Recent prospective longitudinal research has attempted to investigate whether IQ scores at 8 years of age could be predicted from developmental test scores at 12 months in children who underwent surgical correction for cyanotic CHD (TGA) in the first 3 months of life.[339] McGrath and colleagues assessed 135 infants using the BSID and the Fagan Test of Infant Intelligence (FTII – a measure of infant visual information processing), and completed a WISC-III assessment with the children 7 years later. Their analyses revealed that children with poor neurodevelopmental scores at year 1 were at increased risk of achieving lower IQ scores at year 8, but that all three indices of neurodevelopmental status at year 1 (Bayley MDI and PDI scores, and FTII) had low positive predictive values. This result highlights that a substantial proportion of infants who scored within the normal range at year 1 will go on to demonstrate deficits in intellectual functioning at 8 years of age, underscoring the need for more accurate assessments of infant cognitive functioning. New assessment tools need to be sensitive enough to identify the early precursors of the high

prevalence/low severity neurodevelopmental impairments seen later on in children with CHD.

In summary, there is considerable evidence for an effect of congenital heart disease and its treatment on global brain function, typically leading to reduction in full scale IQ with additional specific cognitive deficits. The effect of any additional venous or arterial stroke[340] has received relatively little attention, at least in part because of the diversity of the underlying cardiac disease and necessary surgery.

17.5 Sickle Cell Disease: Cognitive and Behavioural Outcome

Alexandra Hogan

At a time when behavioural abnormality was not routinely associated with sickle cell disease (SCD), Wertham et al[341] related chronic psychopathology, such as psychosis and suicidal intent, to autopsy findings in the brains of five adults with SCD. Despite the implications for cognitive function, the earliest published study of outcome in children with SCD did not report any deficit. Chodorkoff & Whitten[342] administered tests of intelligence (Binet/Wechsler Scales) to 19 children and found no effect on intellectual or psychological functioning (WISC: $N=11$ sibling pairs – full scale IQ 78 vs 84). Similarly, in the 1970s, Logothetis et al[343] administered the Porteus Maze and Wechsler IQ tests to 138 children and adults with homozygous β-thalassaemia (a disease with genetic and clinical similarities to SCD) and found that performance was not significantly impaired in patients compared to controls, for example Full Scale IQ 95 and 93, respectively. There was, however, an association between IQ and indices of illness severity, i.e.: total amount of blood transfused since birth; size of spleen; degree of cephalofacial deformity. In addition, 'abnormalities in character' and 'behaviour' were reported in 96 cases, suggesting a high incidence of psychopathology. While interest in possible cognitive deficits waned, support for an association between SCD and behavioural abnormality gathered momentum, and there followed reports of anxiety and low self-esteem in children with SCD,[344,345] with some evidence to suggest that the onset of pain ('crisis') may actually be preceded by a depressive episode.[346]

Despite the increasing realization that SCD is associated with a high incidence of stroke and the less severe covert or 'silent' brain infarction, there were only sporadic reports of cognitive outcome through the 1980s, and presence or absence of stroke was not consistently documented. The more systematic studies that followed during the 1990s made use of the increasing availability of brain imaging technology to demonstrate an association between the presence and location of brain lesions (Fig. 17.11) and the severity and nature of cognitive impairment. This served to re-focus interest in cognitive function.

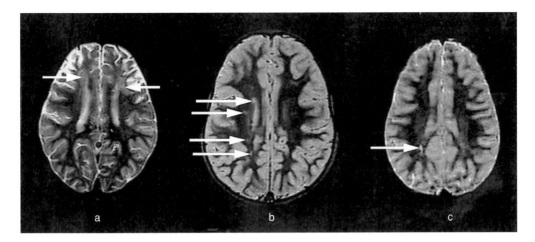

Fig. 17.11. Magnetic resonance T2-weighted images in the axial plane in children with sickle cell disease who underwent cognitive testing showing the range of infarcts in terms of site, size and number.[80] (a) Large bilateral lesion of frontal lobes showing cortical atrophy (not arrowed) and underlying white-matter changes (arrows). (b) Medium lesion (or several small lesions as indicated by arrows) in central white matter of right hemisphere. (c) Small lesion (arrow) in right parietal white matter.

The majority of data have been obtained as part of the American Co-operative Study of Sickle Cell Disease (CSSCD), and from Jamaican,[347] French[348] and East London cohorts.[80]

In children with SCD (as in many without SCD) an acute stroke event does not occur in isolation of chronic derangement in blood oxygenation, and/or chronic neurological conditions such as cerebrovascular disease. It may not be assumed, therefore, that a child with SCD was developing normally before the stroke occurred, or indeed that there is a return to normal function after the child is discharged from hospital often with a positive prognosis. In consideration of this, attention is shifting towards investigation of the extent to which aetiologies such as anaemia and hypoxaemia influence the pattern of cognitive outcome irrespective of acute infarct lesions, and sophisticated neuroimaging techniques have recently identified subtle brain abnormality in those without brain infarct.[349–352]

Our understanding of cognitive deficit in children with SCD has thus progressed, and this is demonstrated in those representative studies described below. By comparison, studies of socio-emotional function showed limited progression during the 1990s, and there are conflicting data. With a few notable exceptions, measures of social, emotional and behavioural function typically appear to be secondary to cognitive assessments, rather than serving as a focus of investigation in their own right. Nevertheless, these data are also discussed.

In general, our experience with the East London cohort resonates with that of American investigators: while the majority of children with SCD cope well with mainstream education, many are vulnerable to subtle cognitive deficits and to psychopathology. It is of concern that this risk is not always communicated to those working with children with SCD on a day-to-day basis.

Sickle cell disease phenotypes

Children with the homozygous form (sickle cell anaemia, HbSS) are more vulnerable to most SCD complications (e.g.

frequent episodes of pain; chest crisis; stroke[353]) and delayed growth[354] than compound heterozygotes with HbSC or HbSβ thalassaemia. In general, however, intellectual deficit may be observed in all common SCD genotypes (HbSS, HbSC, HbSβ[0] thalassaemia, HbSβ[+] thalassaemia),[79,80,354–358] although the majority of studies have focused on those with HbSS, and there are few datasets from compound heterozygotes that take into account social and environmental background.[357]

In the relatively small studies that have been conducted, heterozygotes with HbAS (sickle cell trait) do not appear to have significant intellectual and cognitive deficits compared to sibling controls with HbAA,[79,359] although they have a mild anaemia, and a slightly increased risk of vasculopathy and brain damage.[360] While there were sporadic early reports of lower scores on neuropsychological tests in children with trait compared to children with normal haemoglobin status,[361,362] these findings have not been consistently replicated,[363,364] and more recent studies have typically included children with and without trait as one control group.[365]

Cognitive outcome

As more has been discovered about the nature of cognitive deficit in SCD, three important findings have emerged. Firstly, the relatively high incidence of brain lesions is associated with cognitive impairment.[366,367] Secondly, children without brain lesions, who may be considered to be less severely affected, may nevertheless be impaired relative to controls, and this might result from more subtle neuropathology that begins to emerge in infancy. Thirdly, the pattern of cognitive impairment appears to reflect the greater involvement of the frontal lobes in SCD neuropathology.

While some studies have reported the results of large batteries of neuropsychological assessments,[79,80,365,368,369] or looked specifically for deficits in attention,[370,371] memory[372,373] and language,[374] assessment of intellectual function (IQ) is common to the majority of studies and these data are considered first.

INTELLECTUAL FUNCTION

In contrast to the findings of the original study by Chodorkoff and Whitten,[342] the results of a study by Swift et al[359] indicated that intellectual function is lowered in children with SCD. Swift and colleagues compared the neuropsychological performance of 21 children with SCD to 21 controls (aged between 7 and 16 years) and found that the mean full scale IQ of children with SCD was approximately 16 points lower than that obtained by children without SCD (this is approximately one Weschler IQ standard deviation (15)). An association between SCD and intellectual deficit was also made by Knight et al.[347] In this relatively large Jamaican study, Wechsler IQ tests were administered to 60 patients with SCD and age- and sex-matched controls, aged between 15 and 18 years. The groups were divided by age to take account of the change from child to adult IQ scale. The SCD group obtained mean full scale IQ scores of 72 (WISC-R (child), *N*=28) and 80 (WAIS-R (adult), *N*=32). The mean IQ score obtained from older adolescents ('WAIS-R' group) was significantly lower than controls (73 and 89, 'WISC-R' and 'WAIS-R' SCD groups respectively), and the overall group difference of 5.6 IQ points was small but also statistically significant. Indeed, this difference is smaller than that reported in American children by Swift et al.[359] Neuroimaging was not available to the authors of these studies, so it is possible that a higher incidence of silent infarct might account for the larger group difference in the American study; despite the lack of association between 'soft' neurological signs and IQ reported by Swift et al.[359] In the Jamaican children, differences in IQ were not accounted for by parental occupation, school absenteeism, school drop out or reported levels of 'overactivity'. Instead, pre-pubertal height made a large contribution to the difference in IQ, leading the authors to speculate that early factors, possibly nutritional, contributed to impaired mental development.

A number of studies have associated intellectual impairment with the occurrence of stroke (determined by medical history and/or neurological examination) in children with SCD. An early report by Hariman et al[119] documented a lower mean full scale IQ in children with SCD who had a clinical history of stroke (68) than in age- and gender-matched patients with SCD without clinical stroke (91). More recent studies have utilized MRI techniques to determine the presence of covert (silent) brain infarcts in children who may have been otherwise considered as neurologically normal.

During the 1990s a number of reports were published by the American CSSCD. One of the first to describe IQ data in a large cohort of SCD children (*N*=194; 135 HbSS, 59 HbSC; 6–12 years) revealed a step-wise decrease in IQ scores with disease severity.[375] Children with a normal MRI brain scan obtained the highest mean score (90, *N*=161), those with clinical stroke obtained the lowest (70, *N*=9 all HbSS) and those

with a silent infarct were interim (82, *N*=24; 21/24 HbSS). Similar values were obtained by Watkins et al,[80] in British Children, 41 with SCD, but, importantly, this study included 15 sibling controls.* Children with SCD were categorized according to presence or absence of lesion determined by MRI: five children had suffered a clinical stroke ('symptomatic'), four children had a lesion on MRI but had no history of stroke ('asymptomatic') and 30 children did not have a lesion ('SCD/nrm'). Full scale IQ was lowest in the Symptomatic group (67), and highest in the Control group (92), with the Asymptomatic (79) and SCD/nrm (86) groups obtaining mean scores in between; only the Symptomatic group obtained a significantly lower mean full scale IQ compared to either the SCD/nrm or Control groups. Verbal IQ was higher than performance IQ in all groups, but this difference was not significant.

Subsequent reports from the CSSCD presented the results of longitudinal assessment, but control data were lacking. Wang et al[377] published the results of serial IQ assessments that had been carried out in 373 patients (255 HbSS; 118 HbSC), 89 of whom had MRI evidence of either clinical stroke (27) or a silent lesion (62). Two types of analysis were performed. The first (cross-sectional) analysis compared performance between the three groups (no lesion vs silent lesion vs clinical stroke) in order to determine the extent to which IQ was associated with MRI status. At an average age of 13 years, clinical stroke was associated with significantly lower mean verbal IQ (79) and performance IQ (77) scores compared to children without brain lesions whose verbal and performance IQs were within the low average range but nevertheless one standard deviation below the normative mean of 100 (verbal IQ 85, performance IQ 86). Children with silent lesions were also impaired relative to children without brain lesions, although this difference was significant for verbal IQ (77) but not performance IQ (81). Thus, IQ was significantly lowered in patients with brain lesions, but clinical strokes did not result in greater impairment than silent lesions. Additionally, children without brain lesions also obtained scores that were lower than the normative mean. The second level of analysis in this study investigated the possibility of decreasing intellectual function with increasing age. Longitudinal IQ scores obtained from individual children across groups were investigated, but the authors highlighted the fact that the analysis was restricted by the change in IQ scale from the WISC-R to WISC-III mid-way through the study. Nevertheless, the corrected data showed little change in either performance IQ or full scale IQ with increasing age. By contrast, verbal IQ scores decreased by approximately 0.5 points/year; it is important to note, however, that even at the final assessment, mean verbal IQ did not appear to fall below the low-average range (80–89), as relates to the Wechsler categories for clinical interpretation.

---

* A control group is important as ethnic and socio-economic factors may render this population at risk of cognitive and/or behavioural deficits irrespective of SCD.[362,376] Indeed previous studies of SCD have reported full scale IQ scores in relation to ethnic and socio-economic matched controls ranging from 73 to 94,[79,347,359,370] suggesting considerable normal variation in this population.

A CSSCD study by Thompson et al[378] also described intellectual decline with age in children with SCD. Full scale IQ scores were obtained from 222 children (5–17 years), all of whom had at least two assessments (47%), and some of whom completed three (39%) and even four (14%) assessments over a period of 4 years; therefore the design of this study was part longitudinal and part cross-sectional. Once again, children were categorized into three groups according to MRI and neurological confirmation of presence or absence of overt symptoms (normal brain scan), history of cerebrovascular accident (clinical stroke) or silent infarct. Full scale IQ was lowest in children with stroke at all four assessments (72, 73, 69, 68, respectively), highest in children with a normal brain scan (90, 89, 86, 87) and intermediate in children with silent infarcts (85, 82, 77, 78); verbal and performance IQ appeared comparable at all assessments and in all groups (i.e. within 5 points), but this was not formally analysed. Thus this study reported the effect of neurological status (presence or absence of brain lesion) on longitudinal IQ scores, and provided evidence to suggest that children with brain lesions obtain chronically lower scores than children without brain lesions. However, although the authors claim that intellectual decline is more substantive in children with brain lesions, the extent of decline does not significantly differ between groups and is only in the magnitude of a few IQ points which would not normally be considered clinically significant. In addition, this study also failed to include a sibling control group, and therefore did not control for ethnicity and socio-economic status.

A further study of the CSSCD cohort was made by Steen et al,[360] focusing on those children with HbSS SCD in whom there was no history of stroke. All children had a MRI brain scan, revealing abnormality in 16 cases (mostly white matter infarction). While overall full scale IQ did not differ between groups ('MRI normal': 81; 'MRI abnormal': 78), when scores obtained only from those children who had the child WISC-III (rather than the adult WISC-R) were investigated, a significantly lowered verbal IQ was revealed in those with an abnormal MRI study (74 vs 84). In support of earlier studies, the authors concluded that intellectual impairment was associated with structural brain lesions, but that other factors, such as anaemia and hypoxia, may contribute to the lowered IQ in those with a normal brain scan. Indeed, haematocrit values obtained within 3 months of neuropsychological assessment were associated with full scale IQ. IQ was closer to the normative mean (100) in children with higher ($\geq$27: 86) compared to lower ($\leq$26: 76) haematocrit values. Furthermore, MRI abnormality and reduced haematocrit were identified as significant independent predictors of low full scale IQ: haematocrit accounted for 23% of the variance in full scale IQ, but the proportion of variance associated with MRI abnormality was not documented. Similarly, severely anaemic French children with SCD (haematocrit $\leq$20) obtained significantly lower full scale IQ scores compared to those who were less anaemic ($\geq$21): full scale IQ of 74 and 85 respectively.[348] A reduction in the oxygen-carrying capacity of red-blood

cells (anaemia) may therefore play a role in explaining IQ deficit, irrespective of brain infarction.[379]

The vascular system can respond to the challenge of anaemia by altering cerebral circulation to increase blood flow.[380] In support, lowered haematocrit was correlated with enlarged basilar artery volume measured from magnetic resonance angiography (MRA) scans ($r=-0.60$),[355,365] and other studies have reported a correlation between reduced haematocrit and increased cerebral blood flow velocity (CBFV) assessed by transcranial Doppler (TCD).[381] Such adaptive processes may represent short-term compensatory responses of a vulnerable brain; 'short-term' because increased CBFV is associated with a high risk of overt stroke over the subsequent 3 years.[382,383] Indeed, there is evidence that both increased basilar volume and increased CBFV are also associated with lowered IQ. In the study by Steen and colleagues[384] a negative correlation between MRA basilar artery volume and full scale IQ ($r=-0.62$) was found. Similarly, in the large French cohort, full scale IQ decreased stepwise between groups of children with a normal TCD study ($\leq$170cm/s: 85), children with a conditional study (170–200cm/s: 82) and children with abnormally high CBFV (>200cm/s: 75).[348] Later American studies replicated this finding, reporting, for example, that IQ (in particular verbal IQ), and measures of attention, are impaired in SCD children with high compared to low CBFV assessed by TCD.[385] Using path-analysis, Hogan et al[367] have shown that the association between hypoxaemia (indexed by pulse-oximetry) and full scale IQ is fully mediated by increased CBFV, i.e. decrease in oxygen saturation is associated with increase in velocity of blood flow to the brain, and increased velocity of blood flow is in turn associated with lowered full scale IQ. This mediated relationship suggests that lowered IQ may be a function of abnormal oxygen delivery to the brain, however a limitation of this study was that neither haemoglobin nor presence of infarct were entered into the model. Nevertheless, in support of Kral et al,[385] further analyses showed that the association between CBFV and IQ was significant for verbal but not for performance IQ.

In summary, these studies indicate that intellectual function is adversely affected by SCD, although they suggest that in most cases intellectual development may be somewhat lowered compared to ethnic-matched controls, rather than severely impaired as a consequence of a brain infarct. Moreover, there is limited evidence of clinically significant intellectual decline with increasing age, but this small degree of IQ decline may not hold when compared simultaneously to longitudinal performance in ethnic- and age-matched controls. Moreover, studies investigating intellectual function in late adolescence and early adulthood are lacking, so it is not known if intellectual deficit persists, or if such deficit represents a protracted delay in intellectual development that eventually 'catches up'.

Of particular interest is the subtle lowering of IQ in children who are neurologically normal. This was confirmed by a meta-analysis reporting an approximate 4-point IQ difference between controls and children with SCD without a history of stroke.[366] This difference was small but statistically significant, with an estimated effect size (*d*) of 0.39. Subtle grey and white matter changes detected using sophisticated quantitative and volumetric MRI analysis is consistent with this finding. Such changes are not necessarily associated with brain infarction and not always detectable on conventional MRI scans.[349–352] Indeed, a reduction in dorsal white matter volume,[351] and corpus callosum volume,[352] have both been associated with lowered IQ. Thus, it is possible that a degree of intellectual impairment is associated with potentially modifiable risk factors. In addition, volumetric studies suggest that it may be artificial to divide children into 'no lesion', 'silent infarct' and 'clinical stroke' categories, and that comparisons of IQ deficit and brain white/grey matter loss should be more realistically compared by viewing both variables on a continuum. Of more immediate concern for many families, however, is the extent to which intellectual deficit (whatever the degree) affects educational progression.

ACADEMIC PERFORMANCE

Two studies by Fowler et al[386,387] were particularly informative, as the first compared children with SCD to those with other chronic health concerns, and the second included controls matched for socioeconomic status (SES). In the first study, the average number of school days missed by children with SCD (23) in the sampled year (1980–1981) was higher than for children with chronic lung or cardiac disease (10 days for each). Furthermore, national achievement test score (percentile) was 24 in children with SCD, compared to 61 in children with chronic lung disease, and 57 in children with cardiac disease (the state median for North Carolina at this time was 63). In the subsequent study, the authors addressed the possibility that some of these differences might have been due to differences in SES. Children with SCD (*N*=28, 6–17 years) and an equal number of ethnic and SES-matched controls were assessed using the Wide Range Achievement Test (WRAT). Standard scores obtained for reading and spelling were significantly lower in children with SCD compared to controls (91 vs 104, and 89 vs 101, respectively; normative mean = 100), and there was some indication that reading difficulties increased with age. Level of achievement was not related to severity of SCD as indexed by variables including haemoglobin level and the number of days hospitalized. By contrast, Wasserman[79] did not find any significant performance differences on WRAT measures in children and adolescents with SCD (*N*=43, 8–16 years) compared to controls (*N*=30) (reading: 90 vs 94; spelling 89 vs 92; maths: 82 vs 86), and there was no age effect. The children with SCD had missed significantly more school days, but academic performance (grades) and the proportion of children in special education was comparable between groups. Furthermore, no difference was found in academic achievement scores (Woodcock–Johnson Psychoeducational Battery) between children with SCD and controls when level of intellectual function was controlled for,[359] suggesting that

children were performing at a level that was commensurate with their intellectual capacity.

In a later study, Brown et al[365] administered subtests from the Kaufman Achievement Battery (K-ABC) and the Basic Achievement Skills Individual Screener to a subgroup of school-aged children (7–12 years) from their cohort of 70 children with SCD and 18 sibling controls. While a greater percentage of children with SCD were identified as 'learning disabled' (10–13% across subscales of the K-ABC), this proportion did not significantly differ from that recorded in controls, none of whom were identified as learning disabled according to any measure. School absenteeism, as a proxy measure of disease severity, was not related to intellectual function or to academic achievement, although there was a small but significant correlation (*r*=0.31) between K-ABC subscales and haemoglobin. Richard & Burlew[388] also examined school grades and did not find any differences in the academic performance of 42 children with SCD compared with their peers (*N*=26). However, in the same year Sanders et al[389] described lower scores on the Peabody Individual Achievement Test in SCD children with a history of stroke compared to healthy controls (Reading Recognition: 87 vs 94; Reading Comprehension: 81 vs 92; Written Language Comprehension: 78 vs 103), suggesting that presence of stroke in SCD is associated with lower achievement, but the statistical significance of these group differences was not documented.

Longitudinal data are sparse, but in the CSSCD study by Wang et al,[377] a significant decline in maths but not reading (Woodcock–Johnson, Revised) between the ages of 6 and 12 years was found, equivalent to a loss of 0.9 points per year. In partial support of Sanders et al,[389] group comparisons for each age group (6–8 years; 8–10 years; 10–12 years) revealed significantly lower scores in children with silent infarct compared to children with normal MRI findings, but this was not the case in an earlier cross-sectional study by Brown et al;[371] although the results are not directly comparable as their 6–17 year age range was not divided into subgroups of more limited age ranges for analysis.

More recently, evidence of abnormal cognitive function (auditory discrimination) was found in young children with SCD undergoing routine assessment by Memphis City Schools (Developing Skills Checklist) prior to school entry.[390] In addition, significantly larger numbers of school-aged children with SCD required learning assistance (15/50) compared to age, gender, ethnic and SES matched controls (3/36).[391] Both level of cognitive ability and frequency of illness (indexed by the number of missed school days) were associated with level of academic attainment. This supported the previous finding by these authors that poor school performance is frequently found in children with SCD and silent infarct.[366]

In summary, there is little consensus to indicate the extent to which academic achievement is constrained by SCD, and the degree to which any detected deficit is related to disease severity, but it is clear that some children may require additional help in order to progress through school. It is reassuring that at least one American group is starting to address this issue by exploring rehabilitation strategies.[392,393]

EXECUTIVE FUNCTION

There is substantial verification that the frontal lobes are the most common site of neuropathology in children with SCD. Although it may not be assumed that executive function is related to the frontal lobes at this age with the same degree of specificity found in the mature brain, some studies have systematically attempted to associate the locus of lesions with deficits in executive function. In particular, three domains of function have been investigated, and for each there is evidence in adults that the frontal lobes are an important part of the neural network involved: working memory, inhibition and attention.

White et al[372] investigated working memory in children with SCD aged between 7 and 15 years. It was hypothesized that the nature of deficits in an immediate word-list recall task may suggest which component of the working memory model is at risk, and further, that there may be some association with lesion location. The model of Baddeley and Hitch[394] proposed that working memory may be fractionated into a central executive, and two 'slave' systems, the phonological loop for processing of auditory speech-based information and the visuo-spatial scratchpad for processing visuo-spatial information. White et al grouped 31 children with SCD according to MRI confirmed lesion location: anterior (CA territory and anterior MCA territory, basal ganglia, centrum semiovale; N=4), posterior (posterior to 'anterior' structures; N=4), diffuse (including 'anterior' and 'posterior' structures; N=12) and SCD no-lesion (N=11). Supraspan lists of real words with one, two or three syllables were presented and children were asked to immediately recall them. In the anterior group immediate recall was comparable to controls, but there was an effect of word-length which, according to White and colleagues, indicated dysfunction limited to the phonological loop. There was no evidence of reduced immediate recall or impaired word-length effect in the posterior group, which was assumed to indicate an intact central executive and phonological loop. Finally, children in the diffuse group demonstrated an intact word-length effect but reduced immediate recall compared to controls, suggesting to the authors a dysfunctional central executive. It was concluded that these results provided evidence for a variable pattern of performance in children with SCD, dependent on lesion location. A later study by the same research group focused on children with frontal lobe infarcts, revealing a deficit in learning and free-recall of word lists, and in backward digit-span.[395] The former process (word list recall) is commonly associated with short-term memory functions of the temporal lobe, and the latter (digits backwards) being a function that is particularly sensitive to working memory and frontal lobe integrity, although there is limited neuroimaging to support such a distinction.[396] Nevertheless, the predominant location of lesions in the dorsal frontal lobes is reason to expect that working memory may be vulnerable in children with SCD.

In support, Schatz and Roberts[373] reported selective deficit in the backward recall of digits; however, children with SCD (N=25, mean age 11 years) performed similarly to age-matched controls (N=25) on measures of forward digit span, forward and backwards spatial span, and a modified version of the Self-Ordered Pointing Test (SOPT), a measure of working memory in adults for which there is good evidence of an association with activity of the dorso-lateral frontal cortex.[397] Of note, and in contrast to the study by White et al,[372] the children in this study had no history of stroke and/or a normal MRI brain scan. While it may be concluded that significant working memory deficit on the SOPT is not apparent in children with SCD, replication of this study is important as the SOPT yields other measures which were not examined by Shatz and Roberts (e.g. time scores). Indeed, a more recent study found that children with SCD and frontal lobe lesions took significantly longer to complete the SOPT task compared to sibling controls, and children with SCD without brain lesions.[398] However, in support of Shatz and Roberts, no deficits were found for error rate, and children without lesions performed similarly to sibling controls.

The selective effect on time scores is interesting as children with SCD are susceptible to hypoxia which has been independently associated with processing speed,[399] and in the study by Brown[400] another measure of executive function, the Trail Making Test, did not discriminate between SCD (silent infarct, stroke) and control groups when error rate was examined, but a significant group difference was obtained for the time scores. Furthermore, there is evidence that degree of oxygen saturation is associated with processing speed in a measure of very early executive function development.[401] It would be of interest to investigate the individual and relative contribution of executive function deficit and increased processing speed in future studies of cognitive deficit in children with SCD.

Schatz and Roberts[373] hypothesized that the subtle working memory deficit observed in their children may be partly due to auditory processing abnormalities. This is an important consideration as it is well known that children with SCD are vulnerable to sensorineural hearing loss,[402–405] although a more recent Nigerian study placed the prevalence of sensorineural hearing loss at 3.8% for HbSS,[406] with no increased incidence of otitis media which is associated with speech and language delay. However, in American children there is evidence that auditory discrimination problems in children with SCD present early in life.[390] Consistent with this there is evidence for a reduction in auditory event-related potential (ERP) component amplitude in students with HbSS and HbSC SCD compared to patients with β-thalassaemia, and healthy controls; interestingly this occurred alongside an increase in response time to target stimuli. The authors concluded that brain function associated with auditory attention is indeed impaired as a function of SCD severity.[407] However, the extent to which derangement in auditory processing is associated with working memory deficit, such as the backward recall of digits, remains to be determined.

The Wisconsin Card Sorting Test (WCST) provides a measure of perseverative behaviour, which is associated with impaired inhibitory control,[408] and is commonly administered to adults with frontal lobe lesions. Watkins et al[80] found deficits on this test in SCD children and adolescents with frontal lobe pathology aged between 5 and 16 years. The results revealed a significantly greater number of perseverative errors in five children with lesions involving prefrontal areas than in two children whose lesions did not involve frontal areas; one case had a small infarct in parietal white matter and another had a choroidal fissure. Furthermore, a high rate of perseverative responding was not accounted for by age effects as an age-matched sibling control group obtained results comparable to normal adults. The mean number of categories obtained (maximum = 6) was 3.6 in controls, 4.0 in SCD children without stroke, 3.8 in children with silent infarct and 1.9 in children with clinical stroke. Similarly, perseverative error rate was highest in children with clinical stroke (56) compared to controls, SCD children without stroke, and SCD children with silent infarct (27, 32 and 39, respectively). Follow-up of this cohort revealed that one child who did not show evidence of brain abnormality ('SCD/nrm') subsequently had MRI confirmation of frontal lobe perfusion abnormality which was originally predicted on the basis of a worsening in WCST performance.[409] A later follow-up of a proportion of this cohort alongside additional recruits, revealed that adolescents with silent infarct lesions in the frontal lobe were significantly impaired in measures of categories obtained, perseverative error rate and set-maintenance errors (the ability to sort three cards correctly in a row with positive feedback, but with incorrect sorting of the subsequent card). For all three measures, adolescents with frontal lobe lesions obtained significantly impaired scores compared to adolescents with SCD who had no evidence of brain lesions.[398] Interestingly, at this older age (mean age 18 years), adolescents with frontal lobe silent infarcts obtained slightly higher category scores (4.3) and made fewer perseverative errors (24) compared to those obtained in children in the previous study by Watkins and colleagues.[80] This indicates that there may be some improvement in function on the WCST with increasing age, perhaps partly due to the expected increase in neural efficiency occurring during adolescence, but it will be important to confirm this observation with longitudinal analyses.

Schatz et al[410] also administered the WCST and described category and perseverative error scores in children with SCD with 'anterior' lesions (*N*=7, mean age 11 years: 3.6, 91, respectively), children with SCD with 'diffuse' lesions (*N*=18, mean age 13.6 years: 2.7, 75) and sibling controls (*N*=17, 7–21 years: 4.1, 84). With respect to category scores, the children in the 'anterior' group therefore performed similarly to the children with silent infarct in the study by Watkins et al,[80] and the children with 'diffuse' lesions were interim between the 'anterior' group[410] and the clinical stroke group.[80] Compared with the study by Watkins et al,[80] the higher perseverative error rate in the study by Schatz et al[410] is not accounted for by age

differences (although perseverative error rate was lower in the study of older adolescents),[398] but may be partly explained by methodological and/or other clinical differences between groups.

Schatz and colleagues[410] combined their WCST scores with those obtained from other measures of executive function and attention (e.g. Test of Variables of Attention) to create an 'Attention/Executive' domain score. It was found that deficits on this domain score were present in SCD groups with or without posterior injury. In other words, children with small lesions limited to the frontal lobes had a similar level of impairment in this domain as did children with diffuse infarcts. This provides support for an association between frontal lobe injury and WCST/attention deficit in children with SCD. Furthermore, lesion volume influenced spatial and language abilities but less so attention, executive and memory function, which the authors concluded as evidence to suggest that the location of lesion, rather than the extent of lesion, determines the emergence of deficit in these domains.

Attentional processes have been examined in children with SCD using various neuropsychological measures, although the evidence is conflicting. Goonan et al[411] concluded that the results obtained from two tests of attention and inhibitory control 'refute the notion of disease-related neurocognitive impairment'. A total of 24 patients (4–15 years) with SCD and no stroke history, and 11 sibling controls (7–15 years), were administered a test of sustained attention (computerized vigilance task), and a test purported to measure cognitive impulsivity (Matching Familiar Figures Test: MFFT). The authors hypothesized that patients would be impaired on both of these tasks compared to controls because of the high incidence of frontal lobe abnormality associated with SCD. However, as no significant differences were found for either of these measures, it was concluded that the development of attention proceeds normally in the presence of SCD in the absence of overt neurological symptoms.

Brown et al[365] assessed sustained attention using a computerized vigilance task ('CPT'), as well as 'selective attention' using the MFFT, in a subgroup of their cohort of 70 children with SCD and 18 sibling controls, i.e. those between 3 and 17 years. A significant effect of group was only found for the CPT, with patients getting a lower 'correct' score than controls, suggesting that this measure is more sensitive to SCD than the MFFT. However, there was a significant independent positive correlation between age and CPT scores (*r*=0.69), suggesting that the group difference on this task may be partly explained by age.

Without CT or MRI evidence it is impossible to confirm the presence or absence of silent infarcts, the presence of which may have been associated with more marked attentional impairment in a proportion of children in these studies. Thus, categorizing children with SCD according to presence or absence of neuropathology may be an appropriate way to confirm whether or not there is disease-related attentional impairment, and indeed if impairment is dependent on the involvement of the frontal lobes, but it would still be important to consider volumetric frontal lobe grey/white matter loss on a continuum.

Craft et al[370] investigated attentional processes in 29 children with SCD who were categorized by MRI into three groups according to lesion location: anterior (ACA or MCA territory; *N*=6), diffuse ('not confined to anterior regions'; *N*=11) and no detectable lesion (*N*=12). The mean age at assessment in all groups was 10 years. Auditory vigilance (detection of target letter) and the total number of intrusions across trials in the Children's Auditory Verbal Learning Test (CAVLT) were compared between patients and 20 sibling controls. The test of auditory vigilance revealed a greater mean number of errors in the anterior group (7.2), than in the diffuse group (5.7), no-lesion group (4.1) and sibling controls (3.6), but these differences were not statistically significant. However, the mean number of intrusions in the CAVLT was significantly greater in the anterior group (12.0) than the sibling control group (2.4).

Schatz et al[410] studied 28 children and young adults with SCD and stroke, aged between 7 and 21 years, and 17 sibling controls of similar age, and found a different neuropsychological profile for patients with multiple 'anterior' and 'posterior' infarcts (determined by MRI; *N*=18), from that in children with infarcts restricted to anterior regions. Patients with 'anterior' infarcts (anterior to the central sulcus; *N*=7) were more likely to score lower on tests of attention and 'executive' skill, for example Test of Variables of Attention (reaction time), whereas patients with more diffuse damage had additional deficits in a large battery of tests of visuo-spatial function. Furthermore, the volume of lesion was significantly associated with visuo-spatial and language measures, but was not significantly associated with attention, memory or executive functions. Once again, this suggests that the location of lesion within anterior brain regions, rather than the extent of the lesion, may be the critical factor associated with attentional impairment. Another study by these authors[412] described impaired visual-search in the visual field contralateral to brain lesion in children with a unilateral left (*N*=14) and right (*N*=7) infarct; bilateral infarcts disrupted visual-search across visual fields. This finding is consistent with that reported by Craft et al,[370] namely that children with bi-frontal infarct lesions due to SCD have deficits in orienting and disengaging visual attention. Moreover, children with SCD without brain infarct were not impaired relative to controls, leading the authors to conclude that it is the presence of a frontal lobe infarct, rather than SCD per se, that leads to visual attention deficit; a similar conclusion was reached by Nabors & Freymuth[413] in their study of attention in children with SCD, with and without stroke.

More direct confirmation of this finding was provided by a study of event-related potentials. Specifically, the error-related negativity component occurs within 200ms of an error response in a choice response task, and has been associated with medial frontal lobe function.[414] This component is significantly attenuated in adolescents with white matter lesions in the dorsal frontal lobes compared to a non-lesion

group.[415] The authors hypothesized that the lesions disconnected the lateral frontal cortex from the ERN generator in the anterior cingulate cortex. This meant that only an impoverished template for successful task performance was available to the error-detection system. The implication is that abnormal performance-monitoring may underpin poor performance in executive function tasks in children with SCD and frontal lobe lesions.

In summary, there is a widely held belief that executive function (particularly attention) is abnormal in children with SCD, and there is evidence to support this assertion. Particularly pertinent is a study by DeBaun et al.[369] In a sample of 28 children with SCD (seven with silent infarct, 21 with overt stroke) and 17 sibling controls, it was found that the Test of Variables of Attention (TOVA) was the most robust neuropsychological measure across a number of domains tested for detecting presence of silent infarct (86% sensitivity).

VISUAL-MOTOR FUNCTION

There is little evidence for significant deficit in this functional domain, and when deficits do occur they may sometimes be associated with processing/motor speed abnormality rather than perceptual deficit per se.

In the early study by Fowler et al,[387] children with SCD obtained a standard score of 71 on the test of Visual-Motor Integration (VMI). This is lower than the normative mean of 100, but not significantly lower than case-controls (75). However, low scores were mostly found in older (>12 years: 71) compared to younger (6–11 years: 93) SCD children, suggesting a decline in visuo-motor skills with increasing age. A similar level of VMI performance (78) was obtained by the children with SCD in the study by Swift et al,[359] but as before, this was not significantly different compared to controls (84). More recently, Noll et al[416] provided further confirmation that the VMI is not sensitive to SCD.

Evidence that there may be a (non-motor) visual deficit was provided by Wasserman et al,[79] although this was only in young children. A total of 43 children with SCD and 30 controls were assessed using the motor skills and visual subscales of the Luria-Nebraska Neuropsychological Battery. Visual but not motor scores significantly differed in young children with SCD compared with controls (8–12 years), but neither significantly differed in the older groups (13–16 years). A similar lack of fine-motor deficit was reported by Brown et al[371] and Noll et al[416] using the Purdue Pegboard; the former study did not report deficit in children with clinical or silent stroke compared to children with a normal MRI scan.

DeBaun et al[369] concluded that visual and motor tests were not sensitive to silent infarct (although attention was). However, children with diffuse infarcts, encroaching on posterior brain regions, reportedly have difficulties with copy and recall conditions of the Benton Visual Retention Test, and the Spatial Relations subtest of the Woodcock Johnson Psychoeducational Battery.[370] Moreover, in a later study by Schatz et al,[410] children with SCD with diffuse lesions (*N*=18) performed poorly compared to those with lesions confined to anterior regions (*N*=7) and sibling controls (*N*=17) on measures of 'Spatial Domain', including position discrimination, judgement of line orientation, pattern construction, visual form discrimination and shape discrimination. The differences between the 'diffuse' group and controls were significant, but the 'anterior' group was not significantly impaired relative to controls. The authors used regression analysis to assess the contribution of lesion location (anterior vs posterior) and lesion volume to spatial performance. Lesion location accounted for 2% of the variance in spatial scores, whereas lesion volume accounted for 13% of the variance. Thus, there was a relationship between lesion volume and spatial scores ($P<0.01$), whereas the location of the lesion only influenced scores via an association with lesion volume. It appears, therefore, that while executive function in children with SCD is sensitive to location of lesion (within the frontal lobes), spatial deficit, when it occurs, is due to the extent of tissue damage rather than the location of damage.

SPEECH AND LANGUAGE

One American group in particular has published multiple studies of speech and language function in children with SCD (Arkansas).[374,417] Three speech and language screening measures were evaluated by Gentry and Dancer[418] in a sample of 50 children with SCD, aged between 3 and 21 years: the Fluharty Preschool Speech & Language Screen in the 3–6 year age group; the Joliet 3-Minute Screen in the 7–14 year age group; and, a 'reading passage' and 'speech sample' in the 15–21 year age group. A pass/fail criterion was determined across these measures. In total, 10% of children obtained a 'fail' score, suggesting an articulation or fluency disorder, which was higher than the authors' anticipated, but this finding should be replicated using an appropriate control group. The other two studies did have a control group. Expressive and receptive language scores obtained using the Clinical Evaluation of Language Fundamentals (CELF) were significantly lower in children with SCD and stroke (*N*=10; mean age 13.3 years) compared to age-sex- and race-matched controls (Expressive: 77 vs 93; Receptive: 76 vs 96; the normative mean is 100, SD 15).[419] However, SCD children without stroke (*N*=9; 3–5 years) did not obtain significantly lower scores compared to controls on measures of auditory comprehension, expressive communication, mean length of utterance or articulation skills ('Preschool Language Scale'; Goldman-Fristoe Test of Articulation) in the study by Gentry and Dancer.[418]

Other investigators have reported a similar lack of deficit in SCD children without a history of stroke. Wasserman et al[79] found no significant difference in language scores between older (13–16 years) 'SCD and no stroke history' and control groups using the Receptive and Expressive Speech scales from the Luria-Nebraska Neuropsychological Battery. However, in the younger children (8–12 years) significantly higher scores (indicative of abnormality) were obtained by the SCD group compared to controls (66 vs 54). Brown et al[365] also found

no difference between SCD children without a history of stroke and controls on the Peabody Picture Vocabulary Test, a measure of receptive language ability, or the Expressive One Word Picture Vocabulary Test, a measure of expressive language ability.

Children with SCD and stroke may be expected to show greater language deficit. In support, 10/14 children with SCD and stroke had 'borderline-retarded' Test of Language Development (TOLD) scores, but it is not clear if these scores were significantly different to controls.[119] In children with SCD with unilateral left (*N*=4) and right (*N*=6) hemisphere stroke, determined by CT or MRI, there was no difference between groups for picture naming (Boston Naming Task), verbal fluency or receptive vocabulary (Peabody Picture Vocabulary Test-Revised), although the sample sizes were small and children with a left hemisphere infarct did obtain lower scores on each measure as may be expected from the adult stroke literature.[368]

Interestingly, the Boston Naming Test did not discriminate between SCD (*N*=30 'no CVA pathology'; *N*=11 silent infarct; *N*=22 'CVA') groups, but the Rapid Automized Naming Test yielded a significantly higher error rate in those with clinical stroke (CVA group) compared to those with no CVA pathology.[371] This suggests that some language difficulties may arise when children with SCD are under pressure of time, providing further support for the hypothesis that processing speed is affected by SCD. It would be informative to conduct further studies investigating speech and language function in relation to both current hearing thresholds (audiometry), and to individual history of ear infection, for example using the Childhood Middle Ear Disease and Hearing Questionnaire (CMEDHQ; see Hind et al[420]).

Overview of cognitive function across early development
The possibility exists that brain function may be compromised from early in life before the peak-incidence of stroke which occurs in mid-childhood.[33] One early survey of parents of 16 infants and toddlers with SCD found that parents commonly reported slow physical development, but that speech and language development appeared normal.[421] However, there are only a few studies reporting the results of developmental assessments in infants with SCD. Wang and colleagues[422] administered the Denver Developmental Screening Test to 344 children with SCD aged between 6 and 60 months, and concluded that development is 'relatively normal' before the age of 3 years. 'Questionable' and 'abnormal' test results were more common in children aged 3–5 years. In a later study, these authors investigated the extent to which early developmental delay (assessed by the Bayley's Scales) was related to neurological abnormality in seven infants with SCD,[422] but only a small number of infants had evidence of pathology (7/39) and half of these also had seizures; nevertheless two children with significant developmental delay had pathology (one posterior cerebral artery stenosis without infarction and one infarction without CVD in the context of seizures).

These studies were cross-sectional, meaning that the opportunity to determine the age at which brain abnormalities start to have an effect on development may have been missed. Thompson and colleagues[423] administered the Bayley Scales of Infant Development longitudinally to a total of 89 infants at 6, 12, 24 and 36 months, and reported a significant decrease in cognitive but not psychomotor functioning from the second year of life. The lack of age- and ethnicity-matched controls in these cohorts is problematical considering that these infants may have been at risk of developmental delay due to social and environmental risk factors, irrespective of SCD.[424]

In order to address these two limitations, another study[415] assessed 14 infants with HbSS SCD and a similar number of age- and ethnic-similar controls, using the Bayley Infant Neurodevelopmental Screen longitudinally during the first year of life (3, 9, 12 months). At each age, infants with SCD obtained scores indicative of significantly greater risk of neurodevelopmental delay compared to controls. Moreover, at 9 months, raw scores significantly correlated with cerebral-blood flow velocity assessed by transcranial Doppler and with haemoglobin; greater risk of neurodevelopmental delay was associated with increased MCA cerebral-blood flow velocity (indicative of brain vulnerability to hypoxaemia) and low haemoglobin count (indicative of anaemia). This suggests that cognitive deficits may start to appear from infancy as the main haemoglobin changes from fetal to sickle, and that SCD might more appropriately be viewed as a neurodevelopmental disorder, a view supported by other researchers.[425] An increasing number of studies indicates the validity of this hypothesis, expanding exploration of early SCD development to other domains of cognitive function, including, importantly, early precursors of executive functions.[426,427]

Of particular interest, recent brain MRI data from the American BABY HUG trial of hyrdroxyurea treatment reported the presence of frontal lobe silent brain infarcts in 13% (3/23) of infants with HbSS SCD, at a mean age of only 13.7 months,[428] confirming the importance of early monitoring.

Behavioural outcome

There is limited evidence that children with SCD are at risk from internalizing and externalizing behaviours. Internalizing behaviours manifest as increased anxiety,[344,345] low self-esteem[345] and depression.[429] Externalizing behaviours may present as hyperactivity, aggression and conduct problems.[400] Social skills and adjustment may also be impaired.[358,430] Moreover, negative thinking has been identified as a potential factor in aggravating painful crises, specifically by compromising the individual's ability to adapt to SCD.[431]

Despite earlier evidence for internalizing behaviours in children with SCD, Swift et al[359] did not find any significant abnormality in 21 children with SCD compared to sibling controls using the Achenbach Social Competence Scales (parental interview). Academic competence was rated as lower in children with SCD, but the authors attributed this to more general cognitive deficit. In support, Goonan et al[411] did not find any

significant differences between children with SCD (*N*=24) and controls (*N*=11) on the Child Behaviour Checklist (CBCL). However, Brown et al[400] studied a larger sample of children with SCD (*N*=63), and found significant group differences for both internalizing and externalizing scales of the CBCL, but not for the Vineland Adaptive Behaviour Scale. The presence of significant findings in the latter study may have been due to the presence of infarct in a proportion of the children. Hariman et al[119] studied children with stroke and also found a trend for abnormal scores compared to controls using the California Test of Personality (self report inventory). This test measures social and personal adjustment.

Longitudinal scores have been provided by a CSSCD study. Thompson et al[378] followed 222 children (5–17 years), approximately half of whom were assessed on two or more occasions over a period of 4 years. The children were categorized into three groups: normal MRI, silent infarct and clinical stroke. At each assessment, mothers completed the CBCL and the Family Environmental Scale (FES), a measure of social environment examining family support style: supportive, conflicted and controlling. All mean 'total behaviour' T scores (CBCL) were below the level of clinical significance (>63), and there were no significant increases or decreases over time: 'normal MRI' group (55, 55, 56, 56); 'silent infarct' group (57, 58, 57, 55); and 'stroke' group (57, 56, 59, 57). Out of 118 children with at least three measures, only 9% were consistently rated as having a behaviour problem. The risk of this problem persisting was significantly increased in those children with a higher baseline level of family conflict, and significantly decreased in those with a higher baseline full scale IQ. Regression analysis showed that full scale IQ did not moderate the effect of family conflict on risk for behaviour problems. Moreover, the risk of behaviour problems was not significantly related to SCD severity. Finally, change in behaviour problem score was sensitive to change in family function, such that behaviour got worse as family conflict increased, a finding that is supported by a more recent study focusing on sibling adjustment.[432]

A study by Kral et al[433] provided ecological verification that neuropsychological evidence of executive dysfunction may also manifest in abnormal everyday behaviour. These authors administered the Behaviour Rating Inventory of Executive Function (BRIEF) to a total of 63 children with SCD without a history of stroke. Children were categorized into three groups on the basis of transcranial Doppler scores; in the absence of cerebrovascular disease, higher cerebral-blood flow velocity is indicative of brain vulnerability to hypoxia. BRIEF scores rated by teachers revealed that children with very high velocities (>200cm/s) had significantly higher incidence of executive dysfunction behaviour ('working memory', 'plan and organize' and 'self-monitor' domains) compared to children with a conditional (170–200cm/s) and a normal (<170cm/s) study. Parents' reported some deficit with behavioural regulation ('inhibiting' and 'shifting' behaviour), but in these measures the conditional group got the least impaired mean score, the abnormal group got the worst score and the normal group were interim. Interestingly, no group differences were reported using the Behavioural Assessment System (BASC), a more general measure of internalizing and externalizing behaviour.

Situational behavioural abnormality, for example at school or at home or both, was also indicated in a study of Nigerian children by Iloeje.[434] Parents and teachers of 84 children with SCD and 84 'classroom controls' aged between 6 and 13 years completed the Rutter Scales. The reported 'psychiatric morbidity' (neuroticism) was significantly higher in the SCD group according to both parents (26% vs 4%) and teachers (22% vs 6%), and teachers noted that boys were more affected; although this may be explained by the higher rate of medical complications in males compared to females.[430,435] Furthermore there was an age effect, such that 15% of children aged 6–8 years had 'psychiatric morbidity', increasing to 30% in children aged 12–13 years, and this was similar in both parents' and teachers' reports. However, only 8% of children were rated as having problems on both parent and teacher scales. The rest were situational, with approximately half showing problems at home only (parent scale) and at school only (teacher scale).

The clinical significance of these behaviour problems is debatable. Cepeda et al[436] used DSM-III-R criteria to identify 31% of their sample of 39 children with SCD as 'positive' for one or more 'mental disorders', but this proportion did not significantly differ from that observed in a group of same-race controls (42%). It was concluded that children with SCD are not at increased risk for clinically significant psychopathology. Indeed Yang et al,[437] reported that 29% of their sample of 38 children with SCD (HbSS; 6–18 years) had scores on the Children's Depression Rating Scale indicating high risk for clinical depression, compared to only 12% of controls (*N*=34). Three domains were particularly affected: somatic; self-esteem; and morbid ideation. However, in support of Cepeda et al,[436] when all children were individually assessed by a psychiatrist, an equal percentage of children in each group were described as having evidence of clinical depression (SCD 13%, controls 15%). The authors suggested that children with SCD may be misidentified by their symptoms, perhaps particularly those symptoms that are somatic, as clinically depressed, but that the true prevalence of clinical depression is not elevated.

Nevertheless, in a study of 89 adults (18–67 years) it was found that there were long-term problems with finding employment and with social relationships.[430] Thus, despite the absence of a clinical diagnosis of psychopathology, subtle behavioural problems may persist into adult life. In an elegant study Boni et al[358] investigated socioemotional processing in children with SCD and stroke (*N*=21) and in children with a normal MRI (*N*=20), aged between 6–17 years, and found that children with SCD and stroke may have difficulty decoding or interpreting certain social situations (verbal and non-verbal cues: facial expressions and emotional prosody in voices), particularly those that are complex or ambiguous. However, these difficulties were subtle and did not impact on caregiver and teacher ratings of social skills competence (Social Skills Rating System), or the child's responses on the Children's Depression Inventory.

Future research
While the studies described herein give some indication of the incidence and nature of cognitive and behavioural deficit associated with SCD, two major limitations have been identified. Firstly, the lack of appropriate control groups is unfortunate, particularly in those studies with large numbers of children with SCD, the results of which have been influential. Secondly, few studies have examined cognitive-behavioural functioning in either very young children or in adults, but the age at which SCD begins to affect development, and the extent to which cognitive deficits improve or persist into adulthood, has implications for our understanding of this condition.

Future research should follow three directions. Firstly, it is important to examine more systematically the impact of cognitive impairment on education and socio-emotional development. Secondly, it is necessary to study longitudinally larger cohorts of infants into childhood. This may provide more information about the age from which cognitive impairment becomes apparent. Thirdly, the investigation of potentially modifiable risk factors in SCD, such as hypoxaemia, may eventually determine the usefulness of intervention during the first few months of life when fetal haemoglobin is replaced by sickle haemoglobin. These three lines of research are not mutually exclusive.

In conclusion, children with SCD and neuropathology are more likely to have a lowered IQ and/or additional cognitive and behavioural deficits, although the possibility has been raised that more modest impairment in children without brain lesions may be related to other processes, such as hypoxaemia, that are evident from early infancy. In order to confirm this hypothesis investigation into SCD will need to be focused on the very young and on the asymptomatic.

17.6 Rehabilitation After Stroke in Children

Anne Gordon and Lucinda Carr

Rehabilitation is the process of alleviating disability[438] and maximizing functional independence. Previous chapters of this text have outlined the breadth and nature of disability arising from stroke in children, and current medical and surgical interventions. In Section 17.2 the outcome of stroke was summarized, and the long-term disabilities that often arise from this condition described. In clinical practice there is limited evidence to guide the clinician in decision making regarding the optimal timing, intensity and nature of rehabilitation for children following acquired brain injury. Generalization of findings from adult stroke intervention studies to children is complicated by developmental considerations both at an individual and environmental level.

In this chapter we will

- review the differences in recovery following stroke in adults and children where it relates to rehabilitation;
- review the models of delivery of paediatric neurorehabilitation and more common modes of therapy provided in current practice;
- make the case for further research in the development of evidence-based interventions for children following stroke.

Rehabilitation – domains of concern

The World Health Organization's International Classification of Functioning, Disability and Health (ICF) (see Section 17.2 for description) is now increasingly used in the arena of rehabilitation practice to frame and define methods and approaches to assessment, intervention and outcomes.[439–441] In rehabilitation practice it is well recognized that the aims of intervention may address body structures and functions, activity, participation and quality of life, and that the focus of intervention may change over time dependent on the stage of recovery, and the needs and priorities of the child and family. Assessment of an individual's functional status is an important component of the rehabilitation process in evaluating intervention.[75,442] Early accurate assessment in adult stroke patients is considered important in predicting outcome, setting realistic and attainable therapeutic goals and facilitating co-ordinated discharge planning.[443]

There are a number of published guidelines for adult stroke rehabilitation.[444–446] In comparison to that for other patient groups such as traumatic brain injury and other types of trauma there is strong evidence for post-acute multidisciplinary rehabilitation[446] (Fig. 17.12), but there is still debate on the performance of rehabilitation services due to inconsistencies (and inherent difficulties) in measuring and comparing heterogeneous services and populations at multiple time points using different measures. It has been suggested that

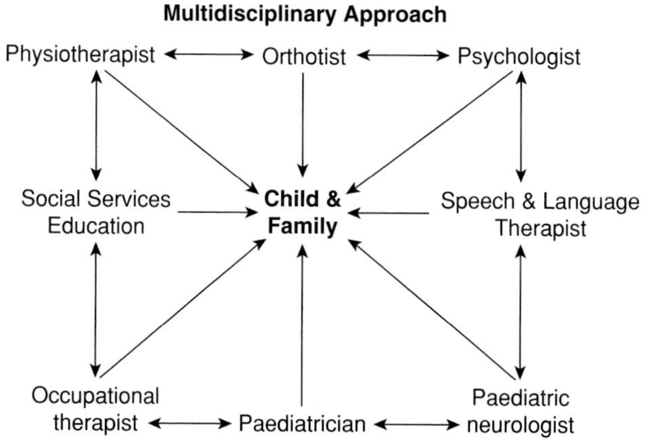

clinical and health policy decision making should be made around the measurement of the quality and outcomes of rehabilitation intervention[447] as well as service structure and process of care.[448] In the smaller field of paediatric rehabilitation, much of this debate also exists, with an even more limited evidence base.

Adult vs child stroke recovery and rehabilitation

The comparative rarity of paediatric stroke, and the ability of the family unit to take on a large part of post-acute care, contrasts with the large numbers of adults requiring rehabilitation following a stroke. A stroke in infancy or childhood presents the possibility of living through adulthood with a chronic disability. Within the first year alone, the healthcare costs following stroke in children are considerable.[78] Over half of the children surviving arterial ischaemic stroke will live with moderate to severe disabilities.[91]

It has been estimated that 90% of adults will have some degree of motor impairment following a stroke, with patients reaching at least half of their eventual best score of motor scales within 2 weeks of stroke and most recovery occurring in the first 3 months.[449] In the long-term approximately half of stroke survivors make a 'good' recovery as measured by Barthel Index scores at 6 months. There are, however, concerns raised in the literature that the consequences of stroke remain underestimated, and that impairments in memory, thinking, mood, emotion and communication skills may also impact functional outcome and quality of life but be under-detected.[450]

Despite the significant resources invested in developing adult neurorehabilitation, there are still wide variations in clinical practice. Most research on rehabilitation focuses on the first 6 months following stroke. Such is the lack of consensus in adult stroke rehabilitation treatments however (in the amount of therapy received and the nature and timing of rehabilitation) that large cross-centre studies have been difficult.[451] There has also been conflicting evidence regarding the effects of duration and intensity of therapy services on outcome.[452] A recent Cochrane review of the literature on community-based rehabilitation more than 1 year following a stroke concluded there was inconclusive evidence of benefits.[453]

Even where guidelines exist resource limitations mean that they are frequently not followed. For example, despite resource allocation in accordance with established guidelines in adult stroke care units, a surprisingly limited amount of therapy and physical activity have been found to take place in the early acute phase of rehabilitation.[454]

It has been found that functional recovery may occur up to 2 years and beyond, following acquired brain injury.[455] A widely held belief is that spontaneous recovery of function occurs during the first 6 months following onset of brain injury. After this period it has been speculated that the gains may be attributed to learning through rehabilitation training.[456] The concept of a recovery plateau following a stroke has remained ambiguous. A recent review of this topic suggested the method of measurement of recovery and consideration

Multidisciplinary Approach

Fig. 17.12. Elements of the multidisciplinary team needed to rehabilitate the child who has had a stroke and to support the family.

of the individual's functioning in addition to external factors such as service provision, physical and social environment, attitudes of professionals and the patient themselves, may influence the perception of a plateau in recovery.[457]

Rehabilitation following acquired brain injury aims to maximize the potential of the brain to change in response to injury, experience or external stimulation.[458] Neuroimaging and neurophysiological techniques have been applied to examine the relationship between brain and behavioural recovery and can therefore inform clinical practice. The cellular changes that occur as the brain recovers from injury are hypothesized to include alteration in the growth of neurones and the strength of synaptic connections; changes in functional representation patterns within the cortex including activation in secondary areas normally connected to the injured area; shift in interhemispheric lateralization to the contralesional hemisphere; and changes in functional maps surrounding the infarcted area.[458,459] Behavioural recovery is thought to be supported by such reorganization of surviving brain tissue, and the best outcomes after stroke in adults associated with the greatest return to the normal state of brain functional organization.[459] Genetics, pre- and post-stroke environmental enrichment, drugs, pre-stroke status, site and size of brain lesion, and demographics have been identified as influencing early spontaneous recovery from stroke in adults.[459]

Of interest to rehabilitation practitioners is the ability to influence this process through the use of external interventions and behavioural training. Functional neuroimaging may have a role in not only improving our understanding of the changes in functional connectivity of the brain over time following injury, but also enabling us to predict recovery, select individuals for intervention and explore the response of the brain to specific interventions.[460] The more commonly applied rehabilitation interventions are summarized later in this chapter.

Paediatric neurorehabilitation

One could argue that paediatric acquired brain injury (ABI) rehabilitation is even more complicated to measure than adult neurorehabilitation. The developmental, educational, family and social considerations through the changing panorama of development from infancy through to adolescence, complicates the ability to measure response to intervention meaningfully. There are fewer specialist rehabilitation facilities for children than adults. Post-acute intervention is more likely to be home or community based in paediatrics, have lesser funds for development of outcome measurement, and address children with wide-ranging illness and disabilities. Despite awareness of the ongoing functional daily life implications of paediatric acquired brain injury, there is limited research investigating the effectiveness of rehabilitation. Children's rehabilitation has until recently been based on evidence from adult rehabilitation. In this rapidly developing field; however, the importance of growth, child development and the occupations of children (i.e. usual activities and participation) are now recognized as central to practice.[461]

When compared with adult populations, there are fewer measures of outcome or functional ability available in paediatrics, particularly measures of response to intervention. Furthermore there is no established uniformity in their application in clinical practice. It is suggested that to sensitively capture all domains of health a combination of measures is indicated.[462] For example, it is unlikely that a single tool could measure an individual's performance from infancy to adolescence in the areas of communication, cognition and mobility, and at the same time capture the amount of assistance required within the child's usual environmental considerations (social, physical, educational, etc.).

Functionally based individualized goal-setting is now mainstream practice in rehabilitation. Tools such as the Canadian Occupational Performance Measure and Goal Attainment Scaling are used in clinical and research practice.[463] Goal setting usually involves interview and observation of the individual (and/or carers) and may meet a number of aims. These include engagement of the individual's active participation and motivation in the rehabilitation process, to improve the outcome of rehabilitation (as evaluated by standard measures), to measure outcome of direct relevance to the individual, and in some settings this may also be required to meet legal or professional standards/requirements.

Models of delivery of paediatric neurorehabilitation

Paediatric neurorehabilitation is now generally family-centred in approach, with the child and family central to the rehabilitation process and actively involved in decision making and goal setting. In clinical practice variations exist in how this philosophy is applied.[464] The optimal duration, nature and timing of rehabilitation remain largely unknown. Rehabilitation often reduces or is discontinued after discharge from inpatient care due to lack of resources or documented progress. In children the concept of recovery itself is somewhat different to that described in the adults, with the focus of rehabilitation not only on recovery of pre-morbid abilities but on continued acquisition of developmentally appropriate skills.

With individual service variation in admission criteria and determination of clinical need, it is challenging to specify optimal service delivery. Many services discharge children from inpatient facilities as soon as practicable and use community-based services to enable the child to return to their usual social and educational setting as soon as possible. Inpatient services vary from paediatric hospital ward-based services, to dedicated rehabilitation facilities on-site or off-site but linked with a paediatric hospital, to community based inpatient or outpatient centres, and home- and school-delivered services. During recovery from brain injury the early acute phase of intervention may consist of stabilization of basic functions/abilities, including neurological status and minimization of early complications such as changes in tone/behaviour/pain/sensory functioning. Following this the post-acute inpatient rehabilitation phase consists of more intensive allied health input, promotion of recovery of pre-existing functioning, ongoing development of new developmentally appropriate skills and compensation for impairments of function.[465] Discharge planning may involve assessment and intervention of home, school and social environments and strategies to facilitate re-integration. Following discharge from inpatient intervention, outpatient care is usually supported by community-based services to facilitate the return of the child into family, social, community and educational environments. Review and intervention may focus on maintenance of function, or trouble-shooting changes in function related to ongoing development and long-term recovery.

INTERVENTION

In the absence of robust empirical evidence for particular intervention types or their optimal pattern of delivery, clinical decision making may be influenced by therapists' clinical experience, that of their peer group and the framework from which they practise. The following are some of the more common clinical interventions applied in isolation or combination to children following stroke and other types of acquired brain injury. Motor interventions are more commonly described than cognitive, behavioural, social or language interventions.

Trombly[466] defines rehabilitation as predominantly a learning process. Treatment therefore should adhere to basic principles of learning, in that the skills being taught are meaningful to the individual, that difficulty be graded and appropriate feedback provided. Practice should be structured to promote learning and encourage transfer between environment and contexts used by the patient. Compensatory strategies may also be applied, and may be physiological, physical, behavioural, environmental, psychological or social. The extent of the impact of compensation on recovery needs evaluation. Paediatric rehabilitation may involve re-education of preexisting skills, compensation for missing functional abilities (when functional deficits persist), and promotion of development of more refined skills within the developmental trajectory appropriate for the individual.

There is as yet little published evidence for the efficacy of intervention (predominantly motor) in the paediatric stroke population. Anecdotally, the motor outcome for children, particularly in the later acquired subgroup, may be one of emerging hemidystonia. Spasticity, the target of most current paediatric rehabilitation techniques, is less common in this group. The following reviews may be of interest to readers in addressing areas allied to paediatric stroke; the medical and therapeutic management of the upper limb in cerebral palsy;[467] early developmental interventions for preterm infants.[468]

THERAPY APPROACHES

The following predominantly motor-oriented approaches are those more widely described in the adult stroke population, and to a lesser extent in the cerebral palsy and child head injury populations. Clinicians working in physiotherapy, occupational therapy and speech pathology aim to restore and promote further development of optimal functional skills. Consideration in these motor-based approaches may include

management of abnormal muscle tone and the prevention of biomechanical changes in muscle. Treatment approaches differ in their particular emphasis with respect to tone and biomechanics, and practice/repetition of functional activities relevant to the individual. Some specific therapy techniques are discussed below:

Bobath/neurodevelopment treatment

The Bobath (Neurodevelopmental Treatment) approach was originally developed in the treatment of adult stroke patients. In children it has been applied mainly to the cerebral palsy population, but also to some children with acquired brain injury. The basis of this concept is that abnormal posture and movement as a result of brain injury may be influenced by therapist handling to alter postural tone and movement patterns. The aim is that through their experience of more normal sensorimotor experiences within a functional context, the child will be able to gain carry-over from therapy for greater functional independence. There is some evidence that increased frequency of general neurodevelopmental therapy may be helpful for children with spastic cerebral palsy;[468] however, this approach requires further evidence of efficacy.

Constraint-induced movement therapy

Constraint-induced movement therapy originally developed to improve activity of the affected upper limb following a stroke and involves restraining the unaffected upper limb during daily sessions of practice using the impaired upper extremity.[469] Recently, modified versions of this approach have been used in the rehabilitation of children with congenital and acquired hemiplegia with good effect.[470-476] There is one study of modified constraint-induced movement therapy in eight children who had had an arterial ischaemic stroke between the ages of 1 month and 7 years. Two withdrew – one because of the development of epilepsy and the other withdrawing consent because of the intensity of the therapy.[477] Of the six who completed 4 weeks of treatment, three each had predominantly spasticity or dystonia. There were no significant improvements in sensorimotor function or quality of upper limb movement with modified constraint therapy, although all children improved in individual therapy goals related to functional performance and children and parents were positive about the intervention.[477] Further investigation is required to determine optimal intervention and definition of which children are most likely to benefit.[478] For example, the relative benefit of the 'shaping' therapy approach taken while wearing a constraint (e.g. mitt or splint) is not yet clear, as opposed to a 'forced-use' approach, i.e. wearing the constraint but without the additional activity-based programme.

Strength training

The literature suggests that progressive resistive exercise of isolated muscle groups improves muscle performance with no adverse effects on muscle spasticity.[479,480] In adult stroke patients and children with cerebral palsy it has been shown that progressive resistance training improves muscle strength without increasing spasticity, but with variable functional gains.[481–484]

Bimanual coordination/training
Based on the principles of motor learning (targeted practice, specific type of practice and structured feedback related to motivation), this is an intensive approach using structured task practice in bimanual play and functional activities.[121,485] Theoretically this approach utilizes the intensive practice component of the constraint therapy, without the need for constraint which impacts bimanual functional hand use during therapy. This approach has shown promising results in a recently published randomized controlled trial;[477] however, larger trials are required to determine optimal population selection and intensity of intervention.

Contralesional repetitive transcranial magnetic stimulation
A pilot randomized controlled trial showed that contralesional inhibitory repetitive transcranial magnetic stimulation (rTMS) was safe and feasible for patients with paediatric subcortical AIS, and seemed to improve hand function in patients with hemiparesis.[486] However, syncope was documented in two patients.[487]

Functional electrical stimulation
Functional electrical stimulation appears to be useful in improving gait after severe hemiplegia in adults, although this is rarely a problem in children. Research on its use in improving function in the upper limb is in progress.

Virtual reality therapy
This new neurorehabilitation approach aims to improve movement performance in children with brain injury. This approach has been shown to improve upper limb function in adults with chronic hemiparesis[488,489] and a pilot in three children with severe congenital hemiparesis showed promise,[490] but further studies are required in paediatric practice. Virtual reality equipment varies, but usually consists of computer-generated surroundings in which the patient is either partly or fully immersed. Some systems require the patient to wear head-mounted visual display equipment. The fundamental premise is that the child is engaged in an audio-visual computer-based program requiring motor responses to participate in the activities presented. The activity protocol can be selected by the clinician to target the patient's clinical needs, for example promotion of range of movement, response speed and strength. Biofeedback frequency can be adjusted to maintain interest and motivation. This intervention has potential in terms of maximizing attention to activity and enabling a variety of settings to progressively challenge an individual to be achieved. A negative element is the cost of the equipment set-up.

Orthotics
Orthoses may be prescribed for a child following stroke. The aim of orthotic prescription may include stabilization and alignment of joints, reduction or prevention of muscle contracture through stretching, and encouragement of more normal and functional movement and sensory feedback. Splinting is an adjunct to treatment, though not a treatment in its own right, and may affect not only the parts splinted but also movement in general.[491] Orthoses are often used in tandem with medical intervention (see below) to maximize functional gains. Optimal regimes of wear for orthoses are not universally agreed. Soft casting (and sometimes thermoplastic splinting) can be used during the acute and subacute phases if spasticity onset places joints and muscles at risk of contractures and deformity. The presence of spasticity, dystonia, or a combination of the two, may, however, place an individual at risk of joint changes, muscle/tendon shortening and/or reduced selective control of a limb. Orthoses may be required long-term to maintain function and maximize range of motion.

The upper limb orthoses commonly prescribed for children with upper limb dysfunction following a stroke are these:

• Thermoplastic/rigid/static for rest (or lower profile for function) – e.g. long finger flexors, wrist, thumb web space
• Neoprene/lycra wrist extension/thumb abduction for function
• Lycra garments for arm/hand.

Lower limb splints include the following:

• Static ankle-foot orthoses
• Hinged/dynamic ankle-foot orthoses/callipers
• Dynamic foot orthoses.

Considerations in the use of orthoses include a rationale for the splint provision (maintain/regain joint range or influence muscle imbalance); how the splint affects movement; do the benefits of wearing the splint (e.g. maintenance of joint range) outweigh the risks (muscle atrophy); whether the carers and child are aware of the regime and precautions; and ensuring regular review is arranged.

OTHER APPROACHES
A number of other approaches are emerging in the literature with an emphasis on context, functional environment and targeted repetition of skills. These approaches combine cognitive, social and behavioural strategies and in some cases share principles with some of the specific motor strategies described above.

Enriched environment/ecological approach
An ecological approach to recovery from brain injury postulates that recovery does not happen spontaneously, but as the result of complex interactions between the child and a stimulating environment (or ecology). This environment may include learning opportunities of appropriate intensity and frequency (e.g. experience of sitting, using hands in play); creating the need in the child to extend their functional abilities in daily life activities (e.g. the peer group in the classroom); facilitating learning of these functions actively; providing regular and appropriate challenges; and providing goal-directed

activities.[492] Using this ecological model of development for children with brain injury, the authors describe a child's rehabilitative environment is thought to consist of external factors (such as a stimulating environment) and internal factors (such as attitude, determination, will, cognitive abilities). While in general terms the fundamental concepts of this approach may seem to be central to standard rehabilitative practice, proponents of this approach state that it extends well beyond time-limited therapies. Further research is required to explore the relationship between brain pathology, the individual and the environment in relation to recovery.

Cognitive and behavioural strategies

This approach uses augmentative information to promote problem solving and learning. While there is limited evidence in the paediatric population, it has been applied to supplement motor learning in children with cerebral palsy.[493]

Our clinical experience is that cognitive strategies are commonly provided during motor skill acquisition activities, especially in grading challenge for an individual through grading of amount and complexity of input. Further research is required to develop this approach. Behavioural strategies include support for positive behaviours and contingency management.[494] While evidence is building there is not yet robust evidence for efficacy of particular approaches.

Medication

There are a number of drugs which by neuromodulation at either central or peripheral levels will reduce spasticity and stretch reflexes, but there is less evidence that they are consistently useful in reducing disability following stroke.[495] Both systemic and focal medications have an important role in the management of abnormal tone following stroke in both the acute and chronic setting.[496] However, in children there are no published guidelines for the 'best use' of medication in children with stroke. Most published studies describe children with cerebral palsy and because of the paucity of robust and meaningful outcome measures it is often difficult to gauge the real effects of intervention on function. Futhermore there is a lack of comparative studies between different medications. Where possible goals should be explicit and outcomes measured.

All medications have potential side-effects so that any trial of treatment needs careful evaluation and the costs and benefits assessed. Any medication given must be considered within the context of the child's overall management, i.e. other medical, social and educational issues. It is important to identify any exacerbating (noxious) factors such as intercurrent illness, epilepsy, gastro-oesophageal reflux, constipation, skin trauma, etc., and to consider the immediate effects of emotion and fatigue, all of which may profoundly affect tone. Discussion with the child and his or her regular carers and therapists is mandatory since the functional impact of abnormal tone and the effects of medication will vary between individuals and the goals of treatment should be clear.

Systemic medication

Systemic medication may be indicated if spasticity or dystonia is widespread and causing discomfort or significant cosmetic or functional impairment. A number of drugs may be considered either alone or in combination. The most commonly used are listed in Table 17.8. In UK practice baclofen, which acts as a $GABA_B$ agonist, is most commonly used for spasticity. It is less sedating than diazepam and does not result in long-term tolerance and dependence,[497] although rebound seizures have been reported with sudden withdrawal (see data sheet). Dantrolene acts directly on peripheral muscle and may have

TABLE 17.8
Drugs commonly used in the treatment of spasticity and dystonia

Drug	Mode of action	Dose	Side effects
Spasticity			
Diazepam	$GABA_A$ agonist at central and spinal cord level	Child: <10kg 2mg twice a day; >20kg 10mg twice a day	Sedation, ataxia, weakness, tolerance and dependence
Baclofen	$GABA_B$ agonist at spinal cord level. Increases inhibition	0.2–1mg/kg three times a day	Sedation, ataxia (central hypotonia), weakness, altered seizure control
Dantrolene[a]	Inhibits calcium release from sarcoplasmic reticulum	0.5–3mg/kg four times a day	Drowsiness, hepatotoxicity[b]
Tizanidine[a]	α_2 adrenergic receptor agonist, inhibits polysynaptic reflex	Adults 2mg three to four times a day	Drowsiness, dizziness, dry mouth, occasional hepatoxicity, hypotension
Dystonia			
Trihexyphenidyl hydrochloride[a] (benzhexol)	Central and peripheral anticholinergic action	Initially 1mg twice a day; increase as tolerated by 1mg every 4 days (often 2–3mg/kg/day)	Dry mouth, pupil dilatation, urinary retention, constipation
L-Dopa[a]	Dopamine agonists	Initially 0.5mg/kg twice a day; may require 8–10mg/kg/day	Nausea, agitation

[a] Not licensed for use in children. [b] Regular check of liver function tests recommended.

fewer central side-effects, but can cause unwanted generalized weakness. In addition to the drugs listed, newer agents such as gabapentin, modafinil and vigabatrin may also have a role.

In adults and children with severe hypotonia after stroke, intrathecal baclofen may be considered if spasticity remains intractable despite conventional therapy.[498,499] Direct administration of baclofen into the intrathecal space enhances local concentration at spinal cord level and minimizes central side-effects. There is clear evidence of reduction in spasticity and spasms and the suggestion of improvement in general function and quality of life in many patients. This treatment is only available at specialized centres.

When managing dystonia, benzhexol is the drug of choice. In contrast to adults, children often tolerate high doses if introduced gradually. The dose should be increased until there is symptomatic relief or side-effects occur. Both baclofen and L-Dopa may also have a role in treating secondary dystonia.

Focal treatment

Motor deficits after childhood stroke are often focal, so that targeted treatment of spasticity and dystonia may be more attractive than systemic medication. The aims of modifying tone may include improvement in function, cosmesis or in provision of care. As with all interventions the goals of intervention need to be clarified before treatment is undertaken. Botulinum toxin A (BTA) is derived from *Clostridium botulinum*. When injected into a muscle it is rapidly taken up at the neuromuscular junction where it prevents vesicle release of acetyl choline, effectively causing chemical denervation. Its effects last around 3 months until a new neuromuscular junction is established by compensatory sprouting. A number of studies have successfully used BTA in the management of spasticity in adults after stroke.[500–503] In paediatric practice BTA is currently only licensed for use in the management of the equinus foot in ambulant children with cerebral palsy. However, it is increasingly used in the management of cerebral palsy in both upper and lower limbs. Whilst definitive best practice still needs to be clarified, published guidelines exist as to its use in this population.[348,504,505] These papers stress the importance of careful patient selection and assessment by a team who have experience of the natural history of the underlying motor disorder. BTA is increasingly used more widely in other chronic spastic and dystonic conditions of childhood. It has a recognized and valuable role in the acute management of the acquired motor disorders such as those resulting from head injury and stroke, where contractures may evolve rapidly. Side-effects are infrequent and transitory, excessive weakness being the most troublesome.[506]

Conclusion

There are many potential sequelae of paediatric stroke. However because of the heterogeneity of the group and the lack of robust measures, the impact of stroke in childhood is almost certainly underestimated. There are significant gaps in our knowledge of the effectiveness of specific interventions in paediatric stroke and allied acquired brain injury populations. Development of valid, standard and reliable measures continues to be crucial in building rehabilitation evidence.

Guidelines for the management of adult and childhood stroke have been produced.[32] In the face of limited evidence for particular rehabilitation frameworks or approaches, and heterogeneous rehabilitation providers and populations, there is a need for further studies of the effectiveness of intervention. This may be achieved on a relatively small scale with non-randomized studies in addition to facilities where randomized controlled trials are possible.

Much remains to be learned regarding patient selection and intensity, duration and type of intervention selection in relation to outcome. Benefits should be evaluated both in terms of functional daily abilities, in addition to quality of life and burden of care to families and society in general.

We would argue that paediatric stroke warrants targeted input, especially during the early period of recovery and rehabilitation, but also beyond. Addressing the rehabilitation needs of children with stroke may also serve as a useful model in considering the needs of other children with acquired brain injury as the natural history in these groups contrasts with the needs of children with congenital pathologies, the largest user group of paediatric therapy services.

REFERENCES

1. DeVivo DC, Holmes SJ, Dodge PR. Cerebrovascular Disease in a Pediatric Population. Ann Neurol 1977; 2(3):261–262.
2. Dusser A, Goutieres F, Aicardi J. Ischemic strokes in children. J Child Neurol 1986; 1(2):131–136.
3. Riikonen R, Santavuori P. Hereditary and acquired risk factors for childhood stroke. Neuropediatrics 1994; 25(5):227–233.
4. Mancini J, Girard N, Chabrol B, Lamoureux S, Livet MO, Thuret I et al. Ischemic cerebrovascular disease in children: retrospective study of 35 patients. J Child Neurol 1997; 12(3):193–199.
5. Abram HS, Knepper LE, Warty VS, Painter MJ. Natural history, prognosis, and lipid abnormalities of idiopathic ischemic childhood stroke. J Child Neurol 1996; 11(4):276–282.
6. Lanthier S, Carmant L, David M, Larbrisseau A, de Veber G. Stroke in children: the coexistence of multiple risk factors predicts poor outcome. Neurology 2000; 54(2):371–378.
7. Chabrier S, Husson B, Lasjaunias P, Landrieu P, Tardieu M. Stroke in childhood: outcome and recurrence risk by mechanism in 59 patients. J Child Neurol 2000; 15(5):290–294.
8. De Schryver EL, Kappelle LJ, Jennekens-Schinkel A, Boudewyn Peters AC. Prognosis of ischemic stroke in childhood: a long-term follow-up study. Dev Med Child Neurol 2000; 42(5):313–318.
9. Steinlin M, Pfister I, Pavlovic J, Everts R, Boltshauser E, Capone MA et al. The first three years of the Swiss Neuropaediatric Stroke Registry (SNPSR): a population-based study of incidence, symptoms and risk factors. Neuropediatrics 2005; 36(2):90–97.
10. Barnes C, Newall F, Furmedge J, Mackay M, Monagle P. Arterial ischaemic stroke in children. J Paediatr Child Health 2004; 40(7):384–387.
11. Chung B, Wong V. Pediatric stroke among Hong Kong Chinese subjects. Pediatrics 2004; 114(2):e206–e212.
12. Brankovic-Sreckovic V, Milic-Rasic V, Jovic N, Milic N, Todorovic S. The recurrence risk of ischemic stroke in childhood. Med Princ Pract 2004; 13(3):153–158.

13. Salih MA, Abdel-Gader AG, Al-Jarallah AA, Kentab AY, Al-Nasser MN. Outcome of stroke in Saudi children. Saudi Med J 2006; 27(Suppl 1):S91–S96.

14. Ganesan V, Prengler M, Wade A, Kirkham FJ. Clinical and radiological recurrence after childhood arterial ischemic stroke. Circulation 2006; 114(20):2170–2177.

15. Fullerton HJ, Wu YW, Sidney S, Johnston SC. Risk of recurrent childhood arterial ischemic stroke in a population-based cohort: the importance of cerebrovascular imaging. Pediatrics 2007; 119(3):495–501.

16. Portnoy BA, Herion JC. Neurological manifestations in sickle-cell disease, with a review of the literature and emphasis on the prevalence of hemiplegia. Ann Intern Med 1972; 76(4):643–652.

17. Powars D, Wilson B, Imbus C, Pegelow C, Allen J. The natural history of stroke in sickle cell disease. Am J Med 1978; 65(3):461–471.

18. Wood DH. Cerebrovascular complications of sickle cell anemia. Stroke 1978; 9(1):73–75.

19. Wilimas J, Goff JR, Anderson HR, Jr, Langston JW, Thompson E. Efficacy of transfusion therapy for one to two years in patients with sickle cell disease and cerebrovascular accidents. J Pediatr 1980; 96(2):205–208.

20. Moohr JW, Wilson H, Pang EJ. Strokes and their management in sickle cell disease. In: Comparative Clinical Aspects of Sickle Cell Disease (ed W Fried). Amsterdam: Elsevier, 1982; 101–111.

21. Balkaran B, Char G, Morris JS, Thomas PW, Serjeant BE, Serjeant GR. Stroke in a cohort of patients with homozygous sickle cell disease. J Pediatr 1992; 120(3):360–366.

22. Russell MO, Goldberg HI, Hodson A, Kim HC, Halus J, Reivich M et al. Effect of transfusion therapy on arteriographic abnormalities and on recurrence of stroke in sickle cell disease. Blood 1984; 63(1):162–169.

23. Njamnshi AK, Mbong EN, Wonkam A, Ongolo-Zogo P, Djientcheu VD, Sunjoh FL et al. The epidemiology of stroke in sickle cell patients in Yaounde, Cameroon. J Neurol Sci 2006; 250(1–2):79–84.

24. Fatunde OJ, Adamson FG, Ogunseyinde O, Sodeinde O, Familusi JB. Stroke in Nigerian children with sickle cell disease. Afr J Med Sci 2005; 34(2):157–160.

25. Dobson SR, Holden KR, Nietert PJ, Cure JK, Laver JH, Disco D et al. Moyamoya syndrome in childhood sickle cell disease: a predictive factor for recurrent cerebrovascular events. Blood 2002; 99(9):3144–3150.

26. Scothorn DJ, Price C, Schwartz D, Terrill C, Buchanan GR, Shurney W et al. Risk of recurrent stroke in children with sickle cell disease receiving blood transfusion therapy for at least five years after initial stroke. J Pediatr 2002; 140(3):348–354.

27. Straeter R, Becker S, von Eckardstein, Heinecke A, Gutsche S, Junker R et al. Prospective assessment of risk factors for recurrent stroke during childhood – a 5-year follow-up study. Lancet 2002; 360(9345):1540–1545.

28. Nowak-Göttl U, Kirkham FJ, Chan AK, Sträter R, Ganesan V, Prengler M et al. Recurrent stroke: the role of prothrombotic disorders. J Thromb Haemostasis 2005; 3(Suppl 1), OR355-http://www.blackwellpublishing.com/isth2005/abstract.asp?id=48021

29. Danchaivijitr N, Cox TC, Saunders DE, Ganesan V. Evolution of cerebral arteriopathies in childhood arterial ischemic stroke. Ann Neurol 2006; 59(4):620–626.

30. Steinlin M, Roellin K, Schroth G. Long-term follow-up after stroke in childhood. Eur J Pediatr 2004; 163(4–5):245–250.

31. Imaizumi C, Imaizumi T, Osawa M, Fukuyama Y, Takeshita M. Serial intelligence test scores in pediatric moyamoya disease. Neuropediatrics 1999; 30(6):294–299.

32. Royal College of Physicians. Stroke in Childhood: Clinical Guidelines for Diagnosis, Management and Rehabilitation. 2004. http://www.rcplondon.ac.uk/pubs/.../childstroke/childstroke_guidelines.pdf

33. Lanthier S, Kirkham FJ, Mitchell LG, Laxer RM, Atenafu E, Male C et al. Increased anticardiolipin antibody IgG titers do not predict recurrent stroke or TIA in children. Neurology 2004; 62(2):194–200.

34. Pegelow CH, Macklin EA, Moser FG, Wang WC, Bello JA, Miller ST et al. Longitudinal changes in brain magnetic resonance imaging findings in children with sickle cell disease. Blood 2002; 99(8):3014–3018.

35. Kenet G, Kirkham F, Niederstadt T, Heinecke A, Saunders D, Stoll M et al. Risk factors for recurrent venous thromboembolism in the European collaborative paediatric database on cerebral venous thrombosis: a multicentre cohort study. Lancet Neurol 2007; 6(7):595–603.

36. Roach ES. Immediate surgery for moyamoya syndrome? Not necessarily. Arch Neurol 2001; 58(1):130–131.

37. Scott RM. Surgery for moyamoya syndrome? Yes. Arch Neurol 2001; 58(1):128–129.

38. Chiu D, Shedden P, Bratina P, Grotta JC. Clinical features of moyamoya disease in the United States. Stroke 1998; 29(7):1347–1351.

39. Yilmaz EY, Pritz MB, Bruno A, Lopez-Yunez A, Biller J. Moyamoya: Indiana University Medical Center experience. Arch Neurol 2001; 58(8):1274–1278.

40. Fung LW, Thompson D, Ganesan V. Revascularization surgery for paediatric moyamoya: a review of the literature. Childs Nerv Syst 2005; 21(5):358–364.

41. Pegelow CH, Adams RJ, McKie V, Abboud M, Berman B, Miller ST et al. Risk of recurrent stroke in patients with sickle cell disease treated with erythrocyte transfusions. J Pediatr 1995; 126(6):896–899.

42. Vichinsky E. New therapies in sickle cell disease. Lancet 2002; 360(9333):629–631.

43. Vernet O, Montes JL, O'Gorman AM, Baruchel S, Farmer JP. Encephaloduroarterio-synangiosis in a child with sickle cell anemia and moyamoya disease. Pediatr Neurol 1996; 14(3):226–230.

44. Smith ER, McClain CD, Heeney M, Scott RM. Pial synangiosis in patients with moyamoya syndrome and sickle cell anemia: perioperative management and surgical outcome. Neurosurg Focus 2009; 26(4):E10.

45. Hankinson TC, Bohman LE, Heyer G, Licursi M, Ghatan S, Feldstein NA et al. Surgical treatment of moyamoya syndrome in patients with sickle cell anemia: outcome following encephaloduroarteriosynangiosis. J Neurosurg Pediatr 2008; 1(3):211–216.

46. Walters MC, Storb R, Patience M, Leisenring W, Taylor T, Sanders JE et al. Impact of bone marrow transplantation for symptomatic sickle cell disease: an interim report. Multicenter investigation of bone marrow transplantation for sickle cell disease. Blood 2000; 95(6):1918–1924.

47. deVeber G. In pursuit of evidence-based treatments for paediatric stroke: the UK and Chest guidelines. Lancet Neurol 2005; 4(7):432–436.

48. Straeter R, Kurnik K, Heller C, Schobess R, Luigs P, Nowak-Gottl U. Aspirin versus low-dose low-molecular-weight heparin: antithrombotic therapy in pediatric ischemic stroke patients: a prospective follow-up study. Stroke 2001; 32(11):2554–2558.

49. Burak CR, Bowen MD, Barron TF. The use of enoxaparin in children with acute, nonhemorrhagic ischemic stroke. Pediatr Neurol 2003; 29(4):295–298.

50. Bowen MD, Burak CR, Barron TF. Childhood ischemic stroke in a nonurban population. J Child Neurol 2005; 20(3):194–197.

51. Herguner MO, Incecik F, Elkay M, Altunbasak S, Baytok V. Evaluation of 39 children with stroke regarding etiologic risk factors and treatment. Turk J Pediatr 2005; 47(2):116–119.

52. Gokben S, Tosun A, Bayram N, Serdaroglu G, Polat M, Kavakli K et al. Arterial ischemic stroke in childhood: risk factors and outcome in old versus new era. J Child Neurol 2007; 22(10):1204–1208.

53. Soman T, Rafay MF, Hune S, Allen A, MacGregor D, deVeber G. The risks and safety of clopidogrel in pediatric arterial ischemic stroke. Stroke 2006; 37(4):1120–1122.

54. Bonduel M, Sciuccati G, Hepner M, Pieroni G, Torres AF, Frontroth JP et al. Arterial ischemic stroke and cerebral venous thrombosis in children: a 12-year Argentinean registry. Acta Haematol 2006; 115(3–4):180–185.

55. Toure A, Chabrier S, Plagne M-D, Presles E, des Portes V, Rousselle C. Neurological outcome and risk of recurrence depending on the anterior vs posterior arterial distribution in children with stroke. Neuropediatrics 2010; 40(3):126–128.

56. deVeber G, Kirkham F. Guidelines for the treatment and prevention of stroke in children. Lancet Neurol 2008; 7(11):983–985.

57. Lyrer P, Engelter S. Antithrombotic drugs for carotid artery dissection. Cochrane Database Syst Rev 2000;(4):CD000255.

58. Arauz A, Hoyos L, Espinoza C, Cantu C, Barinagarrementeria F, Roman G. Dissection of cervical arteries: long-term follow-up study of 130 consecutive cases. Cerebrovasc Dis 2006; 22(2–3):150–154.

59. Fullerton HJ, Johnston SC, Smith WS. Arterial dissection and stroke in children. Neurology 2001; 57(7):1155–1160.

60. Ganesan V, Chong WK, Cox TC, Chawda SJ, Prengler M, Kirkham FJ. Posterior circulation stroke in childhood: risk factors and recurrence. Neurology 2002; 59(10):1552–1556.

61. Rafay MF, Armstrong D, deVeber G, Domi T, Chan A, MacGregor DL. Craniocervical arterial dissection in children: clinical and radiographic presentation and outcome. J Child Neurol 2006; 21(1):8–16.

62. Rosin L. Neurological aspects of patent foramen ovale: in search of the optimal treatment. J Interv Cardiol 2001; 14(2):197–201.

63. Chant H, McCollum C. Stroke in young adults: the role of paradoxical embolism. Thromb Haemost 2001; 85(1):22–29.

64. Cushing KE, Ramesh V, Gardner-Medwin D, Todd NV, Gholkar A, Baxter P et al. Tethering of the vertebral artery in the congenital arcuate foramen of the atlas vertebra: a possible cause of vertebral artery dissection in children. Dev Med Child Neurol 2001; 43(7):491–496.

65. Ganesan V, Prengler M, McShane MA, Wade AM, Kirkham FJ. Investigation of risk factors in children with arterial ischemic stroke. Ann Neurol 2003; 53(2):167–173.

66. Prengler M, Sturt N, Krywawych S, Surtees R, Liesner R, Kirkham F. Homozygous thermolabile variant of the methylenetetrahydrofolate reductase gene: a potential risk factor for hyperhomocysteinaemia, CVD, and stroke in childhood. Dev Med Child Neurol 2001; 43(4):220–225.

67. Health Outcome Indicators: Stroke. Report of a Working Group to the Department of Health (eds A Rudd, M Goldacre, P Amess, J Fletcher, E Wilkinson, A Mason). Oxford: National Centre for Health Outcomes Development, 1999.

68. World Health Organization. The International Classification of Functioning, Disability and Health (ICF). Geneva, Switzerland: World Health Organization, 2001.

69. Bowling A. Measuring Disease. Bubkingham: Open University Press, 1995.

70. Ronen GM, Rosenbaum MP, Streiner DL. Outcome measures in pediatric neurology: why do we need them? J Child Neurol 2000; 15(12):775–780.

71. Hartel C, Schilling S, Sperner J, Thyen U. The clinical outcomes of neonatal and childhood stroke: review of the literature and implications for future research. Eur J Neurol 2004; 11(7):431–438.

72. Duncan PW, Jorgensen HS, Wade DT. Outcome measures in acute stroke trials: a systematic review and some recommendations to improve practice. Stroke 2000; 31(6):1429–1438.

73. Williams LS. Health-related quality of life outcomes in stroke. Neuroepidemiology 1998; 17(3):116–120.

74. Andresen EM. Criteria for assessing the tools of disability outcomes research. Arch Phys Med Rehabil 2000; 81(Suppl 2):15–20.

75. Law M. Evaluating activities of daily living: directions for the future. Am J Occup Ther 1993; 47(3):233–237.

76. deVeber G, The Canadian Paediatric Ischemic Stroke Study group. Canadian Pediatric Ischemic Stroke Registry: analysis of children with arterial ischemic stroke. Ann Neurol 2000; 48(3)526.

77. Gordon AL, Ganesan V, Towell A, Kirkham FJ. Functional outcome following stroke in children. J Child Neurol 2002; 17(6):429–434.

78. Lo W, Zamel K, Ponnappa K, Allen A, Chisolm D, Tang M et al. The cost of pediatric stroke care and rehabilitation. Stroke 2008; 39(1):161–165.

79. Wasserman AL, Wilimas JA, Fairclough DL, Mulhern RK, Wang W. Subtle neuropsychological deficits in children with sickle cell disease. Am J Pediatr Hematol Oncol 1991; 13(1):14–20.

80. Watkins KE, Hewes DK, Connelly A, Kendall BE, Kingsley DP, Evans JE et al. Cognitive deficits associated with frontal-lobe infarction in children with sickle cell disease. Dev Med Child Neurol 1998; 40(8):536–543.

81. North K. Cognitive function and academic performance in children with NF1. In: Neurofibromatosis Type 1 in Childhood (ed K North). Cambridge: Cambridge University Press, 1997.

82. Largo R, Fischer JE, Caflisch JA. Zurich Neuromotor Assessment. Zurich: AWE Verlag, 2002.

83. Mercuri E, Faundez JC, Roberts I, Flora S, Bouza H, Cowan F et al. Neurological 'soft' signs may identify children with sickle cell disease who are at risk for stroke. Eur J Pediatr 1995; 154(2):150–156.

84. Hurvitz EA, Beale L, Ried S, Nelson VS. Functional outcome of paediatric stroke survivors. Pediatr Rehabil 1999; 3(2):43–51.

85. Goodman R, Yude C. IQ and its predictors in childhood hemiplegia. Dev Med Child Neurol 1996; 38(10):881–890.

86. Vargha-Khadem F, Isaacs E, van der Werf S, Robb S, Wilson J. Development of intelligence and memory in children with hemiplegic cerebral palsy. The deleterious consequences of early seizures. Brain 1992; 115(Pt 1):315–329.

87. Ganesan V, Hogan A, Shack N, Gordon A, Isaacs E, Kirkham FJ. Outcome after ischaemic stroke in childhood. Dev Med Child Neurol 2000; 42(7):455–461.

88. Ganesan V, Ng V, Chong WK, Kirkham FJ, Connelly A. Lesion volume, lesion location, and outcome after middle cerebral artery territory stroke. Arch Dis Child 1999; 81(4):295–300.

89. Delsing BJ, Catsman-Berrevoets CE, Appel IM. Early prognostic indicators of outcome in ischemic childhood stroke. Pediatr Neurol 2001; 24(4):283–289.

90. Boardman JP, Ganesan V, Rutherford MA, Saunders DE, Mercuri E, Cowan F. Magnetic resonance image correlates of hemiparesis after neonatal and childhood middle cerebral artery stroke. Pediatrics 2005; 115(2):321–326.

91. Kirton A, Westmacott R, deVeber G. Pediatric stroke: rehabilitation of focal injury in the developing brain. NeuroRehabilitation 2007; 22(5):371–382.

92. Schoenberg BS, Mellinger JF, Schoenberg DG. Cerebrovascular disease in infants and children: a study of incidence, clinical features, and survival. Neurology 1978; 28(8):763–768.

93. Isler W. Stroke in childhood and adolescence. Eur Neurol 1984; 23(6):421–424.

94. Wanifuchi H, Kagawa M, Takeshita M, Izawa M, Kitamura K. Ischemic stroke in infancy, childhood, and adolescence. Childs Nerv Syst 1988; 4(6):361–364.

95. Higgins JJ, Kammerman LA, Fitz CR. Predictors of survival and characteristics of childhood stroke. Neuropediatrics 1991; 22(4):190–193.

96. Keidan I, Shahar E, Barzilay Z, Passwell J, Brand N. Predictors of outcome of stroke in infants and children based on clinical data and radiologic correlates. Acta Paediatr 1994; 83(7):762–765.

97. Fullerton HJ, Wu YW, Zhao S, Johnston SC. Risk of stroke in children: ethnic and gender disparities. Neurology 2003; 61(2):189–194.

98. Fullerton HJ, Chetkovich DM, Wu YW, Smith WS, Johnston SC. Deaths from stroke in US children, 1979 to 1998. Neurology 2002; 59(1):34–39.

99. Blom I, De Schryver EL, Kappelle LJ, Rinkel GJ, Jennekens-Schinkel A, Peters AC. Prognosis of haemorrhagic stroke in childhood: a long-term follow-up study. Dev Med Child Neurol 2003; 45(4):233–239.

100. Al-Jarallah A, Al-Rifai MT, Riela AR, Roach ES. Nontraumatic brain hemorrhage in children: etiology and presentation. J Child Neurol 2000; 15(5):284–289.

101. Meyer-Heim AD, Boltshauser E. Spontaneous intracranial haemorrhage in children: aetiology, presentation and outcome. Brain Dev 2003; 25(6):416–421.

102. Williams AN, Kirkham FJ. Childhood stroke, stroke-like illness and cerebrovascular disease. Stroke 2004; 35:311.

103. Fullerton HJ, Wu YW, Sidney S, Johnston SC. Recurrent hemorrhagic stroke in children: a population-based cohort study. Stroke 2007; 38(10):2658–2662.

104. deVeber GA, MacGregor D, Curtis R, Mayank S. Neurologic outcome in survivors of childhood arterial ischemic stroke and sinovenous thrombosis. J Child Neurol 2000; 15(5):316–324.

105. Andrew M, deVeber G. Pediatric Thromboembolism and Stroke Protocols, 2nd edn. Hamilton, Ontario: BC Decker, 1999.

106. Monagle P, Chalmers E, Chan A, deVeber G, Kirkham F, Massicotte P et al. Antithrombotic therapy in neonates and children: American College of Chest Physicians Evidence-Based Clinical Practice Guidelines (8th edition). Chest 2008; 133(6 Suppl):887S–968S.

107. Roach ES, Golomb MR, Adams R, Biller J, Daniels S, deVeber G et al. Management of stroke in infants and children: a scientific statement from a Special Writing Group of the American Heart Association Stroke Council and the Council on Cardiovascular Disease in the Young. Stroke 2008; 39(9):2644–2691.

108. deVeber G, Andrew M, Adams C, Bjornson B, Booth F, Buckley DJ et al. Cerebral sinovenous thrombosis in children. N Engl J Med 2001; 345(6):417–423.

109. deVeber G, Chan A, Monagle P, Marzinotto V, Armstrong D, Massicotte P et al. Anticoagulation therapy in pediatric patients with sinovenous thrombosis: a cohort study. Arch Neurol 1998; 55(12):1533–1537.

110. Heller C, Heinecke A, Junker R, Knofler R, Kosch A, Kurnik K et al. Cerebral venous thrombosis in children: a multifactorial origin. Circulation 2003; 108(11):1362–1367.

111. Sebire G, Tabarki B, Saunders DE, Leroy I, Liesner R, Saint-Martin C et al. Cerebral venous sinus thrombosis in children: risk factors, presentation, diagnosis and outcome. Brain 2005; 128(Pt 3):477–489.

112. Gold AP, Challenor YB, Gilles FH, Kilal SP, Leviton A, Rollins EI. Report of Joint Committee for Stroke Facilities: IX. Strokes in Children (Part 1). Stroke 1973; 4:835–894.

113. Abram J, Shetty S, Joss CJ. Strokes in the young. Stroke 1971; 2:258–267.

114. Yang JS, Park YD, Hartlage PL. Seizures associated with stroke in childhood. Pediatr Neurol 1995; 12(2):136–138.

115. Goodman R, Yude C. Emotional, behavioural and social consequences. In: Congenital Hemiplegia (eds BG Neville, R Goodman). 1st edn. London: MacKeith Press, 2000; 166–178.

116. Solomon GE, Hilal SK, Gold AP, Carter S. Natural history of acute hemiplegia of childhood. Brain 1970; 93(1):107–120.

117. Giroud M, Lemesle M, Gouyon JB, Nivelon JL, Milan C, Dumas R. Cerebrovascular disease in children under 16 years of age in the city of Dijon, France: a study of incidence and clinical features from 1985 to 1993. J Clin Epidemiol 1995; 48(11):1343–1348.

118. Lanska MJ, Lanska DJ, Horwitz SJ, Aram DM. Presentation, clinical course, and outcome of childhood stroke. Pediatr Neurol 1991; 7(5):333–341.

119. Hariman LM, Griffith ER, Hurtig AL, Keehn MT. Functional outcomes of children with sickle-cell disease affected by stroke. Arch Phys Med Rehabil 1991; 72(7):498–502.

120. Kappelle LJ, Willemse J, Ramos LM, van der Grond GJ. Ischaemic stroke in the basal ganglia and internal capsule in childhood. Brain Dev 1989; 11(5):283–292.

121. Gordon AM, Schneider JA, Chinnan A, Charles JR. Efficacy of a hand-arm bimanual intensive therapy (HABIT) in children with hemiplegic cerebral palsy: a randomized control trial. Dev Med Child Neurol 2007; 49(11):830–838.

122. Tizard JP, Paine RS, Crothers B. Disturbances of sensation in children with hemiplegia. J Am Med Assoc 1954; 155(7):628–632.

123. Novak CB. Evaluation of hand sensibility: a review. J Hand Ther 2001; 14(4):266–272.

124. Krumlinde-Sundholm L, Eliasson AC. Comparing tests of tactile sensibility: aspects relevant to testing children with spastic hemiplegia. Dev Med Child Neurol 2002; 44(9):604–612.

125. Mercuri E, Atkinson J, Braddick O, Anker S, Nokes L, Cowan F et al. Visual function and perinatal focal cerebral infarction. Arch Dis Child Fetal Neonatal Ed 1996; 75(2):F76–F81.

126. Vargha-Khadem F, Isaacs E, Muter V. A review of cognitive outcome after unilateral lesions sustained during childhood. J Child Neurol 1994; 9(Suppl 2):67–73.

127. Lees JA, Neville BG. Acquired aphasia in childhood: case studies of five children. Asphasiology 1990; 4(5):463–478.

128. Gout A, Seibel N, Rouviere C, Husson B, Hermans B, Laporte N et al. Aphasia owing to subcortical brain infarcts in childhood. J Child Neurol 2005; 20(12):1003–1008.

129. Rowan A, Vargha-Khadem F, Calamante F, Tournier JD, Kirkham FJ, Chong WK et al. Cortical abnormalities and language function in young patients with basal ganglia stroke. Neuroimage 2007; 36(2):431–440.

130. Hogan AM, Kirkham FJ, Isaacs EB. Intelligence after stroke in childhood: review of the literature and suggestions for future research. J Child Neurol 2000; 15(5):325–332.

131. Max JE, Robin DA, Taylor HG, Yeates KO, Fox PT, Lancaster JL et al. Attention function after childhood stroke. J Int Neuropsychol Soc 2004; 10(7):976–986.

132. Hetherington R, Tuff L, Anderson P, Miles B, deVeber G. Short-term intellectual outcome after arterial ischemic stroke and sinovenous thrombosis in childhood and infancy. J Child Neurol 2005; 20(7):553–559.

133. Pavlovic J, Kaufmann F, Boltshauser E, Capone MA, Gubser MD, Haenggeli CA et al. Neuropsychological problems after pediatric stroke: two year follow up of Swiss children. Neuropediatrics 2006; 37(1):13–19.

134. Guimaraes IE, Ciasca SM, Moura-Ribeiro MV. Cerebrovascular disease in childhood: neuropsychological investigation of 14 cases. Arq Neuropsiquiatr 2007; 65(1):41–47.

135. Simma B, Martin G, Muller T, Huemer M. Risk factors for pediatric stroke: consequences for therapy and quality of life. Pediatr Neurol 2007; 37(2):121–126.

136. Everts R, Pavlovic J, Kaufmann F, Uhlenberg B, Seidel U, Nedeltchev K et al. Cognitive functioning, behavior, and quality of life after stroke in childhood. Child Neuropsychol 2008; 14(4):323–338.

137. Lansing AE, Max JE, Delis DC, Fox PT, Lancaster J, Manes FF et al. Verbal learning and memory after childhood stroke. J Int Neuropsychol Soc 2004; 10(5):742–752.

138. Westmacott R, Askalan R, MacGregor D, Anderson P, deVeber G. Cognitive outcome following unilateral arterial ischaemic stroke in childhood: effects of age at stroke and lesion location. Dev Med Child Neurol 2009.

139. Chapman SB, Max JE, Gamino JF, McGlothlin JH, Cliff SN. Discourse plasticity in children after stroke: age at injury and lesion effects. Pediatr Neurol 2003; 29(1):34–41.

140. Westmacott R, MacGregor D, Askalan R, deVeber G. Late emergence of cognitive deficits after unilateral neonatal stroke. Stroke 2009; 40(6):2012–2019.

141. Mosch SC, Max JE, Tranel D. A matched lesion analysis of childhood versus adult-onset brain injury due to unilateral stroke: another perspective on neural plasticity and recovery of social functioning. Cogn Behav Neurol 2005; 18(1):5–17.

142. Goodman R, Graham P. Psychiatric problems in children with hemiplegia: cross sectional epidemiological survey. BMJ 1996; 312(7038):1065–1069.

143. Max JE, Fox PT, Lancaster JL, Kochunov P, Mathews K, Manes FF et al. Putamen lesions and the development of attention-deficit/hyperactivity symptomatology. J Am Acad Child Adolesc Psychiatry 2002; 41(5):563–571.

144. Goodman R. The longitudinal stability of psychiatric problems in children with hemiplegia. J Child Psychol Psychiatry 1998; 39(3):347–354.

145. Max JE, Mathews K, Manes FF, Robertson BA, Fox PT, Lancaster JL et al. Attention deficit hyperactivity disorder and neurocognitive correlates after childhood stroke. J Int Neuropsychol Soc 2003; 9(6):815–829.

146. Max JE, Manes FF, Robertson BA, Mathews K, Fox PT, Lancaster J. Prefrontal and executive attention network lesions and the development of attention-deficit/hyperactivity symptomatology. J Am Acad Child Adolesc Psychiatry 2005; 44(5):443–450.

147. Yude C, Goodman R, McConachie H. Peer problems of children with hemiplegia in mainstream primary schools. J Child Psychol Psychiatry 1998; 39(4):533–541.

148. Yude C, Goodman R. Peer problems of 9- to 11-year-old children with hemiplegia in mainstream schools. Can these be predicted? Dev Med Child Neurol 1999; 41(1):4–8.

149. Kirkham FJ, Hogan AM. Risk factors for arterial ischemic stroke in childhood. CNS Spectr 2004; 9(6):451–464.

150. Friefeld S, Yeboah O, Jones JE, deVeber G. Health-related quality of life and its relationship to neurological outcome in child survivors of stroke. CNS Spectr 2004; 9(6):465–475.

151. Ravens-Sieberer U, Gosch A, Abel T, Auquier P, Bellach BM, Bruil J et al. Quality of life in children and adolescents: a European public health perspective. Soz Praventivmed 2001; 46(5):294–302.

152. Hurvitz E, Warschausky S, Berg M, Tsai S. Long-term functional outcome of pediatric stroke survivors. Top Stroke Rehabil 2004; 11(2):51–59.

153. Barry MJ, VanSwearingen JM, Albright AL. Reliability and responsiveness of the Barry–Albright Dystonia Scale. Dev Med Child Neurol 1999; 41(6):404–411.

154. Randall M, Carlin JB, Chondros P, Reddihough D. Reliability of the Melbourne assessment of unilateral upper limb function. Dev Med Child Neurol 2001; 43(11):761–767.

155. Bohannon RW, Smith MB. Interrater reliability of a modified Ashworth scale of muscle spasticity. Phys Ther 1987; 67(2):206–207.

156. Ichord RN, Bastian R, Abraham L, Askalan R, Benedict S, Bernard TJ, Beslow L, Deveber G, Dowling M, Friedman N, Fullerton H, Jordan L, Kan L, Kirton A, Amlie-Lefond C, Licht D, Lo W, McClure C, Pavlakis S, Smith SE, Tan M, Kasner S, Jawad AF. Interrater Reliability of the Pediatric National Institutes of Health Stroke Scale (PedNIHSS) in a Multicenter Study. Stroke. 2011 Feb 11. [Epub ahead of print].

157. Kitchen L, Friefeld S, Anderson P, Sofronas M, Domi T, deVeber G. A validation study of the paediatric stroke outcome measure. Stroke 2003; 34:316.

158. DeMatteo C, Law M, Russell D, Pollock N, Rosenbaum P, Walter S. Quality of Upper Extremity Skills Test. Ontario, Canada: Chedoke-McMaster Hospitals, 1992.

159. Rankin J. Cerebral vascular accidents in patients over the age of 60. II. Prognosis. Scott Med J 1957; 2(5):200–215.

160. Bonita R, Beaglehole R. Recovery of motor function after stroke. Stroke 1988; 19(12):1497–1500.

161. Krumlinde-Sundholm L, Holmefur M, Kottorp A, Eliasson AC. The Assisting Hand Assessment: current evidence of validity, reliability, and responsiveness to change. Dev Med Child Neurol 2007; 49(4):259–264.

162. Bruininks RH, Bruininks BD. Bruininks–Oseretsky Test of Motor Proficiency Manual, 2nd edn. Minnesota: AGS Publishing, 2005.

163. Jebsen RH, Taylor N, Trieschmann RB, Trotter MJ, Howard LA. An objective and standardized test of hand function. Arch Phys Med Rehabil 1969; 50(6):311–319.

164. Haley S, Coster W, Ludlow L, Haltiwanger J, Andrellos P. Pediatric Evaluation of Disability Inventory (PEDI). Boston, NE: New England Medical Centre Hospitals Inc and PEDI Research Group, 1992.

165. Granger CV, Brown SP, Griswold K, Heyer N, McCabe M, Msall ME et al. WeeFIM (Functional Independence Measure for Children), 1991. New York: Centre for Functional Assessment Research.

166. Greer HD, III, Waltz AG. Acute neurologic disorders of infancy and childhood. Dev Med Child Neurol 1965; 7(5):507–517.

167. Aicardi J, Amsili J, Chevrie JJ. Acute hemiplegia in infancy and childhood. Dev Med Child Neurol 1969; 11(2):162–173.

168. Tibbles JA, Brown BS. Acute hemiplegia of childhood. Can Med Assoc J 1975; 113(4):309–314.

169. Schoenberg BS. General considerations of neurological epidemiology. Adv Neurol 1978; 19:11–16.

170. Blennow G, Cronqvist S, Hindfelt B, Nilsson O. On cerebral infarction in childhood and adolescence. Acta Paediatr Scand 1978; 67(4):469–475.

171. Eeg-Olofsson O, Ringheim Y. Stroke in children. Clinical characteristics and prognosis. Acta Paediatr Scand 1983; 72(3):391–395.

172. Mazza C, Pasqualin A, Cavazzani P, Dalla BB, Da PR. Childhood cerebrovascular diseases not associated with vascular malformations. Childs Nerv Syst 1985; 1(5):268–271.

173. Satoh S, Shirane R, Yoshimoto T. Clinical survey of ischemic cerebrovascular disease in children in a district of Japan. Stroke 1991; 22(5):586–589.

174. Inagaki M, Koeda T, Takeshita K. Prognosis and MRI after ischemic stroke of the basal ganglia. Pediatr Neurol 1992; 8(2):104–108.

175. Broderick J, Talbot GT, Prenger E, Leach A, Brott T. Stroke in children within a major metropolitan area: the surprising importance of intracerebral hemorrhage. J Child Neurol 1993; 8(3):250–255.

176. Powell FC, Hanigan WC, McCluney KW. Subcortical infarction in children. Stroke 1994; 25(1):117–121.

177. Visudhiphan P, Chiemchanya S, Wattanasirichaigoon D. Strokes in Thai children: etiology and outcome. Southeast Asian J Trop Med Public Health 1996; 27(4):801–805.

178. Brower MC, Rollins N, Roach ES. Basal ganglia and thalamic infarction in children. Cause and clinical features. Arch Neurol 1996; 53(12):1252–1256.

179. Andrew M, David M, deVeber G, Brooker LA. Arterial thromboembolic complications in paediatric patients. Thromb Haemost 1997; 78(1):715–725.

180. deVeber G, Andrew M, The Canadian Paediatric Ischemic Stroke Study group. The epidemiology and outcome of sinovenous thrombosis in pediatric patients. New Engl J Med 2001; 345:417–423.

181. Williams AN, Davies P, Eunson PD, Kirkham FJ, Green SH. Stroke and Cerebrovascular Disease: Brimingham Children's Hospital 1993–1998. Dev Med Child Neurol 2002; 45:10.

182. Rodrigues SD, Ciasca SM, Moura-Ribeiro MV. Ischemic cerebrovascular disease in childhood: cognitive assessment of 15 patients. Arq Neuropsiquiatr 2004; 62(3B):802–807.

183. Jordan LC, van Beek JG, Gottesman RF, Kossoff EH, Johnston MV. Ischemic stroke in children with critical illness: a poor prognostic sign. Pediatr Neurol 2007; 36(4):244–246.

184. Lee YY, Lin KL, Wang HS, Chou ML, Hung PC, Hsieh MY et al. Risk factors and outcomes of childhood ischemic stroke in Taiwan. Brain Dev 2008; 30(1):14–19.

185. Buompadre MC, Arroyo HA. Basal ganglia and internal capsule stroke in childhood – risk factors, neuroimaging, and outcome in a series of 28 patients: a tertiary hospital experience. J Child Neurol 2009; 24(6):685–691.

186. Merino Arribas JM, de Pablo CR, Grande GT, Sanchez MJ, Gonzalez de la Rosa JB. Nontraumatic hemorrhagic stroke in children after the neonatal period. An Esp Pediatr 1997; 47(4):392–396.

187. Giroud M, Lemesle M, Madinier G, Manceau E, Osseby GV, Dumas R. Stroke in children under 16 years of age. Clinical and etiological difference with adults. Acta Neurol Scand 1997; 96(6):401–406.

188. Jordan LC, Kleinman JT, Hillis AE. Intracerebral hemorrhage volume predicts poor neurologic outcome in children. Stroke 2009; 40(5):1666–1671.

189. Obama MT, Dongmo L, Nkemayim C, Mbede J, Hagbe P. Stroke in children in Yaounde, Cameroon. Indian Pediatr 1994; 31(7):791–795.

190. De Moura-Ribiero MV, Ferreira LS, Montenegro MA, Vale-Cavalcante M, Piovesana AM, Scotoni AE et al. Cerebrovascular disease in children: II. Clinical aspects in 42 cases. Arq Neuropsiquiatr 1999; 57:594–598.

191. Auvichayapat N, Tassniyom S, Hantragool S, Auvichayapat P. The etiology and outcome of cerebrovascular diseases in Northeastern Thai children. J Med Assoc Thai 2007; 90(10):2058–2062.

192. Rasul CH, Mahboob AA, Hossain SM, Ahmed KU. Predisposing factors and outcome of stroke in childhood. Indian Pediatr 2009; 46(5):419–421.

193. Emam AT, Ali AM, Babikr MA. Childhood stroke in Eastern Province, KSA: pattern, risk factors, diagnosis and outcome. Acta Paediatr 2009; 98(10):1613–1619.

194. Tham EH, Tay SK, Low PS. Factors predictive of outcome in childhood stroke in an Asian population. Ann Acad Med Singapore 2009; 38(10):876–881.

195. Bates E, Vicari S, Trauner D. Neural mediation of language development: perspectives from lesion studies of infants and children. In: Neurodevelopmental Disorders (ed H Tager-Flusberg). Cambridge, MA: MIT Press, 1999; 533–581.

196. Muter V, Taylor S, Vargha-Khadem F. A longitudinal study of early intellectual development in hemiplegic children. Neuropsychologia 1997; 35(3):289–298.

197. Kuzniecky R, Andermann F, Guerrini R. Congenital bilateral perisylvian syndrome: study of 31 patients. The CBPS Multicenter Collaborative Study. Lancet 1993; 341(8845):608–612.

198. Vargha-Khadem F, Watkins KE, Price CJ, Ashburner J, Alcock KJ, Connelly A et al. Neural basis of an inherited speech and language disorder. Proc Natl Acad Sci USA 1998; 95(21):12695–12700.

199. Jernigan TL, Hesselink JR, Sowell E, Tallal PA. Cerebral structure on magnetic resonance imaging in language- and learning-impaired children. Arch Neurol 1991; 48(5):539–545.

200. Paulesu E, Frith U, Snowling M, Gallagher A, Morton J, Frackowiak RS et al. Is developmental dyslexia a disconnection

syndrome? Evidence from PET scanning. Brain 1996; 119 (Pt 1):143–157.

201. Bellugi U, Marks S, Bihrle A, Sabo H. Dissociation between language and cognitive functions in Williams syndrome'. In: Language Development in Exceptional Circumstances, 1st edn (eds D Bishop, K Mogford). Edinburgh: Churchill Livingstone, 1988.

202. Bachevalier J. Medial temporal lobe structures and autism: a review of clinical and experimental findings. Neuropsychologia 1994; 32(6):627–648.

203. McFie J. The effects of hemispherectomy on intellectual function in cases of infantile hemiplegia. J Neurol Neurosurg Psychiatry 1961; 24:240–249.

204. McFie J. Intellectual impairment in children with localised post-infantile cerebral lesions. J Neurol Neurosurg Psychiatr 1961; 24:361–365.

205. Basser LS. Hemiplegia of early onset and the faculty of speech with special reference to the effects of hemispherectomy. Brain 1962; 85:427–460.

206. Alajouanine T, Lhermitte F. Acquired aphasia in children. Brain 1965; 88(4):653–662.

207. Lenneberg E. Biological Foundations of Language. New York: John Wiley, 1967.

208. Vargha-Khadem F, Isaacs EB, Papaleloudi H, Polkey CE, Wilson J. Development of language in six hemispherectomized patients. Brain 1991; 114 (Pt 1B):473–495.

209. Woods BT, Teuber HL. Early onset of complementary specialization of cerebral hemispheres in man. Trans Am Neurol Assoc 1973; 98:113–117.

210. Woods BT, Carey S. Language deficits after apparent clinical recovery from childhood aphasia. Ann Neurol 1979; 6(5):405–409.

211. Hecaen H. Acquired aphasia in children and the ontogenesis of hemispheric functional specialization. Brain Lang 1976; 3(1):114–134.

212. Woods BT. The restricted effects of right-hemisphere lesions after age one; Wechsler test data. Neuropsychologia 1980; 18(1):65–70.

213. Dennis M, Kohn B. Comprehension of syntax in infantile hemiplegics after cerebral hemidecortication: left-hemisphere superiority. Brain Lang 1975; 2(4):472–482.

214. Dennis M, Whitaker HA. Language acquisition following hemidecortication: linguistic superiority of the left over the right hemisphere. Brain Lang 1976; 3(3):404–433.

215. Dennis M, Whitaker H. Hemispheric equipotentiality and language acquisition. In: Language Development and Neurological Theory (eds S Segalowitz, F Gruber). New York: Academic Press, 1977; 93–106.

216. Kohn B, Dennis M. Selective impairments of visuo-spatial abilities in infantile hemiplegics after right cerebral hemidecortication. Neuropsychologia 1974; 12(4):505–512.

217. Chomsky N. Reflections on Language. New York: Pantheon, 1975.

218. Chomsky N. Lectures on Government and Binding. Dordrecht: Foris, 1981.

219. Fodor J. The Modularity of Mind. Cambridge, MA: MIT Press, 1983.

220. Geschwind N, Levitsky W. Human brain: left–right asymmetries in temporal speech region. Science 1968; 161(837):186–187.

221. Wada JA, Clarke R, Hamm A. Cerebral hemispheric asymmetry in humans. Cortical speech zones in 100 adults and 100 infant brains. Arch Neurol 1975; 32(4):239–246.

222. Witelson SF, Pallie W. Left hemisphere specialization for language in the newborn. Neuroanatomical evidence of asymmetry. Brain 1973; 96(3):641–646.

223. Molfese DL, Molfese V. Cortical responses of preterm infants to phonetic and nonphonetic speech stimuli. Dev Psychol 1980; 16:574–581.

224. Glanville B, Best C, Levenson R. A cardiac measure of cerebral asymmetries in infant auditory perception. Dev Psychol 1977; 13:54–59.

225. Entus A. Hemispheric asymmetry in processing of dichotically presented speech and nonspeech stimuli by infants. In: Language Development and Neurological Theory (eds S Segalowitz, F Gruber F). New York: Academic Press, 1977; 63–67.

226. Bertoncini J, Morais J, Bijeljac-Babic R, McAdams S, Peretz I, Mehler J. Dichotic perception and laterality in neonates. Brain Lang 1989; 37(4):591–605.

227. Vargha-Khadem F, Corballis MC. Cerebral asymmetry in infants. Brain Lang 1979; 8(1):1–9.

228. Best CT, Hoffman H, Glanville BB. Development of infant ear asymmetries for speech and music. Percept Psychophys 1982; 31(1):75–85.

229. Novak GP, Kurtzberg D, Kreuzer JA, Vaughan HG, Jr. Cortical responses to speech sounds and their formants in normal infants: maturational sequence and spatiotemporal analysis. Electroencephalogr Clin Neurophysiol 1989; 73(4):295–305.

230. Molfese DL, Burger-Judisch L. Dynamic temporal-spatial allocation of resources in the human brain: an alternative to the static view of hemisphere differences. In: Cerebral Laterality: Theory and Research (ed F Kitterle). Hillsdale, NJ: Lawrence Erlbaum Associates, 1991; 71–102.

231. Riva D, Cazzaniga L. Late effects of unilateral brain lesions sustained before and after age one. Neuropsychologia 1986; 24(3):423–428.

232. Aram DM, Ekelman BL, Whitaker HA. Spoken syntax in children with acquired unilateral hemisphere lesions. Brain Lang 1986; 27(1):75–100.

233. Aram DM, Ekelman BL, Whitaker HA. Lexical retrieval in left and right brain lesioned children. Brain Lang 1987; 31(1):61–87.

234. Aram DM, Meyers SC, Ekelman BL. Fluency of conversational speech in children with unilateral brain lesions. Brain Lang 1990; 38(1):105–121.

235. Woods BT, Teuber HL. Changing patterns of childhood aphasia. Trans Am Neurol Assoc 1977; 102:36–38.

236. Vargha-Khadem F, Watters GV, O'Gorman AM. Development of speech and language following bilateral frontal lesions. Brain Lang 1985; 25(1):167–183.

237. Gott PS. Cognitive abilities following right and left hemispherectomy. Cortex 1973; 9(3):266–274.

238. Ogden JA. Visuospatial and other 'right-hemispheric' functions after long recovery periods in left-hemispherectomized subjects. Neuropsychologia 1989; 27(6):765–776.

239. Damasio AR, Lima A, Damasio H. Nervous function after right hemispherectomy. Neurology 1975; 25(1):89–93.

240. Bishop D. Can the right hemisphere mediate language as well as the left? A critical review of recent research. Cognitive Neuropsychol 1988; 5:353–367.

241. Bishop DV. Linguistic impairment after left hemidecortication for infantile hemiplegia? A reappraisal. Q J Exp Psychol A 1983; 35(Pt 1):199–207.

242. Max JE. Effect of side of lesion on neuropsychological performance in childhood stroke. J Int Neuropsychol Soc 2004; 10(5):698–708.

243. Thal DJ, Marchman V, Stiles J, Aram D, Trauner D, Nass R et al. Early lexical development in children with focal brain injury. Brain Lang 1991; 40(4):491–527.

244. Kempler D, Van Lancker D, Marchman V, Bates E. The effects of childhood vs adult brain damage on literal and idiomatic language comprehension. Brain Lang 1996; 55(1):167–169.

245. Reilly JS, Bates EA, Marchman VA. Narrative discourse in children with early focal brain injury. Brain Lang 1998; 61(3):335–375.

246. Bates E, Reilly J, Wulfeck B, Dronkers N, Opie M, Fenson J et al. Differential effects of unilateral lesions on language production in children and adults. Brain Lang 2001; 79(2):223–265.

247. Ballantyne AO, Spilkin AM, Trauner DA. Language outcome after perinatal stroke: does side matter? Child Neuropsychol 2007; 13(6):494–509.

248. Vicari S, Albertoni A, Chilosi AM, Cipriani P, Cioni G, Bates E. Plasticity and reorganization during language development in children with early brain injury. Cortex 2000; 36(1):31–46.

249. Stiles-Davis J, Sugarman S, Nass R. The development of spatial and class relations in four young children with right-cerebral-hemisphere damage: evidence for an early spatial constructive deficit. Brain Cogn 1985; 4(4):388–412.

250. Stiles J, Trauner D, Engel M, Nass R. The development of drawing in children with congenital focal brain injury: evidence for limited functional recovery. Neuropsychologia 1997; 35(3):299–312.

251. Stiles J. The effects of early focal brain injury on lateralization of cognitive function. Curr Dir Psych Sci 1998; 7(1):21–26.

252. Stiles J, Bates EA, Thal DJ, Trauner D, Reilly J. Linguistic, cognitive and affective development in children with pre- and perinatal focal brain injury: a 10 year overview from the San Diego

Longitudinal Project. In: Advances in Infancy Research (ed C Rovee-Collier). Norwood, NJ: Ablex, 1999.

253. Satz P, Strauss E, Whitaker H. The ontogeny of hemispheric specialization: some old hypotheses revisited. Brain Lang 1990; 38(4):596–614.

254. Simos PG, Molfese DL, Brenden RA. Behavioral and electro-physiological indices of voicing-cue discrimination: laterality patterns and development. Brain Lang 1997; 57(1):122–150.

255. Simos PG, Molfese DL. Electrophysiological responses from a temporal order continuum in the newborn infant. Neuropsychologia 1997; 35(1):89–98.

256. Dehaene-Lambertz G, Baillet S. A phonological representation in the infant brain. Neuroreport 1998; 9(8):1885–1888.

257. Naatanen R, Lehtokoski A, Lennes M, Cheour M, Huotilainen M, Iivonen A et al. Language-specific phoneme representations revealed by electric and magnetic brain responses. Nature 1997; 385(6615):432–434.

258. Elman E, Bates E, Johnson M, Karmiloff-Smith A, Parisi D, Plunkett K. Rethinking Innateness: a Connectionist Perspective on Development. Cambridge, MA: MIT Press/Bradford Books, 1996.

259. Banich MT, Levine SC, Kim H, Huttenlocher P. The effects of developmental factors on IQ in hemiplegic children. Neuropsychologia 1990; 28(1):35–47.

260. Isaacs E, Christie D, Vargha-Khadem F, Mishkin M. Effects of hemispheric side of injury, age at injury, and presence of seizure disorder on functional ear and hand asymmetries in hemiplegic children. Neuropsychologia 1996; 34(2):127–137.

261. Brizzolara D, Pecini C, Brovedani P, Ferretti G, Cipriani P, Cioni G. Timing and type of congenital brain lesion determine different patterns of language lateralization in hemiplegic children. Neuropsychologia 2002; 40(6):620–632.

262. Chilosi AM, Pecini C, Cipriani P, Brovedani P, Brizzolara D, Ferretti G et al. Atypical language lateralization and early linguistic development in children with focal brain lesions. Dev Med Child Neurol 2005; 47(11):725–730.

263. Guzzetta A, Pecini C, Biagi L, Tosetti M, Brizzolara D, Chilosi A et al. Language organization in left perinatal stroke. Neuropediatrics 2008; 39(3):157–163.

264. Gadian DG, Isaacs EB, Cross JH, Connelly A, Jackson GD, King MD et al. Lateralization of brain function in childhood revealed by magnetic resonance spectroscopy. Neurology 1996; 46(4):974–977.

265. Feldman HM, Holland AL, Kemp SS, Janosky JE. Language development after unilateral brain injury. Brain Lang 1992; 42(1):89–102.

266. Dall'Oglio AM, Bates E, Volterra V, Di CM, Pezzini G. Early cognition, communication and language in children with focal brain injury. Dev Med Child Neurol 1994; 36(12):1076–1098.

267. Levine SC, Huttenlocher P, Banich MT, Duda E. Factors affecting cognitive functioning of hemiplegic children. Dev Med Child Neurol 1987; 29(1):27–35.

268. Vargha-Khadem F, Isaacs E, Mishkin M. Ontogenetic specialization of hemipheric function. In: Intractable Focal Epilepsy: Medical and Surgical Treatment (eds JM Oxbury, CE Polkey, M Duchowney). London: Harcourt Publishers, 2000; 405–418.

269. Wechsler D. Wechsler Intelligence Scale for children – revised UK edition. Sidcup, Kent: The Psychological Corporation, Harcourt Brace Jovanovich, 1976.

270. Wechsler D. Wechsler Preschool and Primary Scale of Intelligence. Sidcup, Kent: The Psychological Corporation, Harcourt Brace Jovanovich, 1990.

271. Wechsler D. Wechsler Intelligence Scale for Children. UK Version, 3rd ed. Sidcup, Kent: The Psychological Corporation, Harcourt Brace Jovanovich, 1992.

272. Wechsler D. Wechsler Adult Intelligence Scale. New York: The Psychological Corporation, 1955.

273. Liegeois F, Connelly A, Cross JH, Boyd SG, Gadian DG, Vargha-Khadem F et al. Language reorganization in children with early-onset lesions of the left hemisphere: an fMRI study. Brain 2004; 127(Pt 6):1229–1236.

274. Milner B. Sparing of language function after early unilateral brain damage. Neuro Res Prog Bull 1974; 12(2):213–217.

275. Teuber HL. Recovery of function after brain injury in man. Ciba Found Symp 1975;(34):159–190.

276. Ballantyne AO, Spilkin AM, Hesselink J, Trauner DA. Plasticity in the developing brain: intellectual, language and academic functions in children with ischaemic perinatal stroke. Brain 2008; 131(Pt 11):2975–2985.

277. Milner B. Psychological aspects of focal epilepsy and its neurosurgical management. Adv Neurol 1975; 8:299–321.

278. Warrington EK, James M, Maciejewski C. The WAIS as a lateralizing and localizing diagnostic instrument: a study of 656 patients with unilateral cerebral lesions. Neuropsychologia 1986; 24(2):223–239.

279. Riva D, Cazzaniga L, Panaleoni C, Milani N, Fedrizzi E. Acute hemiplegia in childhood: the neuropsychological prognosis. J Pediatr Neurol 1987; 2:239–250.

280. Nass R, deCoudres PH, Koch D. Differential effects of congenital left and right brain injury on intelligence. Brain Cogn 1989; 9(2):258–266.

281. Ricci D, Mercuri E, Barnett A, Rathbone R, Cota F, Haataja L et al. Cognitive outcome at early school age in term-born children with perinatally acquired middle cerebral artery territory infarction. Stroke 2008; 39(2):403–410.

282. Scarvie KM, Ballantyne AO, Trauner DA. Visuomotor performance in children with infantile nephropathic cystinosis. Percept Mot Skills 1996; 82(1):67–75.

283. Hoffman JI. Congenital heart disease: incidence and inheritance. Pediatr Clin North Am 1990; 37(1):25–43.

284. Figueroa JD, Magana BD, Hach JL, Jiminez CC, Urbina RC. Heart malformations in children with Down syndrome. Rev Espan Cardiol 2003; 569:894–899.

285. Delamatar A. Cardiovascular disease. In: Handbook of Pediatric Psychology, 3rd edn (ed MC Roberts). London: The Guilford Press, 2003.

286. Griffin KJ, Elkin TD, Smith CJ. Academic outcomes in children with congenital heart disease. Clin Pediatr (Phila) 2003; 42(5):401–409.

287. Bass JL, Corwin M, Gozal D, Moore C, Nishida H, Parker S et al. The effect of chronic or intermittent hypoxia on cognition in childhood: a review of the evidence. Pediatrics 2004; 114(3):805–816.

288. Linde LM, Rasof B, Dunn OJ. Mental development in congenital heart disease. J Pediatr 1967; 71(2):198–203.

289. Limperopoulos C, Majnemer A, Shevell MI, Rosenblatt B, Rohlicek C, Tchervenkov C. Neurologic status of newborns with congenital heart defects before open heart surgery. Pediatrics 1999; 103(2):402–408.

290. DeMaso DR, Beardslee WR, Silbert AR, Fyler DC. Psychological functioning in children with cyanotic heart defects. J Dev Behav Pediatr 1990; 11(6):289–294.

291. Alden B, Gilljam T, Gillberg C. Long-term psychological outcome of children after surgery for transposition of the great arteries. Acta Paediatr 1998; 87(4):405–410.

292. Feldt RH, Ewert JC, Stickler GB, Weidman WH. Children with congenital heart disease. Motor development and intelligence. Am J Dis Child 1969; 117(3):281–287.

293. Aram DM, Ekelman BL, Ben-Shachar G, Levinsohn MW. Intelligence and hypoxemia in children with congenital heart disease: fact or artifact? J Am Coll Cardiol 1985; 6(4):889–893.

294. Kramer HH, Awiszus D, Sterzel U, van HA, Classen R. Development of personality and intelligence in children with congenital heart disease. J Child Psychol Psychiatry 1989; 30(2):299–308.

295. Smith KM. The innocent heart murmur in children. J Pediatr Health Care 1997; 11(5):207–214.

296. Clarkson PM, MacArthur BA, Barratt-Boyes BG, Whitlock RM, Neutze JM. Developmental progress after cardiac surgery in infancy using hypothermia and circulatory arrest. Circulation 1980; 62(4):855–861.

297. Blackwood MJ, Haka-Ikse K, Steward DJ. Developmental outcome in children undergoing surgery with profound hypothermia. Anesthesiology 1986; 65(4):437–440.

298. Limperopoulos C, Majnemer A, Shevell MI, Rosenblatt B, Rohlicek C, Tchervenkov C. Neurodevelopmental status of newborns and infants with congenital heart defects before and after open heart surgery. J Pediatr 2000; 137(5):638–645.

299. O'Dougherty M, Wright FS, Loewenson RB, Torres F. Cerebral dysfunction after chronic hypoxia in children. Neurology 1985; 35(1):42–46.

300. Newburger JW, Silbert AR, Buckley LP, Fyler DC. Cognitive function and age at repair of transposition of the great arteries in children. N Engl J Med 1984; 310(23):1495–1499.

301. Oates RK, Simpson JM, Cartmill TB, Turnbull JA. Intellectual function and age of repair in cyanotic congenital heart disease. Arch Dis Child 1995; 72(4):298–301.

302. Aisenberg RB, Rosenthal A, Nadas AS, Wolff PH. Developmental delay in infants with congenital heart disease. Correlation with hypoxemia and congestive heart failure. Pediatr Cardiol 1982; 3(2):133–137.

303. Silbert A, Wolff PH, Mayer B, Rosenthal A, Nadas AS. Cyanotic heart disease and psychological development. Pediatrics 1969; 43(2):192–200.

304. Wray J, Sensky T. Controlled study of preschool development after surgery for congenital heart disease. Arch Dis Child 1999; 80(6):511–516.

305. Robertson DR, Justo RN, Burke CJ, Pohlner PG, Graham PL, Colditz PB. Perioperative predictors of developmental outcome following cardiac surgery in infancy. Cardiol Young 2004; 14(4):389–395.

306. Hamrick SE, Gremmels DB, Keet CA, Leonard CH, Connell JK, Hawgood S et al. Neurodevelopmental outcome of infants supported with extracorporeal membrane oxygenation after cardiac surgery. Pediatrics 2003; 111(6 Pt 1):e671–e675.

307. Dittrich H, Buhrer C, Grimmer I, Dittrich S, Abdul-Khaliq H, Lange PE. Neurodevelopment at 1 year of age in infants with congenital heart disease. Heart 2003; 89(4):436–441.

308. McConnell JR, Fleming WH, Chu WK, Hahn FJ, Sarafian LB, Hofschire PJ et al. Magnetic resonance imaging of the brain in infants and children before and after cardiac surgery. A prospective study. Am J Dis Child 1990; 144(3):374–378.

309. Mahle WT, Tavani F, Zimmerman RA, Nicolson SC, Galli KK, Gaynor JW et al. An MRI study of neurological injury before and after congenital heart surgery. Circulation 2002; 106(12 Suppl 1):I109–I114.

310. Olsen P, Vainionpaa L, Paakko E, Korkman M, Pyhtinen J, Jarvelin MR. Psychological findings in preterm children related to neurologic status and magnetic resonance imaging. Pediatrics 1998; 102(2 Pt 1):329–336.

311. Kinney HC, Panigrahy A, Newburger JW, Jonas RA, Sleeper LA. Hypoxic-ischemic brain injury in infants with congenital heart disease dying after cardiac surgery. Acta Neuropathol 2005; 110(6):563–578.

312. Welch RB, Byrne P. Transient changes in neuroimaging appearances of the brain following cardiopulmonary bypass. Am J Dis Child 1990; 144(11):1184.

313. Toet MC, Flinterman A, Laar I, Vries JW, Bennink GB, Uiterwaal CS et al. Cerebral oxygen saturation and electrical brain activity before, during, and up to 36 hours after arterial switch procedure in neonates without pre-existing brain damage: its relationship to neurodevelopmental outcome. Exp Brain Res 2005; 165(3):343–350.

314. Forbess JM, Visconti KJ, Bellinger DC, Howe RJ, Jonas RA. Neurodevelopmental outcomes after biventricular repair of congenital heart defects. J Thorac Cardiovasc Surg 2002; 123(4):631–639.

315. Haneda K, Itoh T, Togo T, Ohmi M, Mohri H. Effects of cardiac surgery on intellectual function in infants and children. Cardiovasc Surg 1996; 4(3):303–307.

316. Bellinger DC, Wypij D, duPlessis AJ, Rappaport LA, Jonas RA, Wernovsky G et al. Neurodevelopmental status at eight years in children with dextro-transposition of the great arteries: the Boston Circulatory Arrest Trial. J Thorac Cardiovasc Surg 2003; 126(5):1385–1396.

317. Sharma R, Choudhary SK, Mohan MR, Padma MV, Jain S, Bhardwaj M et al. Neurological evaluation and intelligence testing in the child with operated congenital heart disease. Ann Thorac Surg 2000; 70(2):575–581.

318. Wells FC, Coghill S, Caplan HL, Lincoln C. Duration of circulatory arrest does influence the psychological development of children after cardiac operation in early life. J Thorac Cardiovasc Surg 1983; 86(6):823–831.

319. Oates RK, Simpson JM, Turnbull JA, Cartmill TB. The relationship between intelligence and duration of circulatory arrest with deep hypothermia. J Thorac Cardiovasc Surg 1995; 110(3):786–792.

320. Bellinger DC, Rappaport LA, Wypij D, Wernovsky G, Newburger JW. Patterns of developmental dysfunction after surgery during infancy to correct transposition of the great arteries. J Dev Behav Pediatr 1997; 18(2):75–83.

321. Settergren G, Ohqvist G, Lundberg S, Henze A, Bjork VO, Persson B. Cerebral blood flow and cerebral metabolism in children following cardiac surgery with deep hypothermia and circulatory arrest. Clinical course and follow-up of psychomotor development. Scand J Thorac Cardiovasc Surg 1982; 16(3):209–215.

322. Bellinger DC, Wernovsky G, Rappaport LA, Mayer JE, Jr, Castaneda AR, Farrell DM et al. Cognitive development of children following early repair of transposition of the great arteries using deep hypothermic circulatory arrest. Pediatrics 1991; 87(5):701–707.

323. Bellinger DC, Jonas RA, Rappaport LA, Wypij D, Wernovsky G, Kuban KC et al. Developmental and neurologic status of children after heart surgery with hypothermic circulatory arrest or low-flow cardiopulmonary bypass. N Engl J Med 1995; 332(9):549–555.

324. Newburger JW, Jonas RA, Wernovsky G, Wypij D, Hickey PR, Kuban KC et al. A comparison of the perioperative neurologic effects of hypothermic circulatory arrest versus low-flow cardiopulmonary bypass in infant heart surgery. N Engl J Med 1993; 329(15):1057–1064.

325. Greeley WJ, Kern FH, Ungerleider RM, Boyd JL, III, Quill T, Smith LR et al. The effect of hypothermic cardiopulmonary bypass and total circulatory arrest on cerebral metabolism in neonates, infants, and children. J Thorac Cardiovasc Surg 1991; 101(5):783–794.

326. Fessatidis IT, Thomas VL, Shore DF, Sedgwick ME, Hunt RH, Weller RO. Brain damage after profoundly hypothermic circulatory arrest: correlations between neurophysiologic and neuropathologic findings. An experimental study in vertebrates. J Thorac Cardiovasc Surg 1993; 106(1):32–41.

327. Karl TR. Developmental and neurologic status of children after heart surgery. N Engl J Med 1995; 333(6):391–392.

328. Hovels-Gurich HH, Konrad K, Wiesner M, Minkenberg R, Herpertz-Dahlmann B, Messmer BJ et al. Long term behavioural outcome after neonatal arterial switch operation for transposition of the great arteries. Arch Dis Child 2002; 87(6):506–510.

329. Wong PC, Barlow CF, Hickey PR, Jonas RA, Castaneda AR, Farrell DM, Lock JE, Wessel DL. Factors associated with choreoathetosis after cardiopulmonary bypass in children with congenital heart disease. Circulation. 1992;86(5 Suppl):118–126.

330. Hovels-Gurich HH, Seghaye MC, Dabritz S, Messmer BJ, von Bernuth G. Cognitive and motor development in preschool and school-aged children after neonatal arterial switch operation. J Thorac Cardiovasc Surg 1997; 114(4):578–585.

331. Kern FH, Ungerleider RM, Schulman SR, Meliones JN, Schell RM, Baldwin B et al. Comparing two strategies of cardiopulmonary bypass cooling on jugular venous oxygen saturation in neonates and infants. Ann Thorac Surg 1995; 60(5):1198–1202.

332. Eke T, Woodruff G, Young ID. A new oculorenal syndrome: retinal dystrophy and tubulointerstitial nephropathy in cranioectodermal dysplasia. Br J Ophthalmol 1996; 80(5):490–491.

333. Mault JR, Ohtake S, Klingensmith ME, Heinle JS, Greeley WJ, Ungerleider RM. Cerebral metabolism and circulatory arrest: effects of duration and strategies for protection. Ann Thorac Surg 1993; 55(1):57–63.

334. Buss MI, McLean RF, Wong BI, Fremes SE, Naylor CD, Harrington EM et al. Cardiopulmonary bypass, rewarming, and central nervous system dysfunction. Ann Thorac Surg 1996; 61(5):1423–1427.

335. Jonas RA, Bellinger DC, Rappaport LA, Wernovsky G, Hickey PR, Farrell DM et al. Relation of pH strategy and developmental outcome after hypothermic circulatory arrest. J Thorac Cardiovasc Surg 1993; 106(2):362–368.

336. Wright M, Nolan T. Impact of cyanotic heart disease on school performance. Arch Dis Child 1994; 71(1):64–70.

337. Fuggle PW, Tokar S, Grant DB, Smith I. Rising IQ scores in British children: recent evidence. J Child Psychol Psychiatry 1992; 33(7):1241–1247.

338. Hynninen KM, Breitve MH, Wiborg AB, Pallesen S, Nordhus IH. Psychological characteristics of patients with chronic obstructive pulmonary disease: a review. J Psychosom Res 2005; 59(6):429–443.

339. McGrath E, Wypij D, Rappaport LA, Newburger JW, Bellinger DC. Prediction of IQ and achievement at age 8 years from neurodevelopmental status at age 1 year in children with D-transposition of the great arteries. Pediatrics 2004; 114(5):e572–e576.

340. Domi T, Edgell DS, McCrindle BW, Williams WG, Chan AK, MacGregor DL et al. Frequency, predictors, and neurologic outcomes of vaso-occlusive strokes associated with cardiac surgery in children. Pediatrics 2008; 122(6):1292–1298.

341. Wertham F, Mitchell N, Angrist A. The brain in sickle cell anemia. Arch Neurol Psychiatry 1942; 47:752–767.

342. Chodorkoff J, Whitten CF. Intellectual status of children with sickle cell anemia. J Pediatr 1963; 63:29–35.

343. Logothetis J, Economidou J, Constantoulakis M, Augoustaki O, Loewenson RB, Bilek M. Cephalofacial deformities in thalassemia major (Cooley's anemia). A correlative study among 138 cases. Am J Dis Child 1971; 121(4):300–306.

344. Whitten CF, Fischhoff J. Psychosocial effects of sickle cell disease. Arch Intern Med 1974; 133(4):681–689.

345. Kumar S, Powars D, Allen J, Haywood LJ. Anxiety, self-concept, and personal and social adjustments in children with sickle cell anemia. J Pediatr 1976; 88(5):859–863.

346. Nadel C, Portadin G. Sickle cell crises: psychological factors associated with onset. N Y State J Med 1977; 77(7):1075–1078.

347. Knight S, Singhal A, Thomas P, Serjeant G. Factors associated with lowered intelligence in homozygous sickle cell disease. Arch Dis Child 1995; 73(4):316–320.

348. Bernaudin F, Verlhac S, Freard F, Roudot-Thoraval F, Benkerrou M, Thuret I et al. Multicenter prospective study of children with sickle cell disease: radiographic and psychometric correlation. J Child Neurol 2000; 15(5):333–343.

349. Steen RG, Langston JW, Ogg RJ, Xiong X, Ye Z, Wang WC. Diffuse T1 reduction in gray matter of sickle cell disease patients: evidence of selective vulnerability to damage? Magn Reson Imaging 1999; 17(4):503–515.

350. Steen RG, Langston JW, Reddick WE, Ogg R, Chen G, Wang WC. Quantitative MR imaging of children with sickle cell disease: striking T1 elevation in the thalamus. J Magn Reson Imaging 1996; 6(1):226–234.

351. Baldeweg T, Hogan AM, Saunders DE, Telfer P, Gadian DG, Vargha-Khadem F et al. Detecting white matter injury in sickle cell disease using voxel-based morphometry. Ann Neurol 2006; 59(4):662–672.

352. Schatz J, Buzan R. Decreased corpus callosum size in sickle cell disease: relationship with cerebral infarcts and cognitive functioning. J Int Neuropsychol Soc 2006; 12(1):24–33.

353. Ohene-Frempong K, Weiner SJ, Sleeper LA, Miller ST, Embury S, Moohr JW et al. Cerebrovascular accidents in sickle cell disease: rates and risk factors. Blood 1998; 91(1):288–294.

354. Stevens MC, Maude GH, Cupidore L, Jackson H, Hayes RJ, Serjeant GR. Prepubertal growth and skeletal maturation in children with sickle cell disease. Pediatrics 1986; 78(1):124–132.

355. Steen RG, Langston JW, Ogg RJ, Manci E, Mulhern RK, Wang W. Ectasia of the basilar artery in children with sickle cell disease: relationship to hematocrit and psychometric measures. J Stroke Cerebrovasc Dis 1998; 7(1):32–43.

356. Grueneich R, Ris MD, Ball W, Kalinyak KA, Noll R, Vannatta K et al. Relationship of structural magnetic resonance imaging, magnetic resonance perfusion, and other disease factors to neuropsychological outcome in sickle cell disease. J Pediatr Psychol 2004; 29(2):83–92.

357. Zafeiriou DI, Prengler M, Gombakis N, Kouskouras K, Economou M, Kardoulas A et al. Central nervous system abnormalities in asymptomatic young patients with Sβ-thalassemia. Ann Neurol 2004; 55(6):835–839.

358. Boni LC, Brown RT, Davis PC, Hsu L, Hopkins K. Social information processing and magnetic resonance imaging in children with sickle cell disease. J Pediatr Psychol 2001; 26(5):309–319.

359. Swift AV, Cohen MJ, Hynd GW, Wisenbaker JM, McKie KM, Makari G et al. Neuropsychologic impairment in children with sickle cell anemia. Pediatrics 1989; 84(6):1077–1085.

360. Steen RG, Miles MA, Helton KJ, Strawn S, Wang W, Xiong X et al. Cognitive impairment in children with hemoglobin SS sickle cell disease: relationship to MR imaging findings and hematocrit. AJNR Am J Neuroradiol 2003; 24(3):382–389.

361. Flick GL, Duncan C. Perceptual-motor dysfunction in children with sickle cell trait. Percept Mot Skills 1973; 36(1):234.

362. McCormack MK, Scarr-Salapatek S, Polesky H, Thompson W, Katz SH, Barker WB. A comparison of the physical and intellectual development of black children with and without sickle-cell trait. Pediatrics 1975; 56(6):1021–1025.

363. Ashcroft MT, Desai P, Richardson SA, Serjeant GR. Growth, behaviour, and educational achievement of Jamaican children with sickle-cell trait. Br Med J 1976; 1(6022):1371–1373.

364. Kramer MS, Rooks Y, Pearson HA. Growth and development in children with sickle-cell trait. A prospective study of matched pairs. N Engl J Med 1978; 299(13):686–689.

365. Brown RT, Armstrong FD, Eckman JR. Neurocognitive aspects of pediatric sickle cell disease. J Learn Disabil 1993; 26(1):33–45.

366. Schatz J, Finke RL, Kellett JM, Kramer JH. Cognitive functioning in children with sickle cell disease: a meta-analysis. J Pediatr Psychol 2002; 27(8):739–748.

367. Hogan AM, Pit-ten Cate, Vargha-Khadem F, Prengler M, Kirkham FJ. Physiological correlates of intellectual function in children with sickle cell disease: hypoxaemia, hyperaemia and brain infarction. Dev Sci 2006; 9(4):379–387.

368. Cohen MJ, Branch WB, McKie VC, Adams RJ. Neuropsychological impairment in children with sickle cell anemia and cerebrovascular accidents. Clin Pediatr (Phila) 1994; 33(9):517–524.

369. DeBaun MR, Schatz J, Siegel MJ, Koby M, Craft S, Resar L et al. Cognitive screening examinations for silent cerebral infarcts in sickle cell disease. Neurology 1998; 50(6):1678–1682.

370. Craft S, Schatz J, Glauser TA, Lee B, DeBaun MR. Neuropsychologic effects of stroke in children with sickle cell anemia. J Pediatr 1993; 123(5):712–717.

371. Brown RT, Davis PC, Lambert R, Hsu L, Hopkins K, Eckman J. Neurocognitive functioning and magnetic resonance imaging in children with sickle cell disease. J Pediatr Psychol 2000; 25(7):503–513.

372. White DA, Salorio CF, Schatz J, DeBaun M. Preliminary study of working memory in children with stroke related to sickle cell disease. J Clin Exp Neuropsychol 2000; 22(2):257–264.

373. Schatz J, Roberts CW. Short-term memory in children with sickle cell disease: executive versus modality-specific processing deficits. Arch Clin Neuropsychol 2005; 20(8):1073–1085.

374. Davis P, Landers A, Gentry B, Montague J, Dancer J, Jackson J et al. Speech and language characteristics of children with strokes due to sickle cell disease. Percept Mot Skills 1997; 85(3 Pt 1):809–810.

375. Armstrong FD, Thompson RJ, Jr, Wang W, Zimmerman R, Pegelow CH, Miller S et al. Cognitive functioning and brain magnetic resonance imaging in children with sickle cell disease. Neuropsychology Committee of the Cooperative Study of Sickle Cell Disease. Pediatrics 1996; 97(6 Pt 1):864–870.

376. Heverly LL, Isaac W, Hynd GW. Neurodevelopmental and racial differences in tactile-visual (cross-modal. discrimination in normal black and white children. Arch Clin Neuropsychol 1986; 1(2):139–145.

377. Wang W, Enos L, Gallagher D, Thompson R, Guarini L, Vichinsky E et al. Neuropsychologic performance in school-aged children with sickle cell disease: a report from the Cooperative Study of Sickle Cell Disease. J Pediatr 2001; 139(3):391–397.

378. Thompson RJ, Jr, Armstrong FD, Link CL, Pegelow CH, Moser F, Wang WC. A prospective study of the relationship over time of behavior problems, intellectual functioning, and family functioning in children with sickle cell disease: a report from the Cooperative Study of Sickle Cell Disease. J Pediatr Psychol 2003; 28(1):59–65.

379. Vichinsky EP, Neumayr LD, Gold JI, Weiner MW, Rule RR, Truran D, Kasten J, Eggleston B, Kesler K, McMahon L, Orringer EP, Harrington T, Kalinyak K, De Castro LM, Kutlar A, Rutherford CJ, Johnson C, Bessman JD, Jordan LB, Armstrong FD;

Neuropsychological Dysfunction and Neuroimaging Adult Sickle Cell Anemia Study Group. Neuropsychological dysfunction and neuroimaging abnormalities in neurologically intact adults with sickle cell anemia. JAMA. 2010; 303(18):1823–1831.

380. Brass LM, Prohovnik I, Pavlakis SG, DeVivo DC, Piomelli S, Mohr JP. Middle cerebral artery blood velocity and cerebral blood flow in sickle cell disease. Stroke 1991; 22(1):27–30.

381. Adams RJ, Nichols FT, McKie V, McKie K, Milner P, Gammal TE. Cerebral infarction in sickle cell anemia: mechanism based on CT and MRI. Neurology 1988; 38(7):1012–1017.

382. Adams R, McKie V, Nichols F, Carl E, Zhang DL, McKie K et al. The use of transcranial ultrasonography to predict stroke in sickle cell disease. N Engl J Med 1992; 326(9):605–610.

383. Adams RJ, McKie VC, Carl EM, Nichols FT, Perry R, Brock K et al. Long-term stroke risk in children with sickle cell disease screened with transcranial Doppler. Ann Neurol 1997; 42(5):699–704.

384. Steen RG, Reddick WE, Glass JO, Wang WC. Evidence of cranial artery ectasia in sickle cell disease patients with ectasia of the basilar artery. J Stroke Cerebrovasc Dis 1998; 7(5):330–338.

385. Kral MC, Brown RT, Nietert PJ, Abboud MR, Jackson SM, Hynd GW. Transcranial Doppler ultrasonography and neurocognitive functioning in children with sickle cell disease. Pediatrics 2003; 112(2):324–331.

386. Fowler MG, Johnson MP, Atkinson SS. School achievement and absence in children with chronic health conditions. J Pediatr 1985; 106(4):683–687.

387. Fowler MG, Whitt JK, Lallinger RR, Nash KB, Atkinson SS, Wells RJ et al. Neuropsychologic and academic functioning of children with sickle cell anemia. J Dev Behav Pediatr 1988; 9(4):213–220.

388. Richard HW, Burlew AK. Academic performance among children with sickle cell disease: setting minimum standards for comparison groups. Psychol Rep 1997; 81(1):27–34.

389. Sanders C, Gentry B, Davis P, Jackson J, Saccente S, Dancer J. Reading, writing, and vocabulary skills of children with strokes due to sickle cell disease. Percept Mot Skills 1997; 85(2):477–478.

390. Steen RG, Hu XJ, Elliott VE, Miles MA, Jones S, Wang WC. Kindergarten readiness skills in children with sickle cell disease: evidence of early neurocognitive damage? J Child Neurol 2002; 17(2):111–116.

391. Schatz J. Brief report: academic attainment in children with sickle cell disease. J Pediatr Psychol 2004; 29(8):627–633.

392. Yerys BE, White DA, Salorio CF, McKinstry R, Moinuddin A, DeBaun M. Memory strategy training in children with cerebral infarcts related to sickle cell disease. J Pediatr Hematol Oncol 2003; 25(6):495–498.

393. King AA, DeBaun MR, White DA. Need for cognitive rehabilitation for children with sickle cell disease and strokes. Expert Rev Neurother 2008; 8(2):291–296.

394. Baddeley A, Hitch G. Working memory. In: The Psychology of Learning and Motivation (ed G Bower). New York, NY: Academic Press, 1974; 47–89.

395. Brandling-Bennett EM, White DA, Armstrong MM, Christ SE, DeBaun M. Patterns of verbal long-term and working memory performance reveal deficits in strategic processing in children with frontal infarcts related to sickle cell disease. Dev Neuropsychol 2003; 24(1):423–434.

396. Sun X, Zhang X, Chen X, Zhang P, Bao M, Zhang D et al. Age-dependent brain activation during forward and backward digit recall revealed by fMRI. Neuroimage 2005; 26(1):36–47.

397. Petrides M. Impairments on nonspatial self-ordered and externally ordered working memory tasks after lesions of the mid-dorsal part of the lateral frontal cortex in the monkey. J Neurosci 1995; 15(1 Pt 1):359–375.

398. Hogan AM, Vargha-Khadem F, Saunders DE, Kirkham FJ, Baldeweg T. Impact of frontal white matter lesions on performance monitoring: ERP evidence for cortical disconnection. Brain 2006; 129(Pt 8):2177–2188.

399. Fowler B, Lindeis AE. The effects of hypoxia on auditory reaction time and P300 latency. Aviat Space Environ Med 1992; 63(11):976–981.

400. Brown RD, Jr. Simple risk predictions for arteriovenous malformation hemorrhage. Neurosurgery 2000; 46(4):1024.

401. Hogan AM, Prengler M, Kirkham FJ, Telfer P, Lane R, Vargha-Khadem F et al. Physiological correlates of neurodevelopmental abnormality in infants with sickle cell anaemia. Dev Med Child Neurol 2004; 47(Suppl 101): 4.

402. Todd GB, Serjeant GR, Larson MR. Sensori-neural hearing loss in Jamaicans with SS disease. Acta Otolaryngol 1973; 76(4):268–272.

403. Sharp M, Orchik DJ. Auditory function in sickle cell anemia. Arch Otolaryngol 1978; 104(6):322–324.

404. Koussi A, Zafeiriou DI, Kontzoglou G, Tsatra I, Noussios G, Athanassiou M. Hearing loss in children with sickle cell disease. Acta Otorhinolaryngol Belg 2001; 55(3):235–239.

405. Burch-Sims GP, Matlock VR. Hearing loss and auditory function in sickle cell disease. J Commun Disord 2005; 38(4):321–329.

406. Alabi S, Ernest K, Eletta P, Owolabi A, Afolabi A, Suleiman O. Otological findings among Nigerian children with sickle cell anaemia. Int J Pediatr Otorhinolaryngol 2008; 72(5):659–663.

407. Hamon JF, Seri B, Sangare A. Auditory event-related potentials and reaction times during simple sensorymotor tasks in subjects with sickle cell disease and related hemoglobinopathies. Ital J Neurol Sci 1990; 11(3):251–258.

408. Luria AR. Towards the mechanisms of naming disturbance. Neuropsychologia 1973; 11(4):417–421.

409. Kirkham FJ, Calamante F, Bynevelt M, Gadian DG, Evans JP, Cox TC et al. Perfusion magnetic resonance abnormalities in patients with sickle cell disease. Ann Neurol 2001; 49(4):477–485.

410. Schatz J, Craft S, Koby M, Siegel MJ, Resar L, Lee R. Neuropsychological deficits in children with sickle cell disease and cerebral infarction: role of lesion site and volume. Child Neuropsychol 1999; 5:92–103.

411. Goonan BT, Goonan LJ, Brown RT, Buchanan I, Eckman JR. Sustained attention and inhibitory control in children with sickle cell syndrome. Arch Clin Neuropsychol 1994; 9(1):89–104.

412. Schatz J, Craft S, Koby M, DeBaun MR. Asymmetries in visual-spatial processing following childhood stroke. Neuropsychology 2004; 18(2):340–352.

413. Nabors NA, Freymuth AK. Attention deficits in children with sickle cell disease. Percept Mot Skills 2002; 95(1):57–67.

414. Hogan AM, Vargha-Khadem F, Kirkham FJ, Baldeweg T. Maturation of action monitoring from adolescence to adulthood: an ERP study. Dev Sci 2005; 8(6):525–534.

415. Hogan AM, Kirkham FJ, Prengler M, Telfer P, Lane R, Vargha-Khadem F et al. An exploratory study of physiological correlates of neurodevelopmental delay in infants with sickle cell anaemia. Br J Haematol 2006; 132(1):99–107.

416. Noll RB, Stith L, Gartstein MA, Ris MD, Grueneich R, Vannatta K et al. Neuropsychological functioning of youths with sickle cell disease: comparison with non-chronically ill peers. J Pediatr Psychol 2001; 26(2):69–78.

417. Gentry BF, Varlik L, Dancer J. Children's perceptions of psychosocial factors related to sickle cell disease. Percept Mot Skills 1997; 85(3 Pt 2):1409–1410.

418. Gentry B, Dancer J. Screening the speech of young patients with sickle cell disease. Percept Mot Skills 1997; 84(2):662.

419. Davis P, Landers A, Gentry B, Montague J, Dancer J, Jackson J et al. Speech and language characteristics of children with strokes due to sickle cell disease. Percept Mot Skills 1997; 85(3 Pt 1):809–810.

420. Hind SE, Atkins RL, Haggard MP, Brady D, Grinham G. Alternatives in screening at school entry: comparison of the childhood middle ear disease and hearing questionnaire (CMEDHQ) and the pure tone sweep test. Br J Audiol 1999; 33(6):403–414.

421. Wang WC, Grover R, Gallagher D, Espeland M, Fandal A. Developmental screening in young children with sickle cell disease. Results of a cooperative study. Am J Pediatr Hematol Oncol 1993; 15(1):87–91.

422. Wang WC, Langston JW, Steen RG, Wynn LW, Mulhern RK, Wilimas JA et al. Abnormalities of the central nervous system in very young children with sickle cell anemia. J Pediatr 1998; 132(6):994–998.

423. Thompson RJ, Jr, Gustafson KE, Bonner MJ, Ware RE. Neurocognitive development of young children with sickle cell disease through three years of age. J Pediatr Psychol 2002; 27(3):235–244.

424. Hess CR, Papas MA, Black MM. Use of the Bayley Infant Neurodevelopmental Screener with an environmental risk group. J Pediatr Psychol 2004; 29(5):321–330.

425. Schatz J, McClellan CB. Sickle cell disease as a neurodevelopmental disorder. Ment Retard Dev Disabil Res Rev 2006; 12(3):200–207.

426. Schatz J, McClellan CB, Puffer ES, Johnson K, Roberts CW. Neurodevelopmental screening in toddlers and early preschoolers with sickle cell disease. J Child Neurol 2008; 23(1):44–50.

427. Schatz J, Roberts CW. Neurobehavioral impact of sickle cell disease in early childhood. J Int Neuropsychol Soc 2007; 13(6):933–943.

428. Wang WC, Pavlakis SG, Helton KJ, McKinstry RC, Casella JF, Adams RJ et al. MRI abnormalities of the brain in one-year-old children with sickle cell anemia. Pediatr Blood Cancer 2008; 51(5):643–646.

429. Morgan SA, Jackson J. Psychological and social concomitants of sickle cell anemia in adolescents. J Pediatr Psychol 1986; 11(3):429–440.

430. Barrett DH, Wisotzek IE, Abel GG, Rouleau JL, Platt AF, Jr, Pollard WE et al. Assessment of psychosocial functioning of patients with sickle cell disease. South Med J 1988; 81(6):745–750.

431. Barakat LP, Schwartz LA, Simon K, Radcliffe J. Negative thinking as a coping strategy mediator of pain and internalizing symptoms in adolescents with sickle cell disease. J Behav Med 2007; 30(3):199–208.

432. Gold JI, Treadwell M, Weissman L, Vichinsky E. An expanded Transactional Stress and Coping Model for siblings of children with sickle cell disease: family functioning and sibling coping, self-efficacy and perceived social support. Child Care Health Dev 2008; 34(4):491–502.

433. Kral MC, Brown RT. Transcranial Doppler ultrasonography and executive dysfunction in children with sickle cell disease. J Pediatr Psychol 2004; 29(3):185–195.

434. Iloeje SO. Psychiatric morbidity among children with sickle-cell disease. Dev Med Child Neurol 1991; 33(12):1087–1094.

435. Leavell SR, Ford CV. Psychopathology in patients with sickle cell disease. Psychosomatics 1983; 24(1):23–29, 32.

436. Cepeda ML, Yang YM, Price CC, Shah A. Mental disorders in children and adolescents with sickle cell disease. South Med J 1997; 90(3):284–287.

437. Yang YM, Cepeda M, Price C, Shah A, Mankad V. Depression in children and adolescents with sickle-cell disease. Arch Pediatr Adolesc Med 1994; 148(5):457–460.

438. Cohen ME, Marino RJ. The tools of disability outcomes research functional status measures. Arch Phys Med Rehabil 2000; 81(12 Suppl 2):S21–S29.

439. Ostensjo S, Bjorbaekmo W, Carlberg EB, Vollestad NK. Assessment of everyday functioning in young children with disabilities: an ICF-based analysis of concepts and content of the Pediatric Evaluation of Disability Inventory (PEDI). Disabil Rehabil 2006; 28(8):489–504.

440. Stucki G, Celio M. Developing human functioning and rehabilitation research. Part II: Interdisciplinary university centers and national and regional collaboration networks. J Rehabil Med 2007; 39(4):334–342.

441. Simeonsson RJ, Leonardi M, Lollar D, Bjorck-Akesson E, Hollenweger J, Martinuzzi A. Applying the International Classification of Functioning, Disability and Health (ICF) to measure childhood disability. Disabil Rehabil 2003; 25(11–12):602–610.

442. Duckworth M. Outcome measurement selection and typology. Physiotherapy 1999; 85:21–27.

443. Kwakkel G, Wagenaar RC, Kollen BJ, Lankhorst GJ. Predicting disability in stroke – a critical review of the literature. Age Ageing 1996; 25(6):479–489.

444. Paediatric Stroke Working Group. Stroke in Childhood: Clinical Guidelines for Diagnosis, Management and Rehabilitation, 2009. Available from: URL:http://www.rcplondon.ac.uk/pubs/books/childstroke/

445. Duncan PW, Zorowitz R, Bates B, Choi JY, Glasberg JJ, Graham GD et al. Management of Adult Stroke Rehabilitation Care: a clinical practice guideline. Stroke 2005; 36(9):e100–e143.

446. Prvu Bettger JA, Stineman MG. Effectiveness of multidisciplinary rehabilitation services in postacute care: state-of-the-science. A review. Arch Phys Med Rehabil 2007; 88(11):1526–1534.

447. Duncan PW, Velozo CA. State-of-the-science on postacute rehabilitation: measurement and methodologies for assessing quality and establishing policy for postacute care. Arch Phys Med Rehabil 2007; 88(11):1482–1487.

448. Donabedian A. The role of outcomes in quality assessment and assurance. QRB Qual Rev Bull 1992; 18(11):356–360.

449. Kreisel SH, Hennerici MG, Bazner H. Pathophysiology of stroke rehabilitation: the natural course of clinical recovery, use-dependent plasticity and rehabilitative outcome. Cerebrovasc Dis 2007; 23(4):243–255.

450. Lai SM, Studenski S, Duncan PW, Perera S. Persisting consequences of stroke measured by the Stroke Impact Scale. Stroke 2002; 33(7):1840–1844.

451. Wade DT, Skilbeck CE, Hewer RL, Wood VA. Therapy after stroke: amounts, determinants and effects. Int Rehabil Med 1984; 6(3):105–110.

452. Cifu DX, Stewart DG. Factors affecting functional outcome after stroke: a critical review of rehabilitation interventions. Arch Phys Med Rehabil 1999; 80(5 Suppl 1):S35–S39.

453. Aziz NA, Leonardi-Bee J, Phillips M, Gladman JR, Legg L, Walker MF. Therapy-based rehabilitation services for patients living at home more than one year after stroke. Cochrane Database Syst Rev 2008;(2):CD005952.

454. Bernhardt J, Chan J, Nicola I, Collier JM. Little therapy, little physical activity: rehabilitation within the first 14 days of organized stroke unit care. J Rehabil Med 2007; 39(1):43–48.

455. Coetzer R, Rushe R. Post-acute rehabilitation following traumatic brain injury: are both early and later improved outcomes possible? Int J Rehabil Res 2005; 28(4):361–363.

456. Tangeman PT, Banaitis DA, Williams AK. Rehabilitation of chronic stroke patients: changes in functional performance. Arch Phys Med Rehabil 1990; 71(11):876–880.

457. Demain S, Wiles R, Roberts L, McPherson K. Recovery plateau following stroke: fact or fiction? Disabil Rehabil 2006; 28(13–14):815–821.

458. Boyd RN, Morris ME, Graham HK. Management of upper limb dysfunction in children with cerebral palsy: a systematic review. Eur J Neurol 2001; 8(Suppl 5):150–166.

459. Cramer SC, Riley JD. Neuroplasticity and brain repair after stroke. Curr Opin Neurol 2008; 21(1):76–82.

460. Carey LM, Seitz RJ. Functional neuroimaging in stroke recovery and neurorehabilitation: conceptual issues and perspectives. Int J Stroke 2007; 2(4):245–264.

461. Helders PJ, Engelbert RH, Gulmans VA, van der Net J. Paediatric rehabilitation. Disabil Rehabil 2001; 23(11):497–500.

462. Grilli L, Feldman DE, Majnemer A, Couture M, Azoulay L, Swaine B. Associations between a functional independence measure (WeeFIM) and the pediatric quality of life inventory (PedsQL4.0) in young children with physical disabilities. Qual Life Res 2006; 15(6):1023–1031.

463. Cusick A, McIntyre S, Novak I, Lannin N, Lowe K. A comparison of goal attainment scaling and the Canadian Occupational Performance Measure for paediatric rehabilitation research. Pediatr Rehabil 2006; 9(2):149–157.

464. Nijhuis BJ, Reinders-Messelink HA, de Blecourt AC, Olijve WG, Groothoff JW, Nakken H et al. A review of salient elements defining team collaboration in paediatric rehabilitation. Clin Rehabil 2007; 21(3):195–211.

465. Anderson V, Catroppa C. Advances in postacute rehabilitation after childhood-acquired brain injury: a focus on cognitive, behavioral, and social domains. Am J Phys Med Rehabil 2006; 85(9):767–778.

466. Trombly C. Clinical practice guidelines for post-stroke rehabilitation and occupational therapy practice. Am J Occup Ther 1995; 49(7):711–714.

467. Boyd RN, Hays RM. Outcome measurement of effectiveness of botulinum toxin type A in children with cerebral palsy: an ICIDH-2 approach. Eur J Neurol 2001; 8(Suppl 5):167–177.

468. Spittle AJ, Orton J, Doyle LW, Boyd R. Early developmental intervention programs post hospital discharge to prevent motor and cognitive impairments in preterm infants. Cochrane Database Syst Rev 2007;(2):CD005495.

469. Taub E, Miller NE, Novack TA, Cook EW, III, Fleming WC, Nepomuceno CS et al. Technique to improve chronic motor deficit after stroke. Arch Phys Med Rehabil 1993; 74(4):347–354.

470. Pierce SR, Daly K, Gallagher KG, Gershkoff AM, Schaumburg SW. Constraint-induced therapy for a child with hemiplegic cerebral palsy: a case report. Arch Phys Med Rehabil 2002; 83(10):1462–1463.

471. Glover JE, Mateer CA, Yoell C, Speed S. The effectiveness of constraint induced movement therapy in two young children with hemiplegia. Pediatr Rehabil 2002; 5(3):125–131.

472. Karman N, Maryles J, Baker RW, Simpser E, Berger-Gross P. Constraint-induced movement therapy for hemiplegic children with acquired brain injuries. J Head Trauma Rehabil 2003; 18(3):259–267.

473. Taub E, Ramey SL, DeLuca S, Echols K. Efficacy of constraint-induced movement therapy for children with cerebral palsy with asymmetric motor impairment. Pediatrics 2004; 113(2):305–312.

474. Charles J, Gordon AM. A critical review of constraint-induced movement therapy and forced use in children with hemiplegia. Neural Plast 2005; 12(2–3):245–261.

475. Charles JR, Wolf SL, Schneider JA, Gordon AM. Efficacy of a child-friendly form of constraint-induced movement therapy in hemiplegic cerebral palsy: a randomized control trial. Dev Med Child Neurol 2006; 48(8):635–642.

476. Taub E, Griffin A, Nick J, Gammons K, Uswatte G, Law CR. Pediatric CI therapy for stroke-induced hemiparesis in young children. Dev Neurorehabil 2007; 10(1):3–18.

477. Gordon A, Connelly A, Neville B, Vargha-Khadem F, Jessop N, Murphy T et al. Modified constraint-induced movement therapy after childhood stroke. Dev Med Child Neurol 2007; 49(1):23–27.

478. Hoare B, Imms C, Carey L, Wasiak J. Constraint-induced movement therapy in the treatment of the upper limb in children with hemiplegic cerebral palsy: a Cochrane systematic review. Clin Rehabil 2007; 21(8):675–685.

479. Damiano DL, Abel MF. Functional outcomes of strength training in spastic cerebral palsy. Arch Phys Med Rehabil 1998; 79(2):119–125.

480. Darrah J, Fran JSW, Chen LC, Nunweiler J, Watkins B. Review of the effects of progressive resisted muscle strengthening in children with cerebral palsy: A clinical exercise. Pediatr Phys Ther 1997; 9:12–17.

481. Ada L, Dorsch S, Canning CG. Strengthening interventions increase strength and improve activity after stroke: a systematic review. Aust J Physiother 2006; 52(4):241–248.

482. Unger M, Faure M, Frieg A. Strength training in adolescent learners with cerebral palsy: a randomized controlled trial. Clin Rehabil 2006; 20(6):469–477.

483. Yang YR, Wang RY, Lin KH, Chu MY, Chan RC. Task-oriented progressive resistance strength training improves muscle strength and functional performance in individuals with stroke. Clin Rehabil 2006; 20(10):860–870.

484. Weiss A, Suzuki T, Bean J, Fielding RA. High intensity strength training improves strength and functional performance after stroke. Am J Phys Med Rehabil 2000; 79(4):369–376.

485. Utley A, Steenbergen B. Discrete bimanual co-ordination in children and young adolescents with hemiparetic cerebral palsy: recent findings, implications and future research directions. Pediatr Rehabil 2006; 9(2):127–136.

486. Kirton A, Chen R, Friefeld S, Gunraj C, Pontigon AM, deVeber G. Contralesional repetitive transcranial magnetic stimulation for chronic hemiparesis in subcortical paediatric stroke: a randomised trial. Lancet Neurol 2008; 7(6):507–513.

487. Kirton A, deVeber G, Gunraj C, Chen R. Neurocardiogenic syncope complicating pediatric transcranial magnetic stimulation. Pediatr Neurol 2008; 39(3):196–197.

488. Page SJ, Levine P. Back from the brink: electromyography-triggered stimulation combined with modified constraint-induced movement therapy in chronic stroke. Arch Phys Med Rehabil 2006; 87(1):27–31.

489. Eng K, Siekierka E, Pyk P, Chevrier E, Hauser Y, Cameirao M et al. Interactive visuo-motor therapy system for stroke rehabilitation. Med Biol Eng Comput 2007; 45(9):901–907.

490. Golomb MR, McDonald BC, Warden SJ, Yonkman J, Saykin AJ, Shirley B et al. In-home virtual reality videogame telerehabilitation in adolescents with hemiplegic cerebral palsy. Arch Phys Med Rehabil 2010; 91(1):1–8.

491. Edwards S. Physiotherapy management of established spasticity. In: Spasticity Rehabilitation (ed G Sheean). London: Churchill Communications Europe, 1998; 71–89.

492. Lebeer J, Rijke R. Ecology of development in children with brain impairment. Child Care Health Dev 2003; 29(2):131–140.

493. Thorpe DE, Valvano J. The effects of knowledge of performance and cognitive strategies on motor skill learning in children with cerebral palsy. Pediatr Phys Ther 2002; 14(1):2–15.

494. Ylvisaker M, Feeney T. Pediatric brain injury: social, behavioral, and communication disability. Phys Med Rehabil Clin N Am 2007; 18(1):133–144, vii.

495. Davidoff RA. Antispasticity drugs: mechanisms of action. Ann Neurol 1985; 17(2):107–116.

496. Gallichio JE. Pharmacologic management of spasticity following stroke. Phys Ther 2004; 84(10):973–981.

497. Roussan M, Terrence C, Fromm G. Baclofen versus diazepam for the treatment of spasticity and long-term follow-up of baclofen therapy. Pharmatherapeutica 1985; 4(5):278–284.

498. Meythaler JM, Guin-Renfroe S, Brunner RC, Hadley MN. Intrathecal baclofen for spastic hypertonia from stroke. Stroke 2001; 32(9):2099–2109.

499. Turner MS. Early use of intrathecal baclofen in brain injury in pediatric patients. Acta Neurochir Suppl 2003; 87:81–83.

500. Brin MF. Spasticity study group: dosing, administration, and a treatment algorithm for use of botulinum toxin A for adult onset spasticity. Muscle Nerve 1997; 6:208–220.

501. Bhakta BB, Cozens JA, Chamberlain MA, Bamford JM. Impact of botulinum toxin type A on disability and carer burden due to arm spasticity after stroke: a randomised double blind placebo controlled trial. J Neurol Neurosurg Psychiatry 2000; 69(2):217–221.

502. Lagalla G, Danni M, Reiter F, Ceravolo MG, Provinciali L. Post-stroke spasticity management with repeated botulinum toxin injections in the upper limb. Am J Phys Med Rehabil 2000; 79(4):377–384.

503. Ozcakir S, Sivrioglu K. Botulinum toxin in poststroke spasticity. Clin Med Res 2007; 5(2):132–138.

504. Carr LJ, Cosgrove AP, Gringras P, Neville BG. Position paper on the use of botulinum toxin in cerebral palsy. UK Botulinum Toxin and Cerebral Palsy Working Party. Arch Dis Child 1998; 79(3):271–273.

505. Heinen F, Schroeder AS, Fietzek U, Berweck S. When it comes to botulinum toxin, children and adults are not the same: multimuscle option for children with cerebral palsy. Mov Disord 2006; 21(11):2029–2030.

506. Bakheit AM, Severa S, Cosgrove A, Morton R, Roussounis SH, Doderlein L et al. Safety profile and efficacy of botulinum toxin A (Dysport) in children with muscle spasticity. Dev Med Child Neurol 2001; 43(4):234–238.

507. Kirkham FJ, Neville BG, Levin SD. Bedside diagnosis of stenosis of middle cerebral artery. Lancet. 1986; 1(8484):797–798.

18
FUTURE DIRECTIONS

Vijeya Ganesan and Fenella J. Kirkham

The period encompassing the gestation of this book has been incontestably the most exciting for those working in the field of paediatric cerebrovascular disease. The field has moved on from being largely descriptive to one that, at last, attempts to understand underlying disease mechanisms and which, therefore, holds real promise of improving the outcomes for affected children. Significant relevant landmarks are an appreciation of the importance of arteriopathy, an explosion in the literature describing the outcome of children affected by vascular stroke syndromes, and unique approaches to deriving aetiological clues that might propel the field forward.

Of these, some deserve special mention. Firstly the International Pediatric Stroke Study (IPSS) group[1] now comprises collaborating centres from more than 10 different countries, achieved with minimal funding. For the first time there is an opportunity to gain a truly international perspective on the disease burden, and also the infrastructure which will be critical to undertake more focused, hypothesis-driven studies. The lack of funding is a relevant point as stroke in adults, so much more prevalent than the paediatric problem, remains a wallflower in research-funding battles. However, this impressive collaboration of committed participants means that the early products of this network are coming into fruition,[1,2] and will support and justify future work.

Secondly, the epidemiological perspective from population-based datasets across the UK, Switzerland, the USA and Kaiser Permanante in Northern California has generated observations which are not reliant on single institution bias. Recent findings from the latter group include those regarding sex, ethnicity[3] and mortality of affected children,[4] the presentation, natural history and outcome of paediatric arterial stroke,[5–8] and the higher incidence of childhood stroke once radiological reports are counted as well as clinical presentations,[9] in addition to the important work showing a much higher incidence of stroke in neonates,[10,11] recently confirmed in Europe[12,13] and Canada.[14]

Thirdly, standardized terminology and evaluation tools[15,16] have significantly contributed hugely to collaboration and Tim Bernard on behalf of the IPSS is currently developing the Childhood AIS Standardized Classification And Diagnostic Evaluation (CASCADE). In a relatively rare condition, where research must span continents, a common language is critical to ensure mutual understanding. The vasculopathy classification,[17] and more recent modifications,[2,18] means that radiologists have been brought into the arena of precise description when reporting neuroimaging. This can only immediately improve patient care and, in the longer term, provide a robust basis for multi-centre research, starting with the Vascular Effects of Infection in Paediatric Stroke (VIPS) cohort recently funded by the National Institute of Neurological Disorders and Stroke. The all-encompassing but vague term 'stroke', coined to describe clinical presentations in adults, is relatively uninformative to the paediatrician, parent or reader of a research paper. 'Stroke' is a clinical term, describing an acute focal neurological syndrome, but in 21st century paediatric practice we should invoke greater precision. At least 20–30% of children with clinical 'stroke' will not have a vascular aetiology;[19,20] amongst those that do, it is so much more helpful to all concerned to use precise terms such as arterial ischaemic stroke, cerebral venous thrombosis (+/– infarction) or intracranial haemorrhage (which can be further subdivided). In the current era of sophisticated neuroimaging it is no longer acceptable to lump all and sundry cerebrovascular disorders together in neonates[21] or in children.[20] Each of the vascular stroke syndromes in children required a focused, targeted approach in the period immediately after presentation, further modified by the age of the affected child. In the era of cost-effective medicine such an investigative approach may yet win favour.

There is now an evidence base for the prevention of arterial ischaemic stroke in children with sickle cell disease, who, worldwide, form the most vulnerable group.[22,23] The STOP and STOP2 studies also serve as a model for paediatric research, illustrating that logistic constraints need not pose a barrier to the highest quality research in children. Although a further trial looking at prevention of progressive silent infarction will publish in 2013, blood transfusion is unlikely to provide a magic bullet for these children and so other, equally well structured studies exploring risk factors and alternative preventative treatments[24–27] are ongoing. The impressive funding record for stroke research in sickle cell disease is especially encouraging to the field as a whole where trials of acute treatment[28,29] and rehabilitative strategies[30–32] are in various stages of evolution.

Finally, there has been a recent proliferation of clinical guidelines relating to childhood stroke. Each of the three currently published (Royal College of Physicians,[33] American College of Chest Physicians[34] and American Heart Association[35]) are derived from the same sparse evidence base, and although there are some differences, the general consensus is encouraging.[36] More importantly, the fact that august bodies are commissioning such guidelines suggests that paediatric 'stroke' is no longer the 'Cinderella' field it once was.

So what does the future hold? Firstly, there is the real prospect of multicentre collaboration and the potential to attract robust funding to answer questions in the laboratory[37–40] as well as in the clinical setting. But both rely on asking the right questions, which are perhaps more difficult to define. The observation that antecedent infection is predictive of the arteriopathy[2] provides a trail which should be followed in an attempt to understand disease mechanisms leading to a logical approach to treatment. At the time of writing, elucidating the trigger of focal cerebral arteriopathy of childhood,[18] be it infective, inflammatory or genetic predisposition, seems an obvious next step, potentially leading to secondary or even primary preventive methods.

Future research might be hampered by the weight of anecdotal evidence underpinning now widely accepted treatments, such as aspirin or anticoagulation for arterial ischaemic stroke, anticoagulation for cerebral venous sinus thrombosis[41] or revascularization for moyamoya.[42,43] There has never been a robust paediatric clinical trial of any of these approaches, although ongoing concerns about recurrence risk, e.g. for posterior circulation stroke,[44] and outcome, e.g. for neonates with venous sinus thrombosis now that it is increasingly diagnosed,[45] mean that there may now be enough momentum to make these studies a priority. Comparison across continents[46,47] and the advent of clinical guidelines,[33–35] which, hopefully, will encourage a more standardized approach to patient management, could provide data that can be critically appraised, so that at least these advocated approaches can be evaluated retrospectively. The wide range of tests needed to examine cognitive, as well as motor, outcome has hampered progress in terms of defining endpoints but good quality data are emerging in neonatal[48] and childhood[49] stroke. In addition to the formal assessment of neurology using the Paediatric Stroke Outcome Measure (PSOM), tools assessing function, such as the PSOM modification for telephone use,[50] the World Health Organization's International Classification of Impairments, Disabilities and Handicaps[49] or appropriate adaptations of the modified Rankin scales,[51] are likely to find a role (Bulder MM, personal communication). Dichotomizing outcome is likely to be important for studies of early predictors,[50,51] and for trials, but drawing the line between good and poor is very difficult and more work is needed to define the currently imprecise categories open to assessor interpretation about 'age appropriate activities' and 'pre-existing disabilities'.[51]

Greater semantic precision should also help to standardize the literature, as well as the clinical approach. The likely underlying disease mechanisms also deserve critical attention. For example, thrombolysis, a proven treatment in atheromatous arterial ischaemic stroke in adults, is unlikely to prove to be a universally applicable approach in children, with the inherent differences in differential diagnosis, risk versus benefit ratio and immaturity of the coagulation system.[52] Although there is much enthusiasm for the pilot paediatric stroke thrombolysis trial (TIPS) recently funded by NINDS,[28,29,52,53]

these are relevant considerations. It is essential that clinical trial design takes the physiology of children and likely disease mechanism into consideration.

A simple, yet fundamental, question, remains about the relevance of patent foramen ovale (PFO) to the genesis of arterial ischaemic stroke in children. PFO is particularly prevalent in this age group, and eminently amenable to treatment, yet there are polarized views in the literature regarding its potential contribution from the fields of cardiology and neurology.[54] Standardized assessment protocols,[55,56] now advocated, can surely only be a prelude to well organized investigations of this association, such as the PFAST study in sickle cell disease.

The promise of modern neuroimaging, in particular magnetic resonance imaging (MRI), in aiding accurate diagnosis and disease characterization has probably not been completely fulfilled. MRI has revolutionized our ability to accurately identify cerebral ischaemia acutely in neonates as well as in children and to distinguish between vascular stroke syndromes and 'stroke mimics'. However, the potential to characterize individual pathophysiology, and to use this to inform treatments, remains limited. MRI has significant advantages in relation to lack of radiation exposure to the developing brain, but there are both logistical and technical challenges remaining which need to be overcome. Especially pertinent to the current discussion are the limitations of interpreting perfusion MRI in patients with cerebrovascular disease.[57]

As already mentioned, future research is likely to lead to treatments more targeted to underlying disease mechanism, taking into account predisposition to poor outcome from the underlying condition,[58] as well as the acute event.[59] However, the wider applicability of existing screening programmes[60] and treatments also deserves consideration. For example, moyamoya in children with sickle cell disease has been shown to be predictive of arterial ischaemic stroke recurrence despite blood transfusion.[61] Revascularization has shown promise in this group[62] but the radiological criteria to identify eligible patients, and the role of surgery in relation to other novel[63] and more established treatments, such as blood transfusion, remain undefined. The potential of interventional neuroradiology, specifically angioplasty and stenting, is also largely unexplored. However, technical developments and an increased skill base means that there are potential treatments which need to be linked with the appropriate patient group.

Intracranial haemorrhage (or 'haemorrhagic stroke') remains a largely unresearched area.[64–68] The existing literature is mainly descriptive and most papers report on specific treatment approaches. Few centres have the expertise to provide holistic evaluation of vascular malformations, encompassing neurosurgery, interventional neuroradiology and radiosurgery, although in the 21st century this should be the standard of care. These are the children at highest risk of mortality, and it is encouraging to see work on assessment of volume of haemorrhage,[64] which is a potential predictor of outcome to be evaluated in prospective studies. These children also face the physical and psychological burden of living with a potentially explosive vascular malformation. The 'paediatric stroke' world should take this group under its wing as there is real potential to critically appraise interventional treatments, as has been successfully achieved in adults.

Finally, a major barrier to adequate care, however flawed it might be currently, is prompt recognition and evaluation of the acutely impaired child. This is not only of relevance to 'stroke' but also a commentary on the inadequacy of acute evaluation, triage and investigation of sick children. Parents realize something is wrong very quickly[69] but they often have to work hard to convince doctors, who in turn face a lack of resources to investigate and refer children on in a timely manner. A hemiparetic 55 year old would be scanned acutely and referred on to a stroke unit; unfortunately, even when resources should not limit access to healthcare, a 7 year old is less likely to receive similar attention. This reflects the lack of general awareness about the vascular stroke syndromes of childhood, and the understanding that the differential diagnosis includes potentially lethal but remediable pathologies. There is a role here for public and professional education, particularly in terms of recognition of the significance of neurological symptoms in children with sickle cell disease, or the need for potential bone marrow donors in this group. There is encouraging evidence for secular improvement in adult stroke care[70] and children with acute neurological presentations may also need to be triaged within hyperacute stroke units with rapid access to emergency imaging before admission to the children's hospital. As diffusion-weighted imaging (DWI) is the most sensitive modality for detection of stroke in the acute phase,[71] as well as playing a role in the diagnosis of mimics, this might allow a DWI sequence only as part of emergency triage (JV Hunter, personal communication), which could probably be achieved without sedation and might enable trials of thrombolytic agents within a 4.5 hour time window, perhaps enhanced by diagnostic/therapeutic transcranial ultrasound.[72,73] Closer links with those caring for adults with stroke may allow research into risk factors, such as lipid profiles, smoking, hypertension and pharmaceutical use,[74–78] across age groups and geographical boundaries,[79] as well as allowing appropriate transition of those with chronic conditions at risk of stroke.[80–82] Further cervical[83,84] and intracranial vascular imaging (including venous) in the acute phase of childhood stroke has a high yield,[85,86] and various imaging techniques are useful diagnostically[87] and prognostically in children[88] as well as neonates,[89,90] but in the current state of knowledge, there is no disadvantage in delaying until paediatric anaesthetic cover for MR, CT or digital subtraction arteriography has been arranged.

The future in paediatric 'stroke' certainly holds exciting promise, both building on blocks recently laid, but also requiring lateral thinking and an appreciation that children are not small adults. This book attempts to encapsulate current knowledge but is written in the hope that in time it will be obsolete due to the much anticipated advances in the field.

REFERENCES

1. Golomb MR, Fullerton HJ, Nowak-Gottl U, deVeber G. Male predominance in childhood ischemic stroke: findings from the international pediatric stroke study. Stroke 2009; 40(1):52–57.
2. Amlie-Lefond C, Barnard D, Sebire G, Friedman NR, Heyer GL, Lerner NB et al. Predictors of cerebral arteriopathy in children with arterial ischemic stroke: results of the international pediatric stroke study. Circulation 2009; 119(10):1417–1423.
3. Fullerton HJ, Wu YW, Zhao S, Johnston SC. Risk of stroke in children: ethnic and gender disparities. Neurology 2003; 61(2):189–194.
4. Fullerton HJ, Elkins JS, Johnston SC. Pediatric Stroke Belt: geographic variation in stroke mortality in US children. Stroke 2004; 35(7):1570–1573.
5. Fullerton HJ, Wu YW, Sidney S, Johnston SC. Risk of recurrent childhood arterial ischemic stroke in a population-based cohort: the importance of cerebrovascular imaging. Pediatrics 2007; 119(3):495–501.
6. Fullerton HJ, Wu YW, Sidney S, Johnston SC. Recurrent hemorrhagic stroke in children: a population-based cohort study. Stroke 2007; 38(10):2658–2662.
7. Ichord RN, Bastian R, Abraham L, Askalan R, Benedict S, Bernard TJ, Beslow L, Deveber G, Dowling M, Friedman N, Fullerton H, Jordan L, Kan L, Kirton A, Amlie-Lefond C, Licht D, Lo W, McClure C, Pavlakis S, Smith SE, Tan M, Kasner S, Jawad AF. Interrater Reliability of the Pediatric National Institutes of Health Stroke Scale (PedNIHSS) in a Multicenter Study. Stroke. 2011 Feb 11. [Epub ahead of print].
8. Mallick AA, Ganesan V, Kirkham FJ, Fallon P, Hedderly T, McShane T et al. A population based study of the outcome one year after childhood arterial ischemic stroke. Stroke 2011; 42 (3) e98 (abstract 188).
9. Agrawal N, Johnston SC, Wu YW, Sidney S, Fullerton HJ. Imaging data reveal a higher pediatric stroke incidence than prior US estimates. Stroke 2009; 40(11):3415–3421.
10. Lee J, Croen LA, Backstrand KH, Yoshida CK, Henning LH, Lindan C et al. Maternal and infant characteristics associated with perinatal arterial stroke in the infant. JAMA 2005; 293(6):723–729.
11. Lee J, Croen LA, Lindan C, Nash KB, Yoshida CK, Ferriero DM et al. Predictors of outcome in perinatal arterial stroke: a population-based study. Ann Neurol 2005; 58(2):303–308.
12. Laugesaar R, Kolk A, Tomberg T, Metsvaht T, Lintrop M, Varendi H et al. Acutely and retrospectively diagnosed perinatal stroke: a population-based study. Stroke 2007; 38(8):2234–2240.
13. Laugesaar R, Kolk A, Uustalu U, Ilves P, Tomberg T, Talvik I et al. Epidemiology of childhood stroke in Estonia. Pediatr Neurol 2010; 42(2):93–100.
14. deVeber G, The Canadian Paediatric Ischemic Stroke Study group. Canadian Pediatric Ischemic Stroke Registry: analysis of children with arterial ischemic stroke. Ann Neurol 2000; 48:526.
15. Wraige E, Pohl KR, Ganesan V. A proposed classification for subtypes of arterial ischaemic stroke in children. Dev Med Child Neurol 2005; 47(4):252–256.
16. Kirton A, Deveber G, Pontigon AM, Macgregor D, Shroff M. Presumed perinatal ischemic stroke: vascular classification predicts outcomes. Ann Neurol 2008; 63(4):436–443.
17. Sebire G, Fullerton H, Riou E, deVeber G. Toward the definition of cerebral arteriopathies of childhood. Curr Opin Pediatr 2004; 16(6):617–622.
18. Braun KP, Bulder MM, Chabrier S, Kirkham FJ, Uiterwaal CS, Tardieu M et al. The course and outcome of unilateral intracranial arteriopathy in 79 children with ischaemic stroke. Brain 2009; 132(Pt 2):544–557.
19. Ganesan V, Prengler M, McShane MA, Wade AM, Kirkham FJ. Investigation of risk factors in children with arterial ischemic stroke. Ann Neurol 2003; 53(2):167–173.
20. Shellhaas RA, Smith SE, O'Tool E, Licht DJ, Ichord RN. Mimics of childhood stroke: characteristics of a prospective cohort. Pediatrics 2006; 118(2):704–709.
21. Chabrier S, Saliba E, Nguyen The Tich S, Charollais A, Varlet MN, Tardy B et al. Obstetrical and neonatal characteristics vary with birthweight in a cohort of 100 term newborns with symptomatic arterial ischemic stroke. Eur J Paediatr Neurol 2010; 14(3): 205–213.

22. Adams RJ, McKie VC, Hsu L, Files B, Vichinsky E, Pegelow C et al. Prevention of a first stroke by transfusions in children with sickle cell anemia and abnormal results on transcranial Doppler ultrasonography. N Engl J Med 1998; 339(1):5–11.

23. Adams RJ, Brambilla D. Discontinuing prophylactic transfusions used to prevent stroke in sickle cell disease. N Engl J Med 2005; 353(26):2769–2778.

24. Kirkham FJ, Lerner NB, Noetzel M, DeBaun MR, Datta AK, Rees DC et al. Trials in sickle cell disease. Pediatr Neurol 2006; 34(6):450–458.

25. Marshall MJ, Bucks RS, Hogan AM, Hambleton IR, Height SE, Dick MC et al. Auto-adjusting positive airway pressure in children with sickle cell anemia: results of a phase I randomized controlled trial. Haematologica 2009; 94(7):1006–1010.

26. Silva CM, Giovani P, Viana MB. High reticulocyte count is an independent risk factor for cerebrovascular disease in children with sickle cell anemia. Pediatr Blood Cancer. 2011;56(1):116–21.

27. Tripathi A, Jerrell JM, Stallworth JR. Cost-effectiveness of adenotonsillectomy in reducing obstructive sleep apnea, cerebrovascular ischemia, vaso-occlusive pain, and ACS episodes in pediatric sickle cell disease. Ann Hematol 2011;90(2):145–50.

28. Amlie-Lefond C, deVeber G, Chan AK, Benedict S, Bernard T, Carpenter J et al; International Pediatric Stroke Study. Use of alteplase in childhood arterial ischaemic stroke: a multicentre, observational, cohort study. Lancet Neurol 2009; 8(6):530–536.

29. Amlie-Lefond C, Chan AK, Kirton A, deVeber G, Hovinga CA, Ichord R et al. Thrombolysis in acute childhood stroke: design and challenges of the thrombolysis in pediatric stroke clinical trial. Neuroepidemiology 2009; 32(4):279–286.

30. Kirton A, Chen R, Friefeld S, Gunraj C, Pontigon AM, deVeber G. Contralesional repetitive transcranial magnetic stimulation for chronic hemiparesis in subcortical paediatric stroke: a randomised trial. Lancet Neurol 2008; 7(6):507–513.

31. Gordon A, Connelly A, Neville B, Vargha-Khadem F, Jessop N, Murphy T et al. Modified constraint-induced movement therapy after childhood stroke. Dev Med Child Neurol 2007; 49(1):23–27.

32. Golomb MR, McDonald BC, Warden SJ, Yonkman J, Saykin AJ, Shirley B et al. In-home virtual reality videogame telerehabilitation in adolescents with hemiplegic cerebral palsy. Arch Phys Med Rehabil 2010; 91(1):1–8.

33. Royal College of Physicians. Stroke in Childhood: Clinical Guidelines for Diagnosis, Management and Rehabilitation. 2004. Available from http://www.rcplondon.ac.uk/pubs/books/childstroke/childstroke_guidelines.pdf

34. Monagle P, Chalmers E, Chan A, deVeber G, Kirkham F, Massicotte P et al. Antithrombotic therapy in neonates and children: American College of Chest Physicians Evidence-Based Clinical Practice Guidelines, 8th edn. Chest 2008; 133(6 Suppl):887S–968S.

35. Roach ES, Golomb MR, Adams R, Biller J, Daniels S, deVeber G et al. Management of stroke in infants and children: a scientific statement from a Special Writing Group of the American Heart Association Stroke Council and the Council on Cardiovascular Disease in the Young. Stroke 2008; 39(9):2644–2691.

36. Gelfand AA, Fullerton HJ, Goadsby PJ. Child neurology: migraine with aura in children. Neurology 2010; 75(5):e16–19.

37. Osredkar D, Sall JW, Bickler PE, Ferriero DM. Erythropoietin promotes hippocampal neurogenesis in in vitro models of neonatal stroke. Neurobiol Dis 2010; 38(2):259–265.

38. Shimotake J, Derugin N, Wendland M, Vexler ZS, Ferriero DM. Vascular endothelial growth factor receptor-2 inhibition promotes cell death and limits endothelial cell proliferation in a neonatal rodent model of stroke. Stroke 2010; 41(2):343–349.

39. Sheldon RA, Osredkar D, Lee CL, Jiang X, Mu D, Ferriero DM. HIF-1 alpha-deficient mice have increased brain injury after neonatal hypoxia-ischemia. Dev Neurosci 2009; 31(5):452–458.

40. Gonzalez FF, Abel R, Almli CR, Mu D, Wendland M, Ferriero DM. Erythropoietin sustains cognitive function and brain volume after neonatal stroke. Dev Neurosci 2009; 31(5):403–411.

41. Moharir MD, Shroff M, Stephens D, Pontigon AM, Chan A, MacGregor D et al. Anticoagulants in pediatric cerebral sinovenous thrombosis: a safety and outcome study. Ann Neurol 2010; 67(5):590–599.

42. Kim SK, Cho BK, Phi JH, Lee JY, Chae JH, Kim KJ et al. Pediatric moyamoya disease: an analysis of 410 consecutive cases. Ann Neurol 2010; 68(1):92–101.

43. Conklin J, Fierstra J, Crawley AP, Han JS, Poublanc J, Mandell DM et al. Impaired cerebrovascular reactivity with steal phenomenon is associated with increased diffusion in white matter of patients with Moyamoya disease. Stroke 2010; 41(8):1610–1616.

44. Mackay MT, Prabhu SP, Coleman L. Childhood posterior circulation arterial ischemic stroke. Stroke 2010; 41(10):2201–2209.

45. Berfelo FJ, Kersbergen KJ, van Ommen CH, Govaert P, van Straaten HL, Poll-The BT et al. Neonatal cerebral sinovenous thrombosis from symptom to outcome. Stroke 2010; 41(7):1382–1388.

46. Jordan LC, Rafay MF, Smith SE, Askalan R, Zamel KM, Deveber G et al; for the International Pediatric Stroke Study Group. Antithrombotic Treatment in Neonatal Cerebral Sinovenous Thrombosis: results of the International Pediatric Stroke Study. J Pediatr 2010; 156(5):704–710.

47. Goldenberg NA, Bernard TJ, Fullerton HJ, Gordon A, deVeber G; International Pediatric Stroke Study Group. Antithrombotic treatments, outcomes, and prognostic factors in acute childhood-onset arterial ischaemic stroke: a multicentre, observational, cohort study. Lancet Neurol 2009; 8(12):1120–1127.

48. Westmacott R, MacGregor D, Askalan R, deVeber G. Late emergence of cognitive deficits after unilateral neonatal stroke. Stroke 2009; 40(6):2012–2019.

49. Cnossen MH, Aarsen FK, Akker SLj, Danen R, Appel IM, Steyerberg EW et al. Paediatric arterial ischaemic stroke: functional outcome and risk factors. Dev Med Child Neurol 2010; 52(4):394–399.

50. Lo W, Zamel K, Ponnappa K, Allen A, Chisolm D, Tang M et al. The cost of pediatric stroke care and rehabilitation. Stroke 2008; 39(1):161–165.

51. Borbone J, Geary M, Keslake J, Prengler M, Ganesan V, Kirkham FJ. Predictors of outcome in paediatric stroke Arch Dis Child 2010; 95(Suppl 1):A11 G9.

52. Ganesan V. Thrombolysis in paediatric arterial ischaemic stroke. Dev Med Child Neurol 2009; 51(2):90–91.

53. Arnold M, Steinlin M, Baumann A, Nedeltchev K, Remonda L, Moser SJ et al. Thrombolysis in childhood stroke: report of 2 cases and review of the literature. Stroke 2009; 40(3):801–807.

54. Kirkham FJ, Salmon AP, Khambadkone S. A hole in the heart: a hole in the head? Arch Dis Child 2011;Feb 21 (epub ahead of print)

55. Bene dik MP, Zaletel M, Megliè NP, Podnar T. A right-to-left shunt in children with arterial ischaemic stroke. Arch Dis Child 2011;Feb 21 (epub ahead of print).

56. Hubail Z, Lemler M, Ramaciotti C, Moore J, Ikemba C. Diagnosing a patent foramen ovale in children: is transesophageal echocardiography necessary? Stroke 2011;42(1):98–101.

57. Calamante F, Ganesan V, Kirkham FJ, Jan W, Chong WK, Gadian DG et al. MR perfusion imaging in Moyamoya syndrome: potential implications for clinical evaluation of occlusive cerebrovascular disease. Stroke 2001; 32(12):2810–2816.

58. Miller SP, McQuillen PS, Hamrick S, Xu D, Glidden DV, Charlton N et al. Abnormal brain development in newborns with congenital heart disease. N Engl J Med 2007; 357(19):1928–1938.

59. Dowling MM, Quinn CT, Plumb P, Rogers ZR, Rollins N, Koral K, Barber R, Buchanan GR. Acute Silent Cerebral Infarction Occurs during Acute Anemic Events in Children with and without Sickle Cell Disease. Stroke 2011; 42(3); e97.

60. Armstrong-Wells J, Grimes B, Sidney S, Kronish D, Shiboski SC, Adams RJ et al. Utilization of TCD screening for primary stroke prevention in children with sickle cell disease. Neurology 2009; 72(15):1316–1321.

61. Dobson SR, Holden KR, Nietert PJ, Cure JK, Laver JH, Disco D et al. Moyamoya syndrome in childhood sickle cell disease: a predictive factor for recurrent cerebrovascular events. Blood 2002; 99(9):3144–3150.

62. Hankinson TC, Bohman LE, Heyer G, Licursi M, Ghatan S, Feldstein NA et al. Surgical treatment of moyamoya syndrome in patients with sickle cell anemia: outcome following encephaloduroarteriosynangiosis. J Neurosurg Pediatr 2008; 1(3):211–216.

63. Hsieh MM, Kang EM, Fitzhugh CD, Link MB, Bolan CD, Kurlander R et al. Allogeneic hematopoietic stem-cell transplantation for sickle cell disease. N Engl J Med 2009; 361(24):2309–2317.

401

64. Jordan LC, Johnston SC, Wu YW, Sidney S, Fullerton HJ. The importance of cerebral aneurysms in childhood hemorrhagic stroke: a population-based study. Stroke 2009; 40(2):400–405.

65. Armstrong-Wells J, Johnston SC, Wu YW, Sidney S, Fullerton HJ. Prevalence and predictors of perinatal hemorrhagic stroke: results from the kaiser pediatric stroke study. Pediatrics 2009; 123(3):823–828.

66. Beslow LA, Ichord RN, Kasner SE, Mullen MT, Licht DJ, Smith SE et al. ABC/XYZ Estimates Intracerebral hemorrhage volume as a percent of total brain volume in children. Stroke 2010; 41(4):691–694.

67. Beslow LA, Licht DJ, Smith SE, Storm PB, Heuer GG, Zimmerman RA et al. Predictors of outcome in childhood intracerebral hemorrhage: a prospective consecutive cohort study. Stroke 2010; 41(2):313–318.

68. Hetts SW, Narvid J, Sanai N, Lawton MT, Gupta N, Fullerton HJ et al. Intracranial aneurysms in childhood: 27-year single-institution experience. AJNR Am J Neuroradiol 2009; 30(7):1315–1324.

69. Beslow LA, Ichord RN, Kasner SE, Mullen MT, Licht DJ, Smith SE et al. ABC/XYZ estimates intracerebral hemorrhage volume as a percent of total brain volume in children. Stroke 2010; 41(4):691–694.

70. McGlennan C, Ganesan V. Delays in investigation and management of acute arterial ischaemic stroke in children. Dev Med Child Neurol 2008; 50(7):537–540.

71. Lakshminarayan K, Borbas C, McLaughlin B, Morris NE, Vazquez G, Luepker RV et al. A cluster-randomized trial to improve stroke care in hospitals. Neurology 2010; 52(11):1033–7.

72. Buerki S, Roellin K, Remonda L, Mercati DG, Jeannet PY, Keller E et al. Neuroimaging in childhood arterial ischaemic stroke: evaluation of imaging modalities and aetiologies. Dev Med Child Neurol 2010; 52(11):1033–7.

73. Tsivgoulis G, Eggers J, Ribo M, Perren F, Saqqur M, Rubiera M et al. Safety and efficacy of ultrasound-enhanced thrombolysis: a comprehensive review and meta-analysis of randomized and non-randomized studies. Stroke 2010; 41(2):280–287.

74. Aylett SE, McShane MA, Kirkham FJ, Connelly A, Kendall B. Comparison of transcranial Doppler and angiography in the assessment of children with cerebrovascular disease. Dev Med Child Neurol 1995; 37(suppl 72): 4.

75. Kopyta I, Sarecka-Hujar B, Emich-Widera E, Marszał E, Zak I. Association between lipids and fibrinogen levels and ischemic stroke in the population of the Polish children with arteriopathy and cardiac disorders. Wiad Lek 2010; 63(1):17–23.

76. Hills NK, Johnston SC, Fullerton HJ. Do classic adult risk factors increase the risk of pediatric arterial ischaemic stroke? Stroke 2011; 42(3) e98 (abstract 186).

77. Christerson S, Strömberg B. Childhood stroke in Sweden I: incidence, symptoms, risk factors and short-term outcome. Acta Paediatr 2010; 99(11):1641–1649.

78. Sharma M, Kupferman JC, Brosgol Y, Paterno K, Goodman S, Prohovnik I et al. The impact of hypertension on the paediatric brain: a justifiable concern. Lancet Neurol 2010; 9(9):933–940.

79. Wong LJ, Kupferman JC, Prohovnik I, Kirkham FJ, Goodman S, Paterno K, Sharma M, Brosgol Y, and Pavlakis SG. Hypertension Impairs Vascular Reactivity in the Pediatric Brain. Stroke 2011; in press.

80. Mackay MT, Wiznitzer M, Benedict SL, Lee KJ, Deveber GA, Ganesan V; on behalf of the International Pediatric Stroke Study Group. Arterial ischemic stroke risk factors: The international pediatric stroke study. Ann Neurol. 2011;69(1):130–140.

81. Strouse JJ, Jordan LC, Lanzkron S, Casella JF. The excess burden of stroke in hospitalized adults with sickle cell disease. Am J Hematol 2009; 84(9):548–552.

82. Mackay M, Cardamone M, Hutchinson D, Barnes C, Coleman L, Cheung M. Arterial Ischaemic Stroke In Children With Heart Disease. Stroke 2011; 42 (3) e97 (abstract 183).

83. Hoffmann A, Chockalingam P, Balint OH, Dadashev A, Dimopoulos K, Engel R et al. Cerebrovascular accidents in adult patients with congenital heart disease. Heart 2010; 96(15):1223–1236.

84. Ganesan V, Cox TC, Gunny R. Abnormalities of cervical arteries in children with arterial ischemic stroke. Neurology 2011;76(2):166–71.

85. Bhattacharya A, Newell H, Evanson J, Kirkham F, Telfer P. Extracranial carotid artery occlusion in children with sickle cell disease. Br J Haem 2007; 137 Suppl. 1; 73: abstract 217.

86. Kirton A, Holland M, Benseler S, Hawkins C, Armstrong D, Wade A, Crous-Tsanaclis A-M, Sebire G, deVeber G; Fibromuscular Dysplasia and Childhood Stroke. Stroke 2011; 42 (3) e97 (abstract 184).

87. Jones BP, Ganesan V, Saunders DE, Chong WK. Imaging in childhood arterial ischaemic stroke. Neuroradiology 2010; 52(6):577–589.

88. Dudink J, Mercuri E, Al-Nakib L, Govaert P, Counsell SJ, Rutherford MA, Cowan FM. Evolution of unilateral perinatal arterial ischemic stroke on conventional and diffusion-weighted MR imaging. AJNR Am J Neuroradiol. 2009;30(5):998–1004.

89. Gordon A, Kirkham FJ. Magnetic resonance perfusion and motor outcome of chronic stroke in childhood. Ann Neurol 2009; 66(suppl 13): S147.

90. Kirton A, Shroff M, Pontigon AM, deVeber G. Risk factors and presentations of periventricular venous infarction vs arterial presumed perinatal ischemic stroke. Arch Neurol 2010; 67(7):842–848.

91. Husson B, Hertz-Pannier L, Renaud C, Allard D, Presles E, Landrieu P, Chabrier S; AVCnn Group. Motor outcomes after neonatal arterial ischemic stroke related to early MRI data in a prospective study. Pediatrics 2010; 126(4):912–918.

INDEX

Note: page numbers in *italics* refer to figures and tables

academic performance, sickle cell disease 374–5
acquired brain injury (ABI) 382
activated protein C resistance 91–2
activity limitations 353
acute chest syndrome (ACS), sickle cell disease 273, *274*
acute disseminated encephalomyelitis *34*, 36–7
  management 331
acute flaccid paralysis 44–5
acute management 319–32
  convalescence *321*
  CT 321–2, *323–4*
  diagnosis 322
  emergency 321
  emergency imaging 321–2, *323–4*, 325
  general measures *319*, 321
  guidelines 319
  haemorrhagic disease of the newborn 325
  haemorrhagic stroke *322*, 325
  intracranial hypertension 330–1
  ischaemic stroke *323*, 325–30
  MRA 322
  MRI 321–2, *323–4*
  MRV 322, 325
  non-vascular stroke syndromes 331–2
  organization 319–21
  rehabilitation *321*
  supportive care *321*
  venous sinus thrombosis *324*
acute myeloid leukaemia (AML) *289*
adenosylcobalamin synthesis defect 238, 239
adenotonsillectomy, sickle cell disease 286
ageing, premature 287–8
air encephalogram 8
Alagille syndrome 253
alpha-actin (ACTA2) mutations 255
alternating hemiplegia of childhood (ACH) 225–31
  atypical forms 228–9
  benign familial nocturnal 230
  bilateral episodes 226–7
  causes 231
  cerebellar ataxia 228
  channelopathies 231
  choreo-athetotic movements 228
  clinical course 228
  clinical findings 225–8
  delayed development 228
  differential diagnosis 229–30
  dyspneic episodes 227
  dystonic attacks 226
  EEG 227
  familial 228–9, 231
  fixed neurological abnormalities 228

hemiplegic episodes 226–7
imaging 229
laboratory findings 229
mechanisms 231
mental retardation 228
MRS 229
non-paroxysmal features 225, *226*, 227–8
ocular motor phenomena 227
onset 225
outcome 228
paroxysmal features 225–7
seizures 227
sleep effects 226
tonic attacks 226
treatment 230
anaemia 261–87
  acquired aplastic 265
  acquired haemolytic 266–7
  congenital aplastic 265–6
  haemolytic
    acquired 266–7
    hereditary 267–87
  iron deficiency 94
  mechanisms of cerebrovascular disease development 262
  neurological complications *263*
  posterior circulation strokes 41
  red cell adhesion 285
  silent infarction *277*
  stroke risk in cancer 289
  vascular system response 373
  see also sickle cell disease
anatomy, historical 3, 7
angiomatous malformations, surgery 171–2
anterior cerebral artery 19
anterior choroidal artery 19
anterior inferior cerebellar artery (PICA) 38
anterior spinal artery syndrome 45
anterior superior cerebellar artery 19, 20
antibiotics, venous sinus thrombosis 151
anticardiolipin antibodies
  perinatal arterial stroke 187
  venous sinus thrombosis 149
anticoagulation
  cardiac disease 251
  cervicocephalic arterial dissection 113
  dolichoectasia 132
  ischaemic stroke 329
    choice of drug 330
    recurrence prevention 339–40
  moyamoya/moyamoya syndrome 126
  Sneddon syndrome 259
  systemic lupus erythematosus 294
  venous sinus thrombosis *32*, 152–3, 248, 286, 294, 329

antiphospholipid antibodies, Sneddon syndrome 259
antiplatelet therapy
  cervicocephalic arterial dissection 113
  dolichoectasia 132
  ischaemic stroke
    choice of drug 330
    recurrence prevention 339–40
  polyarteritis nodosa 293
  see also aspirin
antithrombotic therapy, venous sinus thrombosis prevention 340
aneurysms *see* arterial aneurysms; vein of Galen aneurysmal malformation (VGAM)
anxiety 352
aortic coarctation 39
  spinal cord stroke ischaemic risk factor 46
aortic stenosis 39, *249*
aphasia 8
  expressive 350
  global *351*
aplastic anaemias
  acquired 265
  congenital 265–6
apparent diffusion coefficient (ADC) 52–3, 58–9
  diffusion-weighted imaging 65–6
  DWI change mechanisms following stroke 65
  neonatal stroke *72*
  Sturge–Weber syndrome 213
arginase deficiency 240
aripiprazole 230
arterial aneurysms 172–3
  intracranial haemorrhage 163–4, 168
  location 171
  mycotic 164, 171
  neurofibromatosis type 1 257
  neurological deficits 171
  rupture 171
  sickle cell disease *279*, 280
    management 286
  surgery 170–1
  traumatic 171
  tuberous sclerosis 257–8
arterial disease
  Down syndrome 251–2
  primary 247–8, *249*, *250–1*
arterial spin labelling 63–5
arterial stroke 29, *32*, 35
  beta-thalassaemia 264
arterial tortuosity/arterial tortuosity syndrome 132
arteriopathic stroke 27

arteriovenous malformations *see* cerebral
    arteriovenous malformations (CAVM)
aspirin
    cardiac disease 251
    ischaemic stroke 329, 330
        recurrence prevention 339
    moyamoya/moyamoya syndrome 126
    see also antiplatelet therapy
atherosclerosis
    cryptogenic stroke 87
    infections 87
atherosclerotic vasculopathy 39–40
atrial myxoma 248
attention deficit hyperactivity disorder
    (ADHD) 352
attentional processes, sickle cell disease 376
auditory discrimination, sickle cell disease
    374
autoimmune haemolytic anaemia (AIHA) 266
autoimmunity
    cervicocephalic arterial dissection 108
    moyamoya/moyamoya syndrome 122
Avicenna (Ibn Sina) 3

baclofen, intrathecal *385*, 386
Bacon, Francis 3
bacterial infections
    hypercoagulable state 86
    vasculitis 85–6
Bannayan–Riley–Ruvalcaba syndrome
    259–60
basal ganglia, calcification 291
basilar artery 20
    occlusion 327, 328
behavioural outcomes 352
    congenital heart disease 366
    sickle cell disease 379–80
behavioural problems, perinatal arterial stroke
    193
behavioural strategies 385
behavioural training in rehabilitation 382
Behçet disease 296
benign familial nocturnal alternating
    hemiplegia of childhood (ACH) 230
benign intracranial hypertension 153
benzhexol *385*, 386
Bicêtre group neonatal score for vein of Galen
    aneurysmal malformation 206
bilateral borderzone ischaemia 27
bimanual coordination/training 384
birth trauma 185
Blackfan–Diamond syndrome 265–6, *277*
Blalock–Taussig shunt *249*
Bloch–Sulzberger syndrome 258
blood groups, blood transfusion 325
blood pressure *see* hypertension
blood transfusion
    blood groups 325
    exchange 326
    sickle cell disease 282–3, 285
        emergency management 325–7
        stroke prevention 286–7
    top-up 326
blood–brain barrier, bacterially-induced
    breakdown 86
Bobath approach 383
bone marrow transplantation 286, 287
Bonet, Théophile 3
Bonnet–Dechaume–Blanc syndrome 259
borderzone ischaemia, bilateral 27
Borrelia burgdorferi 86–7
botulinum toxin therapy 386

brain circulation
    arterial supply 17–19
    development 17–21
brain development, congenital heart disease
    364
brain injury
    ontogenic specialization 357–61
    rehabilitation 382
brainstem
    ischaemia in cervicocephalic arterial
        dissection 110–11
    vascular syndromes 38, *39*
Brown–Séquard syndrome, spinal cord
    arteriovenous malformations 47

CADASIL 254
cancer, children with 288–93
    cerebrovascular disease 289
        risk factor reduction 292
    chemotherapy 291–2
    cholesterol level control 292
    cognitive decline 292
    cognitive therapy 292–3
    diffuse brain damage 290–2
    early diagnosis 292
    hormonal deficiency 291
    non-perioperative stroke 288–9
    optimal surgical technique 292
    perioperative stroke 288
    radiotherapy
        dose reduction 292
        effects 290–2
    rehabilitation 292–3
    risk factors for stroke/cerebrovascular
        disease 289
    statin therapy 292
    stroke syndromes 288–9
    vasculopathy prevention 292
capillary telangiectasias, intracranial
    haemorrhage 163, 167–8
carbohydrate deficient glycoprotein (CDG)
    syndromes 254
cardiac arrhythmias 248
cardiac disorders
    anticoagulation 251
    aspirin 251
    central venous thrombosis 248
    embolic 246–7
        Down syndrome 251
    inadequate perfusion/oxygenation in surgery
        246
    Marfan syndrome 253
    posterior circulation strokes 39
    primary arterial disease 247–8, *249*, *250–1*
    stroke recurrence
        prevention 249, 251
        risk 337
    symptomatic stroke 245–9, *250*, 252
    treatment 248–9, 251
    see also congenital heart disease
cardiac failure, vein of Galen aneurysmal
    malformation 204, 205
cardiac surgery
    cooling effects 367
    intellectual function 367–70
    neurodevelopmental outcomes 366–70
    rewarming speed 367
cardioembolic stroke 246–7
cardiomyopathy 248
carer health 353–4
carnitine 240
carotid artery dissection 29–30, 35, 55–6

carotid endarterectomy, internal carotid
    artery *64*
carotid tree 17, *18*
catheter-related thrombosis 91
cavernomas, intracranial haemorrhage 162–3,
    167
cavernous angiomas, surgery 171–2
cavernous sinus thrombosis 85
central venous thrombosis 248
cerebellar ataxia, alternating hemiplegia of
    childhood 228
cerebellar ischaemia, cervicocephalic arterial
    dissection 110–11
cerebral angiography 51
    cerebral infarction 53–4
cerebral arteries, development 17–19
cerebral arteriography 8–9
cerebral arteriovenous malformations (CAVM)
    172, 173–7
    acute management 325
    anatomical predictors of risk 174–5
    Bonnet–Dechaume–Blanc syndrome 259
    clinical manifestations 174
    embolization 173–4, 176–7
    hereditary haemorrhagic telangiectasia 260
    intracranial haemorrhage 161, 162
    intraparenchymal haemorrhage 161
    Leksell gamma knife radiosurgery 178
    LINAC system use 179
    natural history 174
    outcomes 176–7
        of surgery 170
    pathophysiology 174–5
    perioperative management 170
    radiosurgical complications 179
    rebleeding risk 162, 325
    Spetzler–Martin system for classification
        162
    spinal cord 47–8
    treatment 175–7
        stereotactic radiosurgery 177–9
        surgical 169–70
cerebral arteriovenous shunts (CAVS) 172,
    173–7
cerebral artery occlusion, ischaemic lesion
    development 66
cerebral blood flow (CBF) 49, 61
    CT measurement 49
    diffusion-weighted imaging 65–6
    Sturge–Weber syndrome 213
cerebral cavernous malformation (CCM) genes
    163
cerebral hemispheres
    age at injury effects on IQ 359–60, 361
    brain injury effects 357–61
    early specialization 355–6
    equipotentiality 354–5, 356, 357
    function 354–62
    ontogenic specialization 354, 356–62
    side of lesion effects on IQ 359, 361
cerebral infarction
    cerebral angiography 53–4
    computed tomography 51–2
    magnetic resonance angiography 53–4
    magnetic resonance imaging 52–3
    radiological recurrence 338
cerebral ischaemia/infarction
    blood flow restoration 66
    cervicocephalic arterial dissection 110–11
    perfusion imaging 54–5
cerebral perfusion failure,
    moyamoya/moyamoya syndrome 124

cerebral sinovenous thrombosis *see* venous sinus thrombosis
cerebral vascular system, phylogeny 19–20
cerebral vasculitis 127–8, *129*, 130–1
  bacterial infections 85–6
  causes 85–7
  clinical features 127–8
  diagnosis 128
  drug-induced 131
  fungal infections 90–1
  investigations 128, 130–1
  posterior circulation strokes 41
  secondary as systemic disease 131
  treatment 131
  varicella zoster virus 131
  viral infections 87–90
cerebral venous angiomas *see* developmental venous anomalies
cerebral venous sinus thrombosis (CVST) *see* venous sinus thrombosis
cerebral venous thrombosis 5–6
cerebrovascular disease
  children with cancer 289
  sickle cell disease 276–8, *279*
    mechanisms *268*, 276, *279*
cervical artery dissection 116
cervicocephalic arterial dissection 40, 107–15
  aetiology 108–9
  anticoagulation 113
  antiplatelet therapy 113
  autoimmunity 108
  brainstem ischaemia 110–11
  cerebellar ischaemia 110–11
  cerebral ischaemia 110–11
  congenital heart disease 108
  cranial neuropathy 110
  endovascular treatment 113–14
  epidemiology 107
  follow-up 114–15
  genetic risk factors 108–9
  headache 110
  history 109
  Horner syndrome 110
  infections 108
  inflammation 108
  ischaemic stroke 107, 110–11
  ligation for post-traumatic pseudoaneurysm 114
  MRI/MRA 111–13
  neuro-ophthalmic manifestations 111
  neuroradiology 111–13
  oculosympathetic paresis 110
  outcome 114–15
  pain 110
  pathogenesis 109
  pathology 107–8
  presentation 109–13
  recurrence risk 115
  surgery 113–14
  trauma 108
  treatment 113–14
  vasculopathy 108–9
channelopathies
  alternating hemiplegia of childhood 231
  familial hemiplegic migraine 218–19
chemotherapy, children with cancer 291–2
chickenpox 88
  cerebral vasculitis 131
  stroke 131
  transient cerebral arteriopathy 118–19
Chinese medicine, traditional 1
Chlamydia pneumoniae 87

chloral hydrate, alternating hemiplegia of childhood 230
cholesterol, children with cancer 292
choreo-athetotic movements, alternating hemiplegia of childhood 228
choroid plexus 19
citrullinaemia 240
clinical syndromes 27, *28*, 29, *30–4*, 35–8
clinical trials 398, 399
clopidogrel 339
coagulopathy
  inborn errors of metabolism 233, *236*
  intracranial haemorrhage 172
coarctation of the aorta 39, 46
cobalamin
  inborn errors of metabolism 234, 235
  methylmalonic acidaemia 239
Cobb syndrome
  spinal cord arteriovenous malformations 47–8
  vascular naevi 259
coeliac disease, iron deficiency 94
cognitive decline
  children with cancer 292
  radiotherapy 292
  sickle cell disease 270, 287
cognitive outcomes 351–2
  cognitive deficits 352
  congenital heart disease 362
  heart failure/hypoxaemia 362–5
  late-developing effects 352
  sickle cell disease 371–9
cognitive strategies 385
COL4A1 mutations 254, *255*
collagen disorders 39
coma 27
community-based services 382
computed tomography (CT) 49
  arterial dissection 56
  cerebral blood flow measurement 49
  cerebral infarction 51–2
  development 9
  venous sinus thrombosis 57
computed tomography angiography (CTA) 49
  cervicocephalic arterial dissection 112
congenital heart disease 245–6, *247*
  acyanotic lesions 362, 363
  behavioural outcomes 366
  brain development 364
  cervicocephalic arterial dissection 108
  circulatory arrest to deep hypothermia for surgery 367
  cognitive outcome 362
  cyanotic lesions 362, 363, 370
  developmental delay 364
  hypoxia 364–5
  neurodevelopmental outcome 362–70
  neurological abnormalities before surgery 365
  neuropsychological development effects of surgery 366–7
  oxygen saturation 365–6
  preoperative studies 365–6
  surgery effects 366–70
  treatment 249
  types 362, *363*
connective tissue disorders 262
  Marfan syndrome 253
consciousness
  deterioration 321
  see also Glasgow Coma Scale

constrained spherical deconvolution 61, Plate 2
constraint-induced movement therapy 383
continuous arterial spin labelling (CASL) 63, 64
contralesional repetitive transcranial magnetic stimulation 384
convalescence *321*
conventional angiography, cervicocephalic arterial dissection 111, 112
copper, Menkes disease 238
cortical spreading depression (CSD), hemiplegic migraine 220
covert infarctions 27
Cowden syndrome 259–60
cranial neuropathy, cervicocephalic arterial dissection 110
Crohn's disease *295*
cryptogenic stroke *29–30*, 35, 84–99
  atherosclerosis 87
  Fabry disease 37
  head injury 94
  hypertension 94–5
  infections 84–91
  iron deficiency 94
  paradoxical embolism 94–9
  patent foramen ovale 94–9, Plate 3
  thrombophilia 91–3
  trauma 94
Cushing syndrome, hypertension 94
cystathionine β-synthase (CBS) deficiency 234, *237*
cysticercosis 87
cystinosis 236–7, Plate 4
cytokines, proinflammatory 86
cytomegalovirus (CMV) 87

deBarsy syndrome 288
deep vein thrombosis, prevention 321
delivery, perinatal arterial stroke 186
dementia, Down syndrome 252
developmental venous anomalies 133–4
  intracranial haemorrhage 163, 167, 172
diagnosis of stroke 22, 399
Diamond–Blackfan syndrome 265–6, *277*
diencephalic artery *see* posterior choroidal artery
diet, hyperhomocysteinaemia 340
dietary advice, ischaemic stroke 340
differential diagnosis 29, *34*
diffusion anisotropy 68–9
diffusion tensor imaging (DTI) 58–61, Plate 2
diffusion-weighted imaging (DWI) 50, 57–61, 65–8
  acute stroke 66–8
  apparent diffusion coefficient 65–6
  applications 65–8
  cerebral artery occlusion ischaemic lesion development 66
  cerebral blood flow 65–6
  cerebral ischaemia/infarction blood flow restoration 66
  change mechanisms following stroke 65
  directionally encoded colour map 60
  eigenvalues/eigenvectors 59–60
  neonatal stroke *72*
directionally encoded colour (DEC) map 60
disability 353
  alleviation 380–1
  assessment 341
  domains of concern 381
discharge planning 382–3

dolichoectasia 132
Down syndrome *250*, 251–2
    arterial disease 251–2
    dementia 252
    moyamoya 252
    pathophysiology 252
    venous sinus thrombosis 251
drugs
    medications 385–6
    recreational 164, 196
dural sinus
    malformation 173
    occlusion 208
dynamic susceptibility contrast (DSC) 61,
    63
dyslipidaemia 39
dyspnea, alternating hemiplegia of childhood
    (ACH) 227
dystonia 350

educational outcomes 352–3
    sickle cell disease 374–5
Ehlers–Danlos syndrome 253–4
eigenvalues/eigenvectors 59–60
electroencephalography (EEG), historical 10
emotional difficulties 352
endothelial dysfunction 87
enriched environment/ecological approach
    384–5
epidemiology 22–5
    historical 6–7
epilepsy 350
    alternating hemiplegia of childhood
        differential diagnosis 230
    outcome 2
    Sturge–Weber syndrome 213, *214*, 215
Epstein–Barr virus (EBV) 87
equipotentiality model of cerebral hemispheres
    354–5, *356*, 357
evaluation
    early 400
    tools 398
Evans syndrome 266
event-related potentials
    ontogenic specialization 356–7
    sickle cell disease 377
executive function, sickle cell disease 375–7
extracranial arterial dissection, secondary
    prevention 340
extradural haemorrhage 196

Fabry disease 37, 39, *234*, 237
factor IIIc, perinatal arterial stroke 186
factor V (Leiden) G1691A mutation 91, 93
    neurofibromatosis type 1 stroke risk 289
    perinatal arterial stroke 186
    Sneddon syndrome 259
Fallopius, Gabriele 3
familial hemiplegic migraine (FHM) 218–19,
    221
    prevention 222
familial moyamoya disease 122
Fanconi syndrome 236, 265
fetomaternal haemorrhage 185
fibre tractography 68–9, Plate 1
fibroblast growth factor, basic (bFGF) 122
focal neurological deficits, differential
    diagnosis *33*
focal treatment 386
Freud, Sigmund 5, *6*
flunarizine 230
functional electrical stimulation 384

functional outcomes 342, *343*, 344, *345–9*,
    350–4, 382
functional recovery 381–2
fungal infections 90–1
    arterial aneurysms 164, 171
Fusobacterium 85

gabapentin 386
Galen 2
general anaesthesia, imaging 51
Glasgow Coma Scale 321
    ischaemic middle cerebral artery infarct
        outcome 330
gliosis, perinatal arterial stroke *188*, *189*,
    190, 191
globotriaosylceramide 237
glucose utilization, Sturge–Weber syndrome
    213
glutaric aciduria type 1 239–40
glutarylCoA 239
glycosylation, congenital disorders 254
Gowers, William 4, 5, *6*
Grange syndrome 254
great artery of Adamkiewicz 44
    traumatic infarction 46–7
Guglielmi Detachable Coils (GDC) 171
guidelines
    for acute management 319, 321
    for chronic management 319, *320*, 321
    for rehabilitation 381

haematological disorders, venous sinus
    thrombosis 148, *149*
haematopoiesis, intradural extramedullary in
    beta-thalassaemia 265
haemoglobin 267
    assessment in sickle cell disease 325
    congenital disorders 262, 264–5
    sickle cell disease 267
haemoglobin S 325, 326
haemolytic anaemias
    acquired 266–7
    hereditary 267–87
haemophilia, intracranial haemorrhage 164
Haemophilus influenzae, cerebral infarction 85
haemorrhagic disease of the newborn 164,
    325
haemorrhagic parenchymal infarction (HPI)
    183
haemorrhagic stroke 23, 24, 160–79
    acute management 325
    diagnosis *31*
    differential diagnosis *28*, *29*, *30*
    health care costs 25
    hypertension 94
    management *31*, 322
    mortality 344
    non-structural causes 172
    outcome in survivors 344, *348*, *349*
    sickle cell disease 275, 286
    structural lesions 169–72
    surgical treatment 169–72
    beta-thalassaemia 264
    Williams syndrome 252
haloperidol 230
Harvey, William 3
head injury, cryptogenic stroke 94
headache 27, *273*
    cervicocephalic arterial dissection 110
    sickle cell disease *274*, 275, Plate 6
health care utilization 25
health outcomes 340–1

heart failure, cognitive outcomes 362–5
Helicobacter pylori 87
hemianopia, association with hemiplegia 5
hemiparesis 2, 350, *351*
    sickle cell disease *270*, *271*
hemiplegia 350
    acquired 5
    behavioural outcomes 352
    case series of childhood 4–6
    congenital 5
    lesion effects on intelligence 358–61
    perinatal arterial stroke 191–2
    post mortem sequelae *7*
    psychiatric outcomes 352
    Sturge–Weber syndrome 213
    see also alternating hemiplegia of childhood
        (ACH)
hemiplegic migraine 217–22
    acute attack treatments 222
    alternating hemiplegia of childhood
        differential diagnosis 230
    classification 217
    clinical features 218
    cortical spreading depression 220
    cranial vessels 220–1
    EEG *218*
    gene mutations 218–19, *221*
    genotype–phenotype correlation 218
    investigations 221–2
    management 221–2
    MRI *219*, *220*
    neurophysiological/neuroradiological
        features 218
    outcome 222
    pathophysiology 219–21
    prevention 222
    sporadic *221*
hemispheric function
    age at injury effects on IQ 359–60, 361
    brain injury 357–61
        side of lesion effects on IQ 359, 361
    early specialization 355–6
    equipotentiality 354–5, *356*, 357
    ontogenic specialization 354, 356–62
hemolytic uremic syndrome (HUS) 266
Henoch–Schönlein purpura 294, 296
heparin
    ischaemic stroke 329, 330
        recurrence prevention 339
    venous sinus thrombosis 152–3, 329
        prevention 340
hepatitis B virus 88
hepatitis C virus 88
hepatocyte growth factors, moyamoya 122
hereditary haemorrhagic telangiectasia 260–1
    arteriovenous malformations 260
    clinical features 260
    management 261
    pathophysiology 260
    screening 260
    spinal cord arteriovenous malformations 47
hereditary spherocytosis 267
high angular resolution DW imaging (HARDI)
    acquisition 61
Hippocrates 1–2
history of childhood stroke 1–11
    age at injury 7–8
    anatomy 3, 7
    apoplexy connection to brain/cerebral
        vessels 3–4
    case series of childhood hemiplegia 4–6
    early clinical descriptions 1–3

epidemiology 6–7
imaging 8–9
outcomes 7–8
pathology 7
physiology/pathophysiology 10
HIV infection 89–90
homocysteine 37, 233, 234
metabolic pathways *236*
homocystinuria 37, 233–7
classical 234
remethylation defects 234–6
hormone deficiency, children with cancer
291
Horner syndrome *249*
cervicocephalic arterial dissection 110
Hutchinson–Gilford progeria 287–8
hydrocephalus
surgery 171
vein of Galen aneurysmal malformation
206–7
hydroxyurea, sickle cell disease 285–6
hyperammonaemias *235*, 240, *241*
hypercoagulable state
bacterial infections 86
stroke risk 92
beta-thalassaemia 265
hyperdense middle cerebral artery (MCA)
sign *52*
hyperfibrinogenaemia 289
hyperhomocysteinaemia 40, 91
diet 340
hyperlipidaemia 39
hypertension 40
cryptogenic stroke 94–5
haemorrhagic stroke 94
ischaemic stroke 94
moyamoya/moyamoya syndrome 124
neurofibromatosis type 1 257, 289
sickle cell disease 94
Sneddon syndrome 259
transcranial Doppler imaging 94
hypertensive encephalopathy 321
hypoglycaemia 37
hypomelanosis of Ito 259
hypoxaemia
cognitive function effects 362–5
IQ association 373
hypoxia
congenital heart disease 364–5
sickle cell disease 285
stroke risk in cancer 289
hypoxic–ischaemic encephalopathy, perinatal
arterial stroke 186

Ibn Sina (Avicenna) 3
idiopathic thrombocytopenic purpura (ITP)
296
Evans syndrome 266
intracranial haemorrhage 164
imaging of stroke 48–61, *62*, 63–9, *70*,
71, *72*
acute management 321–2, *323–4*, 325
arterial dissection 55–6
cerebral angiography 51
cerebral infarction 53–4
computed tomography 49
arterial dissection 56
cerebral infarction 51–2
venous sinus thrombosis 57
diagnostic difficulties 55–7
diffusion-weighted imaging 50, 57–61,
65–8, *72*

general anaesthesia 51
historical 8–9
magnetic resonance angiography 50
arterial dissection 56
cerebral infarction 53–4
magnetic resonance imaging 49–51
advances 57–61, *62*, 63–9, *70*, *71*, *72*
arterial dissection 56
arterial spin labelling 63–5
cerebral infarction 52–3
diffusion anisotropy 68–9
diffusion-weighted imaging 50, 57–61,
65–8, *72*
dynamic susceptibility contrast 61, 63
fibre tractography 68–9
perfusion imaging 50, 54–5, 61, *62*,
63–5, 69, *70*, *71*, *72*
venous sinus thrombosis 57
magnetic resonance venography 50
venous sinus thrombosis 57
nuclear medicine 51
perfusion imaging 50, 61, *62*, 63–5, 69, *70*,
71, *72*
cerebral ischaemia/infarction 54–5
sedation 51, *52*
ultrasound 48–9
venous sinus thrombosis 56–7, 149–51
immunocompromised patients 89
immunodeficiency 287
stroke risk in cancer 289
immunosuppression
Henoch–Schönlein purpura 294
polyarteritis nodosa *294*
Takayasu arteritis 293
inborn errors of metabolism 37, 233–42
arginase deficiency 240
cerebral haemorrhage predisposition *236*
citrullinaemia 240
coagulopathy 233, *236*
cobalamin 234, 235, 239
cystinosis 236–7, Plate 4
glutaric aciduria type 1 239–40
homocystinuria 37, 233–7
hyperammonaemias 240, *241*
Menkes disease 132, *234*, 238
5,10-methylenetetrahydrofolate reductase
deficiency 235, 236
methylmalonic acidaemia 238–9
mitochondrial encephalopathies 240–2
non-vascular mechanisms *235*, 238–42
organic acidaemias 238–40
ornithine carbamoyl transferase deficiency
37, 240, *241*
propionic acidaemia 239
thrombocytopenia 233, *236*
urea cycle deficits 240, *241*
vascular mechanisms 233–8
see also Fabry disease; mitochondrial
encephalomyopathy, lactic acidosis and
stroke like episodes (MELAS)
incidence of stroke 22–4
incontinentia pigmenti 258
Indian medicine, traditional 2–3
infantile hypotonia and paroxysmal dystonia
230–1
infants, vein of Galen aneurysmal
malformation 209
infections
animal models 85
atherosclerosis 87
bacterial 85–6
cervicocephalic arterial dissection 108

cryptogenic stroke 84–91
hemiplegia association 5
moyamoya 122
posterior circulation strokes 41
sickle cell disease 283
transient cerebral arteriopathy 116
venous sinus thrombosis 148
viral 87–90
see also fungal infections
inferior anterior cerebellar artery 19
inflammation
cervicocephalic arterial dissection 108
moyamoya/moyamoya syndrome 122
sickle cell disease *274*, 283, Plate 6
inflammatory bowel disease 294, *295*
inflammatory vasculopathies 293–4, *295*, *296*
infliximab, Takayasu arteritis 293
instrumental delivery 185
insulin-dependent diabetes mellitus (IDDM)
233
intellectual function
cardiac surgery 367–70
sickle cell disease 372–4
intelligence
hemiplegia-causing lesions 358–61
see also IQ
interleukin 1 (IL-1) 86
internal carotid artery 19
anterior division 20
carotid endarterectomy *64*
division 19–20
migraine 221
moyamoya syndrome 120, 121
occlusion *279*
internal carotid artery dissection (ICAD) *249*
epidemiology 107
Horner syndrome 110
pain 110
International Classification of Functioning,
Disability and Health (WHO) 381,
399
intracerebellar haemorrhage 197–8
intracerebral haemorrhage 223
clinical presentation 27
intraparenchymal 161
magnetic resonance imaging 55
sickle cell disease 280
intracranial arterial dissection 40
intracranial arteriopathy *29–30*, 35
cryptogenic stroke *29–30*, 35
sickle cell disease 35
intracranial haemorrhage
coagulopathy 172
developmental venous anomalies 172
diagnosis 196
extradural haemorrhage 196
future directions 399–400
imaging 196
intracerebellar haemorrhage 197–8
intraparenchymal haemorrhage 161, 197–8
lactic acidosis 196
neonates 194–8
outcome 198
presentation timing 195
risk factors 195–6
sites 195
subdural haemorrhage 196–7
thalamic haemorrhage 197
thrombocytopenia 195
vitamin K deficiency 194, 195
see also intraventricular haemorrhage
(IVH)

intracranial haemorrhage (ICH)
  arterial aneurysms 163–4, 168
  arteriovenous malformations 161, 162
  capillary telangiectasias 163, 167–8
  cavernomas 162–3, 167
  conventional cerebral angiography 166–7
  CT/CTA 164, *165, 166*
  definition *160*
  developmental venous anomalies 163, 167
  epidemiology 160
  imaging 164–9
    recommendations 168–9
  intraventricular 161, 169
  MRI/MRA 165–6, *167*
    vascular lesion features 167–8
  non-traumatic 160–9
  outcome 160–1
  recurrence risk 160
  systemic causes 164
  tumours *161,* 168
  vascular causes 162–4
  see also subarachnoid haemorrhage
intracranial hypertension
  benign 153
  management of intractable 330–1
  spinal cord arteriovenous malformations 47
  vein of Galen aneurysmal malformation
      207
intradural extramedullary haematopoiesis,
      beta-thalassaemia 265
intraparenchymal haemorrhage (IPH) 161,
      197–8
intrauterine growth restriction (IUGR),
      perinatal arterial stroke 185
intraventricular haemorrhage (IVH) 161, 198
  grades 198
  imaging recommendations 169
investigations of focal neurological signs 27,
      28–9
IQ 351, 352, 358–61
  age at insult 359–60, 361
  hemiplegia-causing lesion effects 358–61
  hemispheric side of lesion effects 359, 361
  hypoxaemia association 373
  seizure effects 359
  sickle cell disease 372–4
iron deficiency, cryptogenic stroke 94
ischaemic stroke 27, 223
  acute management *323,* 325–30
  anticoagulation 329
    choice of drug 330
    recurrence prevention 339–40
  antiplatelet therapy
    choice of drug 330
    recurrence prevention 339–40
  cervicocephalic arterial dissection 107,
      110–11
  clinical presentation 24
  diagnosis *32*
  dietary advice 340
  differential diagnosis 29
  dolichoectasia 132
  epilepsy after 350
  health care costs 25
  hyperhomocysteinaemia association 340
  hypertension 94
  management *32*
  mortality 344
  moyamoya 124
  outcome in survivors 344, *345–7,*
      348, 349
  prevention 398

prothrombotic disorders 92–3
recurrence prevention 329, 338–9
sickle cell disease
    blood transfusion 325–7
    management 285–6
    recurrence 339
  silent reinfarction 338
  spinal cord 44–5
  syndromes 29, *32,* 35
  thrombolysis with tPA 327–9
  thrombus propagation prevention *320,* 329
  transcranial Doppler thrombolysis 328
  transient cerebral arteriopathy 115–16
  Williams syndrome 252

Kawasaki disease 296
Klippel–Trenaunay–Weber syndrome 47–8

labour, perinatal arterial stroke 186
lactic acidosis, intracranial haemorrhage 196
language *see* speech and language
Leksell gamma knife radiosurgery 178
Lemierre syndrome 85
  antibiotic treatment 151
leukaemia, intracranial haemorrhage 164
LINAC systems 179
lipopolysaccharide 86
literature standardization 399
Loeys–Dietz syndrome 132
lupus anticoagulant 338

macrocrania, vein of Galen aneurysmal
      malformation 206–7
magnetic resonance angiography (MRA) 50
  arterial dissection 56
  cerebral infarction 53–4
magnetic resonance imaging (MRI) 27, 29,
      49–51
  advances 57–61, *62,* 63–9, *70,* 71, *72*
  apparent diffusion coefficient 52–3, 58–9
    DWI change mechanisms following
      stroke 65
    neonatal stroke *72*
  arterial dissection 56
  arterial spin labelling 63–5
  cerebral haemorrhage 55
  cerebral infarction 52–3
  development 9
  diffusion anisotropy 68–9
  diffusion imaging 57–61
  diffusion-weighted imaging
    acute stroke 66–8
    applications 65–8
    neonatal stroke *72*
  diffusion–perfusion mismatch *70*
  dynamic susceptibility contrast 61, 63
  fibre tractography 68–9
  FLAIR sequence 53
  luxury perfusion 53
  perfusion imaging 50, 61, *62,* 63–5, 69, *70,*
      71, *72*
    cerebral ischaemia/infarction 54–5
    role 69, *70,* 71, *72*
  quantitative diffusion mapping 58–61
  venous sinus thrombosis 57
magnetic resonance spectroscopy (MRS) 50–1
magnetic resonance venography (MRV) 50
  venous sinus thrombosis 57
malaria, venous sinus thrombosis 87
management
  of focal neurological signs 27, *28–9*
  see also acute management

Marfan syndrome 253
McNutt, Sarah 4, 5, *6*
medication 385–6
MELAS *see* mitochondrial
      encephalomyopathy, lactic acidosis and
      stroke like episodes (MELAS)
memantine 230
memory, working 375
meningitis
  cerebral infarction 85–6
  spinal cord stroke ischaemic risk factor 46
Menkes disease *234,* 238
  arterial tortuosity 132
mesencephalic artery 19
metabolic diseases
  management 331–2
  posterior circulation strokes 41–2
metabolic stroke 37–8, 233
  differential diagnosis 29, *30*
methionine synthase (MS) 234
5,10-methylenetetrahydrofolate reductase
      (MTHFR) deficiency 234
  inborn errors of metabolism 235, 236
5,10-methylenetetrahydrofolate reductase
      (MTHFR) gene polymorphism 91,
      92, 93
methylmalonic acidaemia 238–9
methylmalonylCoA 239
middle cerebral artery (MCA) 19
  hyperdense sign *52*
  stenosis in acute myeloid leukemia *289*
middle cerebral artery (MCA) territory
      infarction *185*
  clinical presentation 27
  ischaemic 330, *331*
  occurrence 184
migraine
  aura 219–20
  cranial vessels 220–1
  internal carotid artery 221
  MRA 221
  posterior circulation strokes 41
  Sturge–Weber syndrome 213
  vasospasm 132
  see also familial hemiplegic migraine
      (FHM); hemiplegic migraine
mimics of stroke, management *33*
mitochondrial diseases *235*
  posterior circulation strokes 41–2
mitochondrial disorders 37–8
mitochondrial encephalomyopathy, lactic
      acidosis and stroke like episodes
      (MELAS) 241–2
  posterior circulation strokes 41–2
  stroke mimic 57
mitochondrial encephalopathies *234,* 240–2
mitral valve prolapse 248
modafinil 386
mood disorders 352
Morgagni, Giovanni 3
motor function 350, 381
moyamoya/moyamoya syndrome *29–30,* 35,
      116, 120–2, *123,* 124–7
  aetiology 122, *123,* 124
  Alagille syndrome 253
  angiogenesis 122
  anticoagulation 126
  aspirin 126
  autoimmunity 122
  catheter cerebral angiography 124
  cerebral haemodynamics 124–5
  cerebral perfusion failure 124

clinical presentation 124
diagnosis 124–6
diagnostic criteria 120–1
Down syndrome 252
EEG 125–6
environmental triggers 122, 124
epidemiology 121
extracranial–intracranial bypass 114
familial disease 122
features 120
genetics 122
growth factors 122
hypertension 124
infections 122
inflammation 122
MRI 124
neurofibromatosis type 1 256
outcome 126–7
pathology 121–2
posterior circulation strokes 41
sickle cell disease 279, 286
Sneddon syndrome 259
stroke recurrence risk 337
surgery 126
surgical revascularization 338
transient ischaemic attacks 124, 250
treatment 126
vascular steal phenomenon 124
Williams syndrome 124, 250
multicentre collaboration 399
Mycoplasma pneumoniae 87
myocardial infarction (MI) 248

naevi, pigmented/depigmented and vascular
259
neonates 183–9, 190, 191–8
haemorrhagic disease of the newborn 164,
235
incontinentia pigmenti 258
intracranial haemorrhage 194–8
middle cerebral artery territory infarction
184
seizures 184, 187
thrombotic complications 91
vein of Galen aneurysmal malformation
209
venous sinus thrombosis 147–8
see also perinatal arterial stroke (PAS)
nephrotic syndrome 294
neural tube 18, 19
neurofibromatosis type 1 256–7
aneurysms 257
clinical features 256
hypertension 257, 289
intracranial arterial disease 256
moyamoya 256
pathophysiology 256
radiotherapy 257
risk factors 257, 289
stroke 256
nitric oxide, sickle cell disease 268
Noonan syndrome 253
NOTCH3 gene mutations 254
nuclear medicine 51
nucleus pulposus of intervertebral disc 47

ocular motor phenomena, alternating
hemiplegia of childhood 227
oculosympathetic paresis, cervicocephalic
arterial dissection 110
olfactory artery 17, 18
organic acidaemias 235, 238–40

ornithine carbamoyl transferase deficiency 37,
240, 241
orthotics 384
Osler, William 4–5, 6
Osler–Weber–Rendu disease *see* hereditary
haemorrhagic telangiectasia
osteopetrosis 254
otitis media 5–6
outcome after stroke 340–2, 343, 344, 345–9,
350–4
activity limitations 353
assessment tools 341–2, 343
behavioural 352
sickle cell disease 379–80
cardiac surgery 366–70
carer health 353–4
cognitive 351–2
congenital heart disease 362
heart failure 362–5
hypoxaemia 362–5
late-developing effects 352
sickle cell disease 371–9
disability 353
alleviation 380–1
assessment 341
educational effects 352–3
sickle cell disease 374–5
emotional difficulties 352
epilepsy 350
functional 342, 343, 344, 345–9, 350–4,
382
health 340–1
historical 7–8
measurement 341–2, 343, 382
mortality 342, 344
motor function 350
neurodevelopmental in congenital heart
defects 362–70
parent health 353–4
psychiatric 352
quality of life 353
sensory function 350
sickle cell disease 370–80
social effects 352–3
speech and language 350–1
survivors 344, 345–9, 350–4
oxygen desaturation, sickle cell disease 285
oxygen saturation, congenital heart disease
365–6
oxygen therapy
hyperbaric for radiation necrosis 291
sickle cell disease 286

pain, cervicocephalic arterial dissection 110
paradoxical embolism, cryptogenic stroke
94–9
paragonimiasis 87
parent health 353–4
paroxysmal dyskinesias 230
paroxysmal nocturnal haemoglobinuria 266–7
patent foramen ovale 340, 399
cryptogenic stroke 94–9, Plate 3
imaging 97–9
management 99
pathology, historical 7
pathophysiology, historical 10
perfusion imaging 50, 54–5, 61, 62, 63–5
cerebral ischaemia/infarction 54–5
role 69, 70, 71, 72
perinatal arterial stroke (PAS) 183
aetiology 184–7
behavioural problems 193

blood flow studies 189
circulatory factors 185
classification 184
clinical presentation 187
cognitive impairment 193
compensatory ability 193–4
congenital factors 186
CT 188
delivery 186
diagnosis 187–9, 190, 191
DWI 189, 190, 191
EEG 189
familial factors 186
gliosis 188, 189, 190, 191
haemorrhagic 183
hemiplegia 191–2
hypoxic–ischaemic encephalopathy 186
labour 186
later evolution of lesions 191
maternal factors 185
MRI 188–9, 190, 191
occurrence 183–4
outcome 191–4
placental factors 187
prothrombotic abnormalities 186–7
psychological problems 193
recurrence 191
seizures 187, 192–3
treatment 194
speech and language development 193
treatment 194
ultrasound 187, 190
visual development 193
Wallerian degeneration 191
periventricular leukomalacia 246, 365
perseverative behaviour, sickle cell disease 376
persistent angular structure (PAS) 61
PHACES 251, 256
phaeochromocytoma 94
physiology, historical 10
pial arteriovenous malformations (PAVM)
173–7
anatomical predictors of risk 174–5
clinical manifestations 174
embolization 176–7
natural history 174
outcome 176–7
pathophysiology 174–5
treatment 175–7
placenta, perinatal arterial stroke 187
pneumoencephalography 8
polyarteritis nodosa 293, 294
post-varicella angiopathy (PVA) 118–19
posterior cerebral artery 19
compression 40–1
posterior choroidal artery 19
posterior circulation strokes 38–43
age 38–9
anaemia 41
brainstem vascular syndromes 38
cardiac disorders 39
gender 38–9
hypercoagulable states 41
infections 41
investigations 42
management 42–3
MELAS 41–2
metabolic diseases 41–2
migraine 41
mitochondrial diseases 41–2
moyamoya 41
recurrence prevention 340

posterior circulation strokes (*cont'd*)
  risk factors 38–9
  trauma 40–1
  vascular anatomy 38
  vasculitis 41
  vasculopathy 39–40
posterior communicating artery (PCoA) 18–19
posterior fossa, arterial supply 20
posterior fossa malformation, arterial, cardiac
    and eye abnormalities or a sternal pit
    see PHACES
posterior inferior cerebellar artery (PICA) 38
posterior reversible encephalopathy syndrome
    (PRES) 321, 331
pre-eclampsia, perinatal arterial stroke 185
predisposing conditions 27, *30–1*
premature ageing syndromes 287–8
presumed perinatal stroke (PPERI) 183
preterm infants 184
primary angiitis of the central nervous system
    (PACNS) 127, *129*
  biopsy 130–1
  catheter cerebral angiography 128, 130
  clinical features 127–8
  diagnosis 128
  histopathology 130–1
  investigations 128, 130–1
  MRI/MRA 128, *130*
  neuroimaging 128
  peripheral blood examination 128
  treatment 131
progerias 287–8
propionic acidaemia 239
propionylCoA 239
protein C deficiency 91–2
  beta-thalassaemia 265
protein S deficiency 265
protein Z deficiency 259
prothrombin G20210A mutation 93
prothrombotic risk factors 91–2
pseudoaneurysms, post-traumatic 114
pseudotumour cerebri *see* benign intracranial
    hypertension
pseudoxanthoma elasticum 261, 262
psychiatric outcomes 352
psychological problems, perinatal arterial
    stroke 193
PTEN mutations 259–60
pulmonary atresia *249*
pulsed arterial spin labelling (PASL) 63–4, *70*
pyramidal signs 350
pyruvate kinase deficiency 267

Q-ball imaging 61
quality of life 353
quantitative diffusion mapping 58–61

radiculomedullary feeding vessels 44
radionecrosis, children with cancer 291
radionucleotide imaging 51
radiotherapy, children with cancer 290–2
recognition of stroke, prompt 400
recurrence 337–40
  cervicocephalic arterial dissection 115
  intracranial haemorrhage 160
  perinatal arterial stroke 191
  posterior circulation strokes 340
  prevention
    cardiac disorders 249, 251, 337
    ischaemic stroke 329, 338–9
    posterior circulation strokes 340
    venous sinus thrombosis 153–4, *339*

risk 337–8
  in sickle cell disease 285, 337, 339
  venous sinus thrombosis 153–4, 338, *339*
red cell adhesion, anaemia 285
rehabilitation *321*, 380–6
  adult *vs* child 381–2
  approaches 383–4
  behavioural strategies 385
  behavioural training 382
  bimanual coordination/training 384
  brain injury 382
  cognitive strategies 385
  community-based services 382
  contralesional repetitive transcranial
      magnetic stimulation 384
  definition 383
  delivery 382–6
  discharge planning 382–3
  enriched environment/ecological approach
      384–5
  external interventions 382
  focal treatment 386
  functional electrical stimulation 384
  goal-setting 382
  guidelines 381
  interventions 383
  medication 385–6
  multidisciplinary 381
  orthotics 384
  strength training 383–4
  virtual reality therapy 384
remethylation defects 234–6
renal tubular acidosis 236
research, collaborative 398
retinal vascular malformations,
    Bonnet–Dechaume–Blanc syndrome
    259
reversible posterior leukoencephalopathy
    syndrome (RPLS) *29–30*, 35–6
  clinical presentation 27
  hypertension 94
  stroke mimic 57

Sachs, Bernard 4, 5, *6*
'The Sacred Disease' (Hippocrates) 2
salmonella, cerebral infarction 85
Schimke immuno-osseous dysplasia 254, *255*
sedation, imaging 51, *52*
seizures 27
  acute management 321
  alternating hemiplegia of childhood 227
  IQ effects 359
  middle cerebral artery territory infarction
      185
  neonatal 184, 187
  perinatal arterial stroke 187, 192–3
      treatment 194
  sickle cell disease 275, *276*
  Sneddon syndrome 259
  Sturge–Weber syndrome 213, *214*, 215
  venous sinus thrombosis 148
sensory function 350
sickle cell disease 6, 35, *36*, 267–87
  academic performance 374–5
  acute chest syndrome 273, *274*
  adenotonsillectomy 286
  anaemia 262, 285, 326
  arterial aneurysms *279*, 280
      management 286
  attentional processes 376–7
  auditory discrimination 374
  behavioural outcomes 379–80

blood transfusion 285
  emergency management 325–7
  stroke prevention 286–7
  therapy 282–3
bone marrow transplantation 286
carrier state 267
cerebral blood flow studies 281–3
cerebrovascular disease 276–8, *279*
  mechanisms *268*, 276, *279*
  risk factors 283, *284*, 285
cerebrovascular reserve/autoregulation 282
cognitive decline *270*, 287
cognitive outcome 371–9
complications 268
continuous arterial spin labelling 282
conventional cerebral angiography 280, 285
educational outcomes 374–5
event-related potentials 377
executive function 375–7
genetic predisposition to stroke 283
genotypes 371
haemorrhage risk 279–80
haemorrhagic stroke 275, 286
Hb assessment 325
headache *273*, *274*, 275
hemiparesis *270*, *271*
hydroxyurea 285–6
hypertension 94
hypoxia 285
infarct location 377
infection 283
inflammation *274*, 283, Plate 6
inheritance 267
intellectual function 372–4
internal carotid artery occlusion *279*
intracerebral haemorrhage 280
intracranial arteriopathy 35
intracranial haemorrhage 164
IQ 372–4
ischaemic stroke
  blood transfusion 325–7
  management 285–6
  recurrence 339
molecular sickling 267–8
moyamoya *279*, 286
MRA *278*, *279*, 280–1, 327
MRI 278–80, 327
  perfusion 282
MRV 327
neurological complications 268, *269*, 270,
    273, 275–80
nutritional factors for stroke 283, 285
outcome after stroke 370–80
oxygen desaturation 285
oxygen therapy 286
perseverative behaviour 376
PET 281
phenotypes 371
primary stroke prevention 286–7
red cell adhesion 285
revascularization techniques 286
risk factors for stroke/cerebrovascular
    disease 283, *284*, 285
seizures 275, *276*
silent infarctions *277*, *278*, *280*, Plate 5
  reinfarction 338
situational behaviour 380
SPECT 281–2
speech and language outcomes 378
spinal cord stroke ischaemic risk factor 46
stem cell transplantation 286
stroke incidence 268, *270*

stroke recurrence 285, 337, 339
subarachnoid haemorrhage 280
transcranial Doppler ultrasound *271*, 281,
    282, 285
treatment for stroke 285–7
    early management 285–6
    prevention 286–7
vascular studies 280–1
venous sinus thrombosis 277, 286
visual motor function 377–8
working memory 375
xenon inhalation studies 281
sickle cell trait 267
silent infarctions 27, 29
    radiological recurrence 338
    sickle cell disease *277*, 278, *280*, Plate 5
single photon emission tomography (SPECT)
    51
situational behaviour, sickle cell disease 380
skull fracture 185
sleep
    alternating hemiplegia of childhood 226
    physiology 10
smooth muscle alpha-actin mutations 255
Sneddon syndrome *121*, 258–9
social outcomes 352–3
speech and language
    development with perinatal arterial stroke
        193
    outcome after stroke 350–1
        sickle cell disease 378
Spetzler–Martin system for AVM
        classification 162
spinal cord
    arterial supply anatomy 43–4
    arteriovenous malformations 47–8
    haemorrhage 47
spinal cord stroke 43–8
    haemorrhagic 48
    ischaemic 44–5
        management 48
        risk factors 45–7
    management 48
    prevention 48
spinal epidural haematoma 47
spontaneous spinal epidural haematoma
        (SSEH) 47
statins, children with cancer 292
stem cell transplantation, sickle cell disease
        286
steroid therapy
    radiation necrosis 291
    Takayasu arteritis 293
strength training 383–4
Streptococcus pneumoniae, cerebral infarction
        85
stroke
    subtypes 22–4
    symptomatic 245–97
        anaemia 261–87
        bone marrow transplantation 287
        cardiac disorders 245–9, *250*, 252
        children with cancer 288–93
        genetically determined vasculopathies
            251–61
        immunodeficiency 287
        inflammatory vasculopathy 293–4, *295*,
            296
        premature ageing syndromes 287–8
Strümpell, Ernst von 5, *6*
Sturge–Weber syndrome 212–13, *214*, 215
    apparent diffusion coefficient 213

calcifications 212
cerebral blood flow 213
cognitive outcome 215
CT 212
DWI 213
EEG 215
epilepsy 213, *214*, 215
glucose utilization studies 213
hemiplegia 213
imaging 212–13
management 215
migraine 213
MRI 212–13
neurodevelopmental outcome 215
pathology 212
seizures 213, *214*, 215
surgery 215
subacute bacterial endocarditis (SBE) 164
subarachnoid haemorrhage 23, 161, 197
    arterial aneurysm rupture 171
    clinical presentation 27
    imaging recommendations 169
    sickle cell disease 280
    stroke mimic 57
    surgical treatment 170
    vasospasm 131
subdural haemorrhage 196–7
supratentorial intraparenchymal haematoma
        169
Susac syndrome 296
systemic disease, stroke recurrence risk 337
systemic lupus erythematosus (SLE) 293–4,
        295
    stroke recurrence risk 338

Takayasu arteritis 293
telencephalic artery *see* olfactory artery
temperature, body 321
terminology, standardized 398
thalamic haemorrhage 197
beta-thalassaemia 262, *263*, 264–5, *271*
    hypercoagulable state 265
    pathology 264
    signs/symptoms 262, 264
    silent infarcts 264–5
    treatment 264
thrombocytopenia
    inborn errors of metabolism 233, *236*
    intracranial haemorrhage 195
thrombolysis
    bleeding risk 249
    ischaemic stroke 327–9
    tPA for ischaemic stroke 327–9
    transcranial Doppler 328
    venous sinus thrombosis 32, 153, 286, 329
thrombophilia 91–3
    laboratory evaluation 93
    stroke recurrence risk 337–8
thrombosis
    paroxysmal nocturnal haemoglobinuria 266
    risk factors 91–2
    see also venous sinus thrombosis
thrombotic stroke *see* venous sinus thrombosis
tissue plasminogen activator (t-PA) 327–9
tonsillar prolapse phenomenon 208
top-of-the-basilar syndrome 251
transcranial Doppler (TCD) imaging 48–9
    hypertension 94
    patent foramen ovale 97–9
transcranial Doppler (TCD) thrombolysis 328
transient cerebral arteriopathy 56, 115–20
    aetiology 116

clinical features 117–18
diagnosis 117–18, 118–19
epidemiology 116–17
features 116
genetic factors 116
infections 116
MRA 117–18, *120*
occlusive 118, *119*
outcome 119
pathophysiology 116–17
transcranial Doppler 117–18
trauma 116
treatment 119
varicella zoster virus 116–17, 118–19, 120
transient ischaemic attacks (TIAs) 27
    moyamoya 124, *250*
    shunts 97
    tuberous sclerosis 257
transoesophageal echocardiography (TOE),
        patent foramen ovale 97, 99
transthoracic echocardiography (TTE), patent
        foramen ovale 97, 98, 99
transverse myelitis 44, *45*
trauma
    arterial aneurysms 171
    artery of Adamkiewicz infarction 46–7
    birth 185
    cervicocephalic arterial dissection 108
    cryptogenic stroke 94
    posterior circulation strokes 40–1
    pseudoaneurysms 114
    transient cerebral arteriopathy 116
treatment costs 25
Treponema pallidum 86
tuberculous meningitis 85, *86*
tuberous sclerosis 257–8
tumour necrosis factor α (TNF-)α 86
Turner syndrome 253
twin-to-twin transfusion syndrome 185

ultrasound imaging 48–9
urea cycle deficits 240, *241*
urokinase 327, 329

varicella zoster virus 87–8, *89*
    cerebral vasculitis 131
    transient cerebral arteriopathy 116–17,
        118–19, 120
vascular occlusion, pathophysiology 91
vascular steal phenomenon, moyamoya
        association 124
vascular system response to anaemia 373
vasculitis *see* cerebral vasculitis
vasculopathy
    atherosclerotic 39–40
    genetically determined 251–61
        with neurocutaneous syndromes 256–61
    inflammatory 293–4, *295*, 296
    non-atherosclerotic 40
    prevention in children with cancer 292
vasospasm 131–2
vein of Galen aneurysmal malformation
        (VGAM) 173, 204–11
    arterial supply 204–5
    Bicêtre group neonatal score 206
    calcifications 208
    cardiac failure association 204, 205
    cardiac manifestations 205–6
    choroidal angioarchitecture 205
    developmental delay 207
    dural sinus occlusion 208
    follow-up 209

vein of Galen aneurysmal malformation
(VGAM) (*cont'd*)
  hydrocephalus 206–7
  imaging 205–6
  infants 209
  intracranial hypertension 207
  long-term evolution with patent sinuses
    207–8
  macrocrania 206–7
  morphology 204–5
  mortality/morbidity 209–10
  mural angioarchitecture 205
  natural history 205–8
  neonates 209
  pial congestion/reflux 208
  radiosurgery 210–11
  spontaneous thrombosis 208
  surgery 210
  tonsillar prolapse phenomenon 208
  treatment 175–6, 208–11
  venous drainage 205
  ventricular shunting 207
velocardiofacial syndrome, arterial tortuosity
  132
venous sinus thrombosis *29–30*, 35, 56–7,
  145–55
  acute management *324*
  aetiology 145, *146*
  age at event 154
  anatomy 145, *147*
  antibiotic treatment 151
  anticardiolipin antibodies 149
  anticoagulants *32*, 152–3, 248, 286, 294,
    329
  clinical features *147*, 148–9
  clinical presentation 27
  complications risk 330–1
  conventional angiography 151
  CT 149–50
  diagnosis *32*, 149–51

differential diagnosis 29, *30*
Down syndrome 251
epidemiology 145, *146*
Evans syndrome 266
haematological disorders 148, *149*
haemorrhage 325
imaging 56–7, 149–51
infections 85, 148
iron deficiency anaemia 94
laboratory investigations 149
long-term management 153–4
malaria 87
management *32*
monitoring *152*
mortality 154
MRI/MRV 150, *151*
neonates 147–8
outcome 154–5
pathophysiology 146–7
physiology 145
prothrombotic abnormalities 149
recurrence prevention 153–4, *339*
recurrence risk 338
risk factors 147–8
secondary prevention 340
seizures 148
sickle cell disease 277, 286
signs/symptoms 147–8
surgical decompression 331
systemic lupus erythematosus 294
thrombolysis 286, 329
thrombolytic therapy 153
thrombosis location 151
treatment 151–4
ultrasound 150–1
venous infarction 146–7, 151
venous thrombosis, central 248
ventricular shunting, vein of Galen aneurysmal
  malformation 207
vertebral artery dissection (VAD) 55–6

epidemiology 107
Horner syndrome 110
pain 110
vertebrobasilar artery
  compression 40
  dissection *29–30*, 35
vertebrobasilar circulation stroke 27, 39
vertebrobasilar dolichoectasia 132
vertebrobasilar territory infarction, Fabry
  disease 37
Vesalius, Andreas 3
vigabatrin 386
viral infections 87–90
virtual reality therapy 384
visual development, perinatal arterial stroke
  193
visual hallucinations *273*
visual motor function, sickle cell disease
  377–8
vitamin K deficiency 194, 195

Wallerian degeneration, perinatal arterial
  stroke 191
warfarin
  ischaemic stroke recurrence prevention
    339–40
  venous sinus thrombosis prevention
    340
Wepfer, Johann 3, 4
Werner syndrome 288
Wiedemann–Rautenstrauch syndrome 288
Williams syndrome 252
  moyamoya association 124, *250*
Willis, Thomas 3, *4*
working memory, sickle cell disease 375
World Health Organization International
  Classification of Functioning,
  Disability and Health (ICF) 381,
  399
Wyburn–Mason syndrome 259